V Medical and Surgical Emergencies

VI Special Patient Populations

Sheehy's

Emergency Nursing

Principles and Practice

SHEEHY'S EMERGENCY NURSING

PRINCIPLES AND PRACTICE

Fifth Edition

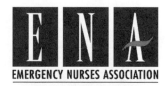

EMERGENCY NURSES ASSOCIATION

Edited By:

Lorene Newberry, RN, MS, CEN

Clinical Nurse Specialist
Emergency Services
WellStar Health System
Marietta, Georgia

With over 583 illustrations

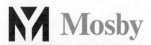

An Affiliate of Elsevier Science

St. Louis   London   Philadelphia   Sydney   Toronto

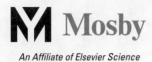

Mosby

An Affiliate of Elsevier Science

11830 Westline Industrial Drive
St. Louis, MO 63146

Notice

Nursing is an ever-changing field. Standard safety precautions must be followed, but as new research and clinical experience broaden our knowledge, changes in treatment and drug therapy may become necessary or appropriate. Readers are advised to check the most current product information provided by the manufacturer of each drug to be administered to verify the recommended dose, the method and duration of administration, and contraindications. It is the responsibility of the licensed prescriber, relying on experience and knowledge of the patient, to determine dosages and the best treatment for each individual patient. Neither the publisher nor the editor assumes any liability for any injury and/or damage to persons or property arising from this publication.

Previous editions copyrighted 1981, 1985, 1992, and 1998

International Standard Book Number 0-323-01684-7

Vice President and Publishing Director, Nursing: Sally Schrefer
Executive Editor: Susan R. Epstein
Senior Developmental Editor: Sharon J. Malchow
Publishing Services Manager: John Rogers
Senior Project Manager: Cheryl A. Abbott
Senior Book Designer: Kathi Gosche

GW/MVB

Printed in the United States of America

Last digit is the print number: 9   8   7   6   5   4   3   2   1

Contributors

SHERRI-LYNNE ALMEDIA, DrPH, MSN, MEd, RN, CEN
Chief Operating Officer
Team Health Southwest
Houston, Texas

SUSAN BARNASON, RN, PhD, CEN, CCRN
Associate Professor
University of Nebraska Medical Center College of Nursing
Lincoln, Nebraska

DARCY T. BARRETT, RN, MSN
Clinical Specialist Critical Care
WellStar Health System
Marietta, Georgia

BILLIE JEAN BARRETT-WALTERS, RN, MSN, ARNP
Unit Coordinator, Emergency Department and Fast Track
Central Baptist Hospital
Lexington, Kentucky

LISA MARIE BERNARDO, RN, PhD, MPH
Associate Professor
University of Pittsburgh School of Nursing
Pittsburgh, Pennsylvania

JULIE BRACKEN, RN, APN, MS, CEN
Director, Nursing Education
Cook County Hospital
Chicago, Illinois

MELINDA GAY BURCH, RN, BSN
Assistant Department Director, Critical Care
Hoag Memorial Presbyterian Hospital
Newport Beach, California

CHRISTINE E. CAMPBELL, RN, MS, CNA
Assistant Director of Patient Care Services
Children's Hospital
Columbus, Ohio

CATHERINE A. CHAPMAN, MSN, CS, FNP, CEN
Director of Clinical Services
Greater Southeast Community Hospital
Washington, District of Columbia

COURTNEY COSBY, RN, MN, MS
Director, Critical Care and Emergency Services
Henrico Doctors Hospital
Richmond, Virginia

LAURA M. CRIDDLE, RN, MS, CEN, CCNS, CFRN
Emergency, Trauma, and Neuro Clinical Nurse Specialist
Oregon Health and Science University
Portland, Oregon

NANCY J. DENKE, RN, MSN, FNP-C, CCRN
Nurse Practitioner, Emergency Department
Poudre Valley Hospital
Ft. Collins, Colorado

NANCY STEPHENS DONATELLI, RN, MS, CEN, CNA
Assessment Coordinator
Shenango Presbyterian SeniorCare
New Wilmington, Pennsylvania

DARCY EGGING, RN, MS, CS-ANP, CEN
Nurse Practitioner
Valley Emergency Care, Inc.
Delnor Community Hospital
Geneva, Illinois

CHRIS M. GISNESS, RN, MSN, CEN, CS, FNP-C
Nurse Practitioner, Associate Provider
Emergency Care Center
Department of Emergency Medicine
Emory University, Grady Campus
Atlanta, Georgia

KATHLEEN FOUNTAIN GRAHAM, MPH, MSN, CPNP
Director of the Alabama Child Death Review System
University of Alabama at Birmingham
School of Public Health
Department of Maternal-Child Health
Birmingham, Alabama

M. LYNN HERMAN, RN, MSN
Associate Professor
Floyd College School of Nursing
Rome, Georgia

RENEÉ SEMONIN HOLLERAN, RN, PhD, CEN, CCRN, CFRN
Chief Flight Nurse
Emergency Clinical Specialist
University Air Care
University of Cincinnati
Cincinnati, Ohio

PATRICIA KUNZ HOWARD, PhD(CAND.), RN, MSN, CEN, CCRN
Staff Development Specialist, Emergency Department
University of Kentucky Hospital
Lexington, Kentucky

BARBARA BENNETT JACOBS, RN, MPH, MS
NIH Fellow
Center for Clinical Bioethics, Georgetown University
Washington, District of Columbia;
PhD Candidate
School of Nursing, University of Connecticut
Storrs, Connecticut

ZEB KORAN, RN, MSN, CEN, TNS
Executive Director
Board of Certification for Emergency Nursing
Des Plaines, Illinois

DEB KOZENY, RN, MS, CEN, CCNS
Trauma Clinical Nurse Specialist/Program Manager
Gwinnett Hospital System
Lawrenceville, Georgia

LINDA L. LARSON, RN, PhD, FNPC
Nurse Practitioner
MayFair Internal Medicine
Littleton, Colorado

SUSAN LAZEAR, RN, MN
Director
Specialists in Medical Education
Woodinville, Washington

N. GENELL LEE, RN, MSN, JD
Nurse Attorney
Montgomery, Alabama

DIANA M. LOMBARDO, RN, MSN, MHA
Family Nurse Practitioner, Urgent Care
Southwest Medical
Las Vegas, Nevada

JOHN R. LUNDE, RNC, MSN, CRNP, NREMT-P
Clinical Director, Emory Flight
Nurse Practitioner, Emergency Medicine
Columbus, Georgia

ESTELLE MacPHAIL, RN, BSN, MS, CEN, CNAA
Nurse Director, Emergency/Trauma Services
Southern New Hampshire Medical Center
Nashua, New Hampshire

ANNE P. MANTON, RN, PhD, FAAN
Associate Professor
Fairfield University, School of Nursing
Fairfield, Connecticut

DELL T. MILLER, RN, MSN, FNP, EMTP, CCRN, CEN
Staff Nurse, Critical Care
Doctors Hospital
Columbus, Georgia;
Nurse Practitioner, Emergency Department
Phenix Regional Hospital
Phenix City, Alabama

SUE MOORE, RN, MSN, CCRN, CFRN, CEN
Clinical Nurse Specialist
REMSA (Regional Emergency Medical Services Authority)- Care Flight
Reno, Nevada

JOAN MORRIS, RN, MSN, APN/CNS
Trauma Care Manager
Lutheran General Hospital
Park Ridge, Illinois

CATHERINE M. OLSON, RN, BSN, TNS
Trauma Nurse Coordinator
Sherman Hospital
Elgin, Illinois

MARY E. O'SHIELDS, RN, MS
Director, Emergency and Trauma Nursing
Saint Francis Hospital
Evanston, Illinois

DEBORAH O'STEEN, RN, MS, CEN
Assistant Manager/Educator, Emergency Center
WellStar Cobb Hospital
Austell, Georgia

ALICA A. PEAVEY, RN-CS, MS, FNP, CLNC
Staff Nurse, Emergency Center
WellStar Kennestone Hosptial
Marietta, Georgia

BARBARA PIERCE, RN, MN
Director, Emergency Services
Huntsville Hospital System
Huntsville, Alabama

BARBARA ANN REED, RN, BSN,
Educator/Staff Nurse, Critical Care
Sentara Healthcare
Norfolk, Virginia;
MSN/ACNP Student
University of Virginia
Charlottesville, Virginia

CHERIE J. REVERE, RN, MSN, CEN, CRNP
Clinical Nurse Specialist, Emergency Department
University of South Alabama Medical Center
Mobile, Alabama

DEBORAH REVIS, RN, PHD
Administrative Director
Emergency, Trauma, and Burn Services
University of Alabama at Birmingham
Birmingham, Alabama

SUZANNE RITA, RN, MSN
Lecturer
Old Dominion University, School of Nursing
Norfolk, Virginia

ANITA RUIZ-CONTERAS
Emergency Staff Developer
Santa Clara Valley Medical Center
Sexual Assault Nurse Examiner
Santa Clara County, California

ELLEN E. RUJA, RN, MSN, CEN, TNCC
Nurse Manager, Emergency Services
Medical University of South Carolina
Charleston, South Carolina

CAROLE RUSH, RN, MED, CEN
Injury Prevention Specialist and Emergency Staff Nurse
Calgary Health Region
Calgary, Alberta, Canada

KATHLEEN SCHENKEL, RN, BSN, CEN
Nurse Manager, Emergency Department
Children's Hospital of Pittsburgh
Pittsburgh, Pennsylvania

S. KAY SEDLAK, RN, MS, CEN
Clinical Nurse Specialist, Emergency Department
St. Mary's Regional Medical Center
Reno, Nevada

DEBORAH E. TRAUTMAN, RN, MSN, CEN
Director of Nursing, Department of Emergency Medicine
The Johns Hopkins Hospital
Baltimore, Maryland

STEVEN A. WEINMAN, RN, BSN, CEN
Director, Office of Continuing Medical Education
Elsevier Health Sciences, Excerpta Medica, Inc.
Hillsborough, New Jersey;
Per Diem Instructor, Emergency Care
New York Presbyterian Hospital
Cornell Medical Center
New York, New York

MARY ELLEN WILSON, RN, MS, CEN, FNP
Clinical Education Specialist, Emergency Services
New Hanover Health Network
Wilmington, North Carolina

KIMBERLY A. WOMACK, RN, MS, ANCP-C, CEN
Emergency Nurse Practitioner
Emerginet, Inc.
Atlanta, Georgia

CHERYL WRAA, RN, MSNC
Trauma Coordinator
University of California, Davis Medical Center
Sacramento, California

Contributors to Previous Edition

Cynthia S. Baxter, RN, BSN, CCRN, CEN
Unit Coordinator
Critical Care Transport
Central Baptist Hospital
Lexington, Kentucky

Doreen K. Begley, RN, BS, CEN
Staff Nurse, Emergency Department
Washoe Medical Center
Reno, Nevada

Lynn M. Feeman, RN, MSN, CEN, CCRN
Trauma Nurse Coordinator
Grady Health Systems
Atlanta, Georgia

Jackie Gondeck, RN, BSN, MHA, CEN
Clinical Education Coordinator, Emergency Department
Brackenridge Hospital
Austin, Texas

Susan L. Hatfield, RN, MS, CEN, FNP
Family Nurse Practitioner—Certified
Internal Medicine
Cartersville, Georgia

T. Randall Huey, RN, MS, CEN
Clinical Nurse Specialist
Emergency Department
Piedmont Hospital
Atlanta, Georgia

Charose James, RN, BSN, CEN
Staff Nurse, Emergency Department
Methodist Hospital
Omaha, Nebraska

Kathleen M. Kearney, RN, MSN, CEN
Clinical Nurse Specialist
Beth Israel Medical Center
New York, New York

Patricia A. Lenaghan, RN, MS, CEN
Service Executive, Emergency Department
Methodist Hospital
Omaha, Nebraska

Sharon K. Mason, RN, CEN, CCRN, CFNP
Staff Nurse, Emergency Room
Cartersville, Georgia

Mary Ellen McNally Pedersen, RN, BS, CPTC
New England Organ Bank
Maine Trasplant Program
Bangor, Maine

Tracy McIntyre Ross, RN, BSN, CEN
Staff Nurse, Emergency Department
Virginia Beach General Hospital;
Staff Nurse, Patient First
Urgent Care Clinic
Virginia Beach, Virginia

Kim M. Rouse, RN, BSN
Manager, Emergency Services
Nebraska Methodist and Children's Hospitals
Omaha, Nebraska

Rebecca A. Steinmann, RN, MS, CEN, CCRN
Clinical Nurse Specialist, Emergency Services
University Hospitals of Cleveland
Cleveland, Ohio

Janet P. Taylor, DSN, RN
Instructor
Associate Degree Nursing
Jones County Junior College
Ellisville, Mississippi

Joe E. Taylor, Jr., PhD, RN, CEN, FNP
Family Nurse Practitioner
Family Medical Associates
Collins, Mississippi

Tener Goodwin Veenema, MS, RN, PNP
Pediatric Nurse Practitioner
Coordinator for Case Management, Emergency Services
University of Rochester Medical Center
Rochester, New York

E. MARIE WILSON, RN, MPA
Chief, System Development
Office of Emergency Medical Services
Connecticut Department of Public Health
Hartford, Connecticut

TRACEY J. WOOD, RN, BSN, CEN
Emergency Center
WellStar Kennestone Hospital
Marietta, Georgia

Reviewers

DONNA MASSEY, RN, MSN
Associate Director of Education
Emergency Nurses Association
DesPlaines, Illinois

LINDA M. SCOTT, RN, MSN, PhD, C-FNP
Professor/Associate Dean
School of Nursing
Marshall University
Huntington, West Virginia

RUSSELL WILSHAW, RN, MS, CEN
Trauma Coordinator
Urban South Intermountain Health Care
Utah Valley Regional Medical Center
Provo, Utah

In memory of Opal . . . mother, nurse, friend . . .
She faced life with laughter, optimism, and common sense.
She faced death with faith, humor, and dignity.
Her life and her death were lessons in courage.

Lorene Newberry

PREFACE

As you peruse this fifth edition of *Sheehy's Emergency Nursing: Principles and Practice,* you will find it new and improved. The best from the previous edition has been continued—organizational structure, powerful visual impact, and effective writing by strong emergency nurses. Contributors again represent the entire spectrum of emergency nursing practice. Practice areas include urban, suburban, and rural emergency departments, with staff nurses, clinical nurse specialists, nurse managers, and nursing instructors well represented.

Specific changes made to the text address changes in practice (e.g., decreasing use of gastric lavage) as well as a change in focus. Content has been intentionally streamlined so that the focus is the emergency nurse at the bedside. Despite this change, the text should still prove beneficial for educators and clinical managers. Across the board, illustrations have been upgraded and content has been enhanced. The chapter on child abuse and neglect includes photographs that speak to the horror of this problem. New photographs add impact to the chapters on pediatric emergencies, pediatric trauma, renal/GU trauma, and many others. New tables and figures add clarity and highlight key information throughout the text.

Quality improvement and case management have been replaced with a chapter on outcomes management that addresses ED-specific issues such as chest pain and asthma management. A chapter on behavioral health emergencies replaces the previous chapter on mental health emergencies. The chapter is essentially new and addresses the most common situations encountered by the ED, such as anxiety and depression. Emergency departments across the country have seen an increase in the number of behavioral emergencies.

General discussion of emergency operations preparedness has been replaced with a chapter on weapons of mass destruction (WMD). The threat of terrorism is an ongoing concern in the wake of the bombings of the World Trade Center and is a potential event for any emergency nurse and emergency department—regardless of location. The chapter provides some common sense tips for dealing with potential WMD events.

But, perhaps the most significant addition to the text is a chapter dedicated to end of life in the ED—a first for an emergency nursing text. Sudden death as well as expected death are realities in our profession. How you convey bad news, deal with grieving families, and many other end-of-life issues are discussed in this chapter. Hopefully, this chapter will provide insight for the frontline nurse.

Enjoy the changes in this latest edition. I hope you find them beneficial to you, your practice, and most importantly to your patients. I know you will recognize the commitment, dedication, and professionalism of those whose work made this book a reality.

Lorene Newberry

ACKNOWLEDGMENTS

Nursing and emergency nursing has been good to me. I have had the opportunity to do many things because I am a nurse. This book is one of those opportunities. But I could not have done it alone . . . just as in nursing we do not practice alone. I acknowledge those individuals who made their mark. The text was finished on time due to the professionalism of the contributors, reviewers, and the editorial and production staff at Mosby/Elsevier Health Sciences. Many thanks for your support and hard work. I am honored to say again that I could not have done it without each one of you.

I recognize and say a special thanks to the following professional groups and individuals who were specifically involved in the creation and publication of the text. I am grateful that the Emergency Nurses Association allowed me to edit a second edition of this text. I am honored to have had the opportunity to contribute to my profession through this text.

Many thanks to all of the 51 chapter writers who reviewed, revised, and researched . . . making sure content was accurate, usable, and reflected current practice. You looked at your practice with a critical eye—not always easy in today's fast-paced world. You make a strong statement for your profession.

One of the many strengths of this book are the reviews by Donna Massey, Linda Scott, and Russell Wilshaw. These individuals with strong clinical backgrounds meticulously read and re-read every chapter . . . for errors, omissions, and linguistic confusion. Their efforts paid off in improved content and clarity.

The publication of this text would not be possible without the work of the staff at Mosby/Elsevier Health Sciences.

Special thanks to the following individuals. Shari Malchow, Senior Developmental Editor, for her assistance in manuscript preparation—correcting references, matching illustrations, and confirming that appropriate permissions were granted. Cheryl Abbott, Senior Project Manager, provided invaluable assistance during the final production. She again demonstrated an ability to see the big picture and the small details. Thanks for catching replications, omissions, and misspellings. And many thanks to all those behind the scenes. They suffered through impossible deadlines, multiple corrections, and the obvious challenge of my penmanship.

It goes without saying that editing a text of this size and magnitude consumes a lot of time and attention. Without the love, support, and caring of family, friends, and co-workers, you become so focused on the task at hand that you forget the importance of your other life. The management team of WellStar Emergency Services continues to challenge me professionally and keep me from stagnating. I benefit from working with the staff of four very different emergency centers—WellStar Cobb Hospital, WellStar Douglas Hospital, WellStar Kennestone Hospital, and WellStar Paulding Hospital. They make me proud of my profession.

And finally, I thank those closest to me for their love and support. My friends who have again tolerated my tendency to work too much and take on too many projects. My family who represents my past and shows me what the future can be. Lastly, to the one who taught me about unconditional love. I am a better person because of you.

Lorene Newberry

Table of Contents

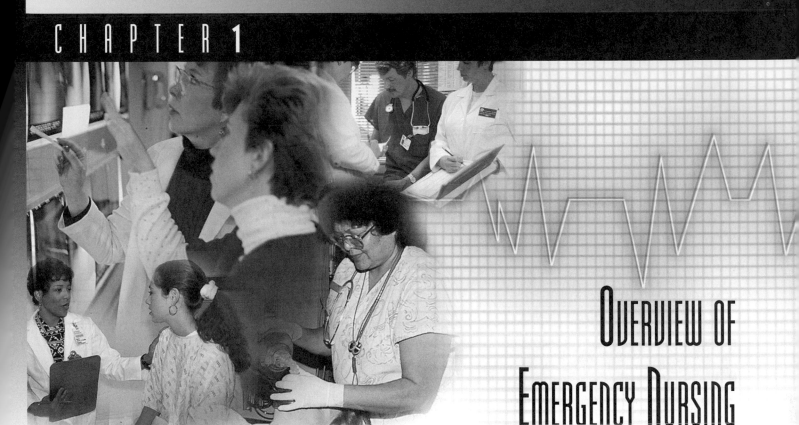

CHAPTER 1

OVERVIEW OF EMERGENCY NURSING

ESTELLE MacPHAIL

Emergency nursing has its origins in the Florence Nightingale era; however, the specialty practice of emergency nursing has evolved only during the past 30 years. By definition, emergency nursing is the care of individuals of all ages with perceived or actual physical or emotional alterations of health that are undiagnosed or require further interventions. Emergency nursing care is episodic, primary, and usually acute.

Alliance or affiliation with a specific body system, disease process, care setting, age group, or population defines most specialty nursing groups. In contrast, emergency nursing is defined by diversity of knowledge, patients, and disease processes. Emergency nurses care for all ages and populations across a broad spectrum of disease, injury prevention, life-saving, and limb-saving measures. Emergency nursing practice requires a unique blend of generalized *and* specialized assessment, intervention, and management skills. The multiple dimensions of emergency nursing specify roles, behaviors, and processes inherent in the practice and delineate characteristics unique to the specialty. Practice area, patient population, and the variety of those who provide care are as diverse in emergency nursing as in the nursing profession as a whole.

The scope of emergency nursing practice encompasses assessment, diagnosis, treatment, and evaluation. The problems that can be perceived are actual or potential, sudden or urgent, physical or psychosocial. They are primarily episodic or acute and occur in a variety of settings. Resolu-

tion of problems may require minimal care or advanced life support measures, patient and/or family education, appropriate referral, and knowledge of legal implications. Care delivery occurs where the consumer lives, works, plays, and goes to school. Box 1-1 identifies just a few practice areas for emergency nursing.

Emergency nursing is multidimensional, requiring knowledge of various body systems, disease processes, and age groups common to other nursing specialties. Processes unique to emergency nursing, such as triage and emergency operations preparedness, are discussed in later chapters. In addition to these recognized processes, emergency nursing is governed by a unique set of unwritten rules that developed as an outcome of the environment and the care of patients (Box 1-2).

Nursing roles include patient care, research, management, education, consultation, and advocacy. Emergency nursing practice is defined through specific role functions as delineated in the Emergency Nurses Association's (ENA) *Standards of Emergency Nursing Practice, Scope of Practice Statement,* and *Emergency Nursing Core Curriculum.* Roles are further defined in ENA's *Trauma Nursing Core Course, Emergency Nursing Pediatric Course, Course in Advanced Trauma Nursing,* and *Prehospital Core Curriculum.* Roles are also determined by the practice arena. The emergency nurse in a teaching institution may function very differently than the emergency nurse in a small rural hospital.

Box 1-1 EMERGENCY NURSING PRACTICE SETTINGS

Hospital emergency department (ED)
Free-Standing ED
Prehospital arena
Air and ground transport units
Military arena
Urgent care center
Health clinic
Health maintenance organization
Ambulatory services
Schools and universities
Business/Industry
Correctional institution
Occupational health clinics

Box 1-2 EMERGENCY NURSING ENVIRONMENT

Unplanned situations that require immediate intervention
Allocation of limited resources
Need for immediate care perceived by the patient or others
Geographic variables
Unpredictable numbers of patients
Unknown patient severity, urgency, and diagnosis
Cultural and language variables

Box 1-3 STANDARDS OF EMERGENCY NURSING PRACTICE

POTENTIAL USES

Criterion-based job descriptions and performance evaluations
Policies and procedures
Standardized care plans
Orientation and education programs
Performance improvement programs
Research projects

Box 1-4 EMERGENCY NURSING FOUNDATION PURPOSE

Enhance emergency health care services to the public by:

Promoting emergency nursing through research and education
Enhancing professional development through research
Providing a means for education of health care professionals in the care and treatment of emergency patients
Educating the general public on emergency-related subjects
Providing research grants and educational scholarships

STANDARDS

A standard is an acknowledged measure of quantitative or qualitative value. It reflects ongoing changes in practice and clarifies the distinction between competence and excellence in practice. The minimally acceptable level of performance is reflected in competency level outcomes. Excellence is practice that surpasses the competency level and, ultimately, contributes to growth and advancement of emergency nursing. Standards are a measure by which the consumer views emergency nursing performance and a measure to which nurses are held accountable.

Standards represent a philosophy and should be considered a collection of recommendations and guidelines that contain outcome criteria to measure and evaluate performance. The original *Standards of Emergency Nursing Practice* (1983) provided a springboard for growth of emergency nursing. Since their development, the *Standards* have been used for a variety of purposes (Box 1-3). In 1992, practice standards from the American Nurses Association were incorporated into the *Standards*. This strengthened the *Standards* by highlighting the depth and breadth of emergency nursing practice.

Emergency nursing practice is systematic and includes nursing process, nursing diagnosis, decision making, and analytic and scientific thinking and inquiry. Professional behaviors inherent in emergency nursing practice are acquisition and application of a specialized body of knowledge and skills, accountability and responsibility, communication, autonomy, and collaborative relationships with others.

RESEARCH IN EMERGENCY NURSING

Promoting research in emergency nursing adds to knowledge of the discipline and contributes to sound clinical decisions. Collaborative research endeavors broaden the scope of emergency nursing knowledge. The *ENA Code of Ethics for Emergency Nursing* (1989) provides a distinctive set of ideals and standards for conduct regarding research activities. Ethical principles are the moral bond linking the profession, the patients served, and the public.

In 1991 ENA established the Emergency Nursing Foundation to promote availability, quality, and effectiveness of emergency nursing practice through education and research. Box 1-4 clarifies the goals of the Emergency Nursing Foundation. Interest from donations and fund-raising activities are invested and distributed for scholarships, research, and special projects. Many nurses have received grants for research and continued education.

SPECIALTY PRACTICE

A characteristic inherent in emergency care is integration of the emergency health care team. In no other area in health care are teamwork and mutual respect more important. Quality of care depends on this team concept. Nurses, nurse practitioners, physicians, physician assistants, paramedics, emergency medical technicians, and first responders must

Table 1-1	EMS PERSONNEL AND RESPONSIBILITIES	
PERSONNEL	**RESPONSIBILITIES**
First responders	Establish basic life support procedures. Include police, fire, and civilian personnel.
EMS dispatchers	Triage, prioritize, and relay call for help. Dispatch essential personnel and equipment. Provide instructions for first responders until advanced help arrives.
Advanced responders	Include emergency medical technicians, paramedics, nurses, respiratory therapists, and physicians. Vary with type of call and community-accepted protocol. Provide advanced care at scene and during transport.

function collegially to provide optimal patient care to the ill or injured.

The outcome of care in the hospital is greatly influenced by the field team's effort during initial stabilization and transfer and through ongoing communication. Personnel needs in the emergency medical service system vary with type of call, community protocol, and available resources. Table 1-1 describes specific emergency personnel and their responsibilities. It is beyond the scope of this text to provide a comprehensive description of each discipline. The brevity of information provided should not be construed as a reflection of the importance of each team member.

Certified Emergency Nurse

The examination for certified emergency nurses (CEN) is a mechanism by which knowledge and skills for safe and competent practice can be measured. It is administered by the Board of Certification for Emergency Nursing to promote the health and welfare of emergency patients by advancing the science and art of emergency nursing through the certification process. A nurse with a CEN credential has demonstrated knowledge in the specialty of emergency nursing. Chapter 2 discusses certification.

Emergency Nurse Practitioner

The nurse practitioner is a professional registered nurse with advanced education in delivery of primary care to adult and pediatric patients. The emergency nurse practitioner is a nurse practitioner who specializes in emergency care because of education and clinical experience. Responsibilities include care of emergency patients under the medical supervision of the attending physician. Certification for a nurse practitioner is provided by professional boards such as the American Nurses Credentialing Center. Nurse practitioner programs are usually a master's level, vary from 44 to 72 weeks, and cover acute and nonacute emergency situations. Practice areas include emergency departments open 24 hours a day, urgent care centers, and rural clinics with minimal or no physician coverage. Some states allow nurse practitioners to have prescription privileges.

Clinical Nurse Specialist

The clinical nurse specialist (CNS) is a registered nurse who, through advanced study of scientific knowledge and supervised advanced clinical practice at the master's or doctoral level, has become an expert in emergency nursing. An emergency CNS demonstrates expertise through innovative, comprehensive, and high-quality performance in emergency nursing. Specific responsibilities include accountability for development and application of practice standards, as well as research to enhance the quality of care for patients, their significant others, communities, and potential consumers of emergency care. Ultimately the emergency CNS strives to improve patient care and enhance treatment outcomes.

The emergency CNS exemplifies professional nursing practice through direct and indirect patient care. Specific role functions are expert clinical practitioner, educator, consultant, researcher, and leader. Within each role, the emergency CNS is a role model, patient advocate, change agent, and cost-effective practitioner. Through application of these responsibilities, the emergency CNS is in a unique position to affect the profession, the specialty, and, most important, the patient.

Case Manager

The case manager role enhances quality patient care while promoting cost effectiveness in the hospital or clinic arena. The case manager crosses departmental lines; therefore, authority and ability to negotiate with multiple providers is essential to ensure optimal care in the most cost-effective manner possible. The case manager has a global focus, covering the continuum of care from patient arrival to discharge and beyond. The objective of the case manager is to provide medically necessary quality care and to ensure access to and continuity of care for a patient.[1]

Specialties Within Emergency Nursing

With the explosion of information and technology, nursing has become more and more specialized. Conventional wisdom that "a nurse is a nurse is a nurse" no longer applies. This is also true for emergency nursing. A subspecialty is, by definition, a group of nurses who work in a specific environment, care for special patient groups, perform special functions, or have special interests related to emergency nursing. Recognized subspecialties within emergency nursing include flight nursing, pediatric emergency nursing, trauma nursing, prehospital nursing, and mobile intensive care nursing. As emergency nursing copes with a changing world, additional subspecialties are emerging. These include groups who deal with infomatics, sexual assault, forensics, telephone triage, and uniformed services. Each subspecialty has unique needs related to education, practice, and networking.

Prehospital Nursing

Prehospital nursing dates back more than 100 years. In the 1970s, nurses staffed mobile advanced life support units. Today nurses in the prehospital arena are an extension of the acute and nonacute settings. In 1992 ENA published the Prehospital Core Curriculum to establish core knowledge and skills pertinent to prehospital nursing practice.

Flight Nursing

Flight nursing requires a strong background in critical care and emergency nursing. Flight nurses provide a high level of care at the scene of an accident, in the referring hospital, and during transport by fixed wing or rotary wing aircraft. The flight nurse integrates knowledge of the nursing process and practice standards set forth by the Air Surface Transport Nurses Association, formerly known as the National Flight Nurses Association. Recognition of the unique and diverse contributions of these groups strengthens the practice of all emergency nurses.

HOSPITAL EMERGENCY DEPARTMENT

Dramatic changes have occurred in the ED during the past 30 years. Emergency rooms became emergency departments (ED), which in turn became emergency centers incorporating prehospital care, flight programs, ambulatory care, occupational health programs, observation units, fast-track/urgent care treatment areas, and satellite units. The Medicare Act of 1965 and Medicaid Act of 1966 gave millions of Americans access to health care. The Vietnam War led to recognition of trauma as a leading cause of death and disability. Federal grants supported development of emergency medical systems. Special centers for the management of trauma, as well as pediatric emergency centers to meet the special needs of children evolved across the country.

EDs care for billions of people each year. Emergency medical evaluation and initial treatment are provided through a well-defined plan based on community need and the defined capabilities of each hospital. The ED is the only provider many people ever know. It serves not only as a receiving center for critically ill and injured people, but also as a 24-hour shelter for people who are frightened and have nowhere else to go. The number of individuals seen in the ED has grown steadily during the past decade. More than 100 billion patients were seen in EDs across the country during 1998. Reasons for these increases are multiple and complex (Box 1-5). In the early 1990s many experts predicted that managed care would reverse this trend by diverting patients to primary care centers. Regrettably, a supporting network of primary care centers failed to material-

BOX 1-5   POTENTIAL CAUSES OF INCREASED EMERGENCY DEPARTMENT CENSUS
No appointment required
Lack of accessibility to private providers
Convenient for those with limited resources
Treatment regardless of ability to pay
Open on weekends, holidays, and after hours
Lack of familiarity with the American health care system

ize, so admissions and ED visits continued to increase at the end of the twentieth century. In 2000, increasing visits and admissions led to development of diversion policies to address this crisis by diverting emergency patients to facilities able to provide care. As the national population increases at a pace beyond the growth of available health care resources, patient volumes will continue to increase in EDs across the country.

Urgent Care Centers

According to the U.S. Census Bureau, the population increased by 32.7 million between 1990 and 2000. This 13.2% increase in the population is reflected in increasing ED visits across the country. The greatest increase in census numbers has been in those patients who fall in the urgent or nonemergent category—patients who could be seen in a primary care physician's office. Fast-track and urgent care centers emerged as a way to manage these patients. Urgent care centers may be part of the existing ED or function as a separate entity outside the ED. Treating patients with minor complaints outside the ED reduces treatment time and enhances patient satisfaction.

SUMMARY

Advances in technology may soon be overshadowed by an increasing demand for emergency care, particularly for critically ill patients. As the ED cares for more critical patients for longer periods, the need for sophisticated monitoring equipment increases. Technology previously reserved for the critical care unit is now commonplace in the ED. As these and other changes occur, emergency nursing becomes more complex and demanding.

As the population ages, health care needs continue to change and become more complex. Preventive medicine is prohibitively expensive for the indigent and most elders. Patients are discharged earlier after surgery, myocardial infarction, and many other conditions. Unfortunately, it means patients are sicker when they arrive in the ED and they stay longer.

This situation is exacerbated by lack of home care and other essential community resources and the recent increase in ED visits. Emergency nurses serve increasingly demanding consumers. The public expects the latest technology and sophistication without loss of "high-touch" care. Insurance companies and employers are looking for the lowest health care cost available. New reimbursement rules such as the Ambulatory Patient Classification system drive decision making. In the past, hospitals received reimbursement from the government and other third-party payers based on cost. In today's health care market, reimbursement is based on a specified number of covered lives rather than actual cost of care provided. Simply put, the hospital is paid what is in its contract, regardless of how much it actually costs to do the procedure or care for the patient. Faced with reimbursement restrictions, health care administrators have tightened their budgetary belts, asking fewer to do more with less.

The year 2000 was marked by the most significant nursing shortage in the past 20 years. Many issues will affect nursing as the health care system undergoes radical change. The nursing profession and how it is perceived will continue to evolve. As nursing becomes more active in the decision-making process and speaks with a single voice, these changes become shining opportunities. Emergency nurses must join together with a new energy, speak with a new voice, and create a new presence for emergency nursing.

References

1. Hammer M: *Case managers make sense of the healthcare system.* Retrieved February 27, 2002 from the World Wide Web: http://healthcare.monster.com/articles/casemanage/

Suggested Reading

Emergency Nurses Association: *Code of ethics,* Chicago, 1989, The Association.

Emergency Nurses Association: *Core curriculum,* ed 5, Philadelphia, 2000, WB Saunders.

Emergency Nurses Association: *Emergency nursing pediatric course,* ed 2, Park Ridge, Ill, 1998, The Association.

Emergency Nurses Association: *Position paper: role of the clinical nurse specialist,* Chicago, 1989, The Association.

Emergency Nurses Association: Position statement, Park Ridge, Ill, 1995, The Association.

Emergency Nurses Association: *Pre-hospital core curriculum,* ed 2, Park Ridge, Ill, 1994, The Association.

Emergency Nurses Association: Scope of practice statement, *JEN* 15(4):361, 1989.

Emergency Nurses Association: *Standards of emergency nursing practice,* ed 4, Des Plaines, Ill, 1999, The Association.

Emergency Nurses Association: *Trauma nursing core course,* ed 5, Chicago, 2000, The Association.

Emergency Nurses Association: *Triage: meeting the challenge,* ed 2, Des Plaines, Ill, 2001, The Association.

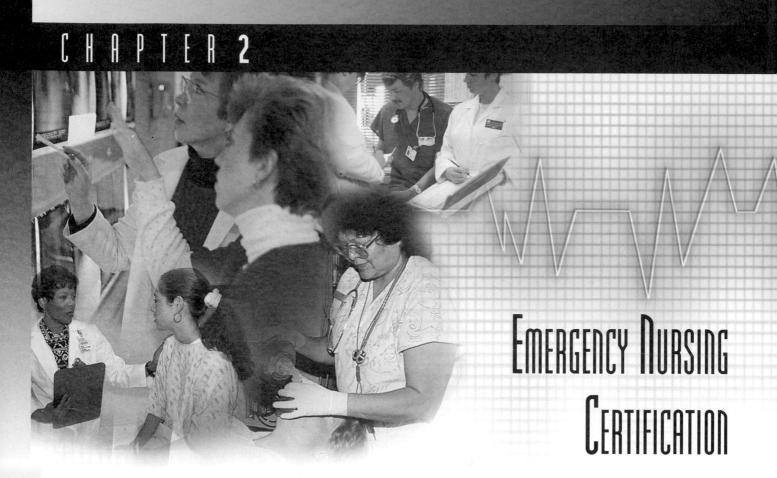

CHAPTER 2

EMERGENCY NURSING CERTIFICATION

ANNE P. MANTON

The opportunity for certification in a nursing specialty dates back to 1945 when the American Association of Nurse Anesthetists first initiated certification. Most certifications in nursing, however, were established within the last three decades. Increase in the number of nursing specialty organizations has been a major factor in proliferation of nursing certifications. More than 70 certifications are currently available. Most specialty organizations offer only a single certification with a second offered as an advanced-level examination in a few cases. The exception to this is the American Nurses Credentialing Center (ANCC), which offers more than 35 specialty and advanced practice certifications.

OVERVIEW

What is the purpose of certification? Why do nurses participate in this process? The primary purpose of certification, whether in nursing or another discipline, is to assure the public that an individual has acquired a specific body of knowledge. The Board of Certification for Emergency Nursing (BCEN) identifies an additional purpose, which is "to provide a mechanism to regularly measure the attainment and simulated application of a defined body of emergency nursing knowledge."[3]

Consequently, certification benefits both the individual nurse and the employer while serving the public interest. Achieving certification may also lead to greater respect from employers and colleagues, salary increases, and perhaps most important, greater self-esteem and a sense of professional accomplishment. Employers and potential employers also benefit from nursing certification. Certification provides an objective measure of an employee's knowledge base, as well as valuable information about prospective employees.

The nursing profession as a whole benefits from certification. Because of the certification process, bodies of specialty nursing knowledge are defined and examined. Certification demonstrates to other health care disciplines that nurses are able to articulate their defined body of knowledge and establish levels of specialty competence based on that knowledge. Another way in which certification benefits nursing is through preparation for the certification examination. Certification requires thorough study of the body of knowledge of the specialty. Certification renewal encourages the practicing nurse to remain current in all aspects of specialty nursing practice.

In a general sense, there are three ways by which nurses can obtain certification. One way is certification by a state or government agency. State certification represents legal endorsement of a nurse's ability to function in certain expanded nursing roles. This process is different from that by which a nurse becomes a registered nurse. Certification by a state usually refers to a specific aspect of nursing practice beyond the level addressed in a state board examination for registration. State certification is often based on prior certification by a nurse certification body, completion of an

6

education program, or both. In some instances, a certifying examination is administered by a state agency. Requirements for state certification vary, so certification by one state may not be recognized by another.

State certification has advantages and disadvantages. Among the advantages are public recognition of specialty nursing and expanded roles in nursing practice. Perhaps most important, state certification allows the state to exercise control over those who perform in specialty or expanded roles. In this way the public is better protected from persons who are not competent to practice in specialty roles.

Disadvantages of state certification include additional responsibilities placed on state boards of nursing, which are usually already overburdened. Effects on other aspects of a board's responsibilities, be it neglect or delay, must be carefully considered. Another possible disadvantage is that regulations may be so narrowly interpreted they restrict dimensions of usual nursing practice. Perhaps the most obvious and ominous disadvantage is that when practice issues are placed in so public a domain, the door is opened for powerful lobbying groups (e.g., third-party payers, medical societies, and other care providers) to influence nursing practice.

Certification can also occur through an institution. The institution may be a health care facility or educational system. This type of certification is usually based on successful completion of an educational offering, often varying in length and characteristics. Most often the state or profession does not control content or requisites for such certification. Because of program variability and lack of oversight by a national body, this type of certification may have limited appeal or applicability outside the particular certifying institution. This is primarily because consumers and professionals alike seem to more highly value academic degrees or certifications based on national standards. Some local triage, trauma nursing, and mobile intensive care nursing certifications (MICN) are examples of this type of certification.

The usual way to obtain certification in a nursing specialty is through a professional organization. Many types of certifications are offered by the ANCC. Most nursing specialty organizations have also developed, or are in the process of developing, a certification process in their specialty. These efforts are testimony to the belief that knowledge beyond the level of safe basic nursing practice is required for specialty nursing practice.

Although mechanisms for certification vary from one specialty to another, certification granted by a specialty organization is nationally and internationally recognized. Certification associated with a specialty nursing organization is also more relevant to that specialty's nursing practice and defined body of knowledge.

SPECIALTY CERTIFICATION

Nursing certifying organizations have various requirements for certification and renewal of certification. Requirements for nursing specialty certification fall into the following cat-

egories: education, practice, demonstration of knowledge, and renewal mechanisms.

All nursing specialty certification organizations require that candidates be registered nurses. This requirement assumes successful completion of the initial licensure examination of nursing (NCLEX). Some specialties require or are considering requiring a bachelor's degree as the minimum for certification eligibility. It is important to note that certification in emergency nursing (CEN) does not require either a bachelor's or master's degree. Completion of a master's degree is a requirement for initial eligibility for ANCC advanced practice certification examinations. The ANCC and other certifying organizations also require specific courses and clinical experience for certifications such as nurse practitioner and nurse midwife.

Some certifications have practice requirements in addition to educational requirements. To be eligible to take the certification examination, the nurse must have spent a minimum number of hours in specialty practice. In areas such as emergency nursing certification, the practice component of the certification process is a strong recommendation, rather than an absolute requirement. It has been demonstrated that nurses with at least 2 years of practice in a specialty are more likely to achieve a passing score on the certification examination than those with less practice time in the specialty.

All nursing specialty certifications require the applicant for initial certification to demonstrate mastery of the body of specialty nursing knowledge by written examination. Certification examinations vary in length and format, but all are sufficient, according to experts within the specialty, to broadly examine the applicant's knowledge base in the specialty. Written examinations (including computer-based examinations) provide the most objective measure of mastery of core knowledge of the specialty. Practical or psychomotor examinations measure the application and attainment of requisite knowledge; however, most certifying agencies find these examinations too cumbersome to conduct with the consistency, objectivity, and integrity necessary for the examination process.

The final component of the certification process that all nursing specialty certification agencies have in common is renewal of certification. In almost all instances, certification is granted for a limited time with the usual range 3 to 5 years. This finite period of certification recognizes the dynamic, always changing, and evolving state of nursing knowledge. Thus, the certified nurse's continued mastery of the knowledge base of the specialty must be verified at regular intervals. The mechanism by which certification is renewed varies with the certifying body. Some opt to require candidates to retake the examination, whereas others choose mandatory continuing education hours. Possible approaches to renewal of certification have broadened considerably in the past several years with such options as portfolio and open-book exams. Regardless of the method used, the purpose of recertification is to ensure competence. Weisfeld and Falk stated that "with the half-life of medical knowledge usually estimated at 5 years, and the pace of obsolescence even faster in some allied occupations, little justification can be found for requiring a demonstration of initial competence, while ignoring the need for continuing competence."[4]

EMERGENCY NURSING CERTIFICATION

The first emergency nursing certification examination was administered in July 1980 and has been offered continually since that time. Originally, the examination comprised 250 questions, all of which were calculated into the score. The number of correct answers necessary for a passing score and certification was consistent at 175. Since 1980 the certification examination has evolved into a more sophisticated measure of emergency nursing knowledge. All question-and-answer sets are now pretested within exams for accuracy, clarity, and reliability before inclusion among those questions that determine the passing score. It is critically important for validity and reliability of the certification examination to have all items pretested. It is because of this pretesting process that the BCEN can know with assurance that each examination has the same degree of difficulty, that no one has an easier or more difficult examination than anyone else. Items being pretested are not included in the test score. Currently each examination contains 25 pretest items and 150 items that are scored.

Examination Content for Certification in Emergency Nursing

To ensure the certification examination reflects current emergency nursing practice, two role delineation studies (RDS) were completed by the BCEN. The first RDS was conducted in 1989-1990. Analysis of that study's findings indicated considerable concurrence between content of the emergency nursing certification examination and emergency nursing practice. Changes were made so the examination closely reflects information from the RDS. A second RDS in 1994 found a high degree of consistency between emergency nursing practice and certification examination content.

Minor adjustments to the content blueprint for the certification examination have been made over time as a result of practice changes reflected in analysis of responses to the latest RDS and changes made in the examination process. The blueprint for the examination is based on clinical categories and is summarized in Table 2-1. Within each of those categories, questions may focus on aspects of assessment, analysis/diagnosis, intervention, or evaluation. The certification examination is constructed according to number of items in each content area as shown in the table.

Certification Renewal

CEN is granted for 4 years. Initial certification can only be accomplished by successfully passing the certification ex-

Table 2-1	**CEN EXAMINATION CONTENT AREAS BY NUMBER OF ITEMS**
NUMBER OF ITEMS	**CONTENT AREA**
13	Cardiovascular emergencies
8	Gastrointestinal emergencies
10	Genitourinary, gynecologic, and obstetric emergencies
9	Maxillofacial and ocular emergencies
10	Neurologic emergencies
15	Orthopedic emergencies and wound management
7	Psychosocial emergencies
14	Respiratory emergencies
21	Patient care management
15	Substance abuse/Toxicologic and environmental emergencies
10	Shock/Multisystem trauma emergencies
12	Medical emergencies
6	Professional issues

amination. Effective with the February 1992 examination, recertification can be accomplished by reexamination or by a renewal option (CEN-RO) that focuses on the nurse's continuing education. CEN-RO can only be used to recertify every *other* time recertification is due. The renewal option cannot be used for two consecutive renewals. For example, a nurse who certified by testing in 1996 and exercised the renewal option (CEN-RO) for certification in the year 2000 must take and pass the certification examination in 2004 to remain a CEN. The CEN-RO option could be used again in 2008. CENs always have the option to renew certification every 4 years by formal testing.

To renew certification via the CEN-RO program option, the nurse must obtain 100 hours of continuing education credit. An accurate record of continuing education credit (CE log) must be maintained and submitted for review with application and appropriate fee by the CE log filing deadline. Of 100 continuing education credit hours, at least 75 of them must be in the clinical category, with up to 25 credits from the other category.

According to the BCEN, the clinical category for continuing education credits "includes any educational offerings that primarily contain information applicable to direct nursing practice in the clinical area. The program content must be primarily focused on the knowledge the nurse can apply in providing direct care to an individual patient or community."[2] The other category "includes any educational offerings related to the professional practice of nursing and the emergency care system."[1] It is the responsibility of the CEN seeking renewal of certification to ensure appropriate categorization of continuing education on the CEN-RO CE log. Questions about clinical versus other categorization should be addressed to the BCEN. Each month, a randomly selected number of CE logs are selected for verification. Those candidates selected for verification must submit documentation of all continuing education activities reflected on the log, including course materials, objectives, outlines, and certificates received. Failure to meet verification requirements of the CEN-RO program means the individuals must take and pass the CEN examination to maintain their CEN credential.

TESTING

Testing provokes anxiety in virtually everyone. It is impressive, then, that to become certified, so many nurses choose to place themselves in this situation. The number of certified nurses is testimony to the confidence nurses have in their mastery of the specialty knowledge base and to their high level of professionalism. Not surprisingly, however, many nurses resist being tested to renew their certification.

Anxiety in the testing situation is normal. Uneasiness and anxiety occur because of the significance we, and others, attach to our success or failure on examinations. Although a certain amount of test anxiety is normal and may even be helpful, such anxiety must be controlled. Uncontrolled test anxiety can interfere with the ability to think clearly and demonstrate knowledge effectively. The following strategies may help nurses reduce that uncomfortable feeling of anxiety.

Foremost among strategies to reduce anxiety is to prepare well for the examination. Confidence in your knowledge base and your ability to respond correctly to a broad variety of questions is essential.

Developing a Study Plan

To study well, first determine your strengths and weaknesses in the material to be tested. Recognize that everyone has weaknesses. Once you identify your particular weaknesses, you can rectify them.

In preparing for the CEN examination, the next step is review of the content outline for the examination, described in the Certification Examination for Emergency Nurses (Candidate Handbook).[3] With the content outline in mind, focus on identification of your specific areas of strength and weakness. Review the Emergency Nursing Core Curriculum or another comprehensive emergency nursing text. As you survey each chapter, ask yourself whether you could answer questions related to that content area. Be honest with yourself. Another resource is the CEN Review Manual[1] or other such book that includes questions and answers for you to try. Armed with your self-assessment results, look once again at the CEN examination content outline. Your studying priorities should be a combination of your relative strength or weakness in content areas and the importance of those content areas; that is, the percentage of questions in that area listed in the examination blueprint.

Creating a list of priorities with timelines for your study plan may be helpful. Areas of your greatest perceived weakness that are identified as areas of high importance in the examination should be studied first. Areas of increasing

---

BOX 2-1   POTENTIAL QUESTIONS RELATED TO THE NURSING PROCESS

How is _____ related to _____?
What do I look for in assessment of _____?
What information leads me to conclude the problem is
_____?
If I see _____ in the presence of _____, what does this tell me?
What is the most appropriate treatment for _____? Why?
How do I know the situation is improving? Deteriorating?

---

strength of knowledge, areas of decreasing importance in the examination, or a combination of these, should be studied next. The last content areas to be studied should be those in which your knowledge base is strong or those in which content importance in the examination is slight. When designing a successful study plan, consider two components. The first consideration is that studying should occur over months, not weeks or days. Cramming does not lead to success. The other component is that some time should be left at the conclusion of your study for review. If you have followed the study plan and prepared well, review may not be necessary; however, reviewing during the week before the examination may increase your self-confidence, an important element of success in most endeavors. Remember, developing a study plan is vital to your success in testing. Failing to plan may mean planning to fail.

Study Techniques

Studying from a book is different from reading a novel; the purpose is different and so is the method. Professional literature includes advice on successful strategies for studying. One common suggestion is to conduct a preliminary survey of the section to be studied. This survey includes a brief preview of the introductory paragraph, headings, definitions, rules, and summary paragraph to identify core ideas. Another suggestion in many books and articles is to develop questions related to the material being studied. Some experts suggest reading the material for ideas and questions after conducting the survey. Others suggest that, once core ideas have been identified through the preliminary survey, the learner should construct questions appropriate to content area and proceed with reading to answer the questions. Whether you read first and then formulate questions to be answered in self-review or generate questions to be answered in subsequent reading of the content, formulation of questions is essential to studying. Although generating questions may seem to consume valuable time, asking and answering questions makes the content meaningful and, therefore, easily retained. When studying for the CEN examination, relate questions to the nursing process—96% of the examination is nursing-process based. Box 2-1 provides examples of questions that might be formulated.

> **Box 2-2**　**SUGGESTIONS FOR EFFECTIVE USE OF TEXTS AND STUDY AIDS**
>
> Look for clues that suggest a larger meaning (i.e., principle).
> Pay close attention to diagrams, graphs, tables, and illustrations. They often summarize an important concept or idea.
> Look for sentences in boldface or italics. Look closely at all sequences of numbered items.
> Look for patterns of relationships. Don't just look at the trees—remember the forest!
> Reduce subject matter to easily remembered divisions such as the nursing process.

As you read each section, concentrate on the content and give attention to ideas and concepts rather than words alone. Conceptualize rather than attempt to memorize. Know and understand basic principles, and reflect on their application as you study various sections. Many principles apply in a variety of instances; for example, airway, breathing, and circulation (ABCs). Keeping these principles in mind as you study each section makes answering those questions about the nursing process easier. Significance of an assessment finding or the value of a particular intervention becomes evident as a point of logic, not as something to be recalled from memory alone.

Visualization is another strategy that may help to increase memory. Think about certain types of patients—what their ideal care entails from assessment through diagnostics and interventions. Finally, how would you evaluate the outcome of all those activities? As you study, try to create pictures in your mind of patient situations.

After in-depth, concentrated reading of each section, attempt to answer questions about that section. This self-questioning often reveals areas for further review. Another strategy is use of a book such as the CEN Review Manual.[1] Use review questions in the book as a self-assessment aid after studying a particular clinical area. There are a number of comparable texts available that can serve as adjuncts for test preparation. If self-questioning identifies areas of knowledge deficits, reread those sections in the Emergency Nursing Core Curriculum or another emergency nursing text until understanding and recollection are achieved. When reading, try to relate or associate ideas or concepts with each other.

Develop "thinking skills" as you study. Establish frameworks or categories for information rather than attempting to memorize details or isolated facts. For example, think of the actions of various drug classifications and when they would be useful rather than when they might be harmful. Rather than memorizing information about laboratory tests, think about what the abnormal values tell you about the patient. Box 2-2 contains more suggestions for effective use of texts and other study aids.

Organizing and implementing a study plan is a matter of individual study style. Some prefer to study alone at an individual pace, while others find studying in a group more beneficial because discussion can generate and answer questions, identify larger issues and principles, and facilitate understanding. To make a study group successful, some guidelines should be considered. It is important to develop a plan and structure to which all group members can agree. Each member should have a role, or responsibility, in presenting and discussing topics. Allow time for socializing, preferably at the conclusion of each planned topical discussion. When socializing is not planned, members often use study time for this purpose. Be selective about group membership and the size of the group. Remember that study groups can be an effective way to prepare for the certification examination or they can waste valuable time.

Another effective study technique is use of audiotapes. Audiotapes are flexible—you can listen in the car, on the beach, or in the health club. These tapes usually appeal more to the person who studies alone or who learns more with repetition. Selection of a specific study technique is dependent on your specific knowledge. If you have a limited knowledge base, review of texts and development of study aids may be the most effective study technique. As you gain experience, question-and-answer books may be more beneficial. Regardless of how you study, use a technique that meets your needs and your existing knowledge base.

Test-Taking Strategies

Perhaps the most influential factor in successful test taking is attitude. It is possible to thoroughly know test material yet fail an examination because of poor attitude. Fear conditions the mind for failure. Fear and anxiety can cause tension and inability to think clearly. Fear can so overwhelm thought processes that what was known only moments before can no longer be recalled. The ability to think logically, solve problems, and determine relationships or associations can be greatly reduced because of fear. Fear can also cause careless mistakes. It is imperative to address fear and determine strategies to manage it before taking a test. Test taking involves skill. A test taker must develop a positive attitude toward his or her ability to master this skill.

The person with a successful attitude anticipates the examination as an opportunity to demonstrate what he or she knows, not a negative situation with potential for failure. The attitude of challenge rather than defeat leads to constructive preparation, which in turn leads to increased self-confidence and a positive attitude toward anticipated outcome of the examination.

Even well-prepared test takers experience some anxiety; therefore, well-internalized test-taking strategies are most helpful. It may be beneficial, especially for poor test takers, to practice these skills on sample test questions. The CEN handbook for candidates includes a number of such practice questions as does the computer software and review manual available from the ENA.

Box 2-3 GENERAL TEST-TAKING TIPS

There is no penalty on the CEN examination for incorrect responses. Your computed score is based only on the number of correct responses. Answer every question, even if you have to guess.

Once you decide on an answer, don't change it without good reason. Your first response is likely to be the correct one. The temptation to change an answer is often caused by reading too much into the question or thinking of the unusual rather than the usual.

You should answer 65 to 70 questions per hour to complete the examination comfortably in approximately 3 hours. Check periodically to make sure you are using your time effectively. Take the time to read the questions carefully and answer them correctly.

Box 2-4 TIPS FOR ANSWERING THE EXAMINATION QUESTIONS

Read the stem of each question carefully. Observe qualifying terms such as always, never, most, usually, not, except, first, initial, primary, next, best, most important, highest, lowest, least, and contraindicated. These words tell you what the question is really asking.

After reading the stem, formulate an answer before looking at your choices. When you think you know the answer, look to see if it is one of your choices. If not, reread the stem. Did you misinterpret what was asked? Is there a choice similar to yours with different terminology? If you are still not sure, rule out any choices you know are incorrect.

When the content is unfamiliar, think of general principles such as the ABCs or the nursing process to choose an answer or eliminate a choice. Think of answers with content that is therapeutic, ensures patient safety, promotes comfort, demonstrates respect, and communicates acceptance. Eliminate responses that are bizarre, hostile, inappropriate, or punitive. Look for terminology in the stem compatible with or suggestive of one particular option.

If the content is familiar but you don't consider any of the choices correct, don't get flustered. Reread the stem to make sure you correctly interpreted the question, then select the best choice, even if it is not the answer you prefer.

Don't read too much into the question. Don't make assumptions about information that is not given. Use only the information provided in the stem of the question. Think in terms of the usual, not the unusual.

If a choice contains a totally unfamiliar term, try to decipher its meaning by considering its roots. If the word remains a mystery, the response is probably incorrect. A totally unfamiliar term is not likely to be part of an idea that is being tested. Unfamiliar terms are often distractors, so don't be fooled.

When it comes time to actually take the examination, remember that extreme fear and anxiety can influence even the most basic test activities. Pay attention to the instructions and follow them carefully. This often helps the test taker overcome initial nervousness. Box 2-3 discusses general test-taking tips relative to the CEN examination, whereas Box 2-4 provides specific tips for answering the examination questions. Throughout the examination, control your fear and anxiety. Periodically stretch and take breaths. It may be helpful to remind yourself that 25 of the questions are pretest questions and do not count toward your final score. Above all, believe in yourself and your ability to successfully pass the CEN examination or any other examination.

SUMMARY

Certification is a relatively new process in nursing. Issues related to certification concern not only emergency nursing, but also all specialty nursing certification. These include educational requirements, practice requirements, certification period, renewal mechanisms, advanced certification options, costs, examination validity and reliability, potential liability, and recognition by professional colleagues and the public. The BCEN has addressed many of these issues as they relate to the CEN exam. Validity and reliability are analyzed for each exam. The test blueprint is revised when appropriate to ensure accuracy of the content areas. Renewal options have been expanded to include a continuing education track.

The future of emergency nursing certification is truly promising. Although the certification examination is taken on a computer, computer experience is NOT necessary to successfully take the examination. It is important to note that, just as with paper and pencil examinations, it is possible to review your test, or return to items that may have been difficult for you before submitting it. Certification is a significant professional accomplishment that benefits the profession, the patient, and the public.

References

1. Barnason S: *CEN review manual,* ed 3, Des Plaines, Ill, 2001, Emergency Nurses Association.
2. Board of Certification for Emergency Nursing: CEN renewal option application brochure, Des Plaines, Ill, 2000, BCEN.
3. Board of Certification for Emergency Nursing: *Certification examination for emergency nurses (candidate handbook),* Des Plaines, Ill, 2000, BCEN.
4. Weisfeld N, Falk D: Chasing elusive competence, *Hospitals* 57(5):68, 1983.

Suggested Reading

Andreoni CP, Klinkhammer B: *Quick reference for pediatric emergency nursing,* Philadelphia, 2000, WB Saunders.
Grossman VGA: *Quick reference to triage,* Philadelphia, 1999, JB Lippincott.
Jordan KS: *Emergency nursing core curriculum,* ed 5, Philadelphia, 2000, WB Saunders.

Kidd PS, Sturt PA, Fultz J: *Mosby's emergency nursing reference,* St. Louis, 2000, Mosby.

Lanros NE, Barber JM: *Emergency nursing with certification preparation & review,* ed 4, Stamford, Conn, 1999, Appleton & Lange.

Proehl JA: *Emergency nursing procedures,* ed 2, Philadelphia, 1999, WB Saunders.

Selfridge-Thomas J, Hall MM, Rea RE: *Challenges in emergency nursing,* ed 2, Philadelphia, 1999, WB Saunders.

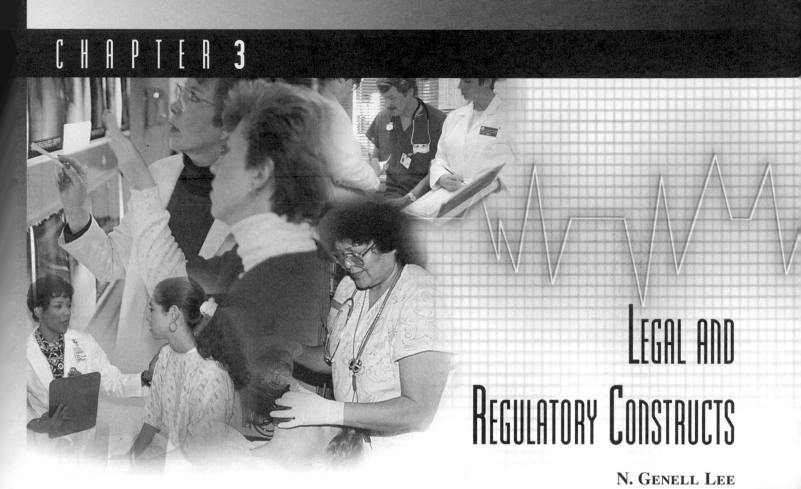

CHAPTER 3

LEGAL AND REGULATORY CONSTRUCTS

N. GENELL LEE

Emergency nursing is a complex blend of skill, experience, knowledge, and personality. In no other area of nursing is a nurse expected to know "cradle-to-grave" information about the pathophysiology of disease, the latest technologic innovations in monitoring and treatment devices, and when to contact the police or health department—all while being an advocate for the patient and family. The emergency department (ED) is like a minihospital, often seeing more patients per year than there are patient days on the hospital's inpatient side. The number of regulations and laws that affect emergency nursing practice is phenomenal. This chapter provides only a snapshot of legal and regulatory constructs that affect the ED the most. Examples of case law, statutes, and regulations are provided for illustration only, not as the definitive word on a particular situation. Hospital legal counsel should be consulted for specific concerns. Discussion covers sources of law, medical records, consent to and refusal of treatment, the Emergency Medical Treatment and Active Labor Act (EMTALA),[30] managed care, preservation and collection of evidence, and mental health issues.

SOURCES OF LAW AND REGULATION

The U.S. Constitution is the supreme law. Through the Bill of Rights, the Constitution guarantees certain individual rights that affect care in the ED. The free exercise clause of the First Amendment affects refusal of care for religious reasons, whereas the free speech clause supports employee or patient statements about care. Right to privacy is not explicitly stated in the Constitution, but has been interpreted by the courts to encompass the right to refuse medical care. Protection against search and seizure and rights of criminal defendants indirectly affects the ED when law enforcement officers request collection of evidence. The emergency nurse is not expected to be a constitutional expert but should remember that an individual entering the ED brings all his or her individual rights and constitutional protections. Table 3-1 summarizes sources of law and regulation.

Congress is designated by the Constitution to make laws. At the state level, each state's constitution designates the state legislature as the source of state laws. A law passed by Congress or a state legislature is a statute. If a statute directly conflicts with a constitutional principle, the courts strike down the statute as unconstitutional. One example of a federal statute is EMTALA. Examples of state statutes are consent laws and licensure of medical professionals.

The Executive Branch of federal and state governments enforces laws through various administrative agencies that develop rules or regulations to enforce applicable statutes. Agencies such as the Occupational Safety and Health Administration (OSHA) can enforce regulations through inspections, fines, and other procedures allowed by law. One example of a regulation established by OSHA is the occupational exposure to bloodborne pathogens regulation, which requires universal precautions if exposure to blood or body fluids is possible.[1] Licensing boards are administrative

Table 3-1   SOURCES OF LAW AND REGULATION

TYPE OF LAW	SOURCE OR ORIGIN	CONTENT OR FOCUS	EXAMPLES
Supreme Law	Constitution	Individual rights	Right to free speech Freedom of religious expression Right to privacy
Statute	Congress or state legislature	Focus varies but cannot conflict with the Constitution	Consent laws Licensure of medical professionals
Common Law	Judicial Branch	Judge-made laws that change as society and its laws change	Abortion laws Drunk driving laws
Regulations	Executive Branch of federal and state government	Enforce federal and state laws	Occupational Safety and Health Administration

agencies in the Executive Branch. Boards of Nursing license qualified individuals, and Nurse Practice Acts specify the nursing practice requirements in each state.

The Judicial Branch interprets the law and develops common law or judge-made law as cases are decided. Various legal analyses are used by the Judicial Branch to interpret federal and state laws. Common law develops over centuries, changing as society and laws change.

COMMUNICATION

The Office of Civil Rights, Department of Health and Human Services (DHHS) reiterated the requirement that health care providers provide translation services for individuals with limited English proficiency (LEP).[7] Any agency, facility, or program that receives federal funds from DHHS is required to comply with the requirements of nondiscrimination against individuals with LEP. In the context of compliance, the four elements in effective programs are (1) assessment of language needs of the population in the service area, (2) comprehensive written policy that ensures language access, (3) training to ensure that staff understands and carries out the policy, and (4) oversight evaluation and monitoring of any language assistance programs.[7] These regulations address oral and written language. Translation of written materials may be necessary if the LEP language group is a significant portion of the population service area. Use of volunteers or family as translators, particularly in health care situations where technical terminology is used, may not meet LEP standards of the Civil Rights Act of 1964.

Notice must be provided to individuals seeking emergency care who have limited English proficiency. Signage, language identification cards, translation of written materials, and telephone communications are some acceptable methods of communicating notice that individuals have a right to free language assistance services. A model plan is included in the *Federal Register* notice.[7] Violations of language translation standards are reported to the Justice Department, Office of Civil Rights, Internal Revenue Service, and the Joint Commission on Accreditation of Healthcare Organizations (JCAHO).

MEDICAL RECORDS

The requirement to maintain medical records on patients treated in the ED comes from state licensure statutes, JCAHO standards, and federal and state regulations.[28] The hospital usually retains the right to control the record, but patients generally have rights to information in the record.[28] Release of information without consent from the patient can lead to criminal and civil liability in some circumstances. Institutional policy, state statute, or federal law may cover confidentiality of medical records. Sensitive areas, often specified in state or federal law, include alcohol and drug treatment, mental health, acquired immunodeficiency syndrome, and the patient's human immunodeficiency virus status. In the absence of a legal or regulatory obligation, a moral or ethical obligation to protect the patient's privacy may exist.[28]

Computerization of medical records raises many sensitive issues. Entry of all or part of the medical record into a hospital information system raises questions of control and access. Systems and personnel security usually limit access to authorized persons.[28] User passwords with differing levels of secured access are the minimum controls in most computerized systems. Developing technology should enhance measures to secure medical record confidentiality. In addition to computerization, transmission of medical information over modems, facsimile (fax) machines, and internal computer networks raises further issues of system and personnel security. The risk of violating patient confidentiality is greater when the communication tool uses public channels. Existing security measures include user verification, retaining transmitted data, and incorporating a confidentiality statement on the fax cover sheet. Current technology allows the sender to verify the telephone number where the fax was received.

The documentation system for the medical record is important, but does not surpass the need to make entries legible, coherent, accurate, and complete. Narrative notes, checklists, SOAP notes, or charting by exception are accepted methods of documentation. A signature identifies the person providing care and ensures authenticity in a legal proceeding. A rubber stamp, written signature, initials, or

---

Box 3-1 REQUIREMENTS FOR PROTECTION OF PATIENTS' MEDICAL INFORMATION

- Patients must consent.
- Consent for release of information requires:
  Plain language
  Purpose of use and disclosure
  Notice of patient's right to review before signing
  Right of patient to restrict information released
  Right of patient to revoke consent
  Copy of signed authorization
- Permitted disclosures of medical information are:
  Public health authorities if state law allows
  To comply with child abuse or neglect laws, domestic violence if state law allows
  As authorized by law for civil, administrative, or criminal proceedings
- Law enforcement disclosures are limited: identification and location purposes.
- Notice of privacy protections: plain language
  Uses and disclosures of protected health information
  Individual's rights and legal duties of covered entity
  Required header: *This notice describes how medical information about you may be used and disclosed and how you can get access to this information. Please review it carefully.*

Table 3-2 TYPES OF CONSENT

TYPE	DESCRIPTION
Consent form	Covers evaluation and treatment such as medications, x-rays, and lab studies. Blanket consent for treatment does not cover invasive or surgical procedures.
Informed	Patient has a full understanding of risks and benefits of the proposed consent for treatment, is not under the influence of mind-altering substances, and has the legal capacity to consent.
Implied consent	Allows treatment in an emergency situation. Based on presumption that a patient would, if able, provide consent for life-saving treatment.

---

computer keys may be used to authenticate an entry into the medical record; however, it is the individual who controls the integrity of any system. Legal implications of various forms of data authentication should be discussed with legal counsel before implementation.[29]

The DHHS promulgated new regulations related to medical record privacy released in December 2000.[6] When President George W. Bush entered office in January 2001, a moratorium was placed on regulations that were released during the final days of the Clinton administration. In April 2001 these regulations were finally released: providers have until April 2003 to comply. The main areas covered are listed in Box 3-1. Consent to release medical record information is much more detailed now that there are regulations specifying the type of disclosures that must occur before release of patient information. Consent for privacy and disclosure of medical records must be signed and dated separately from other consents.[6] DHHS outlined five basic principles reflected in these new regulations: (1) consumer control, (2) boundaries, (3) accountability, (4) public responsibility, and (5) security.[30] The new privacy regulations apply to health plans, clearinghouses, and providers who transmit any health information in electronic form in connection with transactions covered by the regulation. The regulations protect individually identifiable health information. Health information, as defined in the regulation, relates to past, present, or future physical or mental health or payment for such.[6] The regulations also specify that any information, whether oral or recorded in any form, is covered.

CONSENT

Consents are obtained daily in the ED, usually through use of standardized consent forms. If the patient is not given the opportunity to read and question information in the consent form, the courts may later find the patient did not consent.[26] Most ED consent forms used during initial registration provide consent for treatment, consent for disclosure of medical records to third-party payers, and a contractual agreement to assume financial responsibility for any charges not paid by insurance. Many also include consent to fax medical information to the primary care physician. Table 3-2 summarizes types of consent.

Informed consent occurs when the patient has a full understanding of risks and benefits of the proposed treatment, is not under the influence of mind-altering drugs, and has the legal capacity to consent as evidenced by age and competency.[23] Physicians are generally responsible for obtaining informed consent. Nurses frequently witness the patient's signature and assist with treatment; however, questions regarding treatment should be answered by the physician before the patient signs the consent form. The patient can withdraw consent at any time. Verbal withdrawal of consent supersedes written consent.

States generally recognize an emergency exception to informed consent when life- or limb-threatening conditions exist. This doctrine, called *implied consent,* is a legal device created to allow treatment in emergency situations. Implied consent is based on the premise that the patient would, if able, provide consent for lifesaving treatment.[23] Two cases stemming from the emergency exception to informed consent illustrate the difficulties encountered in consent situations.

In *Crouch v. Most,*[13,14] an amateur snake handler was bitten by a rattlesnake on the left index and middle fingers. Initial treatment included ice therapy and injection of antivenin into the fingers. The patient subsequently required amputation of the affected fingers. The patient sued the treating physician, arguing that full disclosure of risks of antivenin should have occurred before its administration. In upholding the trial court's judgment for the physician, the New Mexico Supreme Court stated, "It would indeed be most unusual for a doctor, with his patient who had just been bitten by a venomous snake, to calmly sit down and first fully discuss the various available methods of treating snakebite and the possible consequences, while the venom is being pumped through the patient's body."[13] Although management of snakebites has changed since this case was decided, the principles related to consent are still valid.

Whether a patient under the influence of drugs or alcohol can provide valid consent is a constant source of concern in the ED. In the case of *Miller v. Rhode Island Hospital*,[15,24] an unrestrained passenger with blood alcohol content of 0.233 mg/dl, well above any state's legal limit, arrived in the ED for evaluation after a motor vehicle crash. Trauma surgeons prepared to perform diagnostic peritoneal lavage (DPL) when the patient began questioning what they were doing. After the physicians explained the procedure, the patient attempted to sit up and told the physicians not to perform the procedure. Physicians informed the patient that the extent of injury required evaluation. Because the patient had been drinking, DPL was the standard of care for this evaluation. The patient fought and was ultimately restrained. The patient maintained he was given anesthesia after restraint and woke up with an incision in his abdomen. Physicians admitted the patient for observation. He signed out against medical advice, and brought suit against the hospital and physicians for battery. The trial court granted a judgment in the patient's favor, but the hospital and physicians appealed. The Rhode Island Supreme Court found the trial court judge committed a reversible error in not allowing expert testimony regarding mechanism of injury and indications for DPL. The trial court had not allowed a hospital trauma surgeon to testify on the hospital's protocol regarding nonconsensual DPL, and also instructed the jury not to consider intoxication as a factor in their decision. The appellate court overturned the judgment of the trial court and sent the case back for retrial.[24] Whether intoxication impairs an individual's ability to consent to or refuse treatment is a matter of state law. Sheer numbers of alcohol and drug users in the ED make it essential that every ED have specific policies regarding obtaining consent from these individuals.

The age at which an individual can consent is found in state law. In cases of sexually transmitted diseases, pregnancy, alcoholism, and substance abuse, many states provide that minors below the age of majority can consent for examination and treatment without parental consent.[23] Many states recognize emancipated minors, individuals below the statutory age of consent recognized in the same legal capacity as an adult. The emancipated minor is self-supporting or lives alone without parental supervision or involvement. When an individual who is incompetent or a nonemancipated minor presents to the ED for treatment, state law dictates who has authority to consent. Some states recognize the mature minor doctrine. The criteria for when a minor is considered mature vary between states and are based on the particular facts and circumstances of each case.[23]

Managed care is changing health care delivery in the United States. The ED environment magnifies tension between managed care systems and other forms of health care delivery. Consent and payment issues become intertwined when a patient enrolled in a managed care plan presents to a nonparticipating ED. Patients in managed care plans are usually assigned a primary physician, who serves as the gatekeeper for covered services. The gatekeeper must authorize payment for treatment in a nonparticipating ED; however, consent for treatment must come from the patient. If an emergency exists, most managed care plans will reimburse the nonparticipating ED for initial stabilization. In the absence of specific consent forms for interactions with managed care patients, the prudent approach is to do what is in the patient's best interests.

Individuals in the custody of law enforcement are generally allowed to consent to or refuse treatment. One area of concern is collection of blood or urine specimens for alcohol and drug testing requested by law enforcement. State law determines whether the patient must consent for tests. The nurse or other health care provider is often released from civil or criminal liability if the specimen is obtained in a medically acceptable manner. Legal counsel should approve specific ED policies and procedures related to this issue. As an illustration, Indiana law allows a law enforcement officer to use "reasonable force" to assist the health care provider if the patient in custody refuses to consent and resists obtaining the specimen. Physicians, hospitals, and agents of the hospital including nurses are protected from civil and criminal liability in obtaining the sample if requested by a law enforcement officer.[21]

Consent is an important defense against intentional torts of false imprisonment, assault, and battery. *False imprisonment* occurs when a patient is intentionally held or prevented from moving about freely. Standing in the doorway of a treatment room to prevent a patient from leaving the room raises potential false imprisonment claims. Concise documentation of the patient's behavior, verbal threats or applicable statements, and therapeutic interventions can defend against false imprisonment claims if the patient is impaired and judged a danger to self or others. *Assault* occurs when an intentional threat to inflict injury is coupled with apparent ability to immediately carry out the threat. *Battery* is unconsented touching of another person that results in harmful contact. The emergency nurse who inserts an intravenous catheter despite refusal from a rational adult may be liable for battery in a civil or criminal action. If a patient initially refuses, then later consents after explanation of the procedure, the nurse should document this interaction in the medical record.

Other consent issues include photographs, videotaping trauma resuscitations, disclosure of medical information, and participation in research protocols. Seek advice of legal counsel before implementing a policy covering these issues.

The patient allowed to consent is also allowed to refuse treatment. As Justice Brennan wrote in one Supreme Court opinion, "The right to be free from unwanted medical attention is a right to evaluate the potential benefit of treatment and its possible consequences according to one's own values and to make a personal decision whether to subject oneself to the intrusion."[15] It does not matter if refusal occurs in an emergency situation or is a rational decision in the presence of a terminal condition.

A rational, competent adult can refuse administration of blood even if it is deemed life-saving. Jehovah's Witnesses routinely refuse blood transfusions because of religious objections. In the case of minors and incompetent adults, hospitals usually seek a court order to allow treatment such as blood transfusions. Courts are likely to protect individuals because of the state's interest in protecting life. Waiting for the patient to lapse into unconsciousness and then providing treatment does not provide protection against liability. Proper refusal of treatment does not change because the patient's mental status changed.[23]

Right-to-die cases led Congress to pass the Patient Self-Determination Act in 1990.[6] It requires hospitals to ask patients, on admission, if they have an advance directive and to document this interaction in the medical record. An advance directive includes a living will and durable power of attorney for health care. State law determines the type of advance directive available. When the patient does have an advance directive, communication of its existence to all health care providers is often difficult. Techniques used to ensure dissemination of this information include permanent armbands, a laminated pocket-size copy of the advance directive, or inserting the advance directive in the medical record. Legality of photocopies of living wills should be clarified for specific practice areas.

Patients may refuse treatment by leaving the ED before evaluation, during evaluation, after evaluation but before discharge, or at the time of discharge but before completing necessary paperwork including aftercare instructions. Not every patient who leaves does so against medical advice (AMA). The patient who leaves during evaluation may not inform ED staff. When this occurs, the situation should be clearly documented. If the patient does discuss refusal of treatment and elects to leave AMA, the nurse should ensure the patient understands potential consequences before signing release forms. The medical record should reflect this discussion, patient response, and patient understanding of the consequences of refusing treatment.

EMERGENCY MEDICAL TREATMENT AND ACTIVE LABOR ACT

EMTALA,[2] formerly known as COBRA/OBRA, is a federal statute originally passed by Congress to address patient dumping—transfer of unstable patients for financial reasons. Enforcement and regulation of EMTALA are the responsibility of the DHHS. Regulations identified in EMTALA do not supersede state laws governing medical negligence or simple negligence actions, but do prevail over state law if there is a direct conflict between the provisions of EMTALA and state law. Table 3-3 summarizes specific EMTALA provisions and definitions.

Under EMTALA, all individuals presenting to the ED for examination and treatment are entitled to an appropriate medical screening to determine if an emergency medical condition exists.[3] The statute does not clearly define what constitutes an appropriate medical screening. The Sixth Circuit Court of Appeals, in *Cleland v. Bronson Health Care Group,* described appropriate as "one of the most wonderful weasel words in the dictionary."[12] Studying case law from appellate courts in each circuit provides some direction regarding the courts' definition of an appropriate medical screening. The Eleventh Circuit Court of Appeals said an appropriate medical screening is based on application of the same screening procedures to paying and indigent patients, rather than adequacy of the exam itself.[19]

Regulations require that a zone of 250 yards surrounding the main hospital building be covered by EMTALA. Thus, individuals in the parking structure, public streets, and any other part of the "zone" would be covered by EMTALA. If an offsite location uses the hospital's Medicare provider number, EMTALA applies even if the offsite location is a physician office. Offsite locations covered by EMTALA are required to provide access to a medical screening examination, notice, adherence to financial rules, signage, and patient care standards required of the ED.

Regional referral centers and hospitals with specialized capabilities such as trauma centers, neonatal centers, and burn units are obligated to accept all appropriate transfers of patients who require the care if they have the capacity to treat the individual.[5] An EMTALA violation can result in a civil penalty up to $50,000 per violation for hospitals and physicians. The hospital and physician may also be terminated as Medicare providers.[4] In some hospitals, the triage nurse "triages out" patients with nonurgent complaints after the initial medical screening. "Triaging out" refers to the process of sending patients away from the ED after an initial nursing assessment, but before medical evaluation. This procedure could result in an EMTALA violation if an emergency medical condition exists. The medical screening examination (MSE) is more extensive than triage and if a nonphysician performs the medical screening examination, approval by the governing body of the hospital as well as the medical staff should be documented.

Lawsuits using EMTALA against base station, or resource, hospitals have thus far been unsuccessful. In *Johnson v. University of Chicago Hospitals,*[22] an infant's mother sued, claiming an EMTALA violation. The infant suffered cardiopulmonary arrest. Paramedics contacted the University of Chicago Hospitals (UCH), their designated resource hospital. The "telemetry nurse" directed the paramedics to another hospital because UCH was on "partial bypass." The infant was treated at another hospital and subsequently transferred to Cook County Hospital. Sometime after the

Table 3-3	**KEY EMTALA PROVISIONS**
PROVISION	**DESCRIPTION/DEFINITION**
Medical screening	Applies to any individual who comes to the hospital and requests treatment. Appropriate medical screening determines if an emergency medical condition exists.
Emergency medical condition	Medical condition manifesting acute symptoms of sufficient severity, including pain, that, without immediate medical attention, could reasonably be expected to result in placing the health of the individual, including an unborn fetus, in serious jeopardy; serious impairment to bodily functions; or serious dysfunction of any bodily organ or part. With respect to pregnant women having contractions, there is inadequate time to effect a safe transfer to another hospital before delivery or transfer may pose a threat to the health or safety of the woman or unborn child.
Stabilize	Provide treatment to ensure, within reasonable medical probability, that no material deterioration is likely to result from or occur during the transfer.
Transfer	Movement, including discharge, of an individual outside a hospital's facilities at the direction of any person employed by or associated with the hospital. Does not include movement of a dead individual or an individual who leaves the facility without permission.
Patient refusal	Patients can refuse examination, treatment, and/or transfer. Reasonable steps should be taken to secure written informed consent to refuse.
Physician certification	A physician is required to certify that medical benefits outweigh the risks of the transfer. Certification must contain summary of risks and benefits upon which certification is based.
Appropriate transfer	Transfer is appropriate when the receiving facility has available space, qualified personnel, and agrees to accept the patient in transfer.
Transfer records	Refers to all medical records for the patient and for this specific visit. Includes diagnostic test results, informed written consent or certification, and, when appropriate, the name and address of any on-call physician who refused or failed to appear within a reasonable time to provide necessary stabilizing treatment.
Nondiscrimination	A participating hospital with specialized capabilities or facilities shall not refuse to accept an appropriate transfer of an individual who requires such specialized capabilities or facilities if the hospital has the capacity to treat the individual.
EMTALA claim	A claim must be brought within 2 years of the alleged violation.
Financial inquiries	A participating hospital may not delay appropriate medical screening exams in order to inquire about the individual's method of payment or insurance status. Stabilization must begin before financial inquiries.

transfer, the infant died and the mother sued. The appellate court upheld the trial court's dismissal of the EMTALA complaint, stating that in the plain meaning of the law, the infant never "came to" UCH or its ED. The appellate court further stated, "a hospital-operated telemetry system is distinct from that same hospital's emergency room."[22] The appellate court allowed part of the mother's claims to go forward under state law. In the interim ruling, DHHS stated that "coming to the ED" included property owned by the hospital, including hospital-based ambulance services.[22] If the hospital is not on diversionary status, ambulances en route to a facility may be deemed by the courts as having "come to" the ED.

Regulations found in EMTALA require specific documentation and retention of transfer records. State licensure evaluations and JCAHO often incorporate a review of transfer records into site surveys. Documentation forms and documentation systems are not specified by EMTALA. The only requirement is that the information be maintained.

One goal of managed care is elimination of hospitalization in nonparticipating facilities. Whether the managed care plan is operated privately or by the state, patient transfer from the ED of a nonparticipating facility to a participating facility is definitely covered by EMTALA. The ED often finds itself caught between following managed care policies and complying with federal law. If the patient cannot be stabilized and the nonparticipating facility has the resources to provide care, transfer for financial reasons falls within EMTALA prohibitions. No provisions exist in EMTALA to compensate nonparticipating hospitals for medical screening exams or nonreimbursed hospitalizations of managed care patients. A Special Advisory Bulletin published in 1999 specified that no discussion of financial status should occur until stabilizing treatment has started (after MSE). Although not defined, the Bulletin stated that only "qualified individuals" should discuss financial matters with the patient.[23]

Patients who require transfer must be transported with an appropriate vehicle, equipment, and qualified personnel.[4] This provision applies to every transfer. Transferring a patient who requires advanced life support in a basic life support vehicle with emergency medical technicians violates this provision of EMTALA. Appropriate vehicle and equipment are determined by factors such as time, distance, terrain, geographic considerations such as rush-hour traffic, patient needs, and availability of monitoring devices. Qualified personnel means the providers' scope of practice matches the patient's needs.[10] Scope of practice for nurses, emergency medical technicians, paramedics, and respiratory therapists is determined by state law.

The future promises increased tension between emergency care providers and regulatory constructs. A recent EMTALA case illustrates rising tensions between medical and nursing care and law. The mother of an encephalic infant demanded aggressive management, including mechanical ventilation.[20] Although the mother was advised that mechanical ventilation provided no palliative or therapeutic purpose, she insisted that everything be done to keep her baby alive. She contacted a state agency responsible for enforcing antidiscrimination laws against handicapped or disabled individuals. The agency made it clear to the hospital and doctors it would pursue any remedies available to Baby K. The Fourth Circuit Court of Appeals separated the treatment of acute symptoms from the underlying condition, a position in direct conflict with standard medical and nursing practice. The case has been interpreted by some critics as EMTALA requiring provision of any technologically available treatment to any patient regardless of underlying condition, even if the condition or illness is fatal.[20] The Fourth Circuit Court's decision is not interpreted law in other circuits but demonstrates the impending collision between legal interpretation and emergency patient care.

PRESERVATION AND COLLECTION OF EVIDENCE

Each state identifies specific considerations that must be reported to local or state authorities. These should be listed in the ED policy and procedure manual. Common disclosures include suspected child abuse, elder abuse, communicable diseases, gunshot wounds, stabbings, sexual assault, burns, suspicious deaths, animal bites, and poisonings.[23] The emergency nurse is often required to collect evidence in these and other potential criminal cases. State laws govern the type of evidence needed in each situation; therefore, the emergency nurse must be familiar with local and state laws that govern evidence collection. Medical examiners, local law enforcement, and district attorneys are excellent resources when developing specific policies and procedures for evidence collection and preservation. Legal counsel should be involved to ensure policies and procedures fall within the nurse's and hospital's scope of practice. Placing a forensic kit at the bedside aids in collection and preservation of evidence.[16] Kits should include applicable laws, guidelines, and telephone numbers as a handy reference.[16]

Evidence collection in sexual assault is generally standardized in each state. Rape kits contain instructions, diagrams, evidence containers, and specific documentation requirements. Most states require specific patient consent for evidentiary examination and photographs. Issues discussed in the consent section of this chapter also apply to sexual assault cases.[27] Many states use specially trained sexual assault nurse examiners. See Chapter 54 for further discussion of sexual assault.

As a rule, victims or perpetrators of violent crimes who enter the ED for treatment are candidates for evidence collection. General guidelines for evidence preservation and collection are described in Box 3-2.

BOX 3-2   GUIDELINES FOR EVIDENCE PRESERVATION

Do not discard clothing. Place bloody clothing in a paper bag.
Do not wash the hands of a person with a gunshot wound. Cover with paper bags until the police examine the patient.
Cut around bullet holes and knife cuts in clothing.
Document what the patient says about the incident.
Describe extent of surface wounds and amount of blood present.
Document the patient's behavior.
Delay cleaning until police examine the patient unless it is necessary for essential procedures

---

MENTAL HEALTH PATIENTS

The psychiatric patient presents a unique challenge in the ED and deserves special mention because state and federal laws exist regarding mental health patients. Facilities that do not have inpatient psychiatric services are not exempt from providing emergency psychiatric care. A patient diagnosed with a mental illness is competent to consent to medical care unless a court determines legal incompetence exists. The most pressing issue for these patients is the potential for violence. Patients expressing suicidal or homicidal ideation require immediate intervention to prevent injury to self or others. Each state has laws regarding commitment procedures for psychiatric patients.[23] A psychiatric patient may be held for a time in the ED against his or her express wishes, if state law allows. Policies and procedures should address specific requirements for involuntary holding of psychiatric patients.

Restraint policies should address the decision to restrain, how restraint is accomplished, monitoring the restrained patient, and at what point restraints are removed. Documentation should reflect the patient's behavior and the reason for the intervention. A physician's order is necessary when a patient is restrained. If the situation requires immediate intervention, the physician signature may be obtained after the patient is restrained. Conditions of Participation for hospitals that receive Medicare funds require specific restraint policies and procedures. Orders for restraints must be reevaluated on a regular basis and PRN orders for restraints are prohibited.

MEDICAL NEGLIGENCE

Elements of a medical negligence cause of action are duty, breach of duty, cause in fact, proximate cause, and damages (Table 3-4). Although all elements are important, breach of duty is significant in medical negligence, or malpractice, cases. With some exception, expert witnesses are used in medical negligence actions to define the standard of care and to render an opinion regarding whether the standard of care was met in a particular case. Emergency nurses are generally required to exercise skill and judgment that a reasonably

Table 3-4	ELEMENTS OF MEDICAL NEGLIGENCE	
ELEMENT	DESCRIPTION	
Duty	Exists when a hospital, nurse, or physician establishes a relationship with a patient and volunteers to assume care.	
Breach of duty	Occurs when commission or omission falls below established standard of care.	
Cause in fact	The injury would not have occurred but for the conduct of the nurse. The conduct of the nurse was, more likely than not, a substantial factor in the patient's injury.	
Proximate cause	Determined by foreseeability. The emergency nurse should have foreseen that injury would occur with this particular conduct.	
Damages	Compensation for medical care, lost wages, and pain and suffering. Punitive damages may be asked if the conduct reached the point of willful, wanton, or intentional injury. These damages serve to punish and deter bad conduct.	

prudent emergency nurse would use under similar circumstances.[23]

Sources for the standards of emergency nurses include ED policy and procedure manuals, JCAHO standards, state nurse practice acts, and federal and state law. Professional standards, such as the Standards of Emergency Nursing Practice,[17] authoritative textbooks, and specialty courses may also serve as sources. Certification courses and professional standards documents frequently disclaim legal use of their material; however, attorneys and nurse expert witnesses may use the information to establish the standard of care for a particular patient situation. A word of caution is necessary regarding institutional policies and procedures. Using *all, always, never,* and *shall* turns the policy and procedure into a mandate, rather than a guideline for professional judgment in patient care decisions. If particular conduct is mandated, each nurse should be aware of the policy and follow the policy mandate. The more flexibility afforded the emergency nurse in asserting professional judgment in patient care decisions, the less the likelihood that an internal policy and procedure can be used against the nurse or institution. All ED policies and procedures should be reviewed with an eye toward maximizing clarity. If a policy exists that no one follows, the result can be devastating to the hospital or nurse in a nursing negligence action.

In *Marks v. Mandel,*[9] the ED received notice of the pending arrival of a patient with a gunshot wound to the chest. A moonlighting orthopedic resident did not follow the ED's on-call policy, which required the on-call thoracic surgeon be notified before a thoracic gunshot wound patient arrived in the ED. A delay occurred in reaching the thoracic surgeon and the patient died of his injuries. In the suit that followed, the trial court excluded the ED policy and procedure manual from evidence. Appellate court reversed the trial court, stat-

ing that internal policy and procedure manuals "should be admitted when they contain either (1) evidence of a general industry custom or standard, or (2) evidence that the defendant violated its own policy or an industry standard."[9] The appellate court sent the case back to the trial court for retrial with the direction that the ED policy and procedure manual should be admitted into evidence.

One of the first cases recognizing nursing negligence was *Darling v. Charleston Community Memorial Hospital.*[8] A plaster cast was applied in the ED after an 18-year-old patient broke his leg in a college football game. Shortly after cast application, the patient complained of pain and his toes became swollen and dark. The patient was admitted to the hospital but was subsequently transferred after complications developed. Ultimately the leg was amputated. The court addressed the nursing standard of care, stating that the "jury could reasonably have concluded that nurses did not test for circulation in the leg as frequently as necessary, that skilled nurses would have promptly recognized the conditions that signaled a dangerous impairment of circulation in the plaintiff's leg, and would have known that the condition would become irreversible in a matter of hours. At that point it became the nurses' duty to inform the attending physician, and if he failed to act, to advise the hospital authorities so that appropriate action might be taken."[8] Although the case is criticized in legal literature for the legal analysis of other issues, *Darling* stands for the principle that a nurse can be held liable for nursing negligence.

Managed care physicians and nurses are subject to state laws regarding medical liability or negligence. In *Hand v. Tavera,*[18] the hospital, emergency physician, and on-call managed care physician were sued for medical negligence. Hand, a member of the Humana Health Care Plan 1, arrived in the participating ED complaining of a 3-day headache. The patient had hypertension and his father had died of a brain aneurysm. The emergency physician decided to admit the patient but Dr. Tavera, the Humana physician on call for authorizing admissions, refused, stating the patient could be treated on an outpatient basis. Hand was sent home and suffered a stroke a few hours later. A claim against the hospital, emergency physician, and Dr. Tavera resulted. The hospital settled and the emergency physician was dropped from the case. Dr. Tavera, the remaining defendant, argued that no physician-patient relationship existed and he owed no duty to Hand. The trial court agreed and ruled in favor of Dr. Tavera in a pretrial motion, but the ruling was appealed. The appellate court determined that the Humana managed care plan brought Hand and Tavera together. The appellate court held, "When a patient who has enrolled in a prepaid medical plan goes to a hospital emergency room and the plan's designated doctor is consulted, the physician-patient relationship exists and the doctor owes the patient a duty of care."[18] The case was sent back to the trial court for a determination of other issues in the case. The prudent approach in the ED is for the patient to speak directly to the on-call physician for the managed care plan. Responsibility for disclosure of alternative treatment plans and specifics regarding benefit coverage rests with the managed care plan entity, not the ED.

PRACTICE LOCATIONS

Globalization of the economy is leading to changes in health care. State boundaries are giving way to national and international boundaries. Case management and telephone triage are two examples of changes in health care that are changing the landscape of emergency nursing. About 10 states have entered a mutual recognition compact to facilitate movement of nurses between states.[25] Corporations that provide case management or telephone triage activities are interested in the compact because the regulatory scheme is more consistent than following individual state laws and regulations. Consistency in requirements allows freer movement of nurses between practice locations. Enhanced technology in today's society allows a nurse in one state to assess, manage, and communicate with patients in other states. The Center for Telemedicine Law advocates use of technology in enhancing access of patients to physicians, nurses, and other health care providers.[11] Potential conflict exists between states' rights to protect the health, safety, and welfare of its residents and increasing centralized regulation at the federal level. The final word is yet to be written on this changing area of emergency nursing.

SUMMARY

The essence of liability prevention in all areas of medical and nursing practice is providing and documenting care within accepted standards. Practicing sound medical and nursing principles, including documentation, can reduce the fear of litigation. Education of ED staff on medical-legal issues with frequent review and updating of policies and procedures is essential. Quality improvement processes can ensure correction of deficiencies and strengthen competent practice. The ED patient expects high-quality care that meets medical and legal standards of care, and the competent emergency nurse can and should deliver.

References

1. 29 CFR §1910.1030 (1995).
2. 42 USCA §1395 (Suppl 1995).
3. 42 USCA §1395dd (Suppl 1995).
4. 42 USCA §1395dd (c)(2)(D) (Suppl 1995).
5. 42 USCA §1395dd (d) (Suppl 1995).
6. 45 CFR § 164 et seq. (2000).
7. 65 FR 169 (pp. 52762-52774) (August 30, 2000).
8. 211 NE2d 253 (Ill 1965).
9. 477 So 2d 1036 (Fla Ct Appl 1985).
10. Boyko SM: Interfacility transfer guidelines: an easy reference to help hospitals decide on appropriate vehicles and staffing for transfers, *JEN* 20:18, 1994.
11. Center for Telemedicine Law: Senate Committee on Commerce, Science, and Transportation (Subcommittee on Science, Technology, and Space): hearing on telemedicine technologies (transcript). Retrieved February 27, 2002 from the World Wide Web: http://www.ctl.org.
12. *Cleland v. Bronson Health Care Group Inc.,* 917 F2d 266, 271 (6th Cir 1990).
13. *Crouch v. Most,* 432 P2d 250 (NM 1967).
14. *Crouch v. Most,* 432 P2d 250, 254 (NM 1967).
15. *Cruzan v. Director, Missouri Dept Health,* 110 S Ct 2841, 111 LEd2d 224 (1990).
16. Easter CR, Muro GA: An emergency department forensic kit, *JEN* 21:440, 1995.
17. Emergency Nurses Association: *Standards of emergency nursing practice,* ed 4, Des Plaines, Ill, 1999, The Association.
18. *Hand v. Tavera,* 864 SW2d 678 (Tex Ct App 1993).
19. *Holcomb v. Monahan,* 30F3d 116 (11th Cir 1994).
20. In the Matter of Baby K, 16F3d 590 (4th Cir 1994), cert denied, U.S. 1994.
21. Ind. Code Ann. §9-30-6-6 (Burns Suppl 1995).
22. *Johnson v. University of Chicago Hospitals,* 982 F2d 230, 232 (7th Cir 1992).
23. Lee NG: *Legal concepts and issues in emergency care.* Philadelphia, 2001, WB Saunders.
24. *Miller v. Rhode Island Hospital,* 625 A2d 778 (RI 1993).
25. National Council of State Boards of Nursing, Inc: *Mutual recognition.* Retrieved February 27, 2002 from the World Wide Web: http://www.ncsbn.org.
26. Roach WH Jr, Aspen Health Law Center: *Medical records and the law,* ed 2, Gaithersburg, Md, 1994, Aspen.
27. Rothenberg MA: §2.6, *Emergency Medicine Malpractice,* ed 2, New York, 1994, John Wiley & Sons.
28. Rothenberg MA: §2.10, *Emergency Medicine Malpractice,* ed 2, New York, 1994, John Wiley & Sons.
29. Tomes JP: *Healthcare records: a practical legal guide,* Dubuque, Ia, 1990, Kendall/Hunt.
30. U.S. Department of Health and Human Services: HHS announces final regulations establishing first-ever national standards to protect patients' personal medical records. Retrieved December 20, 2000 from the World Wide Web: http://www.hhs.gov./news/press/2000press/20001220.html.

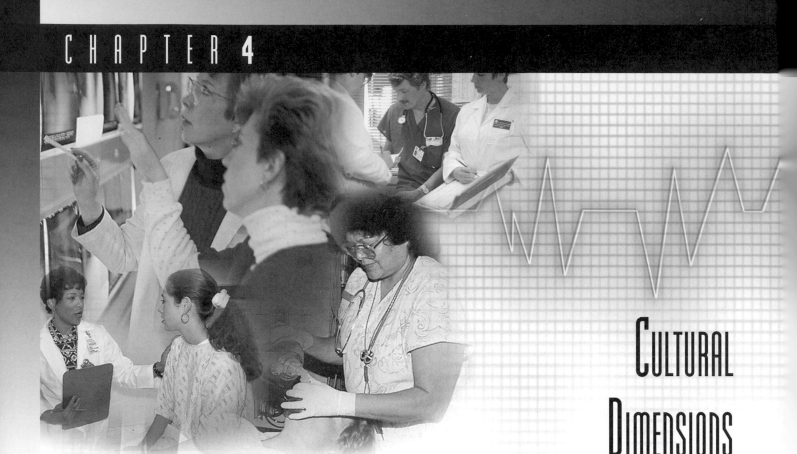

CHAPTER 4

CULTURAL DIMENSIONS

ZEB KORAN

The United States has long been called a melting pot because of the varied ethnic representation in its heritage. Increased affluence and the ease of global transportation have further increased cultural diversity in the United States. In 1992 the U.S. Census Bureau identified more than 30 ethnic designations individually recognized by more than 100,000 people, with numerous other ethnic designations identified by a smaller number of respondents.[2] This diversity challenges the ordinary citizen, as well as the practicing health care professional.

An essential first step toward cultural harmony is understanding what constitutes culture. Culture does not mean the person's social level, racial group, or ethnic heritage. Leininger,[3] a well-known transcultural nursing theorist, defines culture as "values, beliefs, norms, and practices of a particular group that are learned and shared and that guide thinking, decisions, and actions in a patterned way." Six distinct phenomena vary among most cultures—communication, time, space, biologic variations, social organization, and environmental control (Table 4-1).

Styles of communication are a defining characteristic within each culture. Communication is the vehicle for passage of cultural beliefs from generation to generation. Verbal and nonverbal communication is a product of culture. Verbal differences between cultures include language or dialect, definition of specific words, inflections used when speaking, and loudness with which words are spoken. Non-

verbal communication such as touch, eye contact, body posture, and facial expressions also has different meaning in various cultures.

Views of time and personal space are defined by culture. Orientation to the past, present, or future determines normal pace of life within the culture, as well as timing for events such as marriage and adulthood. Personal space represents security, autonomy, privacy, and self-identity and varies between cultures. How an individual responds when stopped on the street for directions or forced to share a room with someone he or she doesn't know is a product of culture.

As the world becomes more culturally diverse, emergency nurses will be confronted by many patients different from themselves and from each other. Immediacy of need inherent in emergency care requires familiarity with many cultural groups to avoid stereotyping. Comprehensive review of all recognized cultures is not possible within the confines of this chapter; readers are encouraged to seek other sources to expand knowledge of major cultures within their practice area. What follows is a brief description of cultures frequently encountered in the United States. Social, familial, and health-related information is included. Table 4-2 highlights select cultural beliefs related to the cause of illness. Brevity of information provided on some cultures is the result of limited available information rather than an opinion on importance of the culture.

Table 4-1	CULTURAL PHENOMENA		
PHENOMENA	**DEFINING CHARACTERISTICS**	**PHENOMENA**	**DEFINING CHARACTERISTICS**
Communication	Language spoken, voice quality, use of silence, physical movements, gestures, eye contact, touch	Time	Orientation is past, present, or future; dictates when certain life events occur (e.g., marriage)
Space	Comfort distance between self and an unknown person	Environmental control	Locus of control is internal or external; belief in witchcraft, voodoo, magic, or prayer; health care beliefs unique to the specific culture
Social organization	Family structure is patriarchal or matriarchal	Biologic variations	Illness prevalent within the specific culture

Table 4-2	PERCEIVED CAUSES OF ILLNESS		
CAUSE	**DESCRIPTION**	**TREATMENT**	**CULTURAL GROUP(S)**
Imbalance between yin and yang	Yin and yang are powers from the universe that control the body. Yin is the female force, inactive and negative; yang is the male force, active and positive.	Restore the balance. Eat yin foods for illness caused by yang forces and yang foods for illness caused by yin forces. *Acupuncture:* Needles inserted in areas of body to treat diseases from yang forces. *Herbal medicines:* Various mixtures used for specific conditions. *Cupping* (Figure 4-1): A substance is heated in a glass to create a vacuum. The glass is immediately turned upside down onto the skin, where it remains until it can be removed easily. It leaves a circular burn. *Coining* (Figure 4-2): A coin is heated and rubbed over the body. The appearance of welts verifies the presence of illness. Also called skin scrapping. *Moxibustion:* Moxa plants are heated and laid near a painful area. The plants leave craters in the skin. *Massage:* Used to concentrate energy on areas of illness.	Chinese Vietnamese
Evil eye	Someone with special powers admires a child but does not touch the child.	That same person should touch the child. Egg mixed with water is laid under the child's head.	Mexican-American
Hot and cold imbalance	Exposure to something with either hot or cold properties.	Exposure to the opposite (e.g., headache is a hot condition so cold herbs are placed at the temples as treatment).	Mexican-American Vietnamese

SPECIFIC CULTURAL GROUPS

Names for cultures change with time and geographic relocation. The name used for each cultural group discussed in the following section reflects the current name in literature and public record.

African-American

African-Americans have been subjected to discrimination in many parts of the country, so many feel angry and powerless. Most prefer being called Mr. or Mrs.; identifying them by their first name without permission is considered disrespectful and demeaning. Most speak standard English, but they may use black English when conversing with others of their cultural group. Black English is a rhythmic, stylized pattern of verbal communication. Individuals may also remain silent rather than speak when they are in a strange environment.

Women are the most important element in the family and are responsible for family health. More than half of all African-American heads of household in the United States are female. The minister also plays a vital role in most African-American households and may influence health care decisions.

Life is viewed as a series of opposites; for example, a birth for a death, with time orientation present or future. A small personal space is accepted without anxiety. Illness is considered the result of disharmony in a person's life. Males generally postpone seeking health care; usually the need for medication is the driving force when an African-American seeks health care. Many believe in folk medicine, voodoo, witchcraft, and magic. There is a high incidence of hypertension, coronary artery disease, sickle cell disease, diabetes mellitus, keloid formation, and lactose intolerance among individuals in this population.

Arabic

Individuals from Arabic countries may be Islamic or Christian; diet and death rites are determined by specific religious affiliation. Arabic culture is patriarchal, with decisions made by elder men. Extended families are common, with members subject to group censorship and pressure. Women have limited rights and must maintain an air of subservience to males. Arabic people often believe in disease-causing entities such as the evil eye. Illness or injury is seen as the will of God, so instruction on prevention is usually unsuccessful. Orientation is to the present, so Arabic people often arrive late for appointments or not at all. Patients may withhold information because the interview is considered intrusive. Arabic people are not expected to engage in self-care or make decisions regarding recovery, but view health care givers as personal employees. Prevalent health problems include urinary infections, cardiovascular disease, diabetes, and thalassemia. Females cannot sign an operative consent form—usually two male family members sign the form.[1] Any display of flesh such as an underwear advertisement is considered pornographic. A female health care provider should care for a female patient. Displaying the sole of the foot to others is considered offensive.

Appalachian

Many Appalachians remain in the Appalachian mountains; however, mobility has increased migration to larger cities in the northeastern and southeastern United States. The people of Appalachia emigrated from countries such as France, Wales, Germany, and Scotland. Various dialects spoken may be difficult to understand. Appalachians are very private, use few adjectives to communicate, and consider direct eye contact rude. This makes obtaining historical information difficult, particularly information related to assessment of pain.

The nuclear and extended families are important in Appalachian culture. The family unit is patriarchal; however, health advice usually comes from the oldest woman or "grandma" of the unit. Folk medicine is important to most. Producing children demonstrates a man is really a man while ensuring the woman is fulfilled, so large families are normal.

Appalachian people tend to focus on the state of their blood (thick or thin; high or low; good or bad). Status of blood is controlled by eliminating or consuming certain foods. High blood means too much blood, as manifested by headaches or dizziness; drinking brine off pickles is an accepted cure. Appalachian people expect others to care for them and wait on them during illness or injury. There is an inherent distrust of hospitals because they are regarded as places to die. Illness is considered the will of God, so fatalism is prevalent in this group. Treatment should be immediate; however, any need for medication or treatments beyond this immediate need is not understood or followed. Consequently Appalachians are typically noncompliant with long-term medication and health care regimens. Geographic poverty and isolation also affect compliance. Common health problems include tuberculosis, diabetes mellitus, and coronary artery disease.

Chinese

Keeping face by not being embarrassed, defeated, or contradicted is extremely important to the Chinese. The culture is very formal, so the first name should not be used unless prefaced with Mr. or Mrs. Demonstrating signs of pain is considered a sign of weakness. The Chinese are very uncomfortable with any physical contact involving strangers. They use high-context communication, messages are sent internally and by physical context; if used, verbal communication is less important than nonverbal. The Chinese believe accepting something when first offered is rude; therefore, pain medication should be offered several times.

Elderly people are highly respected and recognized as authority figures. Consequently grandparents and parents are involved in decisions regarding a child. Moral purity is important to the Chinese, so any public display of affection is strongly discouraged. Needs of the family take priority over individual needs. Marriage is discouraged until after college, with exchange of rings optional. Traditionally the bride retains her own name. The mother plays a more active role than the father in nurturing children. Child abuse is rare in Chinese culture. Shame and guilt are used as forms of discipline.

Hospitals are considered places to die, rather than places to get well. Euthanasia and organ donation are acceptable to the Chinese. They believe blood is the source of life and may resist having blood drawn. The Chinese also believe a person's spirit may escape during surgery. The body is considered a gift from parents and ancestors. Health is a balance between the yin and the yang; illness occurs with an imbalance between the two. Yin represents the female, inactive, or negative force, whereas yang represents the male, active, or positive force. After the birth of a child, a mother does not bathe for 7 to 30 days and is limited to eating certain foods. Soy sauce is thought to make the child's skin darker and may be avoided. Ginseng is used as a strength tonic in pregnant women. Commonly occurring health problems include hypertension, liver and stomach cancer, and lactose intolerance.[4] Hypertension, diabetes, and cancer are the leading causes of death in China.[1] The deceased is buried in a coffin for 7 years, then exhumed and cremated. The ashes are then placed in an urn and returned to a tomb.

Cuban

Cubans are outgoing, friendly, love social events, and are also very hard working. Hand gestures are an important part of communication, used to reinforce emotions and ideas. Interrupting another is not considered impolite. Eye contact indicates sincerity.

Cubans believe some illnesses occur because of supernatural powers such as the evil eye. Amulets worn as a necklace or bracelet, or pinned to clothing are used as protection against these powers and should not be removed without permission. Cubans believe that only magic spells and ethnic treatments can overcome illness that is the result of the evil eye. Health problems include diabetes mellitus and lactose intolerance. A Cuban sees a Do Not Resuscitate (DNR) as giving up hope and even abandonment and may not readily agree to this—despite obvious evidence that it is indicated. Family members remain with the deceased through the night with burial within 24 hours.[1]

Eastern Indian

Many Eastern Indians practice Hinduism, Jainism, Buddhism, or Sikhism, which are religions that believe in reincarnation and the caste system whereby people work their way up the caste levels with each reincarnation. Ultimately individuals reach the highest level, which renders them free from life on Earth so they can continue a better existence.

The term "thanks" is not used or recognized by East Indians. Social acts are duties that do not require recognition. Nods of the head for "yes" and "no" are opposite those used in the United States. Certain gestures such as winking or whistling are considered unacceptable behaviors for women. An apology is necessary if an individual's feet or shoes touch another person. Public displays of affection are not appropriate. Men are allowed direct eye contact with each other, whereas women are expected to keep their eyes cast down when addressing men in their family.

The father is the head of the household, and the elderly are held in high regard and cared for by other members of the family. Decisions are deferred to the elderly, when they are present. Marriage, which is often still arranged by parents, is considered sacred. Divorce is unacceptable because marriage continues past death. Chastity is a virtue of the highest order, so females may refuse treatment from a male health care provider.

Terminal illness should not be discussed with a patient, but deferred to conversations with the family. Illness is thought to occur when an imbalance exists between five essential elements of the body: fire, earth, wind, space, and water. Thalassemia occurs frequently in this population. Vitamin A deficiency is the most common cause of blindness in East Indian children.

Japanese

Japanese consider social rank very important, so those in authority are never questioned. Verbal communication is less important than nonverbal; however, touch as a means of communication is minimal in the Japanese population. Patting on the back is unacceptable. Answers to questions are usually vague and direct eye contact demonstrates lack of respect.

Boys are taught to be assertive and competitive, whereas girls are taught to suppress thoughts and opinions. Husbands

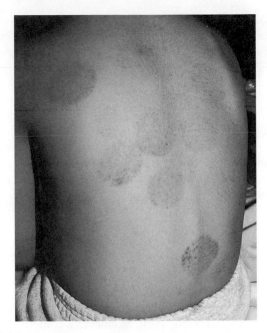

FIGURE 4-1 Cupping. These circular bruises with central petechiae are the sequelae of the Southeast Asian practice of cupping. (Courtesy Dr. Robert Hickey, Children's Hospital of Pittsburgh.)

are the head of the household; however, important decisions are made by the entire family. Families are consulted before the person seeks health care.

Health is considered a balance between the universe and oneself. Illness is thought to occur because energy no longer flows through the body, so treatment focuses on returning energy flow through acupuncture, massage, moxibustion or cupping (Figure 4-1), and acupressure.[4] There is some belief in the supernatural or the evil eye. The Japanese are very stoic with regard to pain. Fevers are managed by application of warm blankets and drinking hot fluids so the person sweats the fever out. There is a high incidence of lactose intolerance, liver cancer, and stomach cancer in this population. The Japanese also have one of the highest incidences of hypertension for all ethnic groups. Isoniazid is inactive in the Japanese population. Succinylcholine takes longer to be inactivated, so muscular paralysis lasts much longer in the Japanese patient.

Laotian

Direct, prolonged eye contact is viewed as lack of respect in the Laotian population. Only parents are allowed to touch the head of a child. Three or four generations typically live together, and health care decisions are made by the oldest man. The family name is always written first, followed by the given name. Males are not circumcised. Women's breasts are used for infant feeding only; however, colostrum is considered poisonous for the newborn, so breastfeeding does not begin until the mother has a milk supply. The lower torso from waist to knees remains covered at all times. To avoid capture by evil spirits, the newborn is never complimented. Laotians have a strong belief in herbal medicine, which leads to a high level of home care. Herbal medicines are considered "cool" medicines, whereas Western medicines are considered "hot" medicines. Laotians believe illness is caused by "bad winds." To release these winds and regain health, the affected body area is scratched or pinched until red lines or marks appear. Loss of soul, another cause of illness, is prevented by wearing strings around the waist, neck, and ankles. Physicians are considered authority figures and are not questioned or expected to explain treatments or care. Pain is usually severe before medication is requested. Tuberculosis occurs frequently in this group.

Mexican-American

Mexican-Americans are very demonstrative; friends may fully embrace as a greeting or kiss each other on the cheek. Many believe touching while bestowing a compliment decreases power of the evil eye. Women do not expose their bodies to males or other women; men may also be extremely modest. Flattering statements to passing females are accepted behavior for Mexican-American males. Coins may be strapped to a newborn's navel to make the child attractive.

Alcohol use is a common way to celebrate life, so alcohol consumption begins at a very early age. Excessive drinking is considered manly as long as the man is able to work and support his family. Men make all family decisions except when health care is needed for a child. Pediatric health care decisions are left to the woman; however, the man signs the consent and receives all instructions.

There is a strong belief in the evil eye and hexes placed by another person. Disease is considered the result of an imbalance between hot and cold, with severity determined by presence of blood and the amount of pain. Folk healers often play an important role in the maintenance of health. Same-sex health care providers are preferred. Pain relief may be refused as a means of atonement. Colostrum is considered unhealthy, so bottled milk is used until the mother can provide breast milk. Warm blankets and hot fluids are used to treat a fever. Mexican-Americans are oriented to the present, so they often do not comply with long-term treatment regimens. Diabetes mellitus, obesity, and lactose intolerance are common health problems.

Native Americans

There are more than 200 tribes of American Indians in the United States, each with unique customs, languages, and beliefs. Dominant characteristics within the majority of Native American groups include orientation to the present, regard for the elderly, strong family ties, belief in herbal or folk medicine, and use of medicine men or women. Native Americans have little regard for the future. Historically, many tribes have had no word for "time," so paying attention to a clock is not a natural instinct. Illness is seen as an imbalance of forces or the result of some violation of taboo or witchcraft. Germ theory is not understood—many tribes do not have a word for germ.

Navajo Indians do not shake hands; they lightly tap the extended hand. The extended family is the family norm with elders acting as the family leader. Wisdom and tradition are very important. Good health is believed to be a balance between the spiritual and social worlds. Health care is a combination of traditional religious practices and Western health care. Explicit explanations are important. The Navajo Indians do not touch the body or belongings of a deceased person. Lactose intolerance is common among Navajo Indians. There is some indication that Native Americans metabolize alcohol differently, which may contribute to the incidence of alcoholism in this group. Common health problems include heart disease, diabetes mellitus, and cirrhosis.

Vietnamese

Vietnamese consider public display of affection inappropriate; however, members of the same sex may hold hands in public while walking. The Vietnamese are uncomfortable with confrontation and may respond to questions with the term "ya," which means merely that they heard what was said. Often mistaken for "yes," ya does not mean they understand or agree with what was said.

Three or four generations usually live in one household, and health care decisions are made by the oldest family member. The family name is always written first, followed by the given name. A woman's breasts are considered functional organs for breastfeeding. The lower torso from waist to knees is considered extremely private and remains covered at all times. Colostrum is considered poisonous to the newborn, so breastfeeding does not begin until the mother produces milk. Males are not circumcised. The Vietnamese believe the head is a spiritual pointer, so they frown on touching the top of a child's head. Complimenting a newborn may lead to its capture by evil spirits. Dating usually begins in the late teens, but marriage is discouraged until people are in their twenties.

The Vietnamese also believe illness is caused by "bad winds." Coin rubbing (Figure 4-2) and other dermal abrasive practices are used to release winds and restore health.[4] There is a strong belief in herbal, or "cool," medicines, so illness is usually managed at home. Physicians are not questioned or expected to explain treatment. Requests for pain medications are usually made only for severe pain. Tuberculosis, hepatitis, and cholera are common health problems.

RELIGION

Spiritual expression is often associated with culture. Major religions recognized around the world include Buddhism,

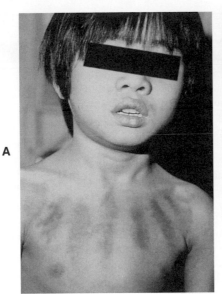
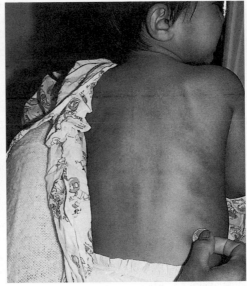

FIGURE 4-2   Coin rubbing. **A,** Vigorous stroking of the skin of a febrile child with a coin produces a peculiar bruising pattern. **B,** Here the father of another child demonstrates the technique. (**A,** Courtesy Dr. Thomas Daley, Bronx-Lebanon Hospital.)

Christianity, Hinduism, Islam, and Judaism, with numerous denominations and other religions also practiced. The emergency nurse cannot assess and treat the patient without consideration for the person's religious or spiritual beliefs. Each religion has specific beliefs and tenets, some of which relate to health and death. Table 4-3 highlights health practices and death rites for select groups. Following is a brief overview of some of the religions that the emergency nurse may encounter.

Buddhism

Buddhists believe in rebirth and karma. Delusions, greed, and hatred lead to an unsatisfactory life and, ultimately, to bad karma. These practices cause future rebirths in worlds that are unsatisfactory.

Karma is based on the theory of cause and effect. If one leads a bad life (cause), the result (effect) will be negative karma with illness the result. This means that illness is the result of actions from either the present life or a past life. Recovery and healing from illness occurs when one gains an awareness or awakens to the wisdom of Buddha.

There are many sects of Buddhism with variations in practice of the religion. Some may chant or use prayer beads, whereas others do not. Specific health care beliefs or practices are as follows:

- Abortion is acceptable in certain situations.
- Blood and blood products are acceptable.
- Organ donation is acceptable if it will assist another that is pursuing Enlightenment.
- Medications may be used to alleviate pain as long as a clear state of mind can be maintained.

- The dying person's state of mind influences rebirth. A calm, clear mind is important, and chanting by others can assist the dying person in maintaining that state of mind.
- Soothsayers, monks, or special rituals may be necessary in suicide, violent death, or death of a small child; however, priests do not routinely visit hospitalized patients.

The nurse's role in care of a patient that practices Buddhism is to provide as calm and peaceful an environment as possible. Maintaining comfort is also important.

Catholicism

Catholicism includes the belief that illness may be a punishment from God for sinful actions or sinful thinking. Catholics believe in life after death. Some Catholics wear a religious medal or hold rosary beads. Fasting occurs at specific times throughout the year; however, the ill are generally exempt from fasting and abstinence. Some specifics related to health care for those who practice Catholicism are as follows:

- Baptism is required in miscarriages and infants when the prognosis is grave.
- Abortion is prohibited and only natural methods of birth control are acceptable.
- Blood and blood products are acceptable.
- Medications are allowed as long as benefits outweigh risks.
- Organ donation is acceptable.
- Amputated limbs should be buried in consecrated ground.
- Patients may request the sacrament of the Annointing of the Sick or the sacrament of Reconciliation (confession).

Table 4-3	RELIGIONS, HEALTH PRACTICES, AND DEATH RITES	
RELIGION	**HEALTH PRACTICES**	**DEATH RITES**
Buddhism	May follow a vegetarian diet.	Donation is a matter of individual conscience.
Catholicism	Abstain from meat on Friday during the Lenten season. Abortion and contraception are condemned.	Donation is considered an act of charity and love. Transplants are morally and ethically acceptable.
Christian Science	Normally rely on spiritual healing, but members are free to choose any form of treatment they desire.	Organ and tissue donation is an individual choice.
Church of Jesus Christ of Latter Day Saints	Do not support tobacco use, alcohol consumption, or caffeine use. Members may wear special garments beneath clothing.	Donation is an individual decision.
Hinduism	May not eat pork, beef, or eggs. May be a strict vegetarian.	Prefer to die at home. Body must be attended until cremation. Nuptial threads or amulets worn by married women should not be removed until just before death. Fetus is treated as discarded tissue before 130 days; after that point it is treated as a fully developed human being. Donation is an individual decision.
Islam	Do not eat pork or pork products. Abstain from all intoxicants. Only, women care for women.	Organ donation and transplantation are accepted.
Jehovah's Witness	Do not accept blood transfusions.	Donation and transplantation are an individual decision.
Judaism	May follow a strict dietary regimen that prohibits consumption of unclean meat as described in the Bible (e.g., pork). Amputated parts must be buried.	Burial should take place within 24 hours. Body should not be left unattended until burial. Cremation is not acceptable. Orthodox, Conservative, Reform and Reconstructionist branch of Judaism support and encourage donation.
Roma (Gypsy)	Illness is a problem shared by the entire clan. Most Roma women will not agree to a pelvic examination unless the procedure is clearly explained as essential to her well-being.	Oppose organ and tissue donation because they believe the body must remain intact for 1 year after death. Tradition holds that the soul retains a physical shape to retrace its steps.
Seventh Day Adventist	Discourage use of alcohol, tobacco, and drugs including stimulants found in coffee, tea, and colas.	Strongly encourage donation and transplantation.

Modified from Ontario Multifaith Council on Spiritual and Religious Care: *Multifaith information manual,* Toronto, Ont, 1995, The Council.

- Use of ordinary means to prolong life is an obligation; however, the person can refuse treatments that would prolong life in a burdensome situation.

It is important to have a religious person present when a patient is dying. To this patient and family, the sacrament of the Annointing of the Sick is important. The nurse should provide privacy if at all possible.

Christian Scientist

Christian Scientists believe that man was created in a state of perfection. Physical illness, along with sins, wants, fears, and emotional disturbances are the result of man's lack of understanding of creation. Prayer is a mechanism to become closer to God, and healing occurs when one manifests both a moral and spiritual change. Christian Scientists may not be completely opposed to physicians but may refuse many of the standard diagnostic procedures because they can lead to unwanted treatments. Other characteristics include the following:

- Abortion is unacceptable.
- Laws for immunizations/vaccines and reporting specific diseases are followed.
- Acceptable health care practices may include care of fractures and delivery of a child.
- Use of medications and blood and blood products is typically not acceptable.
- Surgical procedures are not acceptable.
- Organ donation is an individual's decision but is generally refused.

There are Christian Science nurses that provide care to others of the Christian Science faith. These nurses may carry out health care procedures, such as wound care, in an atmosphere that provides spiritual healing.

Hinduism

The Hindu religion is possibly the oldest religion in the world. The practice of this religion varies greatly because of its variety of beliefs, customs, and practices. Well-being of an individual is assured by following the traditional law of morality and ethics, Dharma. One's karma is a direct result of his or her adherence to the Dharma. Hindus believe in reincarnation and that future lives are contingent on dealing with illness and death. Past actions dictate pain and suffering in one's life. Spiritual mementos include a thread worn around the wrist or torso that should not be removed by health care workers. Hindus also believe that the right hand should be used for eating with the left reserved for personal hygiene. Other beliefs and practices are as follows:

- Beliefs regarding illness vary. Some believe that illness is a punishment for sins, others believe in faith healing.
- Stoicism regarding illness is preferred to resorting to prayer.
- Amputations are a result of sins committed in past lives.
- Blood and blood products as well as medications are acceptable.
- Organ donation and receipt of donated organs are acceptable.
- Care of the sick, both physical and spiritual care, is provided by family members.

Hindus believe it is important to die peacefully to continue to the next life. Friends and family typically offer chants and prayers before and after death. Family and friends express their grief dramatically. A thread may be tied around the neck or wrist of the deceased to signify a blessing. It is customary for a priest to pour water in the mouth of the corpse and for family members to wash the body. Because both of these rites occur immediately after death, it may be necessary for the emergency nurse to provide the appropriate environment to allow completion of this ritual.

Islam

Muslim, Moslem, or Musselman are names of those that practice the Islamic faith. This religion is monotheistic, worshiping one God: Allah. The word Islam means peace; it also means complete submission. Worshipping Allah is the major principle of the faith. Other guiding principles include a judgment day with life after death as well as fasting and prayer five times each day. Life is a gift from Allah, whereas pain, disease, and suffering all manifest Allah's will. Other characteristics of the Islamic faith are presented below.

- Pregnant women and those who are ill are exempt from fasting.
- Female circumcision is practiced by some Moslems.
- An aborted fetus is considered a human being after 130 days.
- Receiving blood or blood products, medications, and organ transplants is acceptable.
- Some of the Islamic faith practice faith healing.

Those of the Islamic faith believe that one should confess their sins and beg for forgiveness in the presence of their family before dying. After death, five steps of burial must occur, with the first being the body washing by Muslim members of the same gender.

Jehovah's Witness

A major focus of this religion is to convert others to the beliefs of the Jehovah's Witness group. People of this religion are expected to devote at least 10 hours of each month to recruiting others. They do not believe in war or ceremonies such as saluting the flag. Jewish holidays, Christian holidays, and birthday celebrations are not recognized. Jehovah's Witness' believe in Jehovah's Kingdom and that the world will someday be restored to a paradise. All those who are beneficiaries of Christ will have healthy, perfect bodies and reside on earth. Factors involving illness and death are as follows:

- Practitioners are opposed to blood and blood products; however, blood expanders and medications can be used as long as they are not derived from blood products.
- Mental and spiritual healing can occur with scripture reading.
- Organ donation is a matter of individual choice.
- Elders of the church and members of the congregation stay with the patient during illness.
- Scriptures and prayer are a major part of recovery from illness.

Judaism

There are three main groups that practice Judaism—Orthodox, Conservative, and Reform. All groups believe that illness may be punishment for sins committed. The Sabbath begins at sundown on Friday and ends with sundown on Saturday. Orthodox Jews limit their activities during the Sabbath. Jews must refrain from working, driving or riding in cars, cooking, and using machinery during the Sabbath. In addition to the Sabbath, there are 13 other holy days for the Jewish faith. Only the rabbi can determine whether surgical procedures are allowed on these days, with the main criterion being preservation of life. Orthodox and Conservative Jews follow strict dietary laws known as Kosher laws, whereas Reform Jews rarely adhere to the Kosher laws. Other characteristics of the Jewish faith are as follows:

- Therapeutic abortions are acceptable; however, aborted fetuses should be buried rather than discarded.
- Birth control is permitted for all but Orthodox Jews.
- Orthodox and Conservative Jews and some Reform Jews circumcise males on the eighth day of life.
- Medications are permitted.
- Amputated body parts are buried per family request with all body parts ultimately buried together.
- Organ donation is acceptable to Orthodox, Reform, and Conservative Jews.
- Life is respected and all efforts to maintain life should be used, including life-prolonging measures.

Hasidic Jews are a separate sect of the Jewish religion. This group's beliefs regarding health care differ from other groups of the Jewish faith. For example, a health care provider of one gender cannot touch a Hasidic Jew of the opposite gender.

The Jewish religion has various prayers for the sick. The common practice with illness is for the rabbi to visit and pray with the patient. With major health care decisions, it is important for the patient and/or family to have access to a rabbi.

Church of Jesus Christ of Latter Day Saints

Church of Jesus Christ of Latter Day Saints (LDS) believe in life after death. They also believe that a major purpose of life is to procreate. Medical treatment is supported; practitioners believe this is one way God has empowered man to heal. They also believe that faith healing, faith in Jesus Christ, and health care should be used together. Many wear a special undergarment that signifies they are worthy to enter a temple. This garment may be removed when caring for the patient; however, some may choose not to remove it. Other practices within the LDS religion are as follows:

- Members are required to fast once each month unless ill.
- Members do not believe in birth control.
- There are no restrictions on use of medications or blood and blood products.
- Organ donation is permitted.
- Healing may include blessing of the sick in which two Elders pray, use oil to anoint, and lay hands on the person's head.
- Herbal folk remedies are an acceptable practice by some.

Members believe in dignified and peaceful deaths. With this religion, various people of the Church play a major role in spiritually caring for the patient. The emergency nurse should provide an environment that is private so various sacraments and prayers can be performed.

Protestant

Many sects are considered within the term Protestant; therefore, there is a wide variety of beliefs regarding illness and health. With most Protestants, conscience is emphasized over tradition or religion when making decisions. Many decisions are based on personal choice (e.g., birth control, use of medications, blood and blood products, and organ donation). Beliefs in prolonging life and euthanasia vary with individuals and with each Protestant Church. Some Protestants believe that only God can take life; others believe that prolongation of life through extraordinary means is inappropriate, and still others support euthanasia. Because of the variety of beliefs within the Protestant religion, it is important that the nurse knows what the patient or family prefers and acts as the patient advocate to ensure their wishes are carried out.

SUMMARY

Cultural groups have unique communication, social, and cultural needs. Recognition of and respect for cultural differences are the first steps toward acceptance and, we hope, cultural harmony. Regardless of personal views, the emergency nurse should treat each patient and family with respect and dignity.

References

1. Geissler, EM: *Pocket guide to cultural assessment,* ed 2, St. Louis, 1998, Mosby.
2. Good D: *Compton's encyclopedia,* New York, 1995, Compton's NewMedia.
3. Leininger M: Transcultural care, diversity and universality: a theory of nursing, *Nurs Health Care* 6(4):209, 1985.
4. Lipson J, Dibble S, and Minarik P: *Culture & nursing care: a pocket guide,* San Francisco, 1996, Regents, University of California.

Suggested Reading

Giger JN, Davidhizar RE: *Transcultural nursing: assessment and intervention,* ed 3, St. Louis, 1999, Mosby.
Ontario Multifaith Council on Spiritual and Religious Care: *Multifaith information manual,* Toronto, Ont, 1995, The Council.
Skabelund GP, Sims SM, editors: *Culturgrams,* Brigham Young University, Salt Lake City, 1995, David M. Kennedy Center for International Studies.

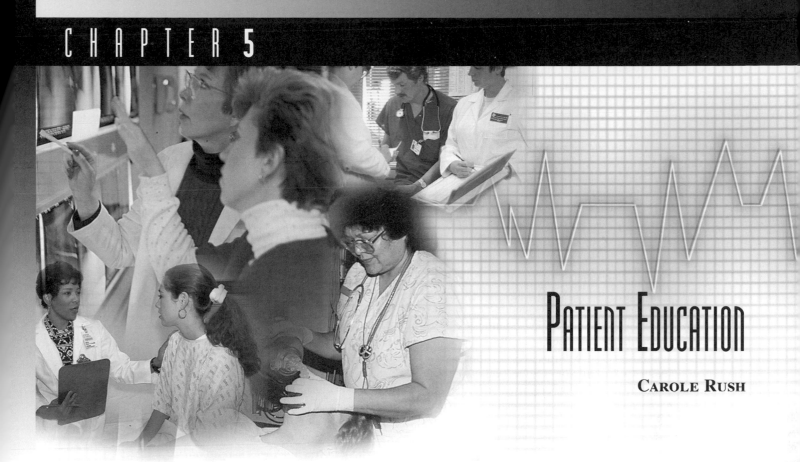

CHAPTER 5

PATIENT EDUCATION

CAROLE RUSH

During the past several years, significant changes have affected the emergency nurse's responsibility for patient teaching. First, patient teaching is explicitly incorporated into the role and responsibilities of the professional emergency nurse as stated in the *Standards of Emergency Nursing Practice* and nurse practice acts of most states, and patient teaching is included in the nursing diagnosis index as "knowledge deficit." Second, documentation of patient teaching is mandated by both quality improvement and accreditation criteria.[4] Third, the variety and sophistication of patient education materials have increased significantly. In the past, most patient education materials were homemade mimeographed copies of information chosen by interested nurses. Now, colorful, humorous, and informative booklets, videotapes, audiotapes, and CD-ROMs are published or produced by patient education departments and companies. Educational materials are also available from medical supply and pharmaceutical companies. Some learning materials are published in languages other than English and in picture format for patients with limited reading abilities. Computerized educational materials are more widely available and have become more affordable.

Although patient education has traditionally been an accepted component of emergency patient care, emphasis on the need for patient teaching has increased dramatically. Influential factors include fear of litigation, cost containment, and restriction of patient admissions. The Joint Commission on Accreditation of Healthcare Organizations (JCAHO) has identified patient and family education as an important function necessary to patient care.[4] Public awareness of the teaching responsibilities of health care professionals has increased significantly. In addition, access to health information on the World Wide Web is contributing to a more assertive consumer. Derogatory publicity regarding errors of omission and commission by health care providers has increased the number of malpractice suits. In an effort to contain rising health care costs, patient admissions have been restricted to those people with illness or injury defined in specific diagnosis-related groups. Because of this economic situation, many patients formerly admitted are now discharged from the emergency department (ED) with specific instructions for home care and referral for follow-up care.

Compounding the fear of litigation and restricted admission is the public's focus on prevention of illness and injury for both personal and financial reasons. Numerous national advertising campaigns focus on cholesterol control, prevention of heart and lung disease, and occupational and vehicular incidents. Many businesses and industries subscribe to health maintenance organizations that promote illness prevention and health maintenance.

All these efforts are aimed at containing escalating health care costs by decreasing use of hospital care. At the same time, the number of patients seen in EDs has increased. Whether this increase is due to lack of personal physicians, limited office hours for nonurgent services, transportation problems, or financial reasons, many people perceive the ED as the only consistently available access to the health care system. Even though numbers and acuity of emergency patients are increasing, staffing restrictions resulting from the nursing shortage have affected the ED as much as other hospital departments. Despite staffing shortages and the increasing numbers of ED patients, effective patient teaching remains one of the top 10 priorities of local, state, and federal governments. Patient education is perceived not only as a patient right but also as a means to contain health care costs and prevent expensive litigation.

Patient teaching in the ED presents a special challenge. Constraints and potential impediments to teaching and learning include varied patient populations, multiplicity of illness and injury, the physician, psychoemotionally compromised conditions of patients, various age-groups of patients, typically tense ED environments, and increased anxiety levels of emergency patients and their families.

To minimize constraints and teach effectively, the emergency nurse must be familiar with the teaching and learning process, maintain current knowledge and skills regarding a large variety of health problems affecting all age-groups, and be able to decrease the patient's anxiety level, thus enhancing the learning opportunity. As with any process involving knowledge and skill, familiarity with the sequential steps increases ease and effectiveness. Recall your first attempt at starting an intravenous infusion: initial attempts are awkward. However, repetition and familiarity with equipment and the process quickly improve skill and confidence.

Regardless of time constraints, number of patients, or the nursing shortage, patient teaching is an integral component of professional emergency nursing care. Because patient teaching in the ED is necessarily "telescoped" (i.e., it focuses on immediate needs while the patient is provided referral for concomitant long-term care), familiarity with the process of patient teaching is essential.

THE TEACHING AND LEARNING PROCESS

Patients benefit from teaching in many ways, including decreased anxiety, reduction in symptoms, increased self-care skills, decreased readmission rates, increased knowledge of their disease process, and increased quality of life.[7] Patient education is a process similar to the nursing process. The steps are[5]:

- Assessing education
- Setting learning goals
- Planning teaching
- Implementing the teaching plan
- Evaluating learning
- Documenting teaching and learning

Teaching and learning are two separate entities. Learning does not necessarily follow teaching. In the most general sense, teaching facilitates learning, whereas learning is evident through changes in behavior. Because time is limited in the emergency care setting, completing the patient education process is a challenge.

Educational Assessment

A comprehensive educational assessment of the patient includes assessing the individual and his or her learning needs, learning styles, and readiness to learn. Assessing the individual focuses on special needs, support systems, health expectations, cultural considerations, economic considerations, and personal factors such as values, interests, and motivations. Assessing learning needs focuses on the patient's current knowledge and personal goals as they affect health and ability to learn. Personal preference, literacy level, and functional ability determine learning style. The patient's readiness to learn can be assessed using life stages identified in Erikson's stages of development, the needs level identified in Maslow's hierarchy of needs, the patient's motivation to learn, and any obvious lack of readiness to learn.

Comprehensive educational assessment is not always possible in the ED; however, interactive discussion with the patient and family throughout the visit will shed light on their educational needs and expectations. The following questions facilitate identification of learning needs and can be adapted to almost any patient education situation.[11]

- Why did you come to the hospital?
- What did you think was happening?
- What has the doctor told you?
- What does it mean to you?
- Do you know what caused your illness or injury?
- How do you think this will change your life?
- How has this illness or injury affected your family?
- How can we help?

Learning Goals

Learning goals should be realistic, patient-centered, written, and flexible. Prioritize objectives based on what the patient "must know," "should know," and what is "nice to know." The essentials are "must know" items and should be taught first.

Planning Patient Teaching

Even when time is limited, it is possible to develop a teaching plan for patients and their families. Use identified learning needs from the educational assessment to determine what the patient should be taught. Focus on items the patient must know. Use moments throughout the entire visit when the patient's interest level is high and questions are asked. Summarize teaching when the patient is discharged. Remove distractions whenever possible. Make the patient comfortable; a patient in pain is not ready to learn.

In most EDs, discharge teaching occurs in the treatment area. However, some high-volume EDs have separate, centralized discharge areas where patients receive prescriptions, written instructions, and specific referrals for follow-up care. There are advantages and disadvantages for both sys-

<table>
<tr><td colspan="2">Box 5-1 COMPARISON OF DISCHARGE TEACHING IN TWO LOCATIONS</td></tr>
</table>

PATIENT CARE AREA	SEPARATE CENTRALIZED DISCHARGE AREA
Teaching done by primary nurse	Teaching done by nurse not familiar with patient, diagnosis, or care given
Nurse more likely to be familiar with what physician has already taught patient	Staff dedicated to discharge process ensure referrals are made
Overall length of stay may increase	
Overall emergency department patient flow slowed by patients occupying treatment space waiting for discharge teaching	Separate discharge area improves overall patient flow and may decrease length of stay

Table 5-1 TEACHING MEDIA

MATERIALS	EXAMPLES OF USE
Objects and models	Model of spine to explain back pain
	Model of heart to explain angina
	Plastic food for diabetic diet teaching
Posters mounted in emergency department (ED) patient rooms or laminated for portable use	Back exercises
	Crutch walking
Videos	Show in waiting room to explain appropriate use of ED
	Injury prevention topics such as child passenger restraints or bicycle helmets
Written discharge instructions with graphics	How to take a child's temperature
	Treatment for vomiting and diarrhea
Toys	Stuffed bear with cast to teach children cast care
Children's storybooks	Popular children's characters can tell stories about visiting the ED and hospital, as well as profile various safety topics such as wearing a bicycle helmet.

tems, which are summarized in Box 5-1. An ideal system for a high-volume ED may be a separate discharge room for each treatment area. The patient is moved to the discharge room to await instructions by the primary nurse. The treatment room is not occupied unnecessarily by a patient awaiting discharge instructions, and the patient can still receive discharge instructions from the primary nurse. A small waiting room provides space for the patient to wait for instructions while maintaining privacy.

Patient teaching in the ED is done by nurses and physicians involved in the patient's care. Patient teaching may also involve physiotherapists, respiratory therapists, and dietitians. In a low-volume ED, team teaching may occur. This type of collaborative teaching is less likely to occur in a high-volume ED. Regardless of how the organization provides patient education, all those involved must document the plan of care and teaching provided in the medical record.

Choosing the best method for patient teaching begins with educational assessment. Discuss what usually works best with the patient and family. Demonstrate psychomotor skills such as crutch walking and dressing changes. Select teaching materials that fit the patient's learning needs, budget, and resources. Table 5-1 provides examples of various teaching media.

Teaching Material

Patient educational material may be developed by staff within the ED, a centralized educational department, or purchased as ready-to-use material from various resource companies including pharmaceutical companies, education groups, or specialty groups such as the American Heart Association, the American Trauma Society, and the American Automobile Association. Figure 5-1 is one example of a preprinted education sheet. Figure 5-2 shows the same sheet in Spanish. Computerized discharge instruction sheets are gaining popularity in many areas. There are advantages and disadvantages to each avenue for obtaining educational material.[9,10] Table 5-2 lists the pros and cons for each source.

When developing your own written material, write for a range of grade levels, usually between the fourth and sixth grade levels.[2,4] Write for the level of the institution's population, if known. Write in the active rather than the passive voice. A conversational style is effective so keep sentences short and express only one idea for each sentence. Use the second person "you" rather than the third person "the patient." Limit the number of words containing three or more syllables; that is, use "doctor" rather than "physician." Present the most important information first, with adequate spacing to prevent eye strain. Keep the eye span to no more than 60 to 70 characters. (This sentence's eye span is 44 characters.) All-capital letter text is harder to read and strains the eyes. Use standard type rather than script or "fancy" type.

Regardless of where educational material is obtained, material should be reviewed before use for applicability to the specific patient population served. Teaching material should be developed with attention to accuracy, reading level, visuals, and referral information. Content should reflect current health care knowledge and practice. What the patient wants to know, as well as what the patient needs to know, should also be included. A question-and-answer format may be useful for patients to sift through and find the topic of interest. Physician involvement in development and approval of teaching materials is recommended. It is also important to include referral information with discharge

Diarrhea can be dangerous. It drains water and salts from your child. If these are not put back quickly, your child can get dehydrated and may need to be hospitalized. To protect your child follow these steps:

MANAGING DIARRHEA

1. As soon as diarrhea starts, give your child fluids. An oral electrolyte solution is the best fluid to give. This will put the water and salts back into your child's body that are lost with diarrhea.

- You can get these solutions at grocery and drug stores.
- If under 2 years old give ½ cup every hour using a small spoon. Call your doctor or public health clinic.
- If over 2 years old give ½ to 1 cup every hour.
- Keep giving the oral electrolyte solution until the diarrhea stops.
- If your child vomits, continue to give the oral electrolyte solution, using a teaspoon. Give one teaspoon every 2—3 minutes until vomiting stops. Then give regular amount.
- Do **not** give sugary drinks such as Gatorade,® cola drinks or apple juice. They can make your child's diarrhea worse.

2. Continue to feed your child as recommended by your doctor or public health clinic. Food will help your child stay healthy.

- If breast-fed continue to breast feed.
- If on formula continue to give formula.
- If on solid foods continue to give regular diet. Good foods to give include cooked meat, cooked cereal or bananas.

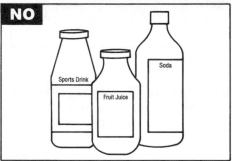

These have the WRONG amounts of water, salts and sugar.

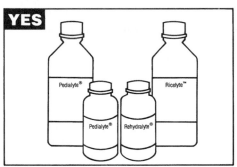

Oral electrolyte solutions have the RIGHT amounts of water, salts and sugar.

Your child may need medical help if the diarrhea is more serious than usual. You should call your doctor or public health clinic immediately if:
- the diarrhea lasts more than 24 hours,
- the diarrhea gets worse,
- there are any signs of dehydration:
    decreased urination
    sunken eyes
    no tears when child cries
    extreme thirst
    unusual drowsiness or fussiness

THE NATIONAL
ORT
Oral Rehydration Therapy
PROJECT

For more information or additional copies, phone (614) 624-7540.

FIGURE **5-1** Preprinted education sheet. (Courtesy The National Oral Rehydration Therapy Project, Ross Products Division, Columbus, Ohio.)

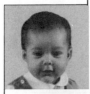

La diarrea puede ser peligrosa. Agota el contenido del agua y de las sales del cuerpo de su hijo. A menos que sean repuestas inmediatamente, su hijo corre el riesgo de deshidratarse y tal vez tenga que ser internado en el hospital. Para evitar esto, haga lo siguiente:

COMO CONTROLAR LA DIARREA

TAN PRONTO COMO empiece la diarrea, déle de tomar líquidos a su hijo. Lo mejor es darle un suero de tomar para la deshidratación (oral electrolyte solution). Esto repone el agua y las sales que ha perdido el cuerpo de su hijo por la diarrea.

- Puede conseguir esta solución en una farmacia o en una tienda de comestibles.
- Si su hijo es menor de 2 años, déle durante cada hora media taza de suero, utilizando una cucharita. Llame a su medico o a la clínica de salud pública.
- Si su hijo es mayor de 2 años, déle al menos la mitad de una taza o la taza entera, durante cada hora.
- Déle de tomar a su hijo el suero hasta que los síntomas de la diarrea desaparezcan.
- No importa si su hijo vomita, siga dándole de tomar el suero en cucharaditas. Déle una cucharadita cada 2 o 3 minutos hasta que deje de vomitar. Vuelva a darle la cantidad indicada según su edad.
- **No le** dé bebidas azucaradas como Gatorade,® refrescos, o jugo de fruta.

SIGA ALIMENTANDO a su hijo de acuerdo a las indicaciones de su médico o de la clínica de salud pública. Una buena alimentación mantiene a su hijo sano.

- Siga dandole pecho.
- Si le da fórmula infantil, siga dándosela.
- Si alimenta a su hijo con comidas sólidas, siga dándole la comida habitual. Entre las comidas indicadas están la carne cocida, los cereales cocidos, fideos o plátanos.

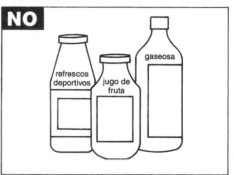

Estos contienen una cantidad INADECUADA de sales y de azúcar.

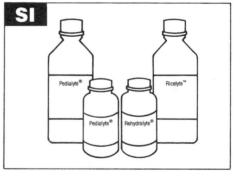

Los sueros de tomar para la deshidratación (oral electrolyte solutions) contienen una cantidad ADECUADA de sales y de azúcar.

SEÑAS DE PELIGRO DE LA DIARREA

Su hijo tal vez necesite atención médica si la diarrea es muy fuerte. Llame al médico o a la clínica de salud pública inmediatamente en caso de:

- diarrea que dura más de 24 horas,
- diarrea que empeora,
- síntomas de deshidratación:
  orinar poco o menos frecuente
  ojos hundidos
  ojos sin lágrimas al llorar
  sed intensa
  demasiado sueño o inquietud

THE NATIONAL
ORT
Oral Rehydration Therapy
PROJECT

Para obtener más información o copias adicionales, llama al (614) 624-7540.

FIGURE 5-2   Preprinted Spanish education sheet. (Courtesy The National Oral Rehydration Therapy Project, Ross Products Division, Columbus, Ohio.)

Table 5-2   COMPARISON OF SOURCES FOR EDUCATIONAL MATERIAL

SOURCE	ADVANTAGES	DISADVANTAGES
Emergency department (ED) staff committee	Small group can accomplish tasks more quickly than large committee Group is familiar with patient population and personnel available	Group may be isolated from rest of hospital and existing materials because of lack of knowledge of that material There may be inconsistency of information with material presented on the same subject by other departments Increased cost to develop small amount of material when compared with bulk order for the institution
Hospital education committee	Eliminates duplication of efforts within the institution Ensures consistency of information within the institution Promotes collaboration and contribution of a large number of health care professionals	Large committee is tedious and takes longer to develop material Increases production costs because of labor hours required to develop the material
Ready-made material	Eliminates duplication of efforts and "reinventing the wheel" May be more cost-effective than developing in-house materials; some companies provide gratuitous materials Institution-wide use of materials helps standardize patient education Some software packages offer information in multiple languages	Information may be too generic or basic Information may conflict with some institutional policies and procedures Some software may not be compatible with existing institution computer systems Some discharge teaching software is only available when an entire package for ED tracking is purchased (cost factor)
Computerized teaching material using purchased software package	Some can be customized with patient name, diagnosis, medication regimen, discharge treatment, referrals, and physician(s) involved Personalized information may increase patient compliance with discharge instructions Some software packages include colorful graphics, which can increase patient understanding and compliance Some software packages offer information in multiple languages	Initial cost of implementation may be prohibitive for some institutions Ideally requires multiple computers to ensure staff access and facilitate simultaneous processing of several sheets Some systems also require physician involvement with the teaching process so the physician must take time to enter the data Some software may not be compatible with existing institution computer systems Some discharge teaching software is only available when an entire package for ED tracking is purchased (cost factor)

instructions. Provide resource information for business hours, evenings, weekends, and holidays.

Reading Level

The average reading level for emergency care patients is between fourth and eighth grade levels.[1,4,8] Figure 5-3 is an example of instructions written at the fourth grade level.[5] Unfortunately many educational materials are printed for higher reading abilities. It is important to determine reading level for any printed materials used for patient education. Computer software programs that measure reading level are available. Two useful programs are Rightwriter and Prose, and the Readability Analyst.[2] Advantages of a computerized program include speed, ease of use, and reliability when multiple formulas are used.[2]

If computerized programs are not available, manual formulas can be used to calculate reading level. The SMOG formula predicts within 1.5 grade levels how difficult a passage is to read.[9] For discharge instructions that contain at least 30 sentences, identify 10 consecutive sentences each from the beginning, middle, and end of the selection. For these 30 sentences, count words containing three or more syllables, including repetitions. Count hyphenated words as one word. For numbers, count the syllables for each numeral. For example, the number 573 counts as seven syllables. Include proper nouns in your syllable count. Avoid sentences with a colon in your count. If you do use one, count it as two sentences. When a word is abbreviated, count the number of syllables for the word when it is spelled out. After you have the total number of words, use the SMOG table (Table 5-3) to determine grade level.

For discharge instructions that contain less than 30 sentences, count the number of sentences in the instructions. Use the conversion table (Table 5-4) to get the conversion number that corresponds to sentences in the instructions. Count words with three or more syllables, then multiply the

Table 5-3 SMOG TABLE	
WORD COUNT (THREE-SYLLABLE WORDS ONLY)	GRADE LEVEL
0-2	4
3-6	5
7-12	6
13-20	7
21-30	8
31-42	9
43-56	10
57-72	11
73-90	12
91-110	13
111-132	14
133-156	15
157-182	16
183-210	17
211-240	18

From Stewart KB: Written patient-education materials: are they on the level? *Nurs '96* 26(1):32j, 1996.

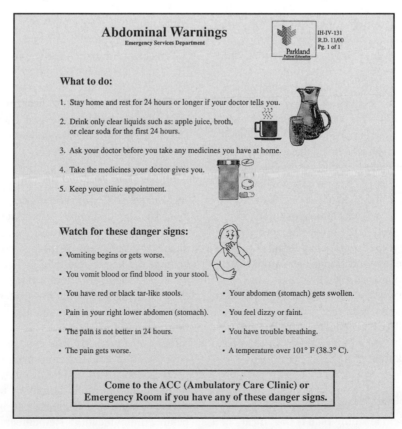

FIGURE 5-3   Instructions written at the fourth grade level. (Courtesy Parkland Memorial Hospital, Dallas, Texas.)

Table 5-4	SMOG CONVERSION TABLE	
NUMBER OF SENTENCES IN SELECTION	**CONVERSION NUMBER**
29	1.03
28	1.07
27	1.10
26	1.15
25	1.20
24	1.25
23	1.30
22	1.36
21	1.43
20	1.50
19	1.58
18	1.67
17	1.76
16	1.87
15	2.00
14	2.14
13	2.30
12	2.50
11	2.70
10	73.00

From Stewart KB: Written patient-education materials: are they on the level? *Nurs '96* 26(1):32j, 1996.

three-syllable word count by the conversion number to get an adjusted word count. Refer to Table 5-3 for the grade level of the material.

Prepurchased patient education materials with inappropriate reading levels can be modified. One suggestion is to highlight the point that patients must know, what symptoms should suggest a call or visit to a health care provider, and follow-up phone numbers.[2]

In addition to ensuring that written words in patient education materials are effective, the author should pay attention to overall patient comprehension. One study evaluated patient comprehension of discharge instructions for a laceration, with and without visuals.[6] Researchers concluded the addition of illustrations improved patient understanding, especially among patients who are nonwhite, female, or have no more than high school education.[8] The age of the audience should be considered when incorporating color into educational materials.[2] The geriatric population may have altered color perceptions and may not respond favorably to certain color combinations. Warm colors such as red, yellow, and orange have more visual appeal than do the cooler colors of violet, blue, and green.[2]

Visuals can be in the form of pictures, cartoons, anatomic diagrams, and photographs. As with the written word, simplicity is effective. Not all patient education materials are easily enhanced with illustrations. Figure 5-4 is an example of instructions with illustrations.

Implementing the Teaching Plan

Implementation of the patient teaching plan is the "meat" of the teaching and learning process; however, patient learning can only take place within the framework of a positive, helping relationship. This type of relationship relies on good communication skills and includes respect, trust, caring, acceptance, sincerity, and patient advocacy. Communication is a process by which information is given and received. Face-to-face communication includes both verbal and nonverbal messages.

Communication

Communication involves not only sending the message but also receiving and understanding the message. It can be verbal or nonverbal. It is the process through which the patient-caregiver relationship develops. The patient may base his or her perception on the nurse's competence level and what the patient sees as the level of communication and interpersonal skills demonstrated by the nurse. Usually the better the communication and the patient's perception of that communication, the more smoothly the therapeutic process goes.

The emergency nurse must be acutely aware of the following facts related to communication:
- Regardless of method, there is some form of communication in any relationship, even if it is nonverbal or does not involve physical contact.
- Communication can be formal or informal.
- All behaviors by the nurse, patient, and patient's family are forms of communication.
- It is impossible not to communicate.
- What you say may not necessarily be what the patient hears.

Verbal Communication. Choose words carefully when communicating with patients or their significant others. Match spoken words with written information the patient will receive. Strategies for teaching patients throughout the life span and teaching patients with special needs will be discussed later in this chapter.

Listening is one way to hear the patient's concerns. Having the patient talk while you listen may relieve anxieties and facilitate information collection. Whenever possible, allow the patient to take the conversational lead. Listening is an active, physically visible process. Being able to listen is a learned skill, acquired through practice.

Nonverbal Communication. Body position is important. The nurse should try to teach from a sitting position facing the patient to avoid being perceived as "talking down" to the patient. If the patient is lying down, raise the head of the bed to maintain eye contact. Patients can sense when staff members are in a hurry. If time is limited, be honest with the patient about how much time is available to discuss his or her condition and aftercare. Allow time to listen. Many nonverbal messages such as those communicated through eye contact, facial expressions, gestures, touch, and body position hold different meanings in different cultures. Cultural sensitivity will be discussed later in this chapter.

Although not often thought of as such, silence as an expressive, nonverbal response can be a useful tool in therapeutic communication. Remember, silence is the absence of words, but not the absence of activity. It may be a natural

How To Use Your Crutches

How to make your crutches fit you:

1. Remove the screw that holds the bottom peg and the top of the crutch together.

2. Place the crutch under your arm.

3. Push the top of the crutch down on the bottom peg so that **3 fingers** fit between the top of the crutch and **under** your arm.

4. Put the screw back in the bottom peg and the top of the crutch to hold them together.

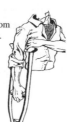

5. Remove the screw in the top of the crutch and the hand grip.

6. When the end of your crutches are 6 inches from the outside of your foot, **move the hand grip so your arm is bent just a little.**

7. Place the screw back into the top of the crutch and hand grip to hold them together.

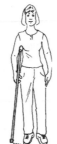

How To Use Your Crutches

Safety:

• Never put more weight on your hurt leg than you have been told to by your doctor. Use your crutches.

• Wipe your crutch tips off after walking over a dusty floor.

• Avoid throw rugs and wet floors. You might slip and fall.

• Do not use your crutches to stop a fall. Use your hands to break the fall. Throw the crutches away from you. Bend at the waist. Using crutches to stop a fall could cause you to hurt yourself.

• **Danger:** If your crutch tips are worn, you may slip. Replace them.

IH-I-32   Parkland
                 Patient Education   R.D. 2/97

How to move around with your crutches:

1. When walking with crutches, the top of the crutch must **not** touch your underarm.

2. Stand up straight.

3. Put the weight of your body on your hands and the hand grips. **Do not** lean on crutches to rest. The pressure can hurt the nerves under your arms.

4. **Stand on your good foot** and move both crutches in front of you.

5. Resting your weight on your hands, **lift and swing your good foot** to where the crutches are.

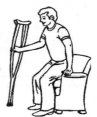

6. **To sit down**, hold both crutches by the hand grip in one hand. Put your other hand on the chair and sit down.

7. **To stand up**, hold both crutches by the hand grip in one hand. **Put your other hand on the chair** and stand up.

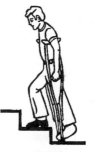

8. **To walk up stairs**, put your weight on the crutches and put your good foot on the step. Then put your weight on your good foot and lift the crutches up to the step that your good foot is on.

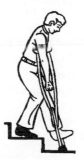

9. **To walk down stairs**, put your weight on your good foot and place the crutches on the step below you. Then put your weight on the crutches and step down with your good foot.

FIGURE 5-4   Instruction sheet with illustrations. (Courtesy Parkland Patient Education, Parkland Memorial Hospital, Dallas, Texas.)

Table 5-5	TEACHING ACROSS THE LIFE SPAN
AGE	**TEACHING CONSIDERATIONS**
Children[11]	Include the parent(s) or caregiver(s) in teaching; they are most familiar with the child.
	Consider the child's stage of physical and cognitive development.
	Be truthful with children when explaining an illness, injury, or procedure. Do not tell a child a procedure does not hurt when it does.
	Allow children to express fears and ask questions.
	Don't explain a procedure too far in advance. This leaves time to imagine scary scenarios.
	Children need to know the reason for the hospital visit and to be reassured it is not because of bad behavior.
Adolescents (ages 13 to 20 years)[5,11]	Include parents with young adolescents, but use judgment with older teens. Parents should be informed of the patient's physical condition and specifics of treatment, but this can be accomplished with separate discussions.
	Any condition that will have an effect on physical appearance requires sensitivity. Body image is an important issue.
	Use peer pressure in a positive way. Often teens come with peers to the emergency department. If appropriate, include peers in teaching because peer pressure may increase compliance.
Young adults (ages 20 to 40 years)[5,7]	Give the patient a practical reason(s) for learning.
	Keep in mind that young adults often take good health for granted.
	If patient has young children, stress the need to recover and/or maintain health to allow care of children.
Middle adults (ages 40 to 60 years)[5,7]	Patients are more aware of possible health problems than young adults.
	Use patients' life experiences as a foundation for new learning.
Older adults (age 60 and older)[5,7]	Motivate patients to learn by showing how acquisition of knowledge and skill will increase their quality of life.
	Use their experiences to relate to current problems.

conclusion of verbally transmitted thoughts. Silence may be useful because it
- Allows time to think.
- May be helpful in finding solutions to problems and answers to questions.
- Is a way to convey your feelings without words.
- May promote acceptance or indicate anxiety in either you or the patient.
- Can be used to pace, time, alienate, resist, or relax when employed carefully.

Barriers to Effective Communication.   Emergency care centers are usually busy, noisy places. Awareness of barriers to effective communication may help eliminate some of these distractions. Try to conduct teaching in a relatively quiet area. Lack of privacy can be an issue because many patient care areas are open. If a patient is in a private room, close the door. Personal attitudes and values about lifestyle, health behaviors, and learning can be projected to the patient, so avoid making judgments.

Teaching Throughout the Life Span

An effective educator is able to individualize teaching strategies to accommodate the entire emergency patient population. Most emergency settings treat adult and pediatric clients. Pediatric facilities should be familiar with adult learning principles when teaching parents and other caregivers. Refer to Table 5-5 for information related to teaching various age-groups.

Teaching in Special Needs Situations

Today's world is a complex blend of individuals with different physical, psychosocial, and cultural distinctions. Aware-

ness of and sensitivity to these differences is essential for effective patient education in the ED. The Americans with Disabilities Act (ADA) of 1990 also has implications for patient education. The ADA speaks to individuals with literacy problems, hearing impairment, and visual impairment. As world travel becomes more common, the emergency nurse must consider cultural differences as they relate to teaching and learning. Refer to Chapter 4 for further discussion of cultural aspects of health and illness.

Literacy.   Illiteracy is a major problem in today's society. Recent estimates place the level of functional illiteracy in the adult population at 13%. Functional illiteracy means the individual can recognize a majority of words but understands only a small percentage of the words. Poor literacy skills are viewed in a negative light in Western culture. Do not assume money, educational level, or color dictate literacy level. Illiteracy does not correlate with intelligence; many self-made business people memorize sufficient information to succeed.[7]

Illiterate or low-literate patients have no clear identifying characteristics. A patient may be very polite, articulate, and willing to sign a document without understanding the written words. To determine the patient's reading ability, observe, listen, and ask questions. A nonthreatening question to ask during assessment is, "Do you like to read?" As a general rule, those who read reasonably well enjoy reading to some extent, whereas those who find reading difficult do not like to read. When given written materials, illiterate patients may give the excuse that their reading glasses are missing. Other patients may pass written materials to a family member or significant others to read.

When teaching patients who cannot read, use short, simple words, avoid medical jargon, and be consistent with chosen words. Teach essential information first, then repeat the information as necessary. Use analogies the patient can understand, with illustrations whenever possible. Have the patient restate, review, or demonstrate the information. Include available family and significant others to reinforce the teaching points.[5]

Hearing Impairment. Many hearing-impaired patients may communicate that fact through gestures, written notes, or through family members. If alone, the patient may be constantly looking over his or her shoulder or appear uneasy. The patient may have a hearing aid, although these devices are not always visible in the external ear. Some hearing aids are designed to be concealed in the ear to avoid embarrassment. Patients' level of frustration may reflect how long they have been disabled and the effectiveness of their coping mechanisms.

When teaching patients who are hearing impaired, ask the patients if they can speech read, formerly called lip reading. If so, face the patient with adequate light on your face and speak slowly and deliberately.[5] Gesturing can increase comprehension. Some patients and families may know sign language. A family member or significant other may be able to sign to the patient. Use a sign language interpreter when necessary. It is important to remember that the ADA requires that health care organizations offer a sign language interpreter to anyone who uses sign language, and at no cost. If the patient uses a hearing aid, make sure it is available. Some patients may not wear the device all of the time, however. Reinforce verbal communication with written instructions and illustrations. Some patients may appreciate a notebook and pencil tied to the bed within easy reach during their ED stay.[5] Be patient; teaching will take more time than with patients who are not hearing impaired.

Visual Impairment. Visual impairment poses obstacles to communication for both the patient and the nurse. The patient may speak only when spoken to because of uncertainty of the presence and location of the other people. Communication can be compared to a telephone conversation. Legally blind persons often carry a white cane or stick, whereas others use a seeing-eye dog to help guide their way. The visually impaired who still have some eyesight may use a magnifying glass to enlarge written words.

When teaching visually impaired patients, announce and identify yourself when you enter the patient's room or cubicle. Remember that verbal communication is more important than nonverbal messages. Maintain normal speech; talking louder will not make the message better understood. Avoid phrases such as "Do you see what I mean?" Explain all steps of a procedure including how the patient will feel.[5] Touch is important to visually impaired people; however, they do not need constant touch. For patients who still have some sight, consider enlarging written instructions and illustrations.[5]

Cultural Diversity and Foreign Languages. Culture consists of values, social and family structure, religion, diet, customs, health beliefs, and expectations.[7] Sensitivity to cultural diversity is essential for the educator. Health care practices in conflict with the patient's values will probably not be followed. It is important to remain open-minded and non-judgmental. Nurses can obtain information about cultures through their human resources department and library. Some institutions discuss basic cultural differences during orientation. If possible, incorporate all nonharmful components of the patient's desired cultural behaviors into the teaching plan. There is no need to speak more loudly, but speech should be slow and clear. Watch for facial expressions and other nonverbal cues that indicate confusion.

When teaching patients who speak a foreign language, try to learn a few words in those languages regularly encountered, and use reference books that translate English medical phrases into various other languages. Use professional interpreters if available; they should be familiar with medical terminology. Keep eye contact with the patient, use short units of speech, and wait for a response. Maintain rapport with the interpreter. Use family or friends to interpret as a last measure.[5] Figure 5-5, *A*, shows an instruction sheet in English; Figure 5-5, *B*, shows the same sheet in Spanish.

Chronic and/or Terminal Illness. The majority of teaching that takes place in emergency care is related to the acute illness or injury surrounding the patient's chief complaint for that emergency visit. Patients can present with an acute manifestation of a chronic illness. New-onset diabetes mellitus and cancerous tumors may be diagnosed in the ED. Most ED discharge teaching materials are related to the immediate care of an acute condition, rather than the long-term management of a chronic illness. If the patient is not admitted to the hospital for further treatment and investigation, the ED nurse can provide an introduction to priorities of care for this new diagnosis and then refer the patient and family to sources of more detailed information. Many hospital libraries have sections for public health care information. Local support groups related to a specific disease or condition can also provide many resources. Patients may be referred to local clinics that specialize in the particular disease.

Evaluation of Learning

The next step in the teaching and learning process is evaluation. Because emergency care teaching sessions are often short, evaluation usually takes place upon discharge. The nurse evaluates whether the process is complete, needs reinforcement, or there are needs that must be referred to an outside agency.[11]

Ask the patient to repeat what has just been discussed and ask him or her questions on the content discussed. Determine if the patient can perform a return demonstration of any skills taught. Other methods of evaluation may be used to evaluate learning. The patient may be telephoned after discharge to evaluate learning. Formal questionnaires on comprehension of written tools may also be used. Focus testing of resources is strongly recommended before introducing new materials to your patient population.

Documentation

Documentation is the final component of the teaching and learning process, but it is no less important than the other

What to do for the Flu

If you have the flu, you will have: **fever, body aches, chills.**

You may also have:

- headache
- weakness
- lack of energy
- sore throat
- vomiting
- loss of appetite
- cough
- nausea (feeling sick to your stomach)

What to do when you have the flu:

1. Wash your hands often. This helps to keep germs from spreading.

2. Stay home and rest as much as possible.

3. Drink plenty of liquids. Water, fruit juice, lemon-lime sodas (like Sprite), and hot tea are good.

4. Eat small meals. Foods like chicken soup or broth, Saltine crackers, plain toast, and gelatin are good.

 Parkland
Patient Education

IH-I-63

5. Take your temperature 3 times a day if you keep feeling hot and sweaty, or chilled.

6. Come to the clinic or ACC (Ambulatory Care Clinic) if you are sick for over 1 week or if your fever goes higher than 100.4° Fahrenheit (38° Centigrade).

7. Take cool baths if you have a fever. This may help you feel more comfortable.

8. Antibiotics will not cure the flu.

   - Take acetaminophen (Tylenol regular strength, Tempra, Panadol, etc for fever, headaches or body aches. Read and follow the directions on the bottle or follow your doctor's advice.

   - Do **not** give Aspirin to babies or children. Ask your child's doctor what to give, how much to give and when to give it.

Lessen your chances of getting the flu:

- Wash your hands often. This is the best way to lessen your chances of getting or passing on the flu.

- Get a good night's sleep every night.

- Eat 3 healthy meals each day.

- Drink plenty of fluids (non-alcoholic).

- Stay away from sick people.

- Consider getting a flu vaccine in October or November. It starts to work in about 2 weeks. The flu season lasts from November through February.

R.D. 11/00

A

FIGURE 5-5   Standardized education sheet in **A**, English, and **B**, Spanish. (Courtesy Parkland Patient Education, Parkland Memorial Hospital, Dallas, Texas.)

Continued

B

Qué Hacer para la Gripe

(What to do for the Flu)

Si tiene la gripe, tendrá: **fiebre, dolor de cuerpo, escalofríos**

También puede tener:

- dolor de cabeza
- vómito
- debilidad
- pérdida del apetito
- falta de energía
- tos
- dolor de garganta
- náusea (sentirse enfermo del estómago)

Qué Hacer Cuando Usted Tiene la Gripe:

1. Lávese sus manos con frecuencia. Esto ayuda a que los microbios no se transmitan.

2. Quédese en la casa y descanse lo más que pueda.

3. Tome bastantes líquidos. El agua, los jugos de frutas, las sodas (gaseosas) de lima-limón (como Sprite) y el té caliente son buenas.

4. Coma pequeñas comidas. Los alimentos como el caldo de pollo y el consomé, las galletas saladas, el pan tostado (sin nada), y la gelatina también son buenos.

5. Tómese su temperatura 3 veces al día si se siente caliente y sudoroso o con frío.

6. Venga a la clínica o a ACC (Clínica de Cuidado Ambulatorio) si se enferma por más de 1 semana o si su fiebre sube a más de 101 grados Fahrenheit (38 grados Centígrados).

7. Si tiene fiebre tome baños de agua fría. Esto puede ayudarle a sentirse mejor.

8. Los antibióticos no curan la gripe.

  - Tome acetaminofén (Tylenol regular strength, Tempra, Panadol, etc.) para la fiebre, dolores de cabeza o del cuerpo. Lea y siga las instrucciones de la botella ó siga las recomendaciones del médico.

  - No le dé Aspirin (Aspirina) a los bebés o a los niños. Pregunte al médico de sus niños qué darles, cuándo darles y cuánto darles..

Reduzca sus Probabilidades de que le Dé la Gripe:

- Lávese sus manos con frecuencia. Esta es la mejor manera de reducir las probabilidades de que le dé la gripe o de pasarla a otros.

- Duerma bien todas las noches.

- Diariamente coma 3 veces alimentos saludables.

- Tome bastantes líquidos (sin alcohol).

- Permanezca retirado de la gente enferma.

- Piense en vacunarse contra la gripe en octubre o noviembre. Esta vacuna comienza a tener efecto en 2 semanas aproximadamente. La temporada de la gripe dura desde noviembre hasta febrero.

IH-I-63 S

Parkland
Patient Education

R.D. 11/00

FIGURE 5-5 cont'd Standardized education sheet in **A**, English, and **B**, Spanish. (Courtesy Parkland Patient Education, Parkland Memorial Hospital, Dallas, Texas.)

Table 5-6 INJURY PREVENTION ORGANIZATIONS		
NAME OF ORGANIZATION	**CONTACT INFORMATION**	**WEBSITE**
Emergency Nurses CARE The Injury Prevention Institute of the Emergency Nurses Association	205 South Whiting Street Suite 403 Alexandria, VA 22304 e-mail: jlencare@aol.com	www.ena.org Click on ENCARE
American Trauma Society	8903 Presidential Parkway Suite 512 Upper Marlboro, MD 20772-2656 (800) 556-7890	www.amtrauma.org
National Highway Traffic Safety Administration	400 7th Street, SW NTS-21 Washington, DC 20590	www.nhtsa.gov
National SAFE KIDS Campaign	1301 Pennsylvania Avenue Suite 1000 Washington, DC 20004-1707	www.safekids.org
International Center for Injury Prevention	5009 Coye Drive Stevens Point, WI 54481 (800) 344-7580	www.cipsafe.org
Consumer Product Safety Commission (CPSC)	Hotline (800) 638-2772	www.cpsc.gov
Centers for Disease Control and Prevention National Center for Injury Prevention and Control	4770 Buford Highway NE Atlanta, GA 30341-3724	www.cdc.gov/ncipc

Box 5-2 INJURY PREVENTION ACTIVITIES

• Discharge teaching information sheets related to injury prevention (Figure 5-6)
• Presentations to school students, teachers, parents, and child case workers on a variety of safety topics and the consequences of injury
    Home safety
    Child passenger restraints
    Bicycle helmets and safety
    Firearms safety
    Traffic safety
• Participation in community safety events such as bicycle festivals and rodeos
• Hosting a Teddy Bear Picnic that features activities to keep teddies (and children!) safe
• Displays and demonstrations at community trade shows
    Installation of child passenger restraints at local automobile events
    Proper fitting of bicycle helmets at local sports and outdoor recreation events

steps. The JCAHO accreditation manual contains a section on patient and family education. The manual specifically describes the institution's responsibility in this area. It is recommended that all nurses involved with patient education be familiar with current JCAHO standards. Basic information to include in documentation includes content taught, method(s) used, the patient's response, adjunct instructions provided, and referrals made. The date, time, and signatures of the patient and the educator should be included. If people other than the patient were included in teaching, document their names and relationship to the patient. All members of the health care team who participate in patient teaching are responsible for documentation. Institutional policies and procedures should be followed for all documentation.

Methods of documentation include written nurse's notes, standardized discharge forms (Figure 5-6), and computer-generated forms. Computerized documentation can also produce a hard copy for the patient and one for the medical record.

OPPORTUNITIES FOR COMMUNITY EDUCATION

Emergency nurses can extend their educational efforts outside the walls of the acute care setting. Experience in caring for ill and injured patients can be used to educate the public about both interventions and preventive measures related to disease processes. Opportunities for community education include:

- Cardiopulmonary resuscitation and other first aid courses
- Blood pressure clinics and other health indicator screenings
- Participation in "wellness fairs" profiling healthy lifestyles
- Institutional open houses, public tours, and community events such as "Teddy Bear Clinics" that introduce the public to the workings of the acute care setting
- Injury prevention activities (See Box 5-2 for a list of examples and Table 5-6 for a list of resources.)

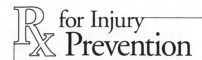 for Injury
Prevention

Protect Your Kids in the Car

The safest place for any child 12 years old and under is in the back seat.

Every child should be buckled in a child safety seat, a booster seat, or with a lap/shoulder belt, if it fits.

Riding with Babies

℞ Babies should ride in rear-facing child seats until they are at least 20 pounds AND at least one year of age. The child seat must be in the BACK seat and face the rear of the car.

℞ Babies riding in a car must never face front. In a crash or sudden stop, the baby's neck can be hurt badly.

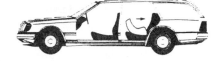

℞ Babies in car seats must never ride in the front seat of a car with air bags. In a crash, the air bag can hit the car seat and hurt or kill the baby.

℞ Never hold your baby in your lap when you are riding in the car. In a crash or sudden stop, your child can be hurt badly or killed.

Riding with Young Kids

℞ Kids over 20 pounds and at least 1 year old should ride in a car seat that faces the front of the car, van, or truck.

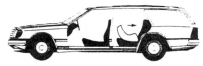

℞ It is best to keep kids in the forward facing car seat for as long as they fit comfortably in it.

℞ Older kids over 40 pounds should ride in a booster seat until the car's lap and shoulder belts fit right. The lap belt must fit low and snug on their hips. The shoulder belt must not cross their face or neck.

℞ Never put the shoulder belt behind their back or under their arm.

Remember...

℞ All kids are safest in the back seat, in a safety seat or seat belt

℞ Always read the child seat instructions and the car owner's manual. Test the child seat to ensure a snug fit by pulling the base to either side or toward the front of the car.

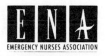
EMERGENCY NURSES ASSOCIATION

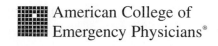 American College of Emergency Physicians®

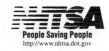
People Saving People
http://www.nhtsa.dot.gov

For additional information, please contact the NHTSA hotline at: 1-888-DASH-2-DOT (1-888-327-4236), or the NHTSA Web site.

U.S. Department of Transportation • National Highway Traffic Safety Administration   September 1997

A

FIGURE 5-6 Examples of discharge teaching information sheets related to injury prevention. **A,** Protecting children in cars. (Courtesy U.S. Department of Transportation and National Highway Traffic Safety Administration.)

Continued

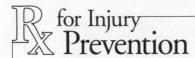

Car Safety

Don't Drink and Drive

℞ More than four out of every ten traffic deaths involve alcohol.

℞ Even small amounts of alcohol affect your judgment, concentration, reaction time *and your ability to drive.*

℞ If you drink, don't drive. If a friend or family member drinks, call them a cab or drive them home.

Wear Your Safety Belt

℞ Wear your lap and shoulder belt correctly, low and snug across the hips, and the shoulder belt across your chest, *not* in front of your neck or face.

℞ Do not put the shoulder belt under your arm or behind your back.

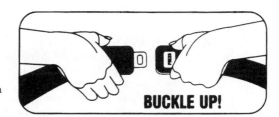

B

℞ If your car has air bags, make sure you wear both the lap and shoulder belt for the best protection. Move the seat back as far as possible from the air bag.

℞ Never place babies under one year old in the front seat of a car with a passenger-side air bag. Always keep babies in the back seat and facing the rear of the car.

℞ All children are safest in the back seat using the safety belt or in a child safety seat.

℞ Pregnant women should always wear the lap and shoulder belt, with the lap belt firmly placed under the belly and across the hips. By protecting Mom, the baby has the best chance of surviving a crash.

℞ *Buckle up every trip, every time, and every body!*

Slow Down - Follow the Speed Limits

℞ Nearly one out of three crashes where someone dies is related to speeding. Speeding makes it hard to steer safely around curves or objects in the roadway.

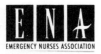

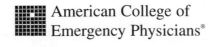 American College of Emergency Physicians®

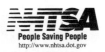 People Saving People
http://www.nhtsa.dot.gov

For additional information, please contact the NHTSA hotline at: 1-888-DASH-2-DOT (1-888-327-4236), or the NHTSA Web site.

U.S. Department of Transportation • National Highway Traffic Safety Administration   September 1997

FIGURE **5-6 cont'd**   Examples of discharge teaching information sheets related to injury prevention. **B,** Car safety. (Courtesy U.S. Department of Transportation and National Highway Traffic Safety Administration.)

Continued

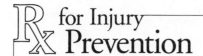 for Injury
Prevention

Kids Riding Bikes

Wear a Helmet

℞ Wearing a helmet is the best thing you can do to be safe when you ride a bike.

℞ Bicycle helmets save lives. Most bike deaths come from head injury. Bike helmets can prevent head injury.

℞ In some states, the law says you have to wear a bike helmet to ride your bike.

℞ Bike helmets should fit like this:
   - sits evenly between ears
   - sits low on your forehead

See and Be Seen

℞ Ride so cars can see you.

℞ Wear bright colors or clothes that reflect light at night so cars, buses, and trucks can see you.

℞ If you ride at night, get a headlight for the front of your bike and "reflectors" on the front and back of your bike.

C

Follow the Rules

℞ Bikes have to follow the same traffic rules and signs as cars.

℞ You must ride in the same direction as the cars are going.

℞ Ride your bike single-file.

℞ Signal when you want to stop or turn.

℞ Look out for holes, wet leaves, or cracks in the street. They can make you crash your bike.

℞ Ride away from the curb in case a car pulls out or someone opens a car door suddenly.

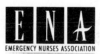 EMERGENCY NURSES ASSOCIATION   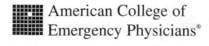 American College of Emergency Physicians®   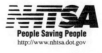 People Saving People http://www.nhtsa.dot.gov

For additional information, please contact the NHTSA hotline at: 1-888-DASH-2-DOT (1-888-327-4236), or the NHTSA Web site.

U.S. Department of Transportation • National Highway Traffic Safety Administration   September 1997

FIGURE 5-6 cont'd Examples of discharge teaching information sheets related to injury prevention. **C,** Bicycle riding. (Courtesy U.S. Department of Transportation and National Highway Traffic Safety Administration.)

Continued

Rx for Injury Prevention

Walking in Traffic

Protect yourself and your family by doing these things:

Walk on the Sidewalk

Rx   Stay on the sidewalk and crosswalks. Avoid walking in traffic where there are no sidewalks or crosswalks. If you have to walk on a road that does not have sidewalks, walk facing traffic.

Cross at Intersections

Rx   Most people are hit by cars when they cross the road at places other than intersections.

Look left, right, and left for traffic

Rx   Stop at the curb and look left, right, and left again for traffic. Stopping at the curb signals drivers that you intend to cross. Cross in marked crosswalks and obey the signal.

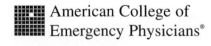

See and Be Seen

Rx   Drivers need to see you to avoid you.
Stay out of the driver's blind spot.
Make eye contact with drivers when crossing busy streets.

Rx   Wear bright colors or *reflective* clothing if you are walking near traffic at night. Carry a flashlight when walking in the dark.

Do not let kids play near traffic or cross the street by themselves. Kids are small, and drivers may not see them if they run into the street.

Watch your kids

Rx   Children should not cross streets by themselves or be allowed to play or walk near traffic. Kids are small, *unpredictable*, and cannot judge vehicle distances and speeds.

Rx   When kids get older, teach them three things to do before they cross the streets:
- Try to cross at a corner with a traffic light
- Stop at the curb.
- Look left. right, then left again to make sure no cars are coming.

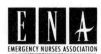 EMERGENCY NURSES ASSOCIATION

American College of Emergency Physicians®

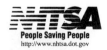 People Saving People
http://www.nhtsa.dot.gov

For additional information, please contact the NHTSA hotline at: 1-888-DASH-2-DOT (1-888-327-4236), or the NHTSA Web site.

U.S. Department of Transportation • National Highway Traffic Safety Administration   September 1997

FIGURE 5-6 cont'd   Examples of discharge teaching information sheets related to injury prevention. **D,** Walking in traffic. (Courtesy U.S. Department of Transportation and National Highway Traffic Safety Administration.)

SUMMARY

To ensure adherence to prescribed therapeutic, restorative, and preventive measures, the emergency nurse is responsible for providing effective, individualized instruction regarding home care measures and the process involved in emergency care. This responsibility necessitates familiarity with sequential steps in the teaching and learning process. The process includes identifying learning needs, assessing learning, establishing realistic goals, selecting and using appropriate teaching methods, allowing for learning time, evaluating results, and documenting instructions. Application of learning and communication principles is a prerequisite to effective teaching. Because all emergency nurses must be familiar with the process involved in carrying out their professional role as nurse teacher, content regarding the patient teaching process is included in orientation and in-service educational programs. In addition, patient teaching is a criterion for quality improvement, clinical ladder, and performance evaluation.

Knowledge of home care is a patient's right. Ensuring this knowledge also benefits the ED by reducing the number of call-backs and return visits. Consequently, patient teaching can be considered an integral component of emergency patient care.

References

1. Austin PE, Matlack R, Dunn KA et al: Discharge instructions: do illustrations help our patients understand them? *Ann Emerg Med* 25(3):317, 1995.
2. Brownson K: Education handouts: Are we wasting our time? *J Nurs Staff Dev* 14(4),176, 1998.
3. Duffy MM, Snyder K: Can ED patients read your patient educational materials? *J Emerg Nurs* 25(4):294, 1999.
4. Joint Commission on Accreditation of Healthcare Organizations: *Comprehensive accreditation manual for hospitals,* Oakbrook Terrace, Ill, 1996, The Commission.
5. Maynard AM: Preparing readable patient education handouts, *J Nurs Staff Dev* 15(1):11, 1999.
6. Pestonjee SF: *Nurses handbook of patient education,* Springhouse, Penn, 2000, Springhouse.
7. Pestonjee SF: *The process of patient education,* Dallas, Tex, 1997, Parkland Memorial Hospital.
8. Spandorfer JM, Karras DJ, Hughes LA et al: Comprehension of discharge instructions by patients in an urban emergency department, *Ann Emerg Med* 25(1):71, 1995.
9. Stewart KB: Written patient-education materials, *Nurs '96,* 26(1):32j, 1996.
10. Vukmir RB, Kremen R, Ellis GL et al: Compliance with emergency department referral: the effect of computerized discharge instructions, *Ann Emerg Med* 22(5):819, 1993.
11. Winthrop E: *Mosby's patient teaching tips,* St. Louis, 1995, Mosby.

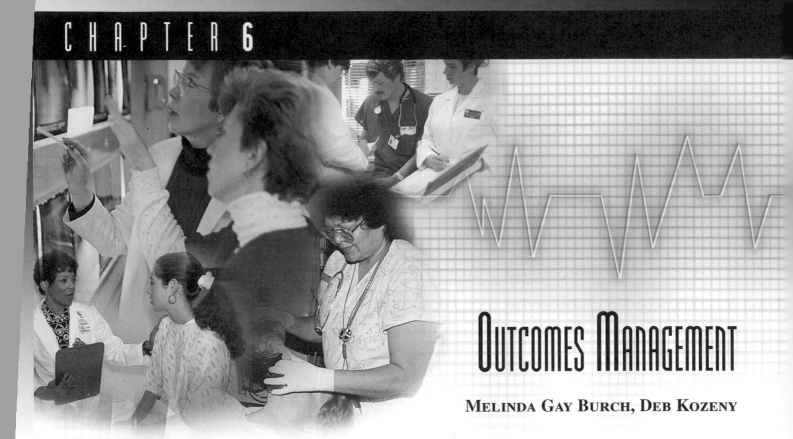

CHAPTER 6

Outcomes Management

MELINDA GAY BURCH, DEB KOZENY

The further we move into the twenty-first century, the more complex care will become as a result of increased technology and expanding knowledge bases. Emergency department (ED) census will continue to increase at an enormous rate and many patients will have difficulty accessing the primary care physician office secondary to health insurance issues or unavailability of appointment times. Availability of the ED on weekends, after hours, holidays, and with no appointment or cash required make it the likely treatment choice for many individuals. Of course, the trauma patient with minor or castrophic multisystem injury will continue to come through our doors. Patients with perceived or real life-threatening medical emergencies such as chest pain, difficulty breathing, and metabolic disorders will still come requiring immediate care whether by referral from their primary care physician or on their own. Exacerbation of chronic illness occurs daily and places a heavy burden on all aspects of health care management. All of these factors, combined with severity of illness, rapid triage/treatment, and patients that are generally unknown to the ED set the stage for poor outcomes.[2]

Companies in the business of health care reimbursement look at each health care facility and evaluate their patient outcomes and benchmark status in the community and nationally. The companies then contract with the facility that provides the best care at the best price. Reimbursement is certainly the driving force from a business standpoint and must be considered for longevity in the health care market. Health care providers must maintain a mindset of patient advocacy, look for ways to measure and improve patient outcomes, and provide care that ranks in the top percentile of established benchmarking. Health care quality appraisal is based on evaluation criteria and specific outcomes.

Continuous quality improvement (CQI) plays a role in outcomes by assisting in reduction and control of variables and measurement of compliance. Quality assurance processes assist with establishing consistent patient care standards while focusing on measuring process performance. These tools used to define and monitor quality during the late 1980s and early 1990s are still the tools required to fully evaluate quality patient care outcomes. Looking at specific patient outcomes has been evolving across health care over the past few years but has developed slowly in the ED. It is difficult to find studies that scientifically and adequately document patient-centered outcomes in an ED. Time frames allotted for patient interaction remain very limited secondary to volume, acuity, and mindset. And, the ED can no longer ignore the patient's health care status after being discharged from episodic intervention. Health care must look across the patient care continuum and evaluate the patient's outcome. For the ED, are there standards or protocols that can be used to measure performance? How does the ED comply with these standards? How does the care provided in the ED affect the outcome of the ED patient?

DEFINING OUTCOMES

The definition of outcomes in health care takes many tracts along all states of illness and wellness but is the result of what occurred during the term of illness or wellness.[5] An outcome can be negative or positive. Some key characteristics of a negative outcome are mortality, morbidity, and readmission to the hospital and repeated ED visits, cost, increased resource utilization, length of stay, and decreased throughput for the system. The desired outcome for the health care consumer is the absence of complication concurrent with increased feelings of wellness, including physical, mental, social, and psychologic aspects. Individuals have their own perception of functional status extending across their life span.[8] Outcomes represent the end result of care. The patient's perception and reported outcome is an excellent indicator for best practice.

Outcomes can be categorized as clinical, or patient centered, and financial. Within these, outcomes may be positive or negative. Historically, health care providers focused on such outcomes as cost, hospital readmissions, morbidity, and mortality. Repeat ED visits, increased resource utilization, and length of stay are outcomes that also have been evaluated and are examples of financially focused outcomes. Examples of positive clinical outcomes in the ED include the cardiac arrest patient who leaves the ED alert and hemodynamically stable or the trauma patient with multiple lower extremity fractures who states pain is controlled with current pain medications.

Outcome management determines desired outcomes, then defines a process to achieve the outcome. Outcome assessment is measurement, monitoring, and evaluation of the outcome. It uses standards, protocols, and guidelines to glean information regarding patient episodes of illness and well-being. Analysis of data correlates the patient's process to patient outcomes. The ED is often the entry point for episodic intervention and a revolving door for acute episodes of chronic illness. In both cases delivery of care and the transition to subsequent levels of care affect outcomes.

Organizational outcomes are measured by improvements in health care and well-being of the population served relative to costs incurred.[5] For example, consider the situation in which an indigent clinic for pediatrics is physically too small and understaffed to accommodate the growing need of the community. The influx of patients begins to have a negative impact on the ED, with increased wait times and overutilization of resources. The follow-up process with the clinic physician after treatment in the ED does not occur because of lack of appointments secondary to space and personnel issues. Now the patients must be followed in the ED or receive no follow-up care at all. Consequently, a negative outcome may occur. The cost of seeing a patient in the clinic is equal to one third the cost of seeing a patient in the ED. Study of visits and cost comparisons in this situation can lead to clinic expansion and an increase to staff. As seen in this example, focus on outcomes is beneficial to the patient and the organization.

BENCHMARKING

Benchmarking is the correlation of specific uniform data to local, regional, and national standards. Institutions are then able to rank themselves comparatively to similar institutions and evaluate where improvements may be needed for them to rank as quality health care providers. Consumers are more educated than ever, with access to information that enables them to make value judgments based on published benchmark data. These consumers go beyond being only a patient to include multidisciplinary health care teams within and outside an institution, governing bodies such as the Joint Commission on Accreditation of Healthcare Organizations (JCAHO) and National Councils, institutions, and entities providing payment.

Benchmarking relies on statistical data such as number of ED visits, number of admissions from the ED, number of return visits to the ED within a certain time frame, and/or return to the ED with the same diagnosis. Additional data for benchmarking includes total number of visits per diagnosis or International Classification of Diseases-9 codes, urgent versus emergent cases, dispositions, cost/charge per visit, gain/loss per visit, length of stay, wait times, complication rate, and satisfaction rating of both the patient and health care providers. These are only a sampling of focus items considered in benchmarking; each one can be related to patient outcome.

The most common benchmarking tool is patient satisfaction scores. By asking the patient for evaluation of care provided, the organization can evaluate whether it met the patient's expectations and needs. A benchmarking study done by the Harvard Emergency Department looked at five urban EDs to determine if feedback of benchmark data was associated with improvement in compliance with process-of-care guidelines and patient-reported measures of quality. They found that the use of benchmarking followed by quality-improvement efforts resulted in some improvements in quality of care. Measures that relied on patient reports of problems with care, rather that patient satisfaction with care, seemed to be more responsive to change. The process of benchmarking, feedback, and quality improvement led to increased compliance with guidelines and fewer patient-reported problems.[2]

OUTCOMES IN THE EMERGENCY DEPARTMENT

Patients in the ED evaluated and treated for episodic care generally have a short length of stay in the department. The patient is sent home, admitted, or transferred to a different level of care. Planning for this transition has become problematic for many EDs. Patients may be given medications, taken to a bed on the floor in a timely manner, or transferred to another facility. Providing consistent standard interventions for and monitoring of the long-term treatment plan that affects response to care or outcome should now be a focus of ED.

Trauma and illnesses with high incidence, high mortality, and significant chronic morbidity should be monitored for patient outcome as a means of managing quality. Illnesses such as congestive heart failure, acute myocardial infarction, and chronic obstructive pulmonary disorder or asthma are usually studied for practice and outcomes in the ED. These studies are summarized later in the chapter.

Collection of data helps define patterns of care and acts as a report card for providers (Box 6-1). Using practice standards or guidelines, care maps, and critical pathways can streamline care delivery.

Expected Outcomes of Care

Quality indicators identify expected outcomes of care and are always specific to a diagnosis or surgical procedure.

Box 6-1 DATA COLLECTION FOR PATTERNS OF CARE

Return visit within 48 hours
Return visit within 72 hours resulting in admission
Admission rates and percentage of patients admitted for 24-hour observation
Deaths within the department
Deaths within 24 hours of emergency department (ED) visit (inpatients or those discharged from the ED)
Lab and x-ray variances
   Requiring an amended plan of care
   Requiring recall to the ED for missed diagnosis
   Requiring call to the primary care physician
Patients requiring transfer to acute facility
Insurance-driven transfers
Length of stay in the department
Triage to admission
Triage to discharge
High-risk patients for discharge

Data from Health Care Resource Group: *Outcomes measurement management: case management focus emergency department/community,* Whittier, Calif, 1998, The Group.

Box 6-2 ASTHMA QUALITY INDICATORS

A. INTERMEDIATE INDICATORS

1. Intravenous (IV) corticosteroid discontinued when peak flow is ≥200-250 L/s
2. IV corticosteroids are changed to prednisone, by mouth; peak flow is ≥200-250 L/s
3. Able to demonstrate the use of metered dose inhaler with spacer

B. DISCHARGE INDICATORS

1. Peak flow is 200-250 L/s
2. Minimal-to-free of shortness of breath or chest tightness
3. Follow-up appointment is arranged
4. Minimal-to-free of wheezing
5. Able to use the metered dose inhaler with spacer
6. Verbalizes understanding of disease process, risk factors, medications, and allergens that cause an asthma attack

From Flarey D, Blancett SS: *Handbook of nursing case management,* Gaitherburg, Md, 1996, Aspen Publishers.

Box 6-3 KEY PARTICIPANTS IN THE DEVELOPMENT OF CLINICAL PATHWAYS

Physicians in the emergency department (ED)
Physician specialists
Staff nurses in the ED
Manager of the ED
Clinical nurse specialist
Case management/social services
Emergency medical services
Pharmacist
Dietitian
Respiratory
Physical therapy
Medical records/billing
Other ancillary departments affected by the pathway
Representation from inpatient services receiving the patient and those responsible for continued care of the patient

---

These indicators are clinical in nature and specific to a plan of care. They reflect the standards of care and best practice. The patient is expected to accomplish certain goals or criteria before discharge. These goals or criteria are intermediate or discharge indicators (Box 6-2).[5] Intermediate indicators are those milestones that the patient must accomplish during his or her stay in the ED; discharge indicators are those that the patient needs to meet at the time of discharge.

Clinical quality indicators are also called clinical outcomes or outcome indicators.[5] They are developed using a multidisciplinary approach and instituted at the time of admission. These can be predetermined by clinical pathways and modified to the patient or can be individually developed for the patient at the time of presentation to the ED.

Clinical Pathways in the Emergency Department

Clinical pathways (CPs) may also be called care maps, clinical paths, or critical paths. The purpose of CPs is to move the patient's care along a designated timeline that allows for specific standards of care, accurate documentation, and a method by which data can be gleaned to determine compliance and variances. Standards of care used in CPs address the expected outcomes for the specific diagnosis or patient type.

For the process of pathway development a multidisciplinary team approach must be taken to ensure that all components of care are addressed. Box 6-3 lists some of the key participants in CP development. Utilization of these participants brings not only expertise to the table but also greatly enhances buy-in for CPs. For example, the development team for a stroke CP should include an ED physician, emergency nurse, neurologist, pharmacist, physical therapist, and the computed tomography technician to ensure that all components of care are addressed. Certain key criteria must exist in an effective CP (Box 6-4).

There are many CPs already established that can be used as a resource. It is important to ensure that the CP used in each ED is customized to the patient population, community needs, resources, and standard of care developed for the institution using national and regional guidelines. What works in one ED may not work in another. The CP should be a tool that actually provides a planned process of care and reflects the patient's movement through the process. The planned process should move care along a time frame that coincides with set standards and is realistic for needs of the patient and the ability of the ED to provide care. The management of outcomes can effectively use the CP when working through variance analysis, outcomes measurement, and outcomes

Box 6-4	**KEY CRITERIA OF EFFECTIVE PATHWAYS**

Triage
Prehospital treatment
Assessment guidelines
High-risk factors
Diagnostic tools
Treatments
Medications
Patient status
Multidisciplinary team intervention
Teaching patient, family, and community
Discharge criteria
Expected outcome

monitoring. Figure 6-1 provides a sample ED chest pain CP; Figure 6-2 is an example of a CP for fever in infants.

Variance Analysis

A variance is anything not consistent with the plan of care or the patient's meeting goals set forth in the expected outcome. A variance is an action that can negatively affect outcome for the patient (e.g., delayed test, delayed procedure, or medication error) (Box 6-5). Positive outcomes include patient progress through the plan of care more quickly than projected or achievement of better-than-predicted results. An example of a positive variance might be when a patient's predicted peak flow on admission is 200 L/s but his or her actual measurement is 280 L/s. The ideal time to collect the data is when the variance occurs; this allows for more complete analysis and is more apt to produce accurate results.

Data Collection Tool Development

Before starting to collect data, tools must be developed that focus on the type of data needed. Such tools should include variance analysis and expected outcomes. A tool must be diagnosis-specific and reflect each outcome met and the reason an outcome is not met.

Outcomes Measurement

The *Handbook of Nursing Case Management* defines outcomes measurement as systematic quantitative observation of variances and outcome indicators, at one point in time, using collection tools that are developed based on a management plan. It serves to identify deficiencies in patient care and noncompliance with standards. To develop a plan to improve care and outcomes, it is necessary to establish a system of outcome measurement.

Outcomes Monitoring

Outcomes monitoring is the continual measurement of variances and outcome indicators along with analysis of what

caused the outcome. This provides data needed to understand what is working and what is not working with patient care. Outcomes monitoring requires assessment, reassessment, and evaluation each time a new plan is formulated.

Outcomes Management

Outcomes management is the analysis and trending of the information collected through outcomes measurement and monitoring. Decision making is done, based on the analysis, to improve the effectiveness of the management plan and the quality of care.[5] As with benchmarking, feedback is key. Feedback must be brought to those involved in the plan's development; when data are not as planned, adjustments must be made. The adjusted data collection tool should then use the same outcomes management process.

Barriers to Positive Outcomes

Many barriers pose problems for the patient, health care provider, and community that affect outcomes. General barriers to all patients include inadequate support systems, poor access to medical care, limited financial resources, poor response to treatment, failure of providers to stay current with treatment methods, educational level, and ability to learn. When looking at a disease-specific population such as those with asthma, barriers that affect outcomes include noncompliance with medication regime, environmental issues, air quality, and inability to accurately self-monitor medications and peak flow rates. Barriers for the caregiver to produce effective outcomes are lack of resources, outdated standards, educational level, and compliance. When developing expected outcomes, potential barriers must be considered to effect change and turn a negative outcome into a positive one. One author recommends that as soon as the patient fails to respond as expected, the plan should be modified.[7]

Effective Outcomes

To reach a goal or outcome requires setting the goal and then working a plan to attain the goal; therefore, specific end points need to be reached with each disease or surgical-specific process. The goal/outcome must be SMART—Specific, Measurable, Achievable, Realistic, and Timely.[10] Establishment of goals and expected outcomes provides direction for care and the health care provider. Outcomes should address quality of life, satisfaction with medical care, functional abilities, compliance with and effectiveness of treatment, and avoidance of or decrease in hospitalizations and ED visits.

THE EMERGENCY DEPARTMENT AND THE COMMUNITY

The ED serves the community and is held to certain state, federal, and local standards of practice. The community depends on the ED to identify barriers to safety and wellness, provide care that reestablishes or promotes wellness, facilitate safe discharges, and make appropriate referrals. This

Text continued on p. 65

♥ GWINNETT HOSPITAL SYSTEM

PROMINA

EMERGENCY DEPARTMENT
CHEST PAIN CLINICAL PATHWAY
INITIAL NURSING ASSESSMENT

Pt. Identification Stamp

Date:	Arrival Time:	Triage Time:

Name:	Age:	DOB:	❑Workers Comp

HX OF PRESENT ILLNESS:
1. Time chest pain began: _____
2. Duration of longest episode of chest pain that prompted ED visit: Hrs._____ Min._____
3. Location of pain:_____
4. Other Hx. of present illness:_____
   _____
   _____
5. What preceded pain...what were you doing when pain began?
   ❑ Resting   ❑ Mild Activity
   ❑ Strenuous Activity ❑ Awakened From Sleep

QUALITY OF CHEST PAIN:
❑ Constant   ❑ Intermittent
❑ Ache   ❑ Numbness
❑ Burning   ❑ Pressure, crushing
❑ Crushing   ❑ Sharp, stabbing
❑ Dull   ❑ Other: _____
❑ Indigestion, gas
                    _____

QUALITY OF CHEST PAIN:

Rating on Scale of   Radiation into:
0-10 _____   ❑ Shoulder(s)
(0 = none   ❑ Arm(s)
10 = most severe)   ❑ Back
                            ❑ Jaw/Neck
                            ❑ Other _____

ASSOCIATED SYMPTOMS:
❑ Diaphoresis   ❑ Nausea
❑ Dizziness   ❑ Vomiting
❑ Dyspnea   ❑ Other _____
❑ Fatigue   _____

CHEST PAIN IS REPRODUCED BY:
❑ Changes in position   ❑ Palpation
❑ Deep breathing   ❑ Activity
❑ Other _____

WEIGHT   Estimated _____ Actual _____

PHYSICAL ASSESSMENT

B/P (R)	B/P (L)	P	R	T ❑ORAL ❑RECTAL ❑TYMPANIC	Pulse Ox:

AIRWAY
❑Clear
  ❑Partially Obstruct
  ❑Obstructed

MONITOR RHYTHM:_____
Skin:
❑Warm and dry   ❑Pale
❑Cool and clammy ❑Cyanotic
❑Diaphoretic   ❑Hot
❑Flushed
❑Other:_____

ABDOMEN:
❑Soft ❑Firm
❑Tender/location _____
❑Flat ❑Distended
❑Bowel sounds
  ❑Present
  ❑Absent

BREATHING
LUNGS: L R   L R
❑Clear ❑ ❑ ❑Rales   ❑ ❑
❑Rhonchi ❑ ❑ ❑Diminished ❑ ❑
❑Wheezes ❑ ❑ ❑Labored · ❑ ❑
                Respirations

NEURO
LEVEL OF CONSCIOUSNESS
❑Alert
❑Oriented:
  ❑Person ❑Place ❑Time
❑Other:_____

LOWER EXTREMITIES:
❑Edema L: ❑Absent ❑Trace
            ❑1+ ❑2+ ❑3+
         R: ❑Absent ❑Trace
            ❑1+ ❑2+ ❑3+
❑Other:_____

CIRCULATION
Heart:
❑S1 S2 Other:_____
CRT ___ secs JVD: ❑Y ❑N
Pulses: L R   L R   L R
Radial ❑ ❑ DP ❑ ❑ PT ❑ ❑

PUPILS:

L=___mm   R=___mm

Sluggish Brisk Non-reactive   Sluggish Brisk Non-reactive

Triage Level ❑A ❑B	Treatment Area: ❑GMC-ED ❑Joan Glancy-ED

RN Signature: _____   page ____ of ____

Seq# 14167
Revised: 4/00
                    page ____of ____

FIGURE 6-1   Sample clinical pathway for chest pain. (Courtesy Gwinnett Hospital System, Lawrenceville, Georgia.)

Continued

EMERGENCY DEPARTMENT CHEST PAIN CLINICAL PATHWAY*

Interdisciplinary Action Plan	PHASE I	Initials	PHASE II	Initials
ASSESSMENT	Initial triage assessment		Complete Initial Nursing Assessment Sheet	
			Nursing reassessment (VS, pain scale, rhythm, neuro status, bleeding)	
INTERVENTIONS	Transport to monitored bed in treatment area		Notify ED physician - Time: _____	
			ED physician evaluation	
			Establish INT site - Time: _____ Site: _____, Gauge: _____	
			Establish additional INT's if needed	
			Site _____ Gauge _____ Time _____	
			Site _____ Gauge _____ Time _____	
DIAGNOSTICS	EKG - Time: _____		EKG completed	
			Order PCXR	
LAB			Cardiac labs and drug levels (if indicated), drawn via INT if possible and sent to lab Time:	
MEDICATIONS			O2 @ 2-4 L / min via NC - Time: _____	
			ASA 160 mg chew & swallow	
			_____ Taken at home _____EMS	
			_____ Given here, Time: _____	
			Pain management initiated (Dose / Time)	
			_____ NTG sublingual x 3 _____ / _____	
			_____ NTG IV (200 mcg / ml) _____ / _____	
			_____ Morphine IV _____ / _____	
			_____ Dilaudid IV _____ / _____	
			Decision to administer tPA - Time: _____ (add tPA Flow Sheet to pathway)	
PSYCHOSOCIAL	Provide emotional support to patient and significant others		Provide emotional support to patient and significant others	
EDUCATION			Orient to ED	
			Pain scale	
			ED course and planned treatment	
			Medications	
OUTCOMES			Verbalizes decrease in pain	
			Cardiac dysrhythmias identified	
			Symptoms and/or EKG suggestive of cardiac etiology	
			Continue Pathway _____ Yes _____ No	

These are guidelines and can be altered at the practitioner's discretion.

Initials	Signature

page _____ of _____

FIGURE **6-1 cont'd**   *Continued*

PHASE III	Initials	PHASE IV	Initials
Nursing reassessment (VS, pain scale, rhythm, neuro status, bleeding)		Nursing reassessment (VS, pain scale, rhythm, neuro status, bleeding)	
Cardiologist/PMD consulted		Cardiologist/PMD evaluation - Time: _____	
CCU/Telemetry bed requested Time: _____		ED physician speaks with patient's significant other	
Establish additional INT		Report called to CCU/Telemetry - Time: _____	
Site _____ Ga _____ Time _____		RN Name: _____	
Site _____ Ga _____ Time _____		Transport to room Time: _____	
Continuous cardiac monitoring		Continuous cardiac monitoring	
Repeat EKG q 30 min x 3 if symptoms persist and initial EKG non-diagnostic [] 1 [] 2 [] 3			
CXR completed			
Lab results obtained and abnormals reported to ED physician			
02 @ 2-4 L / min via NC - Initial: _____		02 @ 2-4 L / min via NC - Initial: _____	
Heparin Weight Based Protocol		Heparin Weight Based Protocol	
IV bolus _____ 70 u kg, _____ u / kg		IV bolus _____ 70 u kg, _____ u / kg	
Maintenance drip _____ 15 u / kg / Hr		Maintenance drip _____ 15 u / kg / Hr	
Lovenox 1 mg/kg _____		Lovenox 1 mg/kg _____	
Aggrastat per protocol		Aggrastat per protocol	
Pain management initiated Dose / Time / Site		Pain management initiated Dose / Time / Site	
_____ NTG sublingual _____ / _____		_____ NTG sublingual _____ / _____	
_____ NTG IV (200 mcg / ml) _____ / _____ / _____		_____ NTG IV (200 mcg / ml) _____ / _____ / _____	
_____ Morphine IV _____ / _____ / _____		_____ Morphine IV _____ / _____ / _____	
_____ Dilaudid IV _____ / _____ /		_____ Dilaudid IV _____ / _____ /	
Decision to administer tPA - Time: _____ (add tPA Flow Sheet to pathway) Time started: _____		Decision to administer tPA - Time: _____ (add tPA Flow Sheet to pathway)	
Provide emotional support to patient and significant others		Provide emotional support to patient and significant others	
Medications		Medications	
		Hospital admission	
Verbalizes pain managed		Verbalizes painfree	
Cardiac dysrhythmias identified		Cardiac dysrhythmias identified	
Hemodynamically stable		Hemodynamically stable	
		Disposition determined	
Continue Pathway _____ Yes _____ No			

*Variation

Initials	Signature

page _____ of _____

FIGURE 6-1 cont'd   (Courtesy Gwinnett Hospital System, Lawrenceville, Georgia.)   *Continued*

EMERGENCY DEPARTMENT
CHEST PAIN PATHWAY
PROGRESS NOTES

Time	BP	P	R	T	Pulse Ox	Pupils L	Pupils R	Pain Scale	Intervention	Progress Notes

page ____ of ____

FIGURE 6-1 cont'd   *Continued*

PHYSICIAN'S ORDERS

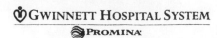

GWINNETT HOSPITAL SYSTEM
PROMINA

INSTRUCTIONS: DETACH SHEET DIRECTLY BELOW
ORIGINAL AND FORWARD TO PHARMACY

PATIENT IDENTIFICATION

☐ ADMIT   ☐ 23 hr OBV Bed   ☐ OUTPATIENT   ☐ DAY SURGERY   Page 1 of 2

EMERGENCY DEPARTMENT CHEST PAIN CLINICAL PATHWAY
PHYSICIAN ORDERS AND DISPOSITION

Date/Time _____

☐ Old chart   ☐ Consult _____ Time Called_____
☐ EKG-STAT (Cardiologist _____)
☐ CXR-Portable
☐ CBC   ☐ PT (Coumadin ☐ Yes ☐ No)
                               ☐ PTT
☐ Chem 7   ☐ Digoxin
                               ☐ CPK ISOS

☐ CMP   ☐ Troponin   ☐ _____
☐ VS with BP in both arms
☐ Pulse Ox on room air
☐ Continuous cardiac monitoring   ☐ May be off monitor for tests
☐ O$_2$ at 2-4 liters/min via nasal cannula
☐ INT
☐ Establish 1 additional IV lines. No further venapunctures, arterial
   punctures, IM or SQ injections.
☐ If not given pta, chewable baby aspirin, two 81 mg tabs po STAT (chew &
   swallow) or, if unable to swallow, ASA 325 mg supp STAT.
☐ **NTG** 0.4 mg SL every 5 min x 3 if systolic BP ≥ 100 m Hg or not pain free
☐ Start NTG (200 mcg / ml) IV at 10 mcg / min NOW; may titrate up to 100 mcg / min to relieve chest pain as long as
   SBP ≥ 100
☐ **Morphine** 2-4 mg IV q 5-10 min. Up to _____ mg maximum dose prn unrelieved with maximal dose IV NTG or SL
   NTG x 3. Hold for excessive sedation
☐ **Dilaudid** 0.5 mg - 2 mg IV q 15-30 min. Up to a maximum dose of 4 mg in 30 min prn unrelieved with maximal
   dose IV NTG or SL NTG x 3. Hold for excessive sedation
☐ r-tPA infusion STAT as follows: Use tPA Flow Sheet
   Reconstitute 100 mg r-tPA in 100 cc Sterile Water. Do not shake vial - swirl slowly
   (IV line for r-tPA should not have filter)
   Administer 15 mg IV over 2 min via pump. Set pump rate at 450 cc / Hr and dose limit at 15 cc
   When infused, follow next step based on patient's weight (may use estimated weight):

☐ ≥ 67 kg   Administer 50 mg IV over 30 min via pump. Set pump rate at 100 cc / Hr and dose limit
   (147 lbs)   at 50 cc. When infused, administer 35 mg IV over 60 min via pump. Set pump rate at 35 cc / Hr
                   and dose limit at 35 cc.

               OR

☐ < 67 kg   When infused, administer 0.75 mg / kg over 30 min not to exceed 50 mg via pump (0.75 mg x #kg x
                   2 = cc / Hr). When infused, administer 0.5 mg / kg over 60 min not to exceed 35 mg (0.5 mg x #kg
                   = cc / Hr). Set pump rates and dose limits accordingly

When infused, hang 50cc Normal Saline to flush tubing. Set pump rate at 35 cc / Hr to clear r-tPA

Seq# 14167
Revised 9/98

PHYSICIAN ORDERS   PHYSICIAN ORDERS   PHYSICIAN ORDERS
White Copy: Chart/Medical Records   Yellow Copy: Pharmacy

Please check all appropriate boxes and fill in blanks.

FIGURE **6-1 cont'd**   (Courtesy Gwinnett Hospital System, Lawrenceville, Georgia.)

Continued

PHYSICIAN'S ORDERS

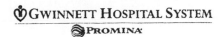

INSTRUCTIONS: DETACH SHEET DIRECTLY BELOW
ORIGINAL AND FORWARD TO PHARMACY

PATIENT IDENTIFICATION

☐ ADMIT   ☐ 23 hr OBV Bed   ☐ OUTPATIENT   ☐ DAY SURGERY   Page 2 of 2

EMERGENCY DEPARTMENT CHEST PAIN CLINICAL PATHWAY
PHYSICIAN ORDERS AND DISPOSITION

☐   **Heparin** Weight Based Protocol Wt. _____ kg Est / Act (Pull inpatient orders to use as guidelines)
IV Bolus   ☐ 70 u / kg   ☐ _____ u / kg
Maintenance drip   ☐ 15 u / kg / Hr   ☐ _____ u / kg / Hr
*Heparin IV infusion to run concomitantly with r-tPA infusion. Follow the weight-based protocol EXCEPT
DO NOT DECREASE OR HOLD heparin infusion with 6 and 12 hour PTTH result unless significant bleeding
occurs; bolus/increase rate per protocol as needed. Begin use of <u>entire</u> standard weight-based protocol with 18
hour PTTH result

☐   Atenolol (Tenormin) 5 mg IV NOW over 5 minutes if SBP $\geq$ 100 and HR $\geq$ 60. Repeat dose 10 min after end
of first dose given if SBP $\geq$ 100 and HR $\geq$ 60. Wait another 15 min and give Atenolol 50 mg po if SBP $\geq$ 100
and HR $\geq$ 60.

☐   Phenergan: _____ mg IV q 1 Hr prn nausea

☐   Other: _____
                      _____
                      _____
                      _____

_____   _____
Date / Time   Physician Signature

DIAGNOSIS:	DISCHARGE INSTRUCTIONS:
	FOLLOW-UP WITH DOCTOR_____ @ _____

CONDITION: ☐UNCHANGED ☐IMPROVED **DISPOSITION:** ☐HOME ☐ADMITTED ☐INPATIENT TRANSFERRED TO:_____ VIA:_____
                                       ☐23 HR. OBV.

MD SIGNATURE:	DATE:	D/C TIME:	D/C WITH:	D/C:☐ AMB	☐ WALK
					☐ WC ☐ CARRIED ☐ POLICE

CLASSIFICATION: ☐CLASS I ☐CLASS II ☐CLASS III ☐CLASS IV ☐CLASS V ☐CLASS VI ☐DICTATION ☐MEDICAL CONTROL ☐TELEMETRY

Seq# 14167
Revised 9/98

PHYSICIAN ORDERS   PHYSICIAN ORDERS   PHYSICIAN ORDERS
White Copy: Chart/Medical Records   Yellow Copy: Pharmacy

FIGURE **6-1 cont'd**   *Continued*

EMERGENCY DEPARTMENT
CLINICAL PATHWAY FOR FEVER IN INFANTS
LESS THAN 60 DAYS POSTTERM
(FEVER > 100.4 RECTALLY NO SOURCE)
INITIAL NURSING ASSESSMENT

WT _____ lb _____ kg   EGA _____ Birthweight _____ lb   C-Section / Vaginal Delivery

MEDICATIONS _____
T _____ P _____ R _____ BP _____
Complications of / During Pregnancy / Maternal Group Beta Strep

Chief Complaint _____

Associated Symptoms _____

RESPIRATION
Airway
❑Clear
   ❑Partially Obstruct
   ❑Obstructed
Breathing
❑Clear/Non Labored
   ❑Labored
   ❑Nasal Flaring
   ❑Expiratory Grunt
   ❑Tachypnea
   ❑Retractions
   ❑Wheezes
   ❑Stridor

CIRCULATION
Pulse
❑Regular
   ❑Irregular
Skin
❑Warm
   ❑Hot   ❑Cool
❑Dry
   ❑Moist   ❑Diaphoretic
❑Color normal
   ❑Pale   ❑Mottled
   ❑Flushed ❑Jaundiced
   ❑Ashen   ❑Cyanotic
   ❑Rash
      ❑Location _____
      ❑Description _____
❑Cap refill < 2 sec
   ❑>2 sec
Mucuos Membranes
❑Pink
  ❑Pale   ❑Cyanotic
❑Moist
  ❑Dry   ❑Sticky
  ❑Cracked

NEURO
❑Alert
❑Active
❑Good eye contact
❑Playful
❑Quiet
  ❑Fussy
❑Not ill appearing
  ❑Ill appearing

Fontanelles
❑Soft
  ❑Firm
❑Flat
  ❑Depressed
  ❑Bulging

ABDOMEN
❑Soft
  ❑Firm
❑Flat
  ❑Distended
❑Bowel Sounds
  ❑Present
  ❑Absent

FEEDING PATTERN
❑Formula _____ oz q _____ hrs
❑Breastfeeding _____ mins q _____ hrs
❑Not eating
Other _____

OUTPUT STATUS in past 6-8 hours
_____ # of wet diapers
_____ # of loose stools
_____ # Emesis
❑Other _____

RN Signature: _____   Date: _____   Time: _____

`Initiated 9/98`
`Seq.# 16227`

FIGURE 6-2 Sample clinical pathway for neonatal sepsis. (Courtesy Gwinnett Hospital System, Lawrenceville, Georgia.)

Continued

EMERGENCY DEPARTMENT PATHWAY FOR FEVER IN INFANTS LESS THAN 60 DAYS POSTTERM

Interdisciplinary Action Plan	PHASE I	Initials	PHASE II	Initials
ASSESSMENT	Initial assessment completed Continued nursing assessment (V/S, neuro status)		Continued Nursing Assessment (VS, neuro status)	
INTERVENTIONS	Notify ED physician - Time: ED physician evaluation INT established		PMD consulted	
DIAGNOSTICS	LP consult obtained by ED physician		LP performed by ED physician Time: _____ CXR completed	
LAB	Lab specimen obtained - via INT if possible UA & C&S obtained by cath Stool obtained for C&S & fecal WBC's (if diarrhea)		Labs received and reviewed	
MEDICATIONS	Fever control medications administered if ordered		Antibiotics as ordered	
PSYCHOSOCIAL	Provide emotional support to patient and significant others		Provide emotional support to patient and significant others	
EDUCATION	Orient to ED ED course and planned treatment		Medications Ongoing patient care explained and taught to family	
OUTCOMES	Infant transported from triage Evaluation by physician Septic workup in progress		Decreased fever Neuro status maintained or improved Disposition received 　Discharge criteria met 　Patient admitted 　　Report called to_____ RN 　　Transferred to floor	
	Continue Pathway ____ Yes ____ No			

These are guidelines and can be altered at the practitioner's discretion.

Initials	Signature

7/98 Revised

FIGURE **6-2 cont'd**

Continued

EMERGENCY DEPARTMENT PATHWAY FOR FEVER IN INFANTS LESS THAN 60 DAYS POSTTERM

Interdisciplinary Action Plan	PHASE I	Initials	PHASE II	Initials
ASSESSMENT	Initial assessment completed Continued nursing assessment (V/S, neuro status)		Continued Nursing Assessment (VS, neuro status)	
INTERVENTIONS	Notify ED physician - Time: ED physician evaluation INT established		PMD consulted	
DIAGNOSTICS	LP consult obtained by ED physician		LP performed by ED physician Time: CXR completed	
LAB	Lab specimen obtained - via INT if possible UA & C&S obtained by cath Stool obtained for C&S & fecal WBC's (if diarrhea)		Labs received and reviewed	
MEDICATIONS	Fever control medications administered if ordered		Antibiotics as ordered	
PSYCHOSOCIAL	Provide emotional support to patient and significant others		Provide emotional support to patient and significant others	
EDUCATION	Orient to ED ED course and planned treatment		Medications Ongoing patient care explained and taught to family	

OUTCOMES	Infant transported from triage
	Evaluation by physician
	Septic workup in progress
			Decreased fever
			Neuro status maintained or improved
			Disposition received
			  Discharge criteria met
			  Patient admitted
			  Report called to _____ RN
			  Transferred to floor	

	Continue Pathway Yes No			

These are guidelines and can be altered at the practitioner's discretion.

Initials	Signature

7/98 Revised

FIGURE **6-2 cont'd**   (Courtesy Gwinnett Hospital System, Lawrenceville, Georgia.)

Continued

EMERGENCY DEPARTMENT
FEVER IN INFANT LESS THAN 60 DAYS POSTTERM
PROGRESS NOTES

Time	T	P	R	Pulse Ox	Pupils		Interventions	Nurse's Notes/ Observations
					L	R		

RN Initial	RN Signature

FIGURE **6-2 cont'd**   *Continued*

**EMERGENCY DEPARTMENT
CLINICAL PATHWAY FOR FEVER IN INFANTS
LESS THAN 60 DAYS POSTTERM
(FEVER > 100.4 RECTALLY NO SOURCE)
PHYSICIAN ORDER AND DISPOSITION**

Page 2 of 2

Discharge criteria for infants 28-60 days postterm, with fever > 100.4F

All low risk criteria met, may discharge home

_____ 28-60 days postterm

_____ Non-toxic appearing with fever improved

_____ Previously healthy (i.e. sickle cell negative, etc)

_____ No significant exposure to communicable diseases

_____ Not previously on antibiotic prior to Emergency Department admission

_____ UA < 10 WBC / HPF spun and few bacteria on cath specimen

_____ LP < 8 WBC per CMM and or rare PMN's, normal protein, and negative gram stain

_____ Stool WBC < 5 WBC / HPF, if diarrhea

_____ CXR negative, if done

Discharge Orders (all low-risk criteria met)

❑   Ceftriaxone 50 mg / kg IV push over 3-5 minutes or IM x 1

❑   Arranged definite F/U in 24 hours

❑   Instruction to caregiver on when to call or return

DIAGNOSIS:	DISCHARGE INSTRUCTIONS:
	FOLLOW-UP WITH DOCTOR _____ @ _____

CONDITION: ☐UNCHANGED ☐IMPROVED   **DISPOSITION:** ☐HOME ☐ADMITTED ☐INPATIENT ☐23 HR OBV   TRANSFERRED TO: VIA:

MD SIGNATURE: DATE: D/C TIME: D/C WITH: D/C:☐ AMB ☐ WALK ☐ WC ☐ CARRIED ☐ POLICE

CLASSIFICATION: ☐CLASS I ☐CLASS II ☐CLASS III ☐CLASS IV ☐CLASS V ☐CLASS VI ☐DICTATION ☐MEDICAL CONTROL ☐TELEMETRY

Initiated 9/98
Seq.# 16226

FIGURE **6-2 cont'd**   (Courtesy Gwinnett Hospital System, Lawrenceville, Georgia.)

Box 6-5   EXAMPLES OF VARIANCES

A. OPERATIONAL VARIANCE

1. Machine breakdown
2. Delay in test or procedure
3. Lost laboratory requisition or specimen
4. Needed service not available on weekends

B. COMMUNITY VARIANCE

1. No nursing home bed available
2. No visiting nurse service available
3. No family available to accompany the patient on discharge
4. Wheelchair, oxygen, suction, etc., cannot be delivered to the home in a timely fashion

C. PRACTITIONER VARIANCE

1. Ordering unnecessary test or procedure
2. Medication error
3. No consent obtained
4. Omission of a test or procedure

D. PATIENT VARIANCE

1. Test refusal
2. Change in condition
3. Patient allergy
4. Signing out against medical advice
5. Noncompliance with care plan

Modified from Flarey D, Blancett SS: *Handbook of nursing case management,* Gaithersburg, Md, 1996, Aspen Publishers.

Box 6-6   COMMUNITY REFERRAL

Crisis intervention
Family and children services
Elderly care assistance programs
Homeless coalitions
Abuse hotlines
Healthy mother/healthy baby agencies
Community clinics offering free to low-cost care
Public health departments
Support groups
Foundations

---

facilitates support for the patient who does not meet admission criteria but needs assistance for safe discharge to his or her environment. Support services include durable medical equipment (e.g., wheelchairs, walkers, beds, humidifiers), home meals, follow-up phone calls, and monitoring systems such as Lifelines. There is also a responsibility for mandatory reporting of communicable diseases, notifying the Department of Motor Vehicle of individuals seen in the ED with uncontrolled seizures, reporting suspected abuse (child, elder, and domestic), and incidences of injury related to criminal offense (stabbing, assaults, and gunshot wounds). Referrals of this nature must be directed to the community agency with the authority to enforce appropriate discharge needs. Other community referrals are noted in Box 6-6.

Working relationships must be established with community agencies for referral of patients. At times the emergency physician and nurse play active roles in community agencies by working at clinics or teaching community classes such as cardiopulmonary resuscitation, effects of drunk driving, and trauma prevention. This community involvement promotes wellness of the community and facilitates appropriate interventions when life-threatening events occur.

The ED is an entry point for health care for many patients in the community. Institutions should remember that first impressions are generally lasting and half of the impression about a facility is from the first contact. The ED must stay focused on ever-changing needs of the community. The health care resource group states that the ED is responsible for accessing and providing for patients' needs efficiently and effectively. The patient must be given explanations, education, and specific information as to where his or her responsibility starts and ends. Effective discharge planning and the community interface prevent inappropriate use of the ED.[7] Knowledge of the community and its expectations of the ED increases the ED's ability to serve the community.

Cost containment and payer sources provide a vital link with the hospital's ability to provide services and the community to provide payment for care rendered. The practices and accountability of the insurance providers can be determined by the community's level of acceptance. Even though a patient generally chooses his or her own insurance provider, the patient has to adhere to rules of referral to an ED and the contract outlining care and home health needs. The insurance carrier in turn has an obligation to assist with care needs and discharge needs.

The ED has specific obligations mandated not only morally but by federal and state regulations to meet medical needs and complete appropriate discharge criteria for patients presenting to the ED. Knowledge of these regulations is imperative for accurate compliance.

Health care providers must educate the community about health care changes and interventions. This leads to the empowerment to focus and reform health and social issues that affect the community. Individuals and institutions must then lend assistance by helping to provide solutions to their issues.

The ED must carry out the patient's care and discharge at the community level as an advocate for the patient and on a patient-by-patient basis. An advocate must know the needs of the patient and the community as a whole. Follow-up phone calls should be done to assess effectiveness of discharge goals; these calls should be recorded and trended to monitor and evaluate the discharge process.

Outcomes Management in the Emergency Department

A case management model is a comprehensive program that encompasses the entire content of this chapter. The case manager is charged with the responsibility for coordinating, negotiating, procuring services and resources for,

> **Box 6-7 CASE MANAGER ROLE RESPONSIBILITIES**
>
> Identifies patients for case management services
>
> Establishes methods for tracking patient progress through the emergency department (ED) and the health care system
>
> Possesses knowledge of community resources for patients and families; is able to activate these services as needed
>
> Develops, implements, evaluates, and revises a case management plan for patients, families, health care team members, payers, and available resources that is based on assessed needs, goals, and outcomes
>
> Collaborates with a multidisciplinary team to develop patient-specific clinical pathways
>
> Gathers feedback and shares the information to facilitate needed change
>
> Educates the patient, family, community, and health care team
>
> Monitors progress and maintains records of patient throughout the ED stay (prehospital treatment to discharge)
>
> Undertakes follow-up calls or visits to evaluate the progress of the care continuum and outcomes
>
> Identifies variance and uses data to facilitate variance reduction and an improved ED quality improvement program
>
> Identifies and carries out methods to reduce cost and unnecessary resource usage

and managing care of complex patients to facilitate achievement of quality and cost:patient outcomes.[3] Documentation of activities and outcomes is vital to improve future interventions.[6]

The ED is fast paced and requires focus on the details of care activities to achieve positive outcomes. In many situations a case management model comprising individual components of this chapter might be inadequate for the facility and community being served. The case manager possesses clinical expertise in the area of care, coordination, and working knowledge of the components in this chapter. Box 6-7 provides a listing of role responsibilities of a case manager in the ED.

Common sense also dictates that no one in the ED would argue the importance of developing procedures and processes to improve quality and decrease cost. However, the promoter of the plan to develop an ED outcomes management program involving use of case managers and clinical pathways is often met with resistance.

Getting Support

Although outcomes management is a multidisciplinary program, it is not surprising that the key supporter, or champion, of the project is frequently an ED nurse manager, clinical nurse specialist, or staff nurse. To get the project from the discussion phase to actual implementation requires someone to be the "project cheerleader" and promote the concept to hospital administrators, ED staff and physicians, and other departments interacting with the ED. It may be beneficial to present a formal proposal with supporting literature and rationale of how the program could improve care and decrease cost for the department.

Steering Committee

After the project is approved, a steering committee is needed to oversee the project. This group should be multidisciplinary and include hospital administrators, ED managers, ED nursing staff, ED physicians, and ancillary services that work closely with the ED (e.g., laboratory and radiology personnel). It is also helpful to involve a representative of the outcomes management/case management program if one exists in the facility. For the program to be successful, members of the steering committee must be empowered to make changes in the ED.

Resources

In these days of limited staffing, some of the questions needing immediate clarification are: "Who will implement the program and make it work on a day-to-day basis?" "Will it be the staff nurse, manager, clinical nurse specialist, or educator?" "Will the role be in addition to what that person is already doing?" "Will the person's role change?" "Will additional personnel be hired to manage this new program?" You may have to start with one person who can demonstrate positive outcomes both clinically and financially. Following this success, showing the impact of not being able to capture the 24-hour influx of patient into the ED can justify the need for 24-hour coverage for the program and increased full-time equivalencies.

Goals and Timelines

To maintain focus, the steering committee must identify goals it wants the program to achieve. Examples include:
- Improving the standard of care
- Standardizing treatment of the most commonly seen ED complaints
- Increasing customer satisfaction
- Enhancing team collaboration
- Reducing costs

Analyzing clinical data, quality assurance, and financial and coding data can assist the team in identifying case types that would benefit from the program. For example, if the ED sees a large volume of patients with abdominal pain and a variety in practice patterns, this might be a patient type that the committee should focus on. Another might be the patient population that carries a high risk for poor outcomes, such as the diabetic patient with frequent ED visits.

When developing a timeline, the group must set realistic goals. The project will probably take longer to implement than anticipated. The timeline must include project implementation and ongoing evaluation.

Education

As with any new project, there will likely be initial resistance to the program. Providing education on managed care, its impact on the ED, and the benefits of an outcomes management program can help overcome resistance. This education process is not a one-time-only inservice or class. It is an ongoing process of effective communication with all disciplines involved with the ED. Special attention should be given to physicians so that there is a clear understanding that the program is not designed to allow non-physicians to practice medicine or to allow non-physicians control over physician practice. The goal of the program is to work in conjunction with the ED physician and attending physician to develop a plan of care that contributes to positive patient outcomes.

STUDIES IN ED OUTCOMES

Research has suggested that patients visiting the ED for asthma care number in excess of 1.2 million dollars. Based on this, the financial impact for these patients in 1997 was more than $280 million.[9] The admission rate for asthma is more than 450,000 with some 5000 deaths reported. It is partially from this information that outcomes of care focus on quality management and reduction of need for hospitalization. Dr. Michael Ackerman and Dr. Richard Sinert championed a study that focused on the improvement of asthma care and outcomes in the ED. Asthma treatment guidelines were implemented through a CQI process, and significant reduction of emergency relapse of asthma patients occurred. Compliance with the guidelines was accomplished through education and patient modification.[1] Another study by Dr. Stephen Edmond and colleagues demonstrated that a guideline-based asthma program changed clinical practice and improved acute asthma care.[4] These studies look at patient outcomes in relation to such things as admission rates, length of stay, peak flow rates, and response to or timeliness of medications, and types of medications used.

Similar studies have looked at acute myocardial infarction with outcomes reflective of door-to-drug studies, medication interventions, triage to electrocardiogram, and treatment times (see Suggested Reading).

SUMMARY

The new millennium of health care challenges the patient, health care provider, and third-party payer to evaluate and redesign health care delivery systems. Focusing on outcomes and continuum of care is the best method to realize optimal health and illness prevention. The outcome-focused model requires monitoring the patient's baseline status, response to ED treatment, and status at time of discharge. No longer do ED personnel have the luxury of looking only at care provided while the patient is in the ED. Emergency staff must look at the big picture and see what effect their actions have on the patient's eventual short- and long-term outcomes. The ED has an opportunity to capture millions of health care consumers. Valuable resources and heath care costs are significantly optimized and contained. A valuable resource to effectively manage this process is a case manager in the ED who uses his or her expertise and working knowledge of emergency medicine, community, outcomes management, and managed care. Outcomes management incorporating clinical pathways and case managers is an effective method for achieving these goals.

References

1. Akerman M, Sinert R, A successful effort to improve asthma care outcomes in an inner-city emergency department, *J Asthma* 36(3): 295, 1999.
2. Burstin HR et al: Benchmarking and quality improvement: the Harvard emergency department quality study, *Am J Med* 107:438, 1999.
3. Center for Case Management, South Natick, Mass, 1996.
4. Edmond SD, Woodruff PG, Lee EY et al: Effect of an emergency department asthma program on acute asthma care, *Ann Emerg Med* 34:321, 1999.
5. Flarey DL, Blancett SS: *Handbook of nursing case management,* Gaithersburg, Md, 1996, Aspen Publications.
6. Frawley M: Managed care corner, *Diplomate Focus, American Board of Quality Assurance and Utilization Review Physicians* 6(2), 1997.
7. Health Care Resource Group: *Case management focus emergency department/community,* Whittier, Calif, 1998, The Group.
8. Landrum P, Schmidt, N, McLean A Jr: *Outcome-oriented rehabilitation,* Gaithersburg, Md, 1995, Aspen Publications.
9. Smith DH, Malone DC, Lawson KA et al: A national estimate of the economic costs of asthma, *Am J Resp Crit Care Med* 156:787, 1997.
10. St. Coeur M: *Case management practice guidelines,* St. Louis, 1998, Mosby.

Suggested Reading

Castro J et al: Research: home care referral after emergency department discharge, *JEN* 24(2):127, 1998.

Gilutz H et al: The "door-to-needle blitz" in acute myocardial infarction: the impact of a CQI project, 24(6):323, 1998.

Markel KN, Marion SA: CQI: improving the time to thrombolytic therapy for patient with acute myocardial infarction in the emergency department, *J Emerg Med* 14(6):685, 1996.

Ornato J: Chest pain emergency centers: improving acute myocardial infarction care, *J Clin Cardiol* 22(IV): IV-3-IV-9, 1999.

Tallon RW, Chest pain observation units, *Nurs Manage J* 27(5): 49, 1996.

Turner C: AMI team buckles down to improve outcomes, *J Hosp Case Manage* 46, 1998.

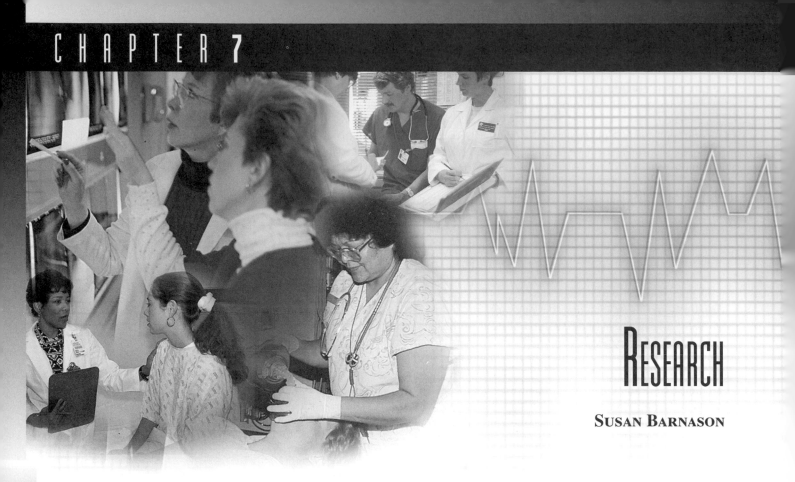

CHAPTER 7

RESEARCH

SUSAN BARNASON

Research has emerged as an essential component for the continuing evolution of professional nursing practice. Research provides a foundation to ensure that nursing actions are based on scientific principles rather than on intuition or traditional practices. Emergency nursing practice strives to achieve optimal patient outcomes; however, it is by development, evaluation, and expansion of nursing knowledge through nursing research that practice and patient care improvements can move forward. The focus of this chapter is to provide an overview of the research process as a basis for emergency nurses to become better consumers of research and to provide a template for formulation of nursing research studies driven by clinical problems and challenges within emergency nursing practice. This chapter will further delineate the role of research in evidence-based practice.

EVIDENCE-BASED PRACTICE

The expectation for clinical practice is to deliver health care based on research-guided clinical decision making. Clinicians need to critically appraise research evidence and integrate research findings with clinical expertise, patient expectations, and within the context of available resources and care delivery.[8] Evidence-based practice strives to close the gap between research and clinical practice realities. Research utilization and other types of knowledge are encompassed within the concept of evidence-based practice. Other types of evidence or "knowledge" include quality improvement data, risk data, standards of care, pathophysiology, benchmarking data and retrospective or concurrent review data from patient records.[3,5,6]

Research utilization was the predecessor to evidence-based practice as a movement from task-oriented to science-based practice.[3,12,16] Research utilization can be broadly defined as the use of a research study in an application unrelated to the original study. All research utilization models are variations of the "change" model (unfreezing, change, and refreezing). Research utilization models include synthesis of research literature on a given topic that summarizes research-based knowledge, which can then be used in clinical practice. In addition, research utilization implies implementation of this summarized knowledge into practice and evaluation of adapted changes in practice.[7] Models of research utilization can vary along a continuum. The initial conceptualization of literature (referred to as *conceptual utilization*) at one end of the contiuum is followed by an evolution of thinking about research ideas and findings on a given topic (referred to as *knowledge creep*). The next marker on the continuum is the action taken to move to a decision about the implications of research synthesis (referred to as *decision accretion*) followed by implementation of research into clinical practice (referred to as *instrumental utilization*).

Research studies, however, may be limited in the number of studies, replication of research, lag in reporting of research, and scope of studies to address a given clinical problem, thereby limiting the impact of a research utilization model.[2,15] Other barriers to research utilization reported in studies have been nurses' knowledge and attitudes toward research, lack of awareness of research results, accessibility of research findings, anticipated outcomes of using research, organizational support to use research, and support from others to use research.[11,14] In general, research studies have limited methodologies and require replication in different settings to provide greater confidence in the generalizability of findings for clinicians to adapt in the clinical setting. Given the limitations of research utilization, the evidence-based practice model is a more comprehensive, realistic approach that integrates multiple sources of knowledge to guide clinical decision-making practices.

RESEARCH PROCESS OVERVIEW

Whether developing a research study or evaluating the merits of published research studies, nurses should proceed through a series of well-defined, logical steps to organize a study. Table 7-1 reflects key components of the research process, which is further summarized in the following sections.

Problem Identification

Nursing research always begins with a question or researchable problem.[9] An identified problem may concern patient care, nursing education, nursing administration, or any issue of nursing interest. Patient care or nursing practice problems generally address practice differences and what is ideal or desirable. Deciding on a specific research question may appear to be difficult for the beginning researcher. However,

nurses should reflect on their own clinical experiences as primary sources for researchable problems in nursing as well as personal experiences. Many times an observation can be turned into a question:

- I wonder whether seeing the dying family member before death helps the family during their bereavement?
- I wonder whether using protocols for laboratory and radiographic examinations can expedite care in the emergency department (ED)?
- I wonder if drawing blood below or above intravenous sites has any bearing on the laboratory values?

Another source for research or problems to be researched is the nursing literature. Most research studies make recommendations for future studies. Often by reviewing several nursing research articles, a nurse may identify research questions based on the state of the science regarding a given area or clinical problem. In addition, several nursing and federal organizations have published recommendations for future research studies. The Emergency Nurses Association, American Association of Critical Care Nurses, American Nurses Association, Sigma Theta Tau, and National Institutes of Health are examples of organizations with research priorities for clinical nursing.

Literature Review

The purpose of the literature review is to explore work conducted in a particular area of interest to formulate or clarify the research problem. After critiquing previous research in a particular area, the researcher summarizes what has been previously studied and delineates how a study contributes to the state of the science.

A good literature review critiques and summarizes other studies to see how they fit into the scope of a study being conducted. A thorough review reinforces the need for the study in light of what has already been done. What is accepted as truth from other studies is the groundwork on which new studies are based. A written literature review should include summaries of articles that differ from the proposed point of view; this indicates that the author conducted an exhaustive review of available knowledge.[9]

Sources of information for literature reviews can include both primary and secondary sources. A primary source of information is the description of an investigation written by the person who conducted it. A secondary source is a description of a study prepared by someone other than the original researcher. Both sources can be helpful, but written literature reviews should be based on primary sources whenever possible. Nonresearch articles that contribute to ideas or theories about the problem may be included, but it is best to focus on primary research articles.[9]

Theoretic and Conceptual Frameworks

Theories and conceptual frameworks provide a structure or blueprint to guide the study of clinical problems. A theoretic framework defines the concepts and proposes relationships

Table 7-1 RESEARCH PROCESS OVERVIEW	
ASPECT OF RESEARCH PROCESS	OVERVIEW OF PROCESS
Problem identification	Identifies the "problem" that will be answered by the research study.
Literature review	Synthesizes current literature and state of the art to summarize how current study can contribute to current body of literature on the topic.
Theoretic or conceptual framework	In theoretically driven studies, sets the context for the propositions or relationships related to the variables in the study.
Purpose and research questions or hypotheses	What is intended to be accomplished in the study.
Methodology • Design • Sampling • Data collection • Data measurement • Data analysis	The methods section communicates what approaches will be or were used by the research to answer the research questions or hypotheses.
Results, conclusions, limitations, and recommendations	Reports the results obtained in the analyses of data. Discussion of the findings includes the drawing of conclusions based on what the results mean, explaining why results were obtained, and how results can be used in practice.

among those concepts. It further enables the researcher to link the findings to a body of knowledge. This framework consists of a definition of concepts and propositions about the relationships of those concepts, helps to organize rules or beliefs about what is observed, and provides a systematic way to organize information about a particular aspect of interest in a research study.

Two components of a theory are concepts and a statement of propositions. Concepts, the building blocks of a theory, are abstract characteristics, categories, or labels of things, persons, or events. Examples of nursing concepts are health, stress, adaptation, caring, and pain. Propositions are statements that define the relationships among concepts. A set of propositions may state that one concept is associated with another or is contingent upon another. Examples of theories used in nursing are psychoanalytic, relativity, evolution, gravity, learning, systems, and homeostasis. Theoretic models of grief and learned helplessness help explain women's responses to battering. The power of theories lies in the ability to explain the relationship of variables and the nature of this relationship. Theories also help stimulate research by giving direction. Questions and ideas formulated about what will occur in specific situations are called hypotheses. Hypotheses are tested in research to determine whether the information fits the theory.[9]

Conceptual frameworks represent a less formal, less well-developed system for organizing phenomena. These frameworks contain concepts that represent a common theme but lack the deductive system of propositions that give the relationship among concepts. Most research in nursing practice uses conceptual frameworks rather than theories. These conceptual frameworks often lay the groundwork for more formal theories.[10]

Research Questions or Hypotheses

Before a problem can be researched, it must be narrowed, refined, and made feasible for study. The research interest can be stated as a research question or a hypothesis. The research question should identify key independent and dependent variables. An independent variable is what is assumed to cause or thought to be associated with the dependent variable. Changes in the dependent variable are presumed to depend on the independent variable's effects. The dependent variable is what a researcher wants to explain or understand. Research questions should be specific and not attempt to measure too much because data analysis may be complex and confusing to interpret. For example, a research question might be, "What effect does the presence of the parent in the child's room have on the child's experience of pain during fracture reduction?" The dependent variable is the child's pain experience and the independent variable is the presence of the parent in the room. The dependent variable is explained through its relationship with the independent variable. It is known that many factors affect a child's perception of pain, but only one independent variable (parent's presence) is intended to be measured in the proposed re-

search question to keep the variables under consideration specific and clear.

Often the dependent variable can have multiple causes. A study may be designed to examine several factors and their influences on a phenomenon. For example, you may want to know whether experience with triage or an educational program concerning triage influences ability to accurately perform triage. Both independent variables (education and experience) can influence triage performance ability (dependent variable).

Several dependent variables can be designated as measures of treatment effectiveness. An example of multiple dependent variables identified in a research question is, "Does a comprehensive triage system influence length of stay in the ED, patient satisfaction, and patient outcome?" Length of stay, patient satisfaction, and patient outcome are all dependent variables by which triage effectiveness is measured.

A hypothesis expands upon a research question because it is a tentative prediction or explanation of the relationship between two or more variables. This prediction of expected outcomes is the basis of the research process. Hypotheses, which often stem from theories, are possible solutions or answers to research problems. The hypothesis is a prediction of the nature of the relationship between several variables, which is intended to be identified before the initiation of the research study. For example, one hypothesis might be that pediatric patients who are promised a reward at the end of a suturing procedure will cooperate and be more compliant than pediatric patients who are not promised a reward. In this example, the researcher is not only delineating whether a relationship between rewards and behavior exists but is also predicting outcomes from this relationship. The null hypothesis indicates that the two populations (samples) have the same mean. Therefore the null hypothesis, stated as "there will not be a relationship between" or "there will be no difference in . . . .," is often generated for statistical purposes, data analysis, and discussion.[9,10,13]

Methodology

The methods section of a research study reflects how the researcher plans to or did implement the research study to answer the research questions or hypotheses. The components of the methodology section include research design, subjects, measures used to collect data, and study procedures. There are two major categories of research designs: quantitative and qualitative. In the context of this chapter, the focus will be quantitative studies. Table 7-2 provides an overview of common types of quantitative research designs.

Subjects

Subjects sampled for a research study depend on the population to be studied and the estimated number of subjects needed to demonstrate a significant difference between experimental and control groups. The definition of a population is not restricted to human subjects. A population can consist of records, blood samples, actions, words, organiza-

Table 7-2   OVERVIEW OF COMMON TYPES OF QUANTITATIVE RESEARCH DESIGNS

RESEARCH DESIGN	CHARACTERISTICS OF RESEARCH DESIGN
Experimental	Manipulation of independent variable
	Randomization of subjects (subjects randomly assigned to control and experimental groups)
	Control or comparison group (one of groups in study does not receive "experimental" treatment but receives normal or routine care)
Quasi-experimental	Manipulation of independent variable
	Lacks control group or randomization
Time-series	Only one group available for study (therefore lacks randomization and control)
	Phenomenon of interest studied over time
	Experimental treatment introduced during the course of the study
Historical	Provides an account of past events
	Performed to test hypotheses or answer questions about causes, effects, or trends relating to past events to shed light on present behaviors or practices
Survey	Provides information about distribution prevalence and interrelationships among variables
	No intervention is performed
	May identify trends and possibly predict future needs
Case study	An in-depth analysis of an individual, a small group, a place, or an organization
	Natural conditions are studies and variables related to history, current characteristics, interaction, or problems
	Usually focus on why the subject feels, thinks, or behaves in a particular manner
Evaluative	Use of scientific research methods and procedures to evaluate a program, treatment practice, or policy
	Program goals or objectives are the focus of evaluative research
Methodologic	A controlled investigation related to ways of obtaining, organizing, or organizing data
	Addresses development, validation, and evaluation of research tools or techniques
Correlational	Design used to examine the relationships between two or more variables
	Cannot imply causal relationships based on findings of correlational studies
Ex post facto or retrospective	Variations of independent variable in the natural course of events
	Also referred to as explanatory, descriptive, causal-comparative, comparative, retrospective ex post facto
Cross-sectional	Examines data at one point in time
Longitudinal	Collects data from the same group at different points in time
Prospective	Explore presumed causes and move forward in time to the presumed effect

tions, numbers, or animals. Whatever the unit to be studied or sampled, a population is always made up of specific elements of interest. Generally, in a research study, it is impossible to include large populations because of expense and time involved for data collection; therefore, a study will usually limit the population sampled to a representative sample. Samples should represent a portion of the entire population to be studied to ensure that the sample is "representative" of the population.

Researchers use probability and nonprobability sampling techniques when designing studies. Probability sampling is the use of some form of random selection to choose the subjects or units to be sampled. Statistical measures, known as "power analyses," can be used by researchers to estimate the sample size needed. Nonprobability sampling is a method based on convenience. Three types of nonprobability sampling are accidental, quota, and purposive sampling. Accidental samples are based on convenience of gathering subjects, such as surveying the first 100 patients in the ED on a particular day. Quota samples are used when a researcher knows an element of the population and bases sampling on the known representativeness within the population. For ex-

ample, if a researcher knew 25% of the nurses in the ED setting were males, the researcher makes sure that 25% of the sample of ED nurses comprises males. This increases the representativeness of the population. Purposive sampling occurs when a researcher "hand picks" cases to be included in the sample that represent the "typical" subjects within a given population. A study may use purposive sampling to ensure a variety of responses or because the choices are judged to be typical of the population. In general, it is recommended that a sample size of 30 be selected for each subset of data or "cell" of the design.[1,4,10,13]

Institutional Review Board (IRB) approval of the research study is another facet to be considered related to subjects in a study. The purpose of IRB study approval is to safeguard subjects' rights and welfare, ensure appropriate procedures for informed consent, and allow subjects to make independent decisions about risks and benefits.[9] Briefly, when a patient gives informed consent, the following aspects should be delineated in the consent form:

- Statement involving research, explanation of purposes of the research, delineation of expected duration of subject's participation, description of procedures to be expected, and identification of any procedures that are experimental

- Description of any reasonably foreseeable risks or discomforts to the subject
- Description of any benefits to the subject or to others that may reasonably be expected from the research
- Disclosure of appropriate alternative procedures or courses of treatment, if any, that may be advantageous to the subject
- A statement describing to what extent, if any, confidentiality of records identifying the subject will be maintained
- For research involving more than minimal risk, an explanation as to whether any medical treatments are available if injury occurs and if so, what they consist of or where further information may be obtained
- An explanation of who to contact for answers to pertinent questions about the research and the subject's rights and whom to contact in the event of a research-related injury to the subject
- A statement that participation is voluntary, refusal to participate will not involve any penalty or loss of benefits to which the subject is otherwise entitled, and that participation may be discontinued at any time without any penalty or loss of otherwise entitled benefits.

Data Collection and Data Measurement

Data collection simply refers to a description of the processes used or proposed to be used to implement the study and gather data. The key to successful data collection is choosing or developing appropriate measures that will accurately describe variables in the study. Measurement tools have some common characteristics: (A) objective, standardized measure, (B) standardized structure (uniform items, response, and scoring), (C) items of measurement are unambiguous, (D) types of items on any one test have a limited number of variations, (E) items do not provide irrelevant cues, (F) measures do not require complex operations, (G) measurement tool encompasses the defined variable, and (H) measure demonstrates relationship between performance on tool and subject's behavior.

Some of the more common types of data collection measures include physiologic and biophysical, observational, interviews and questionnaires, scales, and records or available data. Physiologic measurements are those used to measure characteristics such as temperature, weight, height, cardiac output, muscle strength, and biochemical levels (e.g., hemoglobin, blood sugar, potassium). One advantage of physiologic measurements is objectivity because data are not influenced by the person performing the study. Physiologic measurements are relatively precise and sensitive. When researchers observe the research aspect of interest, direct observation measurements are used. For example, a researcher wants to observe the response of parents to casting or suturing procedures performed on their children. The observation method is most useful for entities difficult to measure, such as interactions, nursing process, changes in behavior, or

group processes. A third type of data collection measure is the use of interviews and questionnaire measures that allow subjects to report data for or about themselves. The purpose of questioning participants is to seek direct data, such as age, religion, or marital status, or indirect data, such as level of intelligence, anxiety, and pain. Another type of measure, scales, makes distinctions among subjects concerning the degree to which they possess a certain trait, attitude, or emotion. Scales are measuring instruments that permit comparisons in dimensions of interest. For example, a researcher interested in knowing whether a nerve block or a local injection of anesthetic is more effective for relieving pain during fracture reduction would use a pain scale to measure pain. Finally, use of records or available data refers to the researcher collecting data from existing databases; for example, a patient chart.

Data Measurement Validity and Reliability. When instruments are used for measuring subjects, the validity and reliability of tools need to be addressed by the researcher. Instruments or tools used for research measurement refer not only to physiologic measures, but also to questionnaires and surveys used in studies. Validity is the degree to which an instrument measures what it is intended to measure.[1,4,9,10,13] Validity is content-, construct-, or criterion-related. Although an instrument may appear to measure some aspect of a construct or element, the instrument must be evaluated to determine whether it really does provide such measurement. Content validity is the degree to which an instrument measures the universe of content that it is said to represent or measure. Content validity is often determined by a panel of experts in the field to be evaluated. If a researcher wanted to measure bereavement behaviors in the ED, social workers, members of the clergy, and emergency nurses might be asked to review the instrument to be used to measure bereavement behavior. Construct validity is the degree to which a tool measures the construct in the study. A construct is an abstraction developed for a scientific purpose. Construct validity is usually determined over time after data from research studies support the construct to a greater degree or question it further. An example might be if a research study was implemented to determine the sense of hope in trauma patients' families. The researcher's instrument must discriminate between families who possess hope and families who do not possess hope to ensure construct validity. Criterion-related validity consists of predictive validity and concurrent validity. The subject's performance on one measure is used to infer the likely response on another measure. Predictive validity is a measure used to predict future performance. For example, a nurse's score on a content knowledge test in emergency nursing predicts how well he or she will perform in practice. Concurrent validity is the degree to which an instrument can distinguish subjects who differ on a certain criterion measured at the same time.

Reliability of an instrument refers to its ability to consistently and accurately measure a criterion. A test of reliability is whether the tool produces the same measurement

Table 7-3	OVERVIEW OF STATISTICAL TESTS FOR DATA ANALYSIS				
LEVEL OF MEASUREMENT	ONE SAMPLE	TWO SAMPLES: RELATED	TWO SAMPLES: INDEPENDENT	MORE THAN TWO SAMPLES	CORRELATION INDEXES
NONPARAMETRIC					
Nominal	Chi-squared		Chi-squared Fisher Exact probability test	Chi-squared	Phi-coefficient
Ordinal	One-sample Kolmorgorov-Smirnov test	Wilcoxon matched-pairs signed rank test	Chi-squared Median test Mann Whitney U	Chi-squared	Spearman rank correlations Kendall rank correlation
PARAMETRIC					
Interval or ratio	With before-after measures: Correlated t-tests Repeated measures analysis of variance	With matched pairs: Correlated t-tests	Independent t-tests Analysis of variance	Analysis of variance	Pearson product moment correlation Multiple correlation Factor analysis

when a measurement is repeated several times. The less an instrument varies in repeated measurements, the greater the reliability of the instrument. An example for a physiologic measure might be that a thermometer that measures a temperature at 98.6° F one moment and 102° F the next is not a reliable measure.[1,4,9,10,13]

Data Analysis

After completing data collection, the researcher summarizes the data through statistical procedures. The purpose of analysis is to answer the study questions or hypotheses. Researchers who use quantitative methods for data collection should plan for analysis before the research data are collected. Statistical tests give meaning to quantitative data because they reduce, summarize, organize, evaluate, interpret, and communicate numeric data. One does not need to know all of the statistical tests to understand the common principle; the statistical test will tell if the findings are "statistically" significant. This means the findings are probably valid and replicable with a new sample of subjects. The "level" of statistical significance is an index of the probability of "reliability" of the findings. An example would be, if a study indicates findings were significant at the 0.05 level, 5 of 100 times there is a risk that the result would be different from the reported finding; in other words, 95 of 100 times the findings would be the same.

Statistical tests are referred to as either descriptive or inferential. Descriptive statistics describe and summarize data. Examples are mode, median, mean, average, percentage, and frequency. Inferential statistics are used to draw conclusions about a large population based on a sample from a study, to make judgments, and to generalize information. Inferential statistics are then used to test the hypotheses to determine whether they are correct. Two categories of inferential statistics are nonparametric and parametric. Most statistical tests are parametric tests, which focus on population parameters, require measurements on at least one interval or ratio scale, and make assumptions about distribution

of the variables.[9] Nonparametric tests are used when measured variables are nominal or ordinal. These tests do not make assumptions about distribution of variables. Table 7-3 provides an overview of commonly performed statistical tests, both nonparametric and parametric, based on level of measurement and variables in study.

Results, Conclusions, and Recommendations

Results of the study are usually organized by the research aims or hypotheses of the study. Results are often reported in the form of tables and graphs. Data summarized in graphs and tables can be more easily interpreted and compared with research questions or hypotheses and theoretic framework. Based on the findings of the study, the research draws conclusions, then uses these conclusions as the foundation for the discussion section of the research report or manuscript. The researcher should attempt to give meaning to "why" the findings occurred by interweaving previous related studies that have been done. Recommendations stem from changes the researcher plans in sample, design, or analysis if the study is repeated. Other explanations for results should be discussed so progress can be made in future studies of the research problem. Implications of research, such as how findings can be used to improve nursing or how to advance knowledge through additional research, should be provided.[1,4,9,10,13]

SUMMARY

In summary, this chapter has provided an overview of nursing research processes. The intent was to provide the reader with a perspective to increase his or her level of understanding and sophistication related to research participation. A continuum best depicts the spectrum of participation in research by nurses. At one end, the level of participation can reflect participation as a nurse's understanding of research concepts; at the other end of the spectrum is participation

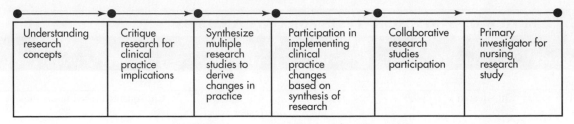

Understanding research concepts	Critique research for clinical practice implications	Synthesize multiple research studies to derive changes in practice	Participation in implementing clinical practice changes based on synthesis of research	Collaborative research studies participation	Primary investigator for nursing research study

FIGURE 7-1   Overview of nursing participation in research.

exemplified by the nurse as a primary investigator in a research study. Refer to Figure 7-1 for an overview of the continuum of nursing research participation. Regardless of the level of participation, all nurses have the opportunity to engage in research.

References

1. Dempsey PA, Dempsey AD: *Using nursing research,* Philadelphia, Penn, 2000, JB Lippincott.
2. Dufault MA, Sullivan M: A collaborative research utilization approach to evaluate the effects of pain management standards on patient outcomes, *J Prof Nurs* 16(4):240, 2000.
3. Estabrooks CA: The conceptual structure of research utilization, *Res Nurs Health* 22:203, 1999.
4. Fain JA: *Reading, understanding and applying nursing research,* Philadelphia, Penn, 1998, FA Davis.
5. Goode CJ, Piedalue F: Evidence-based clinical practice, *J Nurs Admin* 29(6):15, 1999.
6. Hinshaw AS: Nursing knowledge for the 21st century: opportunities and challenges, *J Nurs Scholarship* 32(2):117, 2000.
7. Jones J: Performance improvement through clinical research utilization: the linkage model, *J Nurs Care Qual* 15(1):49, 2000.
8. King KM, Teo KT: Integrating clinical quality improvement strategies with nursing research, *West J Nurs Res* 22(5):596, 2000.
9. Lenaghan PA: Research. In Newberry L, editor: *Sheehy's emergency nursing,* ed 4, Philadelphia, Penn, 1996, Mosby.
10. Mateo MA, Kirchhoff KT: *Using and conducting nursing research in the clinical setting,* Philadelphia, Penn, 1999, WB Saunders.
11. Mullem CA, Burke LJ, Dohmeyer K et al: Strategic planning for research use in nursing practice, *J Nurs Admin* 29(12):38, 1999.
12. Omery A, Williams RP: An appraisal of research utilization across the United States, *J Nurs Admin* 29(12):50, 1999.
13. Polit DF, Beck CT, Hungler BP: *Essentials of nursing research,* Philadelphia, Penn, 2001, JB Lippincott.
14. Retsas A: Barriers to using research evidence in nursing practice, *J Adv Nurs* 31(3):599, 2000.
15. Rodgers SE: The extent of nursing research utilization in general medical and surgical wards, *J Adv Nurs* 32(1):182, 2000.
16. Rosswurm MA, Larrabee JH: A model for change to evidence-based practice, *Image: J Nurs Scholarship* 31(4):317, 1999.

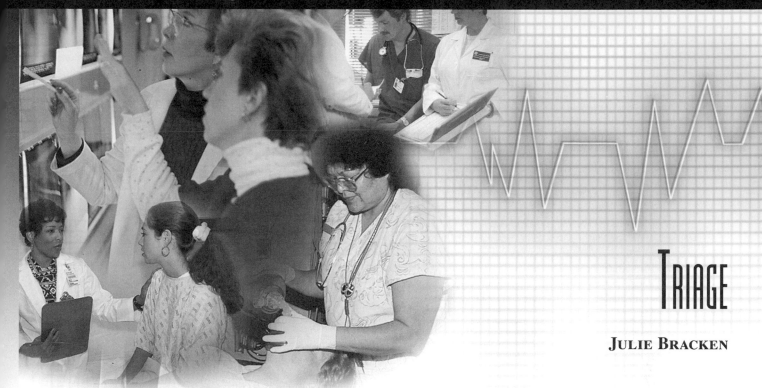

CHAPTER 8

TRIAGE

JULIE BRACKEN

Triage is a process used to determine severity of illness or injury for each patient who enters the emergency department (ED). Putting the patient in the right place at the right time to receive the right level of care facilitates allocation of appropriate resources to meet the patient's medical needs. Ingredients for an effective triage system are adequate space, supplies, a communication system, access to the treatment area, and an experienced professional supported by a multidisciplinary team.[11] In most EDs a registered nurse fulfills this role. Joint Commission on Accreditation of Healthcare Organizations standards identify the registered nurse as the appropriate person to perform patient assessment, which is essential for the triage process.

The word triage is derived from the French verb *trier,* which means "to pick or to sort."[20] Triage dates back to the French military, which used the word to designate a "clearing hospital" for wounded soldiers. The U.S. military used triage to describe a sorting station where injured soldiers were distributed from the battlefield to distant support hospitals. After World War II, triage came to mean the process used to identify those most likely to return to battle after medical intervention. This process allowed concentration of medical resources on soldiers who could fight again. During the Korean and Vietnam conflicts, triage was refined to accomplish the "greatest good for the greatest number of wounded or injured men."[25]

In the civilian arena, triage has two very different uses—disaster triage and daily triage.[4] Disaster triage is similar to military triage in that the goal is the greatest good for the greatest number of injured. Disasters include floods, hurricanes, earthquakes, bombs, collapsed buildings, fires, airline crashes, vehicular crashes, and tornadoes.[11] The primary dif-

ference between disaster triage and military triage relates to patient transport.[4,23] Table 8-1 compares priority categories used for military and disaster triage. During a disaster, transport for some victims is delayed to prevent overloading the receiving ED.

Daily ED use of triage systems began in the early 1960s when demand for emergency services surpassed available resources. Space, equipment, and personnel could no longer handle the explosion in ED visits. From 1958 to the early 1960s, the nation's EDs reported 18 million visits.[20] This figure increased to more than 44 million by 1968 and to more than 99 million by 1990.[11] The greatest increase in patient numbers occurred in the nonurgent category. Reasons cited for increases include lack of available nonemergency services and lack of access to primary or urgent care providers.[11] The number of patients with nonurgent problems increased with the growing number of underinsured or uninsured people using the ED for primary care.[10] The triage process evolved as an efficient way to separate patients requiring immediate medical attention from those who could wait.

TRIAGE SYSTEMS

The primary goal of an effective triage system is rapid identification of patients with urgent, life-threatening conditions.[13] Complementary goals include prioritizing care needs for all patients, regulating patient flow through the ED, and determining the most appropriate area for treatment, whether it is the ED or an outside primary care area.[14]

Any triage system has primary and secondary functions. Primary functions include assessing and reassessing the patient's chief complaint and related symptoms, taking a brief history and physical assessment, and measuring vital signs. Secondary functions include clerical tasks, directions, telephone advice, ambulance patient evaluation, ambulance dispatch, stocking supplies, cleaning, equipment maintenance, crowd control, security, and information.[11] The extent to which a triage system encompasses all these functions depends on daily census, available staff, presence of walk-in clinics or same-day clinics, type and availability of health care providers, availability of specialty treatment areas, and environmental, legal, and administrative constraints.[4,5,20]

ED triage systems vary widely. In 1982 Thompson and Dains identified the three most common triage systems—traffic director (Type I), spot checker (Type II), and comprehensive (Type III).[23] Differences among these systems are related to the depth of triage provided. Table 8-2 compares urgency categories, staffing patterns, documentation requirements, patient assessment and reassessment criteria, and use of diagnostic procedures found in these triage systems.

The comprehensive triage system may be provided as a single-tiered system in which the nurse who first encounters the patient performs the interview, documents triage assess-

Table 8-1 COMPARISON OF MILITARY AND DISASTER PRIORITY CATEGORIES

PRIORITY	MILITARY	DISASTER
1	**Immediate care** Shock, airway problems, chest injury, crush injury, amputation, open fracture	**Class I (emergent) Red** Critical; life-threatening—compromised airway, shock, hemorrhage
2	**Minimal care** Little or no treatment needed	**Class II (urgent) Yellow** Major illness or injury; requires treatment within 30 minutes to 2 hours—open fracture, chest wound
3	**Delayed care** Treatment may be postponed without loss of life; noncritical—simple fracture, nonbleeding laceration	**Class III (nonurgent) Green** Care may be delayed 2 hours or more; minor injuries; walking wounded—closed fracture, sprain, strain
4	**Expectant care** No treatment until immediate and delayed priority patients cared for; requires considerable time, effort, and supplies	**Class IV (expectant) Black** Dead or expected to die—massive head injury, extensive full-thickness burns

Modified from Thompson JD, Dains J: *Comprehensive triage: a manual for developing and implementing a nursing care system,* Reston, Va, 1982, Reston.

Table 8-2 COMPARISON OF TRIAGE SYSTEMS

ELEMENTS	TYPE I: TRAFFIC DIRECTOR	TYPE II: SPOT CHECK	TYPE III: COMPREHENSIVE
ASSESSMENT			
Staff	Nonprofessional	Registered nurse or physician	Registered nurse
Data	Chief complaint	Chief complaint: limited subjective and objective	Thorough assessment: complete, subjective, and objective; education needs; primary health needs
ANALYSIS			
Urgency category	Two categories: emergent, nonurgent	Three categories: emergent, nonurgent, delayed	Four categories: Class I-IV
Nursing diagnosis	None	None	Present
PLAN			
Alternatives	Treatment room, waiting area	Treatment room, waiting area, treat and discharge from triage	Treatment room, waiting area with planned assessment
Diagnostic procedures	None	Inconsistent	Protocol-driven
Documentation	Little, inconsistent	Variable	Systematic
EVALUATION			
Reevaluation	None	None planned, at patient request	Planned, systematic
System	Difficult	Variable	Systematic

Modified from Thompson JD, Dains J: *Comprehensive triage: a manual for developing and implementing a nursing care system,* Reston, Va, 1982, Reston.

ment, assigns triage acuity, and designates treatment areas. This system provides the most customer-friendly triage process because the patient does not feel rushed and the nurse can establish rapport with the patient. The entire triage encounter is documented on a triage record or on the patient's medical record. The triage nurse initiates triage protocols and various interventions.[7] With this system, the triage area should be large enough to allow privacy for the interview without interfering with the triage nurse's ability to see patients as they come through the door. Large-volume EDs may require multiple triage nurses to maintain flow in this type of system.

A multitiered system is used in some large-volume EDs to expedite flow while providing rapid identification of patients with potential threats to life, vision, or limb. In this system, the first triage nurse sees each patient enter the ED, rapidly assesses the patient to determine his or her chief complaint, and identifies immediate threats to life, vision, or limb. Acuity is determined from visual observations, a brief patient interview, and tactile examination of skin and quality of the pulse. The triage interview and vital signs are not obtained in the first tier. If the patient does not require immediate attention, the patient is sent to the second tier of the system for the triage interview, and vital signs are taken before registration. Triage protocols are initiated at the second tier.[7] With a multitiered system, the triage nurse is not occupied with comprehensive triage assessment, has constant visual access to everyone who enters the area, and can rapidly identify patients who require immediate attention.

Regardless of the process used, department structure should support the system. The triage area should be located by the door, so the first professional the patient encounters is the triage nurse. When a multitiered system is used, the first tier should provide immediate visual access to the door without sacrificing security measures or exposing the triage nurse to unnecessary weather conditions. The process should flow from one step to the next without creating unnecessary delay for the patient.

URGENCY CATEGORIES

In the triage process, urgency categories rate patient acuity and prioritize care. Rating systems vary with patient census and available resources. Most rating systems use predetermined criteria to classify patients into two or more categories. The most common system uses three classification levels: emergent, urgent, and nonurgent (Table 8-3).[11,13] The greater the number of urgency categories, the more discriminating an ED can be in meeting a patient's needs. A comprehensive triage system uses four or more classifications. Table 8-4 summarizes these urgency categories by description, reassessment guidelines, and types of patients. Several studies evaluated the reliability of triage rating systems.[3,6,26] The Wuerz study found poor interrater reliability, whereas the Fernandes and Beveridge studies found better reliability with the Canadian rating scales.

Recently a five-level scale called the Emergency Severity Index (ESI) emerged and is used in several academic centers in the United States.[10] This five-level scale stratifies adult patients into defined exclusive categories. Patient acuity, expected resource intensity, and timeliness define the categories. Research by Wuerz demonstrates reliability and validity of the ESI.[27]

TRIAGE STAFFING

Historically, receptionists, ward clerks, nurse aides, emergency medical technicians, licensed practical nurses, registered nurses, physicians, and others performed triage. In 1985, Congress passed the Consolidated Omnibus Reconciliation Act (COBRA) requiring a medical screening for all ED patients before inquiries about finances, insurance, or ability to pay. COBRA, or the Emergency Medical Treatment and Active Labor Act (EMTALA), as it is now known, specifies that medical screening is performed by a qualified

Table 8-3	URGENCY CATEGORIES
CATEGORY	**DESCRIPTION**
Emergent	Immediate care required; condition is threat to life, limb, or vision; "severe"
Urgent	Care required as soon as possible; condition presents danger if not treated; "acute" but not "severe"
Nonurgent	Routine care required; condition minor; care can be delayed

Table 8-4	COMPREHENSIVE TRIAGE: FOUR URGENCY CATEGORIES			
CLASS	**I**	**II**	**III**	**IV**
Descriptor	Immediate; life-threatening	Stable; as soon as possible	Stable; no distress	Stable; no distress
Reassessment	Continuous	Every 15 minutes	Every 30 minutes	Every 60 minutes
Examples	Cardiac arrest, seizures, major trauma, respiratory distress, major burn	Open fracture, pain, minor burn, surgical abdomen, sickle cell, child, and fever	Closed fracture, laceration without bleeding, drug ingestion longer than 3 hours previous with no signs or symptoms	Rash, constipation, impetigo, abrasion, nerves

Modified from Thompson JD, Dains J: *Comprehensive triage: a manual for developing and implementing a nursing care system,* Reston, Va, 1982, Reston.

individual.[10] The definition of a qualified individual is still an area of controversy, left open for interpretation. Use of a registered nurse to provide medical screening and prioritize patient care is widely recommended.[17] The *Standards of Emergency Nursing Practice* specify that a registered nurse should triage each patient.[5] Triage may be performed by a dedicated nurse or by all nurses working in the ED rotating to triage for all or part of a specific shift. As hospitals continually improve triage practices, care must be taken not to back up patients into the waiting room for triage. The goal is to reduce the time before triage. Means of achieving this goal may necessitate additional ED staff to assist at triage during peak flow times. Some EDs allow the registration process to catch up with the patient or modify the triage routine to capture data later in the stay. The most effective system is determined by the individual needs of each ED. However, triage should not encumber care in the ED.[8]

Triage Nurse Qualifications

The triage nurse decides the order in which patients receive medical attention.[14] A hallmark of an effective triage nurse is experience and skill in rapid assessment and correct determination of patient urgency. The ability to recognize who is sick and who is not is a critical success factor for the triage nurse. In-depth knowledge and experience are essential.[11]

Triage areas are often chaotic and demanding. The triage nurse must determine priorities rapidly while under stress from incoming phone calls, multiple patient arrivals, visitors, and other events and people. To function effectively, triage nurses must possess expert assessment skills, demonstrate competent interview and organizational skills, maintain an extensive knowledge base of diseases, and use experience to identify subtle clues to patient acuity. Patients with an obvious critical condition do not present the greatest challenge to the triage nurse. The true test is recognition of subtle clues to a serious problem that can quickly deteriorate without immediate attention.[11,14]

The triage nurse is the first health professional the patient and family encounter in the ED; therefore, highly refined communication skills are essential. Triage nurses must interpret assessment data while providing compassionate support to both the patient and family. In-depth understanding of the human response to crisis helps the triage nurse maintain composure, which improves public image for the ED and hospital.[14]

The complexity of the triage role led to the recommendation from the Emergency Nurses Association that triage should be performed by a registered nurse with a minimum of 6 months' emergency nursing experience.[5] Special training to provide advanced skills and knowledge required in this role is also recommended. A survey by Purnell in 1993 revealed that only 43% of hospitals require special training (i.e., triage course, advanced cardiac life support, assessment, certification in emergency nursing, extended orientation) for nurses working in the triage area. Only 9.5% re-

quire previous ED experience, with a range of 3 months to 3 years reported. Many hospitals acknowledge the desire to provide further education for triage nurses, but list multiple factors that prevent realization of this desire.[18]

Criteria regarding readiness for the triage role vary with each nurse and depend on the institution; sophistication of the triage system; the individual nurse's competence in assessment, clinical judgment, and decision making; and quality of the triage orientation process. Current legislation and legal implications affecting this role are considered when designating new personnel. A risk management approach for the ED identifies strategies for preventing litigation.

Anecdotal information suggests that formal triage orientation and special training improve the triage nurse's effectiveness and comfort in the role. Written protocols to assist decision making and an internship or preceptorship allow the novice to grow with assistance from an experienced triage nurse.

TRIAGE DOCUMENTATION

Documentation with the tiered triage system uses a written triage record or electronic data entry. The triage record is often the first part of the ED nursing record (Figure 8-1). The documentation tool may be comprehensive or reflect only brief patient assessment. Figure 8-2 is an example of a more detailed triage documentation tool.

Another method for standardization of triage data is electronic entry. This method eliminates duplication of information as the data flow throughout the medical record.[15] Regardless of the system, triage documentation provides a "snapshot" of the patient's chief complaint, appearance, and acuity. A focused assessment of the chief complaint is necessary to prioritize care and identify appropriate treatment needs.

PATIENT ASSESSMENT

The goals of the triage process are to gather sufficient data for determining acuity, identify immediate needs, and establish rapport with the patient and family. Use of the nursing process provides the necessary framework for a consistent approach for every patient.

Assessment

This is defined as a rapid systematic collection of data relevant to each patient.[5] Subjective data provide information disclosed by the patient or family whereas objective data are observable, measurable information.[2] Assessment begins with first contact—as the patient walks through the door, by telephone, or during a call from prehospital personnel. The triage nurse is expected to evaluate all patients entering the ED within 2 to 5 minutes of arrival.[5] Current research by Travers suggests the 2-minute standard is met only 22% of the time. This research found the time ranged from 0.5 to 11.1 minutes. The increased time correlated with elderly pa-

Cook County Hospital
Chicago, Illinois

Emergency Nursing - Triage Assessment
Mark appropriate boxes with an X, ☒, fill in information as requested / required.

Date:_____	**SECTION A:**	**Staff Initials**_____

Primary Triage Time_____ in ☐AES ☐PER ☐ASC ☐AHC   Initially seen in ASC/AHC at :Time _____

Patient Name:_____ ☐M ☐F DOB:_____ Age:_____MR #:_____
Last Name, First Name, Middle Initial

Primary Language: ☐English ☐_____ **Information Provided By:** ☐Patient ☐Family Member
Interpreter Used: Name of Interpreter:_____

Mode of Arrival: ☐Walk ☐Wheelchair ☐Cart ☐Carried   **Other:**_____

Accompanied By: CFD #_____ ☐Private ambulance ☐Police/Cermak ☐Self ☐Other:_____
Primary Physician:_____ ☐CCH

Weight:_____ ☐estimated ☐actual	**SECTION B:** Ht/Length:_____	**Staff Initials**_____

CHIEF COMPLAINT(s):

Complaint Codes: ☐☐

SpO₂_____

Capillary Glucose: _____mg/dL

PEFR: _____L/min

Time:_____ **T:**_____ **Pulse:**_____ **Resp:**_____ **B/P:**_____

Mental Status: ☐Alert ☐Oriented X3   ☐Disoriented ☐Lethargic ☐Unresponsive
Respiratory Status: ☐No Problem   ☐Labored ☐Stridor ☐Other:_____
                         Distress: ☐**Mild** ☐**Moderated** ☐**Severe**
Emotional Distress: ☐None   ☐Anxious ☐Crying ☐Pain Scale:_____   ☐Other
Skin Color/Condition: ☐Normal   ☐Pale ☐Flushed ☐Cyanotic ☐Diaphoretic
AW Screen:: ☐Not Applicable ☐Not Assessed ☐Negative ☐Positive *Notified:* ☐Police Star#_____ ☐MSW ☐HCIP ☐RVA

Past Medical History: ☐None H/O: ☐Diabetes ☐Heart problems_____ ☐HTN
☐Asthma ☐Tuberculosis ☐Mental Health Problems ☐HIV+ / AIDS ☐Cancer ☐Seizures ☐Stroke
☐Other:_____ Ob/Gyne: ☐LNMP_____ G___P___A___ Wks Gestation_____ EDD_____
T.B. History: ☐N/A ☐Night Sweats ☐Productive cough ☐Fever ☐Mask Applied   *Pediatric Immunization History:*
Placed in Isolation: ☐Yes   Type / Reason:_____   ☐Up to date ☐Other:_____

Allergies: ☐None ☐Penicillin ☐Sulfa ☐Codeine ☐Dye ☐Other:

Current Medications: ☐None   *Tetanus Status:* ☐< 5 years ☐> 5 years ☐Unknown

_____
_____

Comments: ☐UA ☐UCG ☐Xray_____ ☐EKG   Other:_____

Severity: ☐①Emergent ☐②Semi-Emergent ☐③ Urgent ☐④ Semi-urgent ☐⑤Non-Urgent
Destination:_____ **Time Triage Completed:**_____

No Answer Calls: TIME 1:_____   Addressograph
                     TIME 2:_____
                     TIME 3:_____ ☐CLERK TO LOG OUT
Initials   **Print/Sign Name**   **Title:**
_____
_____
_____

Form#: 1398
August 1997 Rev 5/99
White: Medical Records / Yellow: Unit

FIGURE 8-1   Triage record. (Courtesy Cook County Hospital, Chicago, Illinois.)

tients having complex medical conditions. Travers questions the need to obtain a full set of vital signs on every patient.[24] The ESI rating scale uses vital signs for decision making in only two categories.[27] Some EDs have eliminated the full set of vital signs for lower acuity patients at triage allowing for use of nursing clinical judgment.[12] Facilities should exercise flexibility and care when setting time limits at triage.[9]

In an ideal setting, the triage nurse begins with self-introduction while assessing major threats to airway, breathing, or circulation (ABCs) (i.e., airway compromise,

Wellstar Emergency Services	Initial Nursing Documentation	☐ Cobb ☐ Douglas ☐ Kenn ☐ Paulding

Name	Non-English Speaking? ☐ Spanish Other _____ ☐ Hearing Impaired ☐ Interpreter Requested	ROOM

	Age	Time	Date	PCP	Other Doctor

Chief Complaint

Potential Threat	Assessment ☐ NAD	Skin	Pulse Ox	I Red
☐ None apparent ☐ Life ☐ Vision ☐ Limb ☐ Infant/Child *NOT* Appropriate for age	☐ Resp distress ☐ Chest Pain ☐ Suicidal ☐ OD ☐ Altered LOC ☐ Violent ☐ Obvious fracture ☐ Hemorrhage ☐ Burn/Blisters ☐ Severe Pain	☐ WNL ☐ Pale ☐ Flushed ☐ Cyanotic ☐ Diaphoretic		II Yellow III Green IV Orange

Appearance	Arrival	Disposition	Signature
☐ Alert ☐ Uncooperative ☐ Cooperative ☐ Unresponsive	☐ Ambulatory ☐ WC ☐ Police ☐ Carried ☐ Stretcher ☐ Alone	☐ Exam ☐ Assess ☐ Registration ☐ WR ☐ Fast Track ☐ LBS signed	

Time	Allergies ☐ NKDA ☐ Tape ☐ Latex ☐ Food ☐ Environmental (pollen/bees)	Wt _____ ☐ Measured Ht _____ Asthma > 6yrs	Tetanus ☐ ≤5yrs ☐ > 5 yrs ☐ Peds Immunizations UTD (Info discussed if not current)

Limb/Position	Blood Pressure	Manual	Pulse	Irregular	Resp	Temp	Pulse Ox	LMP_____ ☐ Birth Control Pills
RA LA LL RL → ᛒ ♀								NA→ ☐ Menopausal ☐ Hysterectomy ☐ Depo-Provera
RA LA LL RL → ᛒ ♀								Pregnant? Y N UNK FHT_____ Due Date ____ Visual Acuity ☐ Glasses ☐ Contacts ☐ Implants ☐ Blind Left ____ Right ____ Both ____ Corrected ____

Safety Equip: ☐ No ☐ Seatbelt ☐ Airbag ☐ Child Safety Seat ☐ Helmet ☐ Goggles ☐ Pads ☐ Unknown Treatment PTA: ☐ Denies ☐ See EMS sheet ☐ Immobilized ☐ Medications	Cultural/Religious/Spiritual/Psychosocial/Learning Needs: None identified List:

PPMH: ☐ Denies ☐ Diabetes ☐ Cardiac ☐ High Cholesterol ☐ HTN ☐ Asthma ☐ COPD ☐ Infect Dx ☐ TB ☐ Seizures ☐ Stroke ☐ GB Dx ☐ Ulcers ☐ Thyroid ☐ Cancer ☐ Depression ☐ Chronic Pain ☐ Migraine HA Past Surgical History: ☐ CABG ☐ Cholecystectomy ☐ Appendectomy Other:	Social History: ☐ ETOH _____ (Occ QD) ☐ Cigarettes/cigar/pipe ____ ppd ☐ Chewing tobacco ☐ Snuff ☐ Drugs

CURRENT MEDS (OTC, Rx, Herbal): ☐ See Medication Sheet ☐ Partial listing ☐ Dose/Schedule Unknown	Pain Assessment
	Where? Does it go anywhere? How much does it hurt? When did it start? What makes it better or worse? What does it feel like?

Mark only those systems that apply to complaint or presenting symptoms.

Neurologic	Y	N	Respiratory	Y	N	Cardiac	Y	N	Skin	Y	N	Surface Problems	Scale	Faces
Alert			Cough Prod			Chest pain			Warm/Dry			☐ Laceration ☐ Abrasion	*WORST EVER*	
Oriented X 3			Retractions			Epigastric Substernal			Diaphoretic			☐ Bruises ☐ Deformity	Circle↓	Check↓
+ LOC			Able to speak			Sharp Pressure Dull			Hot Cool Cold			☐ Amputation ☐ Rash	10	
Dizzy			Dyspnea DOE			Radiates to:			Pale Flushed			Where	9	😫
Headache			Shallow			Palpitations			Cyanotic				8	😣
Slurred speech			Stridor			JVD			Jaundice				7	
Facial Asymmetry			Snoring			Pedal edema			Cap Refill ≤ 3 sec > 3 sec			Size	6	😖
MAE			Orthopnea			EENT			GYN/GU				5	
Weakness			PND			Hoarse			Itching			Appearance	4	🙂
RA LA RL LL			Breath Side/Front/Back			Sore Throat			VB pds in last hr:				3	
Sensory changes			Sounds R L A P			R/L/B in appropriate column↓			Dischg V P			Pulses ☐ Present	2	😐
Blurred vision			Clear			Eyes Red			Frequency			☐ Decreased ☐ Absent	1	
Photophobia			Crackles			Eyes Draining			Retention			ROM		
Pupils PERL			Wheezes			Ear Drainage			Gastrointestinal			☐ Normal ☐ Decreased		
Brisk ØPERL R L			Decreasd			Nasal Drainage			N V D			Sensory	0	😄
Sluggish Size			Abnormal			Nose bleed			Color			☐ Normal ☐ Absent		
Fixed									Bleeding					
PPinpoint Rxn			Absent			FB: Eye Ear Nose			Frequency			☐ Decreased ☐ Increased	*NO PAIN*	

Protocols ☐ Fever Adult ☐ Fever Pediatrics ☐ Sprain ☐ Tetanus ☐ UTI ☐ Chest Pain ☐ Respiratory Distress ☐ Eye Injury ☐ Amputation ☐ Fracture

Triage Actions ☐ Cervical collar ☐ Ice ☐ Elevate ☐ Pressure dressing ☐ Splint Other:	Labs	BBG	Time	Updated Acuity Rating ☐ I Red ☐ II Yellow ☐ III Green
To Room @	To x-ray @	Assessed by		Time Date (if different from above)

Form WS0102 Item 17030   Revised 12/00

FIGURE 8-2 Wellstar Emergency Services triage assessment sheet. (Courtesy Wellstar Emergency Services.)

respiratory distress, excessive bleeding, and skin or mentation changes). The triage nurse provides immediate intervention for identified threats to ABCs and transports the patient to the appropriate treatment area. When no immediate threat is identified, the triage nurse proceeds with a brief interview. Eliciting the chief complaint, defined as the reason for seeking emergency care, is the first step.[11] This is a distinct challenge when the patient provides vague or global reasons for the visit. The triage nurse must focus his or her investigation on history of the complaint and related symptoms and signs. The "PQRST" mnemonic is one example of a systematic approach to patient assessment (Table 8-5).

When sufficient information is obtained about the chief complaint and related symptoms, data are collected regard-

Table 8-5	**PQRST MNEMONIC**
COMPONENT	**SAMPLE QUESTIONS**
P (provokes)	What provokes the symptom?
Q (quality)	What makes it better? What makes it worse? What does it feel like?
R (radiation)	Where is it? Where does it go? Is it in one or more spots?
S (severity)	If we gave it a number from 0 to 10, with 0 being none and 10 being the worst you can imagine, what is your rating?
T (time)	How long have you had the symptom? When did it start? When did it end? How long did it last? Does it come and go?

ing medication usage, including prescribed, over-the-counter drugs, herbal medications, and home remedy medications. The triage nurse then evaluates the patient's medical history, including hospitalizations. Immunization history is especially important in children;[13] however, a break in the skin or conjunctiva requires investigation of tetanus immunization status, regardless of age. Allergies to medication and environmental sources are then identified.

At an appropriate time during the interview other subjective data are acquired, including name of the primary health care provider. For female patients, the nurse obtains menstrual and obstetrical history, including gravida and parity. Screening for tuberculosis, child or elder abuse or neglect, and domestic violence is also performed.

Objective data are gathered during the interview. Vital signs (temperature, pulse, respiration, and blood pressure), body weight, and other physical data are acquired by inspection, palpation, percussion, and auscultation. Touching provides information on heart rate, skin temperature, and moisture. Smelling provides information on odors (i.e., ketones, alcohol, infections, hygiene). Hearing provides information on cough quality, hoarseness, stridor, shortness of breath, tone of voice, logical thought, articulation patterns, and "what is not said." A wealth of information from nonverbal cues is obtained visually: facial grimaces, body movements, fear, obvious deformities, skin color, amount of bleeding, cyanosis, use of personal space, appropriateness of clothing, and hygiene.[2,14]

Triage nurses must be highly skilled in asking the right questions and pursuing small details. Triage guidelines, protocols, decision trees, and algorithms aid in this process.[14] Computer programs exist to help structure the enquiry. Advanced interviewing skills support the communication process for giving and receiving information using verbal and nonverbal cues.

Questioning is a useful technique in the interviewing process. A mix of open (eliciting feelings and perceptions) and closed ("yes/no," factual) questions are posed to obtain important data. Reflection, silence, displaying acceptance, showing recognition, verbalizing observations, sharing information, actively listening, and summarizing are all used

in the monumental task of gathering data to make a good health care decision for each patient.[2] The nurse's style varies with each patient and situation.

Barriers to effective communication include language, vocabulary, cultural differences, patient developmental level, gender, age, health status, anxiety, pain, environmental issues, and especially interview interruptions.[1,14] The triage nurse has no control over interruptions during assessment;[14] however, every effort is made to minimize interruptions. Gracious concern, a caring attitude, and willingness to listen help establish rapport with the patient and family.

Diagnosis

Diagnosis is defined as analyzing information collected in the assessment phase to determine acuity needs. Assume a more severe condition exists until proven otherwise to prevent undertriage.[5] Preliminary nursing diagnoses are formulated and an initial database established. Triage nurses must possess a span of knowledge to evaluate a vast array of patient complaints.[14] Critical thinking at this step is mandatory to identify outcomes for each patient.

Planning

Planning is defined as determining a course of action for identified needs to meet the expected outcome.[5] The triage nurse differentiates urgency of problems and prioritizes care by assigning acuity level, designating an appropriate treatment area, communicating pertinent information to other team members, and identifying interventions to meet the expected outcome.[5]

Implementation

Implementation is defined as carrying out the plan of care.[5] The triage nurse initiates nursing interventions, performs diagnostic procedures and treatments defined in established protocols, communicates pertinent information to the patient and family, mobilizes necessary additional resources, and documents all activities in the patient's medical record. Examples of these activities include splinting, ice application, dressings, ordering radiology exams, administering fever or tetanus medications per protocol, stocking emergency supplies and equipment, and ensuring isolation for immunocompromised or contagious patients (i.e., measles, chickenpox, tuberculosis).[13]

Evaluation

Evaluation is defined as interpreting the patient's response to interventions. The triage nurse reassesses the patient based on acuity and within time frames established by the protocol; evaluates effectiveness of interventions; and revises the plan of care, expected outcomes, and acuity based on new or changing patient data.[5] Paying special attention to borderline patients can prevent catastrophic events.

SPECIAL CONDITIONS

Emergency Medical Treatment and Active Labor Act

In 1986 Congress passed COBRA, now called EMTALA, as mentioned previously. This federal mandate applies to every hospital with an ED. A medical screening examination (MSE) to determine presence of an emergency medical condition or active labor is required for all people who come to the ED. If qualified medical personnel determine an emergency medical condition or active labor exists, staff must stabilize the patient within the facility's capability. If transfer to another facility is necessary, specific regulations govern the transfer (see Chapter 10).

Many EDs use the triage encounter to provide the initial MSE required by COBRA/EMTALA.[11,13,14] Facility bylaws must clearly identify individuals approved to complete the MSE. The triage process is then structured to screen the patient before any financial inquiries occur. To ensure a "qualified" medical staff person is present, only an experienced, competent, and trained triage nurse should perform the examination.[14]

Managed Care

More and more consumers choose managed care plans for health care. Many of these plans require authorization before ED treatment; therefore, payment for service becomes contingent on approval. This creates great concern for patients denied authorization for payment. Under EMTALA, the patient is always given the option of ED evaluation before any discussion of payment.

Referrals from Triage

A shortage of community resources and lack of awareness of access to available services are cited as reasons for nonurgent use of EDs. Referring patients to primary care settings, or "triaging out," provides delivery and continuity of care for nonurgent complaints, reduces waiting times, and is cost-effective.[11] Establishing links to primary care settings is a major component in developing a "triage out" program. Specially trained nurses guided by written protocols discuss and identify sources of alternative care. Patient agreement is required for this referral, then appointment information is provided. "Triage out" programs using feedback loops to evaluate patient satisfaction and safety report good results; this feedback is a necessary component to guarantee success.[13] It is also important to remember that the patient must receive an MSE before leaving the ED.

Telephone Triage

Telephone calls eliciting medical information and advice are problematic for EDs because evaluation of patients by phone is difficult.[13] To overcome this problem many facilities and private corporations developed a call center with nurses dedicated to this emerging speciality of nursing.[16,22] Telephone triage is defined as the process of collecting information via phone and determining acuity of the problem and interventions needed.[22] A well-developed program for telephone triage defines use of trend data for the scope of the institutional problem, addresses problem-based protocols consisting of assessment and disposition information, provides documentation of all aspects of the call, possesses a formal orientation for nursing staff with validation of competence, outlines clear policies and procedures, and evaluates the effectiveness of the program via quality improvement.[19]

Rutenberg examined recent research trials involving nurses providing telephone triage. She concludes that protocols are fraught with misinterpretation and that the special skill of interviewing and recognizing variables not considered in a face-to-face encounter is a necessary competence for the telephone triage nurse.[21] Thus, the nurse providing telephone triage must use experience and judgment combined with protocols to provide the best patient outcome.[21,22]

SUMMARY

As the health care system evolves, responsibilities of the triage nurse will continue to change and evolve. The triage nurse remains the initial contact for the patient and family in their emergency experience and, more important, can directly affect patient outcome. Although approaches vary, the common ingredient of a successful program rests with a qualified triage nurse.

References

1. Arslanian-Engoren C: Gender and age bias in triage decisions, *J Emerg Nurs* 26(2):117, 2000.
2. Bellack JP, Edlund BJ: *Nursing assessment and diagnosis,* ed 2, Boston, 1992, Jones & Bartlett.
3. Beveridge R, Ducharme J, James L et al: Reliability of the Canadian emergency department triage and acuity scale: interrater agreement, *Ann Emer Med* 34(2):155, 1999.
4. Emergency Nurses Association: *Emergency nursing core curriculum,* ed 5, Philadelphia, 2000, WB Saunders.
5. Emergency Nurses Association: *Standards of emergency nursing practice,* ed 4, Des Plaines, Ill, 2001, The Association.
6. Fernandes CMB, Wuerz R, Clark S et al: How reliable is emergency department triage? *Ann Emer Med* 34(2):141, 1999.
7. Fry M: Triage nurses order xrays for patients with isolated distal limb injuries: a 12 month ED study, *J Emerg Nurs* 27(1):17, 2001.
8. George JE, Quattrone MS, Goldstone M: Risk management spotlight: increased risk potential of the ED triage nurse, *J Emerg Nurs* 22(3):241, 1996.
9. George JE, Quattrone MS, Goldstone M: Time standards from patient arrival to triage: spotlight on a potentially dangerous practice, *J Emerg Nurs* 22(4):339, 1996.
10. Gilboy N, Travis D, Wuerz R: Re-evaluating triage in the new millennium: a comprehensive look at the need for standardization and quality, *J Emerg Nurs* 25(6):468, 1999.

11. Handysides G: *Triage in emergency practice,* St. Louis, 1996, Mosby.

12. Keddington RK: A triage vital sign policy for a children's hospital emergency department, *J Emerg Nurs* 24(2):189, 1998.

13. Kelley SJ: *Pediatric emergency nursing,* ed 2, Norwalk, Conn, 1994, Appelton & Lange.

14. Kitt S: *Emergency nursing: a physiologic and clinical perspective,* Philadelphia, 1995, WB Saunders.

15. Mason D, Gibson P, Sanders D: Computerized triage: one department's process, *J Emerg Nurs* 23(4):330, 1997.

16. Mohagen M, Hoosier SJ: Telephone triage: an alternative career for emergency nurses, *J Emerg Nurs* 22(6):527, 1996.

17. Molitor L: *Emergency department triage handbook,* Gaithersburg, Md, 1992, Aspen Publishers.

18. Purnell L: A survey of qualifications, special training and levels of personnel working emergency department triage, *J Nurs Staff Devel* 9(5):223, 1993.

19. Robinson DL, Anderson MM, Acheson PM: Telephone advice: lessons learned and considerations for starting programs, *J Emerg Nurs* 22(5):409, 1996.

20. Rund DA, Rausch TS: *Triage,* St. Louis, 1981, Mosby.

21. Rutenberg CD: What do we really know about telephone triage?, *J Emerg Nurs* 26(1):76, 2000.

22. Simonsen, SM: *Telephone health assessment guidelines for practice,* ed 2, St. Louis, 2001, Mosby.

23. Thompson J, Dains J: *Comprehensive triage: a manual for developing and implementing a nursing care system,* Reston, Va, 1982, Reston.

24. Travers D: Triage: how long does it take? How long should it take?, *J Emerg Nurs* 25(3): 238, 1999.

25. United States Department of Defense: *Emergency war surgery,* Washington, DC, 1975, U.S. Government Printing Office.

26. Wuerz R, Fernandes CMB, Alarcon J: Inconsistency of emergency department triage, *Ann Emerg Med* 32(4):431, 1998.

27. Wuerz RC, Milne LW, Eitel DR et al: Reliability and validity of a new five-level triage instrument, *Acad Emer Med* 7(3):236, 2000.

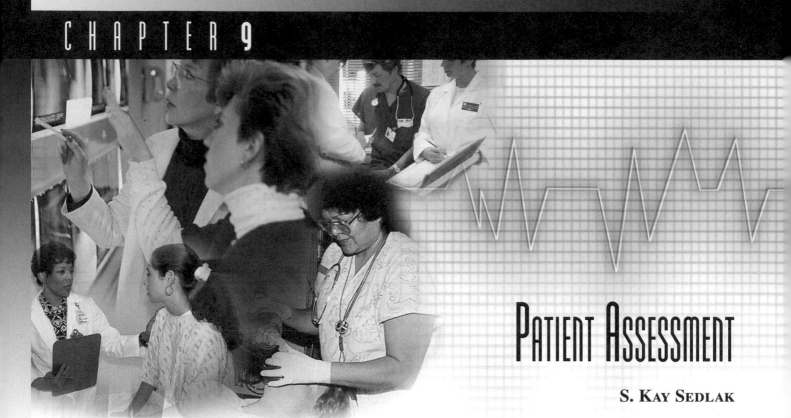

CHAPTER 9

PATIENT ASSESSMENT

S. KAY SEDLAK

The basis of all care delivered to patients in the emergency department (ED) is an accurate and appropriate initial assessment. This is also the first step of the nursing process. When sufficient data are gathered and synthesized, specific patient problems are identified and appropriate therapeutic interventions can be initiated.

Rapid, primary assessment is indicated for all patients presenting to the ED, regardless of initial complaint, to ensure that potentially life-threatening conditions are identified and immediately addressed. The "ABC" (airway, breathing, and circulation) mnemonic is used to direct this initial assessment. Table 9-1 describes this essential process. An experienced nurse automatically assesses the ABCs, promptly recognizes life-threatening conditions, and immediately initiates appropriate therapeutic actions.

All patients without life-threatening conditions receive routine assessment based on facility protocol, identification of chief complaint, vital signs, medications taken, and presence of allergies. The triage nurse should correctly identify the patient's primary problem because this determines priority for care and room placement. Certain complaints and findings support the need for more focused assessment. A systematic approach ensures that important findings are not overlooked. This chapter addresses assessment in detail according to specific body systems. Experience guides the nurse in identifying which systems to evaluate for the patient's complaint. Essential tools for the triage nurse include common sense, knowledge of anatomy and physiology, and ability to apply critical thinking to the situation. For example, the patient who comes to the ED with a laceration to the head may require medical management in addition to placement of sutures to repair disruption in skin integrity. The in-

quisitive nurse may probe further to determine the cause of the laceration and any potential consequences (e.g., a Stokes-Adams attack with injury to brain tissue).

Ongoing assessment is indicated in certain patient conditions to identify response to care rendered or determine deterioration in patient status. No precise rules describe how often repeat assessment should be completed. Facility protocols may offer guidelines for specific situations, such as trauma score calculation for prehospital, on arrival, and 1 hour after presentation; repeat vital sign measurements every 15 minutes for patients receiving thrombolytic therapy; and follow-up pulse oximetry measurements every half hour after intravenous sedation until the value returns to baseline. A high index of suspicion guides the experienced nurse in determining which follow-up measurements to obtain and the appropriate intervals for doing so.

ASSESSMENT TOOLS

Ability to use a variety of assessment tools effectively is the hallmark of experience. Tools may be objective, subjective, verbal, or observed.

Subjective and Objective Data

During the assessment process, two types of information are obtained: subjective and objective. Subjective data are offered by the patient, family, or significant other. This information reflects his or her perception of the problem. Although such information is quite valuable, it may also require clarification based on the patient's culture, feelings, and interpretation of the specific situation. For example, a patient in denial

Table 9-1 ASSESSMENT OF THE ABCs		
COMPONENT	**DESCRIPTION**	**ACTION**
Airway	Represents patent airway	Identify and remove any partial or complete airway obstruction; position airway to maintain patency; insert oro- or nasopharyngeal airway; protect cervical spine
Breathing	Determine presence and effectiveness of respiratory efforts Identify other abnormalities in breathing (e.g., abnormal pattern, abnormal sounds, break in chest wall integrity)	Assist breathing with oxygen therapy, mouth-to-mouth ventilation, or bag-valve-mask ventilation; intubate when necessary
Circulation	Evaluate pulse presence and quality, character, and equality; assess capillary refill, skin color and temperature, and the presence of diaphoresis	Initiate chest compressions, medications, or intravenous fluid resuscitation as appropriate; control bleeding

about a particular health problem may not automatically offer critical information that facilitates identification of the condition. Subjective data are not readily visible to the nurse, but do assist in determining the direction of the focused survey.

Objective data are those that can be observed or measured. Methodologies used to collect objective data include inspection, auscultation, palpation, percussion, smell, and acquisition of laboratory reports and other diagnostic summaries. Objective information is considered factual. Many objective signs are manifestations of specific illnesses and disorders and indicate to the experienced nurse the need for more focused assessment. Gathering objective data offers the health care worker an opportunity to validate the patient's subjective information. Collectively, these data are the basis for identification of patient problems.

A variety of methodologies exist for collecting data, including interviewing the patient, significant other, or bystander; obtaining measurements; performing skilled observations; and consulting other resources. Ideally, all assessment tools can and should be used; although often, particularly in the ED, this is not possible. For example, the patient may have an altered level of consciousness and be unable to give a history, or the patient's condition may not allow sufficient time for complete examination, or appropriate diagnostic tests may not be available at a given facility, particularly during non-business hours. The skilled nurse adapts to such situations, relying even more on ability to identify potential reasons for the patient's condition. Obtaining and interpreting available data become even more critical in such circumstances. The competent nurse anticipates potentially dangerous situations, then determines extent and frequency of the assessment.

Patient Interactions

The general survey proceeds beyond fundamental considerations of the ABCs to a more systematic observation of the patient. This includes observation of the following:
- Affect and mood, including thought organization
- Quality of speech (normal, slurred, silent, unable to speak)
- General appearance (manner of dress, hygiene, color of skin, facial expression)
- Posture and motor activity (observe upright posture and motor activity while the patient walks, sits, undresses)

- Odors (breath, skin)
- Degree of distress, based on preceding observations

The general survey can be conducted simultaneously with the primary survey. Combining the two may be difficult at first but becomes easier with practice. Often, the primary and general survey can be combined with patient history. The determining factor for this interview is the patient's condition at the time. If immediate or unanticipated problems arise, the interview may be delayed and completed during physical examination or after the patient's condition has stabilized.

History

The history interview for the ED patient focuses on the chief complaint. The questions, although open ended, should be directed by that complaint and build on information offered by the patient. The key to obtaining information about chief complaint—why the patient came—is to listen to what the patient says in trying to tell you what is wrong. What the patient tells you is, by definition, subjective and therefore demands objective assessment. The chief complaint should not be recorded as a diagnosis ("possible fractured left arm") but exactly as the patient describes the problem ("fell from step ladder, now pain and swelling in left arm"). Box 9-1 summarizes pertinent historical data.

If the patient initially comes to the triage area and is physically able to proceed through the triage process, history can be completed in the triage area. If the patient enters the ED by ambulance or other vehicle and cannot be processed through triage, the nurse managing the patient in the treatment area obtains history and whatever information prehospital personnel may have regarding status or treatment before arrival. If the patient can respond to questions, any history obtained from others should be validated by the patient. Often, when anxiety from transport diminishes, the patient remembers information he or she could not recall previously.

Sometimes patients cannot describe their symptoms or reason for coming to the ED. When this occurs, attempts should be made to reach someone who can relate history of the present complaint. If a patient is unresponsive and no one is available to provide history, treating the patient becomes more difficult and time consuming. Old medical

PERTINENT HISTORICAL DATA

History of present illness or injury
  How and when injury or illness first occurred
    Influencing factors
    Symptom chronology and duration
    Related symptoms
    Location of pain or discomfort
    What, if anything, the patient has done about the symptoms
Pertinent medical history
  Has this problem ever occurred before?
    If so, was a medical diagnosis made? What was it?
  Has the patient ever had surgery? For what reason? What was the result?
  Is there any family medical history that may influence the patient's present complaint?
  Does the patient have a private physician? (Obtain full name if possible)
Current medication (prescribed or unprescribed, over-the-counter, and recreational)
When was medication taken last?
Allergies
Age and weight
Tetanus immunization history if an injury is involved
Date of last menstrual period, if the patient is female

PQRST ASSESSMENT

P *(Provoking factors)*
  Ask the patient what, if anything, provokes the pain or discomfort. Is there anything that makes it worse or relieves it? What was the patient doing when it began?
Q *(Quality)*
  Ask the patient to describe the pain in his or her own words. It is particularly important to avoid "feeding" descriptive terms to the patient; instead, use open-ended questions to allow a personal description. (Can you tell me how your pain feels to you?)
R *(Region or radiation)*
  Ask the patient to point to the area of pain or discomfort, if possible. Ask if it travels anywhere, if there is pain anyplace else, if the pain moves from the region of onset. A patient may not be able to isolate a single area of pain, particularly if the pain is visceral rather than cutaneous. In this case, ask if the patient can identify the general area for you. Do not touch the patient while he or she shows you where the discomfort is. This may obscure the answers and provide you with incorrect information.
S *(Severity)*
  Ask the patient to describe the severity of the pain using a scale of 0 to 10. On this scale, 0 is equivalent to no pain, and 10 is the most severe pain the patient has ever experienced. Ask if the pain affects normal activity, and if so, how it has affected activities of daily living. Watch while the patient moves or undresses, and assess the degree to which the pain compromises activities.
T *(Time)*
  The time of onset and constancy or duration of symptoms are assessed. Ask if the patient has had these symptoms before, what they were related to, and how they were treated.

---

records, if available, may be helpful; however, treatment should never be delayed until history is available.

The mnemonic "PQRST" (Box 9-2) has been used to great advantage in assessing complaints of pain or discomfort. It helps define the complaint by focusing on essential elements (i.e., provoking factors, quality, radiation, severity, and timing in terms of onset and duration).

Measurements

Vital Signs

Vital signs are an important element of the assessment process and deserve much more than the casual attention they often receive. These readings provide valuable information, which when combined with physical examination findings, can greatly affect management of the patient. When signs and symptoms conflict with one another or with vital signs, meticulous attention must be paid to all elements of the physical examination to determine the cause of the conflict. In the ED where a patient is usually unfamiliar to staff, determining if findings deviate from the patient's normal values is more difficult. Obtaining former medical records may assist in determining what is abnormal for a particular patient.

Vital signs are indicators of the patient's present condition. Serial values should be obtained if vital signs are to have any impact on identification of trends or developments in the clinical situation. Subsequent readings should be considered in light of therapeutic interventions initiated. The body's compensatory mechanisms affect readings, so vital signs must be viewed relative to other clinical findings. What may be considered normal blood pressure might be interpreted differently when considering that the value is only possible because of compensatory mechanisms (e.g., severe peripheral vasoconstriction).

Temperature. Temperature has been referred to as the "forgotten vital sign," particularly in critical patient situations. Practitioners often do not understand the significance of this measurement and consequently neglect to obtain it. Temperature measurement is mandatory for all ED patients to identify hypothermia, hyperthermia, and other febrile conditions. Deviation from normal temperature may be the only clue of a significant medical problem. For most patients, oral measurement is sufficient. The tip of the thermometer must be placed in the pocket of tissue at the base of the tongue against the sublingual artery. Temperature across the buccal cavity changes significantly with distance from this artery. Electronic thermometers, which may not read below 34.4° C, are commonly employed for this purpose. The nurse is also reminded that no single temperature value is normal for all individuals.

Pertinent assessment findings should alert the nurse to obtain the temperature by another method. Rectal temperature may be obtained on pediatric patients and adults unable to cooperate with the oral route (e.g., a patient with altered level of consciousness). This approach does have limitations, such as temperature changes that lag behind core changes, influence of blood temperature returning from the extremities, insulating ability of fecal material, or presence of hard stool limiting insertion of the thermometer to sufficient depth.

Some situations necessitate core temperature measurement. The gold standard for this value is pulmonary artery temperature. Several other approaches that correlate highly with this value but do not carry the same potential for complications include urinary catheter thermistors, esophageal probes, and tympanic thermometers. With tympanic thermometers, placement is critical to ensure accurate readings.

Pulse. Increased dependence on electronic technology has decreased tactile assessment of the pulse. The electronically monitored pulse rate gives no indication of quality and other characteristics of the pulse. Equally important are rhythm disturbances that may not be identified unless these changes are seen on the cardiac monitor. Premature beats may be felt on palpation as missing beats or beats with less amplitude than preceding ones. Irregular rhythms, even subtle ones, can be felt as a chaotic rhythm with varying intensity.

In addition to describing rate and rhythm of the pulse, the nurse should also describe the quality as bounding, normal, weak and thready, or absent. Other characteristic pulse qualities should be determined during cardiovascular assessment by actual palpation of peripheral pulses.

In context with other physical findings, the pulse is an important indicator of cardiac function. Changes in pulse rate are often the first sign that compensatory mechanisms are being used to maintain homeostasis. In early volume depletion, a healthy person with an intact autonomic nervous system can retain normal pressures with only one subtle change—slight increase in pulse rate and amplitude. Any deviation from the normal range for the patient's age that cannot be related to psychologic or environmental factors should be considered an indication of an abnormal physiologic condition until proven otherwise.

Respirations. Assessing respirations as part of the patient's vital signs identifies impairment of ventilatory function, attempts to isolate the cause, and provides timely intervention. When collecting vital signs, the nurse should not count the respiratory rate without completing a respiratory evaluation, in which other factors besides respiratory rate and rhythm are assessed.

Signs of respiratory effort include tracheal tugging, nasal flaring, use of accessory muscles, and retractions. Generally, a healthy person does not make any extra effort to breathe: airway noise is absent, the trachea is midline, nasal cartilage is quiet, and sternocleidomastoid or intercostal muscles are not required to lift the chest cage. Suprasternal, intercostal, or substernal involvement in inspiration indicates increased work of breathing.

Increased anteroposterior diameter can generally be seen on casual observation and indicates chronic alveolar distension. Other changes in chest contour are funnel chest, pigeon chest, kyphosis, and kyphoscoliosis. These particular anatomic changes in contour may interfere with normal lung inflation and exacerbate respiratory conditions.

When a healthy person inspires, the chest expands symmetrically on both sides. When pulmonary or chest wall conditions exist, the chest may rise asymmetrically during ventilation. This asymmetry can be observed with the chest exposed and can also be palpated during inspiration.

The patient's tidal volume can be estimated by observing the rise and fall of the chest during ventilation. Depth of ventilations is described as shallow, normal, or deep. A normal adult moves 300 to 500 ml of air at rest and as much as 2000 ml during exercise, with a corresponding increase in rate. A fast rate is not necessarily indicative of moving more volume, nor is a slow rate necessarily indicative of moving less volume.

Counting the respiratory rate is not measurement enough. All elements of respiration must be evaluated when assessing this vital sign. The days of rapidly calculating a 15-second rate are long over for the nurse in an ED or intensive care unit.

PULSE OXIMETRY. Oxygen saturation measurements have become the standard for patients with respiratory or hemodynamic compromise. Knowledge of the patient's baseline is helpful in determining severity of the situation or response to therapy. The nurse should also be aware of limitations of obtaining values with a finger or ear probe. Inaccurate readings occur with hypotension, anemia, extreme peripheral vasoconstriction, hypothermia, and during administration of certain medications. Readings may also be affected by artificial nails and nail polish, particularly with red polish.

Blood Pressure. Blood pressure varies with numerous factors, including patient condition, age, and gender; therefore, it is not the most reliable indicator of physiologic changes except when considered with pulse and respiration rates and in light of the current clinical situation. Systolic pressure is a measurement of pump integrity; diastolic pressure is a measurement of vascular status. Normal pressures measured in the ED are not necessarily an indication that all is well. As previously mentioned, a healthy person may not exhibit signs of low circulating volume until all compensatory mechanisms have been exhausted. Proper cuff size is essential to obtain accurate measurements. Too small of a cuff leads to falsely elevated readings, whereas too large a cuff causes false low readings.

A change in patient position can cause a precipitous drop in pressure. Thus anyone suspected of volume depletion should be evaluated for postural vital sign (orthostatic) changes. Box 9-3 discusses the procedure for orthostatic or postural vital signs. If significant findings occur during change to the sitting position, this test is considered positive for significant volume deficit. Fluid replacement should begin with volume expanders such as lactated Ringer's solution, normal saline solution, or other solutions appropriate for the situation. The source of volume depletion must be identified and controlled. If the sitting portion of the postural vital sign examination is positive, the standing portion may be deferred, because it will not yield additional information and may prove detrimental to the patient. If equivocal changes occur from ly-

---

Box 9-3 **ORTHOSTATIC VITAL SIGNS**

DESCRIPTION	PURPOSE	INDICATION	SIGNIFICANT FINDINGS
Blood pressure and pulse supine, sitting, and/or standing with less than 1 minute between each value	Identify patients with potential volume deficits that have led to compensatory mechanisms such as severe vasoconstriction	Patients with syncopal episode, dehydration, history of prolonged vomiting, diarrhea, sweating, diuretic therapy, gastrointestinal bleeding, burns, or obvious blood loss	Subjective feeling of dizziness or blurred vision. Decrease in blood pressure ≥20 mm Hg and/or increase in pulse ≥20 beats per minute

---

ing to sitting or no changes occur at all, the patient should be moved to a standing position unless this change is contraindicated (e.g., the patient has a fractured leg). Positive findings are the same as those described for the sitting position.

Whenever evaluating blood pressure values, findings are considered in relationship to the patient's history. If the patient is undergoing antihypertensive therapy, the values obtained during the ED visit may represent significant deviation relative to the patient's "normal" pressure. Pulse pressure (the difference between systolic and diastolic pressures) represents approximate stroke volume when all other variables are constant. Peripheral vascular resistance and elasticity of the vessel walls are critical determinants of pulse pressure; therefore, approximating stroke volume by measuring pulse pressure is more qualitative than accurate. However, pulse pressure provides information about status of the pump and peripheral vessels, and indicates otherwise subtle hemodynamic changes.

Blood pressure can be obtained by auscultation, palpation, or through Doppler imaging, depending on the patient's condition and the environment. Palpation does not provide information about diastolic pressure (i.e., the peripheral vascular system), and the method used for assessment should be communicated so that others use the same method or correlate findings from another method. A single blood pressure recording yields little or no information. Serial pressures must be measured to monitor hemodynamic status. Values are also affected by incorrect cuff size.

All vital signs must be taken and evaluated serially. The patient's condition is a continuum that can be assessed only through constant monitoring. Whenever therapy is instituted, all vital signs should be evaluated to assess efficacy of treatment. Also, vital signs should be repeated when abnormal and before a decision is made about disposition of the patient from the ED (discharged, admitted, or transferred to another facility).

Laboratory and Other Diagnostics

Laboratory and other diagnostic values described in Chapter 12 and elsewhere in this book are additional measurements obtained during patient assessment. They are interpreted in light of other parameters obtained during the assessment process.

Observation

Several techniques are involved in physical examination of any patient. The pattern of use varies with the body system being evaluated. With experience, the emergency nurse develops a routine for performing appropriate assessments in a timely manner.

Inspection

Visual inspection is a key examination technique because observations of the patient as a whole and of each system in particular help integrate what the patient says with what the physical appearance suggests. Inspection must always precede other techniques.

The emergency nurse first evaluates the patient's general appearance. Is the patient unkempt, malnourished, well groomed, or overweight? Does the patient appear to take good care of himself or herself? Or, does he or she exhibit poor hygiene? These observations help relate general appearance to the illness. Checking condition of the mucous membranes gives information about oxygenation and hydration. Observing body movement and posture provides information about pain, mental status, mood, and clues to degree of debilitation. After this "quick look," observations should become specific, focusing on the immediate complaint and specific system being evaluated first.

Auscultation

A stethoscope is used to identify sounds produced by various arteries, organs, and tissues. It does not amplify sounds but transmits them to the user's ear while reducing external noise interference. The diaphragm is useful when auscultating high-pitched sounds; the bell is employed to hear low-pitched sounds. Too much pressure applied to the bell against the skin causes the bell to act like a diaphragm so low-frequency sounds will not be appreciated.

Auscultated sounds are described in terms of pitch, intensity, duration, and quality. Noting presence or absence of sounds or deviation from normal sounds assists in development of a diagnosis. Respiratory, cardiovascular, and gastrointestinal systems are routinely auscultated during examination. Findings for each are discussed in more detail later in this chapter under Review of Systems.

Palpation

Hands become important tools when palpating skin temperature, skin texture, vibrations and pulsations, masses or lesions, muscle tenseness or rigidity, and deformities. When making physical contact with the patient, keep in mind that, depending on the patient's cultural background, touch by a stranger can convey different meanings. Box 9-4 summarizes some common associations with touch by various cultures.

Different parts of the hand are better equipped to feel different sensations. The dorsum of the hand is more sensitive to temperature changes, whereas the palm is more sensitive to vibratory sensations. Fingers are sensitive to touch, but sensation can be diminished by increased pressure on fingertips, so light palpation is generally preferred to deep palpation. Pressure changes are used to palpate and distinguish one organ from another or to define borders of organs. During examination of the abdomen, light palpation is generally followed by deep palpation in the process of identifying abdominal contents.

The preferred technique for light palpation is to use the fingertips of one hand to distinguish hard from soft, rough from smooth, and muscle tone. The preferred technique in deep palpation is to place the fingertips of one hand over and slightly forward of the fingertips of the other hand, which is placed over the area to be palpated. Both hands are used to press firmly and deeply over the area. Palpation with both hands can be employed to fix an organ in place with one hand while palpating borders with the other, or by using one hand to entrap the organ between the fingertips.

Percussion

This is a technique for eliciting vibrations that can be heard and felt when a portion of the body is struck with the examiner's hand or fingers. The extent of the vibration varies depending on density, position, and size of the tissue underlying the area being percussed. Percussion is helpful in outlining borders of an organ, identifying pain and tenderness within an area of the body, identifying fluid within an organ or cavity, and evaluating lung fields for the presence of consolidation, fluid, or air.

Generally, sounds are described in terms of pitch, duration, intensity, and quality. Pitch is determined by the speed with which vibrations travel through the body, strike an organ, and bounce back to the examiner's fingers. When an organ is close to the skin surface, the pitch is high (not to be confused with loud) and is a result of vibrations returning rapidly to the examiner. Duration is the time a vibration lasts and is dictated by distance of the organ from skin surface (i.e., amount of time available for the vibration to exist). A fairly solid tissue transmits a sound of short duration, whereas a hollow organ transmits a sound of reasonably long duration. Intensity of sound is assessed as loudness or softness of the sound heard when an area is percussed. A solid organ transmits a soft sound when percussed because vibrations are traveling little, if at all. The quality of the sound defines what type of organ is making the sound. For example, when the chest is percussed, a certain sound is heard if lungs are normal and the alveoli are inflated with air. This sound is described as resonant and has a different quality than would be heard if the chest were filled with bowel instead of normal aerated lung.

Bone produces a flat percussion note, so percussion is not usually carried out in areas where bone overlies cavities or organs. In addition, the deeper the organ, the more the sound is transmitted by the tissue lying above it, rather than the organ being evaluated. An organ that lies more than 5 cm below the surface is usually not detectable by percussion. Therefore, trying to evaluate a kidney using the anterior approach to percussion is generally not helpful.

Finally, the patient's body must always be compared from side to side when eliciting percussion notes. Comparison makes it much easier to recognize normal sounds for each patient, and helps distinguish changes in quality from organ to organ. If sounds are subtle, moving from side to side helps distinguish and differentiate what is being heard.

Olfaction

Olfaction can provide valuable patient information. Certain conditions are associated with specific odors, such as the smell of ketones on the breath of patients with diabetic ketoacidosis. Abnormal smells may also alert the nurse that the patient has been exposed to various agents (e.g., gasoline, alcohol, smoke, marijuana, cigarettes). Finally, the presence of some odors suggests that the patient has an infection or poor personal hygiene. Again, these findings must be considered in light of other assessment data.

Consultation

Invaluable information regarding the patient's status can be obtained from sources outside the ED. Obtaining previous medical records may provide not only medical history, but also medications, previous assessment findings, abnormalities, and pertinent social information. An additional source of information is health care providers who have interacted with the patient (e.g., private physician, home health nurses, health care workers in clinics, hospital staff who have provided frequent or long-term care for a patient). Health care providers may offer valuable information not necessarily documented anywhere, but known from frequent interactions with the patient.

REVIEW OF SYSTEMS

The final step in the assessment process is a more detailed examination relative to the patient's chief complaint and clinical status. Health care workers find it helpful to develop a routine for this phase of the assessment process, whether it be head-to-toe evaluation or assessment according to systems. Using an organized approach to assessment ensures that key variables are not neglected. Table 9-2 highlights important variables to consider in a head-to-toe assessment. The following discussion describes assessment by the system approach. Assessment of systems is described in detail in applicable chapters.

Cardiovascular System

Physical assessment of patients with cardiac emergencies focuses on identifying their current cardiac status and the presence of potential complications. Symptoms suggestive of cardiac failure include jugular vein distension, crackles, shortness of breath, and peripheral edema. Adequacy of coronary perfusion can be assessed by vital signs and rate and quality of pulses.

Auscultation of heart sounds provides information about the integrity of heart valves, atrial and ventricular muscles, and the conduction system. Normally, each cardiac cycle produces two sounds, the first and second heart sounds. The first heart sound (S1) is generally attributed to closure of the atrioventricular valves after ventricular filling. It signals onset of systole and is heard most loudly at the mitral and tricuspid auscultory areas (Figure 9-1). The pitch of the second heart sound (S2) is slightly higher than that of the first. It represents closure of the aortic and pulmonic valves at the beginning of diastole and is best heard at the pulmonic and aortic auscultatory areas (see Figure 9-1). The third (S3) and fourth (S4) heart sounds are diastolic sounds not normally heard. An S3 is also called a ventricular gallop and may occur in cardiac failure, increased preload, and abnormally slow rates. The term atrial gallop refers to an S4 and indicates poor distensibility of the ventricles when the atria contract and force blood into them. When both S3 and S4 are heard, the sound is called a summation gallop.

Murmurs are produced by turbulent flow, increased flow, or regurgitant flow across valves. The severity of a murmur is described by the Levine scale (Table 9-3). Pericardial friction rub has both a systolic and diastolic component related to cardiac movement. Pericardial friction rub increases in intensity during expiration and with the patient sitting forward. The sound is associated with inflammation of the pericardial sac and may herald pericardial tamponade.

The 12-lead electrocardiogram assists in diagnosing cardiovascular disorders and provides information about

Table 9-2	HEAD-TO-TOE PATIENT ASSESSMENT
COMPONENT	**POTENTIAL ABNORMAL FINDINGS**
Head	Headache, dizziness, seizures, loss of consciousness, syncope, deformity
Eyes	Blurred vision, loss of vision, pain, discharge, conjunctival hemorrhages, jaundice, abnormal eye shape or size, abnormal pupil shape, size, or reactivity
Nose	Drainage, epistaxis, deformity, pain, obstruction
Ears	Discharge, earache, tinnitus, hearing problems, foreign body
Mouth	Bleeding gums, toothache, redness, enlarged tonsils, foul odor, hoarseness
Neck	Pain, enlarged thyroid, bruising, enlarged or tender lymph nodes, distended neck veins, deviated trachea
Chest	Wheezing, dyspnea, rales, use of accessory muscles, retractions, hypertension, angina, murmurs or thrills, abnormal heart tones, implanted devices (i.e., pacemaker, auto-matic implantable cardiovascular defibrillator, venous port)
Abdomen	Constipation, diarrhea, nausea, vomiting, indigestion, abdominal pain/tenderness, bleeding, ascites
Pelvis/perineum	Burning, frequency, hematuria, flank pain, decreased urination, dribbling, vaginal discharge, unilateral perineal swelling
Extremities	Pain, deformity, swelling, redness, cyanosis, abnormal range of motion
Skin	Rash, bruising, poor skin turgor, delayed wound healing; abnormal pigmentation

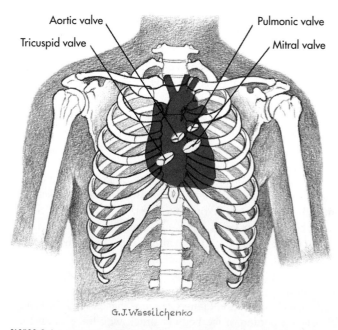

G.J.Wassilchenko

FIGURE 9-1 Anatomic location of cardiac valves. (From Canobbio MM: *Cardiovascular disorders: Mosby's clinical nursing series*, St. Louis, 1990, Mosby.)

rate, rhythm, previous or evolving infarctions, bundle branch blocks, electrical axis, atrial and ventricular enlargement, drug and electrolyte disorders, and pacemaker function. However, it represents only one moment in time. All patients with a suspected cardiac problem should have continuous cardiac monitoring. Different leads may be selected based on what the nurse suspects. Lead II enhances identification of P waves; however, V1 or MCL1 are preferred in most situations. These leads are useful in distinguishing bundle branch blocks, differentiating ventricular and aberrant conduction, and determining pacemaker wire location. During evolution of a myocardial infarction, monitor the lead with the greatest ST segment elevation.

Respiratory System

Breath sounds can change drastically, depending on the degree of pulmonary involvement and time span that the pathologic condition has existed. Auscultation may reveal normal, decreased, absent, or abnormal sounds in various fields. Table 9-4 provides a summary of adventitious or abnormal breath sounds.

Table 9-3	LEVINE SCALE FOR HEART MURMURS	
GRADE	**DESCRIPTION**	
I	Very faint, may not be heard in all positions	
II	Quiet, but heard immediately when stethoscope is placed on the chest	
III	Moderately loud. No thrill (i.e., tactile sensation associated with sound)	
IV	Loud, usually associated with thrill	
V	Very loud, may be heard without placing stethoscope completely on chest	

Table 9-4	ABNORMAL BREATH SOUNDS	
BREATH SOUNDS	**CHARACTERISTICS**	**FINDINGS**
Bronchial when heard over peripheral lung fields	High pitch; loud and long expirations	
Bronchovesicular sounds when heard over peripheral lung fields	Medium pitch with inspirations equal to expirations	
Adventitious	Crackles: discrete, noncontinuous sounds *Fine crackles* (rales): high-pitched, discrete, noncontinuous crackling sounds heard during the end of inspiration (indicates inflammation or congestion)	
	Medium crackles (rales): lower, more moist sound heard during the midstage of inspiration; not cleared by a cough	
	Coarse crackles (rales): loud, bubbly noise heard during inspiration; not cleared by a cough	
	Wheezes: continuous musical sounds; if low pitched, may be called rhonchi *Sibilant wheeze:* musical noise sounding like a squeak; may be heard during inspiration or expiration; usually louder during expiration	
	Sonorous wheeze (rhonchi): loud, low, coarse sound like a snore heard at any point of inspiration or expiration; coughing may clear sound (usually means mucus accumulation in trachea or large bronchi)	
	Pleural friction rub: dry, rubbing, or grating sound, usually caused by the inflammation of pleural surfaces; heard during inspiration or expiration; loudest over lower lateral anterior surface	

Modified from Thompson JM, McFarland GK, Hirsch JE et al: *Mosby's clinical nursing,* ed 5, St. Louis, 2001, Mosby.

Use of accessory muscles is an abnormal finding that indicates increased work of breathing by location of the muscles involved (Figure 9-2).

Specific respiratory patterns offer clues to physiologic abnormalities. Deviant patterns are summarized in Table 9-5.

Neurologic System

The most important indicator of neurologic function is the patient's level of consciousness. Assessing consciousness in the order it may deteriorate is helpful. When cerebral hemispheres are intact, well oxygenated, and functioning normally, the patient responds with purpose to your normal speaking voice. The patient can answer questions readily and remains awake during the interview and examination. In short, the patient is fully conscious, and the nurse can proceed to evaluate degree of orientation, beginning with the one thing the patient is least likely to forget—his or her name. The patient is asked where he or she is, what time or day it is, and what has happened. Allowing for possible patient confusion resulting from stress of the situation or even

from the patient not having been told what hospital he or she was taken to, the patient's answers are assessed to evaluate orientation to person, place, time, and situation. These four areas of orientation are lost in a patient in a progressive order, beginning with disorientation to the situation or amnesia for the situation. As a patient becomes less responsive, orientation decreases.

When the cerebral hemispheres become dysfunctional for any reason, level of consciousness and degree of orientation begin to deteriorate. Changes may initially be extremely subtle. Unless orientation is tested in the same way each time, subtle changes may be overlooked. Pupils, respiratory rate and patterns, and muscle reflexes and tone are assessed next. The Glasgow coma scale (GCS) (Tables 9-6 and 9-7) is used as a standardized objective measurement of neurologic function. It may be necessary to apply noxious or painful stimuli (e.g., press nailbeds or squeeze the trapezius muscle) if the patient does not respond to verbal commands. When evaluating neurologic function, a GCS less than 8 indicates a comatose state. The patient's condition may impose certain limitations, such as with intoxication, inability to move because of paralysis, inability to speak when intu-

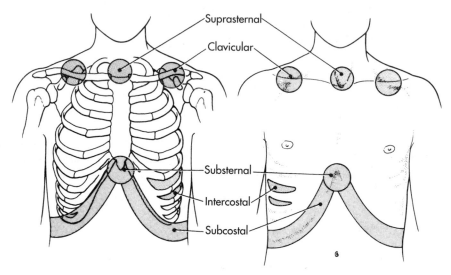

FIGURE 9-2   Areas of respiratory retractions. (From Scipien GM et al: *Pediatric nursing care,* St. Louis, 1990, Mosby.)

Table 9-5   RESPIRATORY PATTERNS

NAME	DESCRIPTION	ETIOLOGY
Eupnea	Normal rate and rhythm	
Tachypnea	Increased respirations	Fever, pneumonia, respiratory alkalosis, aspirin poisoning
Bradypnea	Slow but regular respirations	Narcotics, tumor, alcohol
Cheyne-Stokes	Respirations gradually become faster and deeper, then slower alternating with periods of apnea	Increased intracranial pressure, cardiac and renal failure, drug overdose
Biot's	Faster and deeper respirations with abrupt pauses	Spinal meningitis, other central nervous system conditions
Kussmaul's	Faster and deeper respirations without pauses	Renal failure, metabolic acidosis, diabetic ketoacidosis
Apneustic	Prolonged, gasping inspiration, followed by short expiration	Dysfunction of respiratory center in pons
Central neurogenic hyperventilation	Sustained regular hyperpnea	Midbrain lesions
Ataxic	Completely irregular	Damage to respiratory center in medulla

bated, or language barriers, that can render the total score invalid. Box 9-5 offers a mnemonic for discerning potential causes for an altered level of consciousness.

Head, Ears, Eyes, Nose, and Throat

The head, face, and neck are inspected and palpated for any injuries or deformities, observing for any discharge from natural orifices. Oral mucosa is assessed for color, hydration, inflammation, and bleeding. The uvula should be smooth and pink; redness and swelling may indicate an allergic process. Asymmetry of facial expressions suggests abnormalities in the central nervous system.

The ears are inspected for discharge, foreign bodies, deformities, lumps, or skin lesions. An otoscope is used to examine the tympanic membrane (TM). Pulling the auricle upward and back straightens the canal in an adult, whereas it is pulled downward and back in a child. Using the largest

Table 9-6 GLASGOW COMA SCALE

ACTIVITY	POINTS
BEST MOTOR RESPONSE	
Obeys simple commands	6
Localizes noxious stimulus	5
Flexion withdrawal	4
Abnormal flexion	3
Abnormal extension	2
No motor response	1
BEST VERBAL RESPONSE	
Oriented	5
Confused	4
Verbalizes, inappropriate words	3
Vocalizes—moans/groans	2
No verbal response	1
EYE OPENING	
Spontaneously	4
To speech	3
To noxious stimulus	2
No eye opening	1
TOTAL = 3 to 15	

Box 9-5 CAUSES OF ALTERED LEVEL OF CONSCIOUSNESS: AEIOU-TIPPS

A	Alcohol
E	Epilepsy/electrolytes
I	Insulin (hypoglycemia or hyperglycemia)
O	Opiates
U	Uremia
T	Trauma
I	Infection
P	Poison
P	Psychosis
S	Syncope

Table 9-7 PEDIATRIC COMA SCALE

	EYE OPENING	
SCORE	**>1 YEAR**	**<1 YEAR**
4	Spontaneously	Spontaneously
3	To verbal command	To shout
2	No pain	To pain
1	No response	No response

	BEST MOTOR RESPONSE	
SCORE	**>1 YEAR**	**<1 YEAR**
6	Obeys	Spontaneous
5	Localizes pain	Localizes pain
4	Flexion-withdrawal	Flexion-withdrawal
3	Flexion-abnormal (decorticate rigidity)	Flexion-abnormal (decorticate rigidity)
2	Extension (decerebrate rigidity)	Extension (decerebrate rigidity)
1	No response	No response

	BEST VERBAL RESPONSE		
SCORE	**>5 YEARS**	**2 TO 5 YEARS**	**0 TO 23 MONTHS**
5	Oriented and converses	Appropriate words/phrases	Smiles, coos appropriately
4	Disoriented and converses	Inappropriate words	Cries, consolable
3	Inappropriate words	Persistent crying and screaming	Persistent inappropriate crying and/or screaming
2	Incomprehensible sounds	Grunts	Grunts, agitated, restless
1	No response	No response	No response
TOTAL = 3 to 15			

Modified from Goldberg SJ: *Prehospital pediatric life support,* St. Louis, 1989, Mosby.

speculum that comfortably fits in the patient's ear, the examiner inserts the tip slightly forward and downward into the canal. The TM normally appears shiny and pearl-gray or pale pink. A reddened eardrum suggests inflammation, and blue discoloration suggests blood behind the TM. A tuning fork can be used to distinguish loss of hearing from an anatomic anomaly rather than a sensory abnormality.

A number of causes of eye problems exist: trauma, infection, systemic diseases, degenerative changes, and childhood or inherited disorders. Regardless of etiology, the standard assessment for eye problems includes visual acuity using a Snellen chart. Glasses are used for corrected vision when available. The smallest line the patient can read with each eye individually and then together is noted. Acuity is written as a fraction with the numerator indicating the distance from the chart (generally 20 feet) and the denominator describing the distance at which the line could be read by a person with normal vision. Therefore 20/20 is a normal finding. Other determinations made for a person with an eye problem include presence of pain or discomfort, tearing or secretions, changes in appearance, and integrity of extraocular muscles.

Gastrointestinal System

As with other systems, subjective data offered by the patient provide clues to assessment of the gastrointestinal system. Patients may give a history of nausea, vomiting, food intolerance, abnormal bowel habits, or changes in the character or amount of stool. Emesis or stool should be tested for blood and other laboratory diagnostics as ordered by the physician.

The abdomen is first inspected for symmetry, distension, masses, pulsations, and scars. Listening to bowel sounds in all four quadrants is a key component of the abdominal exam. Hyperperistalsis is suggested by loud, frequent bowel sounds. In contrast, absence of bowel sounds (after listening for 5 minutes) may indicate paralytic ileus. Palpation before auscultation may stimulate bowel sounds.

Palpation of the abdomen is always initiated away from the site of any pain. Sharp pain with rapid removal of your fingers is called rebound tenderness and suggests peritoneal irritability. A rectal examination may be performed to determine rectal tone, character of any stool, and presence of blood.

Genitourinary System

Urinary disorders can be identified by the patient's own subjective interpretation (e.g., changes in output, voiding pattern, location of pain). Obtaining a urine sample for analysis can validate the nurse's suspicions. Gross visual examination for color, clarity, and amount should be done before urine is sent to the laboratory. Palpation of the kidneys may reveal costal vertebral tenderness, structural asymmetry, or the presence of masses.

Female patients, particularly those of reproductive age, warrant additional assessment for a broad spectrum of complaints. One should always consider the possibility of an unknown pregnancy and take a careful menstrual history, in-

cluding use of contraceptives. If the patient is pregnant, fetal heart tones are assessed for presence, location, and rate. When a woman has a specific genital concern, a vaginal exam is indicated. Any discharge or bleeding should be noted and described by character and amount.

Males should be assessed for problems specific to their genitourinary anatomy, including presence of a slow stream, inability to void, penile discharge, or warts.

Musculoskeletal System

Most problems with bones, joints, and muscles are associated with trauma. The skilled clinician, however, considers other possibilities including infectious, degenerative, nutritional, neurologic, and cardiac etiologies. Observation often provides critical data, such as deformity, redness, and swelling. Any effects of the patient's problem on activity and movement must be considered, and range of motion should be compared with normal standards. Other concerns include the impact on distal circulation and sensory changes. Figure 9-3 shows normal movement for various joints.

Integumentary System

The skin is the largest organ in the body and is located externally, so it is an excellent mirror of physiologic changes within the body. Assessment includes breaks in integrity, temperature, turgor, and the presence of rashes or perspiration. Various changes in pigmentation offer clues to patient problems (Table 9-8).

Endocrine System

The endocrine system affects most, if not all, body systems. Complaints most commonly associated with endocrine disorders include fatigue and weakness, weight changes, polyuria and polydipsia, mental status changes, and sexual abnormalities. The focused survey should target the specific presenting complaint. See Chapter 39 for additional discussion.

Hematologic System

Signs of bleeding disorders include easy bruising and ecchymosis, spontaneous bleeding without an identifiable cause, bleeding from multiple sites, evidence of prior bleeding, petechiae, and anemia. Most signs are identified in a variety of other body systems. A detailed history may reveal concurrent diseases or conditions, previous surgeries or illness, medications, hereditary factors, or certain social behaviors (e.g., stress, alcohol, smoking) as potential causes of abnormal bleeding. Laboratory values are key to confirming the cause.

Immune System

Exposure to infectious materials can lead to many different outcomes. Key assessment data include history of immu-

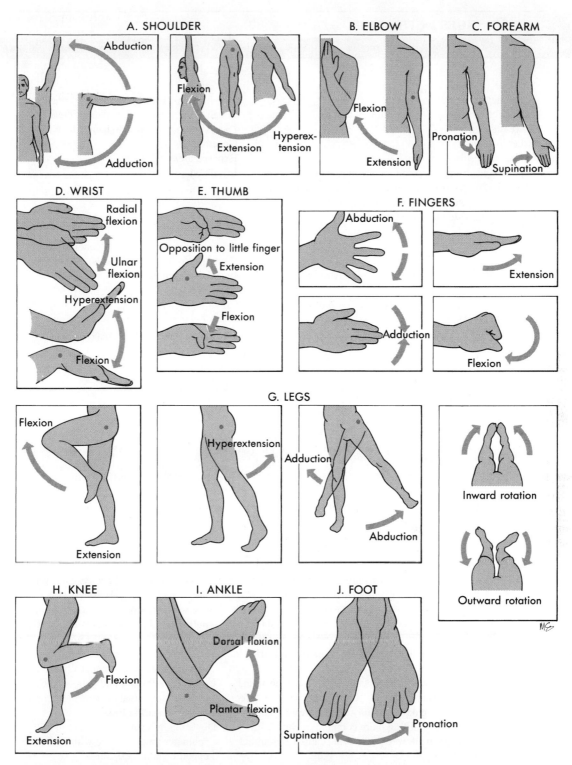

FIGURE 9-3   Range of motion, standards for mobility. **A** to **F,** Upper extremities. **G** to **J,** Lower extremities. (From Beare P, Myers J: *Adult health nursing,* ed 3, St. Louis, 1998, Mosby.)

nizations, prior disease history, and known exposures (including source and time frame). Fever is often an indicator that an infectious process is present; however, infection can occur without an elevated temperature. Because of the lymphatic system's role in fighting disease, lymph nodes can be tender and enlarged.

AGE-SPECIFIC ASSESSMENT

Depending on patient age, variations in assessment can be anticipated. Some of these are summarized in Table 9-9. Attention to these variables can enhance the assessment process and optimize patient outcomes. Refer to

Table 9-8   COLOR CHANGES IN THE SKIN

COLOR	CAUSE	LOCATION
Brown	Generic	Generalized
	Sunlight	Exposed areas
	Pregnancy	Localized (exposed areas, palmar creases)
	Addison's disease and some pituitary tumors	Localized (exposed areas, palmar creases) or generalized
Reddish	Polycythemia	Face, conjunctiva, mouth, hands, feet
	Excessive heat	Generalized
	Sunburn, thermal burn	Exposed areas
	Increased visibility of normal oxyhemoglobin caused by vasodilation from fever, blushing, alcohol, inflammation	Localized
	Decreased oxygen use in skin, as in cold exposure	
	Carbon monoxide poisoning	
Yellow	Increased bilirubinemia caused by liver disease, red cell hemolysis	Exposed areas
		Sclera in initial stages, then generalized
Blue	Hypoxemia	Central (lips, tongue, nailbeds)
	Decreased flow to skin because of anxiety or cold	Localized, peripheral
		Central
	Abnormal hemoglobin from combination with methylene or sulfa drugs	
Pale or white	Obstructive, hemorrhagic, distributive, or cardiogenic shock	Generalized
	Renal failure	Generalized
	Fear or pain	Generalized and self-limiting

Table 9-9   AGE-SPECIFIC ASSESSMENT CONSIDERATIONS

ASSESSMENT PARAMETER	PEDIATRIC	GERIATRIC
History	Consider mother's health during pregnancy; parent-child interactions; developmental level; childhood diseases; child unable to give pertinent data	May be influenced by patient's attitudes about aging; may respond slowly to questions; may be influenced by deterioration of the senses
Vital signs	Faster heart and respiratory rates; blood pressure approximately $70 + (2 \times age\ in\ years)\ 2$ mm Hg; prone to hypothermia	Cardiac irregularities may be a normal variable; influenced by many medications; prone to hypothermia
Cardiovascular	Potential congenital heart problems; murmur and third heart sound may be normal variants	Cardiac output at rest decreases; development of coronary artery disease; heart less able to adapt to stress
Respiratory	Infants are obligate nose breathers; abdominal breathing until age 6 or 7; more susceptible to respiratory infections; airway smaller and more easily occluded	Increased anteroposterior chest diameter; decreased pulmonary function; decreased surface area for gas exchange
Neurologic	Must consider developmental stage; use pediatric coma scale	Degenerative changes; nerve transmission slows; may be affected by changes in other systems
Head, ears, eyes, nose, and throat	20/20 visual acuity not obtained until age 7; anatomic differences in eustachian tube predispose to ear infection; hearing develops fully at age 5 years	Conjunctiva thinner and yellow; arcus senilis may appear, pupil smaller; lens loses transparency; prone to hearing loss
Gastrointestinal	Abdominal guarding more common in child with pain; air swallowed with crying causes abdominal distension	Digestion, gastrointestinal tract motility, and anal sphincter tone decrease with age; prone to loss of appetite and constipation
Genitourinary	Ability to control urination between 2 and 3 years old; consider age of puberty	Renal function decreases after age 40; incomplete bladder emptying
Musculoskeletal	Bones flexible—greenstick fractures; subluxation common	Decreased muscle mass; prone to fractures; degenerative joint disease
Integumentary	Diaper rash; susceptible to contact dermatitis	Decreased mobility leads to stasis dermatitis and ulcers
Endocrine	Growth hormone abnormalities	Thyroid disorders
Hematopoietic	Anemias, leukemias, clotting disorders during childhood	Vitamin B_{12} absorption decreased; reduced hemoglobin and hematocrit
Immune	Passive immunity at birth	Decreased antibody response

specific chapters in this book on pediatric and geriatric emergencies.

SUMMARY

This chapter discusses essential elements of nursing assessment in the ED: purpose, tools, and components of the physical examination. Priority setting through knowledgeable assessment and appropriate intervention contributes significantly to decreasing mortality and morbidity. This is particularly true for the early moments of the patient's visit, but it is also valid for the patient's entire stay in the ED.

Nursing assessment may be brief and confined to a narrow focus or may be a reasonably rapid and efficient evaluation of all systems affected by the current illness or injury. The extent of evaluation is the decision of the emergency nurse based on the patient's condition at that time, chief complaint, and environmental factors. Regardless of the extent of this evaluation, a systematic approach to patient assessment is essential for the best patient care possible.

Suggested Reading

Best RE: Evaluation of a child with altered mental status, *Emerg Office Pediatrics* 12(4):137, 1999.

Cummins RO et al: Guidelines 2000 for cardiopulmonary resuscitation and emergency cardiovascular care: international consensus on science, *Currents Emerg Cardiovascular Care* 11(3):1, 2000.

Jacobs BB, Hoyt KS: *Trauma nursing core course,* ed 5, Chicago, 2000, Emergency Nurses Association.

Jordan KS: *Emergency nursing core curriculum,* ed 5, Philadelphia, 2000, WB Saunders.

Meade DM, Stein L: Follow the signs—patient assessment, *Emerg Med Serv* 26(11):62, 1997.

Perry AG, Potter PA: *Clinical nursing skills and techniques,* ed 4, St. Louis, 1998, Mosby.

Sheehy SB: *Mosby's manual of emergency care,* ed 4, St. Louis, 1995, Mosby.

Werfel PA: The gentle art of pediatric assessment, *JEMS* 23(3):58, 1998.

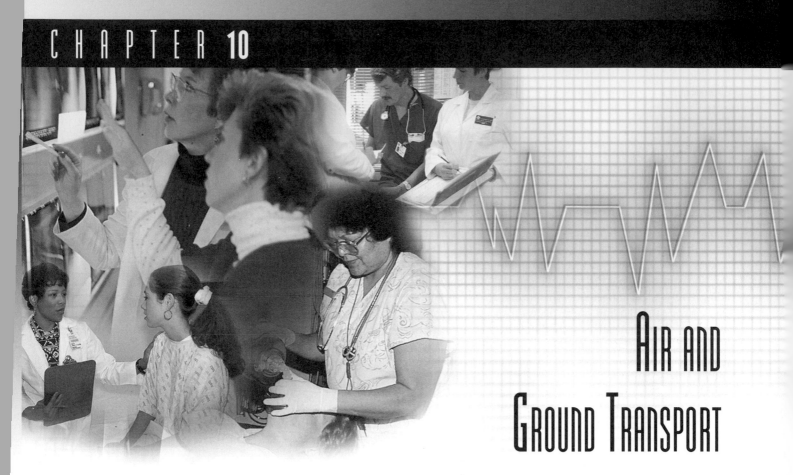

CHAPTER 10

AIR AND GROUND TRANSPORT

SUSAN LAZEAR

Transport of patients, by air or ground, is a unique aspect of emergency nursing. Emergency nurses may be involved in the actual transport or with patient preparation and stabilization before transport. Regardless of role, the emergency nurse must be familiar with (1) how the practice of nursing and medicine differ in the transport environment, (2) how transport affects the patient, (3) equipment used in moving vehicles, (4) communication issues related to transport, and (5) relevant local, state, and federal regulations related to air and ground transport.

As transport systems have developed, so has transport nursing. Transport teams are staffed with a mix of personnel including nurses, physicians, paramedics, respiratory therapists, and emergency medical technicians (EMTs). Transport vehicles include modular and van-type ground ambulances, pressurized and nonpressurized aircraft, and helicopters. The focus of this chapter is the air and ground transport of patients. Prehospital care issues are addressed as they relate to transport.

Transferring patients from one location to another is not a new concept. Throughout the ages, soldiers on the battlefield have been transported in all types of moving conveyances. Military needs provided the impetus for aeromedical evacuation operations. The first patients transported by air were flown in hot air balloons during the Prussian siege

of Paris in 1870. During the 1960s and 1970s, Congress enacted numerous pieces of legislation addressing emergency medical care and transport. As recently as 1995, the Emergency Medical Treatment and Active Labor Act (EMTALA) was established to clarify guidelines for patient transfer. Emergency nurses are an integral part of the transport system—stabilizing patients before transport, providing care during transport, and ensuring patient safety throughout the transport process.

TYPES OF TRANSPORT

Patient transport occurs in two distinct environments: on the ground by ambulance or in the air by a rotor-wing vehicle (helicopter) or fixed-wing vehicle (airplane). Air and ground transport have both advantages and disadvantages; therefore, an informed decision to use air or ground transport must be made on the basis of many factors, such as out-of-hospital time, weather, terrain, work space, equipment, personnel, and proximity of a landing site.

Ground transport is most often accomplished using a modular type vehicle that can easily accommodate two supine patients and a full crew. Access to the patient is excellent, and advanced life support (ALS) measures can be easily performed. These vehicles can also accommodate larger pieces of equipment such as infant isolettes, ventilators, and intraaortic balloon pumps. The level of care during transport varies with training level of transport personnel,

This chapter is dedicated to the memory of Marna Bloom Fleetwood, RN, and Amy Riebe, RN, MN, who lost their lives on September 11, 1995 while performing a job they loved and excelled in—transporting patients.

from basic life support (BLS) to ALS. In choosing a transport vehicle, the referring physician must remember that, legally, quality of care cannot diminish during the transport.

Ground transport is used in large urban areas with short transport times. Many rural areas have long ground transport times but do not always have the luxury of choosing between ground and air transport. Proliferation of air medical services into rural communities is making this choice a reality for many areas.

Adverse weather conditions influence the transport decision. When roads are impassable, air transport is usually the only alternative. Conversely, when weather has grounded air transport vehicles, ground transport is the only option. Another important transport consideration is transit time. For many critically ill or injured patients, the shorter the out-of-hospital time the better the patient's chance for survival. Finally, choice of a transport vehicle depends on needs of the community. Some isolated rural areas have only one ground ambulance for a largely scattered population base. If this vehicle is taken out of service for an interfacility transport, the community is left without coverage for the duration of the transport.

Air transport should not be chosen indiscriminately. It has inherent dangers and is costly. Many third-party providers withhold reimbursement for flights considered nonemergent. Air medical transport should be considered an adjunct to, and not a replacement for, ground-based services. The advantage of fixed-wing transport is the ability to travel long distances at speeds greater than 250 mph. Care is provided in a pressurized cabin with sophisticated on-board medical equipment. Many fixed-wing aircraft can transport multiple patients. In some instances, family members are allowed to accompany the patient. All-weather navigational equipment allows for transfer during inclement weather. Fixed-wing transport requires suitable airfields to ensure safety of the crew and patient. Accessibility to such fields may be a problem in isolated areas.

Rotor-wing vehicles provide rapid point-to-point transport. Helicopters can reach most areas, bypassing difficult terrain. Landing zones can be made at or near the patient to prevent lengthy ground transport time. Most helicopters operate within 150 miles of their base station to allow routine flights without refueling. One disadvantage of helicopters is that their use depends on minimum weather conditions, without which flights can be delayed or canceled. Helicopter cabin size and configuration can restrict access to the patient and limit in-flight interventions. Weight limitations restrict the number of passengers and amount of equipment on board. When transferring by rotor-wing vehicles, comprehensive patient stabilization is required before departure.

TRANSPORT PROCESS

TRANSPORT REGULATIONS

Local, state, and federal regulations affect patient transport in the air and on the ground. Emergency nurses facilitating a patient transfer must be aware of these regulations in terms of choice of transport vehicle. Regulations also specify the emergency nurse's legal responsibilities before, during, and at completion of the transport.

Ground ambulance regulations are developed by each state, usually by the Department (Office) of Emergency Medical Services. Regulations must meet minimum standards outlined in federal regulations (i.e., equipment, personnel, licensure); however, state laws usually exceed these minimum standards. These laws vary significantly from state to state in many aspects. Ambulance capabilities range from BLS to advanced critical care capabilities. Personnel and equipment vary with services rendered. An emergency nurse preparing a patient for transport must assess the patient's needs during transport and then participate in choosing the most appropriate type of transportation for that patient.

Air transport is regulated by the Department of Transportation's Federal Aviation Administration (FAA) and must meet requirements of Part 135 operation. Regulations stipulate qualifications for the pilot-in-command and other flight crew members, maintenance requirements, and aviation management. States may require a transport service to meet minimum requirements of an air ambulance to achieve ambulance licensure in their particular state. Voluntary accreditation, available through the Commission on Accreditation of Air Medical Services, is based on a program's compliance with patient care and safety standards.

Federal regulations for patient transport were first stipulated in 1985 as part of the Consolidated Omnibus Reconciliation Act (COBRA) and subsequently rewritten as EMTALA in 1995. EMTALA states that all patients should have equal access to care and requires hospitals to ensure that proper care is provided. If a hospital cannot provide the care that the patient requires, the patient must be transferred to an appropriate facility. Specific EMTALA mandates for an appropriate transfer are summarized in Box 10-1. The emergency nurse shares responsibility for adherence to these regulations.

Nurses participating in air transport must be cognizant of federal aviation regulations concerning in-flight safety and emergency procedures. The pilot in command of the aircraft is solely empowered with responsibility for safety of the

---

BOX 10-1 EMERGENCY MEDICAL TREATMENT AND ACTIVE LABOR ACT MANDATES FOR APPROPRIATE TRANSFERS[1]

The physician must certify in writing that benefits of transfer outweigh the risks.

The transferring hospital treats the patient within its capacity to minimize patient risk.

The receiving facility accepts the patient and provides appropriate medical treatment.

Copies of all medical records, including treatment, certification, and consents, accompany the patient.

Qualified personnel and appropriate transportation equipment are used for the transfer.

transport, whereas transport personnel are charged with providing the patient with appropriate medical treatment.

Prehospital Transport

In most parts of the country, prehospital transport can be initiated by citizens through the 911 emergency access number. Sophisticated prehospital emergency medical services (EMS) provide patient transport to the nearest appropriate medical care facility. Emergency nurses may function as prehospital care providers, but their capacity to do so varies from state to state. Ground transport can also be initiated for interfacility transport of patients with medical needs that exceed the capabilities of the local hospital.

Helicopters are an integral part of prehospital transport; however, access is generally limited to medically trained personnel in the field. In 1992, the National Association of Emergency Medical Services Physicians (NAEMSP) developed guidelines for helicopter scene response that assist prehospital care providers in determining when a helicopter is appropriate. However, each EMS community is unique, so these recommendations must be adapted to meet the needs of each patient population.

Interfacility Transfers

Every emergency nurse is occasionally involved with organizing and implementing an interfacility transfer. Effective organization includes assessment of the referring facility's capabilities, understanding the receiving facility's capabilities, and an in-depth knowledge of available EMS and transport systems. Implementation of the transport process is expedited if this knowledge is part of a proactive referral strategy developed well in advance. Box 10-2 highlights components of an interfacility transfer.

Development of transfer strategies begins with objective assessment of the referring institution's personnel and facilities. Qualifications and availability of physicians and nurses to care for all patients who come to the emergency department (ED) must be examined. Specific areas that should be considered include the intensive care unit; the operating room; and pediatric, obstetric, neonatal, and psychiatric units. Ability to perform advanced diagnostic testing and provide adequate blood and blood products must also be analyzed. All these factors influence the level of care available to sick or injured patients.

Understanding the capabilities of the receiving institution is a part of the responsibility of the referring institution. Trauma patients are best cared for in centers designated by the American College of Surgeons Committee on Trauma as trauma hospitals. High-risk neonates benefit from care in a neonatal intensive care unit. Other areas of advanced specialized care include burn centers, limb replantation centers, pediatric centers, high-risk obstetric centers, open heart centers, and hyperbaric centers.

The act of transferring a patient from one facility to another should be well documented and fall within legal guidelines identified by each institution. These guidelines must ensure that federal mandates (i.e., EMTALA) have been met. If a patient is unable to give consent because of his or her medical condition, and no family is located, a patient may be transferred under implied consent law. EMTALA assumes that the patient or the family would provide consent if able. A concentrated effort must be made to locate family members before this type of consent is invoked.

Stabilization

Field stabilization of the patient depends on level of training of prehospital care providers. Care can range from basic stabilization to ALS instituted by highly trained paramedics, nurses, or physicians. Regardless of training, management of the airway, breathing, and circulation (ABCs) is paramount, and must be monitored throughout the transfer. Preparation for interfacility transfer of an ill or injured patient depends on the specific illness, injury, age, and circumstances. Potential problems during transport must be identified before departure, and proper interventions undertaken at the referring hospital.

Airway and Breathing

Airway patency during transport is of greatest importance. Potential airway compromise must be anticipated before transport so that proper interventions can be accomplished under controlled circumstances rather than during transport. Endotracheal intubation should be considered in patients who might aspirate, have difficulty with chest expansion, or need ventilatory support (e.g., patients with altered level of consciousness, facial fractures, epiglottitis, inhalation burns). Patients with chest wall injury, spinal cord injury, or neurologic dysfunction may also require ventilatory assistance. Chest tube placement for a possible pneumothorax or hemothorax should be done before transport. A closed drainage system or flutter valve should be in place to avoid recurrence of a pneumothorax. This is critical for transports in unpressurized helicopters and fixed-wing aircraft.

Hemodynamic Stabilization

Interventions to maintain an adequate pulse rate and blood pressure should be initiated before transport. These include control of bleeding, correction of hypovolemia, insertion of

Box 10-2	COMPONENTS OF AN INTERFACILITY TRANSFER

Physician-to-physician communication.
Communication between the transferring facility personnel and the receiving facility personnel.
Selection of appropriate transport vehicle and personnel.
Consent for transfer signed by the patient or relative.
Stabilization to limit effects of transport.
Documentation before, during, and on completion of the transport.

a urinary catheter, and institution of cardiac monitoring. Control of external bleeding sites with pressure or wound closure may be necessary. Splints for long-bone fractures and the pneumatic antishock garment (PASG) for pelvic injuries (if not contraindicated) stabilize fractures and control bleeding. Applying the PASG before loading the patient and inflating the garment as needed is preferable to application in a moving vehicle. Air pressure in the PASG should be monitored carefully during flight—air volume increases with altitude increases.

Proper intravenous (IV) access is needed to replace fluid loss. Large-bore IV cannulas (14-gauge or 16-gauge peripherally or 8.5-gauge subclavian) with blood or trauma tubing provide rapid fluid resuscitation routes. Presence of two or more IV access points during transport obviates the need for restart in a moving vehicle. Use of plastic IV bags for fluid allows use of pressure bags if required. Blood replacement products prepared for transport and placed in a cooler may accompany the patient.

Patients requiring fluid management should have a bladder catheter (if not contraindicated) attached to a urometer to properly measure urinary output. In addition to measuring output, bladder drainage decreases patient discomfort during a long transport.

The cardiac status of the patient must be determined before transport. An electrocardiogram and rhythm strip should be obtained before departure to determine the need for any intervention before transport. Continuous monitoring should take place during transport.

Central Nervous System Stabilization

All attempts should be made to stabilize the patient's neurologic condition (i.e., maintain normal intracranial pressure, control seizure activity, and preserve integrity of the spinal cord).

Maintenance of cerebral perfusion pressure in the head-injured patient includes measures to control increased intracranial pressure. Long-standing therapeutics, which include hyperventilation, elevation of the patient's head if the spine is clear, and limited fluid administration, are now under significant scrutiny by the medical community. Recent studies suggest that hyperventilation may actually worsen cerebral ischemia, and current recommendations suggest maintaining the $PaCO_2$ at 35 mm Hg. The receiving neurologist should be consulted to determine current therapeutics, such as medications (i.e., mannitol, sedation, paralytics), fluid resuscitation, patient position, and ventilation regimen.

Antiseizure medications should be used if a patient has seizure activity. Prophylactic medications to reduce risk of seizures during transport should be determined during the physician-to-physician consultation.

A patient with a suspected or documented spinal cord injury should be placed in a rigid cervical collar and then secured on a long spine board (LSB) with head blocks to prevent movement of the spinal column. Administration of methylprednisolone for spinal cord injury should be initiated before transfer and continued throughout the transport

according to established time dosage guidelines. Treatment should begin within 8 hours of injury. Long transport times are not uncommon, and preventive measures should be undertaken to reduce risk of pressure sore development.

Musculoskeletal Stabilization

Care of the patient with musculoskeletal injuries should include prevention of blood loss, fracture immobilization, wound care, and administration of medications such as pain medications or antibiotics.

Splints should permit assessment of distal pulses during transport. Air splints respond to pressure changes during air transport and should not be used in this environment. Pelvic fractures may be stabilized with a PASG and by placing the patient on an LSB. Traction splints for femur fractures can be used in transport; however, length of the splint must be kept to a minimum so that the transport vehicle door can be closed properly. Free-swinging traction weights are avoided in transport because of risk to medical crew members.

Patients transferred for limb replantation need special care. The amputated part should be preserved by wrapping it in saline-moistened gauze and placing it in a plastic bag. The plastic bag should be placed in a sealed container on ice inside a cooler. The part should not be allowed to freeze—this causes tissue destruction and prevents replantation.

Wound care before transport may be limited to control of bleeding, initial cleansing, and the application of a sterile dressing. Wounds that will be sutured at the receiving facility should be kept moist with saline dressings to ensure tissue viability. Prophylactic antibiotics for open fractures may be ordered to reduce risk of osteomyelitis.

Burn care includes calculation of the percentage of body surface area burned and fluid resuscitation (see Chapter 27). Fluid resuscitation must be continued throughout transport. The transport team must ensure that an adequate supply of fluid is available in the transport vehicle. Burns should be dressed with dry sterile dressings in accordance with local burn center protocols. Application of topical antibiotics is generally avoided. Constricting rings, necklaces, and clothing should be removed. If circulation impairment is present, escharotomy should be performed before transport.

Emotional Stabilization and Psychosocial Support

The patient who will be transferred has many physical and psychologic needs. Nurses can address these needs by recognizing the patient's fears and answering any questions.

Removing patients from home, family, and a familiar environment increases patient stress. Patients may have a fear of flying (if transported by air), fear of dying, and anger, which is often directed at the referring hospital for being unable to care for them. The need for transport is often translated in a patient's mind to mean he or she is dying. Stressors increase the patient's anxiety, causing increased heart rate and respiratory rate, diaphoresis, nausea, vomiting, and a general worsening of condition.

Personnel from the referring hospital and the transport crew should work together to alleviate the patient's fears by thoroughly explaining all procedures, noises, and reasons for the transport. A team member should interact with family members and include the family in all explanations. Transport personnel should work to instill confidence in the patient concerning the referring hospital. This confidence is important. If the patient survives, he or she will be returning to the home community and will be cared for by the referring hospital in the future.

The patient's family also has tremendous fears. If the patient is acutely ill or injured, this interaction may be the last they have with their loved one. The family may not understand the need for the transport. Time must be taken to explain the necessity for immediate transfer. The family may also have what is called the "Mecca syndrome," an inflated idea of what can be done for the patient at the receiving facility. The family may believe the receiving hospital will save the life of a patient, when in fact that may not happen.

A family member may want to accompany the patient. In helicopter transports, this possibility is usually out of the question because of space and weight limitations. However, depending on the type of ground ambulance or fixed-wing aircraft, room may be available for a family member. Transport personnel should make the decision whether to allow the family member to come with the patient during a ground transport, but the final decision in air transport is the responsibility of the pilot in command. If the patient's condition deteriorates during flight, the family member has no place to go, and must watch all interventions. On the other hand, the family member's presence may alleviate some of the patient's anxiety, especially when the patient is a child. The decision should not be made until the time of the transport, because the patient's condition may change and promises cannot always be kept.

To alleviate family anxiety, provide as much information as possible about the receiving hospital. Maps, plans for patient admission, and a telephone contact gives them some direction after the patient departs. The family should be informed of the estimated length of transport and expected time of arrival at the receiving hospital. This time should be calculated taking into consideration weather, unexpected delays, changes in time zone, and other factors. Overestimation of time is always best—if the transport is completed sooner than anticipated, the family will feel relief. On the other hand, if the transport takes longer than expected, the family may fear outcome of the transport itself.

One of the last things that should be done before departure is to allow the family time with the patient. The last remarks and the last kiss goodbye may be the most important few minutes of the transport.

Baseline Diagnostic Studies

Studies necessary for stabilization depend on severity and type of illness or injury. Each situation has different priorities. Baseline studies needed to make proper decisions regarding transfer should be performed while the transfer is being arranged. In severely injured patients, only tests that affect ABCs should be performed.

The American College of Surgeons Committee on Trauma recommends performing the following studies, as time permits:

- Radiographs of the cervical spine, chest, pelvis, and any injured extremity
- Laboratory tests including hemoglobin, hematocrit, arterial blood gases, urinalysis, toxicology screens, blood alcohol content, and blood typing and cross-matching
- Electrocardiogram

Copies of all patient data and radiographs should be properly labeled and sent with the patient. Samples of peritoneal fluid, blood, and spinal fluid should accompany the patient when indicated. Laboratory analysis not completed at the time of transfer should be called or sent by fax to the receiving center.

Documentation

Documentation of the transfer is essential. It confirms adherence to legal mandates, ensures compliance with established standards of care, and protects the caregiver in potential litigious situations. Documentation of prehospital care should include mechanism of injury, time of injury, time of EMS arrival, care provided in the field and during transport, and protocols or orders used during transfer. Documentation related to interfacility transfer includes the prehospital record, the ED record, and documentation of care during the transfer. Box 10-3 summarizes documentation requirements specific to interfacility transfer.

Care During Transport

Assessment and treatment to maintain patient stability during transport is essential. Use of a pulse oximeter and cardiac monitor to monitor oxygenation, pulse rate, and rhythm are extremely beneficial. An ultrasound Doppler and stethoscope are useful when auscultation is difficult. The patient's level of consciousness should be monitored and recorded. Fluid intake and urinary output should also be documented.

Transport personnel should be prepared to implement interventions to maintain patient stability. Protocols and physician orders regarding specific interventions clarify ex-

---

Box 10-3 DOCUMENTATION REQUIREMENTS FOR AN INTERFACILITY TRANSFER

Prehospital care record
Emergency department medical record
Medical history
Lab results
Copies of x-rays
Transfer record
Protocols or orders used during transfer
Signed transfer consent form
Family information including contact person
Contact information at referring hospital

pectations for the transporting team. Interventions that may be needed during transport include securing the airway, suctioning, administering fluids, performing emergency needle thoracotomy, administering medications, and performing ALS measures. In unforeseen emergencies when sophisticated medical equipment and personnel are critical, diversion to a closer facility may be necessary. The location of these facilities should be identified before transport to prevent unnecessary delays.

All care during transport should be documented. A copy of the transport form should be inserted in the patient's chart at the receiving facility. Documentation should include patient assessment, interventions, and the patient's response to these interventions. Unusual events or effects of the transport on patient condition should also be noted.

Communication

Effective communication is the glue that holds the entire transport process together. Each component is essential and dependent on the others. When a call is placed to an emergency operations center, the dispatcher notifies appropriate units to respond. Radio communication is established, and pertinent information is transmitted. Depending on severity and local protocols, the mobile unit can be directly linked to the medical command center or the base station at the receiving hospital. Transmission of pertinent data is necessary so the transport team can receive specific protocols for intervention.

During air transport by helicopter or airplane, the medical crew may be out of range of its base station. However, at no time is the aircraft out of touch with a ground station. The flight team intervenes according to standard protocols at the discretion of flight team members. In the event of an emergency, the pilot in command can contact the ground station and ask to be patched through to medical control of the flight program.

Successful communication includes a complete loop in which all parties are notified and aware of the patient's status. This begins with the physician-to-physician contact that establishes the transport process. Communication is ongoing and should focus on essential information for the transporting and receiving personnel.

Communication techniques, radio codes, and communication technology are too extensive to be included here. The reader is referred to a number of excellent references in the Suggested Readings if more in-depth information is desired. Regardless of technology used, every effort should be made to protect patient confidentiality during any communication. Use of patient names or other identifying factors is discouraged. A standard reporting format may be developed by the transport program to ensure quality assurance for each communication.

Medical Control

Organization of medical control varies from system to system. Online medical control is direct communication be-

tween transport personnel and the physician (or physician-surrogate) via radio or telephone for the purpose of providing orders for patient care. Offline medical control includes those administrative functions necessary to ensure quality of care. Each medical control officer is a physician who is directly responsible for care provided in transport. It is the medical control officer's responsibility to ensure proper training, orientation, and continuing education for those people working under their control.

Transfer of Care

While the patient is in transit, the referring and receiving facilities share responsibility for care of the patient. Only after arrival at the receiving facility is the referring hospital's legal responsibility terminated. Time of arrival at the receiving hospital should be noted in the copy of the chart that remains at the referring facility.

GROUND TRANSPORT

Safety

All transport personnel must develop a positive attitude and a strict policy toward personal safety. Wearing seat belts or other restraining devices should be the first priority. Patient care may be limited during times of high risk to the medical care provider. Providers should consider the risks of potential hazards and take appropriate precautions. Occupational Safety and Health Administration standards regulate minimal requirements for use of protective clothing. Ideal body protection is provided by approved helmets, safety goggles, reinforced boots, and gloves. Some states mandate specific equipment requirements. In some areas, voluntary ambulance specification criteria establish minimum equipment standards.

The risk of infectious disease is high in the prehospital care environment. Barrier protection should be used at all times. Bag-valve masks and pocket masks provide effective ventilation. The incidence of *Mycobacterium tuberculosis* infection is increasing so medical personnel should take every precaution to reduce their risk of exposure. Prehospital care providers also have an obligation to reduce risk of exposure to infectious diseases to other emergency care providers through careful handling of wounds, dressings, and proper disposal of needles and other disposable equipment.

Patient safety is also a priority. Patients must be secured to the stretcher, then the stretcher should be secured to the transport vehicle. Stabilization measures should be undertaken to ensure patient safety throughout the transfer, including use of an LSB, head blocks, restraining belts, and tape.

Personnel

Level of care provided in ground transport depends on level of training for the health care provider. Jurisdiction over these individuals is delegated to the state. However, federal legislation mandates certain minimum levels of care.

Basic EMTs provide BLS. Their basic level of training consists of 100 hours of classroom and field training with 10 hours of in-hospital observation. The EMT may receive additional training in administration of select drugs, use of advanced airway skills, and cardiac defibrillation. People with additional certification may be identified by the following titles: EMT-intermediate, EMT I to VI, cardiac rescue technician, EMT-advanced, EMT-defibrillator, EMT-cardiac, and others. These advanced trained EMTs can provide advanced care.

The EMT-paramedic must complete at least 212 hours of didactic training and 200 hours of hospital-based clinical rotations. Many training programs double this requirement. With successful completion of written and practical examinations, the EMT can be state certified as a paramedic for 2 to 4 years. Paramedics are used extensively in urban emergency medical care systems and are becoming increasingly common in rural areas. Paramedics perform ALS measures and are considered the foundation of ALS care in the prehospital care environment.

Registered nurses are also found in ground transport programs. Training programs for nurses are essentially nonexistent; thus many nurses turn to paramedic training programs to achieve certification. In 1995 the Emergency Nurses Association revised the National Standards Guidelines for Prehospital Nursing Curriculum. These guidelines intend to integrate the nurse's prior education and clinical experience with knowledge and skills needed in the prehospital arena. Although the number of registered nurses working in prehospital care environment remains low, it is increasing. These nurses continually push for recognition of their contribution to emergency care.

Equipment

Statutory law regulates equipment required in ground ambulances. The equipment listed in Box 10-4 is the minimum required for maintaining stability in the ill or injured patient during transport. Medical crew members must be familiar with operation of equipment in the vehicle and any extra equipment brought to provide care for a particular patient. Crew members must also ensure an adequate supply of disposable equipment is available to last throughout the transport, taking into consideration possible delays that may extend the projected transport time. Oxygen must be available for the duration of the transfer. Table 10-1 shows duration of cylinder flow for the two most common sizes of oxygen cylinders.

AIR TRANSPORT

FLIGHT PHYSIOLOGY

Exposure to environmental factors occurs during air transport of patients. Problems encountered depend on changes in atmospheric conditions, vehicle configurations, motion of

---

Box 10-4	**EQUIPMENT NEEDED FOR TRANSPORT**

AIRWAYS

Nasal airway adjuncts
Oropharyngeal airway adjuncts
Endotracheal or nasotracheal tubes

OXYGEN DELIVERY SYSTEM

Oxygen
Oxygen tubing
Oxygen cannulas
Oxygen masks
Bag-valve-mask device
Demand valve
Ventilator
Pulse oximeter

SUCTION EQUIPMENT

Suction catheters
Catheter-tip syringe for gastric tube

INTRAVENOUS EQUIPMENT

IV fluids, pump, and tubing
IV restart equipment
Pressure infusion bag

CARDIAC MONITORING AND RESUSCITATION EQUIPMENT

Cardiac monitor and defibrillator
Defibrillator pads
Recording paper

DOPPLER DEVICE OR SENSITIVE STETHOSCOPE

EMERGENCY MEDICATIONS

RESTRAINTS

IV, Intravenous.

---

the aircraft, and the patient's condition. Some of these can be detrimental to the patient, but with proper nursing care before and during transport, these harmful effects can be minimized or eliminated.

Atmospheric changes occur when the aircraft's altitude changes. Ascending into the atmosphere from sea level causes a decrease in atmospheric pressure, which in turn causes a decrease in the partial pressure of gases, temperature, and expansion of gases. The opposite occurs during descent. Four problems can develop in transport as a result of changes in atmospheric pressure: hypoxia, gas expansion, dehydration, and decreased temperature. Many of these effects are minimal unless the change in altitude is greater than 5000 feet.

Fixed-wing and rotary-wing vehicles are designed according to different principles. Most fixed-wing aircraft used in patient transport are pressurized, which allows for a comfortable cabin atmosphere when flying at high attitudes.

Table 10-1 **DURATION OF CYLINDER FLOW**							
CYLINDER	**2 L/MIN**	**4 L/MIN**	**6 L/MIN**	**8 L/MIN**	**10 L/MIN**	**12 L/MIN**	**15 L/MIN**
E	5.1 hr	2.5 hr	1.7 hr	1.2 hr	1.0 hr	0.8 hr	0.6 hr
H	56 hr	28 hr	18.5 hr	14 hr	11 hr	9.2 hr	7.2 hr

Pressurization differentials allow for different cabin pressures at different atmospheres. Generally, the lower the altitude at which a plane is flying, the lower the cabin pressure that can be achieved. This ability to maintain a physiologically comfortable environment within the aircraft is a benefit when transporting patients who may be affected by atmospheric changes. Although pressurization allows for flights at high altitudes, even subtle changes in the environment may be harmful to a person whose condition is severely compromised.

If the pressurization system fails, pressurization within the cabin might be lost, causing a sudden change in atmospheric pressure. This rapid decompression causes the interior of the cabin to equalize with the pressures outside the cabin, resulting in sudden and often detrimental effects on the human body: rapid loss of oxygen, sudden drop in temperature, and expansion of gas. A healthy person may be able to withstand these changes, but the person in poor health may deteriorate rapidly. Those transporting patients should be aware of these effects and do everything possible before departure to minimize complications.

Rotary-wing vehicles are not pressurized; therefore, these atmospheric changes are felt whenever the helicopter ascends and descends. As a result, patients transported by helicopter may be at greater risk than those transported by fixed-wing aircraft.

Other problems that affect patient outcomes include motion of the vehicle and constraints resulting from vehicle design.

Hypoxia

Many patients transported by air are hypoxic as a result of their condition. This hypoxic state is potentiated when changes in atmospheric pressure occur. As an aircraft ascends in altitude, the partial pressure of oxygen (PO_2) decreases, causing a decreased diffusion gradient for the oxygen molecule to cross the alveolar membrane. Table 10-2 shows the effects of altitude on PO_2.

Simple calculation of the diffusion gradient is accomplished by using the following formulas:

$$(\text{Atmospheric pressure} - \text{Water pressure}) \times (\text{Percentage of oxygen}) = PO_2$$

and

$$\text{Alveolar } PO_2 - \text{Venous } PO_2 = \text{Diffusion gradient}$$

Room air is 21% oxygen. If the patient is receiving oxygen, the fraction of inspired oxygen is used for the patient's oxygen therapy. Assuming that water pressure is equal to 47 mm Hg, the PO_2 at sea level is 150 mm Hg: $(760 - 47) \times (0.21) = 150$.

Table 10-2 **EFFECTS OF ALTITUDE ON PARTIAL PRESSURE OF AMBIENT OXYGEN**		
ALTITUDE (FT)	**ATMOSPHERIC PRESSURE**	**PARTIAL PRESSURE OF AMBIENT OXYGEN (MM HG)**
0	760	150
500	746	146
1000	733	144
1500	720	141
2000	707	138
2500	694	135
3000	681	133
3500	669	130
4000	656	128
4500	644	125
5000	632	123
5500	621	120
6000	609	118
6500	598	115
7000	586	113
8000	564	108
9000	543	104
10,000	523	100

At an altitude of 6000 feet the calculated PO_2 is 118 mm Hg: $(609 - 47) \times (0.21) = 118$ mm Hg.

The decrease in PO_2 that occurs in the respiratory tree is approximately 45 mm Hg; therefore, at the alveolar level, the PaO_2 at sea level is approximately 105 mm Hg and the PaO_2 at 6000 feet is about 73 mm Hg. The PO_2 of venous blood is approximately 40 mm Hg; therefore, the diffusion gradient at sea level is 65 mm Hg ($105 - 40$) and at 6000 feet is 22 mm Hg. Patients with disease-induced hypoxia are severely affected by this drop in diffusion gradient and are at increased risk of compromise during air medical transport. Patients at risk include those with congestive heart failure, adult respiratory distress syndrome, carbon monoxide poisoning, hypovolemic shock, inadequate amount of circulating hemoglobin, and stagnant hypoxia induced by low-flow states such as hypothermia. Altitude-induced reduction in PO_2 causes further deterioration in these patients if interventions are not performed to correct the problems related to hypoxia. Risk for hypoxia is even greater when the patient smokes.

Signs and symptoms of hypoxia include changes in vital signs, tachycardia, pupillary constriction, confusion, disorientation, and lethargy. All of these signs may be caused by a number of other illnesses and injuries, making the diagnosis of hypoxia more difficult. Astute observation of the patient is necessary to detect and correct problems of hypoxia.

Transporting patients by pressurized fixed-wing aircraft can limit complications secondary to this drop in PO_2. Most aircraft used for air transport are able to maintain a sea level cabin pressure when flying below 7000 to 10,000 feet. At higher altitudes, the cabin can be pressurized. Maximum cabin pressure altitude is generally maintained well below 9000 feet. When cabin pressures are controlled, atmospheric changes that occur are limited, controlled, and within a tolerable range.

Before the patient is transported, stabilization measures can be taken to reduce effects of atmospheric changes in oxygenation. Supplemental oxygen can be provided, and if the patient has previously required oxygen, the percentage of oxygen can be increased. This increase in oxygen delivery is prophylaxis, a temporary measure during transport. When the patient arrives at the receiving institution, oxygen can be decreased or terminated pending outcome of arterial blood gas analysis.

Properly positioning the patient combats the effects of hypoxia. Ensuring proper chest excursion by loosening chest restraints on the stretcher allows the patient to breathe easier. In certain aircraft the head of the stretcher can be elevated to an angle of at least 30 degrees; however, in many rotary-wing transports this elevation is not possible because of limited head room.

The hypovolemic patient can receive transfusions to increase hematocrit and oxygen-carrying capacity of the blood. Patients who are alert are generally anxious regarding their outcome, which increases respiratory rate and decreases oxygenation. Providing a calm environment and thoroughly explaining all procedures, noises, and equipment reduce the patient's feeling of helplessness. The case study in Box 10-5 demonstrates the effects of altitude changes on a patient.

Calculating PO_2 of patients in various environments and situations tells only part of the story. The patient described in the case study, whose cardiac history is extensive, may also be anxious about leaving his loved ones and of the final prognosis. Although he may feel most comfortable in the sitting position, he must lie flat during the transport. Assessing vital signs and level of consciousness provides the best indicator of how he is tolerating the transport. All possible interventions to improve the patient's oxygenation status should be initiated. Continuous pulse oximetry should be used to adjust oxygen therapy.

Gas Expansion

According to Boyle's law, the volume of gas is inversely proportional to its pressure. As the transport vehicle ascends, atmospheric pressure decreases and gas expands. One hundred cubic centimeters (cc) of gas at sea level expands to 130 cc at an altitude of 6000 feet, 200 cc at 18,000 feet, and 400 cc at 34,000 feet. Gas expansion is a potential problem in all transports in which the aircraft ascends, but is especially worrisome in an unpressurized fixed-wing aircraft flying above 12,000 feet.

Air is found in many places, including the pleural space when a pneumothorax is present, air splints, endotracheal

---

Box 10-5 EFFECTS OF ALTITUDE CHANGES ON A PATIENT

- A 58-year-old man requires transport from a small rural hospital to a university medical center. He has a long history of cardiac disease and is currently receiving vasopressors for blood pressure support.
- The referring hospital is located at an altitude of 500 feet, whereas the medical center is at 4000 feet. During transport the helicopter must fly over a mountain range with peaks at altitudes more than 6000 feet.
- At the referring hospital, the patient had an oxygen partial pressure (PO_2) of 150 mm Hg when breathing room air. When a nasal cannula was used, PO_2 rose to 178 mm Hg. The patient's pretransport blood gas levels during use of the nasal cannula were adequate.
- During transport, the helicopter must fly at an altitude of 6500 feet to ensure clearance of the mountains. During the time the patient is at this altitude his PO_2 will drop to 138 mm Hg if use of the nasal cannula is continued.
- To ensure that altitude-induced hypoxia does not develop, a nonrebreather mask can be applied. Use of this mask will raise the patient's PO_2 to approximately 400 mm Hg.
- At the medical center, at an altitude of 4000 feet, the patient's PO_2 when a nasal cannula is used is calculated at 152 mm Hg. This PO_2 may be inadequate for his current condition, necessitating the use of other oxygen delivery systems.

---

tube cuffs, intravenous fluid bottles, and in the PASG. Table 10-3 lists various conditions and situations in which gas can expand and nursing measures that can reduce the risk of complications.

If measures are taken during ascent to prevent gas expansion, such as removal of air from the PASG, an opposite measure must be taken during the aircraft's descent. For example, a patient with multiple trauma requires long-distance transport from a village in Alaska to a trauma center in Washington. The patient has been stabilized with the PASG before transport. As the aircraft departs from Alaska and ascends to a cruising altitude of 28,000 feet, the cabin pressure rises to approximately 8000 feet. Air volume in the PASG is now increased by at least one third. The PASG pants may now be too tight and compromise circulation to the patient's lower extremities. By monitoring the patient's blood pressure, transport personnel can decrease air volume in the garment to ensure maximal benefit. During transport, the PASG should be monitored continually for changes in pressure to detect underinflation or overinflation. As the aircraft descends for landing at the receiving airfield, the PASG should be evaluated once again for effectiveness; usually, air must be added.

Rotary-wing vehicles that fly low over flat terrain encounter few problems with gas expansion during transport. However, if transport requires traversing high-altitude areas, the aforementioned interventions are essential.

Table 10-3	EFFECTS OF GAS EXPANSION ON PATIENT CONDITION AND MEDICAL EQUIPMENT	
	COMPLICATIONS	**THERAPEUTIC INTERVENTIONS**
PATIENT CONDITION		
Pneumothorax	Air expansion within pleural cavity, causing dyspnea	Insert flutter valve, chest tube with water seal drainage
Bowel obstruction	Air expands, causing rupture	Insert nasogastric tube to suction; elevate head of bed
Plugged middle ear	Unable to equalize pressure	Valsalva maneuver in awake patient; ascend and descend slowly
Congested sinuses	Trapped air expands, causing pain	Vasoconstrictor sprays
Open skull fracture	Air in cranial cavity expands, causing herniation	Implement hyperventilation measures to reduce intracranial pressure
Colostomies, iliostomies	Air in bowel expands, causing increased motility	Insert rectal tube for decompression; change bag frequently
Gas gangrene	Air expands within tissues, leading to necrosis	Incision and drainage
Dental caries	Pain caused by air expansion	Administer local anesthetic
EQUIPMENT		
Air splints	Air expands: pressure within garment or splints increases	Decrease volume at altitude
IV bottles	Air within bottle expands: fluid does not flow	Use plastic IV bags
Endotracheal tube cuffs	Air expands, causing tracheal necrosis	Decrease volume at altitude
Urinary catheters	Air within drainage system expands: urine does not flow	Use a vent system / Irrigate catheter
Oxygen flowmeters	Flow is increased under pressure	Monitor oxygen supply frequently
Volume ventilators	Volume of gas delivered increases	Measure tidal volume

IV, Intravenous.

Dehydration

Another problem encountered during an increase in altitude is a drop in ambient humidity. Loss of humidification is magnified in a pressurized fixed-wing aircraft, because system pressurization is achieved by recycling air and removing moisture from it. Patients who are dehydrated or diaphoretic are at increased risk for dehydration and possible fluid volume deficits. Supplemental IV fluids should be administered to prevent dehydration.

Other patients affected by dehydration include mouth-breathers and those who are intubated. These patients have lost the natural respiratory humidification mechanisms, so secretions become tenacious and difficult to mobilize. Providing humidified oxygen not only prevents drying of the respiratory tree but counters the effects of hypoxia.

Decreased Temperature

As altitude increases, temperature decreases. For each 1000-foot gain in altitude, temperature drops 2° C until it reaches −55° C. During ascent, this temperature drop cools the aircraft. Although transport vehicles are heated, the fuselage becomes quite cold and radiates cold into the cabin interior. The coldest area of the aircraft is against the outside walls. This cooling, although most significant during cold-weather months, is noticeable at all times of the year.

In addition to altitude-induced temperature changes, a number of environmental conditions affect air transport of patients. Of particular importance is a drop in environmental temperature. Interhospital transports require patient movement outside the hospital, transport outside to the helipad or into an ambulance for transfer to the airfield, and subsequent transfer into the transport vehicle. The opposite occurs at the receiving end of the transfer. These multiple transfers expose the patient to changing environmental conditions, including cold weather. A patient requiring transport is less able to tolerate these stresses and can exhibit signs and symptoms of cold stress, including decreased level of consciousness, increased heart rate, and shivering. These symptoms increase the patient's oxygen demands. Mild hypoxia now worsens significantly.

Awareness of an environmental drop in temperature allows adequate stabilization before the transport. Minimizing exposure to environmental conditions is of utmost importance. The interior temperature of the transport vehicle can be controlled in accordance with the patient's needs rather than needs of the transport crew. Maintaining an adequate supply of linen and wrapping the patient in a rescue (Mylar) blanket is useful in cold environments. Caution should be used with Mylar blankets because they reflect any radiated heat back to the patient, which can lead to overheating if the patient is wrapped too tightly. A cap can be put on the patient's head to reduce radiated heat losses.

When ambient air cools, changes in temperature cause gas molecules to contract. This change in gas molecules is similar to that which occurs with a decrease in altitude, leading to subsequent gas expansion within body cavities and equipment. This effect is most notable in the PASG and air splints. When the patient is transferred from a warm hospital interior to the cold outdoors, the volume of gas within the garment decreases, and peripheral vasoconstriction effect on the venous system can decrease. As ambient temperature increases, the garment expands, causing an increase in the patient's blood pressure. Change in gas volume must be compensated for during each change in environmental conditions.

Other problems that develop with cold environments include cooling IV solutions and crystallization of medications, most notably mannitol. A patient with cold stress resulting from changes in the environment requires warm IV fluids. Solutions stored in the aircraft or solutions exposed to the environment are quite cold and must be warmed before administration. If possible, solutions should be stored in the warmest spot in the cabin. If solutions remain cold, heat packs can be wrapped around the IV bag to warm the fluid. Some transport programs employ heating pads to keep fluids warm. Drawbacks with such a system are the need for electricity to operate the pad and risk of overheating the fluid, which may render it useless. Mannitol should not be stored in an aircraft that is quite cold. Instead, it should be placed in the aircraft immediately before departure.

Acceleration and Deceleration Forces

Acceleration forces occur during takeoff and "climb-out." Blood pools in dependent areas, most commonly the lower extremities, causing fluid shifts that may not be tolerated by the severely compromised patient. Restoration of intravascular volume and proper positioning of the patient can minimize effects of these forces.

Deceleration forces occur during slowing, stopping, or rapid descent. For the patient lying head forward in an aircraft, deceleration forces cause blood to pool in the head and upper body. Pooling produces what is known as "redout" as blood rushes to the head, causing an increase in blood within the ocular cavity. Deceleration forces are most harmful to a patient with increased intracranial pressure. The phenomenon may also adversely affect a patient with congestive heart failure.

Effects of acceleration and deceleration forces vary with speed, angle, and duration. These forces are much more pronounced in a fixed-wing aircraft. In certain instances, pilots can control these effects as long as safety measures and regulations are met. If a patient is known to be severely ill or injured, transport personnel should discuss this problem with their flight crew. A slow descent is often an option. If the airfield is long enough, a longer landing roll can decrease some deceleration forces that occur as the aircraft is slowed to a stop.

Positioning of the patient is crucial to counter these forces. In many aircraft, stretcher restraints are not interchangeable; therefore, the patient must be loaded head-first into the cabin. If the patient can tolerate a head-elevated position, effects of these forces can be minimized, because fluid shifts would be centered at the core of the body rather than in the head.

Rotary-wing vehicles are also subject to acceleration and deceleration forces but to a lesser magnitude than fixed-wing aircraft. In addition to forward and rearward movement, helicopters are capable of lateral movement. Forces resulting from these movements are of little consequence. Because of confined space within the helicopter, positioning the patient to counteract these forces is usually more difficult, if not impossible. Fortunately, pilot control is much greater in the helicopter.

Motion Sickness

Changes in equilibrium caused by excessive motion can cause motion sickness. Nausea and vomiting may develop in the patient, flight crew, and transport personnel. Prophylactic premedication is the best intervention available to limit these complications.

Other causes of motion sickness include hypoxia; excessive visual stimuli, such as blinking lights on the aircraft control panel; stress; fear; unpleasant odors; heat; and poor diet. Gastric gas expansion occurring during ascent can worsen the problem. To prevent or limit these symptoms, transport personnel should provide adequate oxygenation, stare at a fixed visual reference, cool the cabin interior, attempt to limit stressors and fear, and have the patient lie in the supine position.

For crew members with motion sickness, premedication with transdermal scopolamine is the best treatment. However, these patches must be applied at least 30 minutes before departure. Because air medical transports are not usually scheduled, this preventive measure may not be possible. Other preventive measures include eating ginger cookies and using acupressure bracelets. Crew members often "recover" from motion sickness when they focus their attention on the patient; however, residual symptoms may occur after the flight.

Noise

Transport vehicles are inherently noisy. Engine noises create a constant loud hum that is not only distracting but also increases stress. Reducing extraneous noise is often impossible, but limiting sound input can be accomplished by application of earplugs, cotton balls, or headphones. Unfortunately, use of noise reduction devices by the patient reduces communication so he or she is not able to hear. The patient may become increasingly agitated, believing the crew is talking about him or her. It is essential to include the conscious patient in as much conversation as possible. In a helicopter, which is extremely noisy, earpieces of the stethoscope can be inserted into the patient's ears so the crew can speak to the patient by using the stethoscope's diaphragm.

Noise also interferes with ability to hear breath sounds, heart sounds, and blood pressure. Doppler devices are available to assist with detecting blood pressure but are of little use for hearing breath or heart sounds. Other assessment techniques to ascertain adequate ventilation include observing for bilateral chest wall movement, using pulse oximetry, and placing the stethoscope over the trachea to listen for air movement.

The flight crew may be familiar with noises of the aircraft, but the patient should be warned ahead of time. Many aircraft have audible warning signals to prevent accidents, but to the patient these alarms may indicate the aircraft is in danger of crashing. A preflight briefing with the patient should be followed by continual reminders to alleviate these fears.

Long-term noise exposure is also a problem for the flight crew. Protective earplugs should be used to minimize the deleterious effects of noise over time. Periodic hearing tests are recommended to monitor changes in hearing.

Vibration

As a result of vehicle design, aircraft vibrate. The effects of vibration are much more noticeable in a helicopter, especially during takeoff and landing. This constant motion can cause equipment to loosen and become a danger during flight. FAA regulations require that all equipment be secured during takeoff and landing. Equipment should be secured at all times in anticipation of unexpected turbulence.

The patient should be secured to the stretcher at all times. Before loading and unloading, stretcher restraints should be checked for proper fit. During transport, straps may be loosened to allow the patient to move; however, restraints should never be fully released.

Continual vibration can also change equipment settings—constant jostling can cause knobs to slip, changing functioning of the machinery. Ventilators are especially prone to this complication, so settings should be checked frequently during flight.

Immobilization

Long transport times combined with prolonged immobilization of the patient can lead to pressure sores and venous stasis. Space limitations and inability to change the patient's position exacerbate these problems. The patient at greatest risk is one with a suspected spinal injury who is secured to an LSB.

Before departure, all splints, casts, and pressure areas should be padded. A small towel or pad can be placed under the coccyx area of a patient with a suspected cervical spinal injury who is secured to an LSB. In transport, proper positioning and assessment of range of motion should be performed within the space constraints. Assessing for areas of decreased perfusion should be part of assessment of vital signs.

Length of transport includes not only the time it takes to fly from the referring location to the receiving hospital, but also ground transport times, unexpected delays, and transfer times. For example, a patient injured in a motor vehicle crash at a remote site is secured to a backboard to protect the cervical spine. This patient is then transported by ground ambulance to the nearest hospital. After evaluation of injuries, the patient requires care in a major trauma center. Radiographs of the cervical spine are inconclusive, so the patient must remain on the backboard during transport. Subsequently, the patient is taken by

ground ambulance to the nearest airport, flown to the receiving airfield, and again transferred by ground ambulance to the trauma center. Total length of time the patient is secured to the backboard exceeds 6 hours, yet the flight took only 1.5 hours.

Consideration of injuries must take precedence during stabilization of the patient, but using padded splints, traction devices, and protecting bony prominences are a necessary follow-up, limiting preventable problems associated with immobilization.

Safety

Safety in air transport should be the primary concern of all people involved. Most crashes occur in conjunction with helicopter transports; however, risk is also associated with fixed-wing transports. Issues of personal safety, patient safety, and infection control previously discussed for ground transport prevail also apply in air transport.

Fixed-Wing Transports

All equipment must be secured in accordance with FAA regulations. Meeting stringent requirements ensures that passengers and crew are not injured by flying objects during turbulence or if a crash occurs. Equipment not secured to the airframe itself should be kept in soft packs and placed on the floor during takeoff and landing. Emergency exits should never be blocked by equipment or extraneous items.

Ground personnel must be trained and briefed regarding aircraft safety. This briefing should include information on loading and unloading the patient. For instance, weight distribution is critical in aircraft, but ground personnel may not be aware of these requirements. Also, ground personnel should be trained to avoid hazardous areas, such as propellers and the exhaust cowling on a jet engine. No one should approach the aircraft until the pilot in command has given approval to do so.

The pilot in command is responsible for safety of the aircraft at all times and may determine whether to cancel a flight because of weather conditions. Most flight programs do not discuss severity of the patient's condition with the pilot until a decision has been made regarding weather. This relieves the pilot of undue stress when a life-or-death mission is being considered: the pilot should be able to make this decision without feelings of guilt or doubt affecting his or her judgment.

Everyone involved in the transport should be briefed before departure. Pilots should be informed of the patient's condition and specific needs related to takeoff and landing. For example, some patients are adversely affected by a short landing that results in shifts in internal organs and fluids. Family members should be briefed on length of the flight, in-flight expectations, and location and operations of emergency exits. Smoking is prohibited. Seat belts are required on landing and takeoff, although their use is preferred throughout the flight.

Fire extinguishers should be clearly marked, and all personnel should be trained in their use. Emergency procedures for rapid egress should be practiced on a regular basis.

Rotor-Wing transports

Helicopter transports create a sense of drama. Many people assemble to watch a helicopter land and takeoff. Bystanders must be kept away from danger. A safe landing zone (LZ) should be established in a clearing that measures 60 feet × 60 feet up to 200 feet × 200 feet, depending on size of the helicopter. All wires, trees, and possible hazards should be marked and described over the radio to the pilot. Smoke flares can be ignited to assist the pilot in locating the LZ. Flares are blown away from the helicopter during landing, which could ignite a fire. The patient, ground personnel, and bystanders should be at least 500 feet from the LZ and should turn their backs to the helicopter while it is landing. The rotor wash (wind created by the rotor blades) causes swirling dust, dirt, and gravel, which pose hazards to people on the ground.

Ground personnel should not approach the helicopter until the pilot gives the signal it is safe to do so. The helicopter should be approached from the downhill side, never the uphill side. Many crashes occur because people approach the helicopter while the blades are still rotating. When blade rotation begins to slow, the blades drop, which may cause unexpected injury. A "hot" loading or unloading is one that is performed with rotor blades turning at idle power. This procedure should be used only in extreme circumstances and only by experienced personnel. Additional guidelines for helicopter landing safety are listed in Box 10-6. This information should be reviewed frequently and be readily available for review when a helicopter transport is expected.

Ensuring safe transport of the patient is the responsibility of all people involved in the transport. All personnel, whether on the ground or in the air, should remain safety conscious at all times. Safety should be the number one priority.

Personnel

Flight team configurations are many and varied. Emergency and critical care nurses are generally chosen to become flight nurses. They can work alone, as a member of a two-nurse team, or with a paramedic, an EMT, or an emergency physician. Respiratory therapists are also used as a second member or third member of the team, when the patient is intubated and requires ventilatory support.

Flight nursing has developed into a subspecialty of emergency nursing. Flight nurses now go through rigorous training before joining a flight team. The Air Surface Transport Nurses Association (ASTNA), formerly the National Flight Nurses Association, has developed a flight nurse core curriculum to provide standardized training in such areas as flight physiology, stabilization, communications, and medicolegal issues. Initial training includes classroom and clinical experience. Preceptor programs are frequently used

Box 10-6	GUIDELINES FOR HELICOPTER LANDING SAFETY

Landing zone (LZ) size ranges from 60 to 200 square feet, depending on size of the helicopter.

Select an LZ that is easily identifiable, as level as possible, and free of debris and overhead obstructions.

Mark one corner of the LZ with a smoke flare so the pilot can estimate wind speed and direction.

Flashing emergency lights are difficult to see in daylight. Landmarks such as intersections, waterways, distinctive buildings, or baseball or football fields are much easier to find from the air.

Turn off unnecessary lights and white lights such as strobe lights or headlights at night. These lights interfere with the pilot's night vision. Never direct a spotlight at an approaching helicopter.

Flags, cones, safety tapes, ambulance mattresses, poles used for intravenous infusion, other loose equipment, sticks, stones, and broken glass can be drawn into rotor blades or thrown during landing and liftoff.

Only people such as firefighters with proper personal protection, including safety goggles, should be permitted in the vicinity of the LZ.

Assign personnel to guard the area. Prohibit smoking and keep spectators at a safe distance.

Never approach the helicopter unless signaled to do so by the pilot or another air medical crew member. Keep low if the main rotor is still spinning.

Always approach the helicopter within the crew's line of sight and never from the rear or sloped side. If the aircraft is rear loading, approach cautiously with head down after being signaled by the pilot or crew.

Only flight crew members should lock, unlock, or otherwise handle aircraft doors.

Assist the flight crew only as requested. Never attempt to contact the pilot by radio during the helicopter's final approach unless an extreme emergency jeopardizes safety.

to allow the new flight nurse exposure to the transport environment. Recurrent training is also needed to maintain skills, update information regarding current therapies, and review current policies and procedures. Monthly "run" reviews provide performance improvement and promote sharing of learning experiences among staff.

Nurses should be advanced cardiac life support (ACLS) certified and trained in endotracheal intubation, chest tube insertion, and needle thoracotomy techniques. Depending on the capabilities of the program, additional education should include invasive line management, use of intraaortic balloon pumps, and pediatric or neonatal ALS measures if children and neonates are transported. Many programs also require advanced trauma life support (ATLS) credentials. Development of the Flight Nurse Advanced Trauma Course demonstrates ASTNA's commitment to improving educational opportunities available to flight nurses. Development of the certified flight nurse exam encourages flight nurses to achieve certification in flight nursing (CFRN). Flight nursing represents a unique opportunity for nurses to perform emergency care, critical care, and prehospital care during the same patient encounter.

Transport team members have a unique set of circumstances under which to work. Interactions with the patient are short and often rushed. The patients who are transported have an increased mortality because of circumstances necessitating transport. Following the patient's progress in the receiving hospital helps the crew alleviate its anxieties about dealing with patients for the short term. Transport personnel must remember that they are often the only contact the family has with the receiving hospital. The crew can maintain contact with the family, explaining interventions and other procedures. Maintaining contact and follow-up with referring personnel also provides the transport crew with opportunities to communicate about patients and helps instill a sense of commitment and pride in their jobs.

Equipment

Equipment used in air transport must be based on the level and type of medical care the patient requires during the transport. Because of space and weight limitations, not all equipment can be carried in the transport vehicle. Before departure, a decision must be made concerning what equipment and how much should be taken. A limited amount of backup supplies should be on hand in the event of unexpected delays.

All medical equipment must be easily secured during takeoff, flight, and landing. Equipment requiring alternating current should have a backup battery source or an alternative, hand-operated device should be available. All equipment should be protected from electromechanical interference. Equipment with diaphragms such as oxygen analyzers may not function in the pressurized cabin of a fixed-wing aircraft. All equipment should be tested in-flight before it is used on a patient.

Required vehicle equipment and medical equipment is listed in Box 10-7. Specialized equipment is now available for transport vehicles, but before such equipment is purchased, an in-flight test should be performed. Some equipment has specialized accessories that make the equipment difficult to use and costly. For example, some IV infusion pumps require specialized infusion tubing that must be changed before the transport. Time spent repriming tubing can delay transfer.

Expendable items should be placed in soft packs whenever possible. Product packing materials may be removed to eliminate extraneous bulk. Space-efficient equipment packs include burn, neonatal, IV, trauma, and medication packs. Pediatric equipment may be kept in a separate pack to reduce quantity of equipment taken on all transports.

Arranging equipment so that it is ready for use is recommended. Intravenous solutions should be in plastic bags, with tubing secured to the bag with a rubber band. Nasogastric tubes should be banded together with connectors. This organization, completed before transport, expedites inter-

---

| Box 10-7 | EQUIPMENT FOR AIR MEDICAL TRANSPORT |

VEHICLE EQUIPMENT

Communication system
Adequate lighting with ability to isolate pilots from lights
Electrical outlets (110 v AC)
Locking hooks for IV bags and bottles
Fire extinguisher
Survival gear appropriate to environment over which transport occurs
Sharps disposal container
Trash receptacle

MEDICAL EQUIPMENT

Oxygen tanks with flow meters
Air cylinders if ventilator is to be used
Portable and permanent suction devices with regulators
Cardiac monitor with defibrillator
Radio-shielded Doppler device
Stretcher with approved securing mechanisms
Blood pressure cuffs
Emesis basin
Urinal and bedpan
Additional items
    Infusion pumps
    Backboards
    Cervical collars
    Heimlich valves
    Water seal drainage sets
    Cervical spine immobilizer

UNIVERSAL PRECAUTIONS EQUIPMENT

Goggles
Gloves
Gowns
Masks

PATIENT-SPECIFIC EQUIPMENT

IV, Intravenous.

---

ventions and limits the need to open multiple compartments to find additional items.

Equipment of any type should be lightweight and compact. Aluminum cylinders of oxygen, which weigh one third the weight of steel tanks, are available. Pocket-type Doppler devices can be removed from the aircraft and taken with transport personnel.

Adequate equipment should be available to care for the patient during the entire transport and during any unexpected delays. To calculate the amount of equipment necessary, estimate length of the transport, including transfer times, then multiply that figure by one half. To estimate the amount of oxygen remaining in a standard "E" cylinder, the following formula is used:

$$\frac{PSI \times 0.3 \text{ L/min}}{60 \text{ min}} = \text{hr in cylinder}$$

Table 10-4	EFFECTS OF ALTITUDE ON FLOW RATES		
FLOWMETER (L/MIN)	FLOW RATE AT ALTITUDE (CALCULATED)		
	2000 FT	5000 FT	8000 FT
2	2.1	2.4	2.6
4	4.2	4.7	5.3
6	6.3	7.1	7.9
8	8.4	9.4	10.6
10	10.5	11.8	13.2
12	12.6	14.1	15.8

Altitude and pressure changes can change flow rates. Table 10-4 shows the effects of altitude on flow rates.

Medications are commonly carried in hard plastic cases to prevent breakage. The types and amounts of medications carried depend on the types of patients transported and medical protocols of the transport program. Narcotics should be in locked carrying cases that can be secured and should be counted at each shift change.

In-Flight Responsibilities

During transport, vital signs should be obtained at least every 15 minutes. Depending on the patient's condition, vital signs may be taken more frequently. Changes in patient condition usually occur during ascent and descent when pressure changes occur in the aircraft. The patient's response to transport should be closely monitored during these times.

An advantage of air transport is that transport personnel are never farther than a few feet from their patient. This closeness allows astute observation of the patient and the ability to pick up subtle changes in condition. However, noise, distractions, and space limitations within the transport vehicle can distort certain cues. The crew must monitor the patient closely for problems that may develop as a result of changes in atmosphere or the transport itself.

Patients With Respiratory Distress

Warm, humidified oxygen should be administered to all patients. The percentage of oxygen should be increased for those receiving oxygen therapy before the transport. Gas expansion within the pleural cavity can cause the size of a previously undetected pneumothorax to increase, which may lead to respiratory compromise. A flutter valve should be placed to reduce pressure within the chest cavity (Table 10-3). If the patient had a chest tube placed before transport, the tube should never be clamped during flight. A one-way (Heimlich) valve can be placed between the chest tube and the drainage set to prevent air from reaccumulating in the chest cavity with accidental disruption of the system.

Pulmonary secretions become more tenacious with dehydration and decreased ambient humidity. Instillation of sterile saline before suctioning enhances removal of secretions. Hyperventilation can accompany cold stress or may be caused by excessive noise and vibration. Measures should be taken to warm the patient and allay any fears and anxieties.

Immobilizing the patient on the stretcher interferes with chest expansion and can lead to underventilation and subsequent atelectasis. Elevating the patient's head improves oxygenation and gas exchange and helps limit pulmonary congestion that occurs secondary to acceleration and deceleration forces.

Mechanical volume ventilators used in the transport environment should be constantly monitored for delivery of adequate tidal volumes, because gas expansion can affect volume of gas delivered. Oxygen flow rates of at least 15 L/minute are required to operate ventilators, which can rapidly decrease oxygen supply. Should the ventilator fail, the patient must be ventilated with a resuscitation bag.

Patients With Cardiovascular Conditions

Hypoxia presents the greatest risk for the cardiac patient during transport. It can lead to increased myocardial irritability and ventricular ectopy. Providing supplemental oxygen and positioning the patient for optimal gas exchanges is imperative. Interventions to decrease oxygen demand include keeping the patient warm, allaying fears, and preventing motion sickness.

Placing a nasogastric tube can prevent decreased venous return caused by gastric distension. However, placement must be performed with caution because vagal stimulation and bradycardia can develop. The decision to employ a nasogastric tube should be made on a patient-by-patient basis.

Acceleration forces cause pooling of blood in the lower extremities with subsequent poor cardiac return. The opposite effect develops as a result of deceleration forces, in which cardiac congestion and transient fluid overload develop. The patient with congestive heart failure is severely affected by these factors. Pretransport diuresis can help prevent these problems.

Specialized equipment associated with cardiac patients needs special attention. Patients with pacemakers should be monitored for pacemaker malfunction that can occur as a result of radio and navigational equipment signals. Intraaortic balloon pumps are now available for use during transport. Only trained personnel should use these devices, because the risk of balloon dislodgment and equipment malfunction is increased in the transport environment. During transport, close monitoring of pressures within the balloon is imperative to detect changes that may result from gas expansion.

Patients With Multiple Traumatic Injuries

Hypoxia and gas expansion can cause rapid deterioration of the pulmonary and cardiovascular systems. Pulmonary embolus should be considered when increasing dyspnea develops. Thoracic injuries should be identified and stabilized before transporting the patient.

The effect of gas expansion on the PASG, air splints, and endotracheal tube cuffs has been discussed previously. Free air in the peritoneal cavity resulting from bowel injury or peritoneal lavage should be aspirated if possible.

Adequate resuscitation of the trauma patient usually includes fluid and blood support. Measures must be taken to ensure that blood products are properly stored. In the event their use is unwarranted, they can be returned to the blood bank for future use.

Patients With Head Injuries

Patients with an isolated injury or a head injury in conjunction with other injuries are at significant risk from air transport. Increased intracranial pressure decreases the level of arterial oxygen saturation, which may result in hypoxia caused by changes in the partial pressure of oxygen. This hypoxia can cause seizure activity, so seizure precautions should be used at all times.

Noise, vibration, vomiting, and an increased metabolic rate associated with cold stress all increase intracranial pressure. In-flight measures, including hyperventilation, should be used to reduce these untoward effects and prevent unnecessary rises in intracranial pressure. Induction of paralysis can also help control intracranial pressure; however, posturing and other clinical indicators of patient status are forfeited. The patient should be positioned to minimize effects of gravitational forces.

Burn Victims

Burns of the face, head, and neck can cause massive swelling, reducing the airway. Prophylactic intubation before transport eliminates the need for intubation in the poorly lit, cramped interior of the aircraft. Supplemental oxygen should be administered to all patients with suspected smoke inhalation to combat the effects of hypoxia. Providing cool humidified oxygen to the patient with suspected oropharyngeal burns helps reduce swelling.

Loss of the skin causes massive fluid shifts and loss of temperature regulation. Evaporative heat loss increases in the burned area, and the burn victim becomes increasingly dehydrated and cold. All wounds should be covered with absorbent dressings to control heat loss and limit contamination of the wounds. Dressings should not be moistened with saline solution or other fluids, because this enhances hypothermia. Using a Mylar blanket to cover the patient helps limit heat loss.

Patients with burns require large amounts of fluids and dressings; therefore, adequate supplies must be available throughout the transport of a burn victim. Escharotomies may become necessary when fluid shifts occur during take-off and descent.

Maintaining sterility of the transport environment is impossible. Meticulous care to prevent contamination should be taken at all times. Wearing masks and gowns over transport clothing helps limit transfer of bacteria. Topical antibiotic application is discouraged because it delays evaluation of the burn wound when the patient arrives at the receiving hospital.

Patients With High-Risk Obstetric Conditions

Hypoxia and fluid shifts increase uterine irritability and can lead to premature labor. Hypoxia of short duration has little effect on the fetus, but prolonged maternal hypoxia can lead to fetal distress and subsequent fetal demise. Supplemental oxygen should be provided to the patient throughout transport.

Pressure from a distended stomach increases uterine irritability and increases pressure on the diaphragm, which leads to dyspnea. Nasogastric tube placement may be uncomfortable for the pregnant woman, but is necessary to decompress the stomach and decrease the risk of aspiration from delayed gastric emptying.

Pregnancy increases blood volume in the third trimester by approximately 45% to 50%. This increased volume must be replaced if the woman is hypovolemic. Pregnant women can lose a significant portion of their circulating blood volume before hypovolemia is evident. Fluid shifts accompanying acceleration and deceleration forces can decrease uterine blood flow. Proper positioning is essential for the pregnant patient.

The pregnant patient should be placed in the left lateral decubitus position during transport. Safely securing the patient to the stretcher in this position is often difficult. The patient may have to be secured in the supine position during loading and unloading. The woman should be returned to the left lateral decubitus position as soon as the aircraft reaches cruising altitude or with signs of fetal distress. For the pregnant trauma patient, secure the woman to the LSB, then tip the entire board to the left.

Preeclampsia and eclampsia increase nausea and vomiting associated with motion. These patients are also sensitive to extraneous stimulation; noise and vibration may increase blood pressure. Dim lighting and earplugs for the patient help prevent overstimulation.

All personnel who transport high-risk obstetric patients must be familiar with the techniques of childbirth and neonatal resuscitation. Equipment for delivery and resuscitation must be readily available. If delivery is imminent, the transport should reroute to the nearest hospital to avoid in-flight delivery regardless of final destination. Keeping a newly delivered infant warm, dry, and oxygenated is the priority for newborn care.

Pediatric Patients

The problems associated with transport of children are the same as those for adults. However, interventions must take into account the unique anatomic and physiologic features of children. Because equipment of the appropriate size varies with age and weight of the child, a large assortment of choices must be available.

Pediatric patients have smaller vital capacities than adults and are more prone to the effects of hypoxia. Children may not be able to tolerate or cooperate with application of an oxygen mask. In these cases, the oxygen mask can be placed in front of the child's face and oxygen can be blown at the child. A family member accompanying the child can assist with administration of oxygen by holding the mask and encouraging the child to cooperate.

Because the gastric cavity of a child is small, the child has a greater tendency to develop complications from gastric gas expansion. Many nasogastric tubes for children do not have a sump port and should not be used, because absence of the sump port makes emptying the stomach more difficult.

The greater ratio of surface area to body mass in children makes them more susceptible to evaporative heat losses. The proportionally larger surface area of the head and neck also enhance radiated heat loss, which puts the child at great risk for hypothermia. A stocking cap and extra linen help keep the child warm.

Securing children to a standard stretcher is difficult because stretcher restraints are not easily moved to accommodate a smaller size. Extra straps may be necessary to keep the child secured. One method of transporting a child younger than 5 years of age is to place the child in a car seat and secure the car seat to the stretcher restraints.[2] Providing familiar items such as car seats, toys, and security blankets help alleviate the child's fear of the unknown.

If the child's condition is stable, including a family member in the transport may be advantageous. The family member can comfort the child, help explain procedures, and provide diversionary activities as warranted to keep the child occupied.

Other in-flight responsibilities include documentation of all interventions, vital signs, and changes in the patient's condition. Changes in environmental conditions such as with takeoff and landing should also be documented, because changes in the patient's condition may be secondary to the effects of transport rather than to changes in the disease process or condition itself. Throughout the transport, safety must be the number one consideration.

SUMMARY

Air and ground patient transport has improved outcomes for many. Proper stabilization procedures should anticipate potential problems that may be encountered during transport. Employing specialized equipment and personnel trained in transporting patients ensures that the patient is transported in a highly sophisticated environment.

The future may bring consolidation of transport programs. To ensure viability, air transport programs must work together, consolidating and providing a consortium approach to transport. Incorporating ground transport with air transport will improve appropriate utilization of these services.

Newer therapies are being instituted in the prehospital care environment (e.g., thrombolytic therapy). As computer-

ization and information sharing grows, medical control officers can make informed decisions while the patient is still in transport. As these decisions are made, therapies can be instituted immediately rather than waiting for the patient's arrival in the ED. This increased responsibility requires that transport personnel are continually updated in current methodologies. Many studies have confirmed the benefits of early therapy, so transport personnel may assume more responsibility in the future.

Sophistication of air and ground transport is limited by the size and weight of most medical equipment. As miniaturization continues and transport equipment becomes lightweight and truly transportable, transporting patients will develop into an even more specialized aspect of emergency nursing.

References

1. Emergency Medical Treatment and Active Labor Act (EMTALA) (Suppl. 1995). 42 U.S.C.A. § 1395dd.
2. McCloskey K, Orr R: *Pediatric transport medicine,* St. Louis, 1995, Mosby.

Suggested Reading

American Academy of Pediatrics, Task Force on Interhospital Transports: *Guidelines of air and ground transport of neonatal and pediatric patients,* Elk Grove Village, Ill, 1993, The Academy.

Commission on Accreditation of Ambulance Services: *Standards for the accreditation of ambulance services,* Dallas, 1991, The Commission.

Emergency Nurses Association: *Care of the critically ill or injured patient during interfacility transfer,* Des Plaines, Ill, 1999, The Association.

Emergency Nurses Association: *Care of the pediatric patient during interfacility transfer,* Des Plaines, Ill, 1999, The Association.

Guidelines Committee of the American College of Critical Care Medicine, Society of Critical Care Medicine and American Association of Critical Care Nurse Transfer Guidelines Task Force: Guidelines for the transfer of critically ill patients, *Crit Care Med* 21(6):931, 1993.

Jaimovich DG, Vidasagar D: *Handbook of pediatric and neonatal transport medicine,* Philadelphia, 1996, Hanley & Belfus.

National Association of Emergency Medical Services Physicians: Air medical dispatch: guidelines for trauma scene response, *Prehosp Disaster Med* 7(1):75, 1992.

National Flight Nurses Association: *Standards of flight nursing practice,* ed 2, St. Louis, 1994, Mosby.

Youngberg BJ: Medical-legal considerations involved in the transport of critically ill patients, *Crit Care Clin* 8(3):501, 1992.

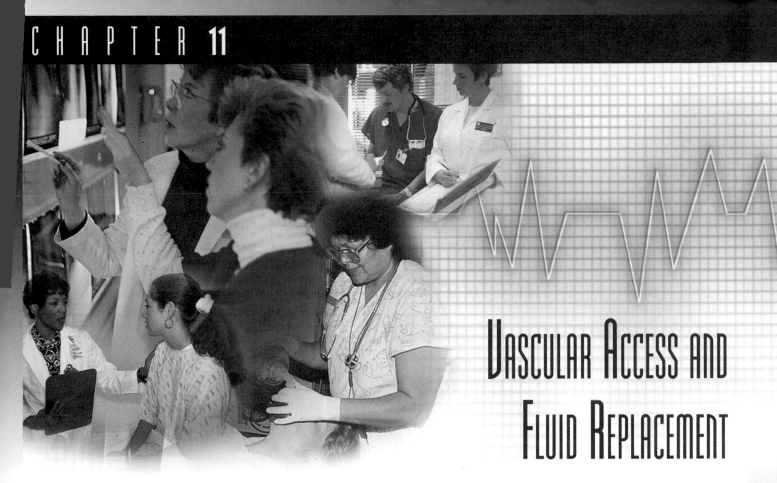

CHAPTER 11

VASCULAR ACCESS AND FLUID REPLACEMENT

ZEB KORAN, LORENE NEWBERRY

Circulatory assessment and related interventions are a cornerstone of interventions for emergency patients, regardless of complaint or symptoms. Patients in the emergency department (ED) often require temporary vascular access for medications, fluid and electrolyte replacement, or transfusion of blood or blood products. Routine vascular access involves inserting catheters into peripheral veins of hands and arms. Site selection depends on the urgency of the situation and the condition of the patient's veins. Central veins may be used for invasive hemodynamic monitoring or when peripheral access is not possible. Needle insertion into bone marrow is also used for emergency fluid replacement. Patients may have catheters or implanted ports for long-term vascular access.

Fluid replacement is used for patients with subtle and overt volume losses. Solution, rate, and amount is determined by patient condition, underlying pathology, and current fluid imbalance. Maintenance fluids are used for patients with no oral intake, whereas aggressive fluid replacement is indicated for patients with significant volume depletion. Patients with hematologic disorders, cancer, or frank blood loss may also require blood or blood product replacement. Vascular access options and various aspects of fluid replacement are described in the following sections.

ANATOMY AND PHYSIOLOGY

Low-pressure vessels located throughout the body receive blood from capillary beds and return it to the heart. Small venules flow into increasingly larger veins, which eventually flow into the inferior and superior venae cavae. Vessel diameter varies among patients and with location on the body. Surface vessels in hands and arms are primary access points; however, vessels in the neck, legs, feet, and head may be used. Figure 11-1 shows the location of major vessels of the body. Valves located along veins prevent backflow (Figure 11-2); therefore, intravenous catheters must be inserted in the same direction as venous flow. Elderly patients lose collagen in vessel walls, which causes significant thinning over time. Vessels may sclerose and become tortuous with aging.

Veins in the upper extremities include digital veins on the dorsal aspect of fingers, metacarpal veins on the dorsum of the hand, cephalic veins, basilic veins, and median veins (Figure 11-3). Figure 11-4 illustrates veins of the hand and fingers. Cephalic veins are located at the radial aspect of the dorsal venous network with the accessory cephalic vein originating from the union of dorsal veins. The basilic vein, which originates from the union of dorsal veins on the ulnar aspect of the arm, can be seen when the elbow is flexed. The union of veins from the palmar aspect of the hand creates the median antebrachial vein. The antecubital fossa, a depression in the anterior elbow, contains the median cephalic vein or median basilic vein.

The dorsal venous network on the foot and saphenous vein on the ankle flow into the larger femoral vein (Figure 11-5). These vessels are rarely used for routine vascular access because of associated complications. The femoral vein

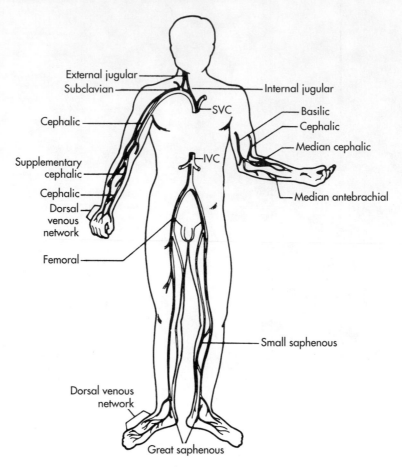

External jugular
Subclavian
Internal jugular
SVC
Cephalic
Basilic
Cephalic
Median cephalic
Supplementary cephalic
IVC
Cephalic
Median antebrachial
Dorsal venous network
Femoral
Small saphenous
Dorsal venous network
Great saphenous

FIGURE 11-1   Major veins of the body.

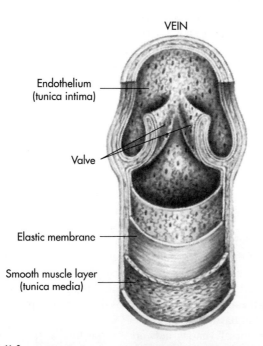

Endothelium (tunica intima)
Valve
Elastic membrane
Smooth muscle layer (tunica media)

VEIN

FIGURE 11-2   Vein cross-section. (Modified from Thompson JM, McFarland GK, Hirsch JE et al: *Mosby's clinical nursing,* ed 5, St. Louis, 2002, Mosby.)

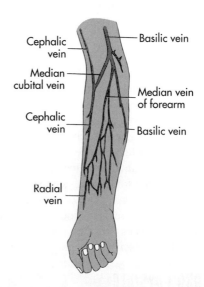

Cephalic vein
Basilic vein
Median cubital vein
Median vein of forearm
Cephalic vein
Basilic vein
Radial vein

FIGURE 11-3   Veins in the upper arm. (Modified from Potter PA, Perry AG: *Fundamentals of nursing,* ed 5, St. Louis, 2001, Mosby.)

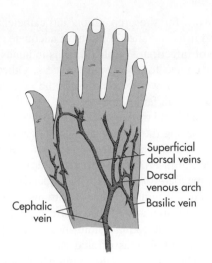

FIGURE 11-4 Veins in the hand. (Modified from Potter PA, Perry AG: *Fundamentals of nursing,* ed 5, St. Louis, 2001, Mosby.)

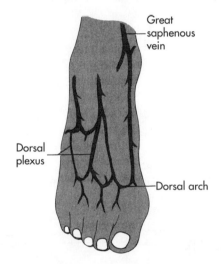

FIGURE 11-5 Veins in the foot and ankle. (Modified from Potter PA, Perry AG: *Fundamentals of nursing,* ed 5, St. Louis, 2001, Mosby.)

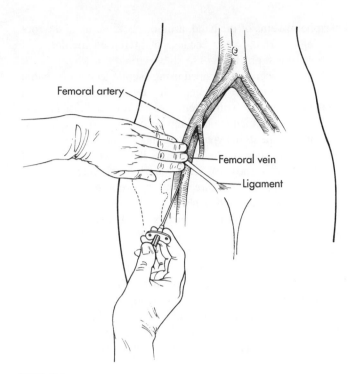

FIGURE 11-6 Femoral vein. (Modified from Meeker MH, Rothrock JC: *Alexander's care of the patient in surgery,* ed 10, St. Louis, 1995, Mosby.)

located medial to the femoral artery is used for access to central circulation in some patients (Figure 11-6).

Peripheral veins of the neck flow into the subclavian vein and can be used for vascular access (Figure 11-7). The external jugular vein is visible in most patients on the lateral aspect of the neck. The internal jugular vein is located beneath and medial to the external jugular. Subclavian veins are used for access to central circulation.

VASCULAR ACCESS

Inserting peripheral intravenous catheters is a routine skill for emergency nurses. Nurses may also insert central catheters; however, this is not a basic skill for the majority of emergency nurses. Nurses use and maintain established vascular access points. Catheters are usually inserted into

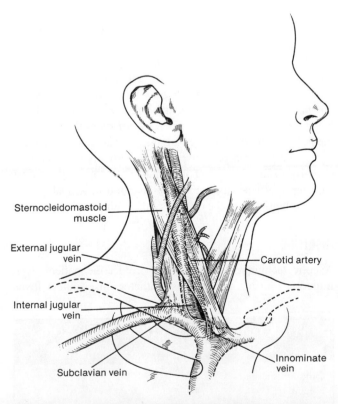

FIGURE 11-7 Veins in the neck. (Modified from Meeker MH, Rothrock JC: *Alexander's care of the patient in surgery,* ed 10, St. Louis, 1995, Mosby.)

peripheral veins of the hand, arm, or neck. Veins in the foot and leg are rarely used because of increased incidence of embolism and phlebitis.

Vascular access is obtained using aseptic technique. Initial insertion attempts should begin with distal veins and progress up the extremity. Proximal veins are not routinely used unless patients need immediate fluid replacement, such as in trauma patients or patients in hypovolemic shock. These veins are also used for patients receiving drugs that have an extremely short half-life (e.g., adenosine). Scalp veins have no valves, so fluid can be infused in either direction; they are also easily visualized, making them an ideal alternative in infants.

Insertion of intravenous catheters is not without risk to the patient and the emergency nurse. Potential complications for the patient include infection and hematoma (Box 11-1). The emergency nurse risks exposure to potentially infectious blood through a needle stick or direct contact with blood or body fluids. Extreme care should be taken to minimize risks through use of universal precautions and appropriate disposal of needles. Intravenous catheters with safety features such as self-capping needles and retracting needles are readily available.

Catheter Selection

The size and type of catheter are determined by urgency of need and patient size, age, and vasculature. Blood should flow easily around the catheter after insertion. Larger diameter catheters are used for administering significant volume, colloid solutions, or blood or blood products, whereas smaller diameter catheters are used for routine vascular access. All intravenous catheters now use a catheter-over-needle design. Intravenous needles without catheters are available, but should not be used. Catheters used for peripheral access include a butterfly or winged catheter (Figure 11-8) and straight catheter-over-needle design (Figure 11-9). Winged catheters are easily inserted and can be stabilized with minimal effort; however, these catheters are not ideal for rapid fluid replacement. Catheters over needles are ideal for aggressive fluid replacement, but can present problems with stabilization, particularly in distal veins of the hand. Dual-lumen peripheral catheters must be flushed before insertion to activate a hydrolytic lubricant on the outside of the catheter.

Insertion

Aseptic technique is essential to protect the patient from infection during intravenous catheter insertion. Gloves

should be worn for site preparation and catheter insertion. The selected insertion site should have adequate circulation and be free of infection. Peripheral veins in hands and arms are the first choice for intravenous access. Other sites include veins of the lower extremities, or the external jugular, internal jugular, and femoral veins.

The external jugular vein is accessible in most patients, but requires turning the patient's neck for access. Lowering the patient's head distends the vein and decreases risk of air embolism during insertion. Use of the external jugular vein is not recommended for patients with suspected neck injury. Use of the internal jugular vein is contraindicated in these patients. Internal jugular access is not used during cardiac arrest because cardiac compressions must be stopped for insertion. Another problem associated with using the internal jugular vein is hematoma development, which compromises respiratory effort. The femoral vein is an excellent choice in cardiac arrest because cardiac compressions can continue. Figure 11-10 shows cannulization of the femoral vein. Femoral access also provides an opportunity for hemo-

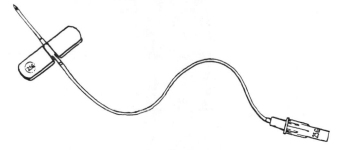

FIGURE **11-8**   Butterfly or winged infusion set.

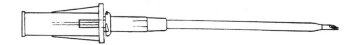

FIGURE **11-9**   Catheter-over-needle design.

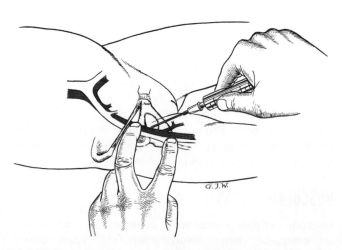

FIGURE **11-10**   Femoral venous catheterization technique. (From Daily EK, Schroeder JS: *Techniques in bedside hemodynamic monitoring*, ed 5, St. Louis, 1994, Mosby.)

Box 11-1	COMPLICATIONS OF INTRAVENOUS CATHETERS

Fluid infiltration
Phlebitis
Embolism of blood, air, or catheter fragments
Infection
Cellulitis

dynamic pressure monitoring. Complications associated with femoral vein access include hematoma and infection.

After a site is selected, a tourniquet is placed proximally to distend vessels for easy insertion (Figure 11-11, *A*). Because veins may be more prominent in elderly patients, a tourniquet may not be required. Tourniquets may actually rupture vessels because of increased pressure in fragile veins. Gently tapping or rubbing vessels below the tourniquet increases vessel size by dilation. When vessels are not easily visualized or palpated, applying warm towels over the vein for 5 minutes causes vasodilation and can facilitate catheter insertion (Figure 11-11, *B*).

Skin preparation begins with initial cleansing using alcohol to remove fat and other residue. Povidone-iodine (betadine) solution is the bactericidal agent of choice unless the patient is allergic to it. The solution is applied directly over the insertion site in a circular pattern moving slowly outward (Figure 11-12). The ideal bactericidal effect requires

that the solution remain on the skin for 30 seconds. The surface is then wiped with sterile gauze.

Local anesthesia is not routinely used for catheter insertion unless time permits. After site preparation, lidocaine 1% may be injected at the insertion site for immediate anesthetic effect. Emla cream applied topically over the insertion site for approximately 15 to 20 minutes is an alternative to injection if time is not an issue.

After the site is prepared, the catheter is inserted by stabilizing the vein to prevent movement during puncture. With the needle bevel up, skin is punctured using the smallest angle possible between skin and needle (Figure 11-13). Veins may be entered on the top or side. The catheter is advanced slowly until blood flashes into the catheter, then the catheter is advanced over the needle into the vein. The tourniquet is removed and intravenous tubing is connected. One-way valves are recommended to prevent bleeding from the catheter during subsequent tubing changes. If fluid therapy is not required, catheters may be capped with a one-way valve and sterile cover. The catheter and tubing should be secured with tape according to hospital policy; however, tape should never be applied directly over the insertion site. Clear, occlusive dressings such as Opsite, Tegaderm, or Bioclusive should be applied over the insertion site. Sites should be labeled with the date, time, catheter size, and initials of the person inserting the catheter.

Central Venous Access

The subclavian, external jugular, and cephalic veins are used for short- and long-term vascular access. Short-term central venous access is indicated when peripheral access cannot be obtained or when the patient's condition requires hemodynamic monitoring. Long-term vascular access is indicated for prolonged intravenous therapy, total parenteral nutrition, extended antibiotic therapy or therapy with caustic drugs such as vancomycin, and in patients with debilitating diseases such as cancer or acquired immune deficiency syndrome. In the ED, central venous access is usually an emergency procedure that uses the subclavian or jugular veins.

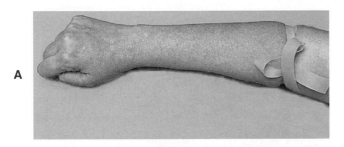

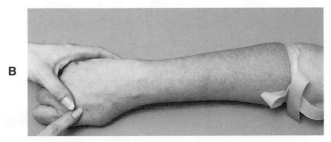

FIGURE **11-11**   **A,** Placement of tourniquet. **B,** Technique for increasing vessel size by dilation. (From Potter PA, Perry AG: *Fundamentals of nursing,* ed 5, St. Louis, 2001, Mosby.)

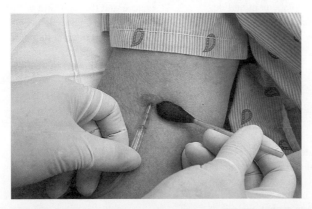

FIGURE **11-12**   Application of solution over insertion site. (From Potter PA, Perry AG: *Fundamentals of nursing,* ed 5, St. Louis, 2001, Mosby.)

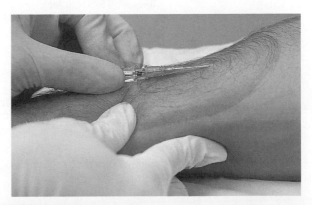

FIGURE **11-13**   Venipuncture. (From Potter PA, Perry AG: *Fundamentals of nursing,* ed 5, St. Louis, 2001, Mosby.)

Figure 11-14 illustrates subclavian vein cannulization. Complications related to initial insertion include infection, hematoma, pneumothorax, and air embolism.[1]

Central venous access catheters are made of silicone or polyurethane and have a radiopaque strip. Silicone is less thrombogenic and becomes pliable with moisture. Disadvantages of silicone include migration of the catheter tip and inability to withdraw blood over time as the catheter softens and collapses inward. Single-lumen and multiple-lumen catheters are available. With a multiple-lumen catheter, the proximal lumen is always used for blood collection.

Nonemergent central lines may be peripherally inserted, tunneled externally, or totally implanted (Table 11-1). Short-term therapy uses a catheter inserted peripherally in the cephalic (Figure 11-15), subclavian, or external jugular vein. Complications include infection and catheter migration. Tunneled external lines (Figure 11-16) and implanted ports (Figure 11-17) are used for long-term access, usually

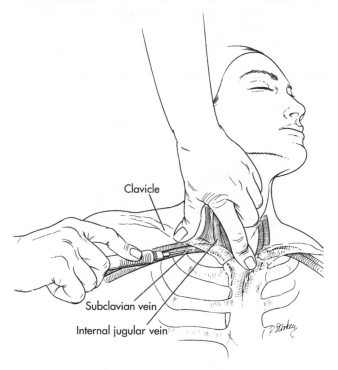

FIGURE **11-14**   Puncture of subclavian vein with needle inserted beneath middle third of clavicle at 20- to 30-degree angle aiming medially. (From Daily EK, Schroeder JS: *Techniques in bedside hemodynamic monitoring,* ed 5, St. Louis, 1994, Mosby.)

Clavicle

Subclavian vein

Internal jugular vein

Table 11-1	VENOUS ACCESS DEVICES		
	NONTUNNELED	**TUNNELED**	**IMPLANTED**
Examples	Peripherally inserted central catheters (PICC) and midline catheters (MLC)	Hickman; Broviac	Hickman Port; Port-a-Cath; Norport; Lifeport
Specific characteristics	Single or multilumen; PICC lines are 60 cm long; MIC lines are 15-20 cm long	Single or multilumen; Dacron cuff where tissue adheres helps ensure placement and decreases infection	Typically implanted in the chest wall; has a self-sealing septum; is accessed through skin with noncoring needle such as Huber needle to prevent damage to septum; special access catheter can be left in place, making repeated sticks unnecessary
Advantages	Do not require surgery for removal; easily removed or replaced	Unlimited use: painless when accessing; easily repaired when damaged; large gauge facilitates blood withdrawal	Less traumatic to body image; less maintenance; decreased chance of infection
Disadvantages	Activity restriction; no sutures so becomes dislodged easily; dressing needed at all times; maintenance costs are high because of frequent heparin flushing and injection cap changes	Mental and physical requirements for managing self-care; high maintenance cost; some patients cannot use this catheter because of body image (tube exiting the body)	High insertion costs; more painful in comparison with tunneled and nontunneled lines

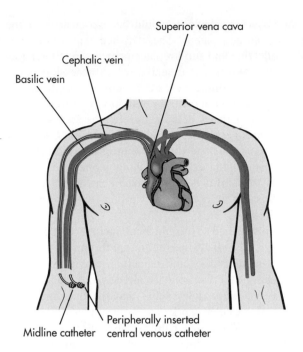

Superior vena cava

Cephalic vein

Basilic vein

Midline catheter

Peripherally inserted central venous catheter

FIGURE 11-15   Placement of peripherally inserted central venous catheter (PICC) and midline catheter (MLC). (Modified from Lewis SM, Collier IC, Heitkemper MM et al: *Medical-surgical nursing: assessment and management of clinical problems,* ed 5, St. Louis, 2000, Mosby.)

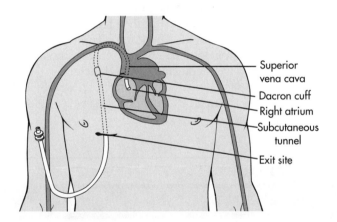

Superior vena cava

Dacron cuff

Right atrium

Subcutaneous tunnel

Exit site

FIGURE 11-16   Silastic right atrial catheter placement with exit in anterior chest wall. (Modified from Lewis SM, Collier IC, Heitkemper MM et al: *Medical-surgical nursing: assessment and management of clinical problems,* ed 5, St. Louis, 2000, Mosby.)

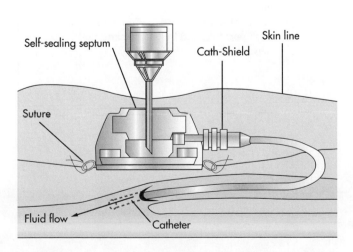

Self-sealing septum

Suture

Cath-Shield

Skin line

Fluid flow

Catheter

FIGURE 11-17   Cross-section of implantable port displaying access of port with Huber needle. Note deflected point of Huber needle that prevents coring of the port's septum. (Modified from Lewis SM, Collier IC, Heitkemper MM et al: *Medical-surgical nursing: assessment and management of clinical problems,* ed 5, St. Louis, 2000, Mosby.

over months or even years. These catheters and ports should be flushed after each use with saline and then heparin. Groshong catheters are a type of tunneled catheter with a unique slit that remains closed unless blood is withdrawn or fluid or medications are given. The slit collapses during blood withdrawal but opens during fluid or medication administration. Because of this unique feature, heparin flush is not required for Groshong catheters.[1] The catheter is still flushed with saline solution after each use, however.

Venous access devices should be used whenever they are available and patent. These devices can be used for blood collection and fluid replacement. Aseptic technique, masks, and gloves are essential when accessing central catheters to minimize risk of infection. Introduction of contaminants into the central circulation represents significant risk for patients with central venous access devices. Box 11-2 lists general guidelines for their use. Central venous catheters must be flushed appropriately after use to ensure patency. Inadequate flushing jeopardizes patency and leads to painful device replacement. Table 11-2 describes flushing guidelines for various central venous access devices.

Problems related to central lines include venous occlusion from a lodged catheter tip, mural thrombus, and fibrin sleeve.[1] Symptoms of occlusion include pain in the insertion area or path of the catheter, facial edema, or edema at the insertion site. Superficial veins may become more pronounced as vascular workload increases around the occluded vessel. The catheter tip can also migrate or become lodged against the endocardium or vessel wall. This problem is usually identified when blood cannot be withdrawn or when the external marker is not in the appropriate location. Turning the patient to the side, raising the arm, or asking the patient to cough may move the catheter.[3]

A fibrin sleeve can develop on the tip of the catheter and prevent blood withdrawal. The fibrin sleeve is confirmed with a chest radiograph. Treatment includes thrombolytic administration with streptokinase or urokinase.

Irritation of the intima lining of the vessel wall by medications, friction from the catheter tip, or bacteria can lead to

---

Box 11-2 GUIDELINES FOR VENOUS ACCESS DEVICES

Wear mask and gloves when accessing central access devices.
Check insertion site for infection.
Use infusion pump to infuse fluids through central lines.
Use injection caps for all ports.
Clamp lines if cap is removed (except for Groshong catheters).
Clamps with teeth can damage the catheter.
Phenytoin and diazepam precipitate in response to silicone and can cause the catheter to clot.
Forceful irrigation may rupture the catheter because of increased pressure.
Insert a noncoring needle into an implanted port until the posterior wall is felt.
Use noncoring needles to prevent damage to septum of the port.

Table 11-2 FLUSHING GUIDELINES FOR VENOUS ACCESS DEVICES

FLUSHING TYPE	TUNNELED/ NONTUNNELED DEVICE	GROSHONG CATHETER	IMPLANTED PORTS	PICC
General flushing	Heparin 10-100 units/ml, use 2.5-5 ml after use and/or every 12 to 24 hr	No heparin; 5 ml of saline after use or once per week	Flush one time per month (if not in use) with 500 units heparin (5 ml); use same amount each time	Heparin 10-100 units/ml, use 1-2.5 ml after use and/or once every 12 hr
After blood withdrawal	Stop infusion for 1 min before blood draw; withdraw and discard 10 ml of blood, draw blood for laboratory tests with syringe, flush with 5 ml saline before heparinizing as above	20 ml saline	Use 10 ml saline to flush port followed by heparin	Flush with saline before heparin flush
Before medication administration	Flush with 5 ml saline before medication administration	5 ml saline	5 ml saline	
After medication administration	Flush with 5 ml saline before heparinizing	5 ml saline	10 ml saline followed by heparin	Flush with saline before heparin flush

PICC, Peripherally inserted central catheter.

a mural thrombus in the vessel in which the catheter is inserted. When this occurs, blood cannot be withdrawn from the device.

Intraosseous Infusion

This method is used for rapid venous access in adults and children; however, most references describe use in children 6 years and younger. An intraosseous needle, bone marrow aspiration needle, or spinal needle is inserted into the marrow cavity of the anterior tibia, medial malleolus, sternum, distal femur, or iliac crest. Figure 11-18 shows

needles used for intraosseous infusion. There is at least one device on the market for adult use that instills fluids into the sternum; however, its use is not widespread. Fluids, blood and blood products, and medications can be safely infused with this technique. The tibia is preferred for infusion in children, whereas the thin sternum is rarely used. Figure 11-19 shows preferred sites. Intraosseous infusion is contraindicated in lower extremity fractures and bone disorders such as osteoporosis.[3] Complications related to this technique include fat emboli, osteomyelitis, and subcutaneous abscess (Figure 11-20). Epiphyseal damage can occur in children.

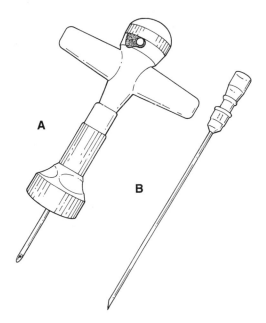

FIGURE **11-18** **A,** Disposable 16-gauge bone marrow aspiration needle (Illinois Sternal). **B,** Three-inch, 18-gauge spinal needle (Becton, Dickenson and Co., Rutherford, NJ). (Modified from Manley L: *J Emerg Nurs* 14(2):66, 1977.)

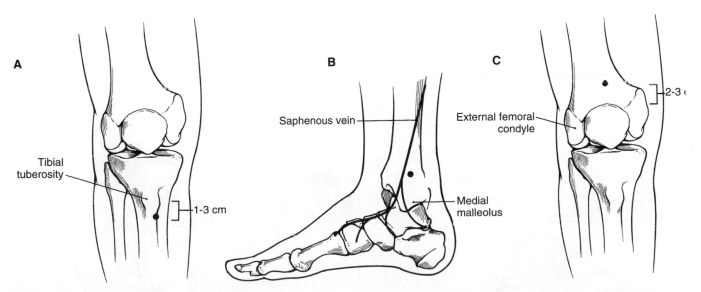

FIGURE **11-19**   Schematic diagram demonstrating IO insertion sites. **A,** The proximal tibia. The IO needle is inserted 1 to 2 cm distal to the tibial tuberosity and over the medial aspect of the tibia. The bevel of the needle is directed away from the joint space. **B,** The distal tibia. The IO needle is inserted on the medial surface of the distal tibia at the junction of the medial malleolus and the shaft of the tibia, posterior to the greater saphenous vein. The needle is directed cephalad, away from the growth plate. **C,** The distal femur. The IO needle is inserted 2 to 3 cm above the external condyles in the midline and directed cephalad, away from the growth plate.

Uenous Cutdown

Vascular access may be obtained surgically when a large volume of fluid is required or when peripheral access cannot be obtained. The procedure is used more often in children than in adults, but has lost favor with increased use of intraosseous needles. Venous cutdown involves surgical isolation of the basilic vein or saphenous vein (Figure 11-21) followed by insertion of a large bore catheter, intravenous tubing, or feeding tube (5 Fr or 8 Fr), which is

sutured in place (Figure 11-22).[3] Disadvantages of this technique include time and skill required to complete the procedure.

FLUID REPLACEMENT

Intravenous fluids may be given to maintain fluid requirements or in an effort to replace fluid losses. Normal metabolic processes in the body and insensible fluid losses through the skin and respiratory tract account for more than

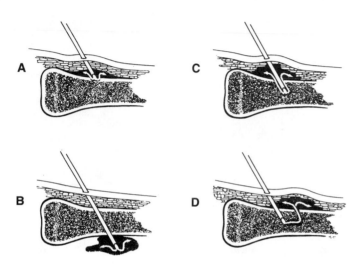

FIGURE **11-20** Schematic diagram of possible problems encountered with IO infusion. **A,** Incomplete penetration of the bony cortex. **B,** Penetration of the posterior cortex. **C,** Fluid escaping around the needle through the puncture site. **D,** Fluid leaking through a nearby previous cortical puncture site. (From Roberts J, Hedges J: *Clinical procedures in emergency medicine,* ed 3, Philadelphia, 1998, WB Saunders.)

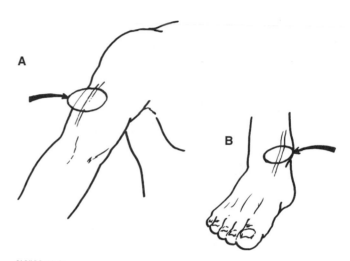

FIGURE **11-21** Common sites for venous cutdown. **A,** Cephalic vein. **B,** Saphenous vein.

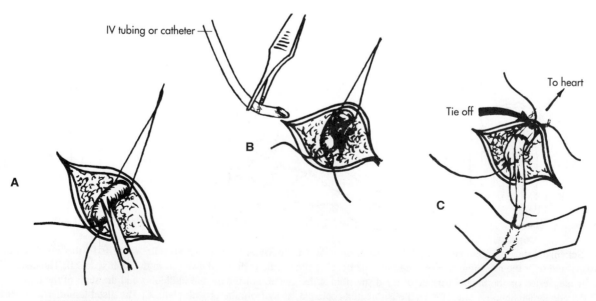

FIGURE **11-22** Venous cutdown. **A,** Isolating and cutting vein. **B,** Inserting cannula. **C,** Suturing cannula in place.

1500 ml/day of fluid loss. Calculation of basal fluid needs is based on patient size calculated as body surface area. Box 11-3 gives formulas for maintenance fluids and for volume replacement. Isotonic, hypotonic, and hypertonic fluids may be used as maintenance fluids. Isotonic fluids provide greater intravascular volume because more fluid remains in the vascular space. Hypotonic fluids shift fluid into intracellular spaces and are more useful for preventing cellular dehydration. Hypertonic fluids move fluid from cells to the extravascular space and may be used to promote diuresis.[2] Table 11-3 gives examples and describes use of these maintenance fluids.

Crystalloid and colloid solutions are used for volume replacement. These fluids may be isotonic, hypotonic, or hypertonic. Crystalloid solutions increase intravascular volume through actual volume administered, whereas colloids pull fluid into the vascular space through osmosis. Synthetic and natural colloid solutions are available. Examples of crystalloid and colloid solutions and actions for each are presented in Table 11-4.

Blood and Blood Products

These naturally occurring colloid solutions are used to replace blood losses and replenish clotting factors. Blood loss depletes the body of blood cells and clotting factors, so whole blood replacement is ideal in frank blood loss. However, whole blood is expensive, not readily available, and has greater risk for transmission of infectious diseases. Packed red blood cells are used more often for blood replacement. Other blood products used for component replacement include platelets, fresh frozen plasma, and albumin. Table 11-5 summarizes administration of these and other blood products in adults; Table 11-6 summarizes administration of these products in children. Blood products are always administered using normal saline. Dextrose solutions cause cellular edema as fluid shifts into the intracellular space. A blood warmer is recommended for large volume blood transfusions.[3]

Before blood administration, a blood sample should be obtained for type and cross-match. Two specimens should be obtained if large-volume replacement is anticipated. Ide-

---

Box 11-3	**FORMULAS FOR FLUID ADMINISTRATION**

BASAL FLUID MAINTENANCE

1500 ml/m^2 BSA/24 hr = ml/24 hr (calculate as ml/hr)
General guidelines: Up to 10 kg = 100 ml/kg/24 hr
   11-20 kg = 50 ml/kg/24 hr plus 100 ml/kg for first 10 kg
   > 20 kg = 20-25 ml/kg/24 hr plus 50 ml/kg for each kg 11 through 20 plus 100 ml/kg for first 10 kg

VOLUME REPLACEMENT WITH CRYSTALLOIDS

Administer 3 ml for each ml lost. Fluid challenges/options are:
   IV bolus 20 ml/kg D5% LR in children
   IV bolus of 200-300 ml LR in adult surgical patients
   IV bolus of 200-300 ml NS in adult medical patients

VOLUME REPLACEMENT WITH COLLOIDS

Administer 1 ml for each ml lost

VOLUME REPLACEMENT FOR MEASURED LOSSES

Gastric losses: Replace 1 ml for each ml lost every 4 hr. Use D5 1/2NS plus 30 mEq K/L
Intestinal losses: Replace 1 ml for each ml lost every 4 hr. Use D5% LR

BASAL URINE OUTPUT

Up to 30 kg = 40 ml/kg/24 hr (2 ml/kg/hr)
>30 kg = 1200 ml/24 hr (17-18 ml/kg/hr)

Modified from Kidd PS, Sturt P, Fultz J: *Mosby's emergency nursing reference*, ed. 2, St. Louis, 2000, Mosby.
NS, Normal saline; *LR*, Lactated Ringer's solution; *BSA*, body surface area.

Table 11-3	**MAINTENANCE IV FLUIDS**	
SOLUTION TYPE	**EXAMPLES**	**USES**
Isotonic	0.9% Normal saline (NS)	Expands intravascular volume. Used for dehydration (e.g., diabetic ketoacidosis, hyperosmolar nonketotic coma) and packed red blood cell administration.
	Lactated Ringer's solution	Expands intravascular volume. Used for maintenance fluid when patient is at risk for free water loss.
Hypotonic	NS 0.45%	Shifts water into intracellular spaces.
	NS 0.2%	Useful in preventing dehydration and assessing renal status.
	Dextrose 5% and water (D$_5$W)	D$_5$W may be used in adult patients for mixing intravenous medications. Used for maintenance fluid when patient is at risk for free water loss.
Hypertonic	Dextrose 5% in NS	Shifts fluid from intracellular to extracellular space.
	Dextrose 10% in NS	Used in water intoxication states created by too much hypotonic fluid administration.
	Dextrose 10% in water	Used for maintenance fluid to promote diuresis.
	Dextrose 5% in 0.45 NS	
	Dextrose 20% in water	

Modified from Kidd PS, Sturt P, Fultz J: *Mosby's emergency nursing reference*, ed 2, St. Louis, 2000, Mosby.

Table 11-4 FLUID RESUSCITATION SUMMARY*

CRYSTALLOIDS	DESCRIPTION/INDICATION	ACTION(S)
0.9% Normal saline†	Isotonic	• May produce fluid overload and hypernatremia • 25% of volume administered remains in vascular space
0.45% Normal saline	Hypotonic, moves fluid from vascular space to interstitial and intracellular spaces	• Decreases blood viscosity • May promote hypovolemia • May promote cerebral edema
5% Dextrose	Hypotonic	• 7.5 ml/100 ml infused remains in vascular space • Inadequate for fluid resuscitation
Lactated Ringer's solution	Isotonic, contains multiple electrolytes and lactate	• May produce fluid overload • May promote lactic acidosis in prolonged hypoperfusion with decreased liver function • Lactate metabolizes to acetate, may produce metabolic alkalosis when large volumes are transfused
Hypertonic saline (7.5%)	Hypertonic, pulls fluid from interstitial and intracellular spaces into vascular space	• Requires smaller amount to restore blood volume • Increases cerebral oxygen drive while decreasing ICP • May promote hypernatremia • May promote intracellular dehydration • May promote osmotic diuresis • Controversial

SYNTHETIC COLLOIDS	DESCRIPTION	ACTION(S)
Dextran‡	(Comes in 40, 70, and 75 molecular weight)	• Associated with anaphylaxis • Reduces factor VIII, platelets, and fibrinogen function, so increases bleeding time • May interfere with blood type and cross-match, glucose, and erythrocyte sedimentation level • Risk of fluid overload
Hetastarch‡		• May increase serum amylase levels • Associated with coagulopathy • Risk of fluid overload

NATURAL COLLOIDS	DESCRIPTION	ACTION(S)
Fresh frozen plasma	Contains all clotting factors	• Potential to transmit blood-borne infection • Can cause hypersensitivity reaction • Blood volume expander
Plasma protein fraction (Plasmanate)	Does not contain clotting factors	• May cause hypersensitivity reaction • May cause hypotension with rapid infusion • Blood volume expander
Albumin‡	5% iso-oncotic 25% hyperoncotic "salt poor"	• Preferred as volume expander when risk from producing interstitial edema is great (e.g., pulmonary and heart disease) • Hypocalcemia
Whole blood	Can be administered without normal saline; reduces donor exposure	• Hyperkalemia, hypothermia, and hypocalcemia • May require greater amount than packed RBCs to increase oxygen-carrying capacity of blood • Rarely used, not cost-effective
Packed RBCs	Administer with normal saline	• Deficient in 2, 3-diphosphoglycerate and may increase oxygen affinity for hemoglobin and decrease oxygen delivery to tissue • Hypothermia, hyperkalemia, and hypocalcemia

EXPERIMENTAL AGENTS	DESCRIPTION	ACTION(S)
Liposome encapsulated hemoglobin hypertonic saline (7.5%)	NOT APPROVED BY FDA	• Improves skeletal muscle oxygen tension • Expands vascular volume quickly • Improves tissue oxygenation
Hypertonic saline (7.5%) with Dextran 70	Combined crystalloid and colloid therapy	• Promotes rapid expansion of blood volume and promotes retention of volume in vascular space • Controversial

Modified from Kidd PS, Sturt P, Fultz J: *Mosby's emergency nursing reference,* ed 2, St. Louis, 2000, Mosby.

ICP, Intracranial pressure; *RBCs,* red blood cells; *FDA,* Food and Drug Administration.

*Dosages are not listed because of variability in patient response and need.

†Fluid overload using these agents may occur because of large amount required (3:1 ratio fluid to volume lost).

‡Fluid overload using these agents may occur in cases of preexisting pulmonary and/or heart disease.

Table 11-5 BLOOD COMPONENT ADMINISTRATION IN ADULTS

BLOOD COMPONENT	USES	BLOOD TYPE	INFUSION RATE	FILTER	VOLUME	COMMENTS
Whole blood	Acute or chronic anemia, aplastic anemia, bone marrow failure, congestive heart failure, chronic renal failure, hepatic coma	*Must* be ABO compatible	2-4 hr Max: 4 hr	Required	500 ml	Rapid infusion if need is urgent. Clotting factors deteriorate after 24 hr.
Packed RBCs	Acute massive blood loss, hypovolemic shock	*Must* be ABO compatible	2-4 hr Max: 4 hr	Required	250 ml	Hgb rises 1 g/dl; Hct rises 3% after 1 U.
Leukocyte-poor RBCs	Thrombocytopenia, platelet function abnormality	Need *not* be ABO compatible	2 hr	Required	Variable	
Fresh frozen plasma	Hypovolemia combined with hemorrhage caused by deficiencies	*Must* be ABO compatible	1-2 hr, rapidly if bleeding	Use component filter	250 ml	Notify blood bank— plasma takes 20 min to thaw; use within 6 hr of thawing. Do not use microaggregate filter.
Platelets	Hemophilia, von Willebrand's disease, hypofibrinogenemia, factor XIII deficiency	Need *not* be ABO compatible	Rapidly as patient tolerates	Use component filter	35-50 ml U	Usually 6-10 U are ordered. Request that blood bank pool all units. Do not use microaggregate filter.
Albumin	Shock caused by burns; maintains blood volume in patients with hypovolemia; hypoproteinemia	Need *not* be ABO compatible	1-2 ml/min in normovolemic patients	Special tubing	Varies	Comes in 5% and 25%; can increase intravascular volume quickly; infuse cautiously.
Cryoprecipitate	Repeated febrile reaction; reaction from leukocyte antibodies and patients who are candidates for organ transplants	*Must* be ABO compatible	30 min	Use component filter	10 ml U	Usually 6-10 U ordered; request that blood bank pool units. Unstable to heat and storage.
Granulocytes			2-4 hr	Use component filter	300-400 ml	VS every 15 min during infusion. Granulocytes have a short life span. Transfuse as soon after collection as possible.

Hgb, Hemoglobin; *Hct,* hematocrit; *RBCs,* red blood cells; *VS,* vital signs.

Table 11-6   BLOOD COMPONENT ADMINISTRATION IN CHILDREN

BLOOD COMPONENT	USUAL DOSE	INFUSION RATE	COMMENTS
Whole blood	20 ml/kg initially	As rapidly as necessary to restore volume and stabilize the child.	Administration is usually reserved for massive hemorrhage.
Packed RBCs	10 ml/kg, not to exceed 15 ml/kg	5 ml/kg/hr or 2 ml/kg/hr if congestive heart failure develops	1 ml/kg will increase Hct approximately 1%. Infuse within 4 hr. If necessary, divide the unit into smaller volumes for infusion. Replace platelets after 6-8 units of RBCs are given.
Platelets	1 unit for every 7-10 kg	Each unit over 5-10 min via syringe or pump	The usual dose will increase platelet count by 50,000/mm³.
Fresh frozen plasma	Hemorrhage: 15-30 ml/kg Clotting deficiency: 10-15 ml/kg	Hemorrhage: rapidly to stabilize the child Clotting deficiency: over 2-3 hr	Monitor for fluid overload.
Granulocytes	Dependent on WBC counts and clinical condition, 10 ml/kg/day initially	Slowly over 2-4 hr because of fever and chills, side effects commonly associated with infusion	Granulocytes have a short life span. Transfuse as soon after collection as possible.
Albumin 5%	1 g/kg or 20 ml/kg	1-2 ml/min or 60-120 ml/hr	Monitor for fluid overload. Type and cross-match are not required.
Albumin 25%	1 g/kg or 4 ml/kg	0.2-0.4 ml/min or 12-24 ml/hr	Monitor for fluid overload. Type and cross-match are not required.

Modified from Kidd PS, Sturt P, Fultz J: *Mosby's emergency nursing reference,* ed 2, St. Louis, 2000, Mosby.

RBCs, Red blood cells; *Hct,* hematocrit; *WBC,* white blood cell.

Table 11-7   TYPE AND CROSS-MATCH PROCEDURES

PROCEDURES	TESTS	TIME REQUIRED (MIN)
Complete type and cross-match	ABO-Rh typing Full cross-match Antibody screening*	30-45
Incomplete type and cross-match†	ABO-Rh typing Saline–immediate-spin cross-match	15-20
Group†	ABO-Rh typing‡	5-10
Group and screen	ABO-Rh typing Antibody screening*§ (Saline–immediate-spin cross-match when ordered for transfusion)	30-45

Modified from Rosen P et al: *Emergency medicine: concepts and clinical practice,* ed 4, St. Louis, 1998, Mosby.

*Additional time is required if antibodies are found.

†Physician requesting the incomplete type and cross-match must take full responsibility for adverse effects.

‡Most blood banks will not release type-specific blood without saline–immediate-spin cross-match.

§After release, screening is completed for less common antibodies.

ally, complete type and cross-match should be done on all blood before administration; however, this procedure can take 40 minutes or more. Type-specific blood or blood that is not completely cross-matched may be given in patients with critical blood loss. Type O blood may be given for patients with extreme blood loss who cannot wait for type-specific blood. Table 11-7 summarizes type and cross-match procedures. Type O-negative blood is given to females, and type O-positive blood is given to males. However, many facilities give type O-negative blood to females and males.

Blood administration is not without risk. Blood processing procedures have reduced risk for transmission of infectious diseases; however, transfusion reactions can occur because of transfusion of incompatible blood, patient allergy, or depletion of clotting factors (Table 11-8). Unrecognized transfusion reactions represent a significant threat to the patient's life. Before transfusion, blood and patient identification should be checked carefully. During the transfusion, the patient should be carefully monitored for signs of reaction including fever, chills, urticaria, breathing difficulty, back pain, and hematuria.

SUMMARY

Intravenous lines provide a route for administration of medications, fluids, blood, and blood products. Venous access and fluid replacement can save the patient's life or create significant threats to health if vigilance is not used with catheter insertion and fluid administration. Consistent use of universal precautions, sharps disposal, and aseptic technique pro-

Table 11-8 TRANSFUSION REACTIONS

REACTION	CAUSE	PREVENTION	ASSESSMENT	INTERVENTION
Hemolytic	Blood incompatibility	Type and cross-match; infuse first 50 ml slowly	Fever, chills, dyspnea, tachypnea, lumbar pain, fever, oliguria, hematuria, tightness in chest; collect blood and urine samples	Discontinue immediately; fatality may occur after 100 ml infused Start NS or LR Consider diuretics; monitor BUN, serum creatinine
Allergic	Antibody reaction to allergens	Screen donors for allergy; administer antihistamines before transfusion	Hypersensitivity, chills, hives, wheezing, vertigo, angioneurotic edema, allergic itching Anaphylaxis, dyspnea, bronchospasm, hypotension, decreased responsiveness, generalized edema	Stop infusion; give antihistamine, steroids, and antipyretics Stop infusion; give epinephrine, start NS; administer LR Anticipate intubation
Pyrogenic	Infusing chilled blood	Screen donors; use aseptic technique in administration	Fever, chills, nausea, lumbar pain	Stop infusion
Hypothermic	Infusing chilled blood	Give at room temperature; use warming coils for rapid infusion	Chills	Slow infusion; cover client
Circulatory overload	Infusion of large amounts of blood, especially to clients with cardiac disease or extremes of age	Infuse slowly; check drip rate frequently	Rales, cough, dyspnea, cyanosis, pulmonary edema, increased CVP	Stop infusion; treat pulmonary edema
Air embolism	Entry of air into vein	Use proper infusion technique; avoid giving under pressure; check connections to tubings; avoid Y-tubes; use filter; use plastic containers	Chest pain, dyspnea, hypotension, venous distension	Stop infusion; position on left side; give oxygen; embolectomy may be performed
Hypocalcemic	Precipitate from acid citrate dextrose Calcium dilution with massive transfusions	Use blood immediately	Numbness, tingling in extremities May contribute to development of diffuse intravascular coagulation	Stop infusion; give calcium as ordered
Hyperkalemic	Hemolysis of red blood cells releases potassium	Use blood immediately	Nausea, vomiting, muscle weakness, bradycardia	Stop infusion

Modified from Barber J, Stokes L, Billings D: *Adult and child care: a client approach to nursing,* ed 2, St. Louis, 1977, Mosby.
NS, Normal saline; *LR,* lactated Ringer's solution; *BUN,* blood urea nitrogen; *CVP,* central venous pressure.

tect the patient and the emergency nurse. Assessment and reassessment during fluid replacement can identify symptoms related to fluid overload, anaphylaxis, and other side effects.

References

1. Kitt S, Selfridge-Thomas J, Proehl J et al, editors: *Emergency nursing: a physiologic and clinical perspective,* ed 2, Philadelphia, 1995, WB Saunders.
2. Lewis SM, Collier IC, Heitkemper MM et al: *Medical-surgical nursing: assessment and management of clinical problems,* ed 5, St. Louis, 2000, Mosby.
3. Proehl JA: *Adult emergency nursing procedures,* Boston, 1999, WB Saunders.

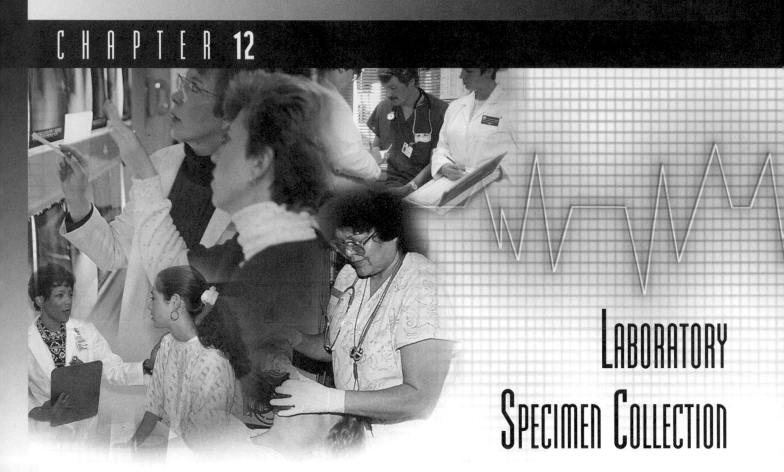

CHAPTER 12

LABORATORY SPECIMEN COLLECTION

DELL T. MILLER, JOHN R. LUNDE

The act of obtaining blood specimens has been practiced since antiquity. Specimens are used to diagnose and monitor the disease process to determine patient treatment. Appropriate diagnosis and treatment of acute disorders in the emergency department (ED) depend on accurate collection and interpretation of laboratory data. A viable specimen is the key to the entire practice of laboratory medicine and vital to the practice of emergency care. Emergency personnel are often called on to obtain specimens for laboratory analysis. The process is not complicated but does require attention to detail and accuracy.

BLOOD COLLECTION

Blood for analysis may be collected from the venous, arterial, or capillary system. In general the majority of blood specimens are venous samples. Collection of blood from the arterial system has a higher risk for complications; therefore, collection of arterial samples is usually limited to arterial blood gas (ABG) analysis. Capillary specimens are collected primarily from infants and children. Regardless of collection site or specimen type, the specimen must be collected using aseptic technique to minimize the risks of infection to the patient and to avoid contaminating the specimen. Personnel collecting the specimen should always use standard precautions and review laboratory orders before specimen collection to ensure that the proper tube is used for

each test. Box 12-1 identifies general rules of safety for specimen collection.

Collection Systems

Venous or arterial blood may be collected from a primary venipuncture or may be withdrawn from existing access points such as venous access ports, central venous catheters, or arterial catheters.

Evacuated Blood Collection System

The evacuated blood collection system (EBCS) is the most widely used and recognized collection system available. EBCS allows collection of multiple specimens with a single venipuncture (Figure 12-1).[2] The key element in the system is an evacuated specimen tube. Vacuum in the tube pulls blood into the tube after the blood vessel has been cannulated. Tubes have color-coded stoppers to indicate additives present. Table 12-1 lists tubes by color, the additives present in the tube, and what the additive does. As with intravenous (IV) and intramuscular needles, venipuncture needles are color-coded for length and diameter.

Nonevacuated Collection System

The nonevacuated collection system is not used as frequently as the EBCS but is a valuable collection system in certain circumstances. This system uses manual pressure

Box 12-1 GENERAL GUIDELINES FOR SPECIMEN COLLECTION

Use standard precautions.

Use aseptic technique.

Review laboratory orders before collection to confirm tests and tubes required for each test.

Identify the patient before specimen collection. Confirm medical record identification number.

Tell the patient what you are going to do.

Position the patient for safety and specimen collection.

Label all specimens with patient name and identification number.

Do not collect the specimen from a site proximal to an intravenous catheter.

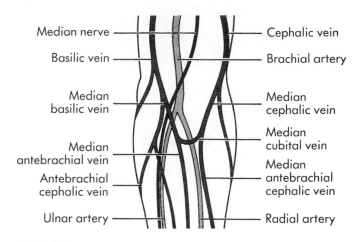

FIGURE **12-2** Superficial arteries and nerves in antecubital fossa.

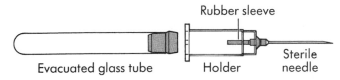

FIGURE **12-1** Evacuated blood collection system.

Table 12-1 COMMONLY USED EVACUATED SPECIMEN TUBES

STOPPER COLOR	ADDITIVE	ACTION, NOTES
Red	None	—
Gold	Inert silicon gel	Acts as a separator between red blood cells and serum after centrifuging
Purple	Ethylenediamine tetraacetic acid (EDTA)	Chelates calcium from the blood, thus preventing clotting; the potassium salt of EDTA is usually used
Blue	Sodium citrate	Same action as for EDTA; the anticoagulant of choice for coagulation studies
Black	Sodium citrate	Same action as for EDTA; used for red blood cell sedimentation studies
Gray	Potassium oxalate	Same action as for EDTA; is also a glycolytic inhibitor for glucose determinations
Green	Heparin	Prevents clotting by deactivating thrombin and thromboplastin; both sodium and lithium salts are used

rather than vacuum to withdraw blood. Use is recommended when vacuum in the EBCS causes the vein to collapse, preventing blood collection, such as in the very young or very old. One example of this system is a butterfly needle attached to a syringe.

Venous Collection

The venous system is the primary source of blood specimens used for laboratory testing. Only a few of the many veins in the human body are actually accessible for venipuncture or intravenous (IV) cannulation, so care must be exercised to guard limited resources for future specimen collection and IV therapy. Most venous specimens are obtained from primary puncture in the antecubital area. Figure 12-2 highlights veins in this area. The vein is selected after visual inspection; however, this should never be the sole method for selection. Palpating for location, size, fullness, and softness of the vein wall is also performed. The tourniquet is never left on for more than 2 minutes because hemoconcentration below the tourniquet can affect test results. The tourniquet is released and reapplied before preparing the puncture site.

With the exception of coagulation tubes, which must be filled completely, most tubes contain an adequate volume of blood when they are half full. A general rule of thumb is that the tube should contain one part additive to nine parts blood. Tubes that do not contain an adequate amount of blood proportionate to the additive can lead to erroneous results. Also, tubes should be filled in a specific order to prevent specimen contamination from additives in the tubes. Blood for blood cultures is collected first, then red-top tubes, blue-top coagulation tubes, and finally purple-top hematology tubes. The patient's condition is always a determinant of which tests are most important; therefore, the priority of collection should reflect this.

Failure to obtain blood may be caused by several problems. If the needle goes through the vein, it must be withdrawn slowly, watching for blood in the tube. If the needle did not puncture the vein, venipuncture must be attempted at another site; however, multiple sticks are not recommended. If the specimen cannot be obtained after two attempts, someone else should stick the patient. Tubes can lose vacuum because of age or a puncture that opens the tube to outside air. When this occurs, another tube must be inserted. If

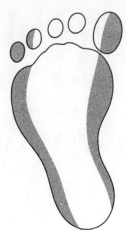

FIGURE **12-3** Shaded areas represent areas on infant's foot used for obtaining blood specimen.

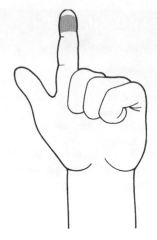

FIGURE **12-4** Shaded area represents area commonly used for obtaining blood specimen from fingertip.

the vein is small and fragile, the vacuum may cause the vein to collapse. In this situation, a needle and syringe are the best alternative. Alternative sites for specimen collection, such as the femoral vein, should be considered. Blood may also be collected when an IV catheter is inserted. A catheter can be used to withdraw the blood or a Luer-lock adapter can be used to fill tubes directly from the IV.

Capillary Collection

Capillary specimens are obtained from infants, children, and adults when multiple blood samples must be taken over a period of time (e.g., glucose testing in diabetic patients). The basic capillary collection system uses a lancet to puncture the skin and a container to collect the specimen. The containers are similar to blood tubes for venous samples in that they contain various additives; however, the requisite volume is smaller.

In children younger than 1 year of age, the heel or great toe is preferred.[7] Figure 12-3 illustrates preferred sites in the foot. The index finger of the nondominant hand is preferred for capillary sticks on children and adults (Figure 12-4). Lancets are designed to minimize depth of penetration. Penetration greater than 2.4 mm has been associated with development of osteomyelitis and sepsis. The area is warmed for 3 to 5 minutes with a heel warmer or cloth soaked in warm water to increase circulation and facilitate specimen collection. Povidone iodine affects results, falsely elevating potassium, phosphorus, uric acid, and bilirubin levels, and should be avoided. The first drop of blood is discarded because it contains fluids from the tissues rather than the capillaries. Moderate pressure is adequate because excessive pressure can cause hemolysis, bruise the heel, and contaminate the specimen with tissue fluids. Collection from the finger is the same procedure as collection from the heel or toe. The lancet should puncture the pulp of the finger.

For blood sugar analysis, the finger is held over the analysis strip and blood is dropped onto the strip. This provides the best sample for the test. If a platelet count is or-

dered, this test is drawn first. Platelets clump, so the count is often lower in capillary specimens.

Venous Access Devices

In addition to primary venipuncture, venous samples may also be collected from intermittent infusion catheters, indwelling central venous catheters, and implanted central venous access devices.[4] General rules of asepsis and use of standard precautions also apply to collection from these access points.

Intermittent Infusion Catheters

If a patient has an intermittent infusion catheter, blood may be collected from this site provided that collection does not endanger integrity of the catheter. The process is the same as that for blood collection from a primary venipuncture with a few exceptions. If the catheter has an access port that must be punctured by a needle, the port must be carefully cleaned before use. After the port is punctured, 3 to 5 ml of blood are withdrawn and discarded before the venous specimen is collected.[6] Blood cultures are never drawn from an indwelling catheter because of the risks for contamination.

Central Venous Access Devices

Many patients have long-term indwelling central venous catheters. The catheter tip is located in the superior vena cava or other large vessel. Access ports may be located subcutaneously or externally. Catheters located in the central circulation are at greater risk for systemic complications if contamination occurs. In addition to gloves and aseptic technique, masks are recommended to prevent droplet contamination.

External Devices. Hickmann and Groshong catheters are long-term devices with external ports (Figure 12-5). The ports for these catheters are usually located at the fourth or fifth intercostal space. When blood is collected from these ports, 3 to 5 ml of blood are withdrawn and discarded before the sample is obtained. After the specimen is obtained, the

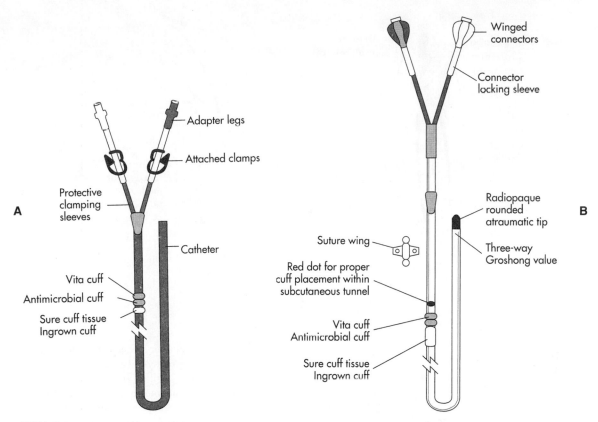

FIGURE **12-5** External central venous access devices. **A,** Hickman dual-lumen catheter. **B,** Groshong dual-lumen catheter. (From Kidd PS, Sturt P, Fultz J: *Mosby's emergency nursing reference,* ed 2, St. Louis, 2000, Mosby.)

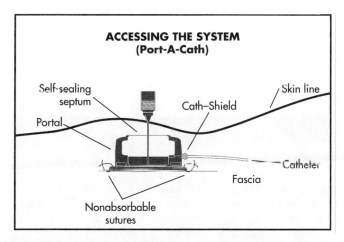

FIGURE **12-6** Implanted access device. (Modified from Kandt KA: An implantable venous access device for children, *Am J Mat Child Nurs,* Jan/Feb 1991.)

catheter should be flushed with saline. A dilute heparin solution can be used to flush the Hickman catheter; however, heparin should not be used with the Groshong catheter.

Internal Devices. The Port-a-Cath, Mediport, and Bard Implanted Port are examples of an internal central venous access device surgically implanted in subcutaneous tissue with the tip in the superior vena cava. The device has a self-sealing diaphragm ideal for multiple sticks (Figure 12-6). A

90-degree, noncoring needle is used to access the device. Locate the device by palpating the chest, and then stabilize it with the thumb and forefinger. The needle is inserted into the center of the device at a 90-degree angle until it touches the bottom of the device. The device is then flushed with 5 ml of saline to ensure patency, and then 5 ml of blood are withdrawn and discarded.

Arterial Systems

Arterial blood is usually obtained for ABG analysis. Blood may be collected from the radial, brachial, and femoral arteries. The radial artery is the preferred site for arterial puncture (Figure 12-7, *A*) because there is collateral circulation to the hand via the ulnar artery, the vessel is easily accessible for palpation and stabilization, and surrounding tissue is relatively insensitive. The brachial artery (Figure 12-7, *B*) is the second choice for arterial collection. Disadvantages include lack of collateral circulation, vessel instability, and proximity to the brachial nerve. The femoral artery (Figure 12-7, *C*) is used when no other site is available. Special precautions must be taken when collecting blood from this site because of the increased risk for hematoma formation and other complications. Figure 12-8 illustrates collection in the pediatric patient.

Before the radial artery is punctured, an Allen's test is usually performed to ensure collateral circulation to the hand.[6]

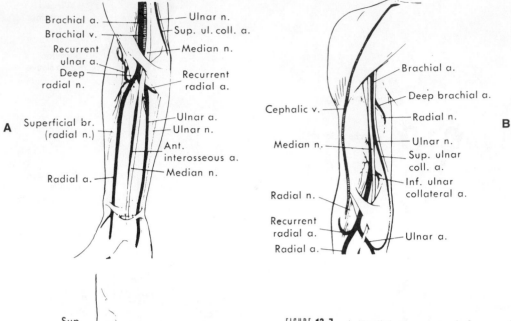

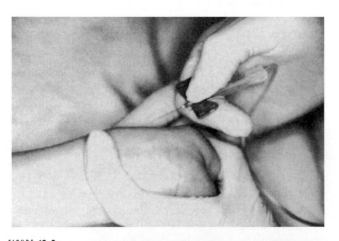

FIGURE 12-7 **A,** Radial artery extends from neck of radius to median side of styloid process. **B,** Brachial artery, continuation of axillary artery. **C,** Femoral artery branches from abdominal aorta and branches to superficial epigastric, superficial circumflex iliac, external pudendal, deep femoral, and descending geniculate arteries. (Modified from Budassi SA: *J Emerg Nurs* 3(2):24, 1977.)

FIGURE 12-8 For arterial blood sampling, the needle should be inserted under the skin at a 30° to 45° angle. A butterfly needle and syringe are used if larger volumes of blood are required. The wrist is held dorsiflexed by the nondominant hand. (From Roberts J, Hedges J: *Clinical procedures in emergency medicine,* ed 3, Philadelphia, 1998, WB Saunders.)

Box 12-2	**PROCEDURE FOR ALLEN'S TEST**

Flex patient's arm with hand above level of the elbow.
Have patient clench fist to force blood from the hand.
Place pressure on both arteries simultaneously, then ask the patient to open the hand. The hand should appear blanched.
Remove pressure from the ulnar artery. The blanched area flushes within seconds if collateral circulation is adequate.
If the area flushes quickly, this is recorded as a positive Allen's test. The test is negative if the blanched area does not flush quickly.
A negative Allen's test means collateral circulation is inadequate to support circulation to the hand; therefore, an alternative site should be selected.

Box 12-2 and Figure 12-9 describe this test. If the test is positive, collateral circulation to the hand is present and the specimen can be collected.[1] Hyperextending the wrist moves the artery closer to the surface and aids stabilization and puncture. The needle is inserted at a 45-degree angle to the skin.

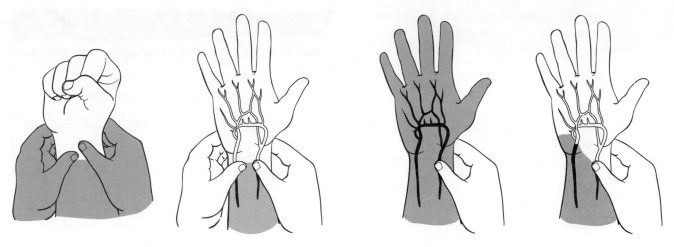

FIGURE **12-9**   Allen's test. (From May JL: *Emergency medical procedures,* New York, 1984, John Wiley & Sons.)

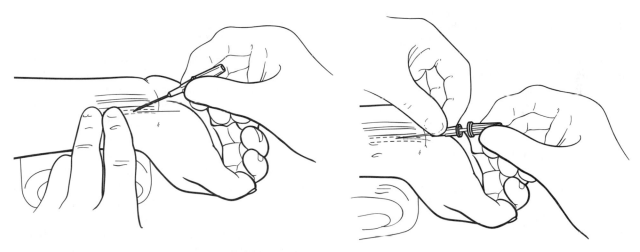

FIGURE **12-10**   Radial artery cannulization.

This minimizes the actual opening into the arterial wall and promotes closure after the needle is removed. Brachial punctures may be performed at a 45- to 60-degree angle, whereas the femoral vein is punctured at a 90-degree angle. Figure 12-10 shows needle placement for radial artery puncture. After the specimen is collected, pressure should be applied to the puncture site for at least 5 minutes, or 10 minutes if the femoral artery is punctured or the patient is on anticoagulants. The specimen is placed on ice if analysis is delayed. Most venous blood tests can be collected from an arterial stick.

Arterial specimens may also be drawn from an existing arterial line. Similarly, a discard sample of 3 to 5 ml is collected before collection of the actual specimen. Care should be taken to prevent introduction of air into the system during the process. In some institutions the discard sample is returned to the patient after the actual specimen is collected; however, this is more common with neonates and infants.

URINE SPECIMENS

Urine testing is one of the world's oldest laboratory tests. Ancient Greeks used a "taste" test to determine the presence

of sugar in the urine. Urine tests are used to assess renal function, diagnose disease, and confirm pregnancy. Urine normally contains numerous metabolic end products and water. Obtaining a good urine specimen is just as important as obtaining a good blood specimen.

The basic urine specimen is a clean-catch, midstream specimen. Catheterization or a percutaneous bladder tap may also be used. A specimen collection bag used for infants is placed on the infant before any procedure that would cause the infant to become upset. Catheterization is often recommended for female patients to minimize contamination from the vagina. A small female catheter, available in size 5 or 8 Fr, is recommended to minimize discomfort. When catheterization is necessary in infants, a size 5 or 8 Fr catheter is recommended. If sexual assault is suspected, the genitalia should not be cleaned before specimen collection. The specimen should be placed in a dry, sterile container and analyzed within 1 hour of collection. Specimens more than 2 hours old should not be submitted for analysis. Accelerated chemical changes, decomposition of cellular contents, and growth of bacteria can alter test results. When toxicologic screening is required, 30 to 50 ml of urine are necessary. Special regulations apply to collection of specimens in the case of a criminal action or on-the-job injury.

BODY FLUID SPECIMENS

In addition to blood and urine, laboratory analysis is done on pleural, synovial, amniotic, peritoneal, gastric, and cerebrospinal fluids. If a cell count is required on body fluid, it should be placed in a tube containing ethylenediamine tetraacetic acid or heparin to prevent clotting. Fluid for chemistry analysis is put in a red-top tube. Synovial fluid for crystal analysis should be placed in tubes containing heparin. If the fluid will be cultured, it is usually left in the collection syringe. The syringe should be capped to ensure an anaerobic environment. Emesis and gastric fluids are used primarily for toxicologic analysis. Complete information about suspected substances should be provided along with the specimen. Amniotic fluid must be protected from light as soon as the sample is obtained and during transport to the laboratory to prevent light breakdown of bilirubin in the specimen.

Cerebrospinal fluid may be submitted in three to five tubes containing 0.5 to 1 ml of fluid each. Tubes are filled in order with Tube 1 filled first. Facilities and physicians often prefer to submit particular tubes for specific tests. In general Tube 1 is used for chemistry analysis, Tube 2 for cell and differential counts, and Tube 3 or 4 for microbiology (i.e., culture, gram stain). Tube 5 is held for any special testing that may be required. When obtaining a sample is difficult, microbiology testing is usually given priority over other tests. Cerebrospinal fluid should be transported promptly to the laboratory for processing.

SPUTUM SPECIMENS

Sputum may be collected for culture, gram stain, and other tests but should be obtained before giving antimicrobial therapy. Many institutions have a high fail rate for sputum collection, collecting saliva and oral secretions more often than sputum. Delays in definitive therapy caused by these inappropriate specimens create a significant financial burden, because cultures must be repeated. Also, broader spectrum antibiotics are ordered when the organism is not identified, which leads to longer therapy while the test is repeated. Box 12-3 describes the procedure for sputum collection.[6]

STOOL SPECIMENS

Stool specimens may be collected for cell counts, presence of ova and parasites, and cultures. A fresh, warm stool is preferred for a culture. A small amount of stool is collected from a bedpan and placed in a dry, sterile container. Care is taken not to contaminate the sample with urine. Therapy should be withheld until specimens are obtained. Specimens for parasitology should be submitted as soon as possible. Unpreserved specimens must be examined for trophozoites within 1 hour. A specimen can be preserved for later examination by dividing it into three portions: one unpreserved, one mixed

---

Box 12-3 **SPUTUM COLLECTION**

Explain the procedure and purpose of sputum collection to the patient.
Remind the patient that sputum must be coughed up from the lungs and that saliva is not the specimen required.
Provide a sterile container.
Ask patient to rinse mouth before collection to decrease specimen contamination.
A total of 5 ml sputum is required.
Instruct the patient to take several deep breaths and cough to expectorate the specimen.
Aerosolized warm saline solution may be given if the patient is unable to produce a specimen.

---

with polyvinyl alcohol, and the third mixed with 10% formalin. Stool samples are usually obtained for 3 consecutive days.

MICROBIOLOGY SPECIMENS

Microbiology specimens are referred to as aerobic or anaerobic specimens. Aerobic specimens are obtained when the organism to be identified can be grown in the presence of oxygen (e.g., *Streptococcus, Staphylococcus* organisms). Anaerobic specimens are obtained when the organism to be identified grows without oxygen. Examples include the *Clostridia* species that cause gangrene and botulism.

Specimens are placed on a designated transport medium after collection. Various swabs with transport media are available commercially for aerobic and anaerobic cultures. Specimens, particularly anaerobic specimens, should be transported to the laboratory as soon as possible after collection. When rapid monoclonal antibody testing for *Streptococcus* organisms is available, two throat swabs should be submitted—one swab for a confirmatory culture and one for rapid testing.

GUIDE TO SELECTED LABORATORY RESULTS

Evaluation of laboratory results is based on comparison of the patient's results to a range of normal values for a given test. A range is usually plus or minus two standard deviations from the mean result for a representative, healthy population. Most health care facilities publish ranges of normal values for the area and population they serve. Normal ranges discussed in this text are generally accepted values for the identified test. Values for a specific institution may vary.

Arterial Blood Gases

Results reported for ABGs are a combination of measured values and calculated values. The pH, partial pressure of carbon dioxide, and partial pressure of oxygen (PO_2) values are measured, whereas bicarbonate, oxygen saturation, and base excess values are calculated. Normal values are identified in Table 12-2.[6] Normal PO_2 values vary with elevation above sea level.

Actual interpretation of ABG results is a two-step process. The acid-base status is determined first, then the pa-

Table 12-2 NORMAL ARTERIAL BLOOD GAS VALUES

COMPONENT	NORMAL RANGE
pH	7.35 to 7.45
pCO_2	35 to 45 mmHg
PO_2	80 mmHg
HCO_3	22 to 28 mEq/L

pCO_2, Partial pressure of carbon dioxide; PO_2, partial pressure of oxygen; HCO_3, bicarbonate.

Table 12-3 ASSESSMENT OF ARTERIAL BLOOD GAS VALUES

CONDITION	pH	pCO2	HCO3
Acute metabolic acidosis	<7.30	<30	Depressed
Chronic metabolic acidosis	Normal	Depressed	Depressed
Acute respiratory acidosis	<7.30	>50	Normal
Chronic respiratory acidosis	Normal	>50	Elevated
Acute metabolic alkalosis	>7.50	Elevated	Elevated
Chronic metabolic alkalosis	Normal	>50	Elevated
Acute respiratory alkalosis	>7.50	<30	Normal
Chronic respiratory alkalosis	Normal	<30	Depressed

pCO_2, Partial pressure of carbon dioxide; HCO_3, bicarbonate.

tient's oxygen status is determined. Acute and chronic acid-base disturbances include metabolic and respiratory acidosis and metabolic and respiratory alkalosis. Table 12-3 highlights ABG results associated with these acid-base disturbances. Common causes of acid-base disturbances are identified in Table 12-4.

Electrolytes

Body fluid is composed primarily of water and dissolved substances called electrolytes, which carry a negative or positive charge. An anion carries a negative charge, whereas a cation carries a positive charge. Electrolytes are measured in milliequivalents per liter (mEq/L) with a balance of cations and anions in the body. Normal ranges for intravascular electrolytes are listed in Table 12-5. The amount of each electrolyte within the cells varies. Table 12-6 lists causes for major electrolyte imbalances (see Chapter 38 for more discussion on electrolytes).

Complete Blood Cell Count

The complete blood cell count (CBC) is used to determine the patient's hematologic status. Historically, a CBC has been

Table 12-4 COMMON CAUSES OF ACID-BASE DISTURBANCES

ACID-BASE DISTURBANCE	CAUSES
Metabolic acidosis	Renal failure, diabetic ketoacidosis, starvation, lactic acidosis, hepatic collapse, ingestion of methanol, ASA, or other acids
Metabolic alkalosis	Extended IV therapy, diuretics, diarrhea, gastric suction or vomiting, steroid therapy, excessive use of NaHCO₃
Respiratory acidosis	COPD, respiratory arrest, primary alveolar hyperventilation, pulmonary edema
Respiratory alkalosis	CNS trauma, CNS infection, carbon monoxide poisoning, anemia, anxiety, psychosis, pain, hyperventilation, hypoxia

ASA, Acetylsalicylic acid; *IV*, intravenous; *NaHCO₃*, sodium bicarbonate; *COPD*, chronic obstructive pulmonary disorder; *CNS*, central nervous system.

Table 12-5 NORMAL RANGES OF ELECTROLYTE VALUES

ELECTROLYTE	SERUM	URINE
Sodium (Na)	136 to 142 mEq/L	80 to 180 mEq/24 hr
Potassium (K)	3.8 to 5.0 mEq/L	40 to 80 mEq/24 hr
Chloride (Cl)	93 to 105 mEq/L	110 to 250 mEq/24 hr
Carbon dioxide (CO₂)	24 to 30 mM/L	—
Magnesium (Mg)	1.8 to 3.0 mg/100 ml	6.0 to 8.5 mEq/24 hr
Calcium (Ca)	8.5 to 10.5 mg/100 ml	100 to 250 mg/24 hr

pCO_2, Partial pressure of carbon dioxide; PO_2, partial pressure of oxygen; HCO_3, bicarbonate.

Table 12-6 CAUSES OF ELECTROLYTE IMBALANCE

IMBALANCE	CAUSES
Hyponatremia	Excess sweating, excess intake of water, diuretics, adrenal insufficiency, renal failure
Hypernatremia	Diarrhea, decreased water intake, salt water ingestion, impaired renal function, febrile illness, inability to swallow, burns, diabetes insipidus
Hypokalemia	Diarrhea, vomiting, diuretics, burns, heat stress, ulcerative colitis, potassium-free IV fluids, metabolic acidosis, steroids
Hyperkalemia	Acute/chronic renal failure, burns, crush injuries, metabolic acidosis, potassium-sparing diuretics

Table 12-7	COMPONENTS OF COMPLETE BLOOD CELL COUNT	
COMPONENT	NORMAL VALUES	COMMENTS
White blood cell count	5000 to 10,000/mm³	
Red blood cell count	Male: 4.6 to 6.2 ml/mm³	
	Female: 4.2 to 5.4 ml/mm³	
Hemoglobin level	Male: 14 to 18 g/100 ml	A conjugated protein responsible for oxygen and carbon dioxide
	Female: 12 to 16 g/100 ml	transport in the blood
Hematocrit	Male: 40% to 54%	Percentage (volume) of red blood cells in a volume of blood, generally
	Female: 37% to 47%	equal to the hemoglobin level $\times$ $\beta 3 \pm 2$
Mean corpuscular volume	82 to 92 μm^3	Average volume of red blood cells in a sample
Mean corpuscular hemoglobin content	27 to 37μg	Average hemoglobin content of red blood cells in a sample
Mean corpuscular hemoglobin concentration	32% to 36%	Average hemoglobin content in 100 ml of blood
Platelets	150,000 to 400,000/μl	Platelets aid in hemostasis and maintenance of vascular integrity

reported in two parts: the cell count and the differential count. The cell count was done by machine, with the differential count done manually. Electronic particle counters have made this process almost obsolete, providing an automated cell count and differential count; however, if the automated differential count reported is abnormal, a manual count is then done.

The cell count of the CBC provides normal values for leukocytes, erythrocytes, hemoglobin, and hematocrit (Table 12-7). Normal CBC values vary with age and sex of the patient. The differential count provides information on red cell morphology and the percentage distribution of leukocytes (see Chapter 42 for discussion of these cell types). The differential is also helpful in evaluation of malaria and other parasites as well as in identification of abnormal cells.[3]

Urinalysis

Urine is composed of 95% water and 5% solutes. Solutes normally found in urine include nitrogenous wastes such as creatinine, uric acid, and urea. Urine also contains electrolytes and pigments derived from bile. A urinalysis tests for the presence of abnormal constituents such as protein, glucose, white blood cells, red blood cells, and ketones. Protein in the urine may indicate glomerulonephritis, whereas glucosuria may be caused by insulin deficiency, stress, or renal disease. White blood cells indicate infection; red blood cells are seen with inflammation, trauma, kidney stones, or posturethral catheterization. Incomplete oxidation of fat leads to ketones in the urine, often seen with diabetes or starvation.

The most commonly used form of urine testing is a reagent tablet or a dipstick. Each strip contains pads that show reactions to specific components of the urine, such as protein, bilirubin, ketones, and glucose. Urinary pH, specific gravity, color, and appearance are also included in the urinalysis.

POINT-OF-CARE TESTING

Point-of-care testing evolved from a demand for rapid lab results. When using point-of-care testing, lab specimens may be collected at the bedside using much smaller specimen sizes. This may be especially beneficial in the very young or very old. A shorter turnaround time on specimens facilitates an earlier therapeutic diagnosis. Expense of point-of-care testing is controversial. The cost is often higher per test than that of the traditional lab; however, point-of-care testing does provide a shorter length of stay, is relatively easy to use, does not require additional personnel, and facilitates earlier intervention.[5] Point-of-care tests include but are not limited to troponin I and myoglobin.

SUMMARY

Analysis of various laboratory tests is the foundation for many diagnostic and therapeutic challenges. Without the benefit of sound specimen collection, diagnosis and treatment for many patients is needlessly delayed. This can place the patient's life in danger, increase potential complications, and add to overall cost of health care. A certificate of waiver for ED laboratory testing covers urine dipstick, urine pregnancy, glucose, and stool hematocrit; however, positive results must be confirmed by laboratory analysis.

References

1. Emergency Nurses Association: *Emergency nursing core curriculum,* ed 5, Philadelphia, 2000, WB Saunders.
2. Fischbach F: *A manual of laboratory and diagnostic tests,* ed 6, Philadelphia, 2000, JB Lippincott.
3. Ignatavicius DD, Workman ML, Mishler MA: *Medical-surgical nursing: a nursing process approach,* ed 2, Philadelphia, 1995, WB Saunders.
4. Kitt S, Selfridge-Thomas J, Proehl J et al: *Emergency nursing— a physiologic and clinical perspective,* Philadelphia, 1995, WB Saunders.
5. McConnell E: Getting up to speed with point of care blood testing, *Crit Care Choices 1999,* p. 7, 1999.
6. Society of Critical Care Medicine: *Fundamental critical care support course text,* ed 3, Des Plaines, Ill, 2001, The Society.
7. Wong DL: *Whaley & Wong's essentials of pediatric nursing,* ed 5, St. Louis, 1997, Mosby.

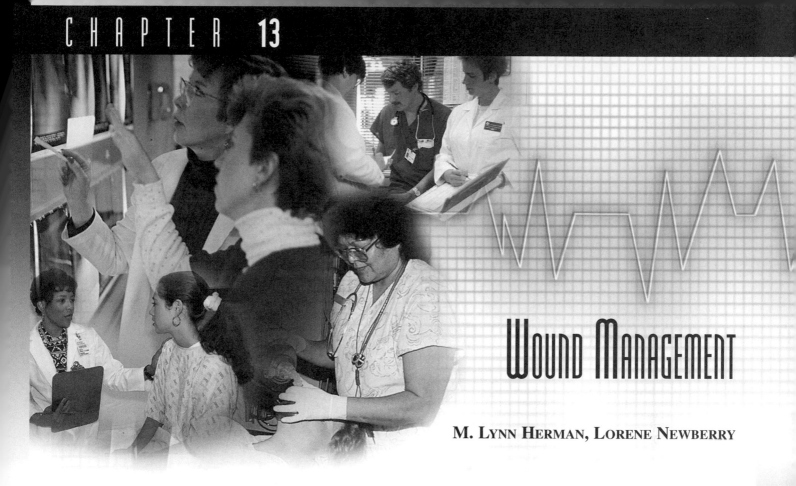

Wound Management

M. Lynn Herman, Lorene Newberry

A wound is described as a disruption of normal anatomic structure and function from a pathologic process beginning internally or externally to the involved organ. The goal of emergent wound management is to restore tissue integrity after injury by wound closure and to restore function to damaged tissue. Emergency nurses encounter many patients with wound injuries that can greatly alter their appearance and function. Unless life-threatening bleeding or neurovascular compromise is present, patients with surface trauma are not a triage priority. Wound management in the emergency department (ED) includes careful assessment, cleansing, wound closure, and discharge care. Basic principles of wound care are promotion of optimal healing, prevention of infection, and reduction of scar formation.

ANATOMY AND PHYSIOLOGY

Skin is the largest organ of the body and is composed of the epidermis, dermis, and subcutaneous tissue (Figure 13-1). The epidermis, or outer layer, generates cells that promote wound healing. Thickness of the epidermis varies with location; it is significantly greater in the soles of the feet and palms of the hand than in the eyelids. Thickening of epidermal layers (calluses) may be caused by poorly fitted shoes, repetitive actions such as plucking guitar strings, or manual labor such as raking the yard. The dermis is a tough connective layer that forms the thickest layer of the skin and contains lymphatic vessels, blood vessels, and nerves. Collagen found in the dermis provides tensile strength, whereas elastin allows skin to resist deformation. Sensory receptors for pain, touch, pressure, heat, and cold are found in the dermis, whereas hair follicles and sweat glands are found between the epidermis and dermis. The subcutaneous layer stores fat below the dermis and provides insulation against heat loss. Heat conduction in fat is one third that of other tissues. Fat also provides protection against injury and acts as an energy storage site.

Skin regulates body temperature through sweating and evaporation. Insensible fluid loss through skin and lungs accounts for 450 to 600 ml/day or 12 to 16 calories/hr of heat loss.[5] Skin also provides innate immunity because macrophages, mast cells, and Langerhans cells in the skin respond to antigens and pathogens, and because of the presence of normal skin flora (i.e., coagulase-positive and coagulase-negative staphylocci, streptocci, and diptheroids).

WOUND HEALING

Wounds heal by either partial or complete regeneration. In humans the dermis is incapable of responding to injury by regeneration; it is unable to completely reestablish its original tissue structure. The dermis undergoes a process of repair in which original tissue is replaced with nonspecific connective tissue, which ultimately functions less effectively. This tissue can hold together the remaining dermis, but has reduced tensile strength and energy-absorbing capacity.[2]

Healing occurs in three cumulative phases or layers (inflammatory, fibroplasia, and collagen maturation), with each

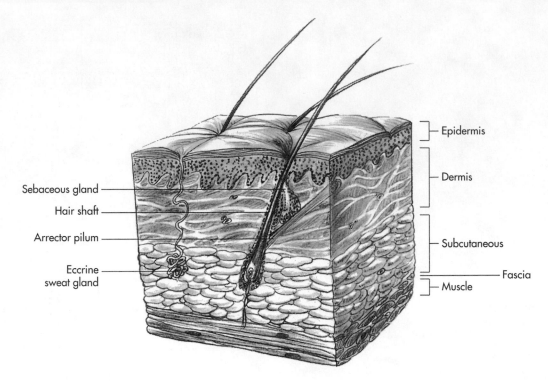

FIGURE **13-1** Epidermis, dermis, and subcutaneous tissue. (From Davis P et al: *Surgery: a problem solving approach,* ed 2, St. Louis, 1995, Mosby).

layer creating the pathway for the next layer to occur (Figure 13-2). After injury, blood flows into the wound and coagulates, forming a clot. Beneath the clot, a network of fibrinogen strands form to unite wound edges. Scab formation begins within 2 hours to minimize fluid loss and prevent bacterial invasion.

After scab formation begins, inflammatory processes start so the wound becomes painful and edematous. Vasodilation in injured tissues leads to protein leakage and antibody release, which create a medium for white blood cells that arrive at the site 6 hours after injury. White blood cells attack bacteria through phagocytosis by using neutrophils to surround and engulf bacteria, providing short-term defense against infection, and monocytes provide long-term defense against infection.

Within 24 hours of injury, fibroblasts generate new epidermis. Fibroblast activity peaks in approximately 6 days during which time lymphatic vessels, blood vessels, and supporting tissues are repaired. New capillary beds form and mesh with damaged tissue, providing oxygen and proteins for tissue growth. During fibroblast activity, collagen is produced for dermal scar tissue. This scar tissue is initially translucent, grayish-red, bleeds easily, and can be damaged with minimal force. Tensile wound strength is weakest 3 days after injury.[4]

Collagen fibers initially develop randomly; however, within 2 weeks, fibers reorganize into thick fibers along stress lines and increase in strength over weeks or months. Heredity, stress, and movement of the affected area determine the amount of scarring. Healing, with increasing collagen density and nerve regeneration, may actually take years. It is significantly affected by conditions such as obesity, infection, diabetes mellitus, and malnutrition.[7] Effects of these and other factors on wound healing are described in Table 13-1.

WOUND EVALUATION

Initial assessment of wounds follows assessment and stabilization of the airway, breathing, and circulation. Mechanisms of injury can provide clues to severity of injury. Wounds caused by small objects may be superficial, whereas crush injuries caused by a large dog's bite can cause significant deep tissue damage. Appearance of the wound provides clues to the difficulty of wound closure. Jagged edges require more skill to close and may not heal as well. The time since injury is critical because delayed care increases the risk for complications such as infection. Special closure techniques are required for wounds more than 12 hours old.

Patient age, physical condition, current health status, and occupation also affect wound healing. Medical conditions such as diabetes mellitus, secondary peripheral neuropathy, morbid obesity, malnutrition, or use of medications such as corticosteroids delay wound healing. Aspirin and nonsteroidal antiinflammatory drugs affect coagulation and healing. Patient occupation influences long-term wound management and compliance with wound care. From an occupational point of view, lacerations on the fingers are more difficult for pianists than for public speakers. Allergy history

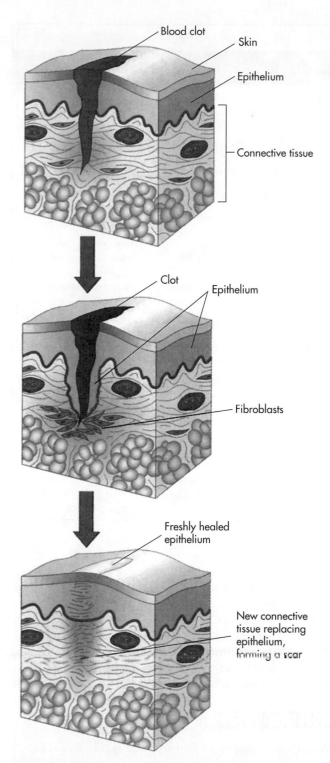

Blood clot
Skin
Epithelium
Connective tissue

Clot
Epithelium
Fibroblasts

Freshly healed
epithelium

New connective
tissue replacing
epithelium,
forming a scar

FIGURE 13-2 Healing of a minor wound. (From Thibodeau GA, Patton KT: *Anatomy and physiology,* ed 3, St. Louis, 1996, Mosby.)

and immunization status should also be evaluated during initial assessment.

The patient should be assessed for associated injuries such as fractures, dislocations, or neurovascular compromise, then possible fractures or dislocations should be splinted. Tendon or ligament injuries, presence of a foreign body, and peripheral nerve damage should also be consid-

Table 13-1	**FACTORS DELAYING WOUND HEALING**
FACTOR	**EFFECTS ON WOUND HEALING**
Nutritional deficiencies	
Vitamin C	Delays formation of collagen fibers and capillary development
Protein	Decreases supply of amino acids for tissue repair
Zinc	Impairs epithelialization
Inadequate blood supply	Decreases supply of nutrients to injured area, decreases removal of exudative debris, inhibits inflammatory response
Corticosteroid drugs	Impair phagocytosis by WBCs, inhibit fibroblast proliferation and function, depress formation of granulation tissue, inhibit wound contraction
Infection	Increases inflammatory response and tissue destruction
Mechanical friction on wound	Destroys granulation tissue, prevents apposition of wound edges
Advanced age	Slows collagen synthesis by fibroblasts, impairs circulation, requires longer time for epithelialization of skin, alters phagocytic and immune responses
Obesity	Decreases blood supply in fatty tissue
Diabetes mellitus	Decreases collagen synthesis, retards early capillary growth, impairs phagocytosis (result of hyperglycemia)
Poor general health	Causes generalized absence of factors necessary to promote wound healing
Anemia	Supplies less oxygen at tissue level

From Lewis SM, Heitkemper MM, Dirksen SR: *Medical-surgical nursing: assessment and management of clinical problems,* ed 5, St. Louis, 2000, Mosby.
WBCs, White blood cells.

ered. A wound culture may be obtained before or after irrigation if wound contamination is present. The wound can be cleaned with isotonic saline or other acceptable solutions (Table 13-2). However, hydrogen peroxide should not be used because it causes absorption of oxygen in the wound, cell destruction, and gives no protection against anaerobes. Soaps with strong cleaning agents or those containing alcohol may cause further tissue damage. Wounds with heavy contamination should be irrigated for 5 minutes or more with local anesthesia injected or applied topically before vigorous scrubbing. Puncture wounds are soaked for 10 to 15 minutes; soaking other wounds should be avoided. The area around the laceration may be shaved; however, eyebrows should never be shaved because the hair may not grow back. Eyebrows also function as landmarks for wound alignment and closure.[8]

Table 13-2 ANTISEPTIC SOLUTIONS

AGENTS	ANTIMICROBIAL ACTIVITY	MECHANICS OF ACTION	TISSUE TOXICITY	INDICATIONS AND CONTRAINDICATIONS
Povidone-iodine solution (iodine complexes) (*Betadine*)	Available as 10% solution with polyvinyl-pyrolidine (povidone) containing 1% free iodine with broad rapid-onset antimicrobial activity	Potent germicide in low concentrations	Decreases PMN migration and life span at concentration >1% May cause systemic toxicity at higher concentrations; questionable toxicity at 1% concentration	Probably safe and effective wound cleanser at <1% concentration 10% solution is effective to prepare skin about the wound
Povidone-iodine surgical scrub	Same as the solution	Same	Toxic to open wounds	Best as a hand cleanser; never use in open wounds
Nonionic detergents *Pluronic F-68* *Shur Clens*	Ethyleneoxide is 80% of its molecular weight Has no antimicrobial activity	Wound cleanser	No toxicity to open wounds, eyes, or intravenous solutions	Appears to be an effective, safe wound cleanser
Hydrogen peroxide	3% solution in water has brief germicidal activity	Oxidizing agent that denatures protein	Toxic to open wounds	Should not be used on wounds after the initial cleaning; may be used to clean intact skin
Hexachlorophene (*pHiso Hex*) (polychlorinated bis-phenol)	Bacteriostatic (2% to 5%) Greater activity against gram-positive organisms	Interruption of bacterial electron transport and disruption of membrane-bound enzymes	Little skin toxicity; the scrub form is damaging to open wounds	Never use scrub solution in open wounds Very good preoperative hand preparation
Alcohols	Low-potency antimicrobial most effective as 70% ethyl and 70% isopropyl alcohol solution	Denatures protein	Kills irreversibly and functions as a fixative	No role in routine care
Phenols	Bacteriostatic >0.2% Bactericidal >1% Fungicidal 1.3%	Denatures protein	Extensive tissue necrosis and systemic toxicity	Never use >2% aqueous phenol or >4% phenol plus glycerol

Modified from Rosen P, Barkin RM, Hockberger RS et al: *Emergency medicine,* ed 4, St. Louis, 1998, Mosby.
PMN, Polymorphic neutrophil.

Devitalized tissue is debrided before wound closure. Wounds may be closed by primary intention, secondary intention, or tertiary intention. The type of closure depends on age of the wound, presence of infection, and amount of contamination present. Figure 13-3 illustrates types of wound healing and closure. Primary intention by sutures, staples, or Steri-Strips within 12 hours of injury is the ideal method of closure because this technique has the least scarring. Table 13-3 describes wound healing with primary intention closure. Secondary intention is used for wounds with devitalized tissue, severe contamination, or infection. Wound edges are not closed initially so the wound granulates to form tissue from the inside out. Tertiary intention, or delayed wound closure, occurs days after injury.

WOUND DRESSINGS

Modern wound dressings are designed to keep the wound moist and therefore enhance epithelialization, clean the wound or keep it clean, and protect the wound from physical trauma or bacterial invasion.[3] Types of wound dressings are described in Table 13-4. Wounds to the face and ears may not require a dressing as long as the area is kept clean.

Depending on the wound, a thin layer of antibiotic ointment (e.g., Bacitracin, Polysporin, Neosporin) may be applied before the dressing.

Use of a silver-coated absorbent dressing is being explored for use with all types of wounds. Early studies show these silver-coated dressings have a much faster bactericidal action against broad-spectrum organisms than does a film dressing.[11] Further research is ongoing.

SPECIFIC WOUNDS

Wounds are categorized into six basic types: abrasions, abscesses, avulsions, lacerations, puncture wounds, and bites. Their severity varies with the cause of injury and amount of tissue damaged; however, patient age, health status, medications, and preexisting conditions affect overall wound severity and healing. Occupation is also a factor in wound care. Wounds may be a minor inconvenience that do not alter lifestyle or affect work requirements. More severe wounds may cause significant discomfort and affect self-care and work. In some cases, lifestyle is permanently altered. Prevention of a chronic wound caused by a treatable acute injury is always a major concern.

Presentation	Closure	Results

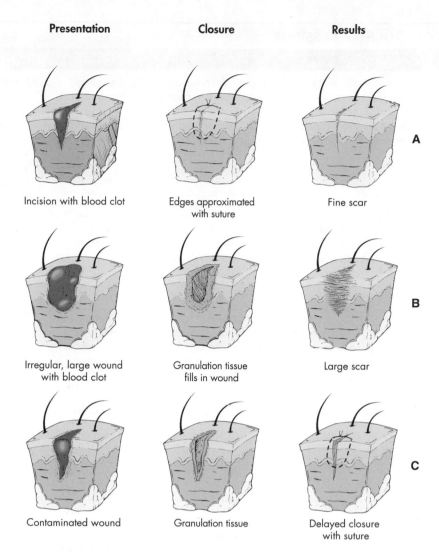

Incision with blood clot	Edges approximated with suture	Fine scar	**A**
Irregular, large wound with blood clot	Granulation tissue fills in wound	Large scar	**B**
Contaminated wound	Granulation tissue	Delayed closure with suture	**C**

FIGURE **13-3**   Types of wound healing. **A,** Primary intention. **B,** Secondary intention. **C,** Tertiary intention. (Modified from Lewis SM, Heitkemper MM, Dirken SR: *Medical-surgical nursing: assessment and management of clinical problems,* ed 5, St. Louis, 2000, Mosby.)

Abrasions

Abrasions occur when skin is rubbed or scraped against a hard surface. Friction removes the epithelial layer and can also remove part of the epidermis so deeper layers are exposed. Examples of abrasions are floor burns, carpet burns, road rash, or brush burns (Figure 13-4). Abrasions have the same physiologic effect as a second-degree burn; thus a significant risk of infection exists from loss of skin and its protective properties. Fluid loss also occurs with loss of surface area.

Foreign bodies left in the skin stain the epidermis and cause permanent scars or a "tattoo." Cleansing is critical in management of abrasions to prevent tattooing. Local anesthesia by topical application or infiltration should be used for abrasions with heavy contamination. Topical antibiotic ointment and nonadherent dressings are used; however, abrasions may occasionally be left open to air. Dressings should be changed daily until eschar forms. Clothing or sunblock should be used for 6 months to prevent discoloration of fragile new tissue.

Table 13-3 **PHASES IN WOUND HEALING**	
PHASE	**ACTIVITY**
Initial (3 to 5 days)	Approximation of incision edges; migration of epithelial cells; clot serving as meshwork for starting capillary growth
Granulation (5 days to 4 weeks)	Migration of fibroblasts; secretion of collagen; abundance of capillary buds; fragility of wound
Scar contracture (7 days to several months)	Remodeling of collagen; strengthening of scar

Modified from Lewis SM, Heitkemper MM, Dirksen SR: *Medical-surgical nursing: assessment and management of clinical problems,* ed 5, St. Louis, 2000, Mosby.

Table 13-4　TYPES OF WOUND DRESSINGS

TYPE	DESCRIPTION	EXAMPLES
Gauze	Provides absorption of exudate; supports debridement if applied and kept moist; can be used to maintain moist wound surface and as filler dressings in sinus tracts	Numerous products available
Nonadherent dressings	Woven or nonwoven dressings may be impregnated with saline, petrolatum, or antimicrobials; minimal absorbency	Adaptic Exu-Dry Sofsorb Telfa Vaseline gauze Xeroform
Transparent film	Semipermeable membrane permits gaseous exchange between wound bed and environment; minimally absorbent so fluid environment created in presence of exudate. Bacteria do not penetrate membrane. Used for dry, noninfected wounds or wounds with minimal drainage.	Acu-Derm Biocclusive Blisterfilm Opsite Polyskin Tegaderm Transeal
Hydrocolloid	Occlusive dressing does not allow oxygen to diffuse from atmosphere to wound bed. Occlusion does not interfere with wound healing; not used in infected wounds; supports debridement and prevents secondary infections; used for superficial and partial-thickness wounds with light to moderate drainage	Comfeel DuoDerm Intact Intrasite Restore Tegasorb Ultec
Polyurethane foams	Moderate to heavy amounts of exudate can be absorbed; can be used on infected wounds; used for partial- or full-thickness wounds with minimal to heavy drainage	Allevyn Epilock Hydrasorb Lyofoam Mitraflex Synthaderm
Absorption dressing	Large volumes of exudate can be absorbed; supports debridement; maintains moist wound surface; placed into wounds and can obliterate dead space; for partial- or full-thickness wounds or infected wounds	AlgiDERM Bard Absorption Debrisan Duoderm Paste Hydragan Kaltostat Sorbsan
Hydrogel	Debridement because of moisturizing effects; maintains moist wound surface; provides limited absorption of exudate; available as sheet or gel; most require a secondary dressing. Used for partial- or full-thickness wounds, deep wounds with minimal drainage, and necrotic wounds	Vigilon Elasto Gel Intrasite Gel Geliperm

Modified from Lewis SM, Heitkemper MM, Dirksen SR: *Medical-surgical nursing: assessment and management of clinical problems,* ed 5, St. Louis, 2000, Mosby.

Abscess

Localized collection of pus beneath the skin causes an abscess. Pus may eventually erupt; however, wound management does not include waiting for this to occur. The wound is cleaned, infiltrated with local anesthesia, and drained. An elliptical area of tissue may be removed to facilitate drainage, then the wound is packed loosely with iodoform or similar material and covered with loose dressing. Antibiotics are indicated when the patient has a fever.

Avulsion

An avulsion is full-thickness skin loss in which approximation of wound edges is not possible. A degloving injury is a severe avulsion injury in which skin is peeled away from the hand, foot, or a greater portion of an extremity. Figure 13-5 shows a degloving injury of the scalp. Degloving injuries of the fingers are more common and involve injury to tendons and ligaments. Management includes local anesthesia by injection or topical application followed by irrigation and debridement of devitalized tissue. A split-thickness skin graft

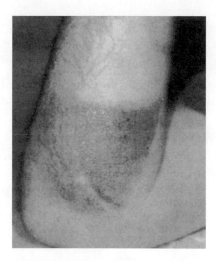

FIGURE **13-4**   Abrasion. (From McSwain Jr, NE, Paturas JL: *The basic EMT: comprehensive prehospital patient care,* ed 2, St. Louis, 2001, Mosby.)

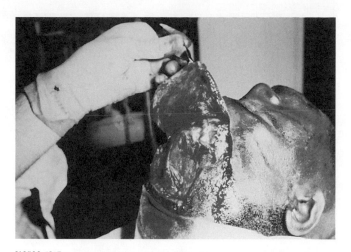

FIGURE **13-5**   Degloving injury of the scalp. (From Auerbach P: *Wilderness medicine,* ed 4, St. Louis, 2001, Mosby.)

is necessary with large avulsions. The wound should be covered with a bulky dressing to protect exposed tissue.

Contusions

Blunt trauma that does not alter skin integrity causes a contusion or bruise. Swelling, pain, and discoloration occur with extravasation of blood into damaged tissues. After assessment of neurovascular status, therapeutic interventions include cold packs and analgesia as necessary. Large wounds or those located in an extremity should be carefully observed for cellulitis or development of compartment syndrome.

Lacerations

Lacerations are open cuts caused by shearing forces through dermal layers. Superficial lacerations involve the epidermis and dermis (Figure 13-6), whereas more severe injuries involve deeper layers including subcutaneous tissue and muscle (Figure 13-7). Initial interventions focus on controlling bleeding and assessing neurovascular function distal to the injury. Anesthesia should be used to facilitate removal of foreign bodies and excision of necrotic or devitalized tissue. Exploration is indicated when damage to underlying structures is possible. Wound closure involves approximation of edges followed by closure with a tape closure, staples, or sutures. Deeper wounds are closed in layers. After the wound is closed, a thin layer of antibiotic ointment is applied followed by a nonadherent dressing.

Puncture Wounds

Puncture wounds are caused by tissue penetration with a sharp object such as knife blade or injection from high-pressure nail guns or paint guns, which can exert pressures up to 2000 psi.[10] Injection injuries cause more severe damage

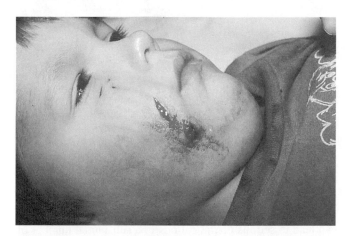

FIGURE **13-6**   Superficial laceration. (Courtesy Thomas Lintner, MD.)

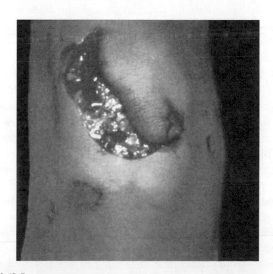

FIGURE **13-7**   Deep laceration. (From Roberts J, Hedges J: *Clinical procedures in emergency medicine,* ed 3, Philadelphia, 1998, WB Saunders.)

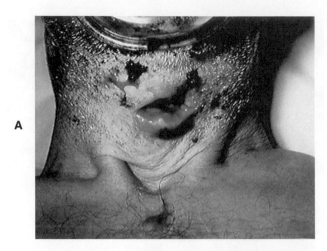

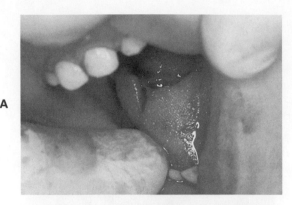

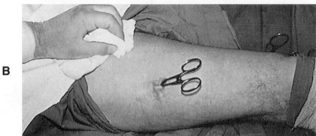

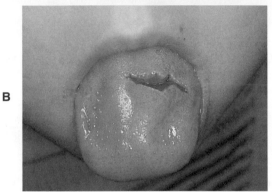

FIGURE **13-8** **A,** Self-inflicted stab wound of the throat. This wound was more than 12 hours old and had entered the pharynx. **B,** An accidental stab wound of the thigh. (From McSwain NE, Paturas JL: *The basic EMT: comprehensive prehospital patient care,* ed 2, St. Louis, 2001, Mosby.)

FIGURE **13-9** Tongue lacerations. **A,** A large gaping tongue laceration in a toddler produced by the upperfront teeth being forced through the tissue by a fall with the tongue protruded. This type of injury usually requires suturing. **B,** This small laceration, though gaping slightly, does not require surgical closure. (From Zitelli B, Davis H: *Atlas of pediatric physical diagnosis,* ed 3, St. Louis, 1997, Mosby.)

to underlying tissues than indicated by the appearance of the surface wound. Lack of consistency in therapeutic approach can lead to serious complications in a substantial number of puncture wounds. Because puncture wounds do not have a dramatic appearance, the wounds are often undertreated. Regardless of appearance, the zone of injury and the wound's proximity to underlying structures should be assessed (Figure 13-8).

Infection is reported in 10% to 15% of puncture wounds. A greater risk for infection exists in wounds that are more than 6 hours old, large and deep, contaminated with foreign matter and debris, occur outdoors, penetrate through footwear, have osseous involvement, and occur in patients with underlying disease such as diabetes mellitus or immunosuppression.[10] Risk for wound contamination increases with high-pressure injuries. Management includes necrotic tissue removal followed by drain placement and sterile dressing application. Impaled objects should be stabilized until safe removal is possible. A foreign body can be removed if the object is small and if removal does not cause further damage. Plain radiographs are helpful to identify the location of embedded objects. Fluoroscopy has also been used successfully to identify foreign bodies such as needles or wires. Standard radiographs may not show objects such as small pieces of glass, wood, or plastic. In these cases, xeroradiography, ultrasonography, computed tomography, or magnetic

resonance imaging can help locate the object. Some objects may be left in place or removed surgically.

Bites

Bites may be caused by animals or humans and involve contusions, avulsions, lacerations, and puncture wounds. Teeth can crush or tear tissue causing extensive damage. An estimated 1 to 2 million people in the United States are bitten by animals each year, with dog bites accounting for 80% to 90% of these injuries and cat bites reported in 5% to 18%. Exotic animals such as primates, felines, alligators, and camels also cause bite injuries. Regardless of the source, bite wounds are considered contaminated. Infection, abscess, cellulitis, septicemia, osteomyelitis, tenosynovitis, rabies, tetanus, and loss of body parts are potential complications of bite wounds.

Human bites usually result from fighting, sexual activity, or can be self-inflicted. Accidental bite injuries of the tongue (Figure 13-9), cheeks, and lips can occur during falls. Surgical closure may or may not be necessary. Box 13-1 identifies bacteria that may be found in human saliva. Infection is the greatest risk with human bites because human saliva contains 10 bacteria per milliliter, including

| Box 13-1 | BACTERIA ISOLATED FROM HUMAN BITES |

AEROBES

Acinetobacter	Neisseria gonorrhoeae
Branhamella (Moraxella) catarrhalis	Other Neisseria spp.
	Nocardia
Corynebacterium	Proteus mirabilis
Eikenella corrodens	Pseudomonas aeruginosa
Enterobacter cloacae	Other Pseudomonas spp.
Other Enterobacter spp.	Serratia marcescens
Escherichia coli	Staphylococcus aureus
Haemophilus aphrophilus	Staphylococcus epidermidis
Haemophilus influenzae	Staphylococcus intermedius
Haemophilus parainfluenzae	Staphylococcus saprophyticus
Klebsiella pneumoniae	α-Hemolytic streptococci
Micrococcus	β-Hemolytic streptococci
Moraxella	γ-Hemolytic streptococci

ANAEROBES

Acidaminococcus	Peptostreptococcus anaerobius
Actinomyces	Peptostreptococcus prevotii
Arachnia propionica	Other Peptostreptococcus spp.
Bacteroides fragilis	Prevotella
Clostridium	Propionibacterium acnes
Eubacterium	Other Propionibacterium spp.
Fusobacterium nucleatum	Veillonella

Modified from Griego RD, Rosen T, Orengo IF et al: *J Am Acad Dermatol* 33:1019, 1995.

| Box 13-2 | BACTERIA ISOLATED FROM DOG AND CAT BITES |

AEROBES

Pasteurella multocida	Other Pseudomonas spp.
Other Pasteurella spp.	Actinomyces
Streptococcus mitis	Brevibacterium
Streptococcus mutans	EF-4a
Streptococcus pyogenes	Weeksella zoohelcum
Streptococcus sanguis II	Other Weeksella spp.
Streptococcus intermedius	Klebsiella
β-Hemolytic streptococci, group G	Lactobacillus
	Citrobacter
β-Hemolytic streptococci, group F	Flavobacterium
	Micrococcus
Other Streptococcus spp.	Proteus mirabilis
Staphylococcus aureus	Stenotrophomonas malto- philia
Staphylococcus epidermidis	
Staphylococcus warneri	Capnocytophaga
Staphylococcus intermedius	Eikenella corrodens
Other Staphylococcus spp.	Flavimonas oryzihabitans
Neisseria weaverii	Acinetobacter
Neisseria subflav	Actinobacillus
Other Neisseria spp.	Alcaligenes
Corynebacterium minutissimum	Enterobacter cloacae
Other Corynebacterium spp.	Erysipelothrix rhusiopathiae
Moraxella (Branhamella)	Reimerella anatipestifer
EF-4b	Rothia dentocariosa
Enterococcus faecalis	Aeromonas hydrophilia
Enterococcus avium	Pantoea agglomerans
Other Enterococcus spp.	Rhodococcus
Bacillus	Streptomyces
Pseudomonas aeruginosa	

ANAEROBES

Fusobacterium	Propionibacterium
Bacteroides fragilis	Peptostreptococcus
Other Bacteroides spp.	Eubacterium
Porphyromonas	Clostridium sordellii
Prevotella	Veillonella

Data from Talan DA et al: Bacteriologic analysis of infected dogs and cats, *N Engl J Med* 340.85, 1999.

Staphylococcus aureus, streptococci, *Proteus, Escherichia coli, Pseudomonas,* and *Klebsielleae* organisms. More than 3% of these organisms are penicillin-resistant *S. aureus.* Hepatitis B virus may also be transmitted through human saliva; however, risk for human immunodeficiency virus infection appears to be low.[10] Management of human bite wounds includes neurovascular assessment, wound exploration, copious irrigation, debridement of devitalized tissue, and application of a bulky dressing. The wound is initially left open. Prophylactic antibiotics should be given within 3 hours of arrival at the ED.

Animal bites carry the risk of infection, tetanus, and rabies. The Centers for Disease Control and Prevention estimate that as many as 4.5 million bites occur annually, almost 800,000 of which require medical attention.[1] Infection occurs in 5% to 15% of dog bite wounds and in a significant number of cat bite wounds. Box 13-2 identifies bacteria that may occur in dog and cat saliva. An increased risk for infection exists in people more than 50 years old and in those with hand wounds, deep puncture wounds, and delayed treatment of more than 24 hours. Up to 33 organisms have been identified in dog saliva. Cat saliva contains *Pasteurella multocida,* an extremely virulent organism that can lead to septic arthritis and bacteremia. Dog bites are more likely to be associated with crush injuries from compressive forces of the canine jaw—up to 400 psi in some breeds. Fifty-seven percent to 86 percent of all cats bites are puncture wounds caused by the

cat's long, slender fangs.[10] Most dog bites occur on the extremities, head, and neck, with fewer bites on the trunk. Children are more likely to have wounds on the head and neck. Most cat bites are found on the arm, forearm, and hand.

Treatment for cat and dog bites is essentially the same: cleaning, debridement, and wound closure for small wounds. It is useful to separate animal bites into high versus low risk when deciding to suture the wound or provide appropriate antibiotic coverage. High-risk wounds include all human and cat bites; hand and foot wounds; wounds surgically debrided; puncture wounds involving joints, ligaments, tendons, and bones; bites with delayed treatment more than 12 hours; and bites in immunocompromised patients. These wounds generally should not be sutured but do require antibiotics. Low-risk wounds include bites involving the extremities, face, or body. These wounds are generally sutured and do not require

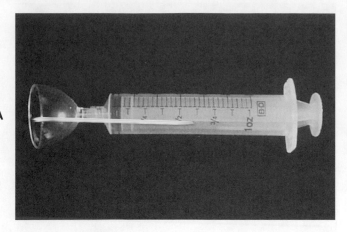
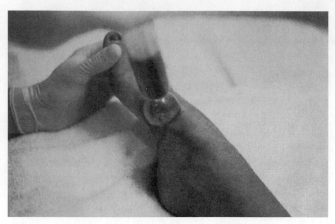

FIGURE 13-10   **A,** ZeroWet Splashield attached to end of a syringe. This device is used in lieu of a needle. **B,** The shield is held near the skin, and the tip of the syringe directs the irrigating solution. (From Roberts J, Hedges J: *Clinical procedures in emergency medicine,* ed 3, Philadelphia, 1998, WB Saunders.)

Table 13-5 EPINEPHRINE USE	
ADVANTAGES	**DISADVANTAGES**
1. Prolongs duration	1. Impairs host defenses—increases infection*
2. Provides hemostasis	2. Delays wound healing*
3. Slows absorption:	3. Do not use for:
Decreases agent toxic potential	Areas supplied by end arteries
Allows increased dose	Patients "sensitive" to catecholamines
4. Increases level of blockade	4. Toxicity—catecholamine reaction†

From Roberts J, Hedges J: *Clinical procedures in emergency medicine,* ed 3, Philadelphia, 1998, WB Saunders.
*Based on laboratory studies.
†For example, in patients taking MAO inhibitors.

antibiotic coverage unless already infected. Rabies and tetanus prophylaxis should be considered for all patients.

WOUND PREPARATION

There are two methods of wound cleaning used in the effort to remove bacteria and contamination of foreign material. High-pressure irrigation, the preferred method, is excellent in removing debris and decreasing the infection rate. Commercial irrigation kits can be purchased or a needle with a syringe can be used. The needle should be as close to the wound as possible without producing trauma to the tissue. Saline or Betadine are used as irrigating solutions. Cleansing the wound by direct contact, although effective for debridement, destroys tissue. Soft brushes may be used. Figure 13-10 shows one type of wound irrigation.

The two most common solutions to clean the wound are Betadine solution and Hibiclens. Although these two cleansing agents are used routinely, they may produce some tissue damage in the wound, including lysis of red cells, damage of white cells, increased possibility of infection, and damage to cartilage.

The practice of shaving the skin is not recommended. Shaving destroys the hair follicles and increases the possibility of infection at the site. Clipping the hair instead of shaving is the alternative method.[9] As mentioned previously, eyebrows are never shaved because they may not regrow in a cosmetically pleasing way, if they grow back at all.

ANESTHESIA

Closure may be accomplished with tape, sutures, or staples. Local anesthesia is required for sutures and staples, with lidocaine preferred for local and regional anesthesia because of greater potency, decreased irritation, and long-lasting anesthetic effect. Lidocaine with epinephrine is used for lacerations in highly vascular areas. Epinephrine solutions should never be used on the nose, penis, ears, or digits. Table 13-5 shows the advantages and disadvantages of epinephrine in wound closure. Disadvantages of lidocaine are dose-related toxicity and include the possibility of an allergic reaction. If a patient is allergic to procaine, he or she will probably not be allergic to lidocaine.[6] Other anesthetic agents are procaine, mepivacaine (Carbocaine), bupivacaine (Marcaine or Sensorcaine), and tetracaine (Pontocaine). Agents may be used to infiltrate the wound area or may be applied topically. Table 13-6 highlights anesthetic agents used for local infiltration and nerve blocks. Mixing sodium bicarbonate 8.4% (Neut) with lidocaine decreases pain associated with infiltration.[8] Warm lidocaine solution also causes less pain. (Warm by running the vial under warm tap water.)

Topical anesthetics are ideal for management of minor lacerations in children. Available solutions include tetracaine, Adrenalin, and cocaine (TAC); Xylocaine, Adrenalin, and Pontacaine (XAP); and lidocaine, epinephrine, and tetracaine (LET). Cocaine solutions should be used cautiously because of potentially deleterious side effects such as central

Table 13-6   PRACTICAL AGENTS FOR EMERGENCY DEPARTMENT USE—LOCAL INFILTRATION

AGENT	CONCENTRATION (%)	MAXIMUM DOSE*† ADULT (MG)	MAXIMUM DOSE*† PEDIATRIC (MG/KG)	ONSET (MIN)	DURATION‡
Procaine	0.5-1.0	500§ (600)	7.0 (9)	2-5	15-45 min
Lidocaine	0.5-1.0	300 (500)	4.5 (7)‖	2-5	1-2 hr
Bupivacaine	0.25	175 (225)	2.0 (3)¶	2-5	4-8 hr

From Roberts J and Hedges J: *Clinical procedures in emergency medicine,* ed 3, Philadelphia, 1998, WB Saunders.
*These are conservative figures; see text for explanation.
†Higher dose for solutions containing epinephrine is in parentheses.
‡These values are for the agent alone; they can be extended considerably with the addition of epinephrine.
§Some authorities recommend up to 1000 mg or 14 mg/kg for procaine.
‖Some authorities recommend up to 7 mg/kg for plain lidocaine in children older than 1 year.
¶Because of lack of clinical trial experience, drug companies do not recommend the use of bupivacaine in children under the age of 12 years.

Table 13-7   PRACTICAL AGENTS FOR EMERGENCY DEPARTMENT USE—MUCOSAL APPLICATION

AGENT	USUAL CONCENTRATION (%)	MAXIMUM DOSAGE*† ADULT (MG)	MAXIMUM DOSAGE*† PEDIATRIC (MG/KG)	ONSET (MIN)	DURATION (MIN)
Tetracaine	0.5	50	0.75	3-8	30-60
Lidocaine	2-10	250-300†	3-4†	2-5	15-45
Cocaine	4	200	2-3†	2-5	30-45

From Roberts J, Hedges J: *Clinical procedures in emergency medicine,* ed 3, Philadelphia, 1998, WB Saunders.
*These are conservative figures; see text for explanations.
†The lower dosage should be used for a maximum safe dose when feasible.

nervous system (CNS) stimulation and vasomotor collapse. These solutions obviate the need for needle infiltration but do require a minimum of 20 minutes for adequate anesthesia. Infiltration is required when the desired anesthetic effect is not achieved. A cotton ball is saturated with anesthetic solution and applied directly to the laceration. A clear dressing such as tegaderm applied directly over the cotton ball holds the cotton ball in place and prevents absorption of the solution when tape is used. The vasoconstrictive effects of epinephrine cause a white ring around the wound. Because of the epinephrine component, these solutions cannot be used in areas of poor circulation. Anesthetic effect varies slightly with each solution because of duration of individual agents (Table 13-7). Solutions containing cocaine are controlled substances and significantly more expensive. Viscous lidocaine may be applied to abrasions before cleaning but is not used as an anesthetic for wound closure.

Regional anesthesia, or Bier block, may be selected when a greater anesthetic effect is desired. A tourniquet is placed proximal to the wound, then the anesthetic agent is injected distal to the injury. After wound repair, the tourniquet is released and the anesthetic agent is slowly absorbed. A local nerve block, or digital block, for anesthesia is accomplished by injecting the anesthetic agent along the nerve to abolish afferent and efferent impulse conduction. The syringe is aspirated before each injection to prevent parenteral lidocaine injection.

One alternative to local and regional anesthesia is nitrous oxide. The patient inhales a 50% mixture of nitrous oxide and oxygen during short, painful procedures such as debridement. Self-administration limits the amount of nitrous oxide used while providing the appropriate level of anesthesia.

WOUND CLOSURE

Primary wound closure uses a tape closure (Steri-Strips), sutures, or staples. Table 13-8 describes advantages and disadvantages for each. The technique chosen depends on wound size, depth, and location. Tape closure is used for superficial linear wounds under minimal tension or as an adjunct after suture removal in patients with thin, frail skin such as the elderly or steroid-dependent patients (Figure 13-11). Tape closure is also more easily accomplished in obese patients because adipose tissue tends to evert wound edges.[8] Tincture of benzoin is applied to skin before tape application to ensure adherence. A tape closure may also be used after deeper layers are closed with sutures. Dressings may or may not be applied over the tape closure. An anesthetic is not necessary, and a lower risk of infection is associated with tape closure. Tape strips remain in place until they fall off. Figure 13-12 illustrates tape closure.

Sutures approximate and attach wound edges, which decrease infection, promote wound healing, and minimize scar formation. A local anesthetic applied by infiltration or topically is required for suturing. Different stitches are used to close various wounds depending on depth, location, and tension of the wound. Figure 13-13 shows various stitches and

Table 13-8 SUTURE MATERIALS FOR WOUND CLOSURE

TYPE	DESCRIPTION	SECURITY	STRENGTH	REACTION	WORKABILITY	INFECTION	COMMENT
NONABSORBABLES							
Silk		++++	+	++++	++++	++	Nice around mouth, nose, or nipples; too reactive and weak to be used universally
Mersilene	Braided synthetic	++++	++	+++	++++		Good tensile strength; some prefer for fascia repairs
Nylon	Monofilament	++	+++	++	++	+++	Good strength; decreased infection rate; knots tend to slip, especially the first throw
Prolene Polypropylene	Monofilament	+	++++	+	+	++++	Good resistance to infection; often difficult to work with; requires an extra throw
Ethibond	Braided coated polyester	+++	++++	++½	+++	+++	Costly
Stainless steel wire	Monofilament	++++	++++	+	+	+	Hard to use; painful to patient; some prefer for tendons
ABSORBABLES							
Gut (plain)	From sheep intima	+	++	+++		+	Loses strength rapidly and quickly absorbed; rarely used today
Chromic (gut)	Plain gut treated with chromic salts	++	++	+++		+	Similar to plain gut; often used to close intraoral lacerations
Dexon	Braided copolymer of glycolic acid	++++	++++	+		++++	Braiding may cause it to "hang up" when tying knots
Vicryl	Braided polymer of lactide and glycolide	+++	++++	+		+++	Low reactivity with good strength; therefore, nice for subcutaneous healing; good in mucous membranes
Polydioxanone	Monofilament	++++	++++	+	Excellent	Unavailable	First available monofilament synthetic absorbable sutures; appears to be excellent

From Swanson NA, Tromovitch TA: *Int J Dermatol* 21:373, 1982.

their uses. Sutures may be absorbable or nonabsorbable, which means they are composed of natural or synthetic material, respectively. Essential qualities of suture material are security, strength, reaction, workability, and infectious potential. Table 13-8 describes these qualities for various suture materials.[10] Ideal suture material is strong, easily secured, resistant to infection, and causes minimal local reaction. Sutures cause minimal discomfort after insertion; however, they also act as a foreign body and can cause local inflammation. A thin layer of antibiotic ointment is applied after suture application, then covered by a nonadherent dressing. Recommendations for suture removal vary with wound location. For wounds in areas of movement or increased surface tension, sutures should remain longer. Table 13-9 provides guidelines for suture removal.

Staples are a fast, economic alternative for closure of linear lacerations of the scalp, trunk, and extremities (Figure 13-14). Wounds closed with staples have a lower incidence of infection and tissue reactivity but do not provide the same quality of closure as sutures. Scars are more pronounced; therefore, staples are only recommended for areas where a scar is not apparent (i.e., scalp). Staples should not be used in areas of the scalp with permanent hair loss because of poor aesthetic results. Local anesthesia is optional when only one or two staples are required because pain from infiltration of anesthetic agents is greater than pain associated

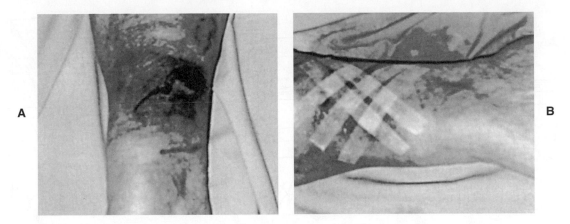

FIGURE 13-11 **A,** A pretibial skin avulsion is an ideal wound to close with closure tapes. **B,** An elderly woman who was on steroids had extremely thin skin that could not be replaced with sutures but healed nicely when closure tapes held the skin in place. A compression dressing, such as an elastic bandage or a Dome paste (Unna) boot dressing, can be applied to minimize flap movement and decrease fluid build up under the flap. (From Roberts J, Hedges J: *Clinical procedures in emergency medicine,* ed 3, Philadelphia, 1998, WB Saunders.)

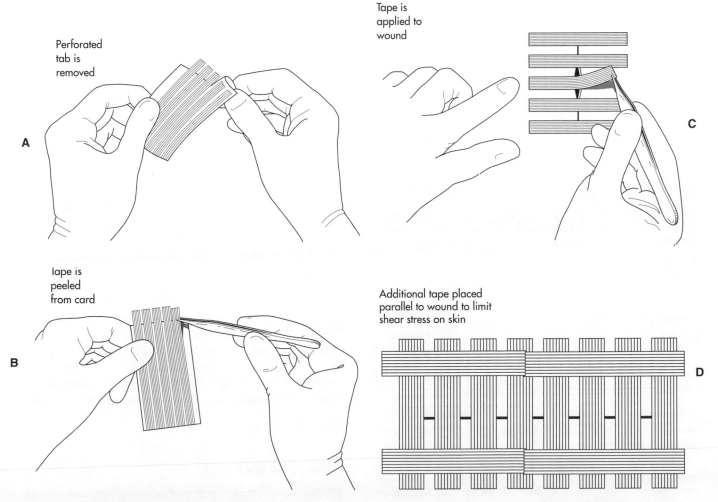

Perforated tab is removed

Tape is applied to wound

Tape is peeled from card

Additional tape placed parallel to wound to limit shear stress on skin

FIGURE 13-12 Tape closure **(A-D)**. (From Meeker MH, Rothrock JC: *Alexander's care of the patient in surgery,* ed 11, St. Louis, 1999, Mosby.)

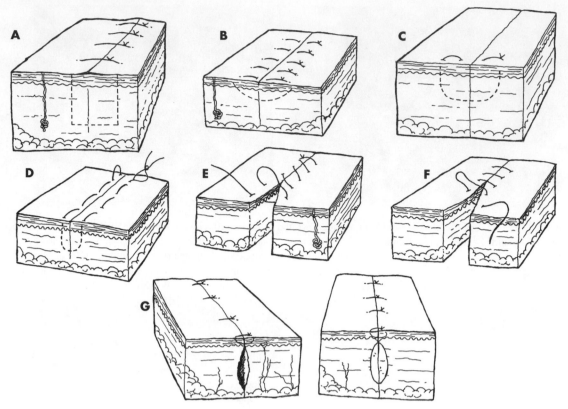

FIGURE **13-13** Stitches for suturing. **A,** Simple interrupted sutures: pairing skin edges together evenly; edges are slightly elevated but flatten with healing. **B,** Vertical mattress suture: assures eversion on healing. **C,** Horizontal mattress suture: closely approximates skin edges and has slight amount of eversion, especially in areas under tension. **D,** Half-buried horizontal mattress sutures: good with flaps, V-shaped wounds, and parallel lacerations. **E,** Subcuticular suture (continuous intradermal suture): good for wounds where sutures should be left in place for longer periods, as in wounds under a great deal of tension. **F,** Continuous suture: good when suture marks will not show, as in scalp. **G,** Buried sutures: reduce dead space and reduce surface tension in wound.

Table 13-9 GUIDELINES FOR SUTURE REMOVAL	
LOCATION	REMOVAL DATE
Eyelids	3 to 5 days
Eyebrows	4 to 5 days
Ear	4 to 6 days
Lip	3 to 5 days
Face	3 to 5 days
Scalp	7 to 10 days
Trunk	7 to 10 days
Hands and feet	7 to 10 days
Arms and legs	10 to 14 days
Over joints	14 days

with insertion of one or two staples. Staples usually remain in place 7 to 10 days. A special staple remover (Figure 13-15) is required for removal.

Dermabond, the newest form of wound closure, is a topical skin glue used to close skin edges that are easily approximated. This type of wound closure should not be used in high skin tension areas or across areas of increased skin tension. Application of three thin layers is more effective than a single thick layer; the Dermabond dries within 2.5 minutes. Discharge teaching should stress not applying liquid or ointment to the closed wound because these substances can weaken the glue, leading to dehiscence. Patients should also be instructed that the adhesive will slough naturally, usually within 5 to 10 days. If removal of Dermabond is necessary, use petroleum jelly or acetone.

WOUND PROPHYLAXIS

Wounds are at risk for local and systemic infection from contaminants, surface organisms, tetanus, and rabies. Protection against these infectious agents begins with cleansing and irrigation. Prophylactic antibiotics are not indicated for most surface injuries unless severe contamination or obvious infection is present.

Tetanus Prophylaxis

Tetanus is a systemic infection caused by *Clostridium tetani,* a gram-positive, spore-forming, anaerobic bacillus. Once activated, the bacillus is extremely resistant to almost any-

Table 13-10 TETANUS PROPHYLAXIS		PATIENT COMPLETELY IMMUNIZED: TIME SINCE LAST BOOSTER DOSE	
TYPE OF WOUND	**PATIENT NOT IMMUNIZED OR PARTIALLY IMMUNIZED**	**5 TO 10 YR**	**10 YR+**
Clean minor	Begin or complete immunization per schedule: toxoid 0.5 ml	None	Tetanus toxoid 0.5 ml
Tetanus-prone	Human tetanus immune globulin, 250 to 500 U; toxoid, 0.5 ml, complete immunization per schedule; antibiotic therapy as indicated	Tetanus toxoid 0.5 ml; antibiotic therapy if indicated	Tetanus toxoid 0.5 ml; tetanus immune globulin, 250 to 500 U; antibiotic therapy if indicated

From Trunkey DD, Lewis FR: *Current therapy of trauma,* ed 3, St. Louis, 1991, Mosby.

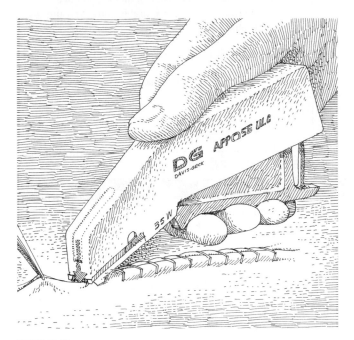

FIGURE **13-14**   Application of skin staples. Staples are centered over incision line, using locating arrow or guideline, and placed approximately one-quarter inch apart. (From Meeker MH, Rothrock JC: *Alexander's care of the patient in surgery,* ed 11, St. Louis, 1999, Mosby.

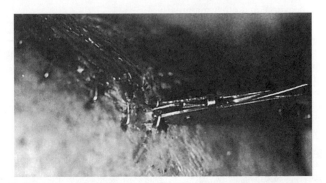

FIGURE **13-15**   Staple remover. (From Potter PA, Perry AG: *Fundamentals of nursing,* ed 5, St. Louis, 2001, Mosby.)

Box 13-3   **TETANUS-PRONE WOUNDS**
More than 6 hr old
Stellate or avulsed
Caused by missile, crushing mechanism, heat, or cold
Obvious signs of infection
Devitalized tissue
Contaminants such as dirt, feces, soil, saliva

thing, including sterilization. The incubation period for tetanus is 2 days to 2 weeks or more. *C. tetani* spores are present in soil, garden moss, and anywhere animal and human excrement are found. Spores may contaminate wounds, but remain dormant in tissue for years. After *C. tetani* enters the circulatory system, bacilli attach to cells in the CNS, causing depression of the respiratory center in the medulla. Symptoms may be mild or severe and include local joint stiffness and mild trismus or inability to open the jaw. Severe tetanus is characterized by severe trismus, back pain, penile pain, tachycardia, hypertension, dysrhythmias, hyperpyrexia, opisthotonos, and seizures.

Prevention of tetanus includes immunization and scrupulous wound care, particularly for tetanus-prone wounds (Box 13-3). Tetanus immunization is part of the childhood immunization regimen that continues with regular tetanus immunizations in adults. Tetanus toxoid provides active immunization, whereas tetanus immune globulin provides passive immunization. People who are inadequately immunized against tetanus should receive active and/or passive protection depending on the type of wound and their individual immunization status. Table 13-10 reviews recommendations for tetanus prophylaxis for clean and tetanus-prone wounds. Prophylaxis should be given within 72 hours to decrease the risk of tetanus.

Rabies Prophylaxis

Rabies exposure can occur with bites from wild and domestic animals. Although rabies is rare in the United States, it should be considered when an animal attack was not provoked, involved a domestic animal not immunized against rabies, or involved a wild animal. Rabies is a neurotoxic virus found in saliva of some mammals. Incubation period is 4 to 8 weeks.

Table 13-11 RABIES POSTEXPOSURE PROPHYLAXIS GUIDE—UNITED STATES, 1999		
ANIMAL TYPE	**EVALUATION AND DISPOSITION OF ANIMAL**	**POSTEXPOSURE PROPHYLAXIS RECOMMENDATIONS**
Dogs, cats, and ferrets	Healthy and available for 10 days' observation	People should not begin prophylaxis unless animal develops clinical signs of rabies*
	Rabid or suspected rabid	Immediately immunize
	Unknown (e.g., escaped)	Consult public health officials
Skunks, raccoons, foxes, and most other carnivores; bats	Regarded as rabid unless animal is proven negative for rabies by laboratory tests†	Consider immediate immunization
Livestock, small rodents, lagomorphs (rabbits and hares), large rodents (woodchucks and beavers), and other mammals	Consider individually	Consult public health officials; bites of squirrels, hamsters, guinea pigs, gerbils, chipmunks, rats, mice, other small rodents, rabbits, and hares almost never require antirabies postexposure prophylaxis

Data from Blazys D: An informal discussion among emergency nurses about their current clinical practice: what's new and what works, *J Emerg Nurs* 27(2):163, 2001.

*During the 10-day observation period, begin postexposure prophylaxis at the first sign of rabies in a dog, cat, or ferret that has bitten someone. If the animal exhibits clinical signs of rabies, it should be euthanized immediately and tested.

†The animal should be euthanized and tested as soon as possible. Holding for observation is not recommended. Discontinue vaccine if immunofluorescence test results of the animal are negative.

Table 13-12 RABIES POSTEXPOSURE PROPHYLAXIS SCHEDULE—UNITED STATES, 1999		
VACCINATION STATUS	**TREATMENT**	**REGIMEN***
Not previously vaccinated	Wound cleansing	All postexposure treatment should begin with immediate thorough cleansing of all wounds with soap and water; if available, a virucidal agent such as a povidone-iodine solution should be used to irrigate wounds
	RIG	Administer 20 IU/kg body weight; if anatomically feasible, the full dose should be infiltrated around the wound(s) and any remaining volume should be administered IM at an anatomic site distant from vaccine administration; also, RIG should not be administered in the same syringe as vaccine; because RIG might partially suppress active production of antibody, no more than the recommended dose should be given
	Vaccine	HDCV, RVA, or PCEC 1.0 ml, IM (deltoid†), one each on days 0‡, 3, 7, 14, and 28
Previously vaccinated§	Wound cleansing	All postexposure treatment should begin with immediate thorough cleansing of all wounds with soap and water; if available, a virucidal agent such as a povidone-iodine solution should be used to irrigate the wounds
	RIG	RIG should not be administered
	Vaccine	HDCV, RVA, or PCEC 1.0 ml, IM (deltoid area†), one each on days 0‡ and 3

From Blazys D: An informal discussion among emergency nurses about their current clinical practice: what's new and what works, *J Emerg Nurs* 27(2):163, 2001.

HDCV, Human diploid cell vaccine; *IM,* intramuscular; *PCEC,* purified chick embryo cell vaccine; *RIG,* rabies immune globulin (human); *RVA,* rabies vaccine absorbed.

*These regimens are applicable for all age-groups, including children.

†The deltoid area is the only acceptable site of vaccination for adults and older children. For younger children, the outer aspect of the thigh may be used. The vaccine should never be administered in the gluteal area.

‡Day 0 is the day the first dose of vaccine is administered.

§Any person with a history of preexposure vaccination with HDCV, RVA, or PCEC; prior postexposure prophylaxis with HDCV, RVA, or PCEC; or previous vaccination with any other type of rabies vaccine and a documented history of antibody response to the prior vaccination.

After inoculation, the rabies virus travels by peripheral nerves to the CNS, causing encephalomyelitis, which is almost always fatal. Sources of rabies in wild and domestic animals are listed in Table 13-11. Carnivorous wild animals are always considered rabid, so immediate rabies prophylaxis should be administered. Domestic animals that show signs of rabies are destroyed, and laboratory analysis is performed. Those animals that appear healthy are observed for 10 days, with pro-

phylaxis required if the animal exhibits signs of rabies. Prophylaxis is always given when the animal cannot be found. Rodents such as rats, chipmunks, hamsters, gerbils, and squirrels rarely carry rabies; however, local authorities should be consulted for confirmation.

Rabies immunization includes administration of rabies immune globulin (RIG) and human diploid cell vaccine (HDCV). RIG provides passive immunization, and HDCV

Box 13-4	NURSING DIAGNOSES FOR SURFACE TRAUMA

Fluid volume, Deficient
Infection, Risk for
Pain
Skin integrity, Impaired
Tissue perfusion, Ineffective

provides active immunization.[12] The best defense against rabies continues to be prevention through vaccinating domestic animals and educating the public about the danger of handling wild animals, especially bats. Table 13-12 summarizes rabies immunization.

SUMMARY

Skin is the first barrier between the body and the rest of the world. Loss of skin integrity affects ability to resist infection, retain fluids, and regulate body temperature. Changes caused by surface trauma such as scarring or tattooing affect body image and can cause significant anxiety for the patient. The emergency nurse can reduce potential complications related to these wounds through assessment, scrupulous wound care, and thorough discharge teaching. Priority nursing diagnoses for patients with surface trauma are listed in Box 13-4.

References

1. Blackman J: Man's best friend, *J Amer Board Fam Prac,* 1998. Retrieved February 18, 2001, from the World Wide Web: http://www.medscape.com/ABFP/JABFP/1998/v11.n02/fp1102.13.blac.html.

2. Calvin M: Cutaneous wound repair, *Wounds* 10(1), 1998. Retrieved from the World Wide Web: http://www.medscape.com/HMP/wounds/1998/v10.n01/w1001.01.calv/w1001.01.calv-01.1.

3. DeLaune S, Ladner P: *Fundamentals of nursing, standards and practice,* Albany, NY, 1998, Delmar.

4. Feliciano DV, Moore EE, Mattox KL: *Trauma,* ed 3, Stanford, Conn, 1996, Appleton & Lange.

5. Guyton AC, Hall JE: *Textbook of medical physiology,* ed 10, Philadelphia, 2000, WB Saunders.

6. Kidd PS, Sturt P: *Mosby's emergency nursing reference,* ed 2, St. Louis, 2002, Mosby.

7. Lewis S, Heitkemper M, Dirksen S: *Medical surgical nursing: assessment and management of clinical problems,* ed 5, St. Louis, 2000, Mosby.

8. Strange GR, Ahrens WR, Schafermeyer R et al: *Pediatric emergency medicine: a comprehensive study guide,* New York, 1996, McGraw-Hill.

9. Schwartz G: *Principles and practice of emergency medicine,* ed 4, Baltimore, 1999, Williams & Wilkins.

10. Tintinalli JE, Ruiz E, Krome RL, *Emergency medicine: a comprehensive study guide,* ed 4, New York, 1996, McGraw-Hill.

11. Wright J, Hansen D, Burrell R: The comparative efficacy of two antimicrobial barrier dressings: in vitro examination of two controlled release of silver dressings, *Wounds,* 1998. Retrieved February 18, 2001 from the World Wide Web: http://www.medscape.com/HMP/wounds/1998/v10.n06/w1006.02.wrig/w1006.02.wrig-01.

12. Centers for Disease Control and Prevention: Human rabies prevention—United States 1999. Recommendations of the Advisory Committee on Immunization Practices, *MMWR* 48(RR-1):1, 1999.

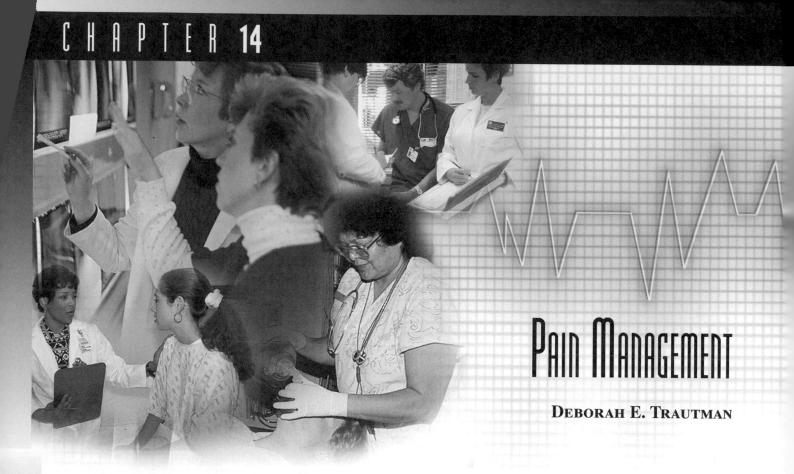

CHAPTER 14

Pain Management

DEBORAH E. TRAUTMAN

Pain is a common complaint that motivates people to seek emergency care. Unfortunately, pain management practices in many emergency departments (EDs) are less than adequate.[2,7,11,12,20] Relief of pain has not been universally adopted as a priority of practice in emergency care. Even with development of clinical guidelines, pain is often underestimated and undertreated.[2,7,10]

Increasing attention has been directed at improving emergency care providers' response to pain management. Assessment and treatment of pain has gained prominence as an important health care issue and has been recognized as a nursing, physician, and organizational responsibility. The 2001 Joint Commission on Hospital Accreditation Standards specify that all patients have the right to appropriate assessment and management of pain (R1.12.8).[14] The standard is intended to ensure that pain management is an important part of health care delivery. In fact, pain assessment has recently been referred to as the "fifth vital sign."

Improving the emergency care providers' response to pain necessitates better understanding of factors that have contributed to inadequate management. Although multiple factors can contribute to ineffective pain management, three barriers often confronted by nurses and physicians include a (1) belief that treating pain early may delay or complicate patient workup or examination; (2) failure to believe or understand the patient's complaint of pain; and (3) fear of oversedation or desire to avoid potential adverse effects of opioids, especially, central nervous system, respiratory, or cardiac depression.[5,17]

Despite existence of these barriers, safe, effective, and early control of pain is a realistic goal for emergency care.

Nurses can be advocates for effective pain relief for their patients. Increasing one's knowledge of pain, assuming a more prominent role in helping patients and physicians manage acute pain, and monitoring treatment plans to ensure safe, effective pain management are among a few of the important contributions the nurse can make in promoting effective pain management.

DEFINITION OF PAIN

Attempts at defining pain vary widely; however, the definition most commonly accepted in nursing is "whatever the experiencing person says it is, existing whenever he or she says it does."[17] Pain is subdivided into two types: acute and chronic. McCaffery[17] defines acute pain as "relatively brief pain that subsides as healing takes place." Chronic pain is usually defined as pain that lasts for 6 months or longer. Acute pain is usually a symptom of an identifiable disease, persisting only as long as the disease itself and responding to adequate pain management. Chronic pain may be associated with chronic tissue disease, may not have an identifiable cause, may last longer than the normal healing period for an acute injury or disease, and may not respond to standard analgesic interventions. Chronic pain management is beyond the scope of this chapter. This chapter focuses exclusively on management of acute pain; however, Table 14-1 does provide a comparison of acute and chronic pain for consideration.

To understand acute pain management, the nurse must recognize that acute pain has both physical and nonphysical components.[16] Specific components are the physical stimulus and the patient's cognitive and emotional interpretation

Table 14-1 COMPARISON OF ACUTE AND CHRONIC PAIN

CHARACTERISTIC	ACUTE PAIN	CHRONIC PAIN
Experience	An event	A situation, state of existence
Source	External agent or internal disease	Unknown; if known, treatment is prolonged or ineffective
Onset	Usually sudden	May be sudden or develop insidiously
Duration	Transient (up to 6 months)	Prolonged (months to years)
Pain identification	Painful and nonpainful areas generally well identified	Painful and nonpainful areas less easily differentiated; change in sensations becomes more difficult to evaluate
Clinical signs	Typical response pattern with more visible signs	Response patterns vary; fewer overt signs (adaptation)
Significance	Significant (informs person something is wrong)	Person looks for significance
Pattern	Self-limiting or readily corrected	Continuous or intermittent; intensity may vary or remain constant
Course	Suffering usually decreases over time	Suffering usually increases over time
Actions	Leads to actions to relieve pain	Leads to actions to modify pain experience
Prognosis	Likelihood of eventual complete relief	Complete relief usually not possible

From McCance KL, Huether SE: *Pathophysiology: the biologic basis for disease in adults and children,* ed 3, St. Louis, 1998, Mosby.

Box 14-1 DO'S AND DON'TS OF PAIN CONTROL

Slow down. Don't hurry in and out of the room.
Talk to the patient about the pain.
Don't tell the patient he or she does not have pain.
Avoid casual or flippant comments.
Be realistic about the situation.
Don't ignore the patient.
Don't be callous.
Don't make judgments.

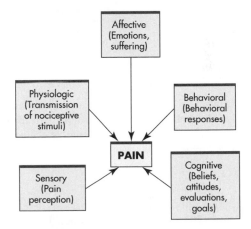

FIGURE **14-1** The five components of pain. (From Lewis SM, Heitkemper MM, Dirksen SR: *Medical-surgical nursing: assessment and management of clinical problems,* ed 5, St. Louis, 2000, Mosby.)

of that stimulus. Pain also has affective and sensory aspects. Removal or treatment of the physical stimulus is the most reliable and therapeutic approach to pain control; however, nursing interventions—and the nurse's role in particular—can influence the patient's interpretation of pain. Interpretation of pain is influenced by such factors as culture, religious beliefs, coping styles, and trust and fear about the ED visit. Handling the subjectivity of pain can prove to be challenging, but a knowledgeable, calm, empathetic nurse can do much to minimize the patient's fears and facilitate early pain management.

How can nurses help the patient better manage their pain? In a study of 148 patients, Copp[8] found that patients frequently shared ideas on how nurses and physicians could help. Box 14-1 summarizes these ideas. These are important points for the nurse to incorporate into the role of assisting with pain management. Not so long ago many nurses considered their role in pain management to be simply administering physicians' orders. This now-antiquated belief minimizes the nurse's contribution to patient care. The emergency nurse's role is vital in facilitating early relief of pain and suffering. The nurse should assure the patient that the health care team acknowledges that the patient is in pain and will treat the pain soon and effectively.

PATHOPHYSIOLOGY

Pain is a multidimensional phenomena consisting of psychologic and physiologic components (Figure 14-1).[1,17] Physical, neurologic, and biochemical properties comprise the physiologic aspect of pain. Somatic sensation is initiated by a variety of somatic receptors. Pain, one type of somatic sensation, is associated with specific receptors known as nociceptors. Stimulation of these nociceptors results in the sensation of pain (Figure 14-2). Mechanical, thermal, or chemical irritation depolarize nociceptors and initiate action potentials in afferent nerve fibers, which conduct impulses toward the brain or spinal cord; efferent nerve fibers carry impulses away from the brain or spinal cord.[16]

Several theories of pain perception exist. Four are discussed briefly in this chapter. The specificity theory postulated by Muller proposes that specific receptors exist for pain. Wolland and Seridan developed the pattern theory,

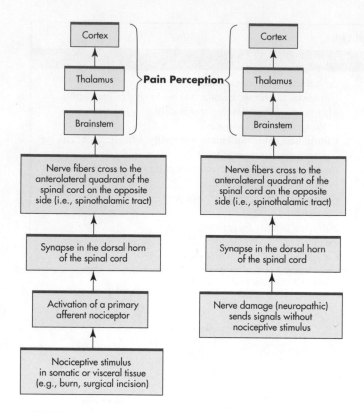

FIGURE 14-2 Mechanisms of nociceptive and neuropathic pain. (From Lewis SM, Heitkemper MM, Dirksen SR: *Medical-surgical nursing: assessment and management of clinical problems*, ed 5, St. Louis, 2000, Mosby.)

which states that multiple receptors form specific patterns of pain sensation. The gate theory developed by Melzak and Wall suggests that sensory input from peripheral fibers is transmitted to the dorsal horn of the spinal cord, where it is modulated and then transmitted to the brain for perception.[18] A recent theory postulates that the classic pain pathway is dual. "The sensation of pain that is experienced arrives in the central nervous system by means of two pathways: (1) a sensory discriminate system that encodes the capacity to analyze the nature (e.g., burning or pricking), location, intensity, and duration of nociceptive stimulation, and (2) an affective, motivational component that gives rise to the unpleasant character of painful sensation."[9] Inhibitory and augmentive controls exist. Prevention and treatment are guided by knowledge of the pathophysiology.

PATIENT ASSESSMENT

Management of acute pain begins with the initial nursing assessment. A concise, comprehensive assessment is essential. Assessment indices include both subjective and objective measures. Because of the broad scope of nursing literature on patient assessment, the following discussion is limited to a brief summarization of nursing assessment of pain. For more detailed assessment techniques, see McCaffery and Pasero.[17]

An initial, focused assessment should be conducted to collect data about the patient's pain. Assessment of pain includes location, quality, intensity, onset, duration, and aggravating or alleviating factors.[15] Not all patients adequately verbalize key components of their pain. Language barriers, cultural differences, fever, and other physiologic or psychosocial factors may interfere with the assessment.

Pain rating scales or use of a pain assessment tool may facilitate gathering pertinent information. If a pain rating scale is used, it is important to use the same scale consistently with the patient. Using the same scale is helpful for the patient and clinicians. It minimizes any confusion or misinterpretation that may occur.[17] Additional data-gathering techniques such as facilitation (saying "mmm-hmm" or "go on"), reflection, repeating key phrases the patient said in a question format, and clarification of ambiguous statements facilitate collection of patient information. Avoid prompting the patient by asking leading questions and making inferences about the patient's pain. Doing so is likely to give rise to an inadequate and perhaps inaccurate assessment.

Objective data include, but are not limited to, physical description of the patient, facial expressions, and measurement of pulse rate, blood pressure, and respiratory rate.[15] Table 14-2 summarizes behavioral responses to pain. After initial assessment, the emergency nurse is responsible for ongoing assessment and evaluation of the patient's pain. This ongoing assessment facilitates evaluation of treatment.

Assessment tools and strategies for the pediatric patient vary from those used for adults.[23] Assessment of pain in the pediatric patient is often difficult because of the child's inability to communicate. Parents can contribute to assessing a child's pain by helping distinguish usual behavior from the child's current reactions. Observing a child for changes in facial expression and body position augments assessment. This is particularly helpful in infants with no verbal skills. Figure 14-3 illustrates the most consistent behavioral indicators of pain in infants.[23] Numeric and visual scales are available for children who are as young as 3 years (Table 14-3). These scales may also be used for individuals with limited cognitive ability. Rating scales and use of numbers expressing severity of pain can be used for older children.

MANAGING PAIN

Managing pain is a multifaceted, multidimensional process. Physical, social, cultural, and psychologic needs, beliefs, and experiences all influence the process. Nursing actions related to pain management are described in Box 14-2 on p. 164. Incorporating these components into the nursing role facilitates an effective nursing approach to and the probability of promoting successful pain management.

Selecting adequate interventions for pain is influenced by a host of factors. Research has shown that tradition, intuition, stereotypes, and ethnicity influence interventions selected for pain management. Burke and Jerrett[4] studied student nurses' perceptions of the best interventions for people

Table 14-2 BEHAVIORAL RESPONSES TO PAIN

AGE-GROUP	VOCALIZATIONS	FACIAL EXPRESSIONS	BODY MOVEMENTS	COPING STRATEGIES
Infants	Crying Fussy Irritable	Lowered brows Drawn together Eyes closed (young infant) Eyes open (older infant) Mouth open	Generalized body responses; rigid or thrashing (young infant) Localized body response; withdraws stimulated area (older infant)	Oral stimulation (sucking) Crying Fetal position
Toddlers/ preschoolers	Crying Screaming Verbalizes "boo-boo," "It hurts" Asks to stop painful stimulus Points to area of pain	Eyes closed or open Furrowed brow	Physical resistance Uncooperative Restless Clinging	Oral stimulation Crying while sleeping (toddlers) Rocking Closing eyes/turning away Lying still or being active (pre-schoolers)
School age	Crying Verbalizing pain quality, location, duration Verbalizing pain	Withdrawn facial expression Furrowed brow	Muscle rigidity Gritted teeth Clenched fists Splinting/guarding Lying still	Verbal stalling Being active or lying still Talking about the pain Using distraction techniques Sleeping Playing or watching television
Adolescents	Crying Groaning	Withdrawn Eyes closed Furrowed brow	Muscle tension and body control Splinting/guarding Lying still	Verbalizing pain Taking medication or initiating actions to relieve pain Sleeping Lying still
Adults	Moaning Sobbing Grunting Shouting Praying Crying out for help Sighing	Frowning Staring Furrowed brow Teeth clenching	Thrashing Tossing Rocking Muscle rigidity	Protective behaviors Posturing Massaging
Elderly	Moaning Grunting Chanting Praying Crying for help	Eyes squeezed closed Withdrawn look Furrowed brow Staring	Rocking Clutching side rails Muscle rigidity	Wandering Rubbing Guarding

Modified from Bernardo L, Conway A: Pain assessment and management. In Sond T, Rogers J, editors: *Manual of pediatric emergency nursing,* St. Louis, 1998, Mosby; Katz E, Kellerman K, Siegel S: Behavioral distress in children with cancer undergoing medical procedures: developmental considerations, *J Consult Clin Psychol* 48(3):356, 1980.

of various ages who were in acute pain. Age was identified as a factor that influenced both the number and type of interventions selected. In this study, student nurses selected more interventions for adolescents and adults, and fewer interventions for infants, toddlers, children, and the elderly. Of eight possible intervention types (Box 14-3), a mean of 3.3 types was selected for infants, 5.0 for adults, and 4.5 for the elderly. More recently, Todd[22] noted that inadequate analgesia for certain conditions was more likely for blacks and Hispanics than for white patients. According to these researchers, oligonalgesia, inadequate prescribing of analgesics for patients in pain, is not the failure to assess pain, but rather the failure to administer analgesics.[22] Further research is needed to advance understanding of factors that contribute to inadequate analgesia.[11,22]

Pain Management Interventions

Pain management interventions include invasive techniques such as medication and noninvasive techniques such as imagery. When selecting a technique for a specific patient, the nurse should recognize that each patient is unique and that no one universally superior pain control method exists for all patients. Patients should be evaluated individually and interventions tailored to each patient and his or her situation. Box 14-4 identifies some general aspects of pain control. The following sections discuss specific aspects of pain management.

Analgesics

Analgesics are divided into three groups: nonopioids, opioids, and adjuvants.[1,17] *Nonopioid* is the term now preferred to nonnarcotic, *opioid* is preferred to narcotic, and *adjuvant*

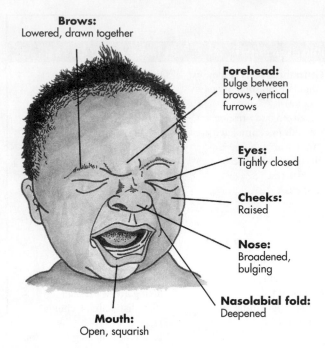

Brows:
Lowered, drawn together

Forehead:
Bulge between brows, vertical furrows

Eyes:
Tightly closed

Cheeks:
Raised

Nose:
Broadened, bulging

Nasolabial fold:
Deepened

Mouth:
Open, squarish

FIGURE 14-3 Facial expression of physical distress is the most consistent behavioral indicator of pain in infants. (From Wong DL, Hockenberry-Eaton M, Wilson D et al: *Wong's essentials of pediatric nursing*, ed 6, St. Louis, 2001, Mosby.)

refers to drugs that have a primary indication other than pain but have an analgesic effect in certain conditions.[17]

Nonopioids. Acetaminophen and nonsteroidal antiinflammatory drugs (NSAIDs) comprise this group of analgesics. Table 14-4 on p. 165 summarizes these agents. Although the exact mechanism of action of acetaminophen is unknown, it is believed to produce analgesia by blocking pain impulses through its effect on the central nervous system.[6,17] Acetaminophen has few adverse effects but also offers very few antiinflammatory effects. Acetaminophen is preferred for patients allergic to aspirin or those with platelet or gastrointestinal problems. The usual recommended daily dose of acetaminophen should not exceed 4000 mg.[17] Acetaminophen may cause liver toxicity and therefore should be used with caution in patients who drink alcohol regularly or have liver disease.

NSAIDs have an antiinflammatory effect on the peripheral tissues. Examples of drugs in this category include aspirin, carprofen (Rimadyl), choline magnesium trisalicylate (Trilisate), choline salicylate (Arthropan), diflunisal (Dolobid), etodolac (Lodine), fenoprofen calcium (Nalfon), ibuprofen (Motrin, Advil), ketorolac (Toradol), ketoprofen (Orudis), meclofenamate sodium (Meclomen), mefenamic acid (Ponstel), nabumetone (Relafen), naproxen (Naprosyn), naproxen sodium (Anaprox, Aleve), piroxicam (Feldene), and salsate (Disalcid). NSAIDs also include the benefit of treating nociceptive (somatic and visceral) pain. These drugs are thought to be particularly effective in treating muscle and joint pain. They are, however, thought to be insufficient in treating severe pain. Drug selection is usually best determined by assessing what has worked well for the

patient in the past. There is a ceiling dose for analgesia but it varies from individual to individual. A general rule is that the dose should not exceed 200% of the recommended daily starting dose.[17]

Opioids. All groups can be used to manage acute pain but opioids are considered the best agents for severe acute pain control.[3,12,17] Opioid analgesics are divided into two categories: mu agonists and agonist-antagonists. Table 14-5 on p. 166 summarizes these agents. The mu agonists (morphine-like) are the largest group and used most often. Examples of drugs in this category include codeine, fentanyl, hydrocodone, hydromorphone, levorphanol, meperidine, methadone, morphine, oxycodone, and propoxyphene.[17] Opioids are believed to relieve pain by action in the central nervous system. It is recommended that only one mu agonist be given by one route of administration. Contraindications to mu agonists include hemodynamic or respiratory compromise, altered sensorium, and inability to monitor the patient and manage side effects.[1] Although little difference is believed to exist among mu agonists and their ability to relieve pain, morphine is often the mu agonist of choice. Adults experience good pain relief with this drug. Dosage recommendations are 5 to 20 mg subcutaneously (SC) or intramuscularly (IM), 2.5 to 15 mg intravenously (IV) every 4 hours or as needed, or 10 to 30 mg by mouth (PO) every 4 hours.[6] Some adverse effects of mu agonists include sedation, somnolence, clouded sensorium, eupohoria, seizures, dizziness, hypotension, bradycardia, shock, nausea, vomiting, constipation, thrombocytopenia, respiratory depression, pruritus, and skin flushing. Physical dependence is expected with regular use for several days or more.

The second group of opioids, the agonist-antagonists, include pentazocine (Talwin), nalbuphine (Nubain), butorphanol (Stadol), and dezocine (Dalgan) and the partial agonist buprenorphine (Buprenex). This group of drugs is indicated for moderate to severe nociceptive (visceral or somatic) pain but is considered inappropriate for severe escalating pain.[6,17] Routes of administration are limited to parenteral with the exception of oral pentazocine and butorphanol nasal spray. These drugs should be used with caution in any patient already receiving mu agonists. Analgesia may be reduced and withdrawal-like symptoms may be precipitated in patients physically dependent on mu agonists.[17]

Adjuvant Analgesics. Adjuvant analgesics are "drugs with other specific indications that have been found to be effective analgesics for selected types of pain."[17] These drugs have analgesic properties, but these properties are not their primary function. Antidepressants, corticosteroids, and psychostimulants are considered adjuvant analgesics. Examples of drugs in this group include:
- Antidepressants: amitriptyline (Elavil), desipramine (Norpramin), nortriptyline (Aventyl, Pamelor)
- Corticosteroids: dexamethasone (Decadron)
- Psychostimulants: dextromamphetamine (Dexedrine), methylphenidate (Ritalin)

Table 14-3 PAIN RATING SCALES FOR CHILDREN

PAIN SCALE/DESCRIPTION	INSTRUCTIONS	RECOMMENDED AGE/COMMENTS
FACES Pain Rating Scale* (Wong and Baker, 1988, 2000): Consists of six cartoon faces ranging from smiling face for "no pain" to tearful face for "worst pain"	***Original instructions:*** Explain to child that each face is for a person who feels happy because there is no pain (hurt) or sad because there is some or a lot of pain. FACE 0 is very happy because there is no hurt. FACE 1 hurts just a little bit. FACE 2 hurts a little more. FACE 3 hurts even more. FACE 4 hurts a whole lot, but FACE 5 hurts as much as you can imagine, although you don't have to be crying to feel this bad. Ask child to choose face that best describes own pain. Record the number under chosen face on pain assessment record. ***Brief word instructions:*** Point to each face using the words to describe the pain intensity. Ask child to choose face that best describes own pain and record the appropriate number.	For children as young as 3 years. Using original instructions without affect words, such as *happy* or *sad,* or brief words resulted in same pain rating, probably reflecting child's rating of pain intensity. For coding purposes, numbers 0, 2, 4, 6, 8, 10 can be substituted for 0-5 system to accommodate 0-10 system. The FACES provides three scales in one: facial expressions, numbers, and words. Use of brief word instructions is recommended.

0	1	2	3	4	5
No Hurt	Hurts Little Bit	Hurts Little More	Hurts Even More	Hurts Whole Lot	Hurts Worst

Oucher (Beyer, Denyes, and Villaruel, 1992): Consists of six photographs of child's face representing "no hurt" to "biggest hurt you could ever have"; includes a vertical scale with numbers from 0-100; scales for black and Hispanic children have been developed (Villaruel and Denyes, 1991)	***Numeric Scale*** Point to each section of scale to explain variations in pain intensity: "0 means no hurt." "This means little hurts" (pointing to lower part of scale, 1-29). "This means middle hurts" (pointing to middle part of scale, 30-69). "This means big hurts" (pointing to upper part of scale, 70-99). "100 means the biggest hurt you could ever have." Score is actual number stated by child. ***Photographic Scale*** Point to each photograph on Oucher and explain variations in pain intensity using following language: first picture from the bottom is "no hurt," second is "a little hurt," third is "a little more hurt," fourth is "even more hurt than that," fifth is "pretty much or a lot of hurt," and sixth is the "biggest hurt you could ever have." Score pictures from 0-5, with the bottom picture scored as 0. ***General*** Practice using Oucher by recalling and rating previous pain experiences (e.g., falling off a bike). Child points to number or photograph that describes pain intensity associated with experience. Obtain current pain score from child by asking, "How much hurt do you have right now?"	For children 3-13 years. Use numeric scale if child can count to 100 by ones and identify larger of any two numbers, or by tens. Determine whether child has cognitive ability to use photographic scale; child should be able to seriate six geometric shapes from largest to smallest. Determine which ethnic version of Oucher to use. Allow child to select a version of Oucher, or use version that most closely matches physical characteristics of child. (Jordan-Marsh and others, 1994).

From Wong DL, Hockenberry-Eaton M: *Wong's essentials of pediatric nursing,* ed 6, St. Louis, 2001, Mosby.
*Wong-Baker FACES Pain Rating Scale Reference Manual describing development and research of the scale is available from the Pain/Palliative Resource Center, City of Hope National Medical Center, 1500 East Duarte Rd., Duarte, CA 91010, (626) 359-8111, ext. 3829; fax: (626) 301-8941; e-mail: mayday_smtplink.coh.org; website: www.mosby.com/WOW/. A compilation of many pain scales, including the FACES, is available free from Purdue Frederick Company, 100 Connecticut Ave., Norwalk, CT 06850-3950, (800) 733-1333 or (203) 853-0123, ext. 7378 or 7314; website: www.partnersagainstpain.com. The use of FACES with children is demonstrated in *Whaley and Wong's Pediatric Nursing Video Series,* "Pain Assessment and Management," narrated by Donna Wong, PhD, RN. Available from Mosby, 11830 Westline Industrial Dr., St. Louis, MO 63146, (800) 426-4545; fax: (800) 535-9935; web site: www.mosby.com.

Continued

Table 14-3	PAIN RATING SCALES FOR CHILDREN—cont'd	
PAIN SCALE/DESCRIPTION	**INSTRUCTIONS**	**RECOMMENDED AGE/COMMENTS**
Poker Chip Tool† Uses four red poker chips placed horizontally in front of child (Hester and others, 1998)	Say to child, "I want to talk with you about the hurt you may be having right now." Align the chips horizontally in front of child on bedside table, a clipboard, or other firm surface. Tell child, "These are pieces of hurt." Beginning at the chip nearest child's left side and ending at the one nearest child's right side, point to chips and say, "This [first chip] is a little bit of hurt, and this [fourth chip] is the most hurt you could ever have." For a young child or for any child who may not fully comprehend the instructions, clarify by saying, "That means this [one] is just a little hurt, this [two] is a little more hurt, this [three] is more yet, and this [four] is the most hurt you could ever have." Do not give children an option for zero hurt. Research with the Poker Chip Tool has verified that children without pain will so indicate by responses such as "I don't have any." Ask child, "How many pieces of hurt do you have right now?" After initial use of the Poker Chip Tool, some children internalize the concept "pieces of hurt." If a child gives a response such as "I have one right now," *before* you ask or before you lay out the poker chips, record the number of chips on the Pain Flow Sheet. Clarify child's answer by words such as "Oh, you have a little hurt? Tell me about the hurt."	For children as young as 4 years.
Word-Graphic Rating Scale‡ (Tesler and others, 1991): Uses descriptive words (may vary in other scales) to denote varying intensities of pain	Explain to child. "This is a line with words to describe how much pain you may have. This side of the line means no pain, and over here the line means worst possible pain." (Point with your finger where "no pain" is, and run your finger along the line to "worst possible pain," as you say it.) "If you have no pain, you would mark like this." (Show example.) "If you have some pain, you would mark somewhere along the line, depending on how much pain you have." (Show example.) "The more pain you have, the closer to worst pain you would mark. The worst pain possible is marked like this." (Show example.) "Show me how much pain you have right now by marking with a straight, up-and-down line anywhere along the line to show how much pain you have right now." With a millimeter rule, measure from the "no pain" end to the mark and record this measurement as the pain score.	For children 4-17 years.

No pain	Little pain	Medium pain	Large pain	Worst possible pain

From Wong DL, Hockenberry-Eaton M: *Wong's essentials of pediatric nursing,* ed 6, St. Louis, 2001, Mosby.

†Developed in 1975 by N.O. Hester, University of Colorado Health Sciences Center, School of Nursing, Denver, CO 80262. Also available in Spanish and French.

‡Instructions for Word-Graphic Rating Scale from Acute Pain Management Guideline Panel: *Acute pain management in infants, children, and adolescents; operative and medical procedures; quick reference guide for clinicians.* ACHPR Pub. No. 92-0020, Rockville, MD, 1992. Agency for Health Care Policy and Research, Public Health Service, U.S. Department of Health and Human Services. Word-Graphic Rating Scale is part of the Adolescent Pediatric Pain Tool and is available from Pediatric Pain Study, University of California, School of Nursing, Department of Family Heath Care Nursing, 2 Kirkham St., Box 0606, San Francisco, CA 94143-0606, (415) 476-4040; e-mail: savedra@Linex.com.

Table 14-3 PAIN RATING SCALES FOR CHILDREN—cont'd

PAIN SCALE/DESCRIPTION	INSTRUCTIONS	RECOMMENDED AGE/COMMENTS
Numeric Scale Uses straight line with end points identified as "no pain" and "worst pain" and sometimes "medium pain" in the middle; divisions along line are marked in units from 0 to 5 or 10 (high number may vary)	Explain to child that at one end of the line is a 0, which means that a person feels no pain (hurt). At the other end is usually a 5 or a 10, which means the person feels the worst pain imaginable. The numbers 1 to 4 or 9 are for a very little pain to a whole lot of pain. Ask child to choose a number that best describes own pain. 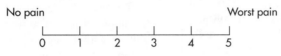	For children as young as 5 years, as long as they can count and have some concept of numbers and their values in relation to other numbers. Scale may be used horizontally or vertically. Number coding should be same as other scales used in a facility.
Visual Analogue Scale Defined as a vertical or horizontal line that is drawn to a certain length, such as 10 cm, and anchored by items that represent the extremes of the subjective phenomenon, such as pain, that is measured (Cline and others, 1992)	Ask child to place a mark on line that best describes amount of own pain. With a centimeter ruler, measure from the "no pain" end to the mark and record this measurement as the pain score.	For children as young as 4½ years, preferably at least 7 years. Vertical or horizontal scale may be used.
Color Tool Uses crayons or markers for child to construct own scale that is used with body outline (Eland and Banner, 1999)	Present eight crayons or markers to child in random order. Ask child to "pick a crayon with a color that reminds you of the most hurt (or pain) that you could possibly have"; once that crayon is selected, separate it from the others. Next, ask child to select a crayon with a color that "reminds you of pain that is a little less than the pain we just talked about"; once the second crayon is selected, separate it from the group and place it with the first crayon selected. Ask child to select a third crayon with a color "that reminds you of only a little pain"; separate this crayon and move it to the selected group. Finally, ask child to select a crayon with a color that "reminds you of no hurt (or pain)" and separate that fourth color. Show the four crayons selected to the child and arrange them in order of "worst hurt (or pain)" to "no hurt (or pain)" and ask child to show on the body outline "where the hurt is." If child offers any verbal comments, note them.	Children as young as 4 years, provided they know their colors, are not color blind, and are able to construct the scale if in pain.

Table 14-6 summarizes these and other agents. The type of pain determines the drug chosen; for example, patients with chronic continuous neuropathic pain have been shown to benefit from first-line treatment with antidepressants.[17] Route of administration for drugs in this group varies but almost all adjuvant analgesics are available orally.

Procedural Sedation

Local sedation is adequate for many procedures in the ED, but systemic analgesics are indicated for more complex procedures. Local and systemic analgesic is reviewed briefly in the following section. Refer to Chapter 13, Wound Management, for additional discussion.

Box 14-2 ESSENTIAL NURSING ACTIONS FOR PAIN CONTROL

Establish an effective, supportive relationship with the patient.

Believe, collaborate with, and respect the patient's response to pain and its management.

Educate the patient about the occurrence, onset, and duration of pain; methods of pain relief; and preventive measures.

Inform the patient what he or she is likely to experience while in the ED to minimize fear of the unknown.

Maintain current knowledge and competencies.

Monitor the patient's response and effectiveness of treatment.

Communicate frequently and effectively with the patient and physician regarding the treatment plan and its effectiveness.

Ensure patient safety at all times. Monitoring the patient facilitates assessment of treatment effectiveness and minimizes potential adverse occurrences.

Maintain a calm, empathetic manner.

Research the multidimensional nature of pain, its assessment, and subsequent management. Use this research in practice.

Box 14-3 PAIN CONTROL INTERVENTIONS

Medication	Distraction
Physical comfort	Relaxation techniques
Verbal reassurance	Breathing techniques
Massage	Imagery

Box 14-4 ESSENTIAL ASPECTS OF PAIN CONTROL

No one universally superior method of pain management exists.

The goal of pain management is to prevent pain whenever possible. Pain relief is more effective if initiated soon after onset of pain.

The underlying cause of pain is an important consideration in selecting analgesia.[14]

A calm, quiet patient does not preclude the presence of pain.

A patient's refusal to accept pain medication may be related to fear of addiction, sedation, loss of control, or method of administration.

A patient's request for specific pain medication does not automatically mean he or she is a drug seeker.[14]

A patient's tolerance for pain is not directly proportional to the amount of analgesia required to relieve pain.

All pain is real. Pain is what a patient says it is.

Local Sedation. Local anesthetics are often used for minor surgical procedures. Onset of rapid nerve block occurs within minutes and reverses within minutes or hours. Lidocaine, bupivacaine, and EMLA—a eutectic mixture of local anesthetics—are often used. The patient's blood pressure, pulse rate, and respiratory rate should be monitored during treatment with injectable agents because systemic toxicity may occur when the dose is too high. Lidocaine and bupivacaine with epinephrine should not be used on the digits, penis, ears, or nose because of vasoconstrictive effects. In explaining the procedure, the ED nurse informs the patient that pain will be blocked but touch and pressure remain intact. Pain management is facilitated if the patient is assisted into a comfortable position before initiating the procedure. Distraction techniques are also beneficial. Research has shown that music provides an effective distraction if used during the procedure.[19]

Systemic Analgesia. Procedural sedation refers to "a technique of administering sedatives or dissociative agents with or without analgesics to induce a state that allows the patient to tolerate unpleasant procedures while maintaining cardiorespiratory function."[5] Procedural pain serves no purpose and should be prevented. Three guidelines for procedural sedation follow.[5]

1. Personnel providing procedural sedation and analgesia must have an understanding of the drugs administered.

2. Personnel attending the patient must have the ability to adequately monitor the patient's response to medications given.

3. Personnel attending the patient must have the skills necessary to manage all potential complications.

Informed consent should be obtained before initiation of analgesia. Patients should be given information regarding the nature of the procedure, risks and benefits, and any potential complications. Contraindications for systemic procedural sedation are clinical instability and refusal by a competent patient.

Although there are risks with systemic analgesia, these can be minimized if the proper agent, dosage, and monitoring are considered. For systemic analgesia, opioids are the drug of choice with the titrated IV route preferred. This is considered the safest approach to rapid analgesia.[1] Opioids are used alone or in combination with other analgesics and sedatives. Before administering a drug it is important to determine the patient's history of drug use. Chemically dependent patients may require higher dosages; patients with low tolerance may require lower doses. Fentanyl is often the drug of choice because of its rapid onset of action and short duration.[17] Fentanyl's onset of action is within 1 to 2 minutes, it peaks within 5 minutes, and usually resolves within 3.6 hours.[17] Fentanyl should be diluted and administered slowly to prevent respiratory muscle rigidity. If respiratory depression occurs from induction with an opioid, it can be reversed with naloxone (Narcan). For adults, Narcan can be administered 0.4 to 2mg IV, SC, or IM and repeated every 2 minutes until 10 mg have been administered. Nalmefene (Revex), a newer opioid antagonist, is also available. The half-life of nalmefene (about 10 hours) is longer than that for naloxene (about 1 hour).[17] It is important to remember that the longer half-life of nalmefene is likely to interfere with postprocedure pain management.

Patient assessment, patient monitoring, and documentation is important before, during, and after the procedure. Emergency nurses and physicians should be cognizant of

Table 14-4   NONOPIOID AGENTS FOR PAIN MANAGEMENT

GENERIC DRUG (TRADE DRUG)	TYPICAL DOSE (MAXIMUM DOSE)	APPROXIMATE EQUIVALENT	ONSET EFFECT (MIN)	PEAK EFFECT (MIN)	DURATION EFFECT (HR)
Acetaminophen (Tylenol, Tempra, others)	600 mg PO 600 mg PR (4000-6000 mg/day)	Aspirin 600 mg	30	60	3-4
Acetylsalicylic acid (aspirin)	600 mg PO 600 mg PR (5200 mg/day)	Morphine 2 mg IM	30	60	3-4
Ibuprophen (Motrin, Advil, others)	200 mg PO (3200 mg/day)	Aspirin 650 mg	30	60-120	4
Choline magnesium trisalicylate (Trilisate)	2000-3000 mg PO (3000 mg/day)		5-30	60-180	3-6
Diflunisal (Dolobid)	500 mg PO (1500 mg/day)	Aspirin 650 mg	60	120-180	8-12
Ketoprofen (Orudis)	25 mg PO (300 mg/day)	Aspirin 650 mg	30	30-120	6
Naproxen (Naprosyn)	250 mg PO (1250 mg/day)	Aspirin 650 mg	60	120-240	6-8
Ketorolac (Toradol)	30-60 mg IM initially (120 mg IM/day × 5 day, max 30 mg IM × 20 doses over 5 days)	Morphine 6-12 mg IM	10	60	3-6
Piroxicam (Feldene)	20 mg/day		60	180-300	>12
Sulindac (Clinoril)	200 mg/day		1-2 days	60-120	Unknown
Indomethacin (Indocin)	25 mg PO (100 mg/day)	Aspirin 650 mg	60	60-120	4
Nabumetone (Relafen)	1000 mg PO (2000 mg/day)	Aspirin 3600 mg/day	1-2 days	Days-2 wk	Unknown
Etodolac (Lodine)	200-400 mg PO (1200 mg/day)	Aspirin 650 mg	30	60-120	4-12

IM, Intramuscular; *IV,* intravenous; *PO,* oral; *PR,* rectal.
Copyright DJ Wilkie, 1998.

their institution's policies on procedural sedation and accept responsibility for ensuring compliance.

Noninvasive Pain Relief Methods

Cutaneous stimulation, distraction, hypnosis, imagery, and relaxation are psychologic approaches to pain management. These approaches are discussed briefly here.

Cutaneous Stimulation. This method applies to cutaneous techniques that stimulate the skin for the purpose of pain relief (e.g., vibration, superficial heat and cold, ice application, massage, methanol application to the skin, and transcutaneous electrical nerve stimulation). Effects of cutaneous stimulation vary; nursing skill and preparation are required before this method is used as a pain management intervention. Emergency nurses should receive an initial orientation and continuing education for these techniques.

Distraction. Distraction facilitates pain management by assisting the patient in focusing on a stimulus other than the pain. Usually distraction minimizes, but does not entirely alleviate, pain. For distraction to be effective, the object of that distraction must be of interest to the patient. Research indicates that music has beneficial pain relief qualities. A study was conducted to determine whether music significantly reduces anxiety and pain associated with laceration repair in the ED.[19] Adult patients 18 years of age and older, who were not under the influence of analgesics, alcohol, or other mood-altering substances, were included. Patients were randomly assigned to one of two groups. A control group received standard laceration repair with lidocaine only. A music group received standard laceration repair with lidocaine and music. Patients in the music group were permitted to select from a variety of audiocassettes and to listen to their choice of music through a headset. Measured psychologic variables included the Spielberger State-Trait Anxiety Inventory, a visual analog pain-rating scale, and a brief questionnaire. Pain scores were significantly lower ($p = 0.001$) in the music group (mean of 2.04) when compared with the control group (mean of 5.92). The authors concluded that music could be a safe, effective, inexpensive, and noninvasive adjunct to pain management in the ED.

Hypnosis, Imagery, and Relaxation. Hypnosis is rarely used in emergency nursing, because few nurses have

Table 14-5 OPIOID AGENTS FOR PAIN MANAGEMENT

GENERIC DRUG (TRADE DRUG)	TYPICAL DOSE (MAXIMUM DOSE)	APPROXIMATE EQUIVALENT	ONSET EFFECT (MIN)	PEAK EFFECT (MIN)	DURATION EFFECT (HR)
OPIOID-AGONIST DRUGS					
Codeine	30-60 mg PO (200 mg PO)	Aspirin 650 mg Morphine 10 mg IM	30-45	20-120	4
Immediate Release	15-60 mg IM	Morphine 10 mg IM	10-30	30-60	4
Oxycodone (Roxicodone, w/aspirin—Percodan, w/acetaminophen—Percocet)	5 mg PO (30 mg PO)	Codeine 60 mg PO Morphine 10 mg IM	10-15	60	3-4
Hydrocodone (Vicodin, Lortab, Lorcet, and others)	5 mg PO (30 mg PO)	Morphine 10 mg IM	10-30	3-60	4-6
Meperidine (Demerol, Pethidine)	50 mg PO (300 mg PO)	Aspirin 650 mg Morphine 10 mg IM Demerol 75 mg IM	15	60-90	2-4
	75 mg IM	Morphine 10 mg IM	10-15	30-60	2-4
	50 mg IV	Morphine 10 mg IM	1	5-7	2-3
Propoxyphene HCl (Darvon, Dolene);	65 mg PO	Aspirin 600 mg	15-60	120	4-6
Propoxyphene napsylate (w/aspirin—Darvon-N, w/acetaminophen—Darvocet-N)	100 mg PO	Aspirin 600 mg			
Tramadol (Ultram)	50-100 mg	Codeine 60 mg PO	60	2 hr	4-6
AGONIST-ANTAGONIST DRUGS					
Pentazocine HCl (Talwin)	60 mg IM	Morphine 10 mg IM	15-20	30-60	2-3
	30 mg PO (180 mg PO)	Aspirin 600 mg Morphine 10 mg IM or Talwin 60 mg IM	15-30	60-90	3
AGONIST DRUGS					
Morphine sulfate	30 mg PO	Morphine 10 mg IM	20-60	120	4-5
Immediate release tablets and liquids	30 mg PR	Morphine 10 mg IM			
Sustained release (MS Contin, Oramorph SR)	30 mg PO	Morphine 10 mg IM		210	8-12
Injectable (Astramorph PF, Duramorph, Infumorph)	10 mg IM	Morphine 10 mg IM	10-30	60	4-5
	5 mg IV	Morphine 10 mg IM	5	20	2-4
Oxycodone					
Immediate release (Roxicodone)	5 mg PO	Codeine 60 mg PO	0-15	60	3-4
	30 mg PO	Morphine 10 mg IM Morphine 30 mg PO			
Controlled release (OxyContin)	30 mg PO	Morphine 30-60 mg PO	30-60	60, 420	12
Methadone (Dolphine)	20 mg PO	Morphine 10 mg IM Methadone 10 mg IM	30-60	90-120	4-6
	10 mg IM	Morphine 10 mg IM	10-20	60-120	4-5
	5 mg IV	Morphine 10 mg IM	5	15-30	3-4
Hydromorphone (Dilaudid)	7.5 mg PO	Morphine 10 mg IM	30	90-120	4
	3 mg PR	Hydromorphone 1.5 mg IM	15-30	30-90	4-5
	1.5 mg IM	Morphine 10 mg IM	15	30-60	4-5
	1 mg IV	Morphine 10 mg IM	10-15	15-30	2-3
Oxymorphone (Numorphan)	1 mg IM	Morphine 10 mg IM	10-15	30-90	3-6
	0.5 mg IV	Morphine 10 mg IM	5-10	15-30	3-4
	10 mg PR	Oxymorphone 1 mg IM	15-30	60	3-6

Copyright DJ Wilkie, 1998.

Table 14-5 OPIOID AGENTS FOR PAIN MANAGEMENT—cont'd

GENERIC DRUG (TRADE DRUG)	TYPICAL DOSE (MAXIMUM DOSE)	APPROXIMATE EQUIVALENT	ONSET EFFECT (MIN)	PEAK EFFECT (MIN)	DURATION EFFECT (HR)
AGONIST DRUGS–cont'd					
Levorphanol	4 mg PO	Morphine 10 mg IM	10-60	90-120	4-5
(Levo-Dromoran)		Levorphanol 2 mg IM		60	4-5
	2 mg IM	Morphine 10 mg IM	10-15	15	3-4
	1 mg IV	Morphine 10 mg IM			
Fentanyl	0.1 mg IM	Morphine 10 mg IM	7-15	20-30	1-2
(Sublimaze,	25-50 µg/hr	Morphine 30 mg	6 hr	12-24 hr	72
Duragesic)	transdermal	sustained-release q8hr			
AGONIST-ANTAGONIST DRUGS					
Butorphanol	2 mg IM	Morphine 10 mg IM	10-30	30-60	3-4
(Stadol); see pentazocine	2 mg IV	Morphine 10 mg IM	2-3	30	2-4
Nalbuphine	10 mg IM	Morphine 10 mg IM	15	60	3-6
(Nubain); see pentazocine	10 mg IV	Pentazocine 60 mg IM	2-3	30	3-4
Dezocine	10 mg IM	Morphine 10 mg IM	30	60-120	3-6
(Dalgan)					
PARTIAL AGONIST DRUGS					
Buprenorphine	0.4 mg IM	Morphine 10 mg IM	15	60	6
(Buprenex)					

Table 14-6 ADJUVANT ANALGESIC AGENTS FOR PAIN MANAGEMENT

GENERIC DRUG (TRADE DRUG)	APPROXIMATE DAILY DOSE	ONSET EFFECT	PEAK EFFECT	DURATION EFFECT (HR)
Carbamazepine (Tegretol, Epitol)	200-1600 mg PO	8-72 hr	2-12	Unknown
Phenytoin (Dilantin)	300-500 mg PO	2-24 hr	1.5-3	6-12
Gabapentin (Neurontin)	900-1800 mg PO	60-120 min	2-4 hr	Up to 24 hr
Sumatriptan (Imitrex)	6-12 mg SC	30 min	Up to 2 hr	Up to 24 hr
Amitriptyline (Elavil and others)	10-150 mg PO	3-4 days	1-2 wk	Days-weeks
Doxepin (Sinequan, Adapin)	25-150 mg PO	3-4 days	1-2 wk	Days-weeks
Imipramine (Tofranil and others)	20-100 mg PO	60 min	2-6 wk	Weeks
Trazodone (Desyrel and others)	75-225 mg PO	2 wk	2-4 wk	Weeks
Paroxetine (Paxil)	20-50 mg PO	3-4 days	1-2 wk	Days-weeks
Hydroxyzine (Vistaril, Atarax, and others)	300-450 mg IM	15-30 min	2-4 hr	4-6 hr
Lidocaine	5 mg/kg IV	2 min	2 min	10-20 min
Mexiletine (Mexitil)	200-400 mg PO	30-120 min	2-3 hr	8-12 hr
Dexamethasone (Decadron and others)	16-96 mg PO/IV	2-4 days	1-2 hr	2.75 days
Dextroamphetamine (Dexedrine and others)	10-15 mg PO	1-2 hr	Unknown	2-10 hr
Methylphenidate (Methidate, Ritalin)	10-15 mg PO	Unknown	1-3 hr	4-6 hr
Nefazodone (Serzone)	200-600 mg PO	3-4 days	1-2 wk	Days-weeks

Copyright DJ Wilkie, 1998.
PO, By mouth; *SC,* subcutaneous; *IM,* intramuscular; *IV,* intravenous.

the knowledge or skills necessary to induce a trancelike state. However, the nurse functioning in the capacity of patient advocate can assist the patient in pursuing this method of pain management by referring the patient to available community resources for continued pain management. Self-hypnosis for pain management is becoming more widely accepted among health care professionals. Nurses interested in

courses on hypnosis can obtain information by contacting the American Society of Clinical Hypnosis.

Using one's imagination to control pain is a form of distraction that produces relaxation. The imagination is used to develop images that promote pleasant sensations and diminish pain perception. For example, a patient may have decreased pain when imagining lying on the beach listening to the sound of waves washing over sand. By assisting in creating this imaginary setting, the nurse can assist the patient with pain management. Effectiveness of imaging depends on familiarity of the image and its pleasantness for the patient.

Relaxation techniques promote a state free from anxiety. When the patient is relaxed, skeletal muscle tension is minimal. Deep breathing is one way to promote relaxation. The nurse can instruct the patient to inhale deeply through the nose and exhale slowly through the mouth. Repeating this sequence several times while concentrating on muscle relaxation is an effective approach for pain management in the ED. It is simple to use and can be taught quickly and easily to most patients.

SUMMARY

Pain is an all-too-often occurrence in any health care arena but is even more so in the ED. "To effectively manage ED patients' pain, an understanding of the basic principles of a pain assessment, actions of pharmacologic agents, and the effectiveness of nonpharmacologic interventions by the emergency nurse is essential."[21] As Dunwoody suggests, "few things we do for patients are more fundamental to the quality of life than relieving pain."[13]

References

1. Abrams B, Benzon HT, Hahn M: *Practical management of pain,* ed 3, St. Louis, 2000, Mosby.
2. Afilialo M, Cantees K, Ducharme J: Pain management: current pain-control practices and research, *Ann Emerg Med* 27(4):404,1996.
3. Agency for Health Care Policy and Research (AHCPR): Acute pain management: operative or medical procedures and trauma, clinical practice guideline No. 1, AHCPR Publication No. 92-0032, February 1992.
4. Burke SO, Jarreet M: Pain management across age groups, *West J Nurs Res* 11:164, 1989.
5. Campbell M: Clinical policy for procedural sedation and analgesia in the emergency department, *Ann Emerg Med* 31(5):663, 1998.
6. Carpenter D: *Nursing 2001 drug handbook,* Springhouse, Penn 2001, Springhouse.
7. Chan L, Verdile V: Do patients receive adequate pain control after discharge from the ED? *Amer J Emerg Med* 16(7):705, 1998.
8. Copp LA: The spectrum of suffering, *Amer J Nurs* 90(8):35, 1990.
9. Cross S: Pathophysiology of pain, *Mayo Clinic Proc* 69:375, 1994.
10. Devine E: AHCPR clinical practice guidelines on surgical pain management: adoption and outcomes, *Res Nurs Health* 22(2): 119, 1999.
11. Ducharme J: Proceedings from the first international symposium on pain research in emergency medicine: foreword, *Ann Emerg Med* 27(4):399, 1996.
12. Durcharme J: Acute pain and pain control: state of the art, *Ann Emerg Med* 35(6):592, 2000.
13. Dunwoody CJ: Patient controlled analgesia: rationale, attributes, and essential factors, *Orthop Nurs* 6(5):31, 1987.
14. Joint Commission on Accreditation of Healthcare Organizations (JCAHO): 2001 Hospital Accreditation Standards, JCAHO, Oakbrook Terrace, Ill., 2001, Joint Commission Resources (JCR).
15. Jordan KS: *Emergency nursing core curriculum,* ed 5, Philadelphia, 2000, WB Saunders.
16. Lewis SM, Heitkemper MM, Dirksen SR: *Medical-surgical nursing: assessment and management of clinical problems,* ed 5, St. Louis, 2000, Mosby.
17. McCaffery M, Pasero C: *Pain: clinical manual,* St. Louis, 1999, Mosby.
18. Paris PM, Stewart RD: *Pain management in emergency medicine,* Norwalk, Conn, 1988, Appleton & Lange.
19. Spurlock P: An emergency nurse's pain management initiative: Mercy Hospital's experience, *J Emerg Nurs* 25(5):383, 1999.
20. Tanabe P, Buschman MB: A prospective study of ED pain management practices and the patient's perspective, *J Emerg Nurs* 25(3):171, 1999.
21. Tanabe P, Buschman MB: Emergency nurses' knowledge of pain management principles, *J Emerg Nurs* 26(4):299, 2000.
22. Todd K, Deaton C, D'Adamo A et al: Ethnicity and analgesic practice, *Ann Emerg Med* 35(1):11, 2000.
23. Wong DL, Hockenberry-Eaton M, Wilson D et al: *Wong's essentials of pediatric nursing,* ed 6, St. Louis, 2001, Mosby.

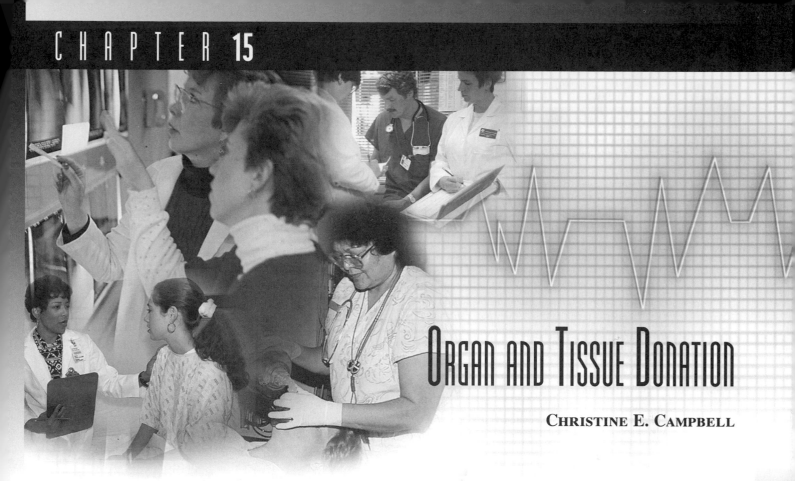

CHAPTER 15

ORGAN AND TISSUE DONATION

CHRISTINE E. CAMPBELL

The shortage of available organs and tissue for transplantation has created a national health care crisis. In the past the emergency nurse was peripherally involved with donation of organs and tissues. However, technology and changes in federal and state legislation have made donation more common in the emergency department (ED). Emergency nurses and other health care providers play a vital role in solving this crisis. Comprehensive discussion of transplantation is beyond the scope of this text; however, Table 15-1 highlights milestones in the evolution of transplantation.

OVERVIEW

Every patient whose death is imminent or who dies in the ED is a potential organ or tissue donor. Box 15-1 summarizes organs and tissues that can be donated. Almost any person who dies can become a tissue donor.[1] Patients with suspected infections are evaluated on an individual basis regarding their potential as a donor. Many needed tissues have been lost because no one remembered to offer the family the option of donation. More important, the family of the person who just died may not have been given the opportunity to carry out the patient's wishes to donate tissues and organs. At a time when family stress is greatest, the wish to donate may not have been considered a priority and was forgotten. The potential donor may have expressed this desire by signing a donor card, completing an advanced directive or living will, or previously discussed these preferences with his or her next of kin. Organ donor wishes are included on the back of driver's licenses in most states.

Health care professionals are required by law to offer organ and/or tissue donation to all who qualify.[2] More than 71,000 people in the United States are waiting for organ transplants, yet fewer than 22,000 received them in 1999. Up to 15,000 people who die annually could be suitable donors. Fewer than 6000 of these deaths result in donation of an organ. Countless people are waiting for a new cornea, bone, or other tissue. Their lives may not hang in the balance, as when one is waiting for a heart, liver, lung, or heart and lung transplantation, but quality of life can be greatly enhanced by tissue transplantation. Table 15-2 gives the number of Americans awaiting transplant.

As common as tissue donation, organ donation is also a possibility when a person suffers a severe brain injury or prolonged anoxic event. Such situations result in eventual death of brain tissue, rendering the patient legally dead and supported only by mechanical means. Potential donors are typically victims of traumatic injuries secondary to a motor vehicle crash, gunshot wound to the head, ruptured cerebral aneurysm, arteriovenous malformation, severe stroke, or severe anoxic event from prolonged cardiac arrest.

A person declared dead by brain-death criteria is a potential organ and tissue donor; however, a patient in asystole is a potential tissue donor only because visceral organ donation requires an intact circulatory system. A donor on a ventilator may require vasopressors to maintain blood pressure, urine output, fluid and electrolyte balance, and alterations of ventilatory settings to maintain adequate ventilation and perfusion. Before a patient is considered for organ donation, he or she must meet criteria for brain death or be in the process of

Table 15-1   MILESTONES IN ORGAN AND TISSUE TRANSPLANTATION

DATE	EVENT
1682	Meekran attempted to replace a portion of a soldier's cranium with the skull bone from a dog.
1800	Corneal graft surgery was performed by Wolfe.
1860s	Grahm developed and used a wooden hoop dialyzer to treat renal failure patients.
1881	Skin grafting was tried as a temporary means for treating a severe burn.
1893	Williams attempted transplanting a sheep's pancreas into a human.
1902	Ullman attempted transplanting kidneys in a goat model.
1940s	Sir Peter Medawar treated skin grafts with cold refrigeration; he also worked on immune response and rejection phenomenon.
1940s	Kolft designed the dialysis machine that is the basis for machines used today.
1954	Merrill and colleagues implemented dialysis therapy.
1954	Murray and Harrison performed the first kidney transplantation between living identical twins.[10]
1963	Starzl performed the first liver transplantation.
1963	Hardy performed the first lung transplantation.
1967	Lillehei performed the first kidney and pancreas transplantation.
1967	Barnard performed the first heart transplantation.
1968	Uniform Anatomical Gift Act of 1968 was adopted as law in all 50 states. The law allows the individual to decide to become an organ or tissue donor, and introduces the option of donor cards that identify the person's wishes.
1968	Harvard Criteria for Determination of Brain Death was published.
1981	Shumway performed the first heart-lung transplantation.
1984	Organ Transplantation Act (PL 98-507) was passed.
1986	Report of Organ Transplantation Task Force was published, which led to the development of the United Network of Organ Sharing (UNOS), a private, nonprofit agency that serves as a clearinghouse for organs and tissues. The United States was divided into 10 UNOS regions with a single Organ Procurement Organization (OPO) designated for each region. Figure 15-1 shows these regions.
1987	Consolidated Omnibus Reconciliation Act of 1986 (PL-99-506) was revised so that hospitals receiving Medicare funding must meet standards for education of patients and staff.
Late 1980s	Uniform Anatomical Gift Act was passed on a state-by-state basis.
1997	National Organ and Tissue Donation Initiative was launched by the DHHS to increase the number of organs and tissues available for donation. The final rule for organ, tissue, and eye donation for hospitals to participate in Medicare and Medicaid was published.
1998	Final rule for donation takes effect, which requires each hospital to contact their OPO in a timely manner about those whose death is imminent or those who die in the hospital. Provisions limit discussion of donation to OPPO staff or trained hospital staff.

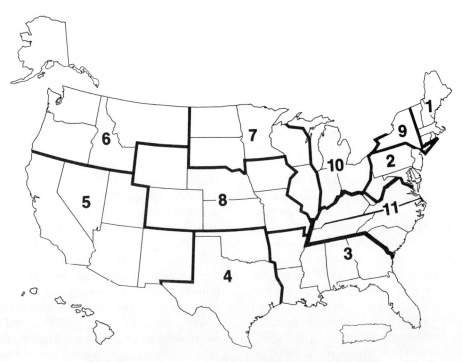

FIGURE 15-1   United Network of Organ Sharing regional map.

Box 15-1	TRANSPLANTABLE ORGANS AND TISSUES	

TISSUES	ORGANS
Cornea	Liver
Bones	Kidneys
Pancreatic islet cells	Heart
Bone marrow	Bones
Ligaments	Lungs
Tendons	Pancreas
Heart valves	Intestines
Skin grafts	Spleen, lymph nodes, vessels
Veins, arteries, nerves	Eyes
Vertebral bodies (bone marrow)	
Soft tissue (e.g., fascia)	

Table 15-2	NUMBER OF PATIENTS IN THE UNITED STATES AWAITING TRANSPLANTS*	

NUMBER IN UNITED STATES	TRANSPLANT NEEDED
51,215	Kidney
17,886	Liver
1,245	Pancreas
270	Pancreas islet cell
2,486	Kidney-pancreas
4,143	Heart
209	Heart-lung
3,824	Lung
178	Intestine
79,125	TOTAL

*United Network for Organ Sharing national patient waiting list weekly update of March 1, 2002.

evaluation for these criteria. Ultimately the patient must be declared dead by brain-death criteria for actual donation to take place.

In the past the family of a patient declared dead according to brain-death criteria was not consistently offered the option of organ and tissue donation. A 1985 Gallup poll described a situation in which 20,000 potential donors were identified but only 3000 became actual organ donors.[7] More recent data support this same phenomenon. In the 1990s, the number of patients awaiting transplant grew 5 times as fast as the number of transplant operations. The most commonly cited reason for this lack in available organs is the health care professional feeling uncomfortable in dealing with death and broaching the subject of donation[11] and wanting to avoid greater suffering for the family. The result of this hesitation, however, is that the supply of organs and tissues does not meet demand. By March 2001 the waiting list for organ transplants had surpassed 75,000.[11]

By the late 1980s this widening gap between potential organ donors and recipients stimulated development and enactment of amendments to the Uniform Anatomical Gift Act on a state-by-state basis.[8,14] These creative adjustments redefined the potential donor in an effort to expand availability of greatly needed organs for transplant. Many states began mandating that health care professionals or a hospital designee offer each family the option of tissue and organ donation as deemed medically appropriate at the time of the patient's death.[2] In response to the need for donors, the U.S. Department of Health and Human Services (DHHS) launched the National Organ and Tissue Donation Initiative in December 1997. Its goals are to increase consent to donation, maximize donation opportunities, and learn more about what works to increase donation and improve transplantation through carefully designed research efforts. To promote best donation practices, DHHS' Health Care Financing Administration published a final rule for organ, tissue, and eye donation as part of revised conditions of participation for Medicare- and Medicare-participating hospitals.[13]

This rule, which took effect August 21, 1998, contains two key provisions. Hospitals must contact their organ procurement organization (OPO) in a timely manner about individuals whose death is imminent or who die in the hospital. Only OPO staff or trained hospital staff—referred to as designated requestors—may approach families about organ donation. A designated requestor is defined in the rule as an individual who has completed a course offered or approved by the OPO. This course is designed in conjunction with the tissue and eye bank community in the methodology for approaching potential donor families and requesting organ donation. Interpretation of this rule does allow some degree of flexibility. Research confirms the importance of training in approaching families for consent and the importance of collaborative relationships among hospitals, OPOs, and tissue and eye banks.[15]

Sensitivity to the family's cultural, religious, and emotional situation must also be considered. More often than not, the family appreciates that the option is offered—something positive can result from the death of a loved one. The family may not wish to hear more about donation and may decline to donate, but at least they are given the opportunity to make that decision. Regardless of the decision regarding donation, the family should be supported in their decision.

Redefinition of the potential cadaver donor population includes expansion of age limits and consideration of patients on a case-by-case basis who have a history of high blood pressure, diabetes, and evidence of minor cardiac and respiratory difficulties. Transplant programs also incorporate the option of a living, nonrelated kidney donation into their programs for those needing a kidney transplant. Kidney transplants are now performed between husband and wife or between a person or significant other in whom a reasonable tissue match exists. The success of organ transplantation has made it routine therapy for many diseases. Work is also being done with a nonheart-beating kidney donor, with differing levels of success. Segmental liver and lung transplants are being done in different areas of the country offering new hope to those who wait.

THE DONATION PROCESS

When a patient dies, the OPO determines if the patient is a potential organ or tissue donor. Four key pieces of information must be documented in the medical record for the donation to take place:

1. Determination and declaration of death
2. Medical examiner's approval (as required by state law)
3. Notification of the OPO
4. Consent from the next of kin

Determination of Death

A patient must be declared dead for the donation process to begin. The Uniform Determination of Death Act (1978) plays an integral role in identifying which criteria must be met to determine death. Death in a person is defined as either of the following criteria[4]:

I. A person with irreversible cessation of circulatory and respiratory function is dead.
   A. Cessation is recognized by an appropriate clinical examination.
   B. Irreversibility is recognized by persistent cessation of functions during an appropriate period of observation, trial of therapy, or both.
II. A person with irreversible cessation of all functions of the entire brain, including the brainstem, is dead.
   A. Cessation is recognized when evaluation discloses two findings:
      1. Cerebral functions are absent.
      2. Brainstem functions (pupillary reflex, corneal reflex, gag reflex) are absent.
   B. Irreversibility is recognized when evaluation discloses three findings:
      1. Reversible conditions such as hyponatremia and hypothermia have been corrected, and the patient is hemodynamically stable.
      2. Cause of coma is established and is sufficient to account for loss of brain functions.
      3. Possibility of recovery of brain functions is excluded.
      4. Cessation of all brain functions persists for an appropriate period of observation, trial of therapy, or both.

These commonly accepted criteria have been adopted as the standard of practice. Traditionally death was believed to occur when a person's heart stopped beating. As technology evolved, a patient could be maintained on mechanical support devices. Consequently, determination of death by brain-death criteria became a recognized practice. It has been described by many neuroscience professional groups, most notably the Harvard Group in the *Harvard Criteria for Determination of Brain Death.*[4] The process of determining death by brain-death criteria when appropriate has become more specific as a result of (1) restating and updating criteria by the President's Commission for the Study of Ethical Problems in Medicine and Biomedical and Behavioral Re-

search, (2) evolution of the definition of brain death, and (3) increased levels of comfort and experience with application of criteria on the part of neuroscience physicians and hospital personnel.

After death has been determined, it must be documented in the patient's medical record, including the time of death. If the OPO has not evaluated the patient for suitability as a donor, then required notification is undertaken at this time, before a designated requestor discusses donation with the family. Criteria used to determine whether a patient is a suitable candidate for donation change frequently.

Medical criteria that may prevent donation of organs and some tissues from a patient include presence of a documented septicemia, communicable disease such as hepatitis, or possibility that the patient is at high risk for human immunodeficiency virus. It is also important to note that those with metastatic cancer are eligible for tissue donation. Almost any person with most forms of cancer, including cancers that have metastasized, is eligible to donate corneas for transplantation or research. Again, the key is to contact the regional procurement agency to determine suitability for donation before discussing donation with the family.

Emergency nurses referring potential donors to the regional procurement agency must employ referral policies approved within their respective institutions. When a nurse calls the local procurement agency, guidelines shown in Figure 15-2 for required information are recommended. A typical referral pattern for tissue or organ donation is outlined in Figure 15-3.

Medical Examiner's Approval

The medical examiner must be notified when a donation takes place under certain circumstances, including:

1. Homicide
2. Suicide
3. Accidental death
4. Death within 24 hours of admission
5. Patient is admitted in comalike state and dies
6. Death of a person 18 years of age or less
   (Medical examiner regulations vary slightly from state to state.)

Each state has specific criteria. Before these criteria are included in a donation policy, the hospital should contact the state medical examiner for more information. For example, the medical examiner's office in Rhode Island requires notification of death and request for approval of donation without exception, for all people who are potential tissue or organ donors. Documentation of this notification is essential for donation to take place. Notation of communication with the medical examiner should be included in the patient's medical record.

Hospital Requirements

Three essential forms in the documentation process are necessary when an organ or tissue donation takes place.[12] First

WORKSHEET
(Does not need to be saved)
ORGAN AND TISSUE DONOR REFERRAL GUIDELINE

(800) _____ - _____
24-Hour Hotline

Name of patient _____ MR# _____

Age _____   Date of birth _____   Admission date _____

Time of death _____   Cause of death _____

Past medical history _____

_____

☐   Ocular history including surgeries _____

☐   Anticoagulation therapy   Yes / No
        What type? (e.g., heparin, coumadin, ASA, TPA, steptokinase _____.)

☐   History of positive blood culture   Date _____

        Name of antibiotic given_____   Date _____

☐   Cancer patient, had   ☐ Chemotherapy   ☐ Radiation therapy
        If so, date and type of last therapy given

        Date _____   Type _____

☐   Social history _____

☐   Family status—Next of kin _____

☐   Attending physician _____

☐   Medical examiner case   Yes / No   Called: ☐ Approve donation
        24-hour phone: (800) _____ - _____   ☐ Disapprove donation

Comments: _____

_____

_____

_____

FIGURE 15-2   Organ and tissue donor referral guidelines.

is the consent form; it must be completed when a family indicates the desire to donate. Usually permission for donation of organs and tissues is written on a specific consent form provided by the local OPO or a state-mandated form with hospital-specific amendments.

Each state and hospital has the option of creating consent forms; however, most procurement agencies provide forms and prefer use of the consent form they developed. This document is modified periodically to comply with changing laws. If consent forms are not available in the ED, the local

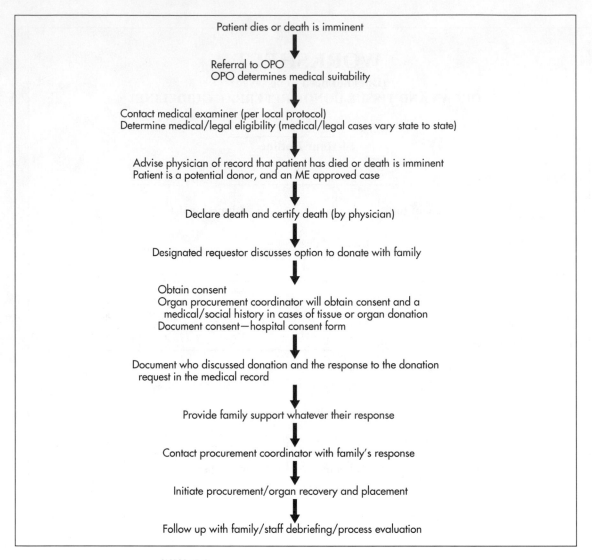

Patient dies or death is imminent

↓

Referral to OPO
OPO determines medical suitability

↓

Contact medical examiner (per local protocol)
Determine medical/legal eligibility (medical/legal cases vary state to state)

↓

Advise physician of record that patient has died or death is imminent
Patient is a potential donor, and an ME approved case

↓

Declare death and certify death (by physician)

↓

Designated requestor discusses option to donate with family

↓

Obtain consent
Organ procurement coordinator will obtain consent and a
  medical/social history in cases of tissue or organ donation
Document consent—hospital consent form

↓

Document who discussed donation and the response to the donation
request in the medical record

↓

Provide family support whatever their response

↓

Contact procurement coordinator with family's response

↓

Initiate procurement/organ recovery and placement

↓

Follow up with family/staff debriefing/process evaluation

FIGURE 15-3   Organ and tissue donation referral pattern.

procurement agency or UNOS provides them promptly (Figure 15-4).

The second is the hospital's internal reporting form that documents the request for donation and the next of kin's response to the request. This document must be completed for every person that dies in the hospital regardless of the family decision to donate, is required for compliance with some state laws, and is helpful with federal law compliance. The internal reporting form can be an extremely helpful tool when attempting to educate staff and determine an area of need within an institution. The form documents patient age, location where death occurred, the offer of donation, reason for not offering donation, family response, next of kin relationship to the deceased, consent for organs and tissues, and what was recovered. Information can be placed in a database so that potential donors and tissues stemming from the donation process can be tracked over the course of the year. Figure 15-5 is an example of this form.

The last form of documentation required is dictated by state law. Many states require an annual report on donation data. Data must be tabulated and submitted to the state de-

partment of health or other state regulatory body for review, licensure, and certification of the institution. This also provides the hospital with much-needed feedback concerning how best to provide donation education within the hospital community. Data can also be reported annually for verification of Medicare and Medicaid funding, as required by federal regulations pertaining to COBRA of 1986 and 1990. (This verification has not yet been mandated.)

Obtaining Consent for Donation

Offering the family or next of kin the option of donation is one of the more difficult yet potentially rewarding responsibilities that emergency nurses assume in their professional careers. Providing a family with the option of donation may give them a measure of comfort and consolation. The comfort is not necessarily experienced at the time of the death, but later when the death has been realized. Knowing that their loved one has been able to help another often helps families cope with the loss and continue their lives.

CONFIDENTIAL DONOR FORM

Lifeline of Ohio Organ Procurement (LOOP)
770 Kinnear Road
Suite 200
Columbus, Ohio 43212
614-291-5667

DONOR IMPRINT

☐ Local   ☐ Non local   ☐ Import organ _____   ☐ Recovered
☐ Organ referral only   ☐ Tissue referral only   ☐ Organ and tissue referral   ☐ Consented but not recovered
Import/Pay back from _____   Telephone number _____

OPO #36P005 Tissue ID number _____   UNOS ID number _____   Coordinator(s) _____
Crossclamp date/time _____   Medical record number _____

Donor Information

Donor hospital _____   Provider number _____   Hospital unit _____
City/State _____   ZIP Code _____   Telephone number _____
Date/Time admission _____   _____
Date/Time of referral _____   _____   Referring person _____
Date/Time of arrival _____   _____   Attending physician _____

Donor name _____   Cause of death (see codes) _____
SSN _____ DOB _____   Mechanism of death (see codes) _____
Address _____   Circumstances of death (see codes) _____
City _____ State _____ ZIP _____   ☐ Brain death   ☐ Asystole
Age _____ Sex ___ Ht. ____ Wt. _____ Race _____   Date/Time _____ _____ _____ MD/DO
Active military   ☐ Yes ☐ No   ☐ Unknown   Date/Time _____ _____ _____ MD/DO
☐ U.S. born   ☐ Not U.S. born   ☐ U.S. citizen   Method(s) used _____
How long lived in U.S. _____ years   M.E./Coroner case   ☐ Yes ☐ No
Donor occupation : _____   Permission for donation ☐ Yes ☐ No Case # _____
Ethnicity ☐ Not Hispanic origin   Restrictions/Denial reason(s) _____
         ☐ Hispanic: Mexican   ☐ Hispanic: Other   _____
HLA A _____ B _____ DR _____ C _____   Name of M.E./Coroner _____
ABO _____ Rh _____ Sub _____   Date/Time of contact _____
                                   Autopsy ☐ Yes ☐ No

Consent Information

Donor card and/or BMV contacted ☐ Yes ☐ No ☐ Unk Date/Time of consent _____ Request made by _____
(NOK) _____   Relationship _____
Address _____   NOK Telephone number _____
_____   Funeral home _____

Organ	Consent requested?	If not requested, write reason.	Consent obtained?	If not, write reason.
Kidney	☐ Yes ☐ No	_____	☐ Yes ☐ No	_____
Liver	☐ Yes ☐ No	_____	☐ Yes ☐ No	_____
Intestine	☐ Yes ☐ No	_____	☐ Yes ☐ No	_____
Pancreas	☐ Yes ☐ No	_____	☐ Yes ☐ No	_____
Heart	☐ Yes ☐ No	_____	☐ Yes ☐ No	_____
Lung	☐ Yes ☐ No	_____	☐ Yes ☐ No	_____
CV tissue	☐ Yes ☐ No	_____	☐ HV ☐ Peri ☐ Saphenous ☐ Femoral	
MS tissue	☐ Yes ☐ No	_____	☐ UE ☐ LE ☐ Skin ☐ Ribs ☐ Tendons	
Eye tissue	☐ Yes ☐ No	_____	☐ Whole eyes	
Consent for research	☐ Yes ☐ No	_____	☐ Other	

Signature _____   Date/Time _____

Revised 6/14/99

FIGURE 15-5   Documentation for hospital management of organ/tissue donation. (Courtesy Lifeline of Ohio, 2000.)

Continued

emergency nurse may participate as a supporter or designated requestor in the process, dependent upon training and hospital protocols. Emergency nurses in supporter roles may need less intense training than individuals in requestor roles. Each institution may have an established protocol for offering donation to a family, and this protocol should be given consideration before proceeding.

Many institutions have a program in collaboration with that of the OPOs who train staff members as designated requestors. These requestors along with OPO staff are the only people who can approach families about their options with

donation. The emergency nurse caring for the patient who has just died may not be familiar with the process of donation. The requestor can be a great resource and can assist with the process. The nurse can also talk to the local OPO for support in this matter; a coordinator from the agency can obtain consent from the family in person or over the telephone. Telephone consent requires two witnesses on the phone to confirm donation. An ED education program can be requested concerning the donation process.

Before the family is made aware of its option, it must be told the patient has died. The family must be comfortable with

---

ANATOMICAL GIFT BY A RELATIVE OR THE GUARDIAN OF THE PERSON OF A DECEDENT

I hereby make this anatomical gift from the body of _____
(Name)

who died on _____ in _____
(Date)   (City and state)

The marks in the appropriate squares and the words filled in the blanks below indicate my relationship to the decedent and my desires respecting the anatomical gift.

1. I survive the decedent as:
    ☐ Spouse
    ☐ Adult son or daughter
    ☐ Parent
    ☐ Adult brother or sister
    ☐ Grandparent
    ☐ Guardian of the person
    ☐ Person authorized to dispose of the body

2. I hereby give the following body parts:
    ☐ Heart
    ☐ Liver
    ☐ Kidneys
    ☐ Pancreas
    ☐ Lungs
    ☐ Small bowel
    ☐ Spleen, lymph nodes, and vessels
    ☐ Heart valves (heart)
    ☐ Skin grafts
    ☐ Long bone segments
    ☐ Iliac crest (hip bone segments)
    ☐ Small bones (humerus, etc.)
    ☐ Soft tissue (fascia, etc.)
    ☐ Eyes
    ☐ Ribs
    ☐ Tendons
    ☐ Ligaments
    ☐ Veins, arteries, nerves
    ☐ Vertebral bodies (bone marrow)

3. To the following person (or institution): _____

4. For the following purposes:
    ☐ Any purposes authorized by law   ☐ Therapy
    ☐ Transplantation   ☐ Medical research and education

5. I give consent for the release of any medical information necessary for these donations.

6. I give consent for infectious disease tests to be performed with blood, spleen, or lymph nodes for the detection of transmissible diseases, including but not limited to: HIV, HTLV, hepatitis, and syphilis. If positive tests are reported, I am aware that I will be notified, as well as appropriate health officials.

7. After the donated organs, tissues, or eyes are removed, the remains of the body shall be disposed in the following manner: _____; at the expense and responsibility of the following persons: _____

_____   _____
Date   City and state

_____   _____
Witness   Signature of survivor

_____   _____
Witness   Address of survivor

Executed in triplicate:
    Original retained on donor's chart
    1 copy accompanies donated organs/tissue
    1 copy available for family at their request

Anatomical Gift by a Relative or the Guardian of the
Person of a Decent, CL-105-2
H:\clinical policies\noteform\105-2.doc
Revised 9/24/2001

FIGURE 15-4   Consent form for donation of anatomical gift. (Courtesy Lifeline of Ohio, 2000.)

The best person to support the family about donation is a professional who has developed rapport with the family, such as the primary nurse, primary care physician, social worker, or member of the clergy who has spent time with the family. The person designated to carry out this responsibility should be familiar with the donation process and comfortable with feelings about death and the donation of tissues and organs. Much thought and knowledge are required to assume this responsibility. Emergency nurses are in an ideal position to support the family during the process of donation. They have been working with the family and patient throughout the admission and have in most situations developed the greatest rapport with the family.

Physicians, emergency nurses, social workers, and pastoral care providers are all examples of team members that contribute to the donation process. The OPO coordinator, designated requestor, and family supporter are key roles in the process. Each hospital will determine who fills theses roles in collaboration with the regional OPO. The person who approaches the family about donation and who provides information about donation to the family must be a trained designated requestor or OPO representative. The

CONFIDENTIAL DONOR FORM

UNOS ID Number _____   LOOP Tissue donor ID Number_____

Admission course/Comments

Admission toxicology screen results:

Please identify any injuries, fractures, incisions, tattoos, social indicators on the diagrams and describe below. Include any operative procedures or invasive lines/tubes.

☐ OR procedures _____
_____

☐ CPR/Downtime _____
Comments _____

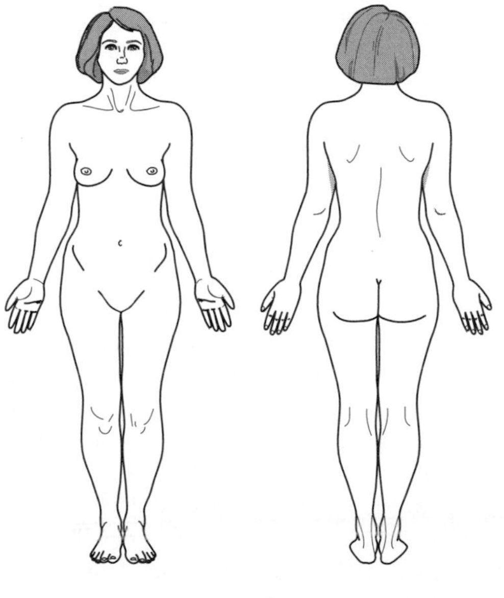

Revised 6/14/99

FIGURE **15-5, cont'd**

the knowledge that everything possible was done to prevent death and that all available treatments were carried out to maintain the life of its family member. The family's sense of devastation is extreme; members are grieving and unlikely to believe that death has occurred. Discussion of anything immediately following the discussion of death may be impossible. The family needs time to grieve and to grasp what has happened before it is asked to make another critical decision.

Waiting until the family gives a verbal or nonverbal cue that it is ready to discuss what is to happen next is essential. In the case of potential brain death, when tissues and organs may be donated, the situation usually involves a sudden, unexpected event, and the person who dies may be young and previously healthy. This patient is usually transferred to an intensive care setting, where a series of tests is administered to establish that criteria for brain death have been met. When death is declared by these criteria, the family can be given a bit more time to adjust to the fact that death has occurred. Understanding death in this instance is difficult for most families: their loved one is breathing, warm, and looks alive. The family must accept that ventilatory support of the patient who is brain dead is strictly mechanical and has nothing to do with life and survival. If the support systems are removed, the patient's heart would stop beating and all signs of life would disappear. Helping the family understand that death has occurred is difficult. Information must be provided for the family by the primary physician in terms it can understand and must be educationally reinforced by the primary nurse and other available health care professionals.

When the patient in the ED is declared dead by the more conventional criterion of cardiac asystole, death is physically more obvious to the family. Grasping the reality of the event is poignant. Death as a result of cardiac arrest is recognized as a tangible end point. Family members have less time to consider possible options or treatments and less time to adjust to their loss.

Emotions can be labile. Adjusting to the idea of death is always difficult. The family will be in shock, engulfed by many different emotions and feelings. Family members may have had little to do with this particular family member recently or they may feel responsible for the death. Families often ask themselves what could have been done to prevent death or how this death might have been made easier. Before the option of donation is broached, family members need time to gain control of their thoughts and adjust, if possible, to the reality that a family member has died and is not going to return. Their lives will never be the same, and as difficult as it may seem, they must continue to live without this loved one.

If family members are in the ED they must be provided a private room or location that is comfortable, quiet, and allows those present an opportunity to share feelings of loss and grief with others or experience that grief alone. Realizing that the family member is dead is the greatest hurdle the family must overcome. Viewing the body of the person who has just died is a critical step in this process.

Assessment of what the family knows or what it has been told is of great importance in offering the option of donation. Until the family can accept that death has occurred, donation should not be discussed. The family must hear the words *death* and *dead* when references are made to the status of its family member. A common error in health care is to refer to the death euphemistically. For example, the nurse may say that the patient "has just expired," "passed on," "will no longer be with us," that "there is no hope," or "it is over." Saying the word dead when talking to the family is straightforward and prevents misinterpretation. Because of shock and denial, the family may not comprehend the impact of the message that there is "no hope for their loved one." This understanding is critical in the case of the family of a patient considered dead by brain-death criteria.

The family essentially "becomes the patient" after death of its loved one. It is important to determine how the family members are working together as a unit. Who is the "strong right arm" of the family? Who is asking the questions? Who is the spokesperson or next of kin? What was the family's relationship to the deceased? How does the family make decisions? General observations of the family's behavior are essential when initiating the process of donation in a way that is comfortable both for the family and for the nurse.

Other goals when assessing the family should include assessment of the family's cultural and religious background and its impact on donation. A decision not to offer donation because of religious and cultural biases based on assumptions about the family's last name and background has no place in the process. The choice belongs to the family.

When a family says no to donation, that response is perfectly reasonable. Donation is not an option for every family or every person. Whatever the decision about donation, it is the right one for that family or person and should be accepted. The nurse's role is to give the family the choice of donation along with the right information about donation, and to support the family's decision.

Family Education

The family needs information about donation so it can decide what is right for the family and what the family member would have wished. Detailed, understandable information is essential. The family must never be coerced into a decision about donation and its benefits.

The family needs to know that if it grants permission for donation, the donation will be carried out promptly. A slight chance exists of changes in physical appearance related to incisions required for different donations. The family should know that this causes no disfigurement that would prevent an open casket or alter funeral arrangements. For example, even after donation of bone, the body can be prepared for an open casket funeral.

The family also needs to know that it will be required to participate in an extensive medical and social history review before donation is possible. This history is carried out in response to U.S. Food and Drug Administration regulations effective July 1, 1995, permitting distribution of tissues and organs for transplant. A typical multitissue donation case study is presented in Box 15-2.

Tissue and organ retrieval occurs after permission is given by the family and when recovery teams can be arranged to recover the tissue. Recovery teams may be in the same facility or they may be 500 miles away, so transportation arrangements may be complex.

Procurement of internal organs and tissue takes place in an operating suite. The multitissue, multiorgan procurement procedure is usually completed in 4 to 5 hours. Delays in the procurement process should be reported to the family promptly. The regional procurement agency provides technical staff to recover the eyes, valves, and skin. If the family made special funeral arrangements, it should inform the

---

BOX 15-2   CASE STUDY: MULTITISSUE DONOR

A 54-year-old man is admitted to the emergency department in cardiac arrest at 2:30 AM. He is in asystole and is declared dead at 3:15 AM. His wife gives permission to donate organs and tissues. "Anything he can donate is fine . . . he always wanted to be an organ donor." The medical examiner approves the donation for corneas, bone, skin, and heart for valves.

emergency nurse or donation coordinator of those plans. Eyes may be recovered in the morgue.

A donation coordinator from the local OPO is available for support in any donation. In most donations of internal organs, the coordinator attends the patient and family at the hospital, obtains consent from the family, explains the process of donation to the family, and coordinates the entire donation from start to finish. In the case of tissue donation only, the coordinator is less likely to be at the hospital but is available for consultation and ensures that necessary support is available. The coordinator works with the emergency nurse, other contact staff at the hospital, and the respective procurement teams.

THE PROCUREMENT PROCESS

Tissue and organ donors are managed differently. The tissue donor has been declared dead, with no heartbeat. The potential organ donor has been declared brain dead, but the heart is still beating. Management of the tissue or organ donor is discussed in the sections below. These patients must be managed carefully to ensure viable tissues and/or organs for transplant.

Tissue Procurement: Eyes, Corneas, Bone, Heart for Valves, and Skin

Tissue procurement is less complex than internal organ procurement. The coordinator from the procurement agency arranges for arrival of recovery teams and works with nursing staff in the operating suite to set up surgery time and conditions convenient for all parties involved.

Maximum time allowed for recovery of tissue after asystole is approximately 10 hours for bone, 6 to 10 hours for heart valves, and 24 hours for corneas and skin. These time limits vary, depending on the procurement agency and availability of refrigeration. The preferred time of recovery is that time closest to asystole.

The process of recovering bones is usually carried out using sterile technique; limbs used include all four limbs, including femur, proximal tibia, fibula, and proximal humerus.[5] Occasionally a mandible, hemipelvis, every other rib, tissues from limbs such as tensor fasciae latae, Achilles tendon with a block of calcaneus, and others are recovered.[3] The surgical procedure lasts approximately $1\frac{1}{2}$ to 4 hours, depending on experience of the team and the number of tissues to be recovered. A single incision is made along each limb so that the respective bones can be extracted. Prosthetic devices made of polyvinyl chloride telescopic tubing or, in some cases wooden dowels, are used to replace bones as a means of reconstruction. Aside from the single incision made along the outer aspect of the limb, no disfigurement associated with the procurement process should be apparent. After bone procurement, bone is stored in a freezer at $-70°$ F, freeze-dried, or processed into chips for later use. The uses of bone are extensive, ranging from replacement of bone invaded by tumor to replacing bone in neurosurgical cases when bone has been removed.

After death the eye donor should be maintained in a refrigerated room if available, with the head elevated at 20 degrees and the eyes taped closed with paper tape. Cool compresses can be placed over the eyes to prevent swelling and ease the procurement process. Recovery of eyes is a clean procedure using sterile technique. It requires 20 to 30 minutes. Two methods of recovery are commonly used: recovery of the entire globe or a corneal punch procedure. The eye tissue is packed in preservative solution, the container is placed on ice, and dispatched to the respective eye recovery center for processing. Corneas are generally transplanted within 24 to 48 hours for treatment of keratoconus and other diseases of the cornea. If the globe has been recovered, the orbit is filled with ample cotton and a cap similar in contour to the eye to eliminate any disfigurement resulting from absence of the globe. Technical staff recovering the eyes must be skilled in these procedures and in many states must be certified in techniques of recovery.

For recovery of the heart for valves, the entire heart is removed from the donor. The chest is opened from the xiphoid process to the sternal notch. The ribs and sternum are retracted and the heart mobilized. Cardiectomy of the heart includes dissection along the great vessels extending distally from the heart as far as possible. The heart is then removed from the chest, placed in sterile lactated Ringer's solution, packed in a sterile container, double-bagged sterilely, and packed on ice for shipping to a processing center. The valves are dissected from the heart, their integrity examined, and the entire heart examined for pathologic conditions. Serologic examinations are performed, and after a brief quarantine, usually 40 days, valves are released for homograft transplant according to size and need. The aortic and pulmonary valves are dissected from the heart and eventually used as replacement valves. Aortic root replacement, repair of tetralogy of Fallot, and pulmonary atresia can also be performed using valve parts. The donor has a single incision on the chest that does not prevent an open casket if the family so wishes.

If the process of skin recovery is available in the region, this procedure can also take place in the morgue. A clean room and sterile technique are required. A dermatome is used to recover skin from the buttocks, thighs, back, and abdomen. A split-thickness graft, removed from the top surface of the body, is barely visible unless the donor has a dark tan or is of high pigment. After skin is recovered it is treated with antibiotics, prepared surgically for grafting, and stored at $-70°$ F. The recovered skin is used for temporary grafts in severely burned patients to provide protection from infection, fluid shifts, and other complications of burns.

Solid-Organ Procurement: Heart, Lungs, Liver, Pancreas, and Kidney

Recovery of solid organs for transplant may be complex and requires cooperation of team members representing many different disciplines. Many hours of hemodynamic mainte-

Box 15-3	HEMODYNAMIC PARAMETERS FOR THE ORGAN DONOR	
PARAMETER		VALUE
Systolic BP		$\geq$100 mm Hg
PaO$_2$		100 mm Hg
SaO$_2$		$\geq$ 95%
CVP		5-15 mm Hg
Urine output		100-500 ml/hr
Hematocrit		$\geq$25%
Temperature		>95 to <102° F

BP, Blood pressure; *PaO$_2$,* partial pressure of oxygen; *SaO$_2$,* arterial oxygen saturation; *CVP,* central venous pressure.

nance of the donor may be necessary before the actual procedure takes place. The donation coordinator works with the family to address its concerns and with the intensive care unit staff to manage the donor until time of the procurement. Hemodynamic parameters of donor management have been worked out and, if met, facilitate procurement of healthy organs for transplant. The hemodynamic parameters of donor management are summarized in Box 15-3. The goals are the same in the pediatric patient but adjusted for weight and size of the potential donor. The potential donor may not necessarily exhibit these parameters, but the patient must still be considered for donation.

After the patient is declared dead by brain-death criteria, management for preservation of organs for transplantation can begin. The donor's blood pressure is extremely labile. Diabetes insipidus resulting from herniation causes an imbalance of fluids and electrolytes. Management of the donor includes balancing fluid and electrolytes, use of vasopressors such as dopamine and dobutamine, and treatment of developing diabetes insipidus. Antidiuretic hormone replacement using a pitressin supplement via intravenous drip, intranasally, or by injection is frequently instituted. Management of pulmonary status should ensure that blood gas levels reflect extremely well-oxygenated organs. Hematocrit is monitored closely to prevent lowered oxygen transport, which may result from excessive bleeding caused by related trauma. All laboratory values must be reviewed, including fluid status, and evaluated for overhydration or underhydration. Numerous laboratory studies, including electrolyte, blood urea nitrogen, creatinine, hematologic studies, liver function tests, cardiac enzyme assessment, electrocardiogram, echocardiogram, transesophageal echocardiography, cardiology consultation, arterial blood gas tests, pulmonary consult, and evaluation of chest radiographs, are carried out to determine health of the organs to be recovered.

After the patient has been accepted as a donor and all organs to be recovered have been assigned to a receiving patient, recovery teams convene. The host hospital has final determination of operating time; however, most donations of organs occur during late hours of the night. The hospital is asked to provide operating room staff and anesthesia support.

The donor is transported to the operating room fully supported by mechanical means and is hemodynamically maintained in the operating room according to goals outlined previously. The donor is maintained throughout the organ dissection and mobilization of the respective tissues until organs and tissues are freed for immediate removal and preservation. After the last aspects of the dissection have been completed, the aorta is clamped, and cardioplegia takes place. Quick cooling and in situ flushing of the organs is then accomplished. After flushing is completed, organs are removed from the donor, examined individually in a sterile back basin, flushed again if required, and packed in a sterile container for transport and immediate transplant (in the case of the heart, heart and lung, and single lung). For kidneys, approximately 24 hours may elapse before transplantation takes place. For the pancreas and liver, this time ranges from 6 to 20 hours, with the preferred time approximately 15 hours. This flexibility of preservation time in the case of the kidneys, liver, and pancreas is largely the result of preservation fluid "U.W." developed by Dr. Folkert O. Belzer of the University of Wisconsin during the late 1980s. This preservation fluid greatly enhances the procurement process, allowing time for transportation of organs and tissue typing of the donor with the recipient. Tissue typing is primarily carried out between kidney donor and recipient and in some cases between heart, heart and lung, and single-lung donor and recipient.

FINANCIAL CONSIDERATIONS

The donation process of tissues and organs is an expensive one. The donor's family does not pay the cost of organ or tissue donation. The recipient, insurance, Medicare, or Medicaid pays all costs related to the donation. The family of the donor should never be issued a hospital bill accrued during the hospital stay until the organ procurement agency has had an opportunity to review charges and take care of all charges related to the donation process. Families must be made aware of this, if at all possible, when they speak with the coordinator. If the family receives a bill, they are encouraged to contact the organ procurement agency to ensure proper payment of the bill.

In the United States, payment for organ transplant is usually made by third-party payers. In 1972 Medicare enacted the End-Stage Renal Disease Act, allowing patients with end-stage renal disease coverage for treatment of dialysis and kidney transplantation. All people were given the opportunity for treatment essential to life. For liver and heart transplantation, most third-party payers cover the cost of the transplantation surgery and postoperative care. However, in many states, third-party reimbursement is not available for heart and lung, pancreas, and lung transplantation; these transplants are still considered experimental. A great deal of controversy exists regarding the expense of transplantation, with emphasis on the number of people helped, cost, and

Table 15-3 SUMMARY OF ESTIMATED CHARGES PER ORGAN AND TISSUE TRANSPLANTATION (1996 DOLLARS)		
ORGAN TISSUE	**ESTIMATED 1ST YEAR CHARGES**	**ESTIMATED ANNUAL FOLLOW-UP CHARGES**	**ESTIMATED TOTAL CHARGES FOR 5 YEARS ADJUSTED FOR SURVIVAL**
Heart	$303,400	$40,000	$434,316
Liver	$244,600	$45,000	$389,091
Kidney	$111,400	$20,000	$196,452
Kidney-Pancreas	$138,300	$20,000	$226,495
Pancreas	$113,700	$7,500	$149,225
Heart-Lung	$301,200	$40,000	$402,188
Lung	$257,700	$40,000	$360,843
Cornea	$8,000	$0	$8,000
Bone Marrow	$217,000	$29,300	$287,300

National Transplant Assistance Fund: Patient & family info. Retrieved from the World Wide Web, January 20, 2002: http://www.transplantfund.org/chart2.html.

life expectancy after the graft and transplantation. Table 15-3 presents the cost estimates for solid-organ transplantations.

Costs vary from center to center but serve as a guideline for actual costs. Many states cannot justify the cost of transplantation in these times of cost containment when so few people benefit. Oregon, for example, reallocated Medicaid monies previously designated for transplantation to other areas of the governmental budget that were felt to better serve a greater number of people (e.g., pregnant mothers, infants, and mothers at high risk). (Kidneys and corneas are an exception to this mandate.)[9] How the money is spent and who pays for these highly specialized, technologically advanced procedures are questions considered daily. The ethics of choosing one cause over another must be grappled with continually.

SUMMARY

Many issues surrounding the role and responsibility of the emergency nurse relate to tissue and organ donors. The emergency nurse has the responsibility to provide the family with the option of tissue and organ donation when a patient dies in the ED. The Emergency Nurses Association Position Statement of 1987[6] clearly indicates this responsibility.

The Emergency Nurses Association believes emergency nurses should be knowledgeable in identification of potential donors, life support of donor patients, and in accessing resource personnel from state or local transplant teams. It is within the role of the emergency nurse, and not mandated by federal law, to initiate discussions regarding organ donation and to facilitate, coordinate, and intervene with families as appropriate.

For too long, the concept of donation has been associated solely with trauma victims: patients maintained and declared dead by brain-death criteria in the intensive care setting. Al-most any person who dies can be a donor of some tissue or organ for transplantation. This is an integral part of the emergency nursing care for patients and families in crisis.

References

1. American Council on Transplantation: *From here to transplant,* Alexandria, Va, 1987, The Council.
2. American Hospital Association, American Medical Association, and United Network for Organ Sharing: *Required request legislation: a guide for hospitals on organ and tissue donation,* Chicago, 1988, The Associations and The Network.
3. DeBoer H: The history of bone grafts, *Clin Orthop* 226:292, 1988.
4. *Defining death: medical, legal, and ethical issues in the determination of death,* Washington, DC, 1981, President's Commission for the Study of Ethical Problems in Medicine and Biomedical Research.
5. Dekker ML: Bone and soft tissue procurement, *Orthop Nurse* 8(2):33, 1989.
6. Emergency Nurses Association: *Role of the emergency nurse in organ procurement: ENA position statement,* Park Ridge, Ill, 1987, The Association.
7. *Gallup Poll 1985: The U.S. public's attitudes toward organ transplant/organ donation, 1985,* Princeton, NJ, The Gallup Organization.
8. Laudicina SS: *Medicaid coverage and payment policies for organ transplants: findings of a national survey,* Washington, DC, George Washington University, 1988, U.S. Department of Health and Human Services.
9. Newberry MA: *Textbook of hemodialysis for patient care personnel,* Springfield, Ill, 1989, Charles C. Thomas.
10. Tilney NL: Renal transplantation between identical twins: a review, *World J Surg* 10(3):381, 1986.
11. United Network for Organ Sharing: *Organ and tissue donation: a reference guide for clergy,* Washington, DC, 1995, U.S. Department of Health and Human Services.
12. United Network for Organ Sharing: *Donation and transplantation nursing curriculum,* Washington, DC, 1996, U.S. Department of Health and Human Services.

13. U.S. Department of Health and Human Services: Hospital participation for organ donation, *Federal Register* 63(119): 33856, Washington, DC, 1998, The Department.

14. U.S. Department of Health and Human Services: *Organ transplantation: issues and recommendations,* report of the Task Force on Organ Transplantation, Washington, DC, 1986, The Department.

15. U.S. Department of Health and Human Services: *Roles and training in the donation process: a resource guide,* Washington, DC, 2000, The Department.

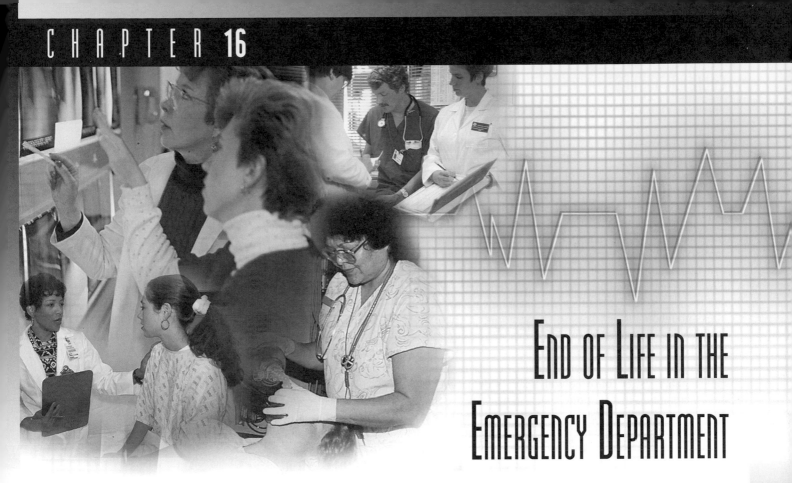

CHAPTER 16

END OF LIFE IN THE EMERGENCY DEPARTMENT

NANCY J. DENKE

Medical decision making in the area of withholding, refusing, or withdrawing life support has become increasingly complex and difficult. We must remember that there is only one person who knows what is best for the individual who is critically ill, and that is the individual. This is absolute. Each individual must be permitted to make all decisions concerning his or her life (or death) as he or she sees fit. No one should have the power to overrule decisions of the individual about his or her own well-being, particularly when it comes to choosing the moment of death.

Most medical professionals are as uncomfortable with the idea of death as everyone else. These individuals are trained to preserve life at all costs. Nowhere else better epitomizes this than the emergency department (ED). The major goal with any patient who presents to the ED is to stabilize a medical crisis and control physical deterioration. Emergency nurses focus on life-saving efforts (i.e., maintaining and stabilizing vital signs in a trauma victim), but are not necessarily expert at helping survivors with the emotional trauma of sudden death. Patient care in the ED involves not only advanced technology and therapy, but also caring for the families of patients. This is an integral part of the emergency nurses' responsibility throughout the patients' stay in the department.

The words "trauma" or "taken to the hospital by ambulance" evoke fear and feelings of helplessness in most people. Admission to the ED is usually sudden and unplanned. The ED is also a busy and intimidating place with sick people, confusing language, and unfamiliar noises and smells. Add this to the severity of illness, uncertainty of the prognosis, and various ethical and cultural dilemmas and it becomes easy to empathize with the families. A variety of stressors (fear of death or disability, a change in role responsibilities) must be faced with any event that brings families to the ED. Many times family members search the faces of nurses and physicians for clues about how their loved one is. The family room can be a hotbed for usual coping mechanisms such as feelings of shock or disbelief and helplessness combined with anger and guilt. These feelings may be so foreign to many families that they lead to frustration or hostility, which may be taken out on ED staff. These feelings can also be heightened when families perceive staff as cold and indifferent. Patients and families may not realize that what appears as cold or callous are often coping mechanisms used to deal with difficult choices, decisions, and patient situations. Hopkins[5] found that failure of the nurse to interact appropriately with families can lead to heightened anxiety and fear, misunderstanding, mistrust, hostility, failure to obtain important information about the patient, and lawsuits. Emergency nurses must give assistance to these families for them to make reasoned and compassionate choices and not to act out their own pain or needs in the confusion of the moment.

CULTURAL ISSUES

The Last Dance by DeSpelder and Strickland provides a comprehensive look at major issues and questions about death and dying.[2] *The Last Dance* reminds us that coping with death was once learned first hand by caring for the dying family member right through to disposition of the body of the loved one.

Different cultures and many great religions around the world consider dying an art to be learned or as essential to a good passage into the next life. Cultural traditions also vary significantly when it comes to telling the patient he or she is dying, whether to remove that person from life support, and how to express grief at the time of death. Geography, religion, and social systems have affected disposition customs of cultures throughout history. These disposition customs have been traditionally determined by four elements: air (exposure), water (ocean burial), earth (burial), and fire (cremation).

Many cultures have sacred rituals or mourning ceremonies that must be followed with death of one of its members. Ceremonies that a culture enacts to mark the passing of an individual use symbols that express how death is perceived within that particular culture. Health care providers must be sensitive to the survivors' needs for these different symbols and rituals and allow people to grieve in their own ways. Hospitals in areas with an ethically diverse population may benefit from protocols customized for different cultures. For example, Hasidic Jews pray continuously on deathbeds, so caregivers should make arrangements that accommodate this ritual. Concern for the ability of the spirit to leave the body is common in many cultures, so rituals may involve moving the patient outside, lighting candles (as in the Roma Culture), or opening a window at the moment of death. These and other sacred death rituals can be difficult in busy EDs. Buddhists have a complex philosophy on how to prepare for death and how to make one's way after death. In the *Tibetan Book of Death,* there is an elaborate set of instructions to be read after an individual dies. Native Americans believe that dying is part of the natural cycle and should not to be feared. Their ceremonies symbolize separation of the dead from the living, transition to an afterlife, and allowing communities to reincorporate after loss of a loved one. If we can understand some of these rituals and beliefs, we can then assist families in their time of grief.

The roles learned long ago for care of the dying have changed significantly in today's modern culture. Families no longer play an active role as caregivers. Rather, this role has been delegated to strangers—health care providers—while the family waits in the waiting room. As the use of hospice care increases for the terminally ill, this trend of less family involvement may be reversed. Caring for the dying can be stressful for both family and health care providers.

Perhaps no other place in the hospital has the frequency of exposure to death as the ED. Although frequent and familiar there, death is no less stressful. The thought that everyone can be saved may a desirable objective, but in reality it is not one always obtained. There are many "what ifs" that go through the minds of ED staff on a daily basis. These "what ifs" lead to personal conflict between emotional and professional responsibilities contributing to guilt, confusion, and even avoidance of any situations that may lead to death.

To decrease these stress producers, emergency professionals must be flexible and have confidence in their responses to circumstances surrounding a patient's death. Only when the emergency nurse is confident about a patient's care and believes the care was beneficial to the patient is the nurse able to cope with repeated exposure to death and dying in the ED. Box 16-1 highlights resources related to transcultural nursing.

Box 16-1 RESOURCES RELATED TO TRANSCULTURAL NURSING

INTERNET	JOURNALS
Transcultural Nursing Society: http://www.tcns.org	Journal of Transcultural Nursing
Resources for Cross Cultural Health: www.DiversityRx.org	Journal of Multicultural Nursing
Transcultural Nursing: http://www.culturediversity.org	Journal of Immigrant Health

DECIDING TO DIE

There has always been a time to live and a time to die! Today, with the ability to prolong life, each one of us will probably have to face this issue ourselves or with someone we love . . . How long is too long?

Billy Graham

Technologic advances have improved health care and provided greater choices in health care, but these advances have also raised questions about the proper use of these options and improvements. Margaret Mead[7] summarizes it well by saying, "The great advances in medicine came about because physicians have taken seriously the Hippocratic obligation to keep people alive." But at whose expense? These very same advances designed to prolong life may also prolong dying. When caregivers understand that death could (and should) be a human act of dignity and not mechanical failure that can be fixed with more technology, they are able to deal humanly with death. Caregivers must know when to keep trying and when to quit. Medical futility is now considered an ethically acceptable reason to discontinue resuscitative efforts. But what is medical futility?

In a presentation on medical and legal implications of cardiac-arrest protocols held in Orlando, Florida, May 2000, Dr. Jorge Martinez[6] addressed this concept of medical futility. He suggested a broad definition of medical futility to include quantitative care (i.e., care that produces no physiologic effect at a given level of probability) and qualitative care (i.e., care that produces effects but no benefit). Box 16-2 provides information about academic and research centers for bioethics in the United States.

ADVANCE DIRECTIVES

"Many people say they do not fear death, but the PROCESS of dying. It's not Destination, but the trip that they dread."

Billy Graham

Since the landmark court case of Karen Ann Quinlan more than 30 years ago, patients have been encouraged to express their thoughts and feelings on end-of-life decisions with an advance directive. Because of this court case, the Patient Self-Determination Act was passed in 1991 to alleviate this fear. This act states that at the time of a patient's admission to the hospital, patients (or parents or guardians of children) must be presented with information about advance directives and their rights in making medical care decisions. These wishes then become a part of the patient's permanent record. Many people fear being kept alive by medical technology beyond what they feel is a meaningful existence. No one should have the power to overrule the decisions of the individual, particularly when it comes to choosing the manner of death. The advance directive should be a guide to the individual's wishes and is based on the concept that the patient is competent and has a right to refuse treatment. These documents become effective only when the patient becomes incapacitated. But what if there is no advance directive? That question has medical ethicists trying to answer despite considerable legal uncertainty in this area.

Advance directives come in three forms: living will, durable power of attorney for health care, and DNR (do not resuscitate; also called DNAR for do not attempt resuscitation). A living will is a legal document in which an individ-

ual can direct treatment modalities against extraordinary measures in the event of irreversible coma and terminal illness. The legality of this document varies from state to state; however, it does not ensure a patient's right to die regardless of geographic location. The durable power of attorney for health care designates a surrogate decision maker when a patient is unable to make decisions. The patient can specify limits or parameters for the type of medical treatment that must be followed by the designated surrogate.

The DNR (or DNAR) is an order that should be documented on the chart. A witness may be required in some areas. The DNR order addresses what life-saving measures should be initiated specifying limits such as cardiopulmonary resuscitation only, medications only, or no defibrillation. Despite the presence of a DNR order, every effort is made in these situations to ease pain and make the patient comfortable. Advance directives vary from state to state, so health care professionals must be familiar with stipulations in their respective states.

Society has obviously done its part by passing this act, forcing health care providers to confront questions that the individual may shy away from and not want to address with patients. Despite written evidence of the patient's wishes, it is still difficult for many caregivers to let go. Most health care providers are as uncomfortable with the idea of death as the families. Health care professionals have been trained to preserve life, not to practice death care. Establishing a good patient-family-health care provider relationship in the ED may be difficult in a crisis situation. Unfortunately, it may be difficult if not impossible to identify the patient's wishes in the ED. Living wills, advance directives, and other documents may not be immediately available in the ED. Families in crisis may not be able to make a decision. It is critical for the emergency nurse to maintain ongoing contact with the patient and family throughout a crisis event. Nurses may appear more visible and many times more approachable than are physicians. Families may find it easier to ask for information and advice from the nurse. Making yourself available to assist families with these difficult issues as they arise is a vital nursing function.

EUTHANASIA

Euthanasia means *good death.* An article by Steinhauser and colleagues[8] in the *Annals of Internal Medicine,* reported on their questions to physicians, nurses, social workers, chaplains, hospice volunteers, patients, and recently bereaved family members at a Veterans Administration hospital. Surprisingly, understanding the concept of good death was lacking in these individuals. They were able to identify six concepts of a good death but were not in agreement about the actual details. They were able to agree on a few concepts such as choices, communication, and pain management,[4] with communication of utmost importance. Moral choice in dying was addressed in a 1998 article in *Christian Bioethics.*[3] In this article Engelhardt looked at physician-assisted suicide and noted that the traditional Christian moral choice of focus at death is on repentance, not on dignity. In contrast, posttraditional Christians are concerned with self-determination, control, and dignity and that voluntary euthanasia is a moral choice. These contrasting opinions make the understanding of good death even more difficult.

There have been numerous writings outlining various rituals in which the elderly or very ill are either allowed or expected to promote the end of life by taking some type of poison. Ancient Greeks and Romans hastened their deaths to avoid humiliation or to escape debilitating illnesses. The Japanese act of hara-kiri is also considered an act of good death with honor. In the early part of the twentieth century, euthanasia was seen as a humane act to end suffering in our own country. It was not until World War II that the stigma of euthanasia as inhumane came into play. At present, Oregon is the only state whose laws allow euthanasia. Worldwide, the Netherlands represents a positive working model of euthanasia with creation of specific criteria and guidelines for performing euthanasia. Euthanasia is also legal in Australia and Colombia.

Because of these moral choices, palliative care and subsequent management of a patient's dying process is often the responsibility of nurses. Ethicists, physicians, and nurses play an active role in the decision making that precedes withdrawal of life support. Ethicists concern themselves with the ethics of the decision-making process; the definition of death and even considerations about giving pain medications that may be thought to shorten the patient's life.[1] Numerous professional organizations[1] have issued guidelines to assist in this decision-making process and give us an avenue to explore with patients and their families when death becomes imminent. But after the decision is made and goals to a good death are obtained, the ethicists leave and care of the dying patient is left up to the nurse. A clear understanding of the goals must be specified for this dying patient so that a "good death" can be achieved. Many times the major and only goal is comfort care with family support.

DEATH OF A CHILD

"A period before the end of a sentence."

Carl Jung

Health care professionals empathize with families who suffer loss of a loved one. Death of a child causes emotional and mental anguish in even the most hardened health care professional. There is a deeply held belief that only old people die so only the old are expected to die. Because of this, health care providers undergo extraordinary efforts in resuscitating children and young people. However, the law states that what is done is in the best interest of the child. When deciding what is in the best interest of a child when resuscitating, health care professionals must ask themselves three questions.

1. Are the measures we are using inhumane?

2. Is the treatment futile?
3. Is the child in an irreversible coma?

If the answer to any of these questions is yes, continued resuscitation should be questioned and current efforts reevaluated.

Parents of children with chronic illnesses may have time to prepare for grieving as they see their child becoming more and more debilitated. Sudden death eliminates the opportunity for any type of preparation. Death of a child is particularly difficult to accept. Parents' fears and guilt are often exacerbated when their child is brought to the ED in a crisis situation. Different grieving processes or reactions are exhibited. It is imperative that caregivers are supportive and not judgmental of these reactions. Disposition rituals such as baptism of a child before pronouncement of death may be critical for the family. Providing an environment that is supportive and comforting is of utmost importance. Caring for the family can be expressed in a number of ways—telling the family how sorry you are for their loss, resting your hand on theirs, sharing their tears. Sit down with them and make eye contact. How this concern is expressed varies with each situation, so the nurse should use his or her instincts for guidance. Answer questions or assist in making decisions. Write pertinent information down and give to a family member who can process it. Offer to cut a lock of the child's hair or make an imprint of the child's hand for the parents.

Surviving siblings should not be forgotten during this time of pain and loss. Siblings may not fully understand the events that have just occurred. Answer questions honestly and give the child only as much information as it seems they need to know. Taking an honest, frank, but sensitive approach will benefit the child greatly. Avoiding terms such as "gone to sleep," "passed away," or "gone away" can decrease confusion that many children encounter when adults talk about death. Because many children are so literal in their thoughts, these phrases can lead to nightmares, fear of sleeping, and even fear that if the parent goes away they will never return. Most important, be sure to tell them that they are not to blame for what has happened. It is important to let them grieve for the family member. Be sure someone is comforting the sibling when the parents are involved in their own grief and "making arrangements." An overview of reactions of siblings is contained in Table 16-1.

Death of a child is not only devastating to the family but can also be difficult for the health care team. A debriefing may be necessary after such an emotionally stressful event. Organizing a critical incident stress debriefing can allow the resuscitation team to recover from these events. Caregivers must also learn to accept peers' reactions to these emotional events and allow for recovery.

FAMILY PRESENCE: THE BENEFITS OF BEING THERE

Traditionally, family members have been prohibited from being present during resuscitation efforts for ethical (patient confidentiality) and practical reasons (interference with staff activity). Other reasons cited are increased litigation and

Table 16-1	REACTIONS OF SIBLINGS TO DEATH	
AGE	CONCEPT	REACTIONS
Birth to 2 years	No real concept of death Has a sense of separation or abandonment; feels a sense of loss; senses that something is different For the small infant, it may be responses related to disruption in routine Beginning to understand reality of death but is confused	May express nonspecific forms of upset: irritability, change in sleep or feeding patterns
2 to 6 years	Realizes that being dead means not being alive—may see death as reversible May believe that the deceased person still physically exists May believe that he or she is responsible for the person's death Fears punishment or that death is a form of punishment Believes that death is contagious	May be curious, confused May ask body-oriented questions Response may be delayed until a time when the child feels safer Adults often miss the relationship between delayed responses to death
6 to 12 years	Learning to think logically and to solve problems. Death is concrete, with specific causes Understands biologic functioning. Death is considered a universal and irreversible event Beginning to deal with possibility of own mortality	Vacillates between emotions—may be angry or curious or may act as if nothing happened May still feel that somehow he or she was to blame May experience intense guilt about having wished his or her sibling were dead at some time in the past May overidentify and fear the future May become excessively demanding Feelings of isolation from family
More than 12 years	Thinks in abstract terms, reality of own death surfaces Denial of own vulnerability	May exhibit exaggerated risk-taking behaviors May become embarrassed to talk about death May become isolated from peers and family

Modified from Emergency Nurses Association: Special patient population: pediatric. In *Orientation to emergency nursing: concepts, competencies, and critical thinking,* Des Plaines, Ill, 2000, The Association.

stress on the staff. Despite these concerns family presence has become increasingly important, with movement over the last decade to provide families this option. Family members who were present when a loved one was in a resuscitative situation reported the experience as a positive and helpful one, even when the individual died. Several studies reported that family members found that it was important and helpful for them to be with loved ones during the event.[6,8] It helped them better understand the seriousness of the patient's condition and that every possible intervention had been undertaken. Most health care providers agreed that the experience helps the family understand the situation and realize the extent to which the health care team had gone in an attempt to save their loved one.

Nevertheless, some staff members report heightened stress during resuscitation when family is present. They felt it was harder for them to remain distant and unemotional. Ironically, they did not feel that their professional function was affected. Even with these thoughts in mind the health care providers felt that the experience was important to the families.

The Emergency Nurses Association (Box 16-3) has developed guidelines for family presence during resuscitation or invasive procedures. For any institution developing a family presence program, it is important that certain factors be included.

- Appropriate staff and facilities, along with staff education
- Preparation of the family for the experience
- Provision of a dedicated person to accompany the family

Box 16-3 ENA POSITION STATEMENT

ENA supports the option of family presence during invasive procedures and/or resuscitation efforts. ENA supports further research related to the presence of family members during invasive procedures and/or resuscitation efforts and the impact it has upon family members, patients, and health care personnel. ENA supports the development and dissemination of educational resources for Emergency Department health care personnel concerning the issues related to family presence. The ENA supports collaboration with other specialty organizations (including, but not limited to nursing, social and family services, pastoral care, physicians, and Prehospital care providers) to develop multidisciplinary guidelines related to family presence during invasive procedures and/or resuscitation.

Emergency Nurses Association: *Family presence at the bedside during invasive procedures and/or resuscitation* (position statement), Des Plaines, Ill, 2001, The Association.

The goal is to keep the clinical mission in focus and the resuscitation area in control without compromising patient integrity and safety. This can be accomplished with a sympathetic and expert nursing staff member or social worker. Appropriate follow-up for the family must be provided, especially when relatives have already witnessed the prehospital part of the resuscitation attempt. Remember, some of the things we do may be profoundly traumatizing to the family.

The family should be prepared for the experience before entering the resuscitation room. Explain to the family what to expect, what they will see, and what they will hear when in the room. Be sure that the family members are not going to add to the chaos already going on in the room. Remind them that this is an option and not something that they have to do. It is important that communication is open and is part of the continuum of caring. Be supportive of the family members if they decline to observe and remind them that they will remain part of the decision process. They should never be pressured. If the family members wants to spend some time with their loved one after he or she has been declared dead, they should be allowed to say goodbye and spend as much time as they need to do this. Provide them with ways to reach closure so they are able to leave the ED.

SUMMARY

More and more people are concerned with quality at the end of their life. Many want the ability to decide when to save their lives and when they should be allowed to die. Technologic advances that have brought about improved health care and greater choices in medical services have also resulted in questions not concerning how, but when, to make use of these choices and improvements. People still want to die with dignity and we as health care providers should enable them to do just that.

The manner in which these issues are handled will influence not only the medical outcome but also the quality of patient care. Having the family present during resuscitation will allow the family to adjust to death of a loved one and manage their grief a bit more easily.

References

1. Chapple HS: Changing the game in the intensive care unit: letting nature take its course, *Crit Care Nurs* 19(3):25, 1999.
2. DePelder LA, Strickland A: *The last dance: encountering death and dying*, Palo Alto, Calif, 2001, Mayfield Publishing.
3. Engelhardt HT: Physician-assisted suicide reconsidered: dying as a Christian in a post-Christian age, *Christian Bioethics* 4(2):143, 1998.
4. Hanson L, Danis M, Garrett J: What is wrong with end-of-life care? Opinions of bereaved family members, *J Amer Geriatr Soc* 45(11):1339, 1997.
5. Hopkins AG: The trauma nurse's role with families in crisis, *Crit Care Nurs* 14(2):35, 1994.
6. Martinez J: Advance directives and family presence during resuscitation: legal and ethical questions, *AACN News* 18(1):14, 2001.
7. Mead M: The cultural shaping of the ethical situation. In Vaux K, ed: *Who shall live? Medicine, technology, and ethics*, Philadelphia, 1970, Fortress Press.
8. Steinhauser K, Clipp E, McNeilly M et al: In search of a good death: observations of patients, families, and providers, *Ann Intern Med* 132(10): 825, 2000.

Suggested Reading

American Heart Association: *Guidelines 2000 for cardiopulmonary resuscitation and emergency cardiovascular care*, Dallas, 2000, The Association.

Dickinson D: Are medical ethicists out of touch? Practitioner attitudes in the US and UK towards decisions at the end of life, *J Med Ethics* 26(4):254, 2000.

Dracup K, Byran-Brown C: Nurses and euthanasia: a tale of two studies, *J Crit Care* 5(4):249, 1996.

Emergency Nurses Association: *Family presence at the bedside during invasive procedures and resuscitation* (position statement), Des Plaines, Ill, 2001, The Association.

Emergency Nurses Association: *Presenting the option for family presence*, ed 2, Des Plaines, Ill, 2001, The Association.

Field MJ, Cassel CK, eds: *Approaching death: improving care at the end of life*, Washington, DC, 1997, Institute of Medicine.

Furukawa M: Meeting the needs of the dying patient's family, *Crit Care Nurs* 16(1):51, 1996.

Haverkate I, van der Wal G, van der Maas P: Guidelines on euthanasia and pain alleviation: compliance and opinions of physicians, *Health Policy* 44(1):45, 1998.

Leininger M: *Transcultural nursing: concepts, theories, research, and practice*, ed 2, New York, 1995, McGraw Hill.

MacDonald W: The difference between blacks' and whites' attitudes toward voluntary euthanasia, *J Sci Study Religion* 37(3):411, 1998.

Meyer EC, Snelling LK, Myren-Manbeck LK: Pediatric intensive care: the parents' experience, *AACN Clin Issues: Adv Pract Acute Crit Care*, 9(1):64, 1998.

Meyers TA, Eichnorn DJ, Guzzetta CE: Do families want to be present during CPR? A retrospective survey, *J Emerg Nurs* 24:400, 1998.

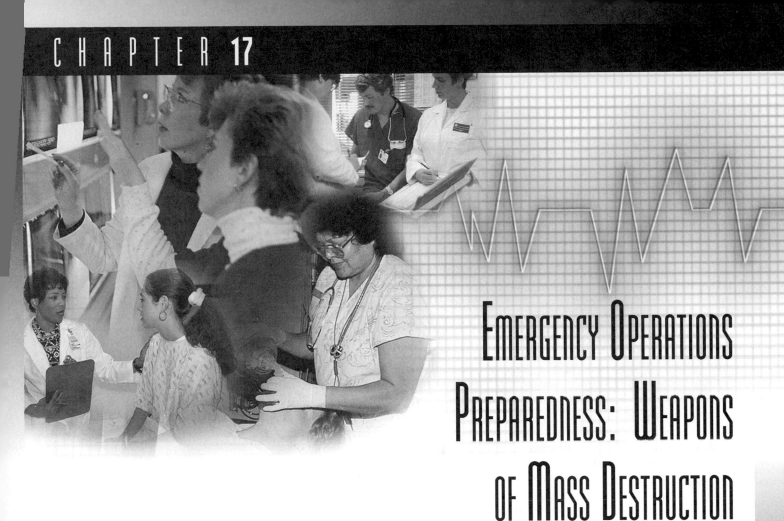

CHAPTER 17

EMERGENCY OPERATIONS PREPAREDNESS: WEAPONS OF MASS DESTRUCTION

MARY E. O'SHIELDS

The twenty-first century has brought new challenges to emergency departments (EDs). Plane crashes into the World Trade Center Towers in New York heightened awareness of the potential for biologic and chemical warfare. Iraq began amassing biologic weapons, including anthrax, botulinum toxin and aflatoxin, which they incorporated into bombs and warheads.[4] Evidence exists that other nations, such as Korea, Iran, Pakistan, Syria, and the Taliban in Afghanistan also have biologic weapons. The Gulf War and anthrax attacks on U.S. Postal Service facilities have made Americans increasingly aware that large-scale chemical or biologic weapons can be directed against the civilian population.

Increased availability of biologic weapons makes these agents a viable option for not only terrorist groups but also individuals. The Office of Technology Assessment has estimated that 100 kg of anthrax spread over Washington DC could kill 1 to 3 million people.[3] To ensure that the United States is prepared for a nuclear, biologic, or chemical weapon attack, Congress passed The Defense against Weapons of Mass Destruction Act of 1996. This Act provides funds to conduct training programs for prehospital and medical personnel. In addition, the Department of Health and Human Services developed metropolitan medical strike teams in 27 cities across the United States that are trained to respond to incidents involving weapons of mass destruction (WMD). These teams will assist in stockpiling antidotes, procuring special equipment, and training personnel in the use of equipment.[6]

Most EDs have sophisticated disaster plans that efficiently mobilize staff, equipment, and supplies when there is an internal or external incident that causes a massive influx of patients or major disruption in hospital services. Over the past two to three decades, EDs across the country have become increasingly sophisticated in caring for victims of mass casualty incidents (MCI) (e.g., victims of earthquakes, tornadoes, floods, bombings). However, recent events highlight the need to concentrate on preparation for biologic and chemical threats. This chapter provides an overview of decontamination, triage, and common biologic and chemical agents. The information presented is limited to weapons available at the time of printing. The number and types of weapons may increase; therefore, the emergency nurse should stay up to date on changes in this area.

PERSONAL PROTECTIVE EQUIPMENT

All personnel who care for patients involved in an WMD incident should wear personal protective equipment (PPE).

The type of agent and concentration of contaminant that remain on the patient determine the appropriate level of PPE that should be worn (Table 17-1). If the agent has not yet been identified, health care workers should use the maximum protection available. Regardless of PPE worn, health care providers should give special consideration to protecting their airway, eyes, and skin. If patients are not decontaminated at the scene before transport, health care providers in the initial triage area may need a full-face respiratory mask; self-contained breathing apparatus (SCBA); and liquid-proof, vapor-impenetrable suits. There are multiple drawbacks to the SCBA. It is bulky, restrictive, and can cause heat-related illness with prolonged use.[1] It can also be difficult to keep staff trained in the correct procedure for use of this sophisticated equipment. Consequently, training and drills for PPE should be held on a regular basis. It may be possible to enlist the help of local fire and disaster management personnel in staff training. The Environmental Protection Agency (EPA) has developed criteria for PPE that can be used in certain biohazardous situations.

It is important for staff to realize that, in most cases, health care providers do not have the necessary equipment or experience to decontaminate victims of chemical warfare. At this time, consensus has not been reached in the medical community regarding the minimum level of required personal protection. After patients have been disrobed, a contaminated patient poses only minimal risk; especially if decontamination takes place in a well-ventilated room.[2] Specialized equipment such as SCBA is expensive to purchase and requires extensive training before staff is comfortable in its use. Using the equipment without proper training can cause equipment failure and injury to the health care provider. In many communities, arrangements have been made with the hazardous material (Haz-Mat) team of the local fire department for assistance in decontamination when a situation involving chemical exposure arises.

DECONTAMINATION

The first priority for the hospital caring for victims exposed to WMD is to protect current patients, ED staff, and the facility. Subsequent priorities include care of the patient and protection of the environment. The ED must be prepared to decontaminate patients and attempt to identify the contaminating agent.

Decontamination procedures are designed to meet the unique challenges faced by each ED. Facilities are unique in terms of entrances, ambulance ramps, surrounding terrain, room layout, personnel, and resources such as Haz-Mat teams. Decontamination is affected by these variables. Some have permanent decontamination rooms, whereas others utilize portable decontamination equipment. Personnel, training, and known hazards within the ED's service area should also be considered. For example, an ED located near a nuclear power plant has different challenges and resources than an ED located in the middle of an agricultural region. Development of decontamination procedures should include assessment of any existing hazards and resources.

A major concern regarding WMD is that unless the attack is widely recognized, as was the case in the Tokyo subway attack, the event may not be recognized until there are multiple casualties. First responders and ED personnel must be able to identify signs and symptoms exhibited by victims, appropriately use PPE, and quickly isolate and decontaminate victims.

It is important to remember that exposed individuals may come to the hospital on their own, without waiting for emergency medical services (EMS). When this occurs, the potential for contamination of the ED increases. Rapid identification of contaminated victims is crucial to prevent contamination of the ED and health care providers. Another concern arises when communication between the Haz-Mat team and EMS breaks down. This occurs when the Haz-Mat team has decontaminated the victims but EMS personnel do not think that the procedure was adequate or they are unaware that decontamination was done. One solution is use of decontamination bracelets. These bracelets are placed on the victim by the Haz-Mat team after decontamination to indicate that the victim has been decontaminated and/or cleared and requires no further treatment. This has proved an effective way to alert EMS personnel and ED staff that patients are 'safe' and do not require further decontamination. The bracelets can also be used by hospitals to indicate walk-in patients that have been decontaminated by the health care decontamination team.

Decontamination for biologic agents (except mycotoxins) may be as simple as manual cleaning or may require other procedures such as disinfection. Decontamination af-

Table 17-1	PERSONAL PROTECTIVE EQUIPMENT FOR CHEMICAL EXPOSURES
Level A	Fully encapsulating chemically-resistant suit and self-contained breathing apparatus (SCBA); worn when highest level of respiratory, skin, eye, and mucous membrane protection is needed
Level B	Provides splash protection by use of chemical-resistant clothing and SCBA; worn when highest level of respiratory protection is needed, but lesser level of skin, eye, and mucous membrane protection is sufficient
Level C	Used when type of airborne substance is known and when skin and eye exposures are unlikely
Level D	Work uniform; should not be used where hazards exist; provides no respiratory protection and minimal skin protection

ter a patient's exposure to an aerosolized biologic weapon lessens the potential for contamination from the patient's body, which prevents reaerosolization and respiratory exposure to health care providers. A warm water rinse, liquid soap for cleansing, and a final rinse can accomplish decontamination. In the nonambulatory casualty area, it is important to remember to wash the patient's back and the backboard before sending him or her to the main triage or treatment area.[10] Removing contaminated clothing eliminates a significant amount of surface contamination, and showering with soap and water effectively removes more than 99.9% of organisms that may be left on the skin.[10]

Conversely, chemical agents pose a risk of secondary exposure for health care providers through dermal contact or inhaling particulates. Patients should be considered chemically contaminated if they present with irritation of mucous membranes, chemical burns, clothing or skin soiled with unidentified liquids or powders, or if a strong, caustic odor is present.[2] Patients should be moved quickly through the decontamination process, because no definitive care is provided in these areas. Patients should undress in the ambulatory decontamination area; this significantly reduces the number of health care providers needed in this area.

Decontamination Stations

Decontamination can be effectively done in permanent decontamination rooms or through the use of portable decontamination equipment. There are advantages and disadvantages to both. Permanent decontamination rooms are costly to build, and it is often difficult to find adequate space in close proximity to the ED. Ideally, a permanent decontamination room has a separate entrance into the hospital, is in close proximity to the ED, has access to water and medical gas, and is large enough for one or two victims on ED or ambulance stretchers and one to two health care workers. The room should not be sealed because this can increase inhalation exposure to health care providers in the room. One viable option in many hospitals is use of the morgue for decontamination. Morgues are usually located near outside entrances and are designed for easy cleaning with hoses overhead and drains in the floor. Some EDs use rooms that are normally used for other purposes, such as stock rooms or casting rooms. When the decontamination room is one of these "multipurpose" rooms, decontamination may be delayed while supplies and equipment are removed and the room is readied for use. These permanent rooms increase the risk for contamination of the facility and staff because the patient comes into the building for decontamination.

Portable decontamination equipment allows for outside decontamination and minimizes the potential for exposure or contamination of additional people. Minimal requirements for a basic outdoor decontamination unit include a hose with an adjustable temperature and low-pressure spray nozzle; liquid soap and nonabrasive brushes; butyl or other

chemical-resistant and splash-resistant aprons, gowns, or jumpsuits; protective eye wear, and large biohazard bags.[12] Advantages of portable equipment are decreased risk of additional contamination, lower inhalation exposure risks, and simultaneous decontamination of multiple victims.[9] Disadvantages are lack of privacy, inclement weather problems, and difficulty collecting run off water. Equipment set-up can also be a problem when it is rarely used. Lighting may be an issue in some areas, so set-up should include lighting that adequately illuminates the decontamination area for nighttime operations. Other procedures are available to overcome some of these difficulties. The shower area can be enclosed with a tent for privacy and to provide protection from the elements. In severe weather, portable heaters can be placed inside the tent to protect against hypothermia. Figure 17-1 shows a portable decontamination system with personnel in Level B protection.

Water temperature for the decontamination area is also critical. Cold water is uncomfortable for the patient, can lead to hypothermia with prolonged decontamination, and creates ice hazards during cold weather decontamination. Extremely hot water causes peripheral vasodilatation that can increase toxin absorption. Water should be heated to a warm temperature comfortable for the patient and staff.

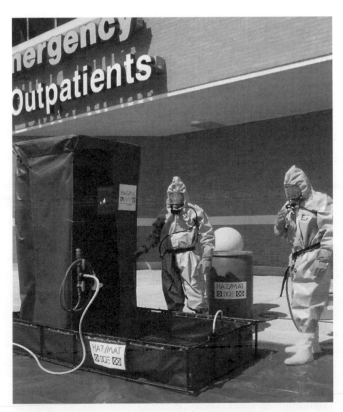

FIGURE 17-1   Portable decontamination system with Level B protection. (Courtesy HAZ/MAT DQE, Indianapolis Indiana.)

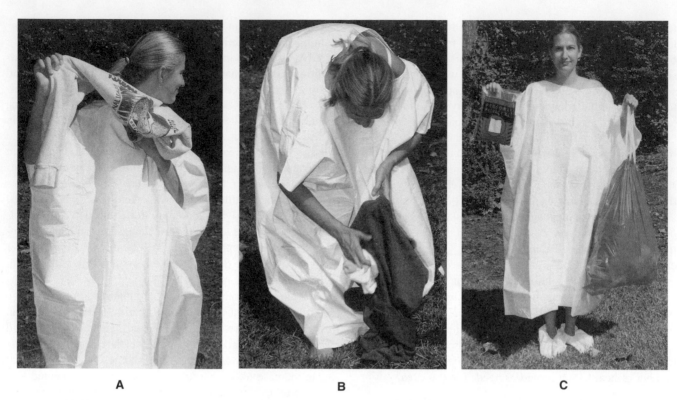

A   **B**   **C**

FIGURE 17-2   **A-C,** Ensuring privacy while using Doffitt kit for clothing removal. (Courtesy HAZ/MAT DQE, Indianapolis, Indiana.)

Decontamination Procedures

One of the easiest but no less critical steps in decontamination is removal of contaminated clothing. Providing a private area for victims to disrobe before decontamination efforts begin is extremely beneficial for decreasing contamination and facilitating the overall decontamination process. All of the victim's belongings should be placed in plastic bags, sealed, and marked with the victim's name and identifying information. Figure 17-2 illustrates the use of a Doffitt kit, which provides privacy for clothing removal.

The U.S. Department of Health and Human Services has stated that although many chemicals can react violently with water, this usually applies when adding water to a large amount of chemical, and not to decontaminating victims whose clothing has been removed and who have little chemical residue on or around their bodies.[14] Therefore after clothing removal, bathing with water is the second critical step in decontamination.

Waste Water.   Containment and disposal of waste water are usually not issues when there is only one patient. However, as the number of patients increases, so does the volume of contaminated water. The type of decontamination set-up that is used determines how waste water is managed. Permanent decontamination rooms usually have self-contained drainage tanks, whereas portable systems collect water in drums (usually 55-gallon). At present, the EPA has not published an official statement regarding containment of waste water by health care facilities after a mass casualty event. Biologic agents in all likelihood pose only a temporary threat, but a chemical incident can result in a more long-term concern. As facilities develop their preparedness plans, local municipalities should be contacted for their expertise regarding contaminated water containment and disposal.

TRIAGE

The intent of triage is to identify those individuals who need immediate assistance, those with less immediate needs, and those with little chance for survival. During a WMD event, all exposed and potentially exposed patients should be directed to the triage team, who will perform a basic assessment. It is important to remember that the first rule in caring for victims of chemical contamination is to prevent further contamination. If the facility is unable to decontaminate victims in a well-ventilated room, or negative pressure room (for chemical agents, smallpox, or plague) within the facility, they should be left outside to prevent contamination of the ED. Unless there is a separate entrance from outside into the decontamination area, all patients should be left outside to prevent contamination of the ED.

Patients may be transported from an incident by ambulance after decontamination or may arrive by private automobile without decontamination. The triage team must wear

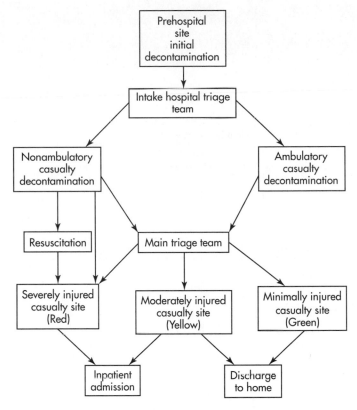

FIGURE 17-3 Emergency department management of contaminated patients.

personal PPE appropriate for the identified agent(s). After decontamination, patients can then be triaged according to established protocols. Figure 17-3 illustrates initial triage, including decontamination by an intake team that determines the patient's care category (red, green, or yellow). Initial triage and other activities that must take place (e.g., securing the health care facility, notification of internal and external authorities) are highlighted in Figure 17-4.

Triage protocols developed for WMD should include agent-specific guidelines, which may be beneficial when caring for patients exposed to chemical or biologic agents. Figure 17-5 outlines treatment protocols for victims exposed to specific chemical agents.[13] Clinical presentation, decontamination procedures, and PPE requirements for specific chemicals are presented in Table 17-2 on p. 199. Table 17-3 on p. 199 identifies clinical presentations, infection control measures, and decontamination procedures appropriate for victims who have been exposed to biologic agents.[5] Figure 17-6 on p. 196 provides quick information regarding isolation and decontamination precautions following biologic weapon exposure.[8]

The triage team should refer incoming patients to the appropriate decontamination area. In the minimally injured treatment area, patients who appear uninjured or minimally injured and do not require medical assistance during decontamination may wash themselves. Throughout the decontamination process, health care providers should be alert for new or evolving symptoms of deterioration secondary to agent exposure.[11] For this reason at least two

health care providers, as well as ancillary personnel, must staff the ambulatory casualty decontamination area.

Patients whose illness or injuries require medical intervention are directed to the nonambulatory decontamination area. The purpose of the decontamination areas is not to provide definitive medical care but to decontaminate patients and subsequently protect other health care providers and the facility from contamination. With a small number of patients, a single decontamination station/set-up may be adequate.

If staffing permits, patients should be sent from the decontamination areas to a main triage team for direction to the appropriate treatment area. Patients who need immediate resuscitation after being decontaminated should be taken to the resuscitation area for intubation and immediate life-saving interventions.

In both decontamination areas, an abbreviated registration is done to capture name, date of birth, and Social Security number. A numbered log is used for all patients seen in the area, and a wristband with the same identifying number is placed on the patient. All belongings should be placed in a large biohazard bag, which is labeled with the same log number as the log sheet and wristband. Using prenumbered forms and belongings bags can decrease the time required for registration and helps with those patients who are unable to give demographic information. Valuables should be placed in a separate, smaller bag and labeled as identified above. If staffing permits, it is beneficial to have valuables cataloged to assist in later return to the owner.

Text continued on p. 201

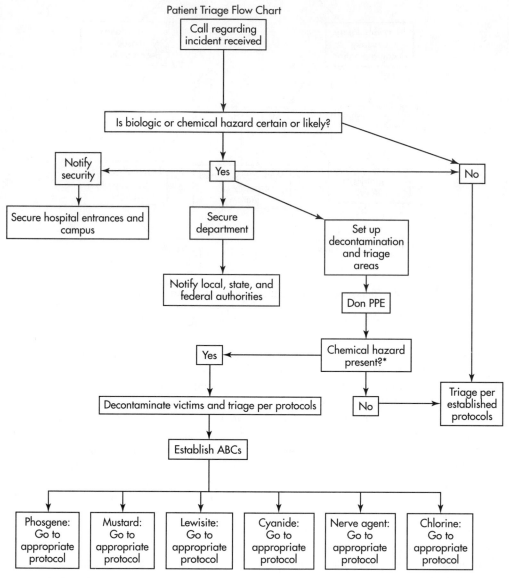

FIGURE **17-4** Patient triage flow chart.

Phosgene Protocol
Restrict fluids
Obtain chest x-rays and blood gases
Oxygen/PEEP

Mustard Protocol
Airway obstruction?
  Tracheotomy
Large burns?
  Establish IV: Do not push fliuds as
    with thermal burns
  Drain vesicules: Unroof large blisters
    and irrigate with topical antibiotics
Treat other symptoms:
  Antibiotic eye ointment
  Morphine PRN

Lewisite Protocol
Treat affected skin with British Anti-
  Lewisite (BAL) ointment, if available
Treat affected eyes with British Anti-
  Lewisite (BAL) ointment, if available
Treat pulmonary symptoms:
  BAL in oil, 0.5 ml/25 lbs/body wgt
  to max. of 4.0 ml. Deep IM; repeat
  q 4 h × 3.
Severe poisoning:
  Shorten interval for BAL injections
    to q 2 hours

Cyanide Protocol
Administer cyanide poisoning kit for
  significant cyanide toxicity and
  persistent high anion gap metabolic
  acidosis
Use clinical response to determine
  administration
Give amyl nitrate until IV access
  obtained, then give sodium nitrite
  followed by sodium thiosulfate
Amyl nitrite:
  Crush 1-2 ampules in gauze and
    hold close to the nose (May also
    place in the lip of the face mask
    or within the Ambu bag.)
  Inhale for 30 seconds per minute
    until IV access is obtained
Sodium nitrite:
  300 mg (10 mls) IV as a 3%
    solution over 5-20 minutes (For
    pediatrics give 0.19-0.33 ml/kg.)
Dilute and infuse slowly if
  hypotensive
May repeat once at half the initial
  dose within 30 to 60 minutes
Sodium thiosulfate:
  12.5 g (50 mls) IV as a 25%
    solution over 10-15 minutes (For
    pediatrics give 0.95-1.85 a
    ml/kg.)
May be given half the initial dose
  after 30-60 minutes

Nerve Agent Protocol
1. Severe respiratory distress?
   No: Go to 6
   Yes: Intubate and ventilate
   Atropine:
     Adults: 6 mg IM or IV
     Infants/Peds: 15-25 ug/kg
   2-PAM C1:
     Adults: 600-1000 mg IM or
       slow IV
     Infants/Peds: 15 mg/kg
2. Major secondary symptoms?
   No: Go to 6
   Yes:
   Atropine:
     Adults: 4 mg IM or IV
     Infants/Peds: 15-25 ug/kg
   2-PAM C1:
     Adults: 600-1000 mg IM or
       slow IV
     Infants/Peds: 15/25 mg/kg
   Open IV line
3. Repeat atropine as needed
4. Repeat 2-PAM C1 as needed:
     Adults: 1.0 gm IV over 20-30
       minutes.
     Repeat q 1 hour × 3 prn
     Infants/Peds: 15 mg/kg
5. Seizures?
   No: Go to 6
   Yes: Diazepam 10 slow IVP
6. Reevaluate q 3-5 minutes; if
     symptoms worsen, repeat from 3.

Chlorine Protocol
Dyspnea?
  Oxygen by mask
  Chest x-ray
Consider phosgene poisoning
Give supportive therapy and treat
  other problems

FIGURE 17-5 Treatment protocols for specific chemical agents.

	BACTERIAL AGENTS								VIRUSES				BIOLOGIC TOXINS			
	Anthrax	Brucellosis	Cholera	Glanders	Bubonic plague	Pneumonic plague	Tularemia	Q Fever	Smallpox	Viral equine encephalitis	Viral encephalitis	Viral hemorrhagic fever	Botulism	Ricin	T-2 Mycotoxins	Enterotoxin B
Isolation precautions																
Standard	!	!	!	!	!	!	!	!	!	!		!	!	!	!	!
Contact		!							!			!				
Airborne				!					!							
Droplet						!					!					
Patient placement																
No restrictions	!							!					!	!	!	!
Cohort patients if no private room available			!		!	!		!	!		!					
Private room		!	!	!	!				!	!		!				
Negative pressure room									!							
Close door at all times				!					!							
Patient transport																
No restrictions	!						!	!			!		!	!	!	!
Limit to essential movement		!	!	!	!	!			!	!		!				
Place mask on patient				!		!			!	!						
Discharge instructions																
No special instructions	!		!	!			!	!		!	!		!	!	!	!
Not discharged until no longer infectious						!			!			!				
Equipment management																
Routine terminal clean			!	!		!		!	!	!	!		!	!	!	!
Disinfect with 10% bleach		!										!				
Dedicated equipment (clean before leaving room)		!							!			!				
Routine linen management	!	!	!	!	!	!	!	!	!	!	!	!	!	!	!	!

FIGURE 17-6 Infection control guidelines: weapons of mass destruction.

Table 17-2	CHEMICAL AGENTS: SYMPTOMS AND CARE		
CHEMICAL AGENT	**CLINICAL PRESENTATION**	**DECONTAMINATION PROCEDURES**	**PERSONAL PROTECTIVE EQUIPMENT**
Phosgene	Ocular: Severe pain, conjunctivitis and keratitis. Dermal: Pain and blanching with erythematous ring, followed by necrosis; absorption through skin can cause pulmonary edema. Respiratory: Immediate upper airway irritation; inhalation and systemic absorption may cause pulmonary edema, necrotizing bronchiolitis, and pulmonary thrombosis. Gastrointestinal: No human data available.	Decontamination immediately after skin and ocular exposure is the only way to prevent or decrease tissue damage because phosgene is absorbed within seconds. Negative pressure room. Patients whose clothing or skin is contaminated with liquid or solid phosgene can contaminate health care providers by direct contact or through off-gassing vapor. Decontaminate before bringing into health care facility. Flush eyes with water 5-10 minutes. Do not cover eyes with bandages. All clothing is removed and skin washed with soap and water. If showers are available, showering with water alone is adequate. Place contaminated clothing and personal belongings in biohazard bag. Contain decontamination runoff.	Pressure-demand, self-contained breathing apparatus. Butyl rubber gloves, eye protection and protective clothing.
Mustard (sulfur and nitrogen)	The sooner after exposure that symptoms occur, the more likely they are to progress and become severe. Ocular: Eyelid swelling and inflammation. Dermal: Erythema. Pulmonary: Laryngitis, shortness of breath, productive cough. Gastrointestinal: Do not induce vomiting.	Decontaminate before bringing into health care facility. Negative pressure room. Contain decontamination runoff. Patients whose clothing or skin is contaminated with liquid or solid mustard can contaminate health care providers by direct contact or through off-gassing vapor. Decontamination within 1-2 minutes after exposure is the only effective way to decrease tissue damage. Place contaminated clothes and personal belongings in biohazard bags.	Pressure-demand, self-contained breathing apparatus. Butyl rubber gloves, eye protection, and protective clothing.
Lewisite and Mustard-Lewisite mixture	Damages skin, eyes, and airways by direct contact. Dermal: Pain and skin irritation within seconds to minutes after contact; erythema and blisters within several hours; starts as small blister in center or erythematous area that expands to include entire inflamed area. Ocular: Vapor causes pain and blepharospasm; edema of conjunctiva and eyelids; high doses may cause corneal damage; liquid Lewisite causes severe eye damage on contact. Respiratory: Burning nasal pain, epistaxis, sinus pain, laryngitis, cough and dyspnea may occur; necrosis can cause local airway obstruction. Gastrointestinal: Inhalation or ingestion may cause nausea and vomiting.	Decontaminate before bringing into health care facility. Negative pressure room. Contain decontamination runoff. To significantly reduce tissue damage, the eyes and skin must be decontaminated within 1-2 minutes after exposure. Place contaminated clothes and personal belongings in biohazard bags.	Pressure-demand, self-contained breathing apparatus. Butyl rubber gloves, eye protection, and protective clothing.

Data from Center for the Study of Bioterrorism & Emerging Infections: Bioterrorism agent fact sheets. Retrieved Decem,ber 18, 2001 from the World Wide Web: www.bioterrorism.slu.edu[4]; McKinney W, Bia F, Stewart C: Bioterrorism: an update for clinicians, pharmacists and emergency management planners. In *Emergency medicine concensus reports,* Atlanta, GA, 2000, American Health Consultants.[11]

Continued

Table 17-2	CHEMICAL AGENTS: SYMPTOMS AND CARE—cont'd		
CHEMICAL AGENT	**CLINICAL PRESENTATION**	**DECONTAMINATION PROCEDURES**	**PERSONAL PROTECTIVE EQUIPMENT**
Lewisite and Mustard-Lewisite mixture—cont'd	Cardiovascular: High-dose exposure may cause capillary permeability and subsequent intravascular fluid loss, hypovolemia, and organ congestion. Renal: High levels of Lewisite may cause renal failure caused by hypotension. Hepatic: High levels may cause hepatic necrosis and hypoperfusion.		
Nerve gases	Respiratory: Bronchial constriction and spasm; severe respiratory distress or apnea; miosis, rhinorrhea. Gastrointestinal: Do not induce emesis.	Decontaminate before bringing into health care facility. Negative pressure room. Contain decontamination runoff. Patients whose clothing or skin is contaminated with liquid or solid nerve agents can contaminate health care providers by direct contact or through off-gassing vapor. If exposed to liquid nerve agent, irrigate eyes 5-10 minutes with water or saline within minutes of exposure to limit injury. If exposed to liquid nerve agent, cut and remove all clothing and wash skin immediately with soap and water. If shower is not available, wash with 0.5% bleach solution. If exposed to vapor only, remove outer clothing and wash exposed skin with soap and water or 0.5% bleach solution. Place contaminated clothes and personal belongings in biohazard bags.	Pressure-demand, self-contained breathing apparatus. Butyl rubber gloves, eye protection, and protective clothing.
Cyanide	Cardiovascular: Dysrhythmias caused by acidosis. Inhalation exposure: Refer to Figure 17.5 for treatment protocols. Dermal: Chemical burns may occur; treat as thermal burns. Ocular: Irrigate for at least 15 minutes; corneal injuries may occur. Abrupt onset of syncope, seizures, coma, gasping respirations, and cardiovascular collapse, causing death within minutes.	Decontaminate before bringing into health care facility. Negative pressure room. Contain decontamination runoff. Patients whose clothing or skin is heavily contaminated with cyanide can contaminate health care providers by direct contact or through off-gassing vapor. Patients exposed only to vapor require no decontamination. Avoid dermal contact with gastric contents that may contain ingested cyanide-containing materials. Remove contaminated clothing and wash with soap and water.	Pressure-demand, self-contained breathing apparatus. Butyl rubber gloves, aprons, eye protection, and protective clothing. Cyanide penetrates most rubbers but butyl rubber provides good, skin protection for a short period.
Chlorine	Acute exposure can cause coughing, eye and nose irritation, tearing. Airway constriction, pulmonary edema and hemoptysis may occur.	Health care providers are at minimal risk of secondary contamination from patients who have been exposed to chlorine gas.	

Table 17-2 CHEMICAL AGENTS: SYMPTOMS AND CARE—cont'd

CHEMICAL AGENT	CLINICAL PRESENTATION	DECONTAMINATION PROCEDURES	PERSONAL PROTECTIVE EQUIPMENT
Chlorine—cont'd	Dermal: Skin irritation, burning pain, inflammation, and blisters. Treat as thermal burns. Liquefied, compressed chlorine can cause frostbite. Treat by rewarming affected areas in a water bath of 102° to 108° for 20-30 minutes. Continue until flush has returned to affected area. Ocular: Do not irrigate frostbitten eyes; if exposed to vapor, irrigate for at least 15 minutes; check for corneal damage.	Clothing or skin soaked with industrial strength bleach or similar solutions may be corrosive to personnel and may release chlorine gas. Remove contaminated clothing and wash with soap and water. Flush exposed skin and hair with plain water for 2-3 minutes; then wash twice with soap and water.	

Data from Center for the Study of Bioterrorism & Emerging Infections: Bioterrorism agent fact sheets. Retrieved December 18, 2001 from the World Wide Web: www.bioterrorism.slu.edu[4]; McKinney W, Bia F, Stewart C: Bioterrorism: an update for clinicians, parmacists and emergency management planners. In *Emergency medicine concensus reports,* Atlanta, GA, 2000, American Health Consultants.[11]

Table 17-3 BIOLOGIC AGENTS: SYMPTOMS AND CARE

DISEASE	CLINICAL FEATURES	INFECTION CONTROL	DECONTAMINATION
Anthrax	Infection begins following inhalation of spores. Prodromal phase: Lasts a few hours to a few days; flulike symptoms including fever, dyspnea, nonproductive cough.	Standard precautions. No private or negative pressure room needed.	Highest risk of infection occurs during initial release, while spores are airborne. Infection following a secondary aerosolization is unlikely. Direct contact with spores should be managed with thorough washing with soap and water; bleach is not necessary. All instruments used in invasive procedures should be sterilized with a sporicidal agent.
Smallpox	Infection begins following inhalation of spores or direct contact between virus and mucous membranes. Patient is asymptomatic during incubation, which is usually 12-14 days. Prodromal phase: Fever, malaise, vomiting, headache, and backache; pustules and scabs appear over 1-2 weeks.	Negative pressure room needed. Gown, gloves, and mask (N-95) needed. Spread via respiratory droplets or through direct contact with contaminated clothing.	If an aerosolization occurs, all virus will be inactivated within 2 days. Standard hospital grade disinfectants are effective in killing the virus and should be used in patient rooms. Linens should be autoclaved or washed in hot water with bleach added. Infectious waste should be placed in biohazard bags and autoclaved before incineration.
Botulism	Inhalation: Onset approximately 72 hours in lab studies; true incubation unknown. Food-borne: 12-36 hours. Wound: 4-18 days. Symptoms: Double or blurred vision, difficulty speaking and swallowing, dry mouth and fatigue; progressive symmetric muscle weakness, beginning in trunk and descending to extremities. Death results from airway obstruction and respiratory paralysis.	Standard precautions only. Respiratory precautions needed if patient is suspected of having flaccid paralysis as a result of meningitis. Human to human transmission does not occur.	Majority of toxin will be inactive within 2 days of release. Following a known exposure, patients and their clothing should be washed with soap and water. Surfaces exposed to an initial release should be cleaned with a 10% bleach solution.
Brucellosis	Incubation period: 5-60 days Nonspecific flulike symptoms: Fever, head and body aches, chills, sweating, weight loss and weakness, anorexia, nausea, vomiting, diarrhea or constipation.	Standard precautions. Person-to-person transmission has occurred from exposure to infected tissue or sexual contact but not through routine care of patients.	Brucella may survive 6 weeks in dust and up to 10 weeks in soil or water but are easily killed by common disinfectants or heat. Standard hospital-approved disinfectants are adequate for cleaning.

Continued

Table 17-3 BIOLOGIC AGENTS: SYMPTOMS AND CARE—cont'd

DISEASE	CLINICAL FEATURES	INFECTION CONTROL	DECONTAMINATION
Cholera	Incubation period: Normally 1-3 days. Patients may either be asymptomatic or have voluminous diarrhea. Abdominal pain and fever are unusual. Symptoms are due to fluid and electrolyte imbalances and may result in hypovolemic shock and renal failure.	Standard precautions unless the patient is incontinent, then contact precautions are necessary. Transmission occurs through the fecal or oral route; proper hygiene is imperative.	Standard hospital approved disinfectants are adequate for cleaning.
Glanders	Incubation period: 1-14 days. May present as either acute or chronic illness. Acute illness most likely in bioterrorism attack. Acute illness presents as either localized disease (pulmonary or mucous membrane) or as fulminant sepsis. Acute septicemia: Fever, headache, night sweats, jaundice, sensitivity to light, diarrhea; generalized redness of skin, often accompanied by necrotizing lesions; acute localized disease. Pulmonary: As above. Mucous membrane: Nasal ulcers and nodules that secrete bloody discharge; papular and/or pustular rash similar to smallpox; liver or spleen abscesses and pulmonary lesions.	Standard precautions unless skin lesions present when contact precautions are necessary. Transmission occurs through inhalation of spores or from contact between nonintact skin and infected tissue.	Standard hospital-approved disinfectants are adequate for cleaning.
Plague	Pneumonic: Most likely to be seen in bioterrorism. Symptoms: Begin in 1-10 days; flulike, including fever, chills, myalgia, weakness, headache, nausea, vomiting, diarrhea, and abdominal pain.	Droplet isolation needed (private room or cohort confirmed cases). Avoid surgery or other aerosol generating procedures. Wear respiratory protection and perform procedure in negative pressure room if invasive procedure is necessary.	Organism remains viable for only 1 hour after aerosol release. Standard hospital-approved disinfectants are adequate for cleaning.
Tularemia	Pneumonic and typhoidal tularemia are the two that are most likely to be seen in a bioterrorism attack. Pneumonic: Nonproductive or minimally productive cough, pleuritic chest pain. Typhoidal: Gastrointestinal symptoms. Both types are likely to lead to sepsis, DIC, and multiorgan failure.	Standard precautions. Tularemia is highly infectious, but there have been no cases of person-to-person transmission.	Can live for weeks in cold, moist conditions. Aerosol release would likely be completely dispersed within a few hours of release. Exposed skin and clothing can be washed thoroughly with soap and water. Contaminated linens should be disinfected via standard hospital procedure.
Q Fever	Incubation period is 2-3 weeks. Symptoms: Begin with sudden onset of fever, chills, headache, weakness, lethargy, anorexia, and profuse sweating.	Standard Precautions. Person-to-person transmission does not occur. Clothing should be handled carefully to avoid reaerosolization.	Resistant to heat and many disinfectants. Exposed individuals should wash skin with soap and water and handle clothing carefully.

Table 17-4 INTERNAL AND EXTERNAL CONTACTS FOR WEAPONS OF MASS DESTRUCTION EVENTS

INTERNAL CONTACTS	EXTERNAL CONTACTS	
Nursing Director	Local EMS Provider	
Medical Director	Local Health Department	
Infection Control	State Health Department	
Administration	FBI Field Office	
	Bioterrorism Emergency Number (CDC)	770/488-7100
	CDC Hospital Infections Program	404/639-6413
	National Response Center	1-800/424-8802
	U.S. Public Health Service	1-800/872-6367

LOCAL, STATE, AND FEDERAL AGENCIES

The reality of a WMD event is that it affects more than the ED. These are community events that require strong relationships between all affected agencies. Preparation should be multidisciplinary and multijurisdictional. Strong collaborative relationships with local, state, and federal agencies improve the collective response to an incident involving WMD.

The ED may be the initial site of recognition for incidents involving biologic warfare. After this occurs, local, state, and federal emergency response systems should be notified. The state office of the Federal Bureau of Investigation, local law enforcement agency, and the Centers for Disease Control and Prevention (CDC) should be notified as soon as determination has been made that an incident has occurred. Table 17-4 on p. 200 identifies those departments that every health care facility should notify. This information should be included in the emergency operations preparedness plan. In addition, nursing and medical directors, internal infection control personnel, and hospital administrators should be notified. A poison control center, if available, can provide valuable information regarding treatment protocols for both chemical and biologic exposures.

When a WMD incident occurs, local and federal authorities should be involved as quickly as possible so the incident can be contained and postexposure protocols can be set in motion. If the event occurs outside the health care facility, such as the Tokyo subway incident, EMS personnel or fire service officials may initiate contact with regulatory and law enforcement agencies. It is critical that ED staff remain vigilant for more covert indications that the community has been exposed to WMDs. Contamination of food supplies, for example, can lead to large numbers of people with symptoms of salmonella poisoning.

Identification of disease presentations that are typical of an endemic process or those that are unusual and raise questions is critical for the public good. Indicators that should alert health care providers of a bioterrorism-related outbreak include a rapidly increasing disease incidence (within hours or days), an unusual increase in patients seeking care with respiratory or gastrointestinal complaints; an endemic disease emerging in an unusual pattern; clusters of patients arriving from a single locale; large numbers of fatal cases; and patients presenting with relatively uncommon diseases, such as anthrax, plague, or tularemia.[7] If any of these indicators are present, the onus of responsibility to notify appropriate agencies rests with the ED.

SUMMARY

Planning and preparation for mass casualties of WMD and smaller numbers of patients involved in industrial exposures are critical to ensure good outcomes for victims and to protect the health care providers. The threat of intentional release of chemical or biologic agents is real, and EDs must begin to develop realistic plans to address this. Regular drills are the only way to acquire the experience and skill necessary to care for contaminated victims and to allay apprehension about the health care facility's ability to treat these patients safely.

References

1. Brennan R, Waeckerie J, Sharp T et al: Chemical warfare agents: emergency medical and emergency public health issues, *Ann Emerg Med* 34(2):191, 1999.
2. Burgess J, Kirk M, Borron S et al: Emergency department hazardous materials protocol for contaminated patients, *Ann Emerg Med* 34(2):205, 1999.
3. Carus WS: *Bioterrorism and biocrime: the illicit use of biological agents in the 20th century,* Washington, DC, 1999, National Defense University.
4. Center for the Study of Bioterrorism & Emerging Infections: Bioterrorism agent fact sheets. Retrieved December 18, 2001 from the World Wide Web: www.bioterrorism.slu.edu.
5. Centers for Disease Control and Prevention: *Bioterrorism references* (2001). Atlanta, 2001, The Centers.
6. Department of Defense Report to Congress: *Domestic preparedness program in the defense against weapons of mass destruction* (1998). Retrieved January 10, 2001 from the World Wide Web: http://www.defenselink.mil/pubs/domestic.html.
7. English J, Cundiff M, Malone J et al: *Bioterrorism readiness plan: a template for healthcare facilities,* Atlanta, Ga, 1999, Centers for Disease Control and Prevention.
8. Johnson S: *Isolation guidelines* (2002). Retrieved February 12, 2002 from the World Wide Web: www.bioterrorism.slu.edu/quick/tables.htm.
9. Levitin H, Siegelson H: Hazardous materials disaster medical planning and response, *Emerg Clin North Amer* 14(2):327, 1996.
10. Macintyre A, Christopher G, Eitzen E et al: Weapons of mass destruction events with contaminated casualties, *JAMA* 283(2):242, 2000.
11. McKinney W, Bia F, Stewart C: Bioterrorism: an update for clinicians, pharmacists and emergency management planners. In *Emergency medicine consensus reports,* Atlanta, Ga, 2000, American Health Consultants.
12. Olson K: Hazmat-o-phobia: why aren't hospitals ready for chemical accidents? *West J Med* 168:32, 1998.
13. Ottawa Fire Department: *Systematic approach to real or potential nuclear, biological or chemical terrorism incidents,* ed 3, Ottawa, Canada, 1999, The Department.
14. U.S. Department of Human Services, Public Health Service, Agency for Toxic Substance and Disease Registry: *Medical management guidelines for acute chemical exposures.* Retrieved February 12, 2002 from the World Wide Web: http://aepo-xdv-www.epo.cdc.gov.

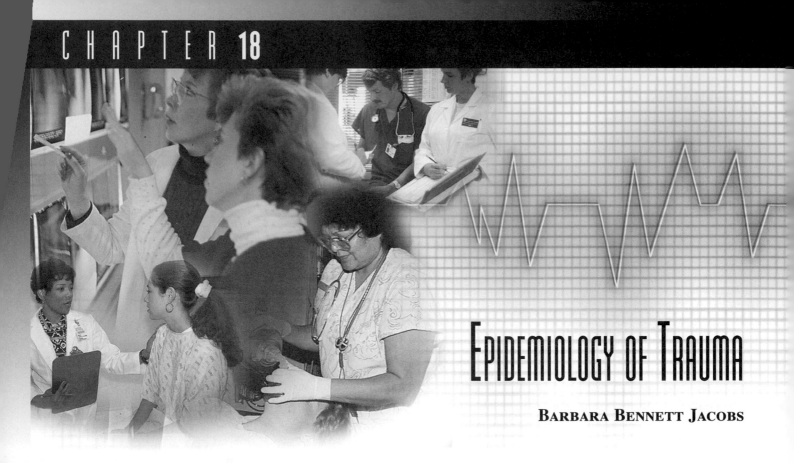

CHAPTER 18

EPIDEMIOLOGY OF TRAUMA

BARBARA BENNETT JACOBS

The "distribution and determinants of disease" is the epidemiology of that disease.[18] The epidemiology of trauma is particularly important because of the implications for social policy, public policy, legislation, and injury prevention programs. Understanding the scope of any problem is central to successful planning and implementation of legal, environmental, and educational remedies. Data elements such as incidence, prevalence, rates, age, sex, race or ethnicity, geographic distribution, and morbidity or mortality are the sources of epidemiologic surveillance and serve to quantify aggregates.

The term "accident" is less frequently used by injury scientists and those involved in prevention because it connotes unexpectedness, random occurrence, and to some extent, inability to be prevented. Researchers examined use of the word "accident" from early writings.[16] Philosophers such as Aristotle and Maimonides used "accident" to describe essential qualities of humans such as one's shape. Use of the word in Biblical, religious, legal, and statistical circles stems from a connotation of random and unexpected reality. Many publications from the U.S. government continue to use the word accident; however, the words "injury" or "trauma" are preferable to describe the significance of this public health problem. Injury comes from the Greek word meaning "wound." Nurses who care for victims of trauma clearly recognize the need for prevention and control strategies to curb trauma mortality and morbidity. Perception of trauma as preventable events rather than acts of random unexpectedness is essential for success of prevention programs. Throughout this chapter the terms "trauma" and "injury" are interchangeable, whereas the term "accident" is used only when the term is used by a reporting agency.

MORTALITY IN THE UNITED STATES

Mortality statistics derived from death certificate data are published annually by the National Center for Health Statistics. Deaths that occur 2 years before the publication date are analyzed. Ten years of data are given in this section to give some perspective on trauma deaths over time because trends in mortality are but one lens used to examine whether prevention, trauma systems of care, or other variables have had an impact. In 1989, 2,150,466 deaths occurred in the United States compared with 2,337,256 deaths in 1998.[28,33] Although these numbers represent a "record high" number of deaths in the United States in 1998, more important, they represent a "record low" in the age-adjusted death rate (471.7/100,000 population). Adjusting for age eliminates distorting effects of areas with a disproportionate percentage of elderly.

Injury Codes and Deaths

The National Center for Health Statistics counts injury deaths by the International Classification of Disease (ICD) "E codes" that describe the external causes of death (i.e., motor vehicle crashes, suicides, homicides). ICD-9 codes in the area of trauma include accidents and their adverse effects (E800-949), suicide (E950-959), homicide and legal intervention (E960-978), and all other external causes (E980-999). All other diseases listed as causes of death, other than trauma, are listed according to N codes or nature codes whereby the actual disease is identified (e.g., diabetes mellitus, meningitis). There is therefore a problem when

Table 18-1	**DEATHS AND DEATH RATES IN THE UNITED STATES FROM 1989 TO 1998**	
YEAR	NUMBER OF DEATHS	DEATH RATE PER 100,000 POPULATION
		CRUDE DEATH RATE	AGE-ADJUSTED DEATH RATE
1989	2,150,466	866.3	523.0
1990	2,148,463	863.8	520.2
1991	2,169,518	860.3	513.7
1992	2,175,613	852.9	504.5
1993	2,268,553	880.0	513.0
1994	2,278,994	875.4	507.4
1995	2,312,132	880.0	503.9
1996	2,314,690	872.5	491.6
1997	2,314,245	864.7	479.1
1998	2,337,256	864.7	471.7*

*Record low.

Table 18-2	**INJURY DEATHS IN THE UNITED STATES FROM 1989 TO 1998**	
YEAR	ACCIDENTS AND ADVERSE EFFECTS (RATE PER 100,000)	SUICIDE, HOMICIDE OR LEGAL INTERVENTION, AND ALL OTHER CAUSES	TOTAL INJURIES
1989	95,028	55,481	150,869
1990	91,983	58,228	150,211
1991	89,347	59,840	149,187
1992	86,777	58,878	145,655
1993	90,523 (35.1%)	60,538 (23.5%)	151,061 (58.6%)
1994	91,437 (34.6%)	59,503 (22.9%)	150,940 (58.0%)
1995	93,320 (35.5%)	57,489 (21.9%)	150,809 (57.4%)
1996	94,948 (35.8%)	55,350 (20.8%)	150,298 (56.6%)
1997	95,644 (35.7%)	54,047 (20.2%)	149,691 (55.9%)
1998	97,835 (36.2%)	52,610 (19.5%)	150,445 (55.7%)

Death rate per 100,000 population.

attempting to identify the actual body system injured that contributed to the death (e.g., spinal cord injury or splenic rupture) because these N codes are not the ones reported in the final death data set. It is possible, however, for researchers to conduct such studies (e.g., in a particular region or state) by requesting death certificate data that contain anatomic locations of injuries.

When E-code categories are combined to identify rate of injury death in the United States, trauma was the fourth leading cause of death for all groups and ages combined in 1998, following diseases of the heart, malignant neoplasms, and cerebrovascular disease. Over the 10 years being examined, deaths from all trauma have been either the third or fourth leading cause of death.[22,25-33]

Table 18-1 depicts the number of all deaths in the United States from 1989 to 1998 and the crude death rate along with the more important age-adjusted death rates. The age-adjusted death rate for 1998 is the lowest rate ever recorded.[33] Table 18-2 presents death rates for those deaths related to injuries in the United States for these same years. In 1998 (the most recent data available), 150,445 deaths from all injuries (accidents and their adverse effects, suicides, homicides or legal intervention, and other external causes) had a combined death rate of 55.7/100,000 population. Death rates for injuries are almost identical to the death rate from all cerebrovascular diseases combined, as seen in Table 18-3.

Age

Comparison of 1994 with 1998 data reveals a slight decrease in the rate of all injury deaths, 57.3 compared with 55.7 (see Table 18-3). The highest death rate from accidents and their adverse effects, suicides, homicides or legal intervention, and other causes continues to be in the age-group 85 years old and older. In 1998, 12,388 total trauma deaths occurred in the 85-year-and-older group, with a death rate of 305.6/100,000 people in that age-group. In comparison, in the 25 to 34 age-group, 22,709 deaths occurred with a cor-

Table 18-3	**DEATH RATES FOR LEADING CAUSES OF DEATH IN THE UNITED STATES FROM 1989 TO 1998**				
YEAR	ALL CAUSES	DISEASES OF THE HEART	MALIGNANT NEOPLASMS	CEREBROVASCULAR DISEASES	ALL INJURIES
1989	866.3	295.6	199.9	58.6	60.8
1990	863.8	289.5	203.2	57.9	60.4
1991	860.3	285.9	204.1	56.9	59.1
1992	852.9	282.5	204.1	56.4	57.0
1993	880.0	288.4	205.6	58.2	58.6
1994	875.4	281.6	206.0	59.2	57.3
1995	880.0	280.7	204.9	60.1	57.4
1996	872.5	276.4	203.4	60.3	56.6
1997	864.7	271.6	201.6	59.7	55.9
1998	864.7	268.2	200.3	58.6	55.7

Death rate per 100,000 population.

Table 18-4	INJURY DEATHS AND DEATH RATES* IN THE UNITED STATES ACCORDING TO AGE FOR 1994 AND 1998†					
AGE-GROUP	DEATH RATE FOR ACCIDENTS AND ADVERSE EFFECTS AND "OTHER"	NUMBER OF ACCIDENTS AND ADVERSE EFFECTS AND "OTHER"	DEATH RATE FOR SUICIDES	NUMBER OF SUICIDES	DEATH RATE FOR HOMICIDE OR LEGAL INTERVENTION	NUMBER OF HOMICIDES OR LEGAL INTERVENTIONS
<1	24.2	936	–	–	8.1	313
<1	22.0	829	–	–	8.5	322
1-4	16.2	2564	–	–	3.0	473
1-4	13	1978	–	–	2.6	399
5-14	9.5	3579	0.9	322	1.5	572
5-14	8.5	3320	0.8	324	1.2	460
15-24	39.9	14,321	13.8	4956	22.6	8116
15-24	36.8	13,691	11.1	4135	14.8	5506
25-34	32.7	14,271	15.4	6354	16.7	6888
25-34	33	12,779	13.8	5365	11.8	4565
35-44	35	14,621	15.3	6375	10.9	4531
35-44	36.9	16,413	15.4	6837	8.0	3567
45-54	31	9231	14.4	4296	6.5	1929
45-54	33.7	11,659	14.8	5131	5.0	1744
55-64	31.6	6638	13.4	2812	4.3	904
55-64	33.3	7554	13.1	2963	3.4	766
65-74	44.9	8403	15.3	2865	3.4	636
65-74	48.9	8999	14.1	2597	2.5	468
75-84	107.1	11,056	21.3	2332	3.6	390
75-85	106.3	12,805	19.7	2355	2.7	318
>85	259.4	9134	23.0	811	3.5	122
>85	282.1	11,436	21.0	851	2.5	101
Unknown	–	118	–	19	–	52
Unknown	–	135	–	17	–	56
TOTAL 1994	35.1	94,872	12.0	31,142	9.6	24,926
TOTAL 1998	36.2	101,598	11.3	30,575	6.8	18,272

*Death rate per 100,000 population.
†Shaded areas represent data for 1998.

responding death rate of 58.6. The greatest number of deaths occurs in the 35 to 44 age-group (26,817) with a corresponding death rate of 60.3, which is 5 times less than in the 85-year-and-older group.[33] Table 18-4 depicts the number of deaths and corresponding death rates for age-groups. Table 18-5 lists the leading causes of death in the United States and ranks them by death rate in the six age-groups. Accidents and their adverse effects are ranked the leading cause of death for all ages from 1 to 44 during 1998. This is slightly different than 1994, in which human immunodeficiency virus was ranked the leading cause of death for those

between the ages of 25 and 44 with accidents and their adverse effects ranked as the leading cause of death for those between ages 1 and 24 in 1994.[30,33]

In 1998 unintentional injury is ranked as the seventh leading cause of death for people 65 years and older.[36] The phrase "unintentional injury" refers to motor vehicle crashes, falls, surgical or medical complications related to injury, ingestions, and fires or burns. Motor vehicle crashes are the leading cause of injury death for people in the 65 to 74 age-group and falls are the leading cause of injury death for those age 75 years and older.[36]

Table 18-5	RANKINGS OF LEADING CAUSES OF DEATH BY AGE-GROUP IN THE UNITED STATES FOR 1994 AND 1998*†					
CAUSE	I TO 4 YEARS	5 TO 14 YEARS	15 TO 24 YEARS	25 TO 44 YEARS	45 TO 64 YEARS	65+ YEARS
Accidents and adverse effects	1	1	1	2	3	7
Accidents and adverse effects	1	1	1	1	3	7
Diseases of the heart	5	5	5	4	2	1
Diseases of the heart	5	5	5	3	2	1
Cerebrovascular diseases			10	8	4	3
Cerebrovascular diseases		10	10	8	4	3
Congenital anomalies	2	4	7			
Congenital anomalies	2	4	6			
Malignant neoplasms	3	2	4	3	1	2
Malignant neoplasms	4	2	4	2	1	2
Homicide	4	3	2	6		
Homicide	3	3	2	6		
Suicide		6	3	5	9	
Suicide		6	3	4	8	
Chronic obstructive pulmonary disease		8	8		5	4
Chronic obstructive pulmonary disease		7	7		6	4
Pneumonia and influenza	7	9	9	10	10	5
Pneumonia and influenza	6	8	8	10	9	5
Human immunodeficiency virus	6	7	6	1	8	
Human immunodeficiency virus			9	5	10	
Chronic liver disease and cirrhosis				7	7	
Chronic liver disease and cirrhosis				7	7	
Diabetes mellitus				9	6	6
Diabetes mellitus				9	5	6

*Death rate per 100,000 population.
†Shaded areas represent data for 1998.

Sex

Sex along with age variances in injury deaths are related to the type of injury incurred. In 1998 there were 104,217 (69%) total injury deaths of males compared with 46,228 (31%) total injury deaths to females, as seen in Table 18-6. In comparison to 1994 there were 107,914 male injury deaths compared with 43,026 female injury deaths, a percentage of 71% to 29%.[30,33]

Race

Race is another variable frequently used to stratify injury deaths. As calculated by the National Center for Health Statistics and using their terms for different races, in 1998 whites had a higher death rate from suicide (12.4) compared

with blacks (5.7) and other races (6.2). The death rate for accidents and their adverse effects demonstrates little differences by race; 36.9 for whites, 37.2 for blacks, and 33.1 for all other races. The homicide or legal intervention death rate for blacks is 24.5 compared with 4.1 for whites, and 19.1 for all other races. The homicide or legal intervention rate for blacks significantly declined in 1998 from 1994 when the rate was 37.4 (see Table 18-7).[30,33]

Geographic Differences

Geographic differences exist in injury mortality. Table 18-8 demonstrates that southern states tend to have higher injury death rates with no change in this trend for the 2 years compared.[30,33] In 1998 the state with the highest death rate from motor vehicle crashes was South Carolina

Table 18-6   Injury Deaths and Death Rates* in the United States for Males and Females for 1994 and 1998†

Injury Category	Male deaths and death rates	Female deaths and death rates	Total injury deaths and death rates
Accidents and adverse effects	60,509 (47.6)	30,928 (23.2)	91,437 (35.1)
Accidents and adverse effects	63,042 (47.7)	34,793 (25.2)	97,835 (36.2)
Suicide	25,174 (19.8)	5,968 (4.5)	31,142 (12.0)
Suicide	24,538 (18.6)	6,037 (4.4)	30,575 (11.3)
Homicide or legal intervention	19,707 (15.5)	5,219 (3.9)	24,926 (9.6)
Homicide or legal intervention	14,023 (10.6)	4,249 (3.1)	18,272 (6.8)
All other injury causes	2,524 (2.0)	911 (0.7)	3,435 (1.3)
All other injury causes	2,614 (2.0)	1,149 (0.8)	3,763 (1.4)
Total 1994	107,914	43,026	150,940
Total 1998	104,217	46,228	150,445

*Death rate per 100,000 population.
†Shaded areas represent data for 1998.

Table 18-7   Injury Deaths and Death Rates* in the United States by Race for 1994 and 1998†

Injury Category	Number of deaths and death rates for whites	Number of deaths and death rates for blacks	Number of deaths for all other races except black or white
Accidents and adverse effects	75,894 (35.1)	12,767 (39.1)	2776
Accidents and adverse effects	82,178 (36.9)	12,801 (37.2)	2856
Suicide	27,976 (12.9)	2271 (7.0)	895
Suicide	27,648 (12.4)	1977 (5.7)	950
Homicide or legal intervention	11,976 (5.5)	12,207 (37.4)	743
Homicide or legal intervention	9241 (4.1)	8420 (24.5)	611
All other causes	2634 (1.2)	719 (2.2)	82
All other causes	2968 (1.3)	709 (2.1)	86
TOTAL 1994	118,480	27,964	4496
TOTAL 1998	122,035	23,907	4503

*Death rate per 100,000 population.
†Shaded areas represent data for 1998.

Table 18-8   Number of Deaths Higher Than 2500 per year and Death Rates* from Accidents and Their Adverse Effects Ranked According to Death Rates in 1994 and 1998

State	Number of deaths 1994	Number of deaths 1998	Death rates 1994	Death rates 1998	Rank in United States 1994	Rank in United States 1998
Tennessee	2449	2627	48.1	48.4	1	1
Georgia	2822	3156	40.9	41.3	2	3
North Carolina	2823	3278	40.6	43.4	3	2
Florida	5155	5877	37.6	39.4	4	4
Pennsylvania	4226	4573	35.1	38.1	5	5
Texas	6218	7421	34.5	37.6	6	6
Illinois	3899	3891	33.4	32.3	7	7
California	9793	9264	31.4	28.4	8	10
Michigan	2866	3133	30.3	31.9	9 (shared)	8
Ohio	3347	3546	30.3	31.6	9 (shared)	9
New York	5118	4676	28.2	25.7	10	11

*Death rate per 100,000 population.

Table 18-9	DEATHS RELATED TO FIREARMS IN THE UNITED STATES FOR 1994 AND 1998				
AGE-GROUPS	DEATHS FROM ACCIDENTS RELATED TO FIREARM MISSILES	DEATHS FROM SUICIDE RELATED TO FIREARMS	DEATHS FROM HOMICIDE OR LEGAL INTERVENTION RELATED TO FIREARMS	DEATHS UNDERMINED WHETHER ACCIDENTALLY OR PURPOSELY INFLICTED BY FIREARMS	TOTAL DEATHS RELATED TO FIREARMS
<1	2	–	11	–	13
<1	–	–	5	–	5
1-4	32	–	60	2	94
1-4	19	–	58	1	78
5-14	151	188	398	28	765
5-14	102	154	254	19	529
15-24	540	3344	6983	189	11056
15-24	260	2510	4559	91	7420
25-34	243	3532	5183	116	9074
25-34	137	2789	3329	54	6309
35-44	155	3264	3025	75	6519
35-44	143	3329	2161	57	5690
45-54	95	2443	1233	45	3816
45-54	77	2652	1005	47	3781
55-64	46	1797	531	30	2404
55-64	63	1873	401	19	2356
65-74	46	2010	282	15	2353
65-74	34	1831	206	10	2081
75-84	32	1684	119	14	1849
75-84	21	1739	85	10	1855
>85	13	497	19	3	532
>85	9	543	20	6	578
Unknown	1	6	22	1	30
Unknown	1	4	19	2	26
ALL AGE-GROUPS 1994					38505
ALL AGE-GROUPS 1998					30708

*Shaded areas represent data for 1998.

(25.9/100,000), and the state with the lowest motor vehicle crash death rate was Massachusetts (7.9/100,000). The state with the highest suicide rate was Nevada (22.7/100,000), and the state with the lowest was New Jersey (7.2/100,000). The area with the highest homicide and legal intervention death rate was the District of Columbia (41.9/100,000). Five states have such few deaths in this category that their rates are not even calculated because they don't meet the standards of reliability or precision. These states and the actual number of deaths resulting from homicide or legal intervention are New Hampshire (19), Vermont (10), North Dakota (11), South Dakota (10), and Wyoming (19).[33]

FIREARM-RELATED DEATHS

The National Center for Health Statistics publishes firearm-related injury deaths as a separate category in its death data reports. Table 18-9 demonstrates that in 2 years (1994 and 1998), 69,213 people died from a firearm-related injury. Firearm-related deaths are more likely to occur in males than in females—regardless of the victim's age. In 1998, 85% of the 30,708 injury deaths by firearms were male. Of the 17,424 suicide deaths from firearms, males accounted for 87%, whereas firearms accounted for 71% of all male suicide deaths. Of the 12,102 homicide and legal intervention deaths by firearms, 83% were male, 51% were black, and 46% were white; 73% of all the black homicide or legal intervention deaths are firearm-related.[33] A special issue of the *American Journal of Preventive Medicine* was devoted to firearm-related injury surveillance.[12] Eight states and New York City reported results of their surveillance systems; sample information from these surveillance systems is depicted in Table 18-10.

Surveillance is a public health tenet—without it, prevention programs cannot be tailored to meet the goal of injury reduction. The Centers for Disease Control and Prevention (CDC) has clearly stated that the same surveillance related to motor vehicle crashes needs to be adopted for firearm violence. Since 1960 the U.S. government has tracked all fatal motor vehicle crashes. According to the CDC, "this science-based public health approach to preventing motor vehicle-related injuries saved hundreds of thousands of lives without ever having to ban automobiles."[41] The implication is that banning firearms may not be a solution to the devastating number of firearm-related deaths and injuries; however, the CDC statement does not suggest that other legal interventions to curb firearm usage are moot. It is chilling to note that during the 33-year period from 1962 to 1994, there was a 130% increase in the number or firearm-related deaths.[21]

GENERAL ESTIMATES OF NONFATAL INJURIES

The incidence of nonfatal injuries is more difficult to determine. Currently, the National Electronic Injury Surveillance System does track injuries related to consumer products. The CDC and the U.S. Consumer Product Safety Commission determined that this system could be expanded to cover all injuries regardless of cause, but such an expansion is not yet in place. However, a few available statistics reflect the wide magnitude of the injury occurrence problem. Excluding newborns, 30.8 million people are discharged annually from short-stay hospitals in the United States; of these 2.6 million are related to injuries and/or poisonings.[23] Annually, 36.9 million visits are made to emergency departments in the United States.[7]

Of the 11 million people age 65 years and older who are hospitalized annually, 8.2% or 943,000 are related to injuries or poisonings. A significant percent (52%) of injury-related admissions are due to fractures.[23] Of interest is that medical costs for the geriatric population is 2.5 times greater than for younger patients with similar injuries; this is due to longer lengths of stays, higher incidence of complications, and more intensive care unit days.[3,44]

Particular Injuries

Falls

It is estimated that 1 of 3 elderly adults fall per year.[42] What is particularly disturbing is that one study concluded that 50% of elder adults hospitalized as a result of a fall are at risk for death within 1 year's time of the fall event.[42] Falls

Table 18-10	FIREARM-RELATED INJURY SURVEILLANCE FACTS
California[14]	There were 5137 deaths in 1994. Assaults accounted for 57% of the above deaths. People ages 15 to 24 are at the highest risk for death. 7,969 people were hospitalized with nonfatal injuries. Between 1990 and 1995 more teenagers died from firearm-related injuries than from vehicle related injuries.
Colorado[11]	In 1994, there were 490 deaths, 400 hospitalizations, and another 100 injuries not requiring hospitalization. 69% of deaths were due to suicide. 85% of deaths resulting from suicide occurred outside a hospital without medical treatment.
Massachusetts[2]	There was a 41% decrease in the number of gun assaults seen in emergency departments: 662 in 1994 and 393 in 1996. Shootings dropped 50% for both blacks and Hispanics, compared with the 25% decrease for non-Hispanic whites.
Missouri[51]	In 1994 84% of gunshot wound victims were male. In 1994 the majority (75%) of male gunshot wound victims were between ages 15 and 34 years.
New York City[51]	A significant decline in the assault death rate occurred between 1990 and 1995, with a 46% decline. In 1995 there were 856 male deaths, 221 female deaths, 6535 male hospitalizations, and 1378 female hospitalizations for weapon-related injuries.

All information related to injuries and deaths is firearm-related.

that result in fractures of the hip in the elderly have some particular characteristics: (1) 84% of them occur at home; (2) 76% occur indoors; (3) 76% occur while the victim is standing; (4) 72% fall in a sideways direction; (5) 47% occur when the victim is moving forward; (6) very few falls (10%) are related to wet or slippery surfaces; and (7) 13% of falls occur as a result of some manifestation of another medical condition such as dizziness, seizures, or sudden paralysis.[38] Research has been replicated that demonstrates that such extrinsic factors as objects in the environment (e.g., furniture, cords, loose mats) are associated with only 25% of falls and that intrinsic factors such as balance and gait are more frequently associated with falls that result in fractures.[37]

Burns

Fortunately, the incidence of serious burns and subsequent hospitalizations has decreased by 50% over the last two decades. Unfortunately, burn injury is the third leading cause of death for children. For those between ages 1 and 4 years, burns are the second leading cause of death.[4] Annually there are approximately 1.25 million burn injuries, of which 51,000 people are hospitalized and approximately 10% die.[4,52] Burns rank as the fifth leading cause of unintentional injury death. The majority of deaths from burns in house fires is due to inhalation of toxic substances.[8,36,40] Those under age 5 and over age 65 are the most susceptible to scald burns from hot liquids; these injuries may lead to hospitalization but rarely lead to death.[40] Those older than age 65 are the group who sustain the majority (75%) of burns from clothing ignition resulting from cigarette smoking or use of stoves and space heaters.

Contact with electrical current leading to electrical burns causes approximately 1000 deaths per year, whereas another 80 deaths per year are due to lightning.[40] It has been estimated that care for a burn victim in a hospital may cost between $36,000 and $117,000. Death of a person in a fire costs between $250,000 and $1.5 million when lost years of estimated productivity are considered in the calculation.[40]

Central Nervous System Injuries

It has been reported by other injury epidemiologists that injury to the central nervous system accounts for 40% to 50% of deaths resulting from trauma.[17] It has also been estimated that the rate of hospitalization for injuries to the brain that are either fatal or nonfatal is 237/100,000 people.[15] It has been reported that subdural hematomas lead to death more frequently than do other lesions and that they are seen more frequently in the older population.[13]

Injuries to the spinal cord are particularly devastating because of effects on neurologic function. The majority (75%) of spinal cord–injured victims are male. The average number of spinal cord injuries is approximately 12,000 per year—of which 40%, or 4800, are fatal. Mechanisms of injury for spinal cord injury include motor vehicle crashes, sports-related events, and violence.[20]

Skeletal Injuries

Injuries to the bony skeleton and the accompanying structures of muscles, tendons, joints, and ligaments are perhaps the most common type of injury. It has been estimated that greater than 50% of admissions to hospitals as a result of trauma are related to fractures, particularly of the lower extremity.[46] The American Association of Orthopedic Surgeons has made available the following information about musculoskeletal injuries[39]:

- Musculoskeletal injuries account for 8000 deaths per year
- 32.7 million musculoskeletal injuries occur annually
- Of the above injuries, 6.1 million are fractures, 14.6 million are dislocations and sprains, 9.4 million have open wounds, and 2.6 million represent "other" injuries

---

Box 18-1 FACTS RELATED TO 1999 MOTOR VEHICLE CRASHES

41,611 traffic-related deaths, with an estimated 3.236 million people injured

35,806 vehicle occupants, 4906 pedestrians, 750 pedalcyclists, and 149 "others" were killed

25,210 (61% of all traffic-related deaths) were drivers; 10,499 were passengers (25%), 5805 were nonmotorists (14%)

2276 operators of motorcycles and another 195 motorcycle passengers were killed; an estimated 50,000 motorcycle-related nonfatal injuries occurred

27,973 of the people killed in traffic-related events were male (67%) and 13,627 (33%) were female

Estimates indicate that 38% of all fatal crashes and 7% of all crashes were alcohol-related

In 1989, 49% of all crashes were alcohol-related; in 1999 there were 15,786 alcohol-related fatalities compared with 22,404 in 1989, a 30% decline

30% of traffic fatalities included at least one driver or nonoccupant with a blood alcohol concentration of 0.10 g/dl or greater; 56% (6960) of the 12,321 total fatalities in this group were drivers and 20% (2443) were passengers

1.4 million drivers in 1998 were arrested for driving under the influence of alcohol or narcotics

Of the 41,611 people killed in traffic-related events, the age-group with the highest rate of death (based on the estimated population of the specific age-groups) is the 16 to 20 age-group at 29.85, followed by those ages 21 to 24 years at 27.49, those older than age 74 years at 24.66, those in the 25 to 34 age-group at 17.98, and those between the ages of 65 and 74 have a death rate of 16.81 (these five age-groups represent the five highest death rates from traffic-related deaths)

Most traffic events that result in deaths occur between midnight and 3:00 AM on both Saturdays and Sundays.

Of the 6.3 million motor vehicle crashes reported to police, close to one third result in injury; less than 1% resulted in a death; the total number of fatal crashes (not persons killed) were 37,043

The majority of fatal crashes occur on undivided roadways (24,374 or 66%), of which the majority of these, 21,552 or 88%, are on two-lane undivided roadways; divided roadways account for 11,853 or 32% of all fatal crashes

51% of the total fatal crashes occur in the daylight, 30% occur in the dark, and the rest occur when it is dark but lighted or at dawn or dusk

49.3% of the 56,668 vehicles involved in fatal crashes are passenger cars and 35.1% are light trucks

Speeding was involved in 30% of all fatal crashes

15 deaths occurred as a result of traffic crashes involving ambulances: 2 ambulance passengers, 2 pedestrians, and 11 occupants of other vehicles

72 deaths occurred as a result of traffic crashes involving police vehicles: 17 police vehicle drivers, 4 police vehicle passengers, 40 occupants of other vehicles, 10 pedestrians, and 1 pedalcyclist

19 deaths occurred as a result of traffic crashes involving fire trucks: five fire truck drivers, three fire truck passengers, nine occupants of other vehicles, one pedestrian, and one pedalcyclist

MOTOR VEHICLE CRASHES

The Fatal Accident Reporting System and the General Estimates System are compiled annually by the National Highway Traffic Safety Administration (NHTSA) and published as a report called *Traffic Safety Facts*.[47] Changes over time reflect interesting issues associated with motor vehicle crashes. In 1966 the fatality rate per 100 million miles traveled in the United States was 5.5. In 1997, 1998, and 1999 the rate has consistently been at the record low of 1.6. Facts related to the 1999 *Traffic Safety Facts* are listed in Box 18-1.[47]

Restraint Use

Since the first mandatory seat belt law was enacted in New York State in 1984, 49 states and the District of Columbia have enacted seat belt laws. Since the first mandatory child restraint use law was enacted in Tennessee in 1978, all 50 states and the District of Columbia have child restraint laws. In 1998, 54.5% of the 15,167 drivers killed in passenger cars were using restraints, as were 51.8% of drivers in light trucks, 70.1% of drivers killed in large trucks, and 73.8% of the drivers killed in buses. Restraint use is even higher in those drivers involved in nonfatal crashes: 80.6% of drivers of passenger cars were using restraints, as were 80.4% of drivers in light trucks, 70.5% of drivers in large trucks, and 77.5% of drivers in buses. Most staggering is that 49.2% of those children under age 5 killed in crashes were not using restraints, 55.2% of those between ages 5 and 9, and 66.5% of those between ages 10 and 15 were also not using restraints. NHTSA has reported that lap and shoulder safety belts "reduce the risk of fatal injury to front seat passenger car occupants by 45% and the risk of moderate-to-critical injury by 50%." More people are using occupant protection. In 1998 NHTSA reported that the observed use of shoulder belts is 68.9% in comparison with a rate of 58% in 1994.[48]

Air Bags

In the United States all new passenger cars of the model year 1998 and later must be equipped with driver and front seat passenger air bags. Air bags, however, are not considered primary restraint systems but are "supplemental" to lap and shoulder belts. An ongoing Special Crash Investigation Program sponsored by NHTSA provides data associated with adult passengers, drivers, and children who sustain fatal or serious injuries in "minor or moderate severity air bag deployment crashes."[34] Table 18-11 reflects the most current data related to this somewhat controversial type of safety mechanism.

The NHTSA Website (http://nhtsa.dot.gov) has a special section devoted to the most updated information on rules and regulations governing on and off switches for air bags. The following points regarding driving in a car equipped with air bags are recommended by NHTSA[35]:

- Children 12 years and younger should ride in the back seat of cars.
- Never use a rear-facing child-restraint seat in a seat with an air bag.
- Always wear a lap and shoulder belt even in vehicles equipped with air bags.
- When driving a car equipped with an air bag, sit at least 10 inches away from the steering wheel and tilt the seat "rearward."
- There are some situations authorized by NHTSA that permit air bag deactivation if the vehicle is not equipped with an air bag off switch.

School Buses

Although the incidence of crashes involving school buses is low, the public is concerned that safety restraints are not standard equipment. Understanding the epidemiology associated with school bus injuries and deaths is an example of how a problem must be identified before implementing

Table 18-11 CONFIRMED NUMBER OF PEOPLE IN THE UNITED STATES WITH A FATAL INJURY OR A LIFE-THREATENING INJURY RELATED TO AN AIR BAG*		
OCCUPANT TYPE	NUMBER OF PEOPLE WITH FATAL INJURY	NUMBER OF PEOPLE WITH NONFATAL INJURY
Children in rear-facing child safety seats	19	8
Children in forward-facing child safety seats	5	2
Children unrestrained or improperly restrained	71	17
Children wearing lap and shoulder belt	6	3
Children injured by driver air bag	3	1
Drivers belted	18	1
Drivers misused belt	3	0
Drivers not belted	42	6
Drivers unknown belt use	1	0
Adult passengers belted	2	4
Adult passengers misused belt	0	0
Adult passengers not belted	5	1
Adult passengers unknown belt use	0	1
TOTAL	**175**	**44**

*Data as of April 1, 2001.

Box 18-2 **NUMBER OF VEHICLES AND NUMBER OF DEATHS INVOLVING BUSES IN THE UNITED STATES IN 1999**

TYPE OF BUS	NUMBER OF BUSES	NUMBER OF OCCUPANT FATALITIES
School bus	138	8
Intercity/cross-country bus	38	32
Transit bus	105	5
Other bus	20	4
Unknown type of bus	16	9
TOTAL	318	58

those strategies that will have the most effect on prevention of such injuries. The majority of deaths involving school buses are not to the buses' occupants. The people who were passengers on school buses involved in fatal crashes from 1989 to 1999 represent only 10% of all fatalities (bus drivers represent 2% and passengers 8%), nonoccupants such as pedestrians and bicyclists represent 25%, and the majority (65%) were occupants of other vehicles involved in the crash. Of the 411,000 fatal traffic crashes in the United States since 1989, 0.31% or 1291 were school bus-related and led to the deaths of 1445 people. Fifty percent of all the school-age pedestrians killed by school buses were between ages 5 and 7. School buses are used to transport passengers other than school children. In the 11 years from 1989 to 1999, there have been 21 people killed in such crashes (5 drivers, 16 passengers). However, one crash in 1987 claimed the lives of 27 occupants. These data indicate that promoting safety around school buses being used for transport of children is one of the necessary prevention strategies.[49] NHTSA has a free school bus safety program for teaching children how to be cautious and vigilant around school buses. Box 18-2 contains information related to traffic crashes involving all buses, not just school buses, in 1999.

THE UNPOWERED SCOOTER

The new lightweight aluminum unpowered scooters hit the commercial market in the year 2000; an older version was sold in the years 1998 and 1999. The CDC and the Consumer Product Safety Commission (CPSC) have published a report estimating that 27,600 injured people were treated in emergency departments for scooter-related injuries between 1998 and 2000.[6] The majority (85%) are children younger than 15 years of age, 23% were older than age 8, and 66% were male. Injuries from using these scooters were fractures or dislocations (29%), lacerations (24%), contusions and abrasions (22%), and strains and sprains (14%). Injuries are predominately of the arms and hands (42%), the head and face (27%), and to the leg and foot (24%). Two deaths during this time were reported; one to an adult who sustained a head injury and the other a 6-year-old boy struck by a car. The CDC has made the following recommendations for scooter use[6]:

- Scooter riders should wear helmets that meet CPSC standards.
- Scooter riders should wear knee and elbow pads.
- Scooters should be used on "smooth, paved surfaces without traffic."
- Scooters should not be used on "water, sand, gravel, or dirt."
- Scooter riding should be avoided at night.
- Supervision should be provided for young children using scooters.

VIOLENCE-RELATED TRAUMA

Research supported by the National Institute of Justice and the CDC was published in the year 2000 under the title, *Extent, Nature, and Consequences of Intimate Partner Violence*.[45] Findings were the results of a national telephone survey of 8000 women and 8000 men in the United States. Using the phrase "intimate partner violence" the study concluded that:

- 25% of the women surveyed admitted to being "raped and/or physically assaulted by a current or former spouse, cohabiting partner, or date at some time in their lifetime."
- 7.6% of men surveyed admitted to the same.
- Using the figures above to estimate the prevalence of intimate partner violence, the researchers concluded that:

  In the United States, 1.5 million women and 834,732 men "are raped and/or physically assaulted by an intimate partner" annually.

  Because victims often are abused more than once, researchers estimated that 4.8 million "intimate partner rapes and physical assaults are perpetrated against U.S. women annually and approximately 2.9 million intimate partner physical assaults are committed against U.S. men annually."

  Of the 4.8 million rapes and assaults to women, it is estimated that 2 million result in injury to women.

  Of the 2.9 million assaults to men, 581,391 result in an injury.

- Only 20% of rapes, 25% of physical assaults, and 50% of stalkings against females are reported to the police.

Perhaps one of the more devastating injuries to children that requires the care of emergency nurses is maltreatment. Three million children annually are estimated to be maltreated with the resulting deaths of three children per day.[19] Violence also extends to the elderly, and an estimated 700,000 to 1.1 million elderly people are being abused.[1] See Chapters 49 through 51 for further discussion of child abuse and neglect, intimate partner violence, and elder abuse and neglect.

COMPARISON WITH OTHER COUNTRIES

The 1998 report from the International Collaborative Effort on Injury Statistics, which studied the injury problem in 10 countries, found that the United States death rate from injuries is approximately 56 to 57 per 100,000. This rate was similar to rates in New Zealand and Norway, but the country with the highest rate was France at 75 per 100,000. England, Wales, Israel, and The Netherlands reported the lowest death rates from injuries.[24] The most troublesome data indicated that the firearm death rate in the United States was twice the rate of all other countries studied. A report from the World Bank determined that of 26 industrialized countries, the United States had a homicide death rate 5 times greater for children younger than age 15 years, a suicide rate twice as great, and a firearm-related death rate that approximated 12 times the rates of other countries for the same age-group.[53]

NATIONAL CENTER FOR INJURY PREVENTION AND CONTROL AT THE CDC

In 1986 the CDC established the Division of Injury Epidemiology and Control in the Center for Environmental Health. In 1992 this division became an official center—the National Center for Injury Prevention and Control (NCIPC). The NCIPC has approximately 140 staff. (The entire CDC has more than 6000 staff with an annual budget of $2.5 million.) It is divided into three divisions: acute care, rehabilitation, research and disability prevention; unintentional injury prevention; and violence prevention. The Center operates five offices including the Office of Research Grants. Annually, approximately $15 million is used to fund extramural grants. There are 10 funded injury control research centers in the United States: Seattle, San Francisco, Los Angeles, Fort Collins, Iowa City, Birmingham, Chapel Hill, Baltimore, Pittsburgh, and Cambridge (Harvard). These centers may focus research on the three phases of injury control (prevention, acute care, or rehabilitation) or in the areas of epidemiology or biomechanics.[43]

INJURY PREVENTION

William Haddon, the first Director of NHTSA, is credited with developing the most widely used epidemiologic model of injury prevention.[9] The Haddon Injury Matrix can be used to construct injury prevention programs that target the preevent, event, or postevent phases. The phases are viewed from the perspective of human factors, vehicle or vector factors, and environmental factors that could contribute to injuries or death. Table 18-12 describes possible injury prevention strategies to reduce falls in the elderly. In general most injury control strategies can be classified according to the three Es. For example, programs to prevent injuries from falls in the elderly address engineering and technologic interventions such as specially designed padded underwear; enforcement and legislative interventions such as regulations related to restraint use; and education and behavioral interventions such as the CDC's *Check for Safety: a Home Fall Prevention Checklist for Older Adults* that is free from the Center.

Haddon is credited with developing the 10 strategies for injury prevention depicted in Table 18-13, which also provides examples related to reducing the incidence of motorcycle-related injuries.[10] Some suggestions may appear unrealistic, yet they are used as examples of strategies that are practically possible but may not be politically attainable.

Not all injury prevention programs work. The key is to implement an evaluation system that measures the impact of all prevention programs. Some may view prevention of one death or one injury as a success, but when scarce resources are used in public health, the impact of expense must be justified. It is difficult to determine the effect of some programs; for example, a red ribbon tied around one's side-mounted mirror or educational programs for teens and drunk-driving prevention. The CDC has *A Primer on Evaluation for Programs to Prevent Unintentional Injury* that describes in detail the qualitative and quantitative research methods to evaluate programs.[5] Its evaluation method is divided into four stages: formative evaluation, process evaluation, impact evaluation, and outcome evaluation.

Access to the Internet is access to a gold mine of sources for prevention programs, such as the free *Campaign Safe and Sober Program* that can be obtained from each state's department of transportation. The entire program provides posters, planning guides, and event calendars. Since 1992 the *Traffic Safety Digest* has been available to any interested injury prevention planner; it is a quarterly digest of traffic

Table 18-12	THE HADDON INJURY MATRIX TO PLAN PREVENTION STRATEGIES		
PHASES	HUMAN FACTORS	VEHICLE OR VECTOR FACTORS	ENVIRONMENTAL FACTORS
Preevent	Reduce use of sedatives	Correct defects in safety equipment (e.g., walkers, wheel chairs)	Use of safety bars, handrails, side rails on beds
Event	Consider reduction in severity of preexisting medical conditions (e.g., vertigo, imbalance)	Cover exposed skin areas with protective barriers to reduce severity of injury (e.g., elbow and knee pads)	Reduction of clutter in the patient's environment
Postevent	Consider if patient is on anticoagulants or other medications and their effects on subsequent bleeding or physiologic response to shock and trauma	Have patients avoid areas where they could become trapped after a fall and where access to help is minimal	Implementation of comprehensive emergency response protocols and systems

Table 18-13	HADDON'S STRATEGIES FOR INJURY PREVENTION RELATED TO MOTORCYCLE CRASHES	
STRATEGY	**APPLICATION TO MOTORCYCLE INJURIES**
Prevent creation of the hazard	Do not manufacture motorcycles
Reduce amount of the hazard	Reduce the amount of motorcycles manufactured that are associated with significant injury
Prevent release of an existing hazard	Ban certain types of motorcycles (e.g., similar to the ban on all-terrain three-wheel vehicles
Modify rate or spatial distribution of the hazard	Use engineering strategies to limit the speed at which motorcycles can accelerate
Separate hazard in time and space from that which is to be protected	Do not allow motorcycle use on highways
Separate hazard by material barrier from that which is to be protected	Wear helmets
Modify relevant basic qualities of the hazard	Use engineering expertise to construct motorcycles in such a way that there is more protection for the occupant
Make what is to be protected more resistant to damage from the hazard	Wear protective garments
Counter damage already done by the hazard	Implement 911 emergency call systems
Stabilize, repair, and rehabilitate the subject of the damage	Implement area-wide, region-wide, and state-wide trauma systems

safety projects from around the country. Typically, a quarterly digest addresses a specific project such as Alcohol and Other Drugs, Buckle Up America, Occupant Protection, ONE DOT, Pedestrian/Bicycle Safety, Police Traffic Services, and Safe Communities.

SUMMARY

In the fourteenth century "accident" meant "to happen by chance; a misfortune; an event that happens without foresight or expectations." This meaning is associated with the French word "accidence" from the Latin verb "accidere" meaning to fall down or to fall to. Emergency nurses face the challenge of caring for injury victims and their families and focusing their expertise and energies on reducing the number of victims of trauma. The data tell us that injury and trauma is still a major public health problem that needs expert attention from health planners, health care professionals, elected public officials, the market arena, and all those interested in reducing the tragedy caused by exchanges with forces in our environment.

References

1. American Nurses Association: *Culturally competent assessment for family violence,* Washington, DC, 1998, The Association.
2. Barber CW, Ozonoff VV, Schuster M et al: Massachusetts weapon-related injury surveillance system, *Am J Prev Med* 15(3S):57, 1998.
3. Battistella FD, Adnan MD, Perez L: Trauma patients 75 years and older: long-term followup results justify aggressive management, *J Trauma,* 44:618, 1998.
4. Brigham PA, McLoughlin E: Burn incidence and medical care use in the United States: estimates, trends, and data sources, *J Burn Care Rehab* March/April:95, 1996.
5. Centers for Disease Control and Prevention: *Demonstrating your program's worth: a primer on evaluation for programs to prevent unintentional injury,* Atlanta, Ga, 2000, The Centers.
6. Centers for Disease Control and Prevention: Unpowered scooter-related injuries: United States, 1998-2000, *MMWR* 49(49):1108, 2000.
7. Committee on Injury Prevention and Control, Division of Health Promotion and Disease Prevention, Institute of Medicine, National Academy of Sciences: *Reducing the burden of injury,* Washington, D.C., 1999, National Academy Press.
8. Dimick A, Wagner R: Burns. In Schwartz GR, Cayton CG, Mangelsen MA et al, editors: *Principles and practice of emergency medicine,* ed 3, Philadelphia, 1992, Lea & Febiger.
9. Haddon W: A logical framework for categorizing highway safety phenomena and activity, *J Trauma* 12:197, 1972.
10. Haddon W: Advances in the epidemiology of injuries as a basis for public policy, *Public Health Rep* 95:411, 1980.
11. Hedegaard H, Wake M, Hoffman R: Firearm-related injury surveillance in Colorado, *Am J Prev Med* 15(3S):38, 1998.
12. Ikeda RN, Mercy JA, Powell KE, editors: Firearm-related injury surveillance, *Am J Prev Med* 15(3S):6, 1998.
13. Jane JA, Francel PC: Age and outcome of head injury. In Narayan BK, Wilberger JE, Povlishock JT, editors: *Neurotrauma,* New York, 1996, McGraw-Hill.
14. Kim AN, Trent RB: Firearm-related injury surveillance in California, *Am J Prev Med* 15:3S,31, 1998.
15. Kraus JF, McArnthur DL, Silverman TA et al: Epidemiology of brain injury. In Narayan RK, Wilberger JE, Povlishock JT, editors: *Neurotrauma,* New York, 1966, McGraw-Hill.
16. Loimer H, Driur M, Guarmiere M: Accidents and acts of God: a history of the terms, *JAMA* 86(1):101, 1996.
17. Mackensie EJ, Fowler CJ: Epidemiology. In Mattox KL, Feliciano DV, Moore EE, editors: *Trauma,* ed 4, New York, 2000, McGraw-Hill.
18. Mahon B, Pugh T: *Epidemiology principles and practice,* Boston, 1970, Little, Brown.
19. McCurdy M, Daro P: *Current trends in child abuse reporting and fatalities: the results of the 1993 annual fifty state survey,* Chicago, 1994, National Committee to Prevent Child Abuse.
20. Mermelstein LE, Keenen TL, Benson DR: Initial evaluation and emergency treatment of the spine-injured patient. In Browner BD, Jupiter JB, Levine AM et al, editors: *Skeletal trauma: fractures, dislocations, ligamentous injuries,* Philadelphia, 1998, WB Saunders.

21. National Center for Injury Prevention and Control: *Fatal firearm injuries in the United States 1962-1994,* Violence Surveillance Summary Series, No. 3, Atlanta, 1997, National Center for Injury Prevention and Control, Centers for Disease Control and Prevention.

22. National Center for Health Statistics, U.S. Department of Health and Human Services: *Deaths: final data for 1996* 47(9), 1998.

23. National Center for Health Statistics, U.S. Department of Health and Human Services: *Hospital discharge survey: annual summary, 1995,* Hyattsville, Md, 1998, Centers for Disease Control and Prevention, Series 13 (133).

24. National Center for Health Statistics, U.S. Department of Health and Human Services: *International comparative analysis of injury mortality: findings from the ICE on injury statistics,* Hyattsville, Md, 1998, National Center for Health Statistics, PHS 98-1250.

25. National Center for Health Statistics, U.S. Department of Health and Human Services, Public Health Service: *Monthly vital statistics report: advance report of final mortality statistics 1989* 40(8), 1992.

26. National Center for Health Statistics, U.S. Department of Health and Human Services, Public Health Service: *Monthly vital statistics report: advance report of final mortality statistics 1990* 41(7), 1993.

27. National Center for Health Statistics, U.S. Department of Health and Human Services, Public Health Service: *Monthly vital statistics report: advance report of final mortality statistics 1991* 42(2), 1993.

28. National Center for Health Statistics, U.S. Department of Health and Human Services, Public Health Service: *Monthly vital statistics report: advance report of final mortality statistics 1992* 43(6), 1995.

29. National Center for Health Statistics, U.S. Department of Health and Human Services, Public Health Service: *Monthly vital statistics report: advance report of final mortality statistics 1993* 44(7), 1996.

30. National Center for Health Statistics, U.S. Department of Health and Human Services, Public Health Service: *Monthly vital statistics report: advance report of final mortality statistics 1994* 45(3), 1996.

31. National Center for Health Statistics, U.S. Department of Health and Human Services, Public Health Service: *Monthly vital statistics report: report of final mortality statistics* 45(11), 1997.

32. National Center for Health Statistics, U.S. Department of Health and Human Services: *Deaths: final data for 1997* 47(19), 1999.

33. National Center for Health Statistics, U.S. Department of Health and Human Services: *Deaths: final data for 1998* 47(9), 2000.

34. National Highway Traffic Safety Administration: *Cases from the special crash investigation program.* Retrieved April 26, 2001 from the World Wide Web: http://www.nhtsa.dot.gov.

35. National Highway Traffic Safety Administration: *Questions and answers regarding air bags, new occupant protection technology in 1998 vehicles, and supplemental questions and answers regarding air bags.* Retrieved April 26, 2001 from the World Wide Web: http: www.nhtsa.doc.gov.

36. National Safety Council: *Injury facts,* Itasca, Ill, 1999, The Council.

37. Northbridge ME, Nevitt MC, Kelsey JL et al: Home hazards and falls in the elderly: the need to consider the health and functioning of the individual, *Am J Public Health* 85:509, 1995.

38. Norton R, Campbell AJ, Lee-Joe T et al: Circumstances of falls resulting in hip fractures among older people, *J Am Geriatr Soc* 45:1108, 1997.

39. Praemer MA: *Musculoskeletal conditions in the United States,* Chicago, 1992, American Association of Orthopedic Surgeons.

40. Pruit BA, Mason AD: Epidemiological, demographic, and outcome: characteristics of burn injury. In Herndon DN, editor: *Total burn care,* Philadelphia, 1996, WB Saunders.

41. Rosenberg ML, Hammond R: Surveillance the key to firearm injury prevention, *Am J Prev Med* 15(3S):1, 1998.

42. Schwab CW, Shapiro MD, Kauder DR: Geriatric trauma: patterns, care and outcomes. In Mattox KL, Feliciano DV, Moore EE, editors: *Trauma,* ed 4, New York, 2000, McGraw-Hill.

43. Sleet D, Bonzo S, Branche C: An overview of the national center for injury prevention and control at the Centers for Disease Control and Prevention, *Inj Prev* 4:308, 1998.

44. Stamatos CA, Sorensen PA, Tefler KM: Meeting the challenge of the older trauma patient, *Am J Nurs* 96:40, 1996.

45. Tjaden P, Thoennes N: *Extent, nature, and consequences of intimate partner violence. Findings from the national violence against women survey,* Washington, DC, 2000, U.S. Department of Justice, Office of Justice Programs, National Institute of Justice, NCJ 181867.

46. Trafton PG: Lower extremity fractures and dislocations. In Mattox KL, Feliciano DV, Moore EE, editors: *Trauma,* ed 4, New York, 2000, McGraw-Hill.

47. U.S. Department of Transportation, National Highway Traffic Safety Administration: *Traffic safety facts 1999,* Washington, DC, 2000, National Center for Statistics and Analysis, DOT HS 809-100.

48. U.S. Department of Transportation, National Highway Traffic Safety Administration: *Traffic safety facts 1999, occupant protection,* Washington, DC, 2000, National Center for Statistics and Analysis, DOT HS 809-090.

49. U.S. Department of Transportation, National Highway Traffic Safety Administration: *Traffic safety facts 1999, school buses,* Washington, DC, 2000, National Center for Statistics and Analysis, DOT HS 809-095.

50. Van Tuinen M, Crosby A: Missouri firearm-related surveillance system, *Am J Prev Med* 15(3S):67, 1998.

51. Wilt SA, Gabre CS: A weapon-related injury surveillance system in New York City, *Am J Prev Med* 15(3S):75, 1998.

52. Wolf SE, Herndon DN: Burns and radiation injuries. In Mattox KL, Feliciano DV, Moore EE, editors: *Trauma,* ed 4, New York, 2000, McGraw-Hill.

53. World Bank: *World development report,* New York, 1994, Oxford University Press.

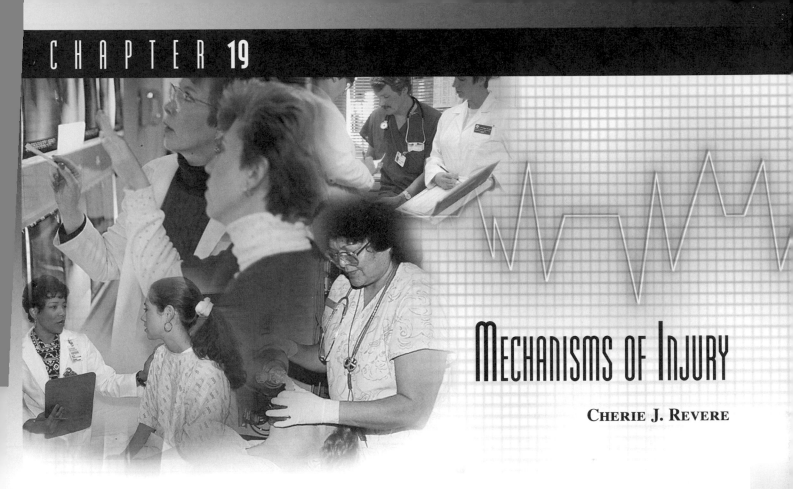

CHAPTER 19

MECHANISMS OF INJURY

CHERIE J. REVERE

Trauma is the most frequent cause of death for children and adults under 45 years of age. The great social, personal, and economic costs associated with traumatic injuries make trauma a major public health problem in the United States. Trauma is also the main cause for loss of work years because the younger population is affected more often than is the older population. An estimated 4 million productive work years are lost each year. One of three people who live in the United States is injured annually, 340,000 are permanently disabled, and more than 150,000 die.[4] Injuries are the number one reason patients seek treatment or see physicians. Treatment of injuries accounts for 25% of hospital, clinic, and emergency department (ED) visits.

Trauma is now recognized as a disease process with mechanisms of injury as part of its etiology. Strong assessment skills are essential for health care providers because treatment of trauma patients is contingent on locating all injuries. Unfortunately, even with strong assessment skills some injuries go undetected if the "index of suspicion" is not sufficient. Providing trauma care without understanding or recognizing the mechanism that produces injuries is not optimal trauma care. Understanding mechanisms of injury and using a high index of suspicion enable the caregiver to predict and locate occult injuries more quickly and save time initiating essential treatment. Injury should be considered present until definitively ruled out in the hospital setting.

Injury is defined as trauma or damage to some part of the body. Injury occurs when an uncontrolled or acute source of energy makes contact with the body and the body cannot tolerate exposure to that acute energy. Energy originates from several sources, including kinetic (motion or mechanical), chemical, electrical, thermal, and radiation. Absence of heat and oxygen causes injuries such as frostbite, drowning, or suffocation. Kinetic energy is defined as energy that results from motion.[10] A basic component in producing injury is absorption of kinetic energy. Box 19-1 defines essential concepts for understanding mechanisms of injury.

Severity of trauma depends on the wounding agent. Velocity and missile mass affect severity of gunshot wounds, whereas deceleration injuries depend on rate of deceleration, victim body mass, and area of energy dissipation. Burn severity is determined by duration of contact and temperature. Personal and environmental factors that affect injuries include sex, age, underlying disease processes, and nutrition. Risk factors amenable to prevention measures are sex, age, alcohol, race, income, geographic region, and temporal variation.

Males are 2.5 times more likely to be injured or involved in an accident than females because of their participation in more hazardous activities and greater risk taking. The high rate of injury in people between 15 and 24 years of age may be caused by experimentation with drugs and alcohol in combination with poor judgment. Elderly people (more than 75 years of age) have the highest death rate from injuries that may be associated with existing medical conditions.

Alcohol is a major factor in all types of trauma, including motor vehicle crashes (MVCs), family violence, suicides, homicides, and altercations. Alcohol alters judgment and

Box 19-1	ESSENTIAL CONCEPTS FOR MECHANISMS OF INJURY
Acceleration	Increase in velocity or speed of a moving object.
Acceleration/deceleration	Increase in velocity or speed of object followed by decrease in velocity or speed.
Axial loading	Injury occurs when force is applied upward and downward with no posterior or lateral bending of the neck.
Cavitation	Creation of temporary cavity as tissues are stretched and compressed.
Compression	Squeezing inward pressure.
Compressive strength	Ability to resist squeezing forces or inward pressure.
Deceleration	Decrease in velocity or speed of a moving object.
Distraction	Separation of spinal column with resulting cord transection, seen in legal hangings.
Elasticity	Ability to resume original shape and size after being stretched.
Force	Physical factor that changes motion of body at rest or already in motion.
High velocity	Missiles that compress and accelerate tissue away from the bullet, causing a cavity around the bullet and the entire tract.
Inertial resistance	Ability of body to resist movement.
Injury	Trauma or damage to some part of the body.
Kinematics	Process of looking at an accident and determining what injuries might result.
Kinetic energy	Energy that results from motion.
Low velocity	Missiles that localize injury to a small radius from center of the tract with little disruptive effect.
Muzzle blast	Cloud of hot gas and burning powder at the muzzle of a gun.
Shearing	Two oppositely directed parallel forces.
Stress	Internal resistance to deformation, or internal force generated from application load.
Tensile strength	Amount of tension tissue can withstand and ability to resist stretching forces.
Tumbling	Forward rotation around the center; somersault action of the missile can create massive injury.
Yaw	Deviation of bullet nose in longitudinal axis from straight line of flight.

coordination, so it causes or contributes to injury-producing events. Injury and death rates vary with race and income. For blacks and whites, the higher the income, the lower the death rate. The number of MVCs decreases in a depressed economy, whereas homicide and suicides increase. The highest homicide rate occurs in the black population, the highest suicide rate is seen in whites and Native Americans, and the lowest death rates occur in Asian Americans.

Physical environment or geographic area also characterizes injury rates. Homicides and suicides occur more in urban areas, whereas unintentional injuries or accidents are more numerous in rural areas. Injury and death rates are greater on weekends with the peak on Saturday. More injuries are seen in July—probably as a result of summer recreation activities.

Along with wounding force, recognition of subsequent tissue response is important to evaluating injuries. When tissue limits are surpassed, the resultant injury causes physiologic or anatomic damage. A central nervous system (CNS) injury is a physiologic injury that may cause permanent damage despite healing. Skeletal fractures are anatomic damages that can heal without permanent disability. Understanding mechanisms of injury affects outcome because common injury patterns can be predicted, identified, and treated.

KINEMATICS

Kinematics is the process of looking at an event and determining what injuries are likely to occur given the forces and motion involved. Physics is the foundation on which kinematics is based. Understanding essential laws of physics is the first step toward understanding kinematics.

Newton's first law of motion states that a body at rest remains at rest and a body in motion remains in motion unless acted on by an outside force. Stationary objects set in motion by energy forces are illustrated by pedestrians struck by a vehicle, blast victims, and people with gunshot wounds. Moving objects interrupted or acted on to stop their motion are the same as people falling from a height, vehicles hitting a tree, or vehicles braking to a sudden stop.

The second essential law of physics, the Law of Conservation of Energy, states that energy is neither created nor destroyed but changes form. As a car decelerates slowly, the energy of motion (acceleration) is converted to friction heat in braking (thermal energy).

Trauma may be penetrating or blunt. Penetrating trauma causes a break in the skin that communicates to the outside. The injury pattern associated with penetrating trauma is related to the energy created and dissipated by the wounding agent and the surrounding area. Damage is contingent on the velocity of the wounding agent and underlying structures that are damaged. With blunt trauma in which trauma occurs without communication to the outside, injuries are less obvious, so the extent of injury is difficult to diagnose.

Patient Assessment

Initially trauma patients may not appear seriously injured because of strong compensatory mechanisms that maintain adequate vital signs. All members of a trauma team must anticipate injuries by recognizing potential patterns of injury related to the energy and force of the accident. Assessment, resuscitation, and stabilization efforts based on patterns and mechanisms recognized in each patient enable health care providers to recognize hidden or internal injuries and avoid potentially harmful diagnostic interventions.

Health care providers should match injuries to reported mechanisms. Patients, family, and friends may have reasons to fabricate, falsify, or deny the actual event. Consequently, injuries identified in the examination must match the reported mechanism. Eliciting a careful history of the injury during initial assessment of a trauma patient is vital. Accurate information, especially about mechanisms surrounding injuries, can reduce morbidity and mortality in many circumstances.

When assessing a trauma patient, the emergency nurse should note mechanisms associated with major force or energy transfer (e.g., pedestrian hit by vehicle traveling faster than 20 mph, falls from more than 20 feet, MVC with major vehicular damage, speed change of more than 20 mph, vehicle rollover, ejected occupant, death of occupant). Some injuries are significant because of potential complications, such as two or more long bone fractures; flail chest; penetrating trauma to the head, neck, chest, abdomen, or groin; and any combination of these patterns with burns over more than 15% of the head, face, or airway.[2] Patients with significant injuries require close monitoring for complications or changes in hemodynamic stability.

Certain questions elicit valuable information regarding the mechanism of injury and are helpful in assessing potential injuries. What type of vehicle was the patient driving (large or small)? What was the estimated speed at the time of the crash? Were seat belts or restraint devices used? Were the devices applied appropriately? Were airbags installed and did they deploy? Where was the patient in the vehicle (driver, front passenger, or rear seat passenger)? If ejected, how far was the patient thrown or found from the vehicle? How much damage was done to the vehicle? Where was the majority of damage? Occupants have injuries on the same side as the vehicle damage.[3] The emergency nurse should ask about steering wheel deformity for all drivers. If the patient fell, what was the approximate height of the fall? Were any objects struck during the fall? What was the surface where the patient landed? In what position was the patient found after the fall?

With penetrating injury, the wounding agent (e.g., knife, gun, arrow, ice pick) must be ascertained. What was the size and length of the agent? With guns, what was the caliber (millimeter for European guns) and distance from the weapon to the patient? Patients with penetrating trauma must be assessed for other types of trauma such as falls or assaults. Patients may be exposed to more than one type of energy.

A detailed history is not always possible and is often impractical. Valuable information can be obtained from family members, emergency medical service (EMS) personnel, police, fire fighters, bystanders, or eyewitnesses; however, these resources are often overlooked in a hectic ED. Management of life-threatening injuries must take priority over obtaining a detailed history; however, every effort should be made to obtain as much historic data as possible.

After resuscitation is accomplished, rapid examination or assessment should be performed. Patients with penetrating trauma are easier to assess than those with blunt trauma because injuries are usually focused in one area. Surface trauma may or may not be present with blunt injuries; therefore, assessment tends to be more difficult. During secondary survey, missed injuries can be found by systematically examining the patient who is completely undressed. Maintaining a high index of suspicion for probable injuries for certain mechanisms and performing a detailed physical assessment minimize risks of missed injuries.

BLUNT INJURY

Blunt trauma is an injury with no opening in the skin or communication to the outside environment. Definitive diagnosis of blunt trauma is difficult. The extent of injuries is less obvious than penetrating ones; however, these injuries may be more life-threatening. Depending on the tissue injured and properties associated with this tissue, certain diagnostic studies are more helpful than others. Air-filled organs, such as lungs and bowel, are subject to explosion injuries. Crush injuries to solid organs (liver and spleen) may present with minimal external signs of injury, but blunt trauma energy is transmitted in all directions, so organs or tissues burst or break if pressure is not released.[6]

Automobiles are responsible for at least half of blunt injuries. Blunt abdominal trauma accounts for 1% of all trauma admissions, but is associated with a 20% to 30% mortality rate resulting from chest and head injuries.[2]

Examples of blunt force events include MVCs, falls, contact sports, and assaults. Direct impact, when a wounding agent and body surface make contact, causes the greatest injury. Injuries result when energy is released on impact with the body. Various body tissues respond differently; tissue may move and displace with impact or rupture from the force.

Common forces in blunt trauma are acceleration or deceleration, shearing, and compression. Acceleration or deceleration injuries occur with increased velocity or speed of a moving object followed by a sudden decrease. Shearing injuries occur when two oppositely directed parallel forces are applied to tissue. Compression injuries occur with a squeezing inward pressure applied to tissues. An example of these forces is seen with blunt injury to the thoracic aorta. Rapid deceleration causes the aorta to bend and stretch. Shearing damage occurs when vessel elasticity is exceeded by stretching forces. Shearing damage causes the aorta to dissect, rupture, tear, or form an aneurysm.

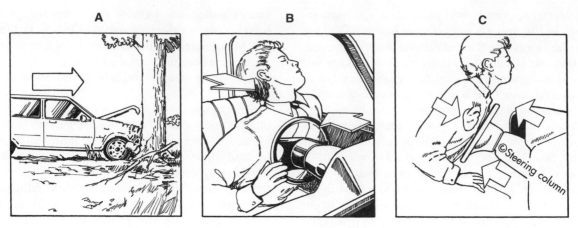

FIGURE **19-1** The three collisions of a motor vehicle collision. **A,** Auto hits tree. **B,** Body hits steering wheel, causing broken ribs. **C,** Heart strikes chest wall, causing myocardial contusion.

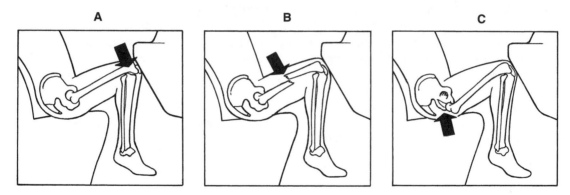

FIGURE **19-2** Down and under pathway. **A,** Dislocation of the knee. **B,** Fracture of the femur. **C,** Dislocation from the acetabulum.

Motor Vehicle Collisions

Before collision the occupant and vehicle are moving at the same speed. At the time of collision the vehicle and the occupant decelerate to a speed of zero, but at different rates. Deceleration forces are transferred to the body in three points of collision (Figure 19-1).[2] The first collision occurs when the automobile strikes another object. As the vehicle stops, the unrestrained driver or occupant continues to move forward. The second collision occurs when the driver or occupant strikes the steering wheel, windshield, or other structures in the car. The body stops; however, internal organs continue to move until they collide with another organ, cavity wall or structure, or they are restrained suddenly by vasculature, muscles, ligaments, or fascia—the third collision point. Different damage occurs with each collision; therefore, each point must be considered separately to avoid missed injuries.

One way to estimate injuries in an MVC is to look at the vehicle. Because this is not possible in the ED, the emergency nurse should ask prehospital providers about vehicular damage—interior and exterior. Some EMS providers take instant snapshots, allowing hospital personnel to see vehicular damage first hand. The picture showing mechanisms of injury can then become a permanent part of the medical record.

Frontal Impact. This type of impact occurs when the vehicle front impacts another object (e.g., another vehicle, tree, bridge abutment). The first collision results in damage to the front end. The more severe the damage and the faster the car was traveling, the greater the probability for severely injured victims because of the high level of energy involved.

Multiple injuries are produced when an unrestrained body comes to a sudden stop. Interior structures, such as the windshield, steering wheel, dashboard, or instrument panel, injure the occupants when contact is made. After the vehicle stops, occupants in the front seat continue to move down and under, or up and over, the dashboard.

DOWN AND UNDER. The first path an occupant may travel after frontal impact is down and under. With this path the occupant continues forward movement downward and into the steering column or dashboard. The knees impact the dashboard; however, most energy is absorbed by the upper legs. This mechanism causes patella dislocations, midshaft femur fractures, and posterior dislocations or fractures of acetabulum or femoral head. This classic knee-femur-hip injury is caused by the transfer of energy from the knee through the femur into the hip (Figure 19-2). When one of these injuries is identified, the patient should be carefully evaluated for the other injuries.

UP AND OVER. Continued forward motion from frontal collision carries the body up and over, so the chest, abdomen, or both strike the steering wheel. Head injuries, such as contusions and scalp lacerations, skull fractures, facial fractures, cerebral hemorrhage or cerebral contusions can occur when the head or face strikes the steering wheel or dashboard.

The brain does not stretch easily, so if one part of the brain moves in one direction, the rest follows. The skull stops suddenly after striking the steering wheel, windshield, or another stationary object, but the brain continues to move forward and strikes the inside of the skull.[5] This area of the brain is compressed and may sustain ecchymosis, edema, or contusion. The other side of the brain continues to move forward and may be disrupted and shear away from tissue and

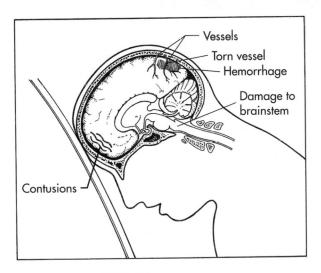

FIGURE **19-3** Brain injury.

vascular attachments (Figure 19-3). This impact can cause two separate injuries, shear injury and compression injury, to the same organ.

When the head collides with an object, injury to the cervical spine can also occur. The spider web effect of the broken windshield suggests the possibility for cervical spine injury. If prehospital providers report a spider web effect, caregivers must maintain a high index of suspicion for occult spinal injury.

Chest injuries occur when the thorax is compressed against the steering wheel. Injuries include fractured ribs and sternum, anterior flail chest, myocardial contusion, and pulmonary contusion. The abdomen may also collide with the steering wheel, causing compression injuries. Ruptured hollow organs such as the stomach and bladder spill contents, whereas fractured or lacerated solid organs such as the liver and spleen are associated with significant blood loss. Organs in the abdominal cavity are attached to the abdominal wall by the mesentery, ligaments, and vasculature. As organs continue their forward motion, attachments are torn or lacerated. Thoracic vertebral injuries occur as energy travels up or down the thoracic spine; however, these injuries are less common because the thoracic vertebrae are so well protected.

The steering wheel is often referred to as a modern day battering ram, the most lethal weapon in the vehicle.[1] When steering wheel deformity is reported, the index of suspicion for neck, face, thoracic, or abdominal injuries should increase significantly. Injuries caused by colliding with the steering wheel may be readily visible, or represent only the tip of the "injury" iceberg. Lacerations of the chin and mouth, contusion and ecchymosis of the neck, traumatic tattooing of the chest and abdomen, and bruising of the chest and abdomen may be obvious or subtle. Internal occult injuries may be secondary to compression forces, shearing forces, and displacement of kinetic energy.[7] Figure 19-4 illustrates injuries commonly seen with steering wheel impact.

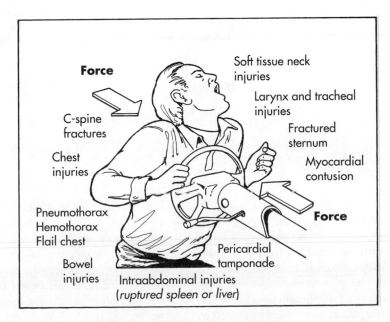

FIGURE **19-4** Steering wheel injuries.

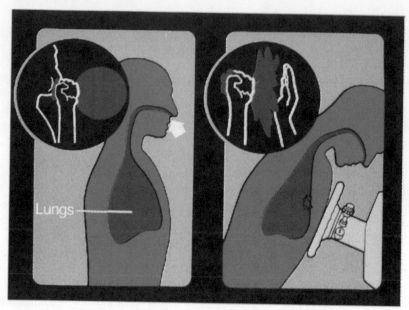

FIGURE **19-5** Compression of lung against closed glottis by impact on anterior or lateral chest wall produces effect like that of compressing a paper bag when opening is closed tightly by hands: the paper bag ruptures and so does the lung. (From Prehospital Trauma Life Support Committee of the National Association of Emergency Medical Technicians in Cooperation with the Committee on Trauma of the American College of Surgeons: *PHTLS: basic and advanced prehospital life support,* ed 4, St. Louis, 1999, Mosby.)

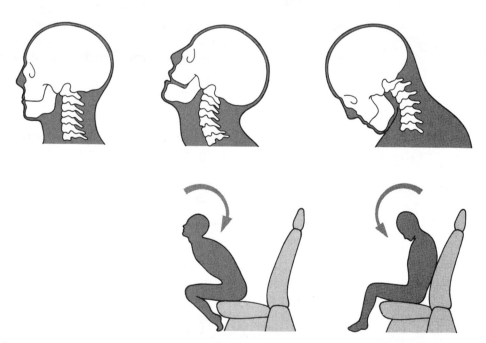

FIGURE **19-6** Rear-impact collision results in hyperextension of neck. (From Neff JA, Kidd PS: *Trauma nursing: the art and science,* ed 2, St. Louis, 1999, Mosby.)

Certain organs are more susceptible to shear injuries because of ligamentous attachments (e.g., liver, spleen, bowel, kidneys, aortic arch). Compression forces commonly injure the lungs, diaphragm, heart, and bladder. Respiratory distress in trauma patients may be caused by injuries such as pneumothorax, flail chest, and pulmonary contusion. A diaphragmatic hernia and ruptured diaphragm also cause respiratory distress in a trauma patient and are characterized by bowel sounds in the chest. If a trauma patient has a contused chest wall, myocardial contusion should be considered.

In frontal and lateral impacts, a mechanism sometimes called the "paper bag effect" leads to pneumothorax. The driver or occupant sees the accident about to happen, inhales deeply, and holds his or her breath. The glottis closes and seals the lungs. As the chest impacts, the lungs burst like paper bags (Figure 19-5).

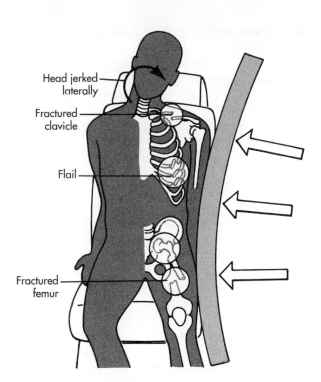

FIGURE 19-7   Potential injury sites in lateral-impact collision. Injury is still possible in lateral crash with airbag inflation; however, injuries are usually fewer with airbag inflation than without. (From Neff JA, Kidd PS: *Trauma nursing: the art and science,* St. Louis, 1993, Mosby.)

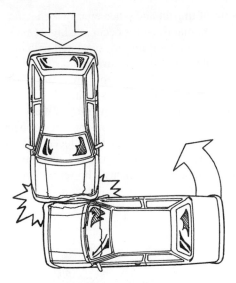

FIGURE 19-8   Rotational impact.

Frontal impacts are also characterized by extremity injuries. Fractures of the lower extremities, ankles, and feet occur when the occupant extends the feet, or are secondary to vehicle intrusion into the passenger compartment. An unrestrained back-seat passenger doubles the risk for injury to front-seat occupants during frontal impact.

Rear Impact.   Rear-impact collision occurs when a stationary object or a slower moving object is struck from behind. Initial impact accelerates the slower moving or stationary object and may force the vehicle into a frontal collision. When the vehicle suddenly accelerates, hyperextension of the neck may occur, especially when head rests are not properly positioned. Strained and torn neck ligaments also occur. Figure 19-6 demonstrates how these injuries occur. If the vehicle strikes another object or is slowed by the driver applying the brake, rapid forward deceleration occurs. The crash then involves two points of impact, rear and frontal, which increases the chance for occupant injuries. Injuries common to each mechanism must be assessed.

Lateral or Side Impact.   When a vehicle is struck on either side, most injuries are dependent on vehicle deformity as the vehicle remains in place or moves away from the point of impact. If the vehicle remains in place, energy is transferred or changed to vehicle damage rather than the energy of motion. Trauma to the occupants can be more severe because of intrusion into the interior compartment.

With side-impact or lateral collisions, occupants generally receive most injuries on the same side of their body as the vehicle impact. A second collision may occur between occupants if another passenger is in the vehicle. The head and shoulder of one occupant may impact the other occupant's head and shoulder. When a patient has an injury on the side opposite impact, caregivers should assess both occupants for associated injuries.

Figure 19-7 illustrates injuries from a side-impact collision. Flail chest, pulmonary contusion, and rib fractures are possible chest injuries. Numerous musculoskeletal injuries can occur. Energy from an impact can pin the occupant's arm against the car, causing injury to the chest wall and clavicle or force the femoral head through the pelvis, causing a pelvic or acetabulum fracture.[3] Strain on the lateral neck can cause spinal fractures or ligament tears. Side impacts can cause spine fractures associated with a neurologic deficit more often than rear collisions. Other injuries include a ruptured liver when impact is on the passenger side and ruptured spleen when impact is on the driver's side.

Rotational Impact.   When the corner of one vehicle strikes another stationary vehicle, a vehicle traveling in the opposite direction, or a slower vehicle, a rotational impact occurs (Figure 19-8). The part that is hit on the second car stops forward motion, whereas the rest of the vehicle rotates around until all energy is transformed. As the car is hit, the occupant's forward motion continues until it impacts with the side of the car as the vehicle begins rotating. Injuries that occur in rotational impacts are a combination of those seen in frontal and lateral impacts.

Vehicle Rollover.   Rollover is when a car flips, regardless of whether the motion is end-over-end, or side-over-side. In rollovers, injuries are sometimes difficult to predict. Occupants frequently have injuries in the same body areas where damage occurs to the vehicle. Just as the vehicle impacts at different angles, several times, so does the occupant's body and internal organs. In the rollover mechanism, the chance for axial loading injuries is increased.

Ejection.   Ejection occurs when an occupant is thrown from the vehicle. Occupants who are ejected sustain injuries at the point of impact and when energy is transferred to the entire body. Spinal fractures occur at a higher rate in ejected people.[4] Increased mortality is associated with ejection, and those at greatest risk are unrestrained occupants.

Restraints. Restraint systems are designed to prevent injuries and decrease the severity of injuries by allowing occupants to decelerate at the same rate as the vehicle rather than being thrown against interior structures or being ejected from the vehicle. Injuries can be reduced with use of restraints. Occupants who are ejected have a much greater chance of dying than occupants who remain in the vehicle.

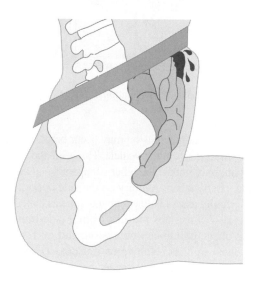

FIGURE **19-9** A seat belt that is positioned above the rim of the pelvis allows the abdominal organs to be trapped between the moving posterior wall and the belt. Injuries to the pancreas and other retroperitoneal organs, as well as blowout ruptures of the small intestine and colon, result. (From McSwain N, Paturas J: *The basic EMT: comprehensive prehospital patient care,* ed 2, St. Louis, 2001, Mosby.)

Restraints also keep occupants from striking each other within the compartment; therefore, restraints worn properly reduce fatalities and the severity of injuries. The most effective restraint system is the three-point restraint, which is a shoulder harness and lap belt. Three-point restraints decrease severity of the "second" collision, reducing facial, head, and abdominal injuries, and long-bone fractures.[2]

Injuries caused by a shoulder-lap belt fastened loosely or worn above the anterior iliac crest (Figure 19-9) include compression to abdominal organs such as pancreas, liver, spleen; possible rupture of the diaphragm with herniation of abdominal organs; and lumbar spine anterior compression fractures. Diaphragmatic rupture occurs from increased intraabdominal pressure from the misplaced lap belt. Figure 19-10 illustrates the consequences of incorrect use of lap belts and shoulder straps. Lap belts worn alone allow injuries to the face, head, neck, and chest, whereas shoulder belts worn without a lap belt can cause neck injuries—even decapitation.

Properly used restraints transfer energy from the impact to the restraint system instead of to the occupant. Injuries received when seat belts are used properly are generally non–life-threatening or the chance of sustaining a life-threatening injury is greatly reduced. Box 19-2 describes injuries that occur even with proper seat belt usage.

AIRBAGS. Newer cars are now equipped with at least a driver-side airbag. Some vehicles also have passenger-side airbags and side impact airbags. Airbags are designed to protect front seat occupants in frontal deceleration collisions by inflating from the center of the steering column or the dashboard or both at impact (Figure 19-11), cushioning the head and chest, and then rapidly deflating. Injuries reported from airbag deployment include facial trauma, such as tattooing, ecchymosis, and corneal abrasions. Episodes of minor trauma from airbags are becoming more commonplace as these life-saving devices are installed in more cars.[2] Tem-

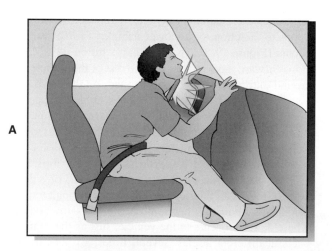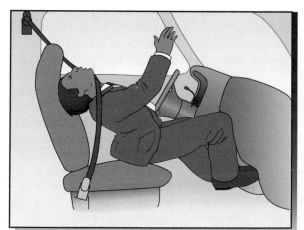

FIGURE **19-10** **A,** Without the diagonal strap the forward motion of the upper body can cause severe injuries to the face, head, and neck. **B,** When worn alone, the diagonal strap retards forward motion but produces an excessive force on the neck. Neck injuries as severe as decapitation have been reported. (From McSwain N, Paturas J: *The basic EMT: comprehensive prehospital patient care,* ed 2, St. Louis, 2001, Mosby.)

SPINAL

Cervical vertebral fractures from flexion forces
Neck sprains secondary to hyperextension
Lumbar vertebral fractures secondary to flexion-distraction forces

THORACIC

Soft tissue injuries of the chest wall associated with belt placement
Sternal fractures with or without myocardial contusion
Fewer than three rib fractures if restrained; more than four if unrestrained
Trauma to breast in females

ABDOMINAL

Soft-tissue injuries (contusions, abrasions, ecchymosis)
"Seat belt" friction burns or abrasion where seat belt rests
Injuries to small bowel secondary to crushing and deceleration
Ruptured aorta secondary to longitudinal stretching of the vessel
Injuries to the liver, pancreas, gallbladder, and duodenum secondary to crushing forces

| Box 19-3 | HIGHWAY DESIGN CHANGES THAT REDUCE MOTOR VEHICLE CRASHES |

Separate opposing streams of traffic.
Eliminate intersections, overpasses, and underpasses.
Create wider shoulders and remove obstacles from roadside.
Install breakaway barriers.
Use road surface materials that decrease skidding.
Increase use of visual barriers to reduce driver distraction (increase height of center dividing wall).

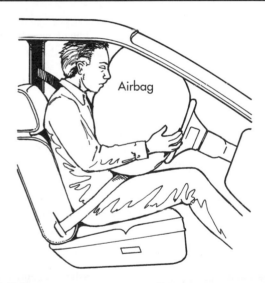

FIGURE 19-11   Inflated airbag.

porary hearing loss has also been reported. Abrasions and ecchymosis from airbag deployment are seen on forearms. Serious injuries have been seen in small drivers who adjust the seat closer to the steering wheel. Drivers and passengers should sit at least 10 inches away from the steering wheel and tilt the seat rearward for vehicles with airbags. Infants and children placed in the front seat have been seriously injured or killed by inflating airbags. Some automobiles are manufactured with airbags in the roof that come down to protect the head and side airbag in the doors. At least one automobile has air bags that protect the legs by inflating from under the dash.

MVC PREVENTIVE MEASURES. Because MVCs account for more than half the injuries associated with blunt trauma,

preventive measures are an ongoing concern. Research has shown that the number of MVCs can be reduced by highway design changes, enforcement of speed limits, and improvements in vehicle design. Box 19-3 shows how changes in highway design can reduce the number of MVCs that occur.

Enforcing the speed limit also reduces injuries from MVCs because speed is a determining factor in the severity of injuries. The greater the speed or velocity, the more energy dissipated and the more severe the injury. The size and design of vehicles also affect injury. Small cars are associated with more injuries and deaths than larger cars. Making all cars larger is not the only answer because a great number of deaths from MVCs occur in single-car crashes involving large and small vehicles. Changes in interior design can decrease injuries seen in occupants. If automobile racing designs were incorporated into all privately owned vehicles, likelihood of escaping a collision without injury would increase dramatically.

Tractor Accidents

The majority of fatalities associated with tractors are crushing injuries when the tractor turns over. When tractors turn over it is generally to the side; however, they can overturn to the rear. Rear overturns do not allow the driver to jump free or be thrown clear. Other mechanisms of injury include thermal burns from ignited fuel or hot engine parts and chemical burns from diesel fuel, hydraulic fluid, gasoline, or battery acid.

Pedestrian Injuries

When a pedestrian is struck by a vehicle, certain injuries can be predicted based on the person's age or size. Children and adults have different injuries because of their size differences and orientation to the vehicle.

In children, frontal impacts usually occur because children tend to freeze and face the approaching vehicle. The femur or chest of the child impacts the bumper or hood depending on the child's size. The child is then thrown backward (rarely clear) with the upper back or head impacting the ground or pavement, where contralateral skull injuries occur. Very small children are rarely thrown clear of the vehicle because of their low center of gravity, size, and weight. A child may be knocked down and under the vehicle, then run over. Multisystem trauma should be suspected in any child hit by a car. A combination of injuries referred

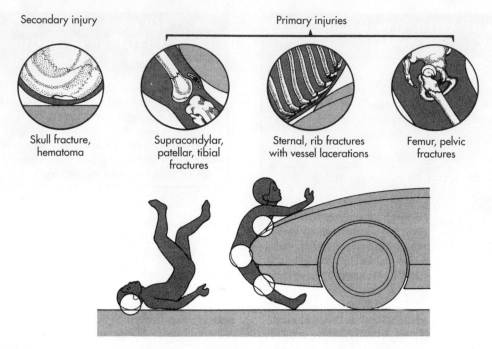

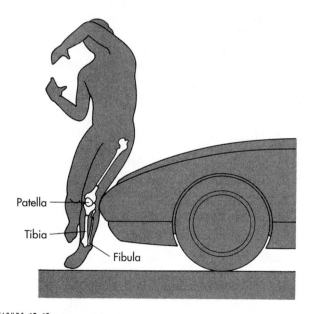

FIGURE **19-12** Potential primary injury sites of child pedestrian. (Modified from Neff JA, Kidd PS: *Trauma nursing: the art and science,* St. Louis, 1993, Mosby.)

FIGURE **19-13** Potential primary injury sites of adult pedestrian. (From Neff JA, Kidd PS: *Trauma nursing: the art and science,* St. Louis, 1993, Mosby.)

to as Waddell's triad often occurs when a child is struck by a car (Figure 19-12). Waddell's triad is characterized by injuries to the chest, head, and femurs.

Adults struck by a vehicle sustain injuries to the lower extremities along with head, chest, and abdominal injuries. Adults try to protect themselves by turning sideways, so the impact is usually lateral. Upper and lower leg impact with the bumper and hood of car causes bowing of both legs with fractures above and below the joint of impact. This may also cause ligament damage to the opposite knee from associated strain. Figure 19-13 shows points of impact when an adult is struck by a vehicle.

Another common injury in an adult pedestrian is a fractured pelvis. As the victim folds over, the upper femur and pelvis strike the front of the hood. The abdomen and chest strike the top of the hood. The victim then travels off the hood and onto the pavement or into the windshield. The victim may be able to protect the face and head with the arms during this forward motion. If the victim is thrown any distance, he or she can be run over by a second vehicle. Tire mark impressions may be found on the clothing or skin of victims who are run over.

Motorcycle Crashes

Injuries occurring from motorcycle crashes depend on the amount and type of kinetic energy and part of the body impacted. Head, neck, and extremity injuries occur more frequently with motorcycle crashes because of a lack of a protective encasement. Clues to the amount of force sustained during a collision include length of skid marks, deformity of the motorcycle, and stationary objects impacted. The condition of a motorcycle driver is often similar to an occupant ejected from a vehicle (Figure 19-14). Three types of motorcycle impacts with predictable injuries are head-on impact, angular impact, and ejection.

Head-on Impact. During a head-on impact, the motorcycle impacts an object that stops the bike's forward motion. The bike flips forward so the rider strikes or travels over the handlebars. As the rider strikes the handlebars, abdominal and chest injuries and shearing fractures of the tibia can oc-

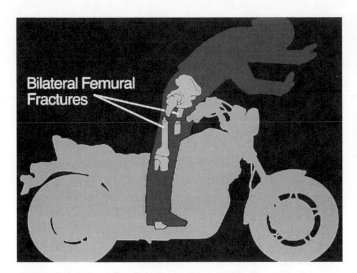

FIGURE **19-14**   The body travels forward and over the motorcycle, impacting the thighs and femurs into the handlebars. The driver can also be ejected. (From National Association of Emergency Medical Technicians: *Prehospital trauma life support,* ed 4, St. Louis, 1999, Mosby.)

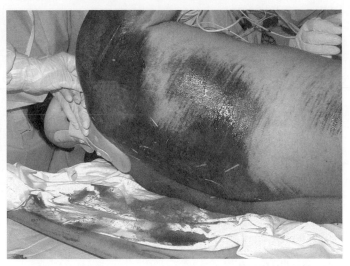

FIGURE **19-15**   Road burns after a motorcycle crash without protective clothing. (From McSwain N, Paturas J: *The basic EMT: comprehensive prehospital patient care,* ed 2, St. Louis, 2001, Mosby.)

cur. Bilateral femur fractures occur if the rider's feet are trapped by the foot pegs at the time of impact. A helmet may protect the rider's head, but does not protect the neck. If the rider impacts the head and neck, injuries may still occur.

Angular Impact.   When a cycle is hit at an angle and collapses on the rider, the angular impact injures the side that is crushed between the rider and ground or the object struck. Injuries tend to occur in lower extremities such as open fractures of the tibia or fibula, crushed legs, ankle dislocation, and soft-tissue injuries.

Ejection.   When a rider is thrown off the motorcycle, injuries occur to whatever body part is hit at the time of impact and the point of impact when the body lands. Energy from the impact is absorbed by the rest of the body. Ejection from a motorcycle has a high potential for severe injuries.

Laying the Bike Down.   Laying the bike down is a maneuver used by professional riders to separate themselves from the bike when they see an impending collision. This maneuver slows the rider as the bike is turned sideways, and the rider drags the inner leg. The most common injuries seen with laying the bike down are minor fractures, abrasions, and crush injuries to lower legs. Figure 19-15 shows road burns that occurred in a rider who was not wearing protective clothing.

Bicycle Crashes

Several mechanisms for bicycle collisions exist; the most common are collisions with a motor vehicle or pedestrian and falling off the cycle. Approximately 90% of all deaths related to bicycles are the result of a collision with a motor vehicle. A rider usually loses control and falls off because of hazardous ground surfaces, performing stunts, speeding, or generalized lack of skill.

Bicycle crashes have certain common patterns of injuries. The spokes of a bicycle wheel can fracture the feet when feet are caught in the wheel. These injuries are generally seen in second riders and may cause the person to be thrown and sustain other injuries. Properly installed wheel guards decrease spoke-related injuries.

When a rider is thrown over the handlebars as a bike impacts an object and tips forward, the rider without a helmet may suffer injuries similar to someone ejected from a car (i.e., head, neck, abdomen, and chest injuries). If the rider impacts the middle bar or seat, straddle injuries such as vaginal tears, scrotal injuries, and perineal contusions occur.

Bicycle-mounted child seats are another cause of injuries with bicycle use. The child may fall from the seat, the seat can detach from the bicycle, the bike can tip over, or the child's extremity may be caught in wheel spokes. Head and facial injuries are common and often severe. Child seats mounted on bicycles do not provide protection to the child's head and face, and the child is not developmentally ready for self-protection; therefore, helmets should be worn by all children in bicycle-mounted seats.

Injuries can occur to bicycle riders from rear-view mirrors that extend from trucks or vans. Significant head, neck, and facial injuries and severe deep lacerations to the head and neck can occur and are often fatal.

Watercraft

Watercraft or boating accidents can occur from colliding with another boat or an obstruction in the water. Occupants of boats are not provided with restraint systems, and the boats are not built to absorb the energy associated with impacts. There is a potential for drowning or hypothermia when occupants are thrown into the water and water temperatures are cold. Other injuries may be similar to those seen in people ejected from a vehicle.

All-terrain Vehicles

All-terrain vehicles (ATVs) have two basic designs: three-wheeled or four-wheeled vehicles. Four-wheeled vehicles offer easier handling and more stability than three-wheeled vehicles, which, when turned sharply, are prone to rollover because of a higher center of gravity. Some states have enacted laws defining the minimum operator age and requiring helmets for all riders.

The three most common mechanisms of injury associated with all-terrain vehicles are rollover, a rider falling off, and the vehicle hitting a stationary object and causing forward deceleration of the rider. Injuries depend on which part of the rider's anatomy is struck and the mechanism involved. Head, spine, and chest injuries involving the ribs, sternum, and clavicles have been reported.

Personal Watercraft

In recent years personal watercraft (PWC), such as wave runners and jet skis, have become popular recreational vehicles. The injury rate is about 8.5 times higher with PWCs than with motorboats. Different styles allow the driver to sit, stand, or kneel while operating the watercraft, with some PWCs large enough to carry two to three passengers. A high speed can be obtained quickly with most PWCs. Collisions can occur with other watercraft or objects in the water. The potential for injury is very similar to the injury patterns seen with ATVs. Rectal, vaginal, and perineal trauma may occur when passengers or drivers hit the water (buttocks first) or seat at high speeds. Drowning is another complication associated with PWC accidents.

Snowmobiles

Snowmobiles are used for work and play. Injuries that are commonly seen are similar to those associated with ATVs. The snowmobile has a low center of gravity and low clearance. Crush injuries are frequently seen because it turns over more easily and is heavier than most ATVs. Significant neck injuries can occur if the rider runs into an unseen wire fence or rope. Patterns of injury depend on the mechanism and part of the body affected. Hypothermia is a significant risk if the rider is not adequately clothed for the weather or is not found immediately after the event.

Falls

Vertical deceleration is the mechanism associated with falls. Severity and types of injuries seen in people who fall or jump depends on height of the fall, area of the body impacted, and the landing surface. Falls are severe when the distance is 3 times greater than victim height; however, any fall greater than the person's standing height has the potential for significant injury. Different patterns of injuries are seen with different types of falls. Small children tend to land on the head because it is the biggest part of their body. Certain injuries occur when a person lands feet first. A trio of injuries, called the Don Juan syndrome, includes bilateral calcaneus fractures, compression fractures of the vertebrae (usually thoracolumbar), and bilateral Colles fractures. Energy initially causes bilateral calcaneus fractures, then displaces upward and causes other injuries including femur fractures, hip dislocations or fractures, vertebral compression fractures, and basilar skull fractures. Wrist fractures occur from acute flexion as the person falls forward onto their outstretched arms. Deceleration forces of this nature can also cause secondary renal injuries.

If a person lands on other areas of the body, injuries occur at those impact points and to the rest of the body. If impact is on the wrist, energy is transferred upward through the elbow and shoulder, whereas impact on the knee transfers energy upward to the hip. Another point of impact may be the head, as seen in diving injuries. With this impact, injuries occur because weight and force of the torso, pelvis, and legs bear down on the head and cervical spine. This type of injury is known as a compression injury or axial loading injury. Vertebral bodies are compressed and wedged, producing vertebral fragments that can pierce the cord.

Sports-Related Injuries

Injuries associated with sports are generally caused by compressive forces or sudden deceleration. Twisting, hyperflexion, or hyperextension can cause other injuries. Factors that affect injury include lack of protective equipment, lack of conditioning, and inadequate training of the participant. Mechanisms associated with recreational sports and sports-like activities are similar to those involved in MVCs, motorcycle collisions, and bicycle crashes. Potential mechanisms associated with individual sports are numerous; however, general principles are the same as with falls and MVCs.

- What energy or forces impact the victim?
- What parts of the body are affected by the energy or force?
- What are the obvious injuries?
- What injuries are associated with the involved energy or force?

Damaged equipment, such as broken snow skis or helmets, can help establish impact. Table 19-1 describes injuries associated with various sports.

PENETRATING TRAUMA

Injuries caused by foreign objects in motion that penetrate the body are called penetrating trauma. Energy created by the foreign object is dissipated into surrounding tissues. Evaluation and assessment of penetrating trauma depend on the wounding agent, how energy is dissipated, distance from victim to weapon, and characteristics of the tissues struck. Examples of penetrating trauma include gunshot wounds, stab wounds, and impalements. The tissue penetrated and underlying structures damaged determine severity of the injury. Victims of penetrating trauma may also suffer blunt injuries, for instance, falling down a flight of stairs after being shot.

A variety of objects can produce penetrating injuries, including those thrown from a lawn mower or industrial machinery. However, in today's society the majority of penetrating injuries are caused by knives and guns.

Table 19-1	SPORTS-RELATED INJURIES[6,9]
SPORT	**POTENTIAL INJURIES**
Boxing	Cumulative brain damage, ocular injuries, lacerations, nasal fractures, hand fractures
Gymnastics	Spinal cord injuries, extremity fractures, sprains, strains
Football	Spinal cord injuries, head injuries, knee strains, fractures, lacerations
Skiing	Head injuries, lower extremity fractures, exposure to elements
Ice hockey	Facial fractures, soft tissue injuries, lacerations
Running	Lower extremity injuries, strains, sprains
Baseball	Head injuries, ocular injuries, fractures, lacerations, sprains, strains
Basketball	Lower extremity sprains, strains, fractures, lacerations, contusions
Horseback riding	Head injuries, bite wounds, crush wounds
Inline skates	Wrist fractures, head injuries, lower extremity fractures
Bungee jumping	Major impact-related injuries, intraoccular hemorrhages, spinal cord injuries, peroneal nerve injuries, soft tissue injuries

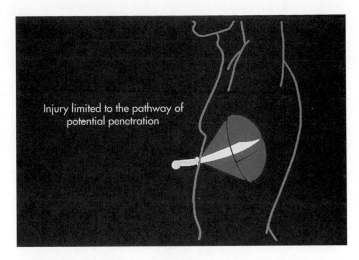

Injury limited to the pathway of potential penetration

FIGURE **19-16**   Movement of knife blade inside victim produces damage, limited to path of penetration. (Modified from Prehospital Trauma Life Support Committee of the National Association of Emergency Medical Technicians in Cooperation with the Committee on Trauma of the American College of Surgeons: *PHTLS: basic and advanced prehospital life support,* ed 4, St. Louis, 1999, Mosby.)

Stab Wounds

Stab wounds are considered low-velocity injuries and therefore low energy. Minimal secondary trauma occurs. Damage is the result of the sharp cutting edge of the wounding agent. For patients with penetrating trauma, knowing the position of the attacker and the victim can identify the projected path of the weapon, weapon used, and gender of the attacker. Women tend to stab downward whereas men tend to stab upward. Determination of gender is not considered absolute because intentional injuries do not always fit a specific pattern.

Damage from a stab wound depends on location of the penetrating object. Tissue damage is generally isolated to the area of penetration (Figure 19-16); however, penetrating injuries with a single wound can penetrate several body cavities, causing lethal injuries. For example, the weapon can enter the thoracic and abdominal cavities with just one penetration. Chest wounds at the level of the nipple or below can involve the abdominal cavity and underlying organs.

More than one wound may exist. It is also important to remember that small entrance wounds can hide extensive internal damage caused by weapon movement. Internal damage is directly proportional to the length of the wounding object and to the density of tissue affected.

Impalements

Impalements are low-velocity injuries that occur as a result of falls, MVCs, or secondary to a flying or falling object. Impaled objects should be stabilized and removed only when the patient is in a controlled environment where surgical support is available.

Gunshot Wounds

Most penetration wounds by firearms are from handguns, shotguns, and rifles. Missile velocity determines tissue deformation and extent of cavitation.[6] Velocity is generally described as low velocity or high velocity. Low-velocity missiles travel at 1000 to 3000 ft/sec and have little disruptive effect on tissues. Injuries are localized at the center of the tract with a small radius of distribution. The temporary cavity is 2 to 3 times the diameter of the missile.[4] Low-velocity missiles push tissues aside along the path.

High-velocity missiles travel more than 3000 ft/sec and cause more serious injuries because of high cavitation and energy transfer.[2] High-velocity missiles create a cavity around the bullet and the bullet tract by compressing and displacing tissue. As kinetic energy is transferred from the bullet to the tissue, the cavity enlarges. A tract temporarily displaces tissue laterally and forward as the missile moves forward. Behind or following the missile, negative pressure contaminates the wound by pulling in foreign material. These cavities can be 30 to 40 times the diameter of the bullet. Wounds often require debridement because of extensive tissue disruption. Figure 19-17 shows the cavitational differences with low-velocity and high-velocity bullets.[3]

Entrance and exit wounds with high-velocity missiles differ with types of tissues and body areas hit.[8] Exit wounds may be larger when the missile travels through smaller structures such as an extremity because all energy has not dissipated by the time the bullet exits; cavitation and missile movement is still occurring. Exit wounds tend to be small in dense tissue because cavitation is complete and most energy is dissipated. If the bullet fragments while traveling through the tissues, no exit wound is found. Figure 19-18 compares entrance and exit wounds.

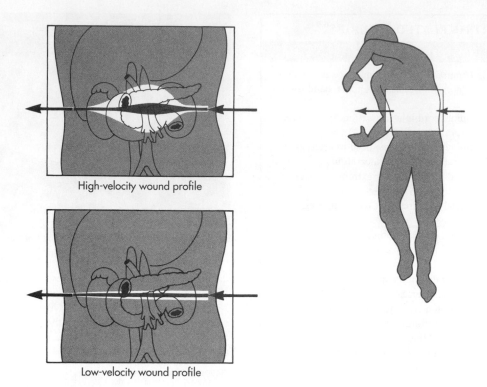

FIGURE **19-17**   Potential injury path of high- and low-velocity bullets. (From Neff JA, Kidd PS: *Trauma nursing: the art and science,* St. Louis, 1993, Mosby.)

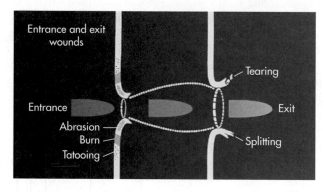

FIGURE **19-18**   A spinning missile produces a 1 to 2 mm abraded edge along wound if it enters straight. If it enters at an angle, abraded side is on bottom of missile, with more skin contact, and covers a much wider area. Difference in entrance and exit wounds is also depicted. Exit wounds are generally longer and more explosive. (Modified from Prehospital Trauma Life Support Committee of the National Association of Emergency Medical Technicians in Cooperation with the Committee on Trauma of the American College of Surgeons: *PHTLS: basic and advanced prehospital life support,* ed 4, St. Louis, 1999, Mosby.)

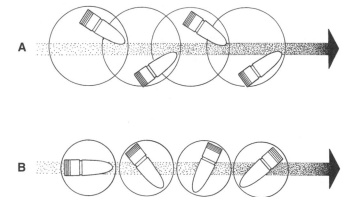

FIGURE **19-19**   Effect of bullet movement on wounding potential. **A,** Yawing. **B,** Tumbling.

Next to velocity, bullet yaw and tumbling are important factors in tissue destruction. Bullets become unstable in flight as velocity increases. Yawing refers to deflection or deviation of the nose of the bullet from a straight path. Tumbling refers to the continuous forward rotation around the center of the bullet causing the bullet to somersault, creating massive tissue destruction. Figure 19-19 demonstrates these movements. Yawing and tumbling increase with impact, producing more damage as temporary and permanent cavity size increases.

Deformation of the bullet is another important factor when assessing gunshot wounds. Energy production increases when missiles change shape on impact. Types of bullets that produce greater kinetic energy include soft-nosed, flat-nosed, and hollow-point bullets that mushroom on impact.

Another feature of gunshot wounds is the muzzle blast seen with close-range wounds or when the gun is pressed

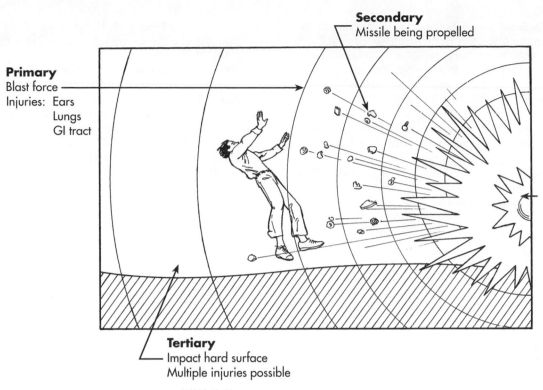

Secondary
Missile being propelled

Primary
Blast force
Injuries: Ears
Lungs
GI tract

Tertiary
Impact hard surface
Multiple injuries possible

FIGURE **19-20**   Effects of an explosive blast.

against the skin. Immediately on firing, a cloud of burning powder and hot gas is released from the muzzle. If a muzzle blast is evident, tattooing from burning particles, abrasions, and burn marks at the entrance wound is seen.

Blast Injuries

Blasts are not as common in the United States as in other countries; however, the potential for hazardous explosions at chemical plants, oil refineries, shipyards, and other industrial settings does exist. Terrorist activity has increased the concern for explosions in urban areas. Explosions can occur anywhere because of the large amount of volatile materials carried by rail or truck. Blasts occur when explosives are detonated and changed to gases. As the gas expands, an equal volume of air is displaced and travels after the blast wave. Disruption of tissue, evisceration, and traumatic amputation can happen from this mass movement of air. When the explosive casing ruptures, the casing fragments become high-velocity projectiles.

The greater density of water means a blast wave travels more rapidly and farther in water than air. Consequently, injuries associated with underwater blasts are usually more severe. Closed-area explosions cause more damage than open-area ones because of the potential inhalation of smoke and toxic gases.

Blast injuries occur in three phases or impact points. Figure 19-20 diagrams how injuries occur from an explosive blast. As explosives change to an expanding mass of heated gas, primary injuries occur because of concussive effects of the pressure wave. Concussion injuries are frequently overlooked because they are not obvious and may occur without external signs of trauma; however, these injuries are usually the most severe. Injuries associated with this mechanism include CNS injuries, rupture of air-containing organs, and tearing of membranes and small vessels. The associated heat wave can also cause burns on areas of the body facing the explosion.

Fragments such as glass, rocks, or metal debris become high-velocity projectiles, causing secondary injuries. Examples of injuries include impalements, fractures, traumatic amputations, burns, and soft-tissue injuries such as contusions, abrasions, and lacerations.

The third point of impact occurs when the victim is thrown through the air and becomes a missile. Tertiary injuries associated with this mechanism are similar to those seen when people are ejected from vehicles or fall from heights, and these injuries generally occur at the point of impact. Structural collapse during the blast can lead to crush injuries.

SUMMARY

Treatment of trauma patients depends on locating all injuries and rapidly intervening to correct those that are life-threatening. Consideration of mechanisms of injury is essential to identify patients with possible underlying injuries who require further evaluation and treatment.

References

1. Creel JH Jr: Scene size-up. In Campbell JE, Alabama Chapter of American College of Emergency Physicians, Editors: *Basic trauma life support for paramedics and other advanced providers,* ed 4, Upper Saddle River, NJ, 2000, Brady.
2. Jacobs BB, editor: *Trauma nursing core course: provider manual,* Des Plaines, Ill, 2000, Emergency Nurses Association.
3. Kidd P: Assessment of the trauma patient. In Neff J, Kidd P, editors, *Trauma nursing: the art and science,* ed 3, St. Louis, 2000, Mosby.
4. Mattox KL, Feliciano DV, Moore EE, editors: *Trauma,* ed 4, New York, 2000, McGraw-Hill.
5. McSwain N: Kinematics of trauma. In McSwain N, White RD, Paturas JL et al, editors: *The basic EMT: comprehensive prehospital patient care,* St. Louis, 1997, Mosby.
6. McQuillan K, Flynn MB, Hartstock RL: *Trauma nursing: from resuscitation through rehabilitation,* ed 3, Philadelphia, 2001, WB Saunders.
7. Porter RS: Blunt trauma. In Bledsoe BE, Porter RS, Cherry RA, editors, *Paramedic care: principles and practice,* Upper Saddle River, NJ, 2001, Prentice-Hall.
8. Porter RS: Penetrating trauma. In Bledsoe BE, Porter RS, Cherry RA, editors, *Paramedic care: principles and practice,* Upper Saddle River, NJ, 2001, Prentice-Hall.
9. Vanderford L, Meyers M: Injuries and bungee jumping, *Sports Med* 20(6):369, 1995.
10. Venes D, editor: *Taber's cyclopedic medical dictionary,* Philadelphia, 2001, FA Davis.

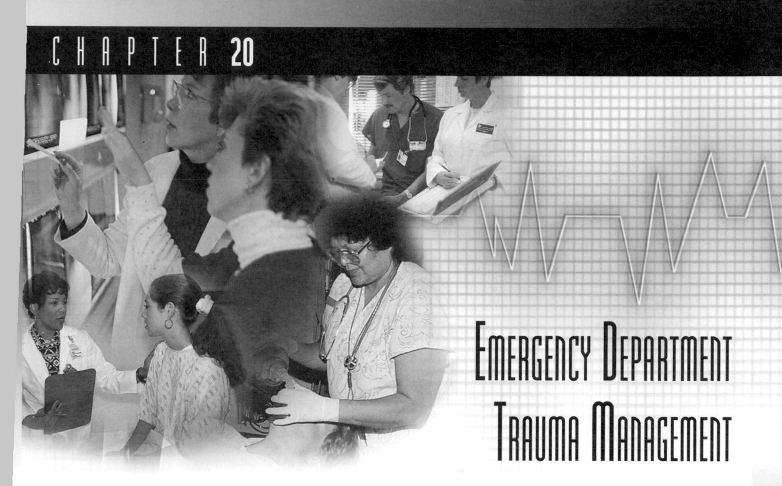

CHAPTER 20

EMERGENCY DEPARTMENT TRAUMA MANAGEMENT

DEBORAH REVIS,
LORENE NEWBERRY

Trauma is the leading cause of death in the United States for people in the first four decades of life. However, death is only the tip of a very large iceberg in the overall devastating effect of traumatic injury in society. Mortality statistics related to trauma death cited to focus on the criticality of injury often neglect to mention morbidity and the lifelong effects of significant injury on the survivor, his or her family, and the community. The fiscal effect of traumatic injury is impressive; the estimated expenditure of total lifetime costs associated with both fatal and nonfatal injuries occurring in any 1 year amount to more than 260 billion (1995 dollars).[6]

The incidence of traumatic injury is not limited to densely populated areas where the majority of designated trauma centers are located. It is therefore incumbent on the emergency nurse to realize that essential clinical competencies and a sound knowledge base in trauma nursing are necessary to provide the highest quality care to this fragile patient population, wherever he or she may practice. Trauma care is ideally provided in institutions that specialize in trauma.[7a] Regional trauma systems were proposed in this country 2 decades ago to reduce injury-related mortality. According to Nathens and colleagues, as of 1995 only 22 states had regional trauma systems. Although states with trauma systems had a 9% lower crude injury mortality rate

than those without,[11] trauma systems and verified trauma centers have not sustained the growth necessary to provide a national network of trauma care. Based on the fiscal burden of trauma care, many hospitals throughout the country have elected to withdraw from voluntary participation in trauma networks or systems.

Because of the inadequate number of designated trauma centers and the distance from hospitals providing such care, many trauma patients are assessed, stabilized, admitted, or treated in nontrauma centers. Emergency nurses in these facilities are challenged by trauma situations similar to those seen in designated trauma centers. Patients do not choose the location of a traumatic injury (e.g., car wreck, fall, gunshot wound) according to how close the accident may occur to a trauma center. The care that is expected, however, by virtue of a hospital holding itself out to offer emergency services is to save the patient's life and to immediately treat all associated injuries. Although specialized trauma centers have treatment areas, staff, and physicians dedicated to trauma care from resuscitation through rehabilitation, most emergency departments (EDs) must provide trauma care while facing a myriad of other patients presenting with an assortment of ailments from sore throat to heart attack. The volume of trauma patients may not be as great as in trauma centers but the intensity faced by the emergency nurse and the requisite knowledge are similar. This chapter describes departmental and staff preparations before trauma patient arrival, management of a trauma patient during the resuscitative phase, transfer criteria to the appropriate level of care, and a critique of the care delivered. Many of the principles presented in this chapter are drawn from the successes of an organized trauma system and designated trauma center criteria prescribed by the American College of Surgeons.[1a]

Table 20-1	COMPONENTS FOR IDEAL EMERGENCY DEPARTMENT TRAUMA RESUSCITATION AREA
COMPONENT	**DESCRIPTION/COMMENTS**
Treatment space	Allow sufficient space for exam stretcher, trauma team, supplies, and traffic around the bed
	Walls should be leaded for stationary x-ray unit
	Locate supplies logically around the room (e.g., airway supplies at head of bed, splinting supplies near foot of bed)
Overhead radiograph capabilities	Ceiling tracks facilitate use and eliminate need for portable machine
	Tracks may interfere with ceiling-mounted IV holders
	May not be able to provide adequate oblique films in some situations
	Adjacent dark room provides best turn-around time for films
Procedure tables	Maintain large procedure tables for trays (e.g., thoracotomy, venisection, peritoneal lavage)
	Create storage space under counters when tables are not used
Surgical light	Choose a model that provides adequate lighting for gross surgical procedures (i.e., ED thoracotomy)
	Two midsized lights might be preferable to one large OR light
	Positioning can be a challenge with radiograph tracks
Wall suction	One suction unit for each bed for gastric, nasotracheal, and two pleural drainage systems
Scrub sink	Foot controls and plaster trap increase effectiveness
Radiograph view box and hot light	Build in hot light to decrease counter clutter
Hemodynamic monitoring	Hardwire units for each bed to monitor cardiac rhythm, NIBP, and pulse oximetry as a minimum
	ICP, arterial pressure, and PA pressure monitoring should be available

ED, Emergency department; *IV,* intravenous; *OR,* operating room; *NIBP,* noninvasive blood pressure; *ICP,* intracranial pressure; *PA,* pulmonary artery.

PREPARATION

Trauma patients arrive in the ED by private automobile, ambulance, helicopter, or police vehicle. The amount of time it takes for a trauma patient to reach an ED or trauma center after injury varies by accident location, length of rescue, availability of an emergency medical services (EMS) system, time it took to report the injury, and other variables. The worst enemy of a trauma patient immediately after an injury is time, thus the often-coined term the *golden hour of trauma.* To decrease mortality and morbidity, ED preparation is an essential element for the maxim of "do no further harm" cited in Advanced Trauma Life Support.[11]

Preparation includes many facets of trauma care, including facility design for the trauma suite or ED room where trauma resuscitations are done, trauma team presence on patient arrival, and necessary drugs and equipment to handle a potentially complicated injury or injuries. The first thing to consider is where the patient will be placed to initiate the resuscitation. Given unlimited funds all EDs can create an ideal trauma resuscitation area. However, this is not realistic for most facilities. Each ED has architectural strengths and weaknesses that require creative solutions for maximum use of space and efficiency of personnel.

The primary objective of a trauma resuscitation area is rapid assessment of a severely injured patient supported by adequate lighting, space, and equipment to identify and treat life-threatening insults (Table 20-1). Before dedicating a specific area of the ED to trauma resuscitations, consideration should be given to community needs related to trauma, ED volume, institutional resources, and number of treatment bays in the ED. It may not be practical to reserve a room solely for trauma victims in a small ED. The charge nurse

Box 20-1	ESSENTIAL SUPPLIES, INSTRUMENTS, AND TRAYS

Crash cart containing ACLS drugs
Intubation supplies with blades, handles, and tubes easily accessible
Chest tube insertion trays with chest drainage systems
Thoracotomy tray including rib spreaders, vascular clamps, long-handled instruments, pledgets, and cardiac sutures
Autotransfusion supplies
Blood and fluid warmer (preferably high-volume devices)
Venous access supplies for peripheral, intraosseus, and central access with range of sizes
Diagnostic peritoneal lavage tray
Defibrillator with pediatric and internal paddles
Transport monitor with ECG, NIBP, pulse oximetry, and end tidal CO_2
Dressings, suture supplies, splinting material, restraints
Gastric tubes, urinary drainage system
Rapid sequence induction medications
Ventilator
Tracheostomy and cricothyrotomy supplies

ACLS, advanced cardiac life support; *ECG,* electrotroencephalogram; *NIBP,* noninvasive blood pressure; CO_2, carbon dioxide.

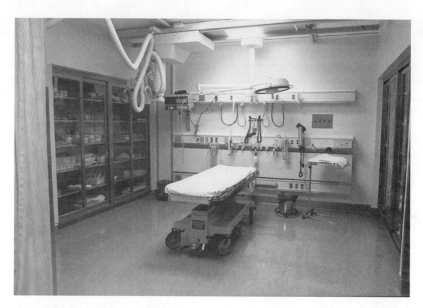

FIGURE 20-1   Emergency department trauma resuscitation bay. Note overhead x-ray and surgery light. (Courtesy WellStar Kennestone Hospital, Marietta, Ga.)

should have the ability to move patients out of an area to accommodate a severely injured patient requiring resuscitation. This space, although used by more than one type of patient, should have equipment located and stored in such a way to facilitate rapid deployment of staff to the room and supplies organized to allow ease in setting up. Equipment should be available to assess and treat life-threatening emergencies such as a compromised airway, a tension pneumothorax, or blood loss (Box 20-1).

Figure 20-1 is an example of a single-patient resuscitation area that can accommodate two patients if necessary. This example provides a more sophisicated arena for trauma care in a larger volume ED than may be found in most facilities. Components considered in creation of a trauma resuscitation area include, first of all, enough space. For effective organization and visualization of supplies and equipment, enough square footage is critical. Unless a storage room is adjacent to the trauma suite, the room may house large equipment such as a Level I Rapid Infuser, Bair Hugger, Bovie, or blanket warmer. Additional space is needed for supplies, carts, cabinets, area for a scribe, computers, and physician documentation area. The right amount of space and organization of supplies decreases tension in an environment ripe for conflict.

Location of the trauma resuscitation room is also important. Given the luxury of placing the room anywhere in the ED, the best choice is unique depending on the location of ambulance portals, trauma elevators, operating room, computed tomography scanner, radiology suite, intensive care unit, special procedures, blood bank, and helipad. Additional structural considerations include adequate metal framing in the ceiling to suspend radiologic equipment, booms for gases versus headwalls, and surgery-quality lighting. If the trauma resuscitation area is not staffed as an independent area, shifting nurses to accommodate this func-

tion is also a critical factor in deciding where the trauma area should be located. A pneumatic tube system may assist in rapid transport of blood samples to the lab. There should be an attempt to locate the room in an area least likely to be compromised by unnecessary observers, such as the press. Wherever the room is located, functionality and patient safety should always be the key deciding factors.

The most sophisticated trauma suite is useless without a well-trained and organized trauma team. A team approach has proven most efficient in reducing valuable seconds that may save the patient's life. Team composition varies with available human resources, but a multidisciplinary team with medical, nursing, and other specialties represented is ideal (Table 20-2). Team members may originate in the ED or come from other areas such as helicopter crews, intensive care units, or the postanesthesia care unit. Notification of team members may include overhead paging and dedicated pagers. Designated trauma centers enhance communication to the team by establishing "trauma alert" criteria for level of patient acuity for team notification.

Team member responsibilities may be identified by procedures, such as establishing intravenous access or focus on a specific anatomic area for assessment (e.g., head, left side of the patient's body). Responsibilities should be clearly defined whether the trauma resuscitation is accomplished in a Level I trauma center or small rural ED.

Trauma protocols are recommended to ensure ongoing quality and to delineate staff responsibilities before the patient arrives. Trauma drills executed before receiving critically injured patients are an effective way to achieve an advanced level of communication. It is too late to practice when a patient is exsanguinating on the table. Trauma critiques after the resuscitation allow the team to identify areas that went well during resuscitation and areas for improvement. Figure 20-2 is an example of a form that may be used

Table 20-2	MULTIDISCIPLINARY TRAUMA TEAM
DISCIPLINE	**ROLE**
Emergency nursing	Assesses patient and provides ongoing care
	Prepares trauma suite
	Documents and coordinates care
	Administers medications
Emergency medicine	Provides initial assessment in many institutions
	Determines notification priority for other specialties (e.g., surgery, neurosurgery, orthopedics)
	Intubates and provides initial airway management
	Maintains awareness of need to complete essential tests such as cervical spine films
Surgery	Acts as team leader in trauma centers
	Focuses on surgical management and diagnosis of traumatic injuries
Pulmonary services	Provided by anesthesiology in some institutions
	Intubates, manages airway and ventilations
	Collects lab specimens and obtains ECG in some situations
Radiology services	Completes essential radiographs and special procedures
	Provides final interpretation onsite or through use of teleradiography
Laboratory	Collects specimen and analyzes trauma panels
Blood bank	Processes type and cross-match; provides uncross-matched blood when needed
Social services/ patient representative	Contacts family, minister, and others
	Provides immediate support to family during resuscitation
	Obtains vital information and documents valuables
Ancillary staff	Includes nursing assistants, patient care technicians, and other nonlicensed personnel
	Removes clothing, transports patient, and performs procedures (e.g., ECG, splint application, dressing wounds, and urethral catheterization)

ECG, Electrocardiogram.

for a trauma critique. These critiques should follow the trauma resuscitation as soon as possible, regardless of whether the process went exceptionally well or there were problems that need immediate resolution. The focus of the critique is not on staff but on the processes built into the protocol. Outcome of the critique is a stronger team, efficiency, and a focus on overall care.

Preparation begins before the patient arrives. As stated previously, preparation includes an organized area within the scope of the facility's resources to accommodate resuscitation of a severely injured patient. The team should be alerted as rapidly as possible before patient arrival and should communicate with each other in the moments available before the resuscitation begins. This communication can clarify confusion about responsibilities but also helps individual members focus as a team on anticipated injuries. The effectiveness of EDs and trauma centers depends on the entire team working together with a common vision of efficient, skilled, and organized management. In most instances some prior notification is provided by EMS. The person receiving the notification should elicit as much information as possible without compromising rapid transport of the patient. Knowing in advance the mechanism of injury and patient acuity facilitates set-up of special equipment. Knowing for example that a patient with a gunshot wound to the chest was found in an alley in 20° F will help caregivers anticipate and intervene early for hypothermia. It is not financially prudent to open a large number of supplies and trays before patient arrival; however, it is wise to secure necessary equipment ahead of time and have it readily accessible.

Documentation of the trauma resuscitation protects the patient, institution, and staff providing care. The record reflects efforts of the trauma team from the first moments of patient arrival, providing evidence of the patient's physiologic response to treatment. Vital sign changes, decreased urinary output, and decreasing oxygen saturation are examples of indicators that alert the astute nurse to physiologic compromise in the patient's condition. Tools used for documentation vary from institution to institution but generally involve written or computerized documentation tools. Many institutions use trauma flowsheets rather than a narrative script. Figure 20-3 shows a flowsheet used by a busy, designated Level I trauma center. Flowsheets are usually more user-friendly and accommodate documentation in the stressful atmosphere of trauma resuscitation.

Trauma care is intense because of the gravity of the patient's condition. This intensity occurs in spite of extensive planning and preparation. Each trauma patient's presentation is unique, with numerous unknown facts. The appearance of injuries associated with a traumatic event can be overwhelming to even the most seasoned trauma practitioner. Conflicts can arise among team members when faced with life-and-death decisions related to the patient's care. The trauma resuscitation room is often noisy and crowded. Some practical tips for ED trauma management are found in Box 20-2 on p. 238. These tips are offered not to create a perfect environment for trauma resuscitations but to arrest potential irritants in this challenging environment.

Trauma damage control logs are used in some trauma centers (Figure 20-4, p. 239). These logs alert the trauma coordinator, charge nurse, or ED management of conditions existing in the trauma suite that require immediate attention. Examples of entries in a trauma damage control log include broken or missing equipment, a physician request to add a new drug to the formulary, or a suggestion on how to improve a component of the trauma protocols. The trauma damage control log should have an entry on who followed

Text continued on p. 238

Date: _____

University of Alabama at Birmingham (UAB)
Emergency Department
TRAUMA CRITIQUE FORM

Case summary/Brief fact scenario

_____
_____
_____
_____
_____
_____
_____
_____
_____

	Yes	No	Comments
EMS Report			
Met trauma alert criteria – alerted?			
Room prepared?			
Trauma team notified?			
Trauma protocol followed?			
Support staff present?			

Positive aspects of resuscitation

_____
_____
_____
_____
_____

Areas for improvement

_____
_____
_____
_____
_____
_____
_____

Miscellaneous comments

_____
_____
_____
_____
_____

FIGURE 20-2   Example of a trauma critique form. (Courtesy University of Alabama at Birmingham Emergency Department, Birmingham, Ala.)

Grady Health System®
80 Butler Street
Atlanta, GA 30335

Allergies

Date:________________________

Arrival Time:________________________

ED Notification Time:__________ DOB__________ Age:__________ Mechanism of injury:____________________
Time Trauma Team Called:____________________ Sex:__________ ____________________
Stat ☐ Resp ☐ LMP:__________ Approximate time of injury:__________
Transported by:____________________Service LOC duration:_____ Last Tetanus__________
☐ground ☐ air Safety belt: ☐ yes ☐ no ☐ unkown Helmet ☐ yes ☐ no ☐ unknown
Prior Medical Hx:______________________________Current Meds____________________

Emerg. Med. Attending
____

Emerg.Med. Resident
____

	Surgery Attending	Surgery Resident	ORTHO	NSQ.
Called				
Responded				
Arrival				

Morehouse ☐ Emory ☐

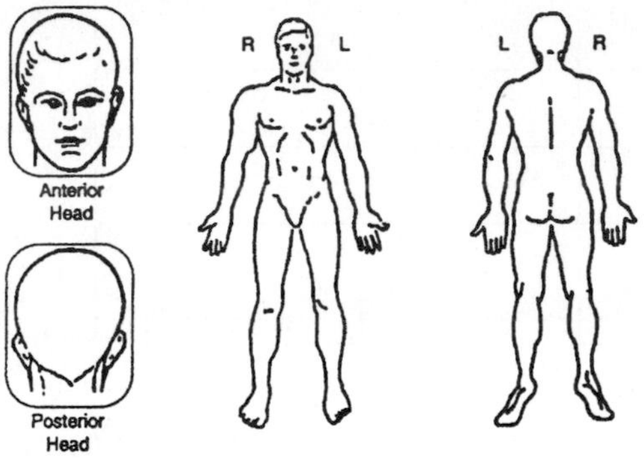

Anterior Head
Posterior Head
R
L
L
R

A. Abrasion
B. Burn
C. Contusion
D. Deformity
E. Ecchymosis
F. Fracture
G. GSW
H. Edema
I. Avulsion
J. Tenderness
K. Scar
L. Laceration
M. Amputation
N. Stab
☐ IV's on arrival

Airway ☐ clear ☐ obstructed
C-spine: ☐ immobilized ☐ cleared
Breathing: ☐ normal ☐ labored
☐ shallow ☐ assisted ☐ intubated
☐ absent ☐ trach deviation
Circulation: ☐ carotid rhythm__________
Skin: ☐ cool ☐ warm ☐ dry ☐ wet
☐ pale ☐ flushed ☐ cyanotic ☐ mottled
Chest: ☐ decreased ☐ R ☐ L
☐ absent ☐ R ☐ L
☐ asymmetrical ☐ symmetrical
Extremities: (Circle if NOT present)
Upper: Moves sensation - pulses ☐ R
: Moves - sensation - pulses ☐ L
Lower: Moves sensation - pulses ☐ R
Moves sensation - pulses ☐ L

Time	BP	Pulse	Resp	Temp	0_2 Sat	GCS	NURSES NOTES

Page 1 of 2 WHITE - Medical Records YELLOW - Trauma Center PINK - Emergency Dept. 12/96

FIGURE 20-3 Emergency department trauma flow sheet. (Courtesy Grady Health System, Atlanta, Ga.)

Continued

TIME PROCEDURE

_____ Rigid C-Collar _____ Headrolls/tape _____ Spineboard
_____ 0_2: Device_____%_____ Device_____%_____
_____ OGT_____
_____ Trauma Labs:

☐ Chem 19   ☐ UDS
☐ Amylase   ☐ UA
☐ PT - PIT   ☐ ABG
☐ CBC   ☐ T & CM
☐ Beta HCG

_____ CT
_____ US   +☐   -☐
_____ Radiology
_____ Peritoneal Lavage:

In_____cc   Out_____cc
Blood: Positive   Negative

_____ Foley #_____   OGT_____
Blood: With dip stick   _____Positive   _____Negative
_____ Chest Tube: Right_____Fr.   Left_____Fr.
_____ Autotransfusion:_____cc
_____ Rectal Tone: Normal   Absent
_____ Stool Guaiac: Positive   Negative
_____ Prostate_____

INTAKE AND OUTPUT

CRYSTALLOIDS   PTA_____cc Total

Time	IV#	Solution	Amount	Site	Total Infused

TOTAL CRYSTALLOIDS ABSORBED

BLOOD COMPONENTS (include autotransfusion)

Time	Unit#	Solution	Amount	Site	Total Absorbed

TOTAL BLOOD PRODUCTS ABSORBED

GLASGOW COMA SCALE - ADULT

1. Eye Opening:
   Spontaneous 4
   To Voice 3
   To Pain 2
   None 1

2. Verbal Response:
   Oriented 5
   Confused 4
   Inappropriate Words 3
   Incomprehensible Words 2

3. Motor Responses:
   None 1
   Obeys Commands 6
   Purposeful Movement (Pain) 5
   Withdraw (Pain) 4
   Flexion (Pain) 3
   Extension (Pain) 2
   None 1

TOTAL _____

GLASGOW COMA SCALE - PEDIATRIC

1. Eye Opening: Spontaneous   4
                  To Speech   3
                  To Pain   2
                  None   1

2. Best Verbal:
   oriented/smiles,cries 5
   confused 4
   inapprop./inapp. cry 3
   incomprehensible/grunts 2
   no response 1

3. Best Motor:
   Spontaneous 6
   Localizes Pain 5
   Withdraws to pain 4
   Decorticate (Flexion) 3
   Decerebrate (Extension) 2
   None 1

REFERENCE TOTAL _____

MEDICATIONS ALLERGIES _____

Time	Med	Dos	Route	Initial
	Tetanus/0.5cc		IM	

MD Signature:

DISPOSITION SUMMARY:

Time family notified:_____   Time out of ED:_____
By whom:_____
Clerk Disposition of: Clothing_____   valuables_____ #

Nurse Signature:_____

Admission: OR ☐   ICU ☐

Admited to: ☐ Surgery   ☐ Ortho
             ☐ Neuro Surg. ☐ Home
             ☐ Morgue   ☐ Other_____

Nurse II:_____

M ONITOR

WHITE - Medical Records   YELLOW - Trauma Center   PINK - Emergency Dept.

FIGURE 20-3 cont'd

Box 20-2	PRACTICAL TIPS FOR EMERGENCY DEPARTMENT TRAUMA MANAGEMENT

PERSONNEL/TRAUMA TEAM

Determine team composition; then post daily assignments.

Decide which physician is in charge.

Designate a primary nurse who is assigned to the patient and is responsible for coordination of care.

Designate a recorder or scribe for initial resuscitation.

Identify a documentation area in a permanent location or flexible area for each room.

Don personal protective equipment (e.g., gown, goggles, gloves) and lead aprons before patient arrives.

Establish protocols for patient assessment, trauma labs, trauma surgeon notification, and trauma surgeon back-up.

Practice and critique protocols.

Provide interpreter services.

Develop a trauma flow sheet.

ROOM/SUPPLIES

Maintain personal protective equipment (e.g., gowns, gloves, masks, shoe covers) for team members.

Keep sufficient lead aprons hanging in the room.

Stock large sharps containers.

Organize supplies by system or process (e.g., abdominal, thoracic, hemodynamic).

Place IV access supplies on both sides of the room.

Place large trash cans and linen containers in room.

Place essential forms and phone numbers at the documentation area.

Install at least one dictation line and two phones in the area.

Put intubation supplies at the head of the bed.

Stock prenumbered trauma charts and forms at the documentation area.

Create a separate pediatric resuscitation area or cart stocked with pediatric supplies.

Do not overstock.

Remove clutter.

Keep critical items visible.

IV, intravenous.

up on a problem and if the problem was resolved. This log should be maintained under the protection of quality improvement safeguards within an institution.

INITIAL RESUSCITATION

This chapter does not lend itself to the details of complete trauma resuscitation. Rather, an approach to the multisystem traumatized patient is discussed. It is highly recommended that a nurse employed in the ED take the Trauma Nursing Core Course offered by the Emergency Nurses Association. This 2-day course provides core-level knowledge of trauma nursing care through lectures and teaching stations to facilitate acquisition of requisite psychomotor skills. Most trauma courses and textbooks approach trauma patient care with a primary assessment followed by the secondary assessment.

This approach provides an organized and structured method for assessment of the patient with multiple injuries. The risk in not using such a structured approach is to rush immediately toward obvious wounds (e.g., amputations, open fractures, crushed extremity) and therefore miss subtle but life-threatening injuries. While using a framework of primary and secondary assessment, it is important to realize that a host of interventions may be occurring simultaneously. For example, while the physician in charge is assessing the patient's airway and reporting findings to the scribe, the nurse may be simultaneously inserting an intravenous catheter.

Primary assessment, the first visual impression of the patient, includes evaluation of the airway (with cervical spine immobilization), breathing, circulation (ABCs), and disability or neurologic status (Table 20-3). Primary assessment begins as the patient comes through the door. It should be pointed out that the first primary assessment was conducted in the field when the patient was transported by EMS. Listening to the paramedic's report without delaying care can provide invaluable information about mechanism of injury, injuries, previous vital signs, and prehospital treatment. This information provides comparison data to determine changes in patient condition.

The routine approach with the ABCs of trauma assessment have proven to provide the necessary structure to remain focused in an environment that can distract experienced physicians or nurses. Tables 20-4, 20-5, and 20-6 provide examples of life-threatening problems related to airway, breathing, and circulation problems. Symptoms and interventions are also discussed. These tables are not exhaustive of all life-threatening problems that a patient with traumatic injury can experience. The intent of these tables is to illustrate that problems falling into these categories must be treated immediately in the order in which they are identified—airway, then breathing, then circulation. Treating circulatory problems without ensuring that the patient has a patent airway places the patient's life in immediate danger.

Secondary assessment is a more complete evaluation including vital signs, history, head-to-toe examination, and inspection of the back (Box 20-3, on p. 242). Some potentially life-threatening injuries identified by secondary assessment include hypothermia, pelvic fractures, and spinal cord injury. Certain injuries suggest the presence of concomitant injuries that should alert the emergency nurse to the need for careful assessment and ongoing monitoring (Table 20-7, on p. 243). Obvious fractures should be immobilized and open wounds covered with sterile saline gauze.

Diagnostic studies including laboratory analysis and radiographic examination are obtained following assessment and treatment of life-threatening injuries. Blood work varies with each institution but should include as a minimum a type and cross-match. Table 20-8, on p. 243 identifies common laboratory tests obtained in trauma patients and provides clinical implications for each. Radiographic examinations vary with institutions and patient assessment; however, specific studies and related clinical implications are summarized in Table 20-9, on

University of Alabama at Birmingham (UAB)
Damage Control Log

Date	Problem/ Concern	Suggested solution	Contact person/ Pager #	Date resolved	Comments

FIGURE 20-4   Damage control log. (Courtesy University of Alabama at Birmingham Emergency Department, Birmingham, Ala.)

p. 244. Special procedures such as angiography and diagnostic peritoneal lavage are indicated for some patients (Table 20-10, on p. 244). When the patient must be taken from the ED to the radiology department, a transport monitor, oxygen, and documentation forms should be taken with the patient.

Trauma patients should be carefully monitored throughout resuscitation for changes in condition and development of life-threatening problems. Patients may go directly to surgery after rapid ED management, remain in the ED for extensive diagnostic tests, or be transferred for specialty care. Patients transferred usually include those with burn injuries, pediatric trauma, and spinal fracture. Transfer to a trauma center should be considered for patients with multiple injuries, cardiac injury, and comorbid factors. Table 20-11, on p. 245, reviews criteria for early transfer to a trauma center.

Text continued on p. 245

Table 20-3 PRIMARY ASSESSMENT

ASSESSMENTS	INTERVENTIONS
A = AIRWAY WITH SIMULTANEOUS CERVICAL SPINE STABILIZATION AND/OR IMMOBILIZATION	
While maintaining spinal stabilization:	Position the patient
Vocalization	Jaw thrust or chin lift
Tongue obstruction	Suction or remove foreign objects
Loose teeth or foreign objects	Oro/nasopharyngeal airway
Bleeding	Cervical spine stabilization
Vomitus or other secretions	Endotracheal intubation
Edema	Needle or surgical cricothyrotomy
B = BREATHING	
Spontaneous breathing	Supplemental oxygen
Chest rise and fall	Bag-valve-mask ventilation
Skin color	Needle thoracentesis
General rate and depth of respirations	Chest tube
Soft tissue and bony chest wall integrity	Nonporous dressing taped on 3 sides
Use of accessory and/or abdominal muscles	
Bilateral breath sounds	
Jugular veins and position of trachea	
C = CIRCULATION	
Pulse general rate and quality	Direct pressure over uncontrolled bleeding sites
Skin color, temperature, degree of diaphoresis	Two large-bore intravenous catheters with warmed lactated Ringer's solution or normal saline
External bleeding	Infuse fluid rapidly with blood tubing
	Blood sample for typing
	Pericardiocentesis
	ED thoracotomy
	Cardiopulmonary resuscitation and advanced life support measures
	Blood administration
	Surgery
D = DISABILITY (NEUROLOGIC STATUS)	

Modified from Emergency Nurses Association: *Trauma nursing core course provider manual,* ed 5, Des Plaines, Ill, 2000, The Association.

Table 20-4 LIFE-THREATENING AIRWAY PROBLEMS

PROBLEM	SIGNS AND SYMPTOMS	INTERVENTIONS

Airway obstruction (complete or partial)	Dyspnea, labored respirations
	Decreased or no air movement
	Cyanosis
	Presence of foreign body in airway
	Trauma to face or neck
	Breathless
	Agitation
	Combativeness
		Airway opening maneuvers
		  Jaw thrust
		  Chin lift
		  Suction
		Airway adjuncts
		  Nasal airway
		  Oral airway
		  Endotracheal tube
		  Laryngeal mask airway (LMA)
		Surgical airway
		  Cricothyrotomy
		  Tracheostomy

Inhalation injury	History of enclosed space fire, unconsciousness, or exposure to heavy smoke Dyspnea Wheezing, rhonchi, crackles Hoarseness Singed facial or nasal hairs Carbonaceous sputum Burns to face or neck	Provide high-flow oxygen (100%) via nonrebreather mask or bag-valve device Prepare for endotracheal intubation as soon as possible

Modified from Kidd PS, Sturt P, Fultz J: *Mosby's emergency nursing reference,* ed 2, St. Louis, 2000, Mosby.

Table 20-5 **LIFE-THREATENING BREATHING PROBLEMS**

PROBLEM	SIGNS AND SYMPTOMS	INTERVENTIONS
Tension pneumothorax	Dyspnea, labored respirations Decreased or absent breath sounds on affected side Unilateral chest rise and fall Tracheal deviation away from affected side Cyanosis Jugular venous distension Tachycardia and hypotension History of chest trauma or mechanical ventilation	Provide high-flow oxygen (100%) via nonrebreather mask or bag-valve device Perform rapid chest decompression by needle thoracotomy Place chest tube on affected side
Pneumothorax	Dyspnea, labored respirations Decreased or absent breath sounds on affected side May have unilateral chest rise and fall May have visible wound to chest or back History of chest trauma	Provide high-flow oxygen (100%) via nonrebreather mask or bag-valve device Place chest tube on affected side Place occlusive dressing over any open chest wound and secure on three sides with tape
Hemothorax	Dyspnea, labored respirations Decreased or absent breath sounds on affected side May have unilateral chest rise and fall May have visible wound to chest or back History of chest trauma (usually penetrating)	Provide high-flow oxygen (100%) via nonrebreather mask or bag-valve device Place chest tube on affected side Consider autotransfusion
Sucking chest wound	Dyspnea, labored respirations Decreased or absent breath sounds on affected side Visible, sucking wound to chest or back	Provide high-flow oxygen (100%) via nonrebreather mask or bag-valve device Cover wound with occlusive dressing and secure on three sides with tape Watch for signs of tension pneumothorax and remove dressing during exhalation if they are noted
Flail chest	Dyspnea, labored respirations Paradoxical chest wall movement Chest pain Tachycardia	Provide high-flow oxygen (100%) via nonrebreather mask or bag-valve device Prepare for intubation and mechanical ventilation
Full-thickness circumferential burn of thorax	Dyspnea, labored respirations Shallow respirations Obvious circumferential burns to thorax	Provide high-flow oxygen (100%) via nonrebreather mask or bag-valve device Prepare for immediate escharotomy

Modified from Kidd PS, Sturt P, Fultz J: *Mosby's emergency nursing reference*, ed 2, St. Louis, 2000, Mosby.

Table 20-6 **LIFE-THREATENING CIRCULATION PROBLEMS**

PROBLEM	SIGNS AND SYMPTOMS	INTERVENTIONS
External hemorrhage	Obvious bleeding site	Direct pressure Elevation
Shock	Tachycardia Weak, thready pulses Cool, pale, clammy skin Tachypnea Altered mental status Delayed capillary refill Oliguria or anuria	Provide high-flow oxygen (100%) via nonrebreather mask or bag-valve device Place two large-bore IV lines with warm isotonic crystalloid solution infusing (lactated Ringer's solution or 0.9% NaCl) Administer fluid bolus (2 L in adults or 20 ml/kg in children) Prepare to administer blood

Modified from Kidd PS, Sturt P, Fultz J: *Mosby's emergency nursing reference*, ed 2, St. Louis, 2000, Mosby.
IV, Intravenous.

Box 20-3	SECONDARY ASSESSMENT

E = EXPOSE PATIENT/ENVIRONMENTAL CONTROL (REMOVE CLOTHING AND KEEP PATIENT WARM)

Remove clothing
Use blankets
Use warming lights

F = FULL SET OF VITAL SIGNS/FIVE INTERVENTIONS/FACILITATE FAMILY PRESENCE

In addition to obtaining a complete set of vital signs, consider the five interventions:
  Cardiac monitor
  Pulse oximeter (SpO_2)
  Urinary catheter if not contraindicated
  Gastric tube
  Laboratory studies
  Facilitate family presence

G = GIVE COMFORT MEASURES

Verbal reassurance
Touch
Pain control

H = HISTORY

MIVT
Patient-generated information
Past medical history

H = HEAD-TO-TOE ASSESSMENT

Head and face
  Inspect for wounds, ecchymosis, deformities, drainage from nose and ears, and check pupils
  Palpate for tenderness, note bony crepitus, deformity
Neck
  Remove the anterior portion of the cervical collar to inspect and palpate the neck. Another team member must hold the patient's
    head while the collar is being removed and replaced
  Inspect for wounds, ecchymosis, deformities, and distended neck veins
  Palpate for tenderness, note bony crepitus, deformity, subcutaneous emphysema, and tracheal position
Chest
  Inspect for breathing rate and depth, wounds, deformities, ecchymosis, use of accessory muscles, paradoxical movement
  Auscultate breath and heart sounds
  Palpate for tenderness, note bony crepitus, subcutaneous emphysema, and deformity
Abdomen and flanks
  Inspect for sounds, distention, ecchymosis, and scars
  Auscultate bowel sounds
  Palpate four quadrants for tenderness, rigidity, guarding, masses, and femoral pulses
Pelvis and perineum
  Inspect for wounds, deformities, ecchymosis, priapism, blood at the urinary meatus or in the perineal area
  Palpate the pelvis and anal sphincter tone
Extremities
  Inspect for ecchymosis, movement, wounds, and deformities
  Palpate for pulses, skin temperature, sensation, tenderness, deformities, and note bony crepitus

I = INSPECT POSTERIOR SURFACES

Maintain cervical spine stabilization and support injured extremities while the patient is logrolled
Inspect posterior surface for wounds, deformities, and ecchymosis
Palpate posterior surfaces for tenderness and deformities
Palpate anal sphincter tone (if not performed previously)

Modified from Emergency Nurses Association: *Trauma nursing core course,* ed 5, Des Plaines, Ill, 2000, The Association.
MIVT, Mechanism, injuries, vital signs, treatment.

Table 20-7	SENTINEL INJURIES AND ASSOCIATED FINDINGS	
INJURY	**ASSOCIATED INJURIES**	
First rib fracture	Heart and great vessel injury (i.e., sub-clavian vein and artery), head and neck injury	
Scapula fracture	Brachial plexus injury, pulmonary contusion, great vessel injury, CNS injury	
Sternal fracture	Myocardial contusion, great vessel injury, pulmonary contusion	
Lower rib fractures		
Left	Spleen lacerations	
Right	Liver lacerations	

CNS, Central nervous system.

Table 20-8	COMMON LABORATORY TESTS
LABORATORY TEST	**CLINICAL IMPLICATIONS**
Complete blood count (CBC)	Hematocrit and hemoglobin may be normal or above normal despite acute hemorrhage; normal values do not exclude hemorrhagic shock
Electrolytes	Baseline data
	Rule out electrolyte imbalance
Protime (PT)	Baseline data
Prothrombin time (PTT)	Rule out coagulopathies
Amylase	Baseline data
	Elevated value may indicate possible intraabdominal injury
Lipase	Baseline data
	Elevated value may indicate possible intraabdominal injury; has higher sensitivity for pancreatic injury
Lactate	Baseline data
	Elevated level correlates with acute hemorrhage, shock, and increased anaerobic metabolism
Arterial blood gas (ABG)	Assess ventilatory and respiratory status
	Acidosis, especially in the presence of normal or decreased $PaCO_2$ level correlates with shock
	Base deficit of −6 or greater correlates with acute hemorrhage and shock
	Decreased PaO_2 and SaO_2 and an elevated $PaCO_2$ may indicate an airway or breathing emergency
Liver function tests (LFTs)	Baseline data
	Elevated values may indicate liver damage
Type and cross-match	Prepare for administration of blood and blood products
Urinalysis	Dip for blood; gross hematuria suggests injury

Modified from Kidd PS, Sturt P, Fultz J: *Mosby's emergency nursing reference*, ed 2, St. Louis, 2000, Mosby.

PaCO₂, Partial pressure of carbon dioxide in arterial gas; *PaO₂*, alveolar-arterial difference in partial pressure of oxygen; *SaO₂*, arterial oxygen saturation.

Table 20-9 COMMON RADIOGRAPHIC EXAMINATIONS		
RADIOGRAPHIC EXAMINATION	**INDICATION**	**CLINICAL IMPLICATIONS**
Chest x-ray	Chest trauma or pain Shortness of breath Abnormal breath sounds	Anteroposterior examination with patient in supine position if immobilized Should be taken immediately upon arrival if possible Do not delay treatment of a suspected tension pneumothorax for a chest x-ray
Pelvis x-ray	Blunt trauma Pelvic pain or instability Blood at urethral meatus	Anteroposterior examination with patient in supine position Should be taken early in the resuscitation
Cervical spine x-ray	Blunt trauma Trauma above nipple line Neck tenderness Neurologic deficit	Cross-table lateral film usually obtained early in resuscitation, with three views required to complete the series Immobilization should be maintained until spine is radiographically and clinically cleared
Thoracic and lumbar spine x-ray	Blunt trauma Back pain or trauma Neurologic deficit	Patient should be logrolled until spine is cleared radiographically and clinically
Extremity x-rays	Extremity trauma, deformity, or pain	Suspected fractures should be immobilized before radiographs
Head CT	Head trauma Loss of consciousness Focal neurologic findings Altered level of consciousness	Transfer to a definitive care facility should not be delayed to obtain a head CT
Abdominal CT	Abdominal trauma or pain Altered level of consciousness Unreliable clinical examinations	Transfer to a definitive care facility should not be delayed to obtain an abdominal CT
Abdominal ultrasound	Abdominal trauma or pain	Interference in imaging may occur with obesity, bowel gas, and subcutaneous emphysema

Modified from Kidd PS, Sturt P, Fultz J: *Mosby's emergency nursing reference*, ed 2, St. Louis, 2000, Mosby.
CT, Computed tomography.

Table 20-10 COMMON SPECIAL PROCEDURES		
PROCEDURE	**INDICATION**	**CLINICAL IMPLICATIONS**
Angiography	Suspected vessel injury Cerebral blood flow study	Be prepared to assess and intervene in the event of an anaphylactic reaction to contrast media Insertion site must be watched closely for bleeding after procedure
Diagnostic peritoneal lavage	Abdominal trauma or pain, especially in a hemodynamically unstable patient	Gastric and bladder decompression must be done before performing a diagnostic peritoneal lavage This procedure does not evaluate the retroperitoneal space
Transesophageal echocardiogram	Widened mediastinum Significant chest trauma	Patient is usually rolled on side for procedure Patient may be sedated during procedure

Modified from Kidd PS, Sturt P, Fultz J: *Mosby's emergency nursing reference*, ed 2, St. Louis, 2000, Mosby.
CT, Computed tomography.

Table 20-11	CRITERIA FOR EARLY TRANSFER OF TRAUMA PATIENT	
SYSTEM/ LOCATION	**INJURY**
Central nervous system	Penetrating injury or open fracture with or without cerebrospinal fluid leak
	Depressed skull fracture
	Glasgow Coma Scale (GCS) <14 or GCS deterioration
	Lateralizing signs
	Spinal cord injury or major vertebral injury
Thoracic	Major chest wall injury
	Widened mediastinum or other suggestions of great vessel injury
	Cardiac injury
	Patients receiving prolonged ventilation
Pelvis	Unstable pelvic ring fracture
	Unstable pelvic fracture with shock or continued hemorrhage
	Open pelvic injury
	Acetabular fractures
Major extremity injuries	Fracture or dislocation with loss of distal pulses
	Open long-bone fractures
	Ischemic extremity
Multiple injuries	Head injury with face, chest, abdominal, or pelvic injury
	Burns with associated injury
	Multiple long-bone fractures
	Injury to two or more body regions
Co-morbid factors	Age more than 55 years
	Pediatric patient
	Cardiac or respiratory disease
	Morbid obesity
	Pregnancy
	Immunosuppression

SUMMARY

Patients who survive a traumatic injury long enough to reach definitive care in an ED are fortunate. Aggressive assessment and interventions to sustain the patient's life must be modulated with appreciation for the delicacy of his or her condition. For example, rough transfer from ambulance stretcher to the ED stretcher can exaggerate an existing injury, dislodge vital intravenous catheters, or precipate fibrillation in a hypothermic patient. One of the overlooked roles of the emergency nurse assigned to care for a trauma patient is protection from further harm while assisting with necessary life-saving interventions. The emergency nurse must advocate for appropriate pain management, which may be forgotten during heroic life-saving interventions.

The importance of ED trauma management cannot be overstated. All EDs provide trauma care, with emergency nurses holding a pivotal role. Staff and departmental preparation minimize confusion and decrease time required for definitive care. A systematic approach to assessment and intervention improves patient outcomes through early recognition of potentially life-threatening injuries and intervention for identified problems.

References

1. American College of Surgeons: *Advanced trauma life support provider manual,* ed 6, Chicago, 1997, The College..

1a. American College of Surgeons: Resource document for optimal care of the injured patient, Chicago, 1999, The College.

2. Calleary J, el-Nazir A, el-Sadig O et al: Advanced trauma and life support principles: an audit of their application in a rural trauma centre, *Ir J Med Sci,* 168(2):93, 1999.

3. Conte M: Fluid resuscitation in the trauma patient, *CRNA* 8(1):31, 1997.

4. Emergency Nurses Association: *Trauma nursing core course provider manual* ed 5, Des Plaines, Ill, 2000, The Association.

5. MacKenzie E: Review of evidence regarding trauma system effectiveness resulting from panel studies, *J Trauma* 47 (Suppl 3):534, 1999.

6. MacKenzie E: Trauma. In Mattox K, Feliciano D, Moore EE, editors:*Trauma,* ed 4, New York, 1999, McGraw-Hill.

7. Mann N: Assessing the effectiveness and optimal structure of trauma systems: a consensus among experts, *J Trauma* 47 (suppl 3):S69, 1999.

7a. Mattox KL, Feliciano DV, Moore EE: *Trauma,* ed 4, New York, 2000, McGraw-Hill.

8. May A, McGwin G, Lancaster L et al: The April 8, 1998 tornado: assessment of the trauma system response and the resulting injuries, *J Trauma* 48(4):666, 2000.

9. Mikhail J: Resuscitation endpoints in trauma, *AACN Clin Issues* 10(1):10, 1999.

10. Mikhail J: The trauma triad of death, hypothermia, acidosis, and coagulopathy, *AACN Clin Issues* 10(1):85, 1999.

11. Nathens A, Jurkovich G, Rivara F et al: Effectiveness of state trauma systems in reducing injury-related mortality: a national evaluation, *J Trauma* 48(1):25, 2000.

12. Podnos Y, Wilson S, Williams R: Effect of surgical panel composition on patient outcome at a level 1 trauma center, *Am Med Assoc* 133(8):847, 1998.

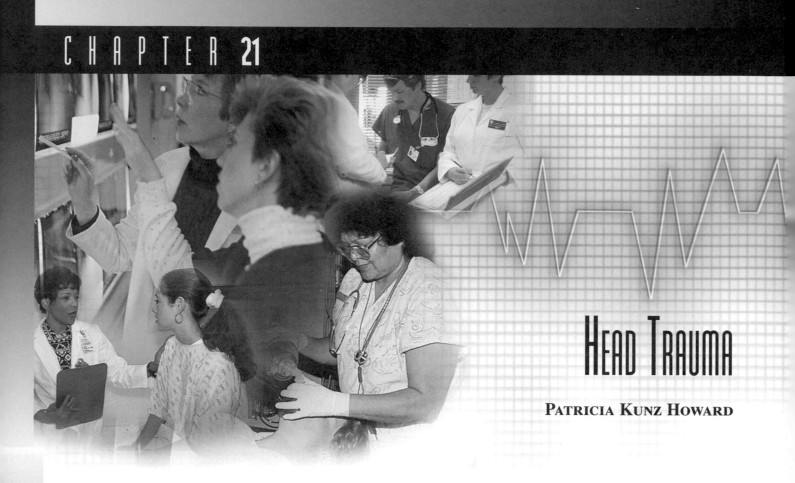

CHAPTER 21

HEAD TRAUMA

PATRICIA KUNZ HOWARD

Epidemiology of traumatic brain injury in the United States has shown that these injuries are most likely to cause death or permanent disability. Approximately half of the annual trauma deaths in the United States can be attributed to head injuries. Annually in the United States more than 1 million people sustain head injuries, 230,000 are hospitalized and survive, while yet another 50,000 die from traumatic brain injury.[6,12,14] The cost of traumatic brain injuries to our society is devastating from a financial and psychosocial impact. Annual expenditures for direct care of victims with traumatic brain injury (TBI) exceed $4.5 billion. Injuries permanently change the lives of the victim and the family.

TBIs occur most frequently as a result of motor vehicle crashes, violence, and falls. Changes in momentum cause stress and deformation of brain tissues including neuronal, axonal, and vascular structures.[2] A small percentage of patients with severe TBI have concomitant fracture of the cervical spine. Alcohol is recognized as a contributing factor in the incidence of TBI, placing the victim at greater risk for injury and making assessment of the head-injured patient more complex. Causes of TBI differ by age: falls are most common for people older than age 65, whereas motor vehicle crashes remain the prevalent cause for people 5 to 64 years of age, with the 15- to 24-year-old age-group at greatest risk. Traumatic brain injuries caused by firearms have a high association with fatality; greater than 90% of the victims die.[12] Approximately two thirds of these deaths are classified as suicides. The high incidence and prevalence of TBI reinforces the need to develop more effective prevention strategies.

This chapter begins with brief review of anatomy and physiology. It also provides an overview of assessment techniques for adult patients with acute head injuries. Current management options for TBI are also discussed. Refer to Chapter 29 for discussion of pediatric trauma.

ANATOMY AND PHYSIOLOGY

The hair, scalp, skull, meninges, and cerebrospinal fluid (CSF) protect the brain from injury (Figure 21-1). The scalp consists of five layers of tissue: skin, subcutaneous tissue, galea aponeurotic, ligaments, and periosteum. The skull is composed of the frontal, parietal, temporal, and occipital bones. Figure 21-2 illustrates the relationship between components of the nervous system. Cranial bones join with facial bones to form the cranial vault, a rigid cavity that can hold 1400 to 1500 ml of material. Other bony structures of import are depressions at the base of the skull called the anterior, middle, and posterior fossae. The frontal lobe is located in the anterior fossae; parietal, temporal, and occipital lobes in the middle fossae; and brainstem and cerebellum in the posterior fossae.

Three layers of meninges surround the brain and provide additional protection. The outermost meninge is the dura mater (meaning "tough mother"), which consists of two layers of tough fibrous tissue. The inner layer of the dura mater forms the falx cerebri and tentorium cerebelli. Potential spaces located above the dura mater (epidural) and below the dura mater (subdural) are at risk for hematoma forma-

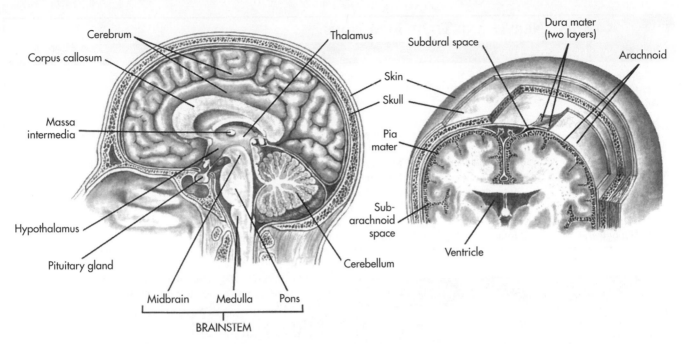

FIGURE 21-1   Brain structures. (From Thompson JM et al: *Mosby's clinical nursing*, ed 5, St. Louis, 2002, Mosby.)

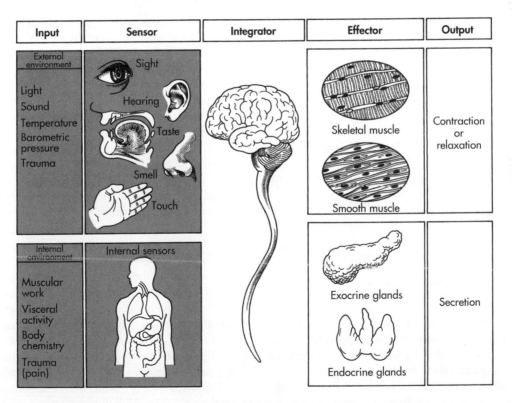

FIGURE 21-2   Components of the nervous system. (From *Mosby's medical, nursing, and allied health dictionary*, ed 5, St. Louis, 1998, Mosby.)

tion because the middle meningeal artery lies in the epidural space, and veins are located within the subdural space. The middle meningeal layer is the arachnoid mater (spiderlike), a fine, elastic layer. Below the arachnoid mater, the subarachnoid space contains arachnoid villi, fingerlike projections that form channels for CSF absorption. Adhering to the surface of the brain is the pia mater (meaning "tender mother").

The cerebrum consists of two hemispheres separated by a longitudinal fissure. Each lobe of the cerebrum is responsible for specific functions. The frontal lobe coordinates voluntary motor movements and controls judgment, affect, and

Table 21-1	CRANIAL NERVES AND THEIR FUNCTIONS	
CRANIAL NERVES	**FUNCTION**	**PHYSIOLOGIC EFFECTS**
I. Olfactory	Sensory	Smell
II. Optic	Sensory	Vision
III. Oculomotor	Motor	Extraocular movement of eyes; raises eyelid; constricts pupils
IV. Trochlear	Motor	Allows eye to move down and inward
V. Trigeminal	Motor and sensory	Facial sensation, mastication and corneal reflex
VI. Abducens	Motor	Allows eye to move outward
VII. Facial	Motor and sensory	Movement of facial muscles; closes eyes, secretes saliva and tears
VIII. Acoustic	Sensory	Hearing and equilibrium
IX. Glossopharyngeal	Motor and sensory	Gag reflex, swallowing, and phonation
X. Vagus	Motor and sensory	Voluntary muscles for swallowing, involuntary to visceral muscles (heart, lungs)
XI. Spinal accessory	Motor	Turns head, shrugs shoulders
XII. Hypoglossal	Motor	Tongue movement for swallowing

Box 21-1	GLASGOW COMA SCALE	
EYE OPENING		
Spontaneously		4
To verbal command		3
To pain		2
No response		1
BEST MOTOR RESPONSE		
Obeys commands		6
Localizes pain		5
Withdraws from pain		4
Abnormal flexion		3
Abnormal extension		2
No response		1
BEST VERBAL RESPONSE		
Oriented		5
Confused		4
Inappropriate words		3
Incomprehensible sounds		2
No response		1
TOTAL		3-15

Data from Teasdale G, Jennett B: Assessment of coma and impaired consciousness: a practical scale, *Lancet* 2:81, 1974.

personality. Hearing, behavior, emotions, and dominant-hemisphere speech are controlled by the temporal lobe. Sensory interpretation occurs in the parietal lobe, whereas the occipital lobe is responsible for vision.

The cerebellum is located in the posterior fossae adjacent to the brain stem and separated from the cerebrum by the tentorium cerebelli. Primary functions of the cerebellum are integration of motor function, maintenance of equilibrium, and maintenance of muscle tone.

The brainstem consists of the midbrain, pons, and medulla. Although each structure has important pathway functions, the medulla contains the cardiac, respiratory, and vasomotor centers. The reticular activating system, also located in the brainstem, is responsible for arousal, the lowest level of consciousness, which is interpreted as awakeness.

Cranial nerves originate in the brainstem. Table 21-1 describes the function of each cranial nerve.

PATIENT ASSESSMENT

After ensuring adequate control of airway, breathing, and circulation (ABCs), the emergency nurse should perform a complete, concise neurologic assessment. A subtle change in level of consciousness is the earliest indication of deterioration in the head-injured patient. Assessment of the level of consciousness should be directed toward acquiring the highest-level response with the least stimulus. The Glasgow Coma Scale (GCS) (Box 21-1) is a universally accepted[1] consistent measure of neurologic assessment.[8,13] Completing the GCS allows assignment of numeric values to clinical findings and assists in recognition of trends in neurologic changes. Interpretation of the GCS must be correlated with other clinical assessment findings. Presence of other physiologic conditions such as hypotension, hypothermia, alcohol, or substance abuse may artificially lower the total GCS score. Patients with a total GCS below 8 have sustained a severe head injury in the absence of previously identified physiologic conditions.

Normal pupillary response to direct light examination is constriction. Consensual reaction (constriction of the opposite pupil) should occur with direct light examination. Unilateral pupil dilation may indicate early compression of the third cranial nerve. Anisocoria or unequal pupils are a normal finding in 20% to 25% of the population, so assessment of reactivity in the dilated pupil is critical. Bilateral fixed and dilated pupils are indicative of impending transtentorial herniation. Figure 21-3 illustrates pupil reactions at different levels of consciousness.

Abnormal motor responses include inequality in movement from side to side and posturing. Decorticate posturing is rigid flexion with arms flexed toward the core and lower extremities extended. This type of posturing is associated with lesions above the midbrain. Rigid extension of the arms with wrist flexion and rigid extension of lower extremities is decerebrate posturing. This type of posturing is associated with an insult to the brainstem. Figure 21-4 illustrates de-

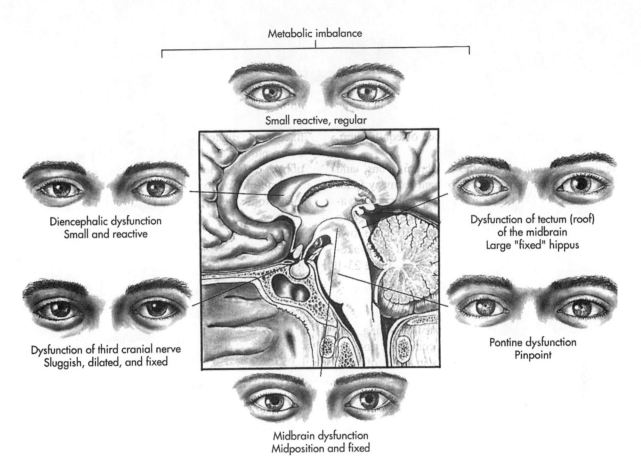

Metabolic imbalance

Small reactive, regular

Diencephalic dysfunction
Small and reactive

Dysfunction of tectum (roof)
of the midbrain
Large "fixed" hippus

Dysfunction of third cranial nerve
Sluggish, dilated, and fixed

Pontine dysfunction
Pinpoint

Midbrain dysfunction
Midposition and fixed

FIGURE 21-3   Pupils at different levels of consciousness. (From Huether SE, McCance KL: *Understanding pathophysiology,* ed 2, St. Louis, 2000, Mosby.)

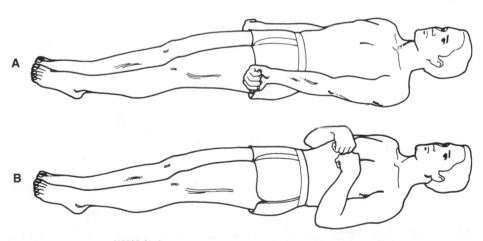

A

B

FIGURE 21-4   **A,** Decerebrate and **B,** decorticate posturing.

cerebrate and decorticate posturing. Lateralization occurs when patients with TBI present with unilateral decorticate and decerebrate posturing. Posturing may be spontaneous or elicited by verbal or painful stimuli.

Additional Assessment Parameters

Integrity of the brainstem is evaluated by the oculocephalic (Doll's eye) reflex and the oculovestibular reflex with the ice water caloric test. A Doll's eye examination is performed to evaluate brainstem integrity only after the cervical spine has been cleared. To perform the Doll's eye examination, briskly rotate the patient's head to the right or left. If the brainstem is intact, the patient's eyes deviate away from the direction the head is rotated (normal examination). Loss of brainstem integrity is presumed when eyes remain midline with rotation of the head or move in a dysconjugate manner with rotation. Figure 21-5 illustrates these three responses.

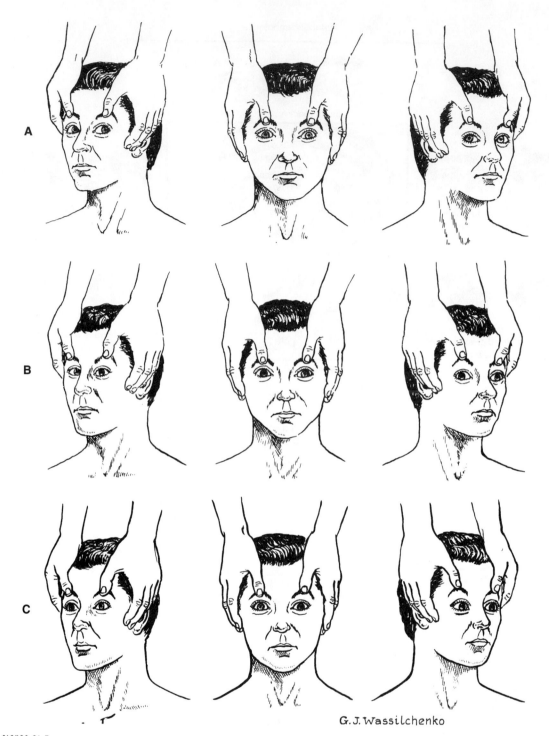

G. J. Wassilchenko

FIGURE 21-5   Test for oculocephalic reflex response (Doll's eye phenomenon). **A,** Normal response—eyes turn together to side opposite from turn of head. **B,** Abnormal response—eyes do not turn in conjugate manner. **C,** Absent response—eyes do not turn as head position changes. (From Rudy EB: *Advanced neurological and neurosurgical nursing,* St. Louis, 1984, Mosby.)

Oculovestibular response is evaluated by injection of ice water in the ear of an unresponsive patient. Normal response is conjugate deviation of eyes. No movement, dysconjugate movement, or asymmetric movement indicates interruption in the functional connection between the medulla and mid-brain. Figure 21-6 illustrates evaluation of this reflex. Severe dizziness and vomiting occur with this test in a conscious patient, so the ice water test is contraindicated in semiconscious or conscious patients. Another contraindication is tympanic membrane rupture.

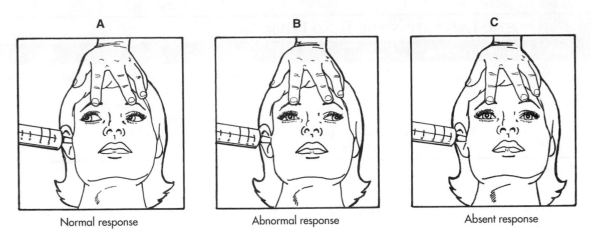

A Normal response **B** Abnormal response **C** Absent response

FIGURE 21-6   Test for oculovestibular reflex (ice water caloric test). **A,** Normal response—conjugate eye movements. **B,** Abnormal response—dysconjugate or asymmetric eye movements. **C,** Absent response—no eye movements. (From Huether SE, McCance KL: *Understanding pathophysiology,* ed 2, St. Louis, 2000, Mosby.)

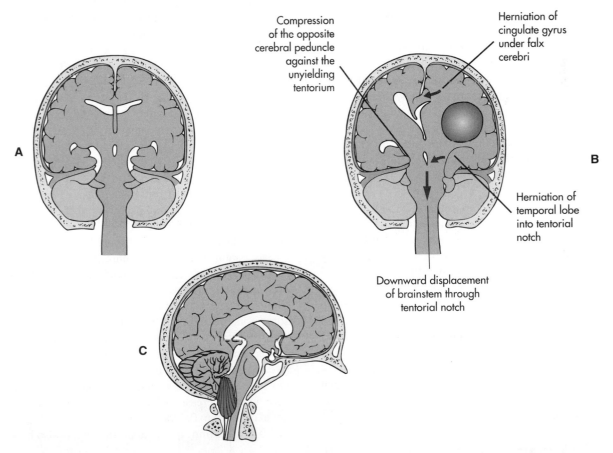

Compression of the opposite cerebral peduncle against the unyielding tentorium

Herniation of cingulate gyrus under falx cerebri

Herniation of temporal lobe into tentorial notch

Downward displacement of brainstem through tentorial notch

FIGURE 21-7   Herniation. **A,** Normal relationship of intracranial structures. **B,** Shift of intracranial structures. **C,** Downward herniation of the cerebellar tonsils into the foramen magnum. (From Huether SE, McCance KL: *Understanding pathophysiology,* ed 2, St. Louis, 2000, Mosby.)

PATIENT MANAGEMENT

Initial stabilization of the head-injured patient is directed toward maintenance of blood pressure, oxygenation, ventilation, and as restoration of circulating volume. The first priority of care for the head-injured patient is rapid resuscitation. Current recommendations for treatment of severe head injury specify that treatment for increased intracranial pressure should be initiated only in the presence of signs of transtentorial herniation (i.e., unilateral or bilateral pupillary dilatation, asymmetric pupillary reactivity, motor posturing, or continued neurologic deterioration after physiologic stability has been restored).[4] Figure 21-7 illustrates the mechanism that causes herniation. Because of the frequency of concomitant

Table 21-2   DIAGNOSTIC EVALUATION FOR HEAD INJURY

DIAGNOSTIC EXAMINATION	PURPOSE	COMMENTS
Cervical spine radiographs	Visualization of all seven cervical vertebrae to rule out injury	Tomograms or CT scans of the cervical spine may be necessary to completely rule out injury
Skull radiographs	Evaluate for skull fractures	Bone windows from CT scan may give more definitive evidence of basilar skull fractures
CT scan	Detect intracranial injuries—bleeds, hematomas, cerebral edema	Patients may require sedation to obtain adequate CT scan

CT, Computed tomography.

cervical spine trauma, cervical spine stabilization should be maintained until adequate radiographic examinations have ruled out cervical spine trauma. Prevention of secondary injuries begins with recognition of factors that correlate with further brain injury, such as hypoxia, hypercapnia, hypotension, and cerebral ischemia secondary to increased intracranial pressure. Hypoxia during the immediate postinjury period, reported in more than one third of all head-injured patients, substantially increases morbidity and mortality associated with head injury.[1] Presence of a secure airway, adequate ventilatory rate, and volume resuscitation decrease the incidence of hypoxia, hypercapnia, and hypotension. Diagnostic evaluation for head injury is initiated after stabilization of the ABCs. Available resources often determine tests performed; however, most emergency departments have access to radiographs and computed tomography (CT) scan. Table 21-2 discusses these diagnostic tests with regard to purpose and advantages.

After initial stabilization the emergency nurse should consider other interventions that promote return of optimal neurologic function. General guidelines for care of the head-injured patient include ensuring a patent airway, ventilatory support as indicated, hemodynamic stability (systolic blood pressure [SBP] above 90 mm Hg), ongoing neurologic assessment, administration of pharmacologic agents as needed (i.e., neuromuscular blocking agents, anticonvulsants), and other interventions based on patient condition. An integral component of caring for head-injured patients is inclusion of the family or significant other in the plan of care. Head injuries can be overwhelming for the family; psychosocial support and education regarding the injury cannot be overemphasized.

Intracranial Pressure

In the adult patient the skull is a closed box containing the brain, CSF, and blood. For intracranial pressure (ICP) to remain within normal limits (0 to 15 mm Hg) an increase in blood, CSF, or brain mass must be accompanied by a reciprocal decrease of one of the other components. Sustained ICP greater than 20 mm Hg represents intracranial hypertension. Failure to reduce ICP may cause ischemia and necrosis of brain tissue. Cerebral blood flow is maintained through autoregulation as cerebral blood vessels dilate and constrict to preserve adequate blood flow to the brain. Cere-

bral perfusion pressure (CPP) is calculated by subtracting ICP from mean arterial pressure (MAP).

Recommended indications for invasive management of intracranial hypertension include abnormal admission CT scan with GCS of 3 to 8. Indications in the presence of normal CT scan are two of the following: age greater than 40 years, abnormal posturing, or SBP less than 90 mm Hg. ICP monitoring aids in detection of intracranial mass lesions, limits unnecessary use of adjunctive therapies to control ICP, maintains normal ICP by draining CSF, helps determine prognosis, and may improve outcome.[1] The ultimate goal of ICP monitoring is to optimize cerebral perfusion while preventing secondary brain injury. Studies have shown that ventricular catheters with an external strain gauge are the most accurate means of monitoring ICP. Intraparenchymal catheters with a fiber-optic tip can drift and may not be as accurate. Many facilities use a fiber-optic monitor and external strain gauge device simultaneously to ensure accurate ICP monitoring (Figure 21-8).

Management of elevated ICP includes measures that ensure adequate cerebral blood flow. Scientific evidence has clearly established that maintaining cerebral perfusion pressure above 70 mm Hg is necessary to prevent primary cerebral ischemia and the resultant secondary injury that may occur.[1] Treating refractory intracranial hypertension with vasopressors to augment CPP has demonstrated improved clinical outcomes. Augmented CPP has demonstrated enhanced cerebral blood flow. The vasopressors phenylephrine (Neo-Synephrine) and norepinephrine (Levophed) are the most frequently used agents to augment CPP by elevating SBP, which increases MAP. Norepinephrine dosing should not exceed 0.2 to 0.4 mcg/kg/min. Low-dose Dopamine (1.5 to 3.0 mcg/kg/min) for renal perfusion has also been used.[11]

Hyperventilation

Recent studies have shown that chronic prophylactic hyperventilation should be avoided during the first 5 days after severe TBI. Cerebral blood flow studies illustrate substantial reduction in cerebral blood flow within the first few hours of injury in which absolute blood flow values are consistent with ischemia.[1,4] Hyperventilation reduces cerebral blood flow without consistently decreasing ICP. In addition, autoregulation may be interrupted and further compromise blood flow to the injured area. Hyperventila-

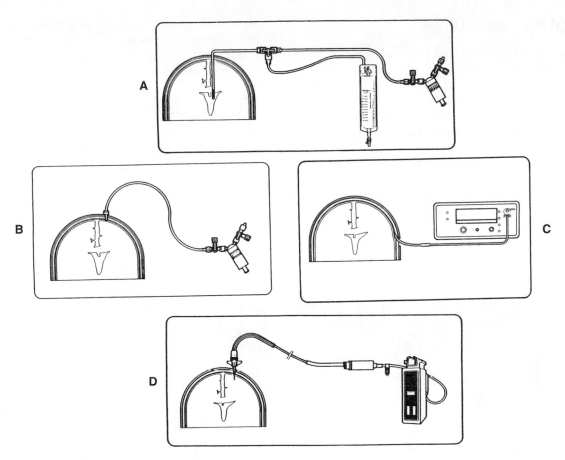

FIGURE 21-8 **A,** Ventricular pressure monitoring system. **B,** Subarachnoid pressure monitoring system. **C,** Epidural pressure monitoring system. **D,** Intraparenchymal pressure monitoring system. (From Thelan LA et al: *Critical care nursing: diagnosis and management,* ed 3, St. Louis, 1998, Mosby.)

tion should be instituted when other means do not control ICP and should be employed to minimize adverse effects. When hyperventilation is used, maintain pCO_2 at 30 mm Hg.

Mannitol

Mannitol is an osmotic diuretic that reduces ICP by changing the osmotic gradient, which causes fluid to leave cerebral extracellular tissues and move to intravascular beds. Movement of fluid reduces total brain mass, therefore decreasing ICP. Mannitol should be administered at doses of 0.25 to 1 gm/kg when signs of transtentorial herniation are present or progressive neurologic deterioration is evident. The patient's overall volume status should be assessed before administration of mannitol.

Neuroprotective Agents

Neuroprotective agents believed to protect the brain from secondary injury remain the subject of scientific scrutiny and controversy across the United States. Pharmacologic adjuncts are believed to affect three key mediators of reperfusion injury: oxygen-free radicals, lipid peroxidation, and excitatory amino acids. For each of these mediators, neuroprotective agents are being used to counteract secondary injury effects. (See Chapter 35 for additional discussion of neuroprotective agents.)

Oxygen-free radical scavengers synthesize with oxygen-free radicals to produce a less harmful substance. Reduction in circulating oxygen-free radicals provides better control of ICP, subsequently lessening cerebral ischemia.

Lipid peroxidation is inhibited by lazaroids, synthetic nonglucocorticoid steroids that suppress cellular membrane breakdown. Lazaroids assist in stabilization of cell membranes, impede neuronal deterioration, and deter secondary brain injury.

Excitatory amino acids (EAAs) are liberated during an ischemic event. Presence of EAAs produces a hypermetabolic state that extends the injury by overwhelming neurons.[9] N-methyl-d-aspartate antagonists restrict the effects of EAAs at an injury site. This action reduces metabolic activity and protects tissues from ischemia. Additional theories about the role and effect of cytotoxic changes will continue to emerge as neuroprotective strategies are evaluated.

Additional Treatment Modalities

Intravenous fluids of choice for TBI patients are 0.9% NaCl or lactated Ringer's solution. Dextrose solutions should be avoided because of increased cerebral edema. Barbiturate therapy may be considered for patients with refractory intracranial hypertension. Hemodynamic stability should be confirmed before induction of barbiturate coma. Early seizure activity should be treated with appropriate anticonvulsants. Prophylactic use of anticonvulsants is not recommended for prevention of late postinjury seizure activity. Paralytics in conjunction with sedation may help control ICP. No evidence exists to support routine use of glucocorticoids in head injury. Follow-up of patients who received steroids after a head injury reveals no difference in outcomes. If cervical spine injury has been ruled out and the patient is hemodynamically stable, elevating the head of the bed 30 to 45 degrees may decrease ICP. Maintaining the head in neutral alignment also facilitates venous drainage.

SPECIFIC HEAD INJURIES

Head injuries may be grouped into focal injuries or diffuse injuries. Focal injuries have an identifiable area of involvement, whereas diffuse injuries involve the entire brain. Examples of focal injuries include skull fractures and hematomas. Diffuse injuries include concussion and diffuse axonal injury. Firearms or other projectiles frequently cause penetrating injuries to the head. These injuries typically result in significant focal injuries along the path of entry (Figure 21-9).

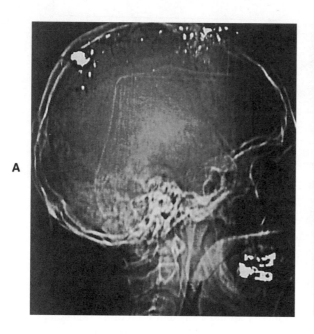

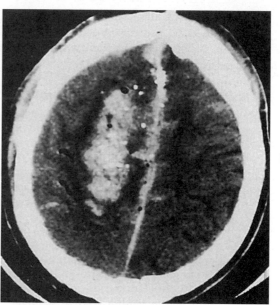

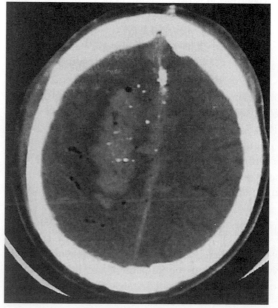

FIGURE 21-9   **A,** Lateral skull radiograph showing evidence of penetrating head injury and skull fracture. **B** and **C,** Regular and soft tissue computed tomography scans showing tract of missile, along with intracerebral hematoma, intracranial air, subarachnoid hemorrhage, and interhemispheric blood. (From Parrillo JE, Bone RC: *Critical care medicine: principles of diagnosis and management,* St. Louis, 1995, Mosby.)

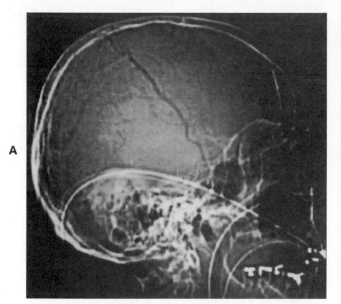
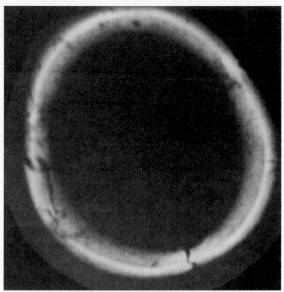

A

B

FIGURE 21-10 **A,** Lateral computed tomography (CT) showing extensive linear skull fracture. **B,** Bone windows of CT scan of same patient showing fracture. (From Parrillo JE, Bone RC: *Critical care medicine: principles of diagnosis and management,* St. Louis, 1995, Mosby.)

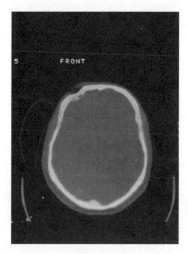

FIGURE 21-11 Computed tomography scan of depressed skull fracture right frontal region.

Focal Head Injuries

Scalp Lacerations

The scalp protects the brain from injury by acting as a cushion to reduce energy transmission to underlying structures. Excessive force applied to the scalp often causes a laceration; the scalp has an extensive vascular supply with poor vasoconstrictive properties, causing lacerations to bleed profusely. Bleeding can be controlled with direct pressure to the affected area followed by wound repair and tetanus prophylaxis as indicated. Staples or clips may also be used for rapid closure.

Skull Fractures

Skull fractures occur when energy applied to the skull causes bony deformation. Clinical presentation of skull frac-

tures is directly correlated to type of fracture, area involved, and damage to underlying structures. A linear skull fracture is nondisplaced and associated with minimal neurologic deficit (Figure 21-10). Supportive care is usually all that is required for optimal neurologic recovery.

When energy displaces the outer table of bone below the inner table of the adjoining skull, a depressed skull fracture occurs (Figure 21-11). Surgical elevation is required when depressed bone fragments become lodged in brain tissue. Open depressed skull fractures are surgically elevated and repaired as soon as possible because of increased risk of infection.

A basilar skull fracture develops when enough force is exerted on the base of the skull to cause deformity. The base of the skull includes any bony area where the skull ends and is not limited to the posterior aspect of the skull. A basilar skull fracture may be visualized on a radiograph; however, this is not always true. Approximately 25% of basilar skull fractures are not seen on radiograph; therefore, diagnosis is usually made on the basis of clinical findings. Basilar skull fractures that overlay the middle meningeal artery may cause a subgaleal hematoma. Disruption of the middle meningeal artery is the cause of more than 75% of epidural hematomas. A basilar skull fracture may also cause intracerebral bleeding.

Neurologic changes that occur with a basilar skull fracture range from mild changes in mentation to combativeness and severe agitation. Combative behavior is often considered a hallmark of a basilar skull fracture. Clinical manifestations of basilar skull fracture include periorbital ecchymoses (raccoon eyes) (Figure 21-12, *A*) from intraorbital bleeding, Battle's sign (ecchymosis over the mastoid process) (Figure 21-12, *B*) 12 to 24 hours after initial injury, hemotympanum (blood behind the tympanic membrane

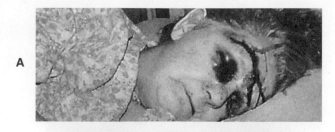

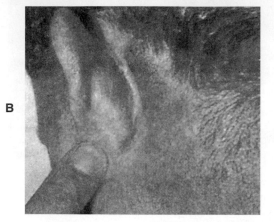

FIGURE 21-12   **A,** Raccoon eyes. **B,** Battle's sign. (From London PS: *A colour atlas of diagnosis after recent injury,* London, 1990, Wolfe Medical Publications.)

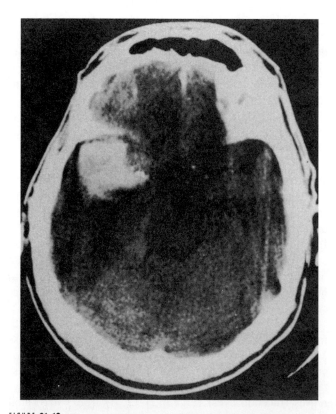

FIGURE 21-13   Computed tomography: contusion. (Courtesy of Laurence Cromwell, MD, Department of Radiology, Dartmouth-Hitchcock Medical Center.)

caused by a fracture of the temporal bone), and CSF leak from the nose or ear caused by temporal bone fracture. If the tympanic membrane is intact, fluid drains through the eustachian tube and appears as CSF (rhinorrhea). However, absence of visible CSF does not eliminate the possibility of a basilar skull fracture. If a CSF leak is considered, test the fluid draining from the nose on filter paper. Formation of two distinct rings is called the "halo" or "ring" sign and indicates presence of CSF. Clear fluid should be tested for glucose, a normal finding in CSF.

Diagnostic interventions include skull radiographs and a CT scan in some patients. Additional interventions focus on protecting the patient from injury, preventing infection, and using nasal drip pads as needed for rhinorrhea. Nasal packing is not recommended. Frequent neurologic assessment with ongoing reassessment is essential for early identification of deterioration in neurologic function.

Contusion

Cerebral contusion is a bruise on the surface of the brain that occurs from movement of the brain within the cranial vault (Figure 21-13). When an acceleration-deceleration injury occurs, two contusions may result, one at the initial site of impact (coup) and one on the opposite side of the impact (contracoup).[2,3] The clinical presentation varies with size and location of the contusion. Commonly occurring symptoms include altered level of consciousness, nausea, vomiting, visual disturbances, weakness, and speech difficulty. Interventions focus on preservation of neurologic function, control of pain, and adequate hydration.

Epidural Hematoma

Epidural hematoma is bleeding between the skull and dura mater (Figure 21-14) resulting from a direct blow to the head. A skull fracture and injury to the middle meningeal artery may also be present. A torn middle meningeal artery with arterial bleeding leads to a rapidly forming hematoma, with associated morbidity and mortality of more than 50%. Approximately half of the patients with an epidural hematoma have no evidence of skull fracture. Signs and symptoms include a brief period of unconsciousness followed by a lucid period, then another loss of consciousness. This brief lucid period is considered a hallmark of an epidural hematoma; however, it does not occur in all patients. If alert, the patient with an epidural hematoma complains of severe headache and may exhibit hemiparesis and a dilated pupil on the side of injury.

Subdural Hematoma

Subdural hematomas occur more frequently than other intracranial injuries and have the highest morbidity and mortality of all hematomas. Bleeding into the subdural space between the dura mater and arachnoid leads to subdural hematoma (Figure 21-15). A subdural hematoma may be acute, subacute, or chronic. When acute the hematoma usually results from dissipation of energy that ruptures bridging veins in the subdural space. Clinical features are loss of con-

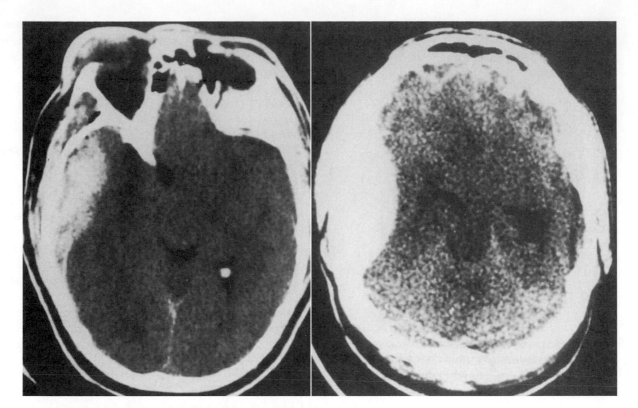

FIGURE 21-14 Nonenhanced head computed tomography scan displaying right ventricular epidural hematoma in a young male, resulting from motor vehicle collision. (From Parrillo JE, Bone RC: *Critical care medicine: principles of diagnosis and management*, St. Louis, 1995, Mosby.)

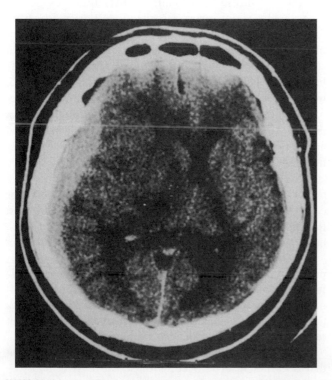

FIGURE 21-15 Computed tomography: acute subdural hematoma. (Courtesy of Laurence Cromwell, MD, Department of Radiology, Dartmouth-Hitchcock Medical Center.)

sciousness; hemiparesis; and fixed, dilated pupils. Surgical intervention within 4 hours of injury has the best potential for neurologic recovery.

Subacute subdural hematomas develop 48 hours to 2 weeks after injury. The clinical presentation is progressive decline in level of consciousness as the hematoma slowly expands. The brain compensates as a result of slow blood collection over time, so decline in neurologic function occurs gradually. After the subdural is drained, the patient improves quickly with little or no lasting neurologic deficit.

Chronic subdural hematomas, seen frequently in the elderly, progress slowly. Blood collects over 2 weeks to months; by the time a person is examined, the causative mechanism may have been forgotten. Chronic subdural hematomas are initially tolerated by the elderly because of brain atrophy associated with aging. As the brain decreases in size, the space within the cranial vault increases. A hematoma collects over time without obvious changes in neurologic status until its size is sufficient to produce a mass effect. Treatment of a chronic subdural consists of burr holes and a subdural drain. Patients become more alert after the subdural is drained.

Other Focal Injuries

Intraventricular hemorrhage (Figure 21-16) and intracerebral clots (Figure 21-17) are types of focal injuries. Management depends on the size of the clot and source of bleed-

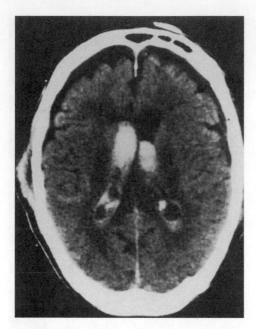

FIGURE 21-16   Computed tomography scan of head showing intraventricular hemorrhage secondary to motor vehicle collision. (From Parrillo JE, Bone RC: *Critical care medicine: principles of diagnosis and management,* St. Louis, 1995, Mosby.)

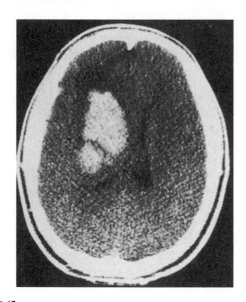

FIGURE 21-17   Nonenhanced head CT scan showing large right hemispheric clot in 26-year-old male patient who sustained closed-head injury from a motor vehicle collision. Note mass effect on right lateral ventricle. (From Parrillo JE, Bone RC: *Critical care medicine: principles of diagnosis and management,* St. Louis, 1995, Mosby.)

ing. Surgical evacuation may be necessary in concert with medical management of increased intracranial pressure.

Diffuse Brain Injuries

Concussion

A concussion can occur as a result of a direct blow to the head or from an acceleration or deceleration injury in which the brain collides with the inside of the skull. Brief interruption of the reticular activating system may occur, causing transient amnesia. Amnesia usually requires no therapeutic intervention other than observation for development of potential complications. A classic concussion is characterized as loss of consciousness followed by transient neurologic changes such as nausea, vomiting, temporary amnesia, headache, and possible brief loss of vision.

Care for the patient with a concussion includes observation, especially with prolonged loss of consciousness (greater than 2 to 3 minutes). With protracted nausea and vomiting, hospital admission may be considered to avoid dehydration. Nonnarcotic analgesia may be administered for headache. Narcotics affect the level of consciousness and interfere with ongoing patient assessment. Patients with a concussion may be discharged with a responsible adult who will observe the patient overnight for possible complications, such as confusion, difficulty walking, altered level of consciousness, projectile vomiting, and unequal pupils. Discharge teaching includes instructions on how to assess neurologic status in the home and when to contact the primary care provider.

Headache, memory loss, and difficulty with activities of daily living are characteristic of postconcussion syndrome, which can occur up to 1 year after the patient's initial injury. Interventions include supportive treatment and recognition that this is a true physiologic consequence of what was perceived as a minor head injury.

Diffuse Axonal Injury

The phrase "diffuse axonal injury" (DAI) illustrates the major pathophysiologic event associated with the most severe form of TBI. This injury is almost always the result of blunt trauma that causes shearing and disruption of neuronal structures, predominantly white matter. Prognosis for diffuse axonal injuries depends on the degree of injury (mild, moderate, or severe) and severity of damage from any secondary injury. The terms mild, moderate, and severe reflect the clinical presentation of diffuse axonal injury and should not be confused with the grading system indicating the actual underlying pathophysiology of DAI.[5]

Mild DAI is characterized by loss of consciousness for 6 to 24 hours. Initially the patient may exhibit decerebrate or decorticate posturing but improves rapidly within 24 hours. Return to baseline neurologic status may occur over days, but periods of amnesia may be present.

Moderate DAI is a coma lasting longer than 24 hours, possibly extending over a period of days. Brainstem dysfunction (decorticate/decerebrate posturing) is evident almost immediately and may continue until the patient begins to wake. Patients with moderate DAI usually recover but rarely return to full preinjury neurologic function.

Severe DAI is characterized by brainstem impairment that does not resolve. Victims of severe DAI remain comatose for days to weeks. Autonomic dysfunction may also be present. Overall prognosis for severe diffuse axonal injury is extremely poor. Early CT scans may be unremark-

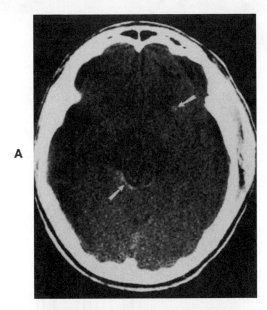

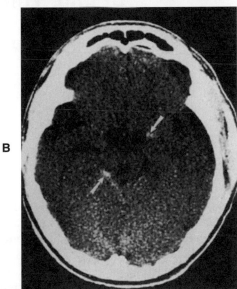

FIGURE 21-18   **A and B,** Computed tomography scans of head in a patient with coma secondary to motor vehicle collision. Scans show punctate hemorrhage in left frontal lobe and midbrain and subarachnoid hemorrhage in perimesencephalic cisterns. This picture is suggestive of diffuse axonal injury. (From Parrillo JE, Bone RC: *Critical care medicine: principles of diagnosis and management,* St. Louis, 1995, Mosby.)

able; however, serial examinations reveal areas of edema and microvascular hemorrhage (Figure 21-18). Treatment for all degrees of DAI includes general supportive care, prevention of further brain injury, and support for the family.

SUMMARY

Head injuries are a major cause of traumatic deaths in the United States and cause significant long-term disability. Recognition and prevention of secondary injuries related to

ischemia, increased ICP, and hypoxia are essential components of care. Box 21-2 summarizes nursing diagnoses for these challenging patients.

References

1. American Association of Neurological Surgeons Joint Section on Neurotrauma and Critical Care: *Guidelines for the management of severe head injury,* Park Ridge, Ill, 2000, The Association.
2. Bandak F: On the mechanics of impact neurotrauma: a review and critical synthesis, *J Neurotrauma* 12(4):635, 1995.
3. Cruz J et al: Severe acute brain trauma. In Cruz J, editor: *Neurologic and neurosurgical emergencies,* Philadelphia, 1998, WB Saunders.
4. Fortune J et al: Effect of hyperventilation, mannitol, and ventriculostomy drainage on cerebral blood flow after head injury, *J Trauma* 39(6):1091, 1995.
5. Graham DI: In Rosenthal M, Griffith ER et al: *Rehabilitation of the adult and child with traumatic brain injury,* Philadelphia, 1999, FA Davis.
6. Guerrero J, Thurman DJ, Sniezak JE: Emergency department visits association with acute traumatic brain injury: United States, 1995-1996, *Brain Inj* 14(2):181, 2000.
7. Hansen M: *Pathophysiology: foundations of disease and clinical intervention,* Philadelphia, 1998, WB Saunders.
8. Hickey JV: *Neurological and neurosurgical nursing,* ed 4, Philadelphia, 1997, JB Lippincott.
9. Hilton G: Experimental neuroprotective agents: nursing challenge, *Dimens Crit Care* 14(4):181, 1995.
10. McQuillan KA, Von Rueden KT, Hartstock RL et al: *Trauma nursing from resuscitation through rehabilitation,* ed 3, Philadelphia, 2001, WB Saunders.
11. Rosner MJ, Rosner SD, Johnson AH: Cerebral perfusion pressure: management protocol and clinical results, *J Neurosurg* 83:949, 1995.
12. Sosin D, Sniezek J, Waxweiler R: Trends in death associated with traumatic brain injury, 1979 through 1992, *JAMA* 273(22):1778, 1995.
13. Teasdale G, Jennett B: Assessment of coma and impaired consciousness: a practical scale, *Lancet* 2:81, 1974.
14. Thurman DJ, Guerrero J: Trends in hospitalization associated with traumatic brain injury, *JAMA* 282(10):954, 2000.

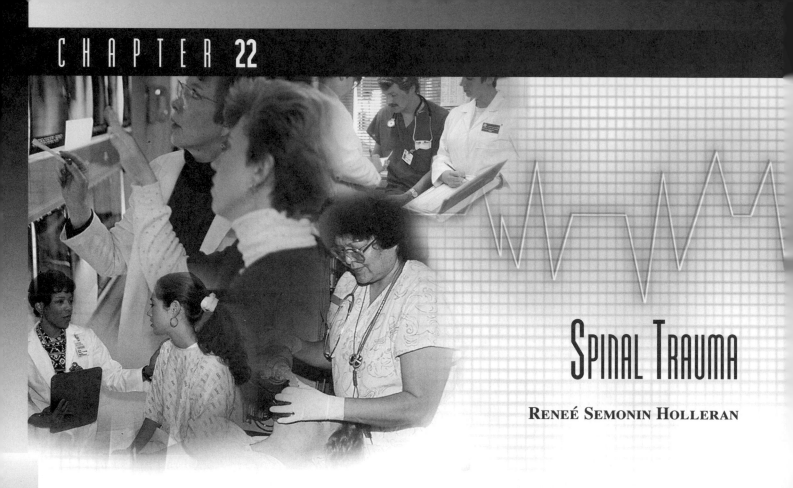

CHAPTER 22

SPINAL TRAUMA

RENEÉ SEMONIN HOLLERAN

Trauma to the spinal column and the spinal cord can result in devastating and life-threatening injuries. Each year approximately 10,000 acute spinal cord injuries occur in the United States. The majority of those injured are males under age 30. The estimated cost for care ranges from $162,000 to more than $540,000 during the first year after the patient's injury. Lifetime costs will vary based on age of the patient and site of the injury. High cord injuries in young patients cost over $2,000,000 per year. Spinal cord injuries cost close to $10 billion dollars per year in the United States.[7] Prehospital care, rapid transport, medical, surgical, and technologic advances have all contributed to increasing the life expectancy of those who have suffered a spinal cord injury.[15]

The spinal cord may be injured in a number of ways. The most common mechanism of injury is a motor vehicle crash, accounting for more than 30% of acute spinal cord injuries.[15] Motor vehicle crashes cause spinal cord injuries by rollovers, occupant ejection, and collisions with pedestrians. Other mechanisms include falls, direct blows to the head or neck, penetrating wounds from guns or knives, and sports injuries. The increase in outdoor activities such as inline skating, snowboarding, and bicycling have contributed to additional sources of spinal cord injuries.[15] Unfortunately, since the 1970s, there has been an increase in violence, such as gunshot wounds to the neck and chest areas, that has caused spinal cord injuries.[15]

In the past, many people with acute spinal cord injuries died from respiratory complications such as aspiration and pneumonia. At present, establishment of spinal cord injury care systems have decreased complications from acute spinal cord injuries and improved survival of those injured.[7] Spinal cord patients need to be transferred to the appropriate care facility as soon as possible to decrease complications and costs that may occur related to the injury.

Care of the patient with spine trauma begins in the prehospital environment with rapid identification of injury or potential for injury based on the mechanism of injury followed by appropriate patient immobilization. Five percent of patients with major trauma have an unstable cervical spine injury, and two thirds of these patients have neurologic deficits.[5] After patients are in the emergency department (ED), the patient should be fully evaluated to rule out concomitant life-threatening injuries such as tension pneumothorax or intraabdominal bleeding.

Emergency care of the patient with spine trauma requires an organized, multidisciplinary approach. Patient survival and quality of life from the acute injury depend on emergency care a patient receives. This chapter discusses anatomy and physiology of spine trauma, mechanisms of injury, patient assessment and initial interventions, specific injuries, and current research related to management of acute spine injury.[6]

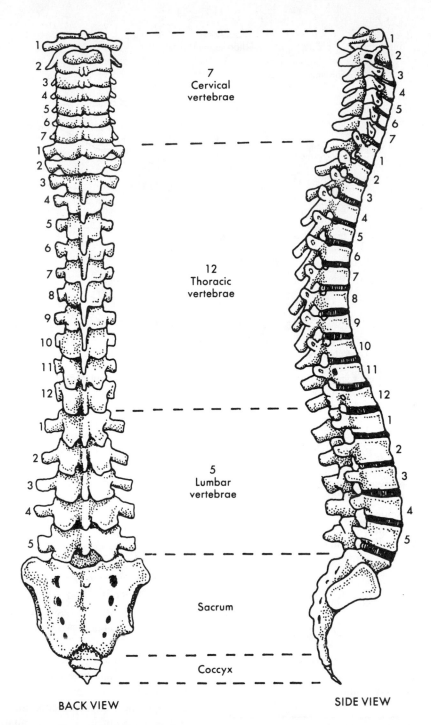

FIGURE 22-1 Vertebral columns. (From Rosen P, Barkin RM, Hockberger RS et al: *Emergency medicine: concepts and clinical practice,* ed 4, St. Louis, 1998, Mosby.)

ANATOMY AND PHYSIOLOGY

ANATOMY

The spinal cord regulates body movement and function through transmission of nerve impulses. It is an integral part of the central nervous system, extending from the superior border of C-1 to the superior border of L-2. It tapers in the lower thoracic area and terminates in a cone-shaped structure known as the conus medullaris. The cauda equina contains the spinal nerve roots that exit below the conus medullaris. The spinal cord travels through a canal within the vertebrae and is covered by three layers of meninges: the pia, the arachnoid, and dura.[1,6,9,9a,12]

The human body has 7 cervical, 12 thoracic, 5 lumbar, and 1 sacral vertebrae (Figure 22-1). The vertebral column provides support for the head and trunk and protection for the spinal cord. A vertebral body is composed of the body, a vertebral arch, and a vertebral foramen. The arch of the vertebra is composed of two pedicles, two laminae, four facets, two transverse processes, and the spinous process, which can be palpated.[6]

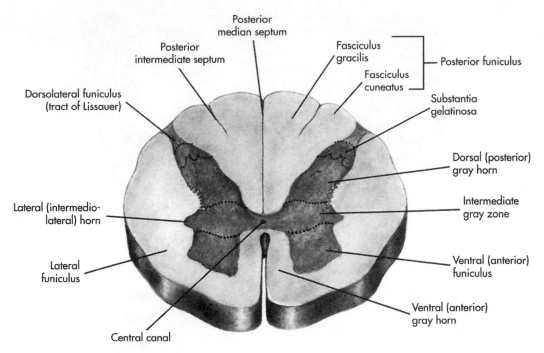

FIGURE 22-2   Cross-section of spinal cord illustrating subdivisions of white and gray matter. (From Rudy EB: *Advanced neurological and neurosurgical nursing,* St. Louis, 1984, Mosby.)

Table 22-1	EXAMPLES OF SPINAL TRACTS AND THEIR FUNCTIONS	
SPINAL TRACT	**FUNCTION**
Dorsal columns (ascending)	Conscious muscle sense, touch, vibration
Lateral spinothalamic tract (ascending)	Pain and temperature
Ventral spinothalamic tract (ascending)	Light touch
Ventral pyramidal tract (descending)	Voluntary control of skeletal muscle
Extrapyramidal tract (descending)	Automatic control of skeletal muscle
Dorsal spinocerebellar tract (ascending)	Unconscious muscle sense
Lateral pyramidal tract (descending)	Voluntary control of skeletal muscle

Data from Jaworski M, Wirtz K: Spinal trauma. In Kitt S et al, editors: *Emergency nursing,* Philadelphia, 1995, WB Saunders; and Walleck C: Central nervous system II: spinal cord injury. In Cardona V et al, editors: *Trauma nursing,* ed 2, Philadelphia, 1994, WB Saunders.

The cervical vertebrae are the most mobile part of the spine, so this area is the most frequent site of injury. The rib cage keeps the vertebrae from T1 to T10 stable and relatively immobile. The second most common site of injury is the thoracolumbar junction at T11 to L2. This is a transition area between the rigid thoracolumbar region and the more mobile lumbar region.[5]

Ligaments connect the vertebral bodies and provide support and stability to the vertebral column. They also keep the spinal column from excessive flexion and extension. Between the vertebral bodies are discs that act as shock absorbers and articulating surfaces for the adjacent vertebral bodies.[1,6,9a,12]

Physiology

The primary function of the spinal cord is to regulate function and movement of the body by transmitting nerve impulses between the brain and the body. The spinal cord is an extremely delicate collection of nervous tissue. A cross-sectional view of the spinal cord (Figure 22-2) reveals an H-shaped core composed of gray matter. The gray matter is divided into posterior, horizontal, and anterior columns and nine laminae. The posterior gray matter mediates sensory impulses for processes, such as proprioception, pressure sense, vibratory sense, and movement. The horizontal gray matter contains interconnecting neurons that form the first part of a two-neuron pathway for the sympathetic nervous system. The central canal pierces the horizontal gray matter. The anterior part of the gray matter contains the motor cell bodies that form the final common pathway for all impulses going to skeletal muscles. The motor cell axons pass out of the spinal cord by way of the ventral root and end at the muscles' motor end plates.[1]

The white matter of the spinal cord is formed by axons of the cells within the gray matter, axons of sensory cells in the dorsal ganglia, and descending tracts from the brain, brainstem, and cerebellum. These fibers are organized into tracts in the white matter and run parallel to the spinal cord's vertical axis. The tracts ascend to and descend from the brain to

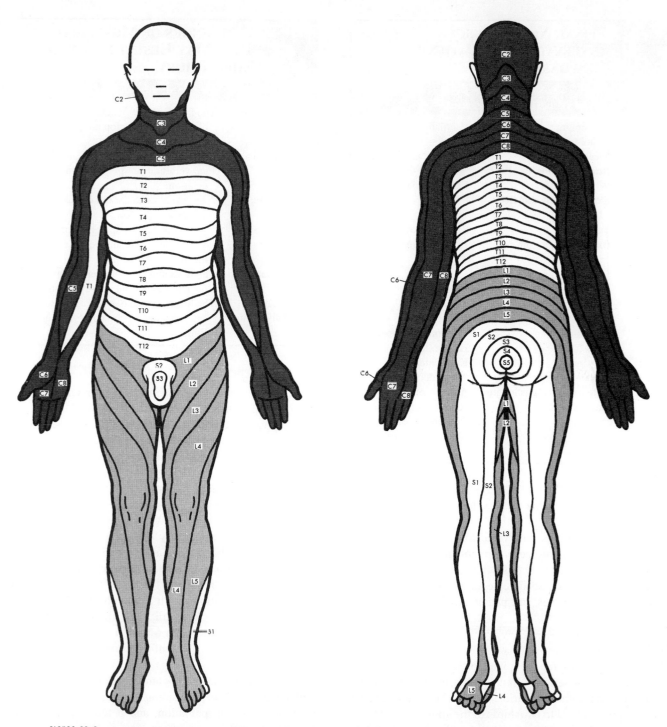

FIGURE **22-3** Sensory dermatomes. (From Rosen P, Barkin RM, Hockberger RS et al: *Emergency medicine: concepts and clinical practice,* ed 4, St. Louis, 1998, Mosby.)

other parts of the spinal cord. The spinal cord is composed of multiple tracts. Table 22-1 lists some of these tracts and describes their functions.[1,2,9a]

Spinal Nerves

The spinal cord has 31 pairs of spinal nerves that provide pathways for involuntary responses to specific stimuli. They innervate voluntary striated muscle. Each of these

nerves has a posterior root that transmits sensory impulses and an anterior root that transmits motor impulses. The nerves are paired and correspond to specific spinal cord segments. The nerves are identified as follows: 8 cervical nerves, 12 thoracic nerves, 5 lumbar nerves, 5 sacral nerves, and 1 coccygeal nerve. The dorsal root of these nerves supplies a distinct region of the body surface known as a *dermatome* (Figure 22-3). Assessment of the 28 dermatomes

Table 22-2	SPINAL NERVE MUSCLE INNERVATION AND PATIENT RESPONSE	
NERVE LEVEL	MUSCLES INNERVATED	PATIENT RESPONSE
C-4	Diaphragm	Ventilation
C-5	Deltoid	Shrug shoulders
	Biceps	Flex elbows
	Brachioradialis	
C-6	Wrist extensor	Extend wrist
	Extensor carpi radialis longus	
C-7	Triceps	Extend elbow
	Extensor digitorum communis	Extend fingers
	Flexor carpi radialis	
C-8	Flexor digitorum profundus	Flex fingers
T-1	Hand intrinsic muscles	Spread fingers
T-2 to	Intercostals	Vital capacity
L-1	Abdominal	Abdominal reflexes
L-2	Iliopsoas	Hip flexion
L-3	Quadriceps	Knee extension
L-4	Tibialis anterior	Ankle dorsiflexion
L-5	Extension hallucis longus	Ankle eversion
S-1	Gastrocnemius	Ankle plantar flexion Big toe extension
S-2 to S-5	Perineal sphincter	Sphincter control

Table 22-3	CATEGORIES OF MOVEMENT THAT MAY RESULT IN SPINAL CORD INJURY	
CATEGORY	MECHANISM OF INJURY	
Hyperextension	The head is forced back, and the vertebrae of the cervical region are placed in an overextended position.	
Hyperflexion	The head is forced forward, and the cervical vertebrae are placed in an overflexion position.	
Axial loading	A severe blow to the top of the head causes a blunt downward force on the vertebrae and the spinal column.	
Compression	Forces from above and below compress the vertebrae.	
Lateral bend	The head and neck are bent to one side, beyond the normal range of motion.	
Overrotation and distraction	The head turns to one side, and the cervical vertebrae are forced beyond normal limits.	

provides information about injury to sensory areas of the spinal cord.

A group of muscles innervated by a single spinal segment, known as myotomes, contains the distribution of spinal cord motor activity. As with the dermatome, these fibers correspond to a specific segment of the spinal cord. The innervated muscles and patient response are summarized in Table 22-2.[9,9a]

Vascular Supply

The vascular supply for the spinal cord comes from the vertebral artery and a series of spinal rami arteries that enter the intervertebral foramina at various levels.[9] The anterior spinal artery supplies blood to two thirds of the spinal cord. The remaining one third of the spinal cord's blood supply is carried by the two posterior arteries, which originate from the vertebral artery. Unlike other structures in the body, spinal cord arteries cannot develop adequate collateral blood supply when they are blocked or injured.[9,9a]

PATIENT ASSESSMENT

The emergency nurse with initiation of critical interventions as appropriate performs primary and secondary assessment of an injured patient. Because all patients with multisystem injuries or significant mechanisms of injury may have a spinal injury, each patient should be completely immobi-

lized. Spinal immobilization involves manual immobilization of the patient's head until a hard cervical collar, lateral head support such as head blocks or rolled sheets, and backboard have been applied (Figure 22-4). The entire spine should be immobilized with a backboard and straps across the chest, abdomen, and knees. After the patient's critical needs have been met, the emergency nurse may then perform a more focused assessment related to spinal injury.

It is important that after the initial assessment and resuscitation have been safely completed, the patient is removed from the backboard and placed on the appropriate bed. Patients who have sustained neurologic injury, particularly those with sensory loss, are at great risk of developing complications such as decubitis, which may put the patient at risk for additional injury and infection. Backboards have also been found to cause headaches and other types of back discomfort unrelated to the mechanism of injury.[6]

Initial assessment of the patient with spine trauma begins with obtaining history including the mechanism of injury, as well as inspection, palpation, and percussion of the spine and spinal cord.

Mechanisms of Injury

Mechanisms of spine injury may come from blunt or penetrating forces. The vertebrae, spinal cord, and nerve roots may be injured as a result of fractures, dislocations, or subluxation. The cord may also be injured through direct penetration by a bullet, knife, or other sharp object. Six basic types of movement can injure the spinal cord. These are illustrated in Figure 22-5 and summarized in Table 22-3.

When obtaining information from the patient with a suspected spine injury, the emergency nurse should ask the pa-

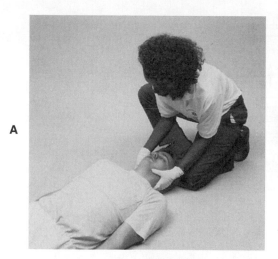

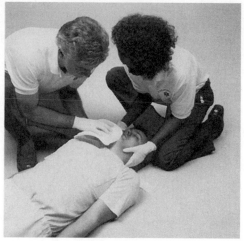

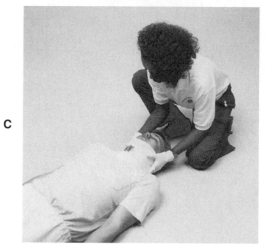

FIGURE 22-4 Spinal immobilization. **A,** Manual inline immobilization is applied and this position is maintained throughout the procedure. **B,** A collar is positioned and secured with Velcro straps. **C,** Support is maintained for the patient with spread fingers until the patient is secured to a short or long spine board. (From Sanders M: *Mosby's paramedic textbook,* ed 2, St. Louis, 2000, Mosby.)

tient about neck pain, changes in sensation or movement since the accident, and loss of consciousness. If the patient is unconscious, prehospital history may be the only source of information about the patient immediately after the accident. The emergency nurse should acquire as much history as possible from prehospital care providers.

History

Spinal cord injury should be suspected with any of the following: history of significant trauma and altered mental status from intoxication; history of seizure activity since the accident; any complaint of neck pain or altered sensation in their upper extremities; complaint of neck tenderness; history of loss of consciousness; injury above the clavicle; fall greater than three times the patient's height; fall that results in fracture of the heels; an unrestrained (no seat belt) person with facial injury; significant injuries in a motor vehicle crash that causes chest and intraabdominal injuries; and a motorcycle crash.[8] The patient may complain of feeling an "electric shock" or "hot water" running down the back. A history of incontinence before arrival in the ED may be reported. Priapism may be noted in male patients.

Inspection

The emergency nurse should observe the patient for obvious signs of spinal injury including abnormality in the vertebral column, cervical edema, and entrance or exit wounds in the neck, chest, or abdomen. The patient's ventilatory pattern and effort can indicate a cord injury. Injuries to the spinal cord above C-6 interfere with ventilation. Use of abdominal muscles rather than the diaphragm to breathe suggests injury to the cord at level C-3 to C-5.

The emergency nurse should observe the patient's ability to move and perceive pain during procedures such as intravenous catheter insertion or arterial punctures. The patient may be holding his or her head forward, suggesting a level C1 to C2 injury, or may have his or her arms folded across the chest indicating a level C5 to C6 injury. Priapism indicates a cervical spine injury because it occurs with loss of sympathetic nervous system control and parasympathetic stimulation.[6]

The emergency nurse should observe the patient for a cerebral spinal fluid (CSF) leak from the nose or ears. Confirm the presence of CSF with a halo test or dextro stick. The patient must be carefully checked for ecchymosis, tracheal deviation, or hematoma in the posterior pharyngeal area,

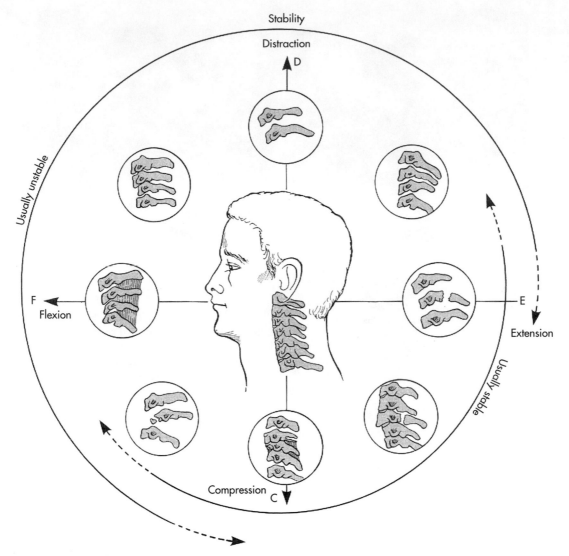

FIGURE 22-5   Mechanisms of injury to the spine. The mechanism of cervical injury (flexion versus extension) determines the type of cervical spine fracture or dislocation. (From Moore EE, editor: *Early care of the injured patient,* ed 4, Philadelphia, 1990, Decker.)

which may indicate spinal injury, particularly in penetrating neck trauma.

Palpation

The patient's spinal column should be palpated for pain, tenderness, and deformity. If the cervical collar is removed for this procedure, manual immobilization must be maintained. Skin temperature can be assessed by palpation. A patient with a spinal cord injury becomes poikilothermic because of loss of sympathetic tone, assuming the temperature of the surroundings. This can leave the patient at great risk of becoming hypothermic.

Injury above the T-4 level usually disrupts the sympathetic nervous system, causing vasodilatation below the level of the injury. If the patient is diaphoretic, diaphoresis is present above rather than below the level of the injury.

Strength and equality of movement of all four extremities should be evaluated. Table 22-2 summarizes specific responses and their relationship to spinal motor nerve innervation. A quick motor evaluation should include flexion and extension of the arms, flexion and extension of the legs, flexion of the foot, extension of the toes, and sphincter tone.[6]

Sensory status may be assessed by evaluation of dermatomes (Figure 22-3). A brief assessment includes using a safety pin or cotton swab so that the patient can distinguish between sharp and dull. Test the top of the shoulder, at the nipple line, the umbilicus, and the great toe on each side.[6]

Percussion

The emergency nurse can assist with or perform an assessment of the patient's reflexes. Reflexes are summarized in Table 22-4.

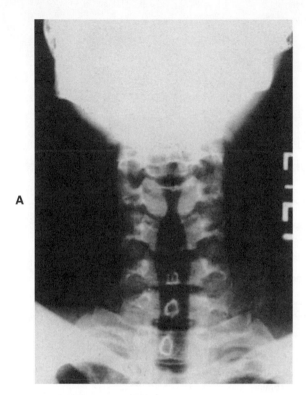

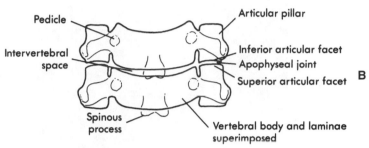

FIGURE 22-6 Anteroposterior view of cervical spine. (Modified from Rosen P, Barkin RM, Hockberger RS et al: *Emergency medicine: concepts and clinical practice,* ed 4, St. Louis, 1998, Mosby.)

Table 22-4	REFLEXES TESTED IN SPINAL TRAUMA	
REFLEX	**SPINAL CORD LEVEL**
Biceps	C5-6
Brachioradialis	C5-6
Triceps	C7-8
Superficial abdominal (above umbilicus)	T7-T10
Superficial abdominal (below umbilicus)	T11-L1
Cremasteric	T12-L1
Knee jerk	L3-L4
Ankle jerk	S1
Anal wink	S2-S4
Bulbocavernosus	S3-S4
Plantar response	Brain-cord continuity

Radiographic Evaluation

Radiographic evaluation of the injured patient is performed to assess alignment, identify fractures or ligamentous injuries, and identify spinal cord compression by bone or soft tissues.[5] Anteroposterior (Figure 22-6) and lateral (Figure 22-7) x-ray views of the spine show all seven cervical vertebrae and the C7-T1 junction. When a satisfactory cross table is obtained, the C-spine series should be completed. A swimmer's view (Figure 22-8) is performed when all the cervical vertebrae cannot be visualized, whereas an open-mouth series is used to evaluate integrity of the odontoid body and C-1 and C-2 vertebrae.[9] Any patient with a history of a fall or significant chest and abdominal trauma should have films of the thoracic and lumbosacral spine.

Computed tomography (CT) facilitates evaluation of soft tissue damage, patency of the neural canal, and compression of the spinal cord. A CT scan is indicated for patients with subluxation, fractures, neurologic deficits with no apparent abnormalities, severe pain without obvious injury, and when C-7/T-1 junction cannot be visualized.[5,9]

Magnetic resonance imaging (MRI) has emerged as an excellent diagnostic tool for spinal cord injury. An MRI does not show bone well, so it should be used in conjunction with a CT scan. In a study done by Schroder and colleagues,[14] the CT scan revealed all acute bony injuries but did not consistently identify longitudinal ligament lesions, intramedullary hemorrhages, and vertebral disk herniations. The MRI, however, identified all medullary and paravertebral soft tissue changes, dislocations, and spondylophytes narrowing the spinal channel.[14] Schroder and colleagues thought that when the patient's condition allowed, an MRI should be performed before a CT scan. However, an unstable patient should not be taken for an MRI. The MRI is of particular importance in a pediatric patient who has suffered a spinal cord injury without radiographic abnormality (SCIWORA).[5,10]

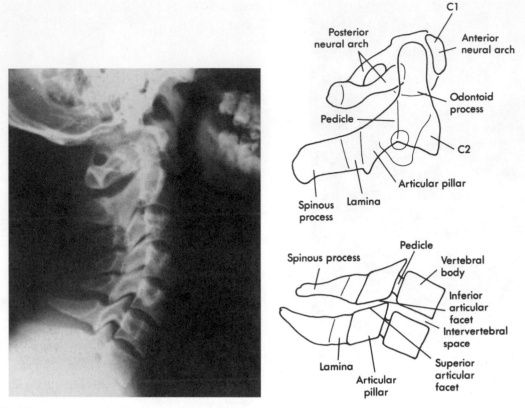

FIGURE 22-7 Lateral view of cervical spine. (Modified from Rosen P, Barkin RM, Hockberger RS et al: *Emergency medicine: concepts and clinical practice,* ed 4, St. Louis, 1998, Mosby.)

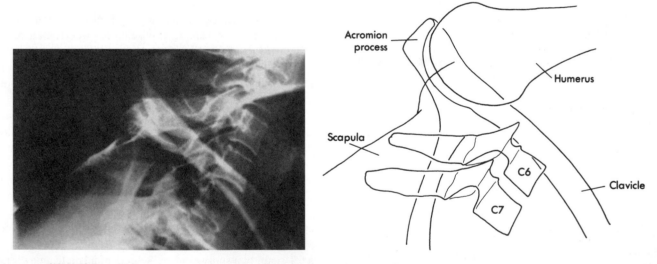

FIGURE 22-8 Swimmer's view of cervical spine. (Modified from Rosen P, Barkin RM, Hockberger RS et al: *Emergency medicine: concepts and clinical practice,* ed 4, St. Louis, 1998, Mosby.)

STABILIZATION

Initial stabilization of a patient with trauma to the spine begins with recognition and treatment of life-threatening injuries such as airway and vascular compromise. The airway is evaluated while maintaining C-spine control. Therapeutic interventions are directed at ensuring an adequate airway, maintaining ventilations, supporting adequate circulation, and preventing further injury.

Airway Management

The patient with cervical spine trauma is at risk for hypoxia, respiratory arrest, and aspiration. The emergency care team

Box 22-1	CERVICAL SPINE IMMOBILIZATION PROCEDURE

Cervical spine immobilization should be performed as a team. Generally, four people should work together.

1. Leader is positioned at the head of the patient and positions his or her hands on each side of the patient's head, with thumbs along the mandible and fingers behind the head on the occipital ridge. Maintain gentle but firm stabilization of the patient's neck throughout the entire procedure.
2. Assess the patient's motor and sensory level by asking the patient to wiggle his or her toes and fingers. Touch the patient's arms and legs to determine sensory response.
3. Apply and secure appropriate fitting cervical collar. Follow the directions for sizing that comes with each collar. An ill-fitting collar can cause pain, occlude the patient's airway, or fail to give appropriate immobilization.
4. Straighten the patient's arms and legs and position team members so that the patient may be rolled on the backboard as a unit.
5. The patient's head should be immobilized until the straps are correctly placed. The straps should be placed so that the patient is secured to the backboard at the shoulders, hips, and proximal to the knees.
6. The patient's head should be further immobilized with head blocks or towel rolls. Tape or straps should not be placed across the chin.
7. The patient's head should be manually immobilized until the head and neck are immobilized.
8. The patient's motor and sensory function should be reassessed after the patient is immobilized.
9. Some patients such as those with a compromised airway or neck deformities may not be able to tolerate laying flat.
10. Massive neck swelling that may result from a penetrating injury may prohibit the use of a cervical collar. Towel rolls and tape may be a safer method of securing the patient to the board and allow for evaluation of the patient's injury.

Modified from Emergency Nurses Association: *Trauma nursing core course provider manual,* ed 5, Des Plaines, Ill, 2000, The Association.

Box 22-2	HELMET REMOVAL PROCEDURE

Various helmets are available for those sports in which head protection is recommended. Motorcycling, bicycling, kayaking, ice hockey, football, and auto racing are just a few. The careful removal of this gear is imperative for protection of the cervical spine.

PROCEDURE

A quick examination of the helmet to determine its construction before attempting removal may save time, effort, and risk to the patient. Some sport helmets have air bladders that can be deflated to make space in the helmet, some have removable parts, and some are made of molded plastic that can be safely cut with a cast saw. Creating enough space to allow hands for cervical spine immobilization is the objective in altering the helmet, and all procedures should be explained to the patient as removal progresses.

1. Never attempt to remove a helmet alone; airway protection can be achieved with most helmets in place, and the potential for complicating an injury with a difficult removal is great.
2. One person should apply in-line stabilization by placing one hand behind the head, resting on the occiput, and the front hand on the angles of the mandible, thumb on one side, fingers on the other. (This person is in control of the head and neck.)
3. The second person should then remove the helmet by pulling laterally on the sides and sliding it off in caudad maneuver. If the helmet has full face protection, special consideration must be given to the eye and mouth covering, which must be removed first. If it cannot be removed, tilt the helmet (not the head) back to pass the face protector over the patient's nose.

From Sheehy SB et al: *Manual of clinical trauma care: the first hour,* ed 3, St. Louis, 1999, Mosby.

must also initiate interventions to minimize postinjury edema. The airway may be at risk from a spinal cord injury that compromises muscles of respiration or from localized edema that can cause airway obstruction, particularly in penetrating neck trauma. Advanced airway management such as endotracheal intubation should be considered early. The emergency care team must be prepared for alternative airway management such as cricothyrotomy if endotracheal intubation attempts fail. Any airway maneuvers require that the cervical spine remains adequately immobilized.

Cervical Spine Immobilization

The emergency nurse must ensure that the patient is correctly immobilized. Box 22-1 summarizes this procedure. The equipment required to immobilize the cervical spine includes a rigid cervical collar, lateral head immobilizer, and backboard.

A rigid cervical collar is applied to decrease head and neck movement. When applying a cervical collar, the emergency nurse should follow directions for size selection and application. Inline immobilization should be maintained during application of the cervical collar. Rigid cervical collars should not obstruct the patient's mouth or airway or interfere with ventilations. These collars should be applied after the patient's head has been placed in a neutral inline position.[6]

Placing the patient on a backboard does not completely immobilize the spine. The head must be stabilized laterally with a commercial head immobilizer, towel rolls and tape, or by taping the patient's head to the backboard. Tape or straps should never obstruct the patient's airway. The patient should be secured to the backboard at the chest, abdomen, and knees.

If the patient has a helmet in place, it should be removed. Box 22-2 and Figure 22-9 illustrate this procedure. ED

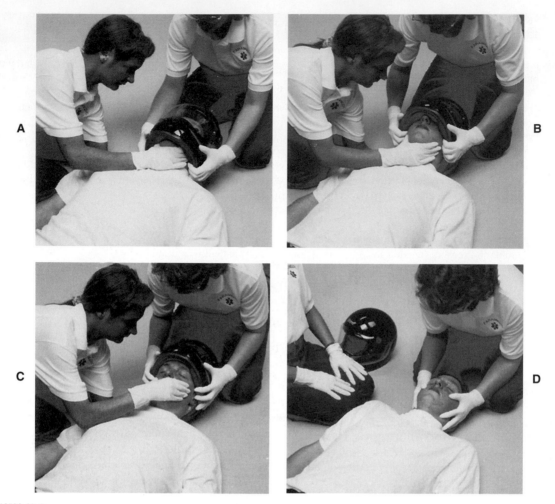

FIGURE 22-9   Helmet removal. **A,** The helmet and the head are immobilized in an inline position. The patient's mandible is grasped by placing the thumb at the angle of the mandible on one side and two fingers at the angle on the other side. The other hand is placed under the neck at the base of the skull, producing inline immobilization of the patient's head. **B,** The side of the helmet is carefully spread away from the patient's head and ears. **C,** The helmet is then rotated to clear the nose and removed from the patient's head in a straight line. **D,** After removal of the helmet, inline immobilization is applied as is a rigid cervical collar. (From Sanders M: *Mosby's paramedic textbook,* ed 2, St. Louis, 2000, Mosby.)

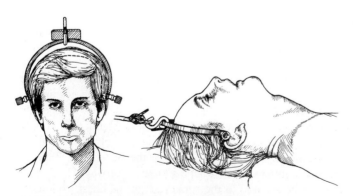

FIGURE 22-10   Gardner-Wells tongs. (From Stauffer ES: In Evarts CM, editor: *Surgery of the musculoskeletal system,* New York, 1983, Churchill Livingstone.)

personnel should practice this procedure for safe and efficient performance.[8]

Circulation Management

Hypotension may be directly related to spinal shock. Injury to the spine cord may cause loss of sympathetic vasomotor tone, leading to hypotension and bradycardia. With disruption of the sympathetic nervous system in spinal trauma, a drop in blood pressure from vasodilatation does not cause a compensatory increase in the heart rate. When hypotension is present, injuries such as a tension pneumothorax or intraabdominal bleeding, which also cause hypotension, should be ruled out.

In the patient with a spinal cord injury, hypotension may be the result of spinal shock or secondary to hypovolemia from other injuries. If the cause of the patient's hypotension is not clear, intravenous crystalloid solutions should be used

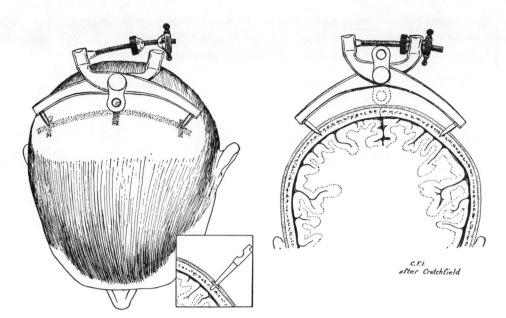

FIGURE 22-11   Crutchfield tongs for skeletal traction in fractures or fracture-dislocations of cervical spine. *Inset:* Special drill constructed with flange that allows it to penetrate outer table only. (From Crenshaw AH, editor: *Campbell's operative orthopedics,* ed 7, vol 4, St. Louis, 1987, Mosby.)

to correct hypovolemia.[6] A pulmonary artery catheter may be inserted to monitor fluid resuscitation and prevent complications from excessive fluid administration. Fluid and blood loss should be corrected before vasoactive medications are considered to maintain the circulation.

Pharmacologic Management

If the patient arrives in the ED within 8 hours of injury, high-dose methylprednisolone (MP) should be administered. In 1990 Bracken and colleagues[4] demonstrated neurologic improvement in patients with spinal cord injury who received MP within 8 hours of injury. The patient receives an initial bolus of MP of 30 mg/kg over 15 minutes followed 45 minutes later by a continuous infusion of 5.4 mg/kg/hr for 23 hours. Administration of MP is the current standard of care for spinal cord injury; however, recent research has begun to question its effectiveness.[8] George and colleagues found that patients who received high-dose MP were at greater risk for pneumonia, decubitis ulcer formation, and urinary tract infections. Administration within 8 hours of injury did not improve the functional status of the patient as assessed by mobility and the functional independence measures.[8] Further research is needed to determine whether high-dose MP is effective or may actually place the patient at risk for postinjury complications. However, administration of MP remains the standard of care. See Box 22-3 for an example of MP dosing. A two-tiered approach has been used in some areas. Patients who receive MP within 3 hours of injury are given a 24-hour regimen, whereas those with MP started between 3 and 8 hours of injury are given an additional 24-hour infusion.[4]

Additional Interventions

The patient with an acute spinal cord injury needs a urinary catheter to decrease bladder distention and to monitor urinary output during resuscitation. A gastric tube should be inserted to protect the patient from aspiration. A histamine blocker is given to prevent development of gastric ulcers.[6]

The emergency nurse needs to remember that the patient with a spinal cord injury has lost the ability to control body temperature. The patient should be kept warm and protected from unnecessary exposure. Warm blankets or a commercial warmer such as a Bair Hugger should be used to keep the patient warm and prevent cold stress— particularly if the patient receives a large amount of intravenous fluids. Fluids should be warmed before administration.

Cervical Tongs and Skeletal Fixation

Unstable cervical fractures may initially be stabilized in the ED with application of cervical tongs, which provide consistent traction and minimize cord compression. Two types of tongs currently used are Gardner-Wells tongs (Figure 22-10) and Crutchfield tongs (Figure 22-11).

In some EDs halo fixation devices (Figure 22-12) are applied, which provide the most rigid immobilization of all cervical orthotic devices and have been used since 1959.[3] A halo device may be used for stabilization of Jefferson (C1) fractures, type III odontoid fractures, type II hangman's fractures (C-2), single-column cervical spine injuries, and management of cervical fractures in patients with ankylosing spondylosis. Halo traction devices are contraindicated

Box 22-3   METHYLPREDNISOLONE THERAPY OF SPINAL CORD INJURY

Purpose: To standardize and facilitate the preparation and administration of high-dose methylprednisolone in cases of acute spinal cord injury.

Time sequence: This therapy has been found to be of benefit only if begun within 8 hours of injury and completely administered over 24 hours.*

Preparation of drug:

1. Reconstitute two 2-g vials of Upjohn brand Solu-Medrol, using the diluent provided with the product (30 ml of diluent per 2-g vial). The result is 4 g (4000 mg) in 61.2 ml.

2. From a 250 ml bag of normal saline (Abbott), withdraw 91.2 ml (this is equal to the volume of the methylprednisolone 4 gm to be added, plus 30 ml of overfill).

3. Add the 4 g methylprednisolone to the bag; resultant solution is 16 mg/ml of methylprednisolone. The same method is used to prepare loading and maintainence doses. Most patients will require more than one bag to complete therapy.

4. If using products other than Solu-Medrol, 2-g vials, and Abbott brand 250 ml normal saline bags, prepare a 16 mg/ml solution to use the dosing table accurately. Reconstitute 4 g of drug according to product direction and remove from a 250-ml bag a volume equal to the drug volume plus the overfill before adding the drug. Contact the pharmacy for specific information on overfill amounts for the manufacturer of IV solutions.

Loading dose: A loading dose of 30 mg/kg is given over 15 minutes. Using the prepared solution, infuse loading dose at the rate appropriate for patient's weight (see dosing table).

Caution: Rate is in ml/hr but *infuse for 15 minutes only!*

WAIT 45 MINUTES AFTER LOADING DOSE IS COMPLETED.

Maintenance dose: A dose of 5.4 mg/kg/hr is infused for 23 hours. Using the same prepared solution, begin the 23-hour drip at the rate specified on the dosing table.

Patient Weight (kg)	Loading Dose (30 mg/kg)	Loading Dose (Rate in ml/hr for 15 minutes)	Maintenance Dose (5.4 mg/kg/hr)	Maintenance Dose (Rate in ml/hr for 23 hrs)
30	900 mg	225	162 mg/hr	10.1
35	1050 mg	262.5	189 mg/hr	11.8
40	1200 mg	300	216 mg/hr	13.5
45	1350 mg	337.5	243 mg/hr	15.2
50	1500 mg	375	270 mg/hr	16.9
55	1650 mg	412.5	297 mg/hr	18.6
60	1800 mg	450	324 mg/hr	20.2
65	1950 mg	487.5	351 mg/hr	21.9
70	2100 mg	525	378 mg/hr	23.6
75	2250 mg	562.5	405 mg/hr	25.3
80	2400 mg	600	432 mg/hr	27
85	2550 mg	637.5	459 mg/hr	28.7
90	2700 mg	675	486 mg/hr	30.4
95	2850 mg	712.5	513 mg/hr	32.1
100	3000 mg	750	540 mg/hr	33.7
105	3150 mg	787.5	567 mg/hr	35.4
110	3300 mg	825	594 mg/hr	37.1
115	3450 mg	862.5	621 mg/hr	38.8
120	3600 mg	900	648 mg/hr	40.5
125	3750 mg	937.5	675 mg/hr	42.2
130	3900 mg	975	702 mg/hr	43.9

Remember:

Table assumes preparation of methylprednisolone as a 16 mg/ml solution as outlined previously. The tubing may be primed with drug solution before delivery of the required volume via an infusion pump. The tubing then will *not* need to be flushed to deliver the entire dose.

Loading dose rate is in ml per hour; total loading dose is run in over 15 minutes.

Wait 45 minutes after completion of loading dose, then begin maintenance dose. Maintenance dose is administered at the appropriate hourly rate for 23 hours.

Therapy should be started within 8 hours of injury and administration completed within 24 hours from start of therapy.

*Note that the infusion may run for 48 hours in patients with initial bolus given between 3 and 8 hours after injury.

Modified from Bracken MB, Shepard MJ, Collins WF et al: A randomized controlled trial of methylprednisolone or naloxone in the treatment of acute spinal-cord injury: results of the Second National Acute Spinal Cord Injury Study, *N Engl J Med* 322:1405, 1990; and The Upjohn Company: *Solu-Medrol brand methylprednisolone,* Kalamazoo, Mich., Upjohn (package insert).

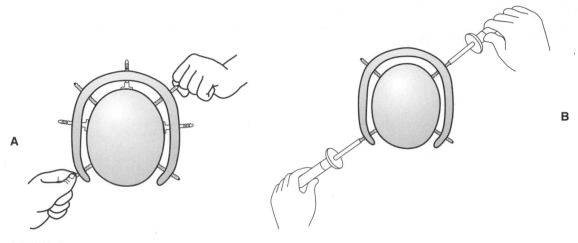

FIGURE 22-12 Halo traction. An open-back halo device is applied in the ED and can later be fitted to a vest for early patient mobility. **A.** Pins are inserted by hand until each pin is tight. **B.** A torque wrench is used to completely secure the pins. The wrench stops when 8 lbs per inch of torque is reached. (Courtesy ACC Medical Company, El Segundo, Calif.)

Box 22-4 PROCEDURE FOR APPLICATION OF HALO TRACTION

1. Determine the ring's crown size by holding it over the crown of the patient's head.
2. Measure the patient's chest circumference to determine the size of the vest.
3. Identify sites for pin insertion on the patient's head. Evaluate for trauma to these areas.
4. Shave pin site areas and cleanse the skin with antiseptic solution.
5. Assist the physician in anesthetizing the pin site area. This is usually done with injection of 1% lidocaine.
6. Administer sedation if the patient's condition permits it.
7. Assist the physician in insertion of the pins.
8. Ensure that the appropriate weight has been added to the traction. Weight may vary from 5 to 10 lb depending on stability of the injury or the presence of a dislocation, which must be reduced.
9. Tape tools to the halo vest for emergency use.
10. Obtain cervical spine films after application of the halo device.

From Botte MJ et al: Halo skeletal fixation: techniques of application and prevention of complications, *Clin Orthop* 239:12, 1989.

---

when the patient has an unstable skull fracture or traumatized skin where the pins are inserted.

When cervical traction is applied in the ED, the emergency nurse may assist with this procedure. The procedure should be explained to the patient, and, if the patient's condition permits, sedation should be administered to decrease anxiety and ensure patient comfort. Box 22-4 summarizes the procedure for application of a halo device.[13]

Complications related to application of a halo skeletal fixation device include pin loosening, which causes loosening of the crown, infection at the pin site, development of pressure sores, loss of cervical reduction, pin-site swelling, difficulty swallowing, and puncture of the dura.[3] Emergency nurses should be familiar with these complications because patients often come to the ED after discharge with some of these conditions.

PSYCHOSOCIAL CARE

Injury to the spine elicits a tremendous amount of anxiety and fear from both the patient and the family. The major concern of many patients and families is whether the patient will be able to move, walk, or "be the same" again. Unfortunately, this cannot be answered fully in the ED. The emergency nurse's discussions with the patient and family should be based on honesty. All questions should be answered and all procedures should be explained. The family should be allowed to see the patient as soon as possible and remain there. Care of these patients can be quite challenging. Being truthful from the beginning and focusing care on prevention of further injury are important emergency nursing interventions.

SPINAL CORD INJURIES

Injuries to the spinal cord are the result of primary and secondary injuries. The primary injury is a direct injury from blunt or penetrating forces. Secondary injury is a consequence of vascular changes; release of catecholamines, endorphins, and enkephalins; lipid peroxidation; lysosomal enzymes; and adenosine triphosphate.[1] Acute spinal cord injury causes physiologic derangement of gray and white matter, which decreases oxygen tension, and disrupts vasomotor tone and autoregulation. Injuries to the spinal cord may be complete or incomplete. Injuries of the vertebral column may occur with or without associated spinal cord injury. Figure 22-13 describes specific injuries of the vertebral column.

Cervical

Jefferson (C-1)	Hangman (C-2)	Odontoid (C-2)

Facet dislocation	Body compression	Burst	Other

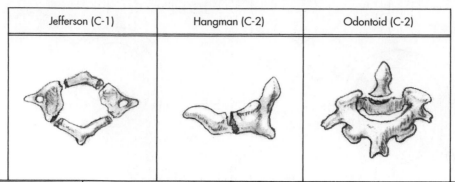

Thoracic/Lumbar

Compression	Slice	Burst (anterior)

Burst (posterior)	Chance	Dislocation	Other

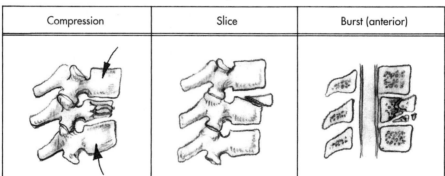

FIGURE 22-13   Common vertebral column fractures. (Modified from *Orthopaedic knowledge update—I*, Chicago, 1984, American Academy of Orthopaedic Surgeons.)

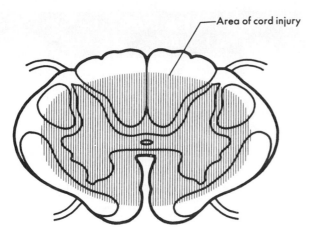

FIGURE 22-14 Central cord syndrome. (Modified from Rosen P, Barkin RM, Hockberger RS et al: *Emergency medicine: concepts and clinical practice,* ed 4, St. Louis, 1998, Mosby.)

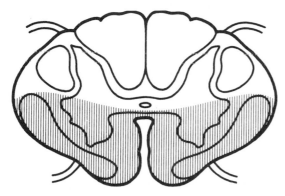

FIGURE 22-15 Anterior cord syndrome. (Modified from Rosen P, Barkin RM, Hockberger RS et al: *Emergency medicine: concepts and clinical practice,* ed 4, St. Louis, 1998, Mosby.)

A new spine classification system[11] has been proposed. This new classification system has five fundamental components: number of columns injured, extent of translatory displacement, anterior vertebral distortion with resulting angulations, canal compromise, and percent loss of vertebral heights. The goal of this classification is development of a realistic and reliable means of universal communication between health professionals in spinal care so that patients receive the best care and have the best chance for rehabilitation as soon as possible after an injury.

Complications related to spinal cord injury are related to location of the injury. An injury to the cervical spine puts the patient at risk for pulmonary and ventilatory problems; injury between T-1 and T-4 causes loss of sympathetic tone. A low-thoracic spine injury causes loss of abdominal muscle functions, decreased respiratory reserves, and gastric distension. Injury to the lumbosacral area of the spinal cord may cause loss of temperature regulation and bowel and bladder function, and put the patient at risk for developing deep venous thrombosis, decubitus ulcers, and pulmonary emboli.[6]

Spinal and Neurogenic Shock

When a complete injury occurs, motor and sensory functions cease below the level of injury. Pain, touch, temperature, and inhalation are evaluated as part of a sensory evaluation. Neurogenic shock is generally seen with injuries above the T-6 level. Disruption of the sympathetic nervous system causes flaccid paralysis, loss of sphincter tone, bradycardia, and hypotension. Other signs of neurogenic shock include cool, dry skin and bounding peripheral pulses.

If the patient's injury indicates the potential for neurogenic shock, the emergency team should quickly rule out other potential causes of shock. Blood loss from thoracic and abdominal injuries may be the cause of the patient's shock state, particularly if the patient's spinal cord injury is not the only injury. Management of neurogenic shock is discussed in the initial management section of this chapter.

Spinal shock is characterized by temporary loss of reflexes, flaccid paralysis, and areflexia.[6] Intensity and duration are determined by level of injury.

Incomplete Spinal Cord Injury

The most common type of incomplete cord injury is a complete cord lesion with lumbar-root sparing.[13] Other types of incomplete spinal cord lesions are central cord syndrome, anterior cord syndrome, posterior cord syndrome, Brown-Séquard syndrome, and nerve root injuries. Confirmation of an incomplete lesion is based on evaluation of sensory and motor functions as defined by the American Spinal Injury Association.

Central Cord Syndrome

Central cord syndrome (Figure 22-14) is caused by hyperextension and is seen most often in elderly patients after a fall. This syndrome causes loss of function in the upper extremities, whereas lower extremity function is not affected. Bowel and bladder function are maintained.

Anterior Cord Syndrome

Anterior cord syndrome (Figure 22-15) usually results from occlusion of the anterior spinal artery, a herniated nucleus pulposus (rupture disk), or transection of the anterior portion of the cord. The patient has hyperesthesia, hypoalgesia, and incomplete or complete paralysis. The patient is able to feel vibrations and has proprioception because the posterior column is preserved.

Brown-Séquard Syndrome

Hemisection of the cord in the anteroposterior plane is known as Brown-Séquard syndrome (Figure 22-16). The most common cause is a penetrating injury such as a gunshot, knife, or a missile fragment penetration. Brown-Séquard syndrome is characterized by ipsilateral (same side) paresis or hemiplegia and contralateral (opposite side) decreased sensation to pain and changes in temperature. A per-

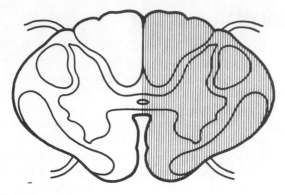

FIGURE 22-16   Brown-Séquard syndrome. (Modified from Rosen P, Barkin RM, Hockberger RS et al: *Emergency medicine: concepts and clinical practice,* ed 4, St. Louis, 1998, Mosby.)

son can feel one side of the body but not the other and can move that side but not the other.

Nerve Root Injuries

Injuries to nerve roots often occur as a result of spinal cord trauma. Common symptoms include hypoalgesia, pain, or referred pain.

Penetrating Injuries

Penetrating injuries to the spinal cord are usually the result of gunshot wounds and stab wounds. The emergency nurse should look for entrance and exit wounds. Presence of CSF indicates spinal cord perforation. If the missile passes through the abdominal viscera into the spinal cord, the patient is at great risk of central nervous system infection.

If the patient is brought to the ED with the wounding object in place, the emergency nurse should leave the object in place and stabilize it. Bullets and wounding objects such as a knife are evidence and should be handled carefully to maintain integrity of the evidence.

Swelling from soft-tissue injury secondary to penetrating injury can put the patient in danger of airway obstruction. Soft-tissue injury to abdominal and thoracic structures can produce life-threatening complications in the patient with a penetrating neurologic injury. Many of these patients go to the operating room for resuscitation and stabilization.

Spinal Cord Injury Without Radiographic Abnormality

Spinal cord injury is relatively uncommon in young children because anatomic differences allow for more laxity in the child's neck ligaments. However, more common in the pediatric population than in adults is SCIWORA. This injury usually occurs at the cervical or thoracic levels of the cord. The child has spinal cord injury with neurologic deficits; however, no evidence of bony injury exists. As previously discussed, an MRI has been found invaluable in diagnosing this injury.[10]

Autonomic Dysreflexia

Autonomic dysreflexia is a complication of spinal cord injury above the T-6 level. This life-threatening emergency is seen in patients after spinal shock has resolved. Multiple stimuli below the level of injury can trigger this response. Stimuli include a full bladder, full rectum, or decubitis ulcer. When triggered, the sympathetic nervous system overreacts below the lesion because of a lack of control from higher nerve centers.

Signs and symptoms of autonomic dysreflexia include sudden severe headache, hypertension, sweating, cardiac dysrhythmia (tachycardia or bradycardia), flushing above the level of injury, and coolness below the level of injury. The patient may also complain of nasal stuffiness and appear quite anxious.

Treatment of autonomic dysreflexia begins with identifying the cause of the sympathetic response. Assessing for a full bladder or constipation, the nurse can begin to rapidly relieve the problem. Medications that may be administered are ganglionic blockers such as apresoline. When these medications are used to lower a patient's blood pressure, the patient must be closely monitored to quickly identify any serious complications such as cerebral hemorrhage. All these drugs must be given cautiously with close monitoring of the blood pressure to prevent a precipitous drop. After the emergency is over, the emergency nurse should work with the patient and family to develop interventions to prevent another occurrence.[12]

SUMMARY

Spinal trauma is not as common as other types of injury, but its consequences are devastating. It affects approximately 200,000 people each year and is extremely expensive.[6,11] Patients are generally young and require extensive physical and psychosocial care. Emergency care of these patients involves resuscitation and rehabilitation to decrease and prevent further injury to the spinal cord. Box 22-5 identifies pertinent nursing diagnoses for the patient with spinal cord injury.

Current research focuses on treating the effects of any secondary injuries that occur with spinal cord damage and regrowth of the damaged cells. Naloxone, calcium channel blockers, and antioxidants are examples of some of the experimental medications that have been studied. The most successful way to lessen spinal trauma is prevention. Use of seat belts, air bags, new car construction such as reinforced side compartments, helmets, and other safety devices are some methods used to prevent spinal injury. Teaching children, adolescents, and adults the consequences of risky behavior such as snowboarding may eventually help decrease the uncommon but lamentable consequences of this injury.

References

1. Boss B: Alterations in neurologic function. In McCance K, Huether S, editors: *Pathophysiology,* ed 3, St. Louis, 1998, Mosby.
2. Boss B: Concepts of neurologic dysfunction. In McCance K, Huether S, editors: *Pathophysiology,* ed 3, St. Louis, 1998, Mosby.
3. Botte MJ et al: Halo skeletal fixation: techniques of application and prevention of complications, *Clin Orthop* 239:12, 1989.
4. Bracken MB, Shepard MJ et al: Methylprednisolone administered for 24 or 48 hours, or 48 hour tirilazad mesylate, in the treatment of acute spinal cord injury; results of the third National Acute Spinal Cord Injury randomized controlled trial, *JAMA* 277(20):1597, 1997.
5. Chiles BW, Cooper PR: Acute spinal injury, *New Engl J Med* 334(8):514, 1996.
6. Emergency Nurses Association: *Trauma nursing core course provider manual,* ed 5, Des Plaines, Ill, 2000, The Association.
7. *Facts about spinal cord injury and the central nervous system,* Retrieved from the World Wide Web: http://paralysis. apacure.org/progress/facts.html.
8. George et al: Failure of methylprednisone to improve the outcome of spinal cord injuries, *Am Surg* 61:659, 1995.
9. Jaworski M, Wirtz K: Spinal trauma. In Kitt S et al, editors: *Emergency nursing,* Philadelphia, 1995, WB Saunders.
9a. McQuillan KA, Von Rueden KT, Hartsock RL et al: *Trauma nursing: from resuscitation through rehabilitation,* ed 2, Philadelphia, 2001, WB Saunders.
10. Medina FA: Neck and spinal cord trauma. In Barkin R, editor: *Pediatric emergency medicine,* ed 2, St. Louis, 1997, Mosby.
11. Meyer et al: *New spine fracture classification system,* Retrieved March 11, 2001 from the World Wide Web: http://www.nwu.edu/spine/fxclass.htm.
12. Morris G, Taylor W: Modern management of acute spinal cord trauma. In Grenvik G et al, editors: *Textbook of critical care,* ed 4, Phildelphia, 2000, WB Saunders.
13. Proehl J, editor: *Emergency nursing procedures,* ed 2, Philadelphia, 1999, WB Saunders.
14. Schroeder RJ et al: Comparison of the diagnostic value of CT and MRI injuries of the cervical vertebrae, *Aktuelle Radiologie* 5(4):197, 1995.
15. Spinal Cord Injury Information Network: Retrieved June 2000 from the World Wide Web: http://www.spinalcord.uab.edu.

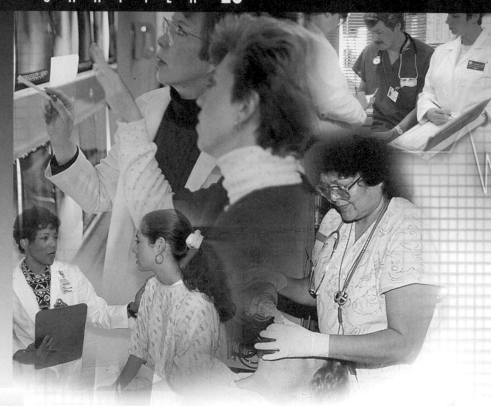

CHAPTER 23

THORACIC TRAUMA

ALICA A. PEAVEY,
LORENE NEWBERRY

Chest trauma is one of the most common injuries, accounting for 20% to 25% of deaths in adults. It is the leading cause of death among children ages 1 to 14.[14] Chest trauma is due to blunt or penetrating forces. Mechanism of injury, force, trajectory, type of weapon, angle of impact, proximity to the victim, secondary factors such as fire, and overall physical attributes of the patient determine degree and type of injury. Emergency nurses should include these data in their initial assessment and diagnostic decision tree. The *index of suspicion* in combination with assessment serves as a framework for clinical decisions. Patients with trauma do not always manifest their injuries immediately and can change rapidly within the first hour after injury.

Blunt trauma may be caused by auto accidents, falls, exploding tires, or any mechanism whereby the force of impact, particularly sudden deceleration, causes internal structural damage. Causative agents for penetrating injury are just as varied and not exclusive to weaponry such as guns and knives. Falls, accidents, or natural disasters that result in impaled tree limbs, fencing, or falls onto fenceposts are not uncommon. Emergency nurses should anticipate that patients can have a combination of blunt and penetrating injuries.

Thoracic injury and treatment has been described for centuries; however, it was not until the end of World War II that a chest tube connected to underwater seal drainage became standard treatment for many thoracic injuries. Endotracheal intubation, anesthesia, and chest roentgenography, developed in the nineteenth and early twentieth centuries, and advances in the past 50 years such as improved ventilatory assistance, antibiotics, blood gas analysis, and specialized nursing care have increased survival in patients with thoracic injuries. Despite these advances thoracic trauma's mortality rate remains second only to brain and spinal cord injuries.

Thoracic trauma requires systematic assessment for potentially lethal injuries followed by rapid intervention. This chapter discusses assessment and treatment of various thoracic injuries. Understanding the anatomy and physiology is essential.

ANATOMY AND PHYSIOLOGY

The thoracic cavity skeleton includes the sternum, ribs, costal cartilages, and thoracic vertebrae (Figure 23-1). The thorax is fairly mobile and expands easily to accommodate respiratory efforts. Ribs attach posteriorly to thoracic vertebrae and anteriorly to the sternum. Seven upper ribs are joined directly to costal cartilages, whereas ribs 8, 9, and 10 interface indirectly with the sternum through fusion of costal cartilage. Ribs 11 and 12 do not interface with the sternum. The diaphragm forms the inferior border of the thorax, whereas the superior border is continuous with structures of the neck.

Internal thoracic structures are composed of organs and structures of the pulmonary, cardiovascular, and gastrointestinal systems (Figure 23-2). Pulmonary structures are located in the pleural space, whereas cardiovascular and

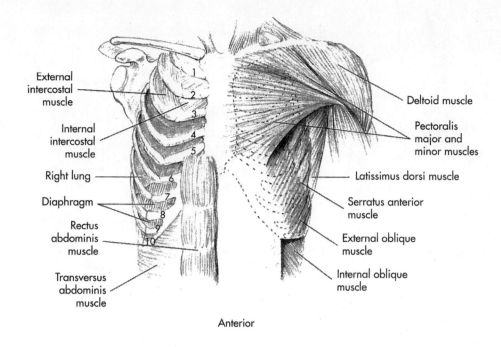

Anterior

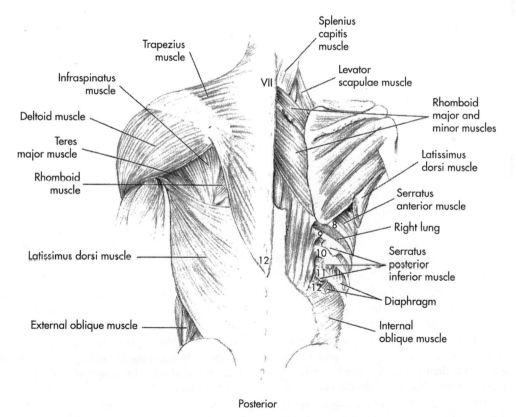

Posterior

FIGURE 23-1   Bony structure of the chest wall and the anterior and posterior musculature. (From Davis JH et al: *Clinical surgery,* St. Louis, 1987, Mosby.)

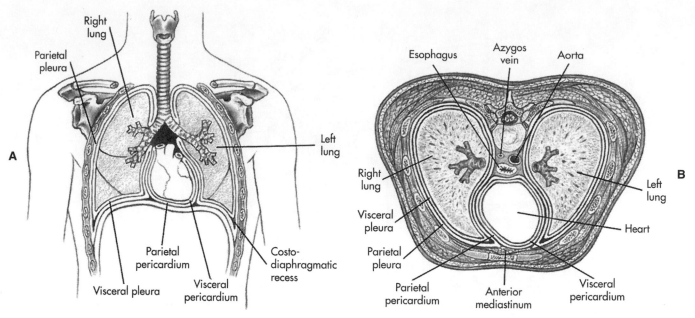

FIGURE 23-2   Chest cavity and related structures. **A,** Anterior view. **B,** Cross-section. (From Thompson JM, McFarland GK, Hirsch JE et al: *Mosby's clinical nursing,* ed 5, St. Louis, 2002, Mosby.)

gastrointestinal structures are located in the mediastinum, a cavity between the two pleural spaces.

Pulmonary System

Lungs are cone-shaped organs above the diaphragm that extend approximately 1.5 inches above the clavicles. Each lung is located in a cavity lined with a serous membrane called the pleura. The visceral pleura covers the lungs themselves whereas the parietal pleura covers the rib cage, diaphragm, and pericardium. A potential space between these layers is the pleural cavity. Pleural cells secrete pleural fluid that separates the lungs but allows membranes to remain in contact and move without creating friction.

Normal breathing occurs through the processes of ventilation (Figure 23-3), which moves air in and out of the lungs, and respiration, which exchanges gases across alveolar capillary membranes. During inspiration, phrenic nerve stimulation causes the diaphragm to contract and pull downward. As the diaphragm pulls downward, external intercostals pull the chest wall out, which enlarges the thoracic cavity. As lung capacity increases, intrathoracic pressure becomes negative (i.e., lower than atmospheric pressure). This negative intrathoracic pressure draws air into the lungs. During expiration this process is reversed as the diaphragm relaxes and moves up. Intercostal muscles compress the chest so that the lungs recoil passively. Intrathoracic pressure becomes more positive as lung capacity diminishes. Increasing positive intrathoracic pressure forces air out of the lungs.[2]

Cardiovascular System

The heart is located in the mediastinum positioned with the right ventricle anteriorly beneath the sternum. The pericardium, a three-layered sac that surrounds and protects the heart, is a fibrous envelope separated from the heart by the pericardial space, a potential space between the parietal pericardium and the visceral pericardium, or epicardium. The heart's middle layer is the endocardium with the inner muscular layer called the myocardium. The pericardium contains pericardial fluid (5 to 30 ml) that prevents friction during contraction. The outer parietal pericardium is the fibrous pericardium, which attaches to the sternum, great vessels, and diaphragm to hold the heart in place.

Four muscular chambers, called atria and ventricles, contract rhythmically as they fill and empty with blood. The right atria and ventricles receive deoxygenated blood and pump the blood to the lungs for oxygenation. Oxygenated blood then enters the left side of the heart, which sends blood to the systemic circulation. The left heart is a high-pressure system, the right heart a low-pressure system. Valves separate chambers to prevent regurgitation of blood back into the atria and ventricles. Cardiac function and output depend on contractility, heart rate, preload (volume achieved during diastolic filling of the ventricles), and afterload (force or resistance against which the heart must pump to eject blood).

The thoracic aorta carries oxygenated blood to various tissues. Three anatomic parts of the aorta are recognized: ascending aorta, aortic arch, and descending aorta. The aortic arch is attached to the pulmonary artery by the ligamentum arteriosum. Near the ligamentum, a portion of the aorta branches off to form the left subclavian artery. At this point of the aorta, just distal to the ligamentum, the aorta is relatively immobile and is at increased risk for disruption. More than 85% of aortic injuries caused by acceleration or deceleration forces occur here.

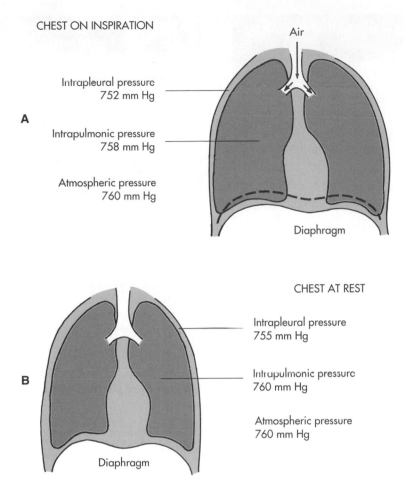

CHEST ON INSPIRATION

Air

A

Intrapleural pressure
752 mm Hg

Intrapulmonic pressure
758 mm Hg

Atmospheric pressure
760 mm Hg

Diaphragm

CHEST AT REST

B

Intrapleural pressure
755 mm Hg

Intrapulmonic pressure
760 mm Hg

Atmospheric pressure
760 mm Hg

Diaphragm

FIGURE 23-3 **A,** Contraction of diaphragm increases vertical dimensions of lungs. **B,** Relaxation of diaphragm decreases vertical dimensions of lungs. (From Wade JF: *Comprehensive respiratory care,* ed 3, St. Louis, 1982, Mosby.)

Also in the mediastinum is the trachea, located posterior to the heart; the esophagus, posterior to the trachea; the phrenic nerve; and the diaphragm. Other thoracic cavity structures include the thymus gland in the anterior mediastinum behind the sternum, the esophagus, and subclavian and common carotid arteries.

PATIENT ASSESSMENT

The patient with an obvious or suspected thoracic injury must be promptly assessed because these injuries can produce death within minutes. Rapid assessment of airway, breathing, and circulation (ABC) followed by rapid, essential interventions is paramount. Control of the cervical spine occurs simultaneously with assessment of the patient's airway. Breathing rate, depth, and effort are assessed after airway patency is ensured. If an open chest wound is present, a three-sided occlusive dressing should be applied. Vaseline gauze, defibrillator pads, or gauze taped on three sides are all effective. After the dressing is applied, the patient must be monitored for

development of tension pneumothorax. Supplemental oxygen should be administered with a nonrebreather mask at 100% or bag-valve mask as appropriate. Circulation is assessed by palpating pulse rate and character. Obvious bleeding is controlled with direct pressure and fluid resuscitation. Two large-bore intravenous lines should be started using lactated Ringer's or other appropriate crystalloid solution. Box 23-1 highlights initial assessment of a patient with thoracic trauma; Box 23-2 presents assessment data that should be obtained during the secondary assessment. Therapeutic interventions are listed in Box 23-3.

SPECIFIC THORACIC INJURIES

Thoracic injuries include injuries of the chest wall, pulmonary system, cardiovascular system, and esophagus. Acuity is determined by the effect of the injury on ventilation and circulation. Figure 23-4 compares normal ventilatory movement seen in the presence of a sucking chest wound with that seen in flail chest.

Box 23-1	INITIAL ASSESSMENT OF THORACIC TRAUMA

AIRWAY WITH C-SPINE CONTROL

BREATHING

Bilateral breath sounds
Respiratory stridor
Shortness of breath
Cyanosis
Tracheal deviation
Sucking chest wounds
Subcutaneous emphysema
Distended neck veins
Pulse oximetry
Paradoxical chest wall movement
Intercostal and accessory muscle use
Upper abdominal injury

CIRCULATION

Skin color and temperature
Heart sounds
Vital signs
Blood pressure equal in upper extremities (equal or asymmetric)
Extremity pulses (equal, diminished, or absent)

ADDITIONAL CONSIDERATIONS

Pattern of abrasions or bruising
Wound size and location

Box 23-2	SECONDARY ASSESSMENT OF THORACIC TRAUMA

Assess pain.
Obtain patient history.
Identify mechanism of injury.
Determine time of the injury.
Determine what the patient remembers about the event.

Box 23-3	THERAPEUTIC INTERVENTIONS FOR THORACIC TRAUMA

Maintain patent airway.
Promote adequate ventilation.
Provide high-flow oxygen.
Prepare for intubation.
Cover open chest wound.
Assist with chest tube insertion or needle decompression.
Monitor bleeding from chest.
Prepare for autotransfusion.
Initiate two large-bore intravenous lines.
Facilitate essential radiographs—cervical spine, chest, and pelvis.
Monitor cardiac rhythm continuously.
Monitor blood pressure, respiratory rate and effort, pulse oximetry, and level of consciousness every hour or more often if indicated by patient condition.
Document urine output and patient response to therapeutic interventions.

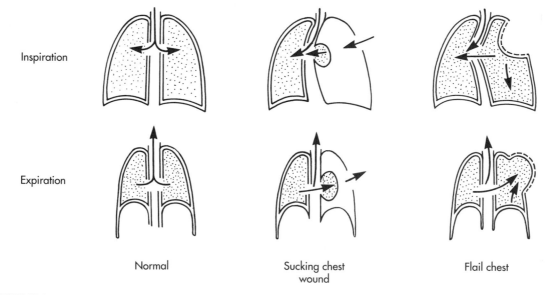

Inspiration

Expiration

Normal   Sucking chest wound   Flail chest

FIGURE 23-4 Comparison of ventilatory movement in normal and injured chests. (From Johnson J, Kirby CK: *Surgery of the chest,* ed 4, Chicago, 1970, Year Book Medical.)

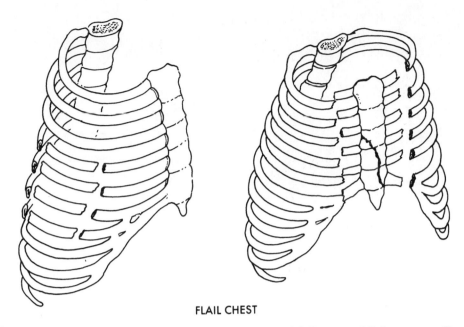

FLAIL CHEST

FIGURE 23-5   Fracture of several adjacent ribs in two places with lateral flail or central flail segments. (From Rosen P, Barkin RM, Hockberger RS et al: *Emergency medicine: concepts and clinical practice,* ed 4, St. Louis, 1998, Mosby.)

Chest Wall Injuries

Rib Fractures

The exact incidence of rib fractures is unknown, but experts estimate a regional trauma center can expect 10% of all trauma admissions to have rib fractures. Fractures result from a direct or indirect blunt force or crush injuries. The most common mechanism of injury associated with rib fractures is a motor vehicle crash.

Rib fractures may occur in a single rib or multiple ribs and occur most often in the fourth through tenth ribs. These fractures are not themselves considered life-threatening. The patient often has tenderness so respirations are shallow to avoid moving the chest wall. Subcutaneous emphysema or crepitus may also be present. Radiographs assist with diagnosis but are only 70% accurate for rib fractures. Fractures that separate the sternum from costal cartilage are not evident on a radiograph.

Treatment for most rib fractures is analgesia and good pulmonary toilet. Pain management is essential because even one or two rib fractures can result in disability from pain and the risk of secondary atelectasis. Oral or intravenous analgesia are used for many patients; however, intercostal nerve blocks may be appropriate for some patients. Good pulmonary toilet, such as coughing and deep breathing, are used to prevent complications, including pneumonia or atelectasis. Incentive spirometry may also be used to prevent these conditions. Patients with multiple rib fractures are usually admitted for observation. Those with severe injuries (eight or more fractured ribs, massive flail injury) may re-

quire internal fixation with plates and screws. First and second ribs are well-protected by the clavicle, so significant blunt force is required to fracture these ribs. Great vessel injuries should be considered when the first or second rib is fractured. Other injuries associated with upper rib fractures are injuries to the clavicles, scapulae, trachea, and lungs. Lower rib fractures (9 through 12) are associated with injuries to the spleen, liver, or other abdominal contents, depending on location of the fracture(s).

Elderly patients with rib fractures are at greater risk for complications because of diminished vital capacity that occurs with aging. Impaired ventilation worsens in all patients during the first few days after injury secondary to increasing chest wall edema and decreasing compliance. In an elderly patient with rib injury and diminished capacity, serial assessment is essential to prevent complications. Patients with decreased pulmonary function from asthma or chronic occlusive pulmonary disease also require careful assessment because vital capacity in this population is also decreased.

Children have thin chest walls, and their bony thorax is more cartilaginous. Consequently, energy is easily transmitted to underlying thoracic structures without fracturing ribs. When rib fractures do occur in children, concurrent thoracic and abdominal injuries may be severe.[8]

Flail Chest

A flail chest is defined as fractures in two or more adjacent ribs in two or more places, or bilateral detachment of the sternum from costal cartilage (Figure 23-5). Flail chest is usually associated with a massive crush injury or

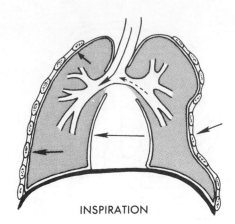 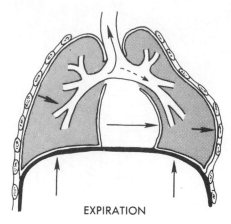

INSPIRATION   EXPIRATION

FIGURE 23-6   Chest wall movement with flail chest. On inspiration flail section sinks in as chest expands, impairing ability to produce negative intrapleural pressure to draw in air. Mediastinum shifts to uninjured side. On expiration flail segment bulges outward, impairing ability to exhale. Mediastinum shifts to injured side. Air may shift uselessly from side to side in severe flail chest (broken lines). (From Rosen P, Barkin RM, Hockberger RS et al: *Emergency medicine: concepts and clinical practice,* ed 4, St. Louis, 1998, Mosby.)

high-speed motor vehicle crash. This injury creates a free-floating, unstable segment that moves in opposition to normal chest wall movement (Figure 23-6). The flail segment moves in when the patient inspires and out with exhalation. A flail chest causes hypoventilation of both lungs followed by atelectasis and eventually hypoxia. The injury is usually associated with an underlying pulmonary contusion that worsens the injury because of loss of compliance, increased airway resistance, and decreased gas diffusion.

Diagnosis of flail chest is usually made by direct observation. The affected area moves paradoxically from the rest of the chest. However, muscular splinting of the chest immediately after injury may mask a flail chest until hours later when muscles become fatigued and paradoxic movement becomes obvious.[1,3] With flail chest the thorax moves in an uncoordinated manner, so air movement is extremely poor. Palpation of the chest wall indicates abnormal motion and crepitus. The patient complains of pain and difficulty breathing. Radiographs may not be helpful because costochondral separation may not appear. Arterial blood gas values reflecting respiratory failure aid in diagnosis.[1]

Treatment consists of ensuring adequate oxygenation, administering fluids carefully, and providing pain relief with intercostal nerve blocks. Fluids are limited because of associated pulmonary contusion and potential development of adult respiratory distress syndrome. Intubation and mechanical ventilation is not required for all patients, but patients should be monitored carefully for any change in respiratory status that indicates a need for more aggressive management (i.e., changes in respiratory rate, arterial oxygen tension, and work of breathing).[1] Patients who require mechanical ventilation are usually managed with continuous positive end expiratory pressure. Continuous positive airway pressure may be used for some patients.

Sternal Fracture

Sternal fractures occur when tremendous force is applied to the chest, as with steering wheel impact. The most common site of fracture is the junction of the manubrium and body of the sternum.[3] In addition to pain a sternal fracture has significant potential for underlying cardiac injury including myocardial contusion and pericardial tamponade.

The patient may experience dyspnea and localized pain with movement and may hypoventilate to avoid chest wall movement. Chest wall ecchymosis, sternal deformity, or crepitus may also occur. Treatment includes pain relief, a baseline electrocardiogram (ECG), and serial patient examinations. If the fracture is displaced, operative reduction may be required. If cardiac symptoms are present, an echocardiogram may be obtained to check for cardiac tamponade. Otherwise patients are treated symptomatically.

Pulmonary Injuries

Laryngeal Injury

Fracture of the larynx is a rare, life-threatening injury. Common mechanisms of injury include striking the anterior neck on the steering wheel or dashboard, karate blows, or "clothesline" injuries when a snowmobiler or motorcycle rider hits a clothesline, wire, or tree limb with direct anterior neck impact. The patient presents with hoarseness, subcutaneous emphysema, and crepitus. Injury is suggested with a history of blunt trauma to the neck; however, initial diagnosis may be difficult if initial presentation is subtle, such as local tenderness or crepitus. A lateral soft-tissue radiograph of the neck or computed tomography (CT) scan may be necessary to confirm diagnosis. Intubation is indicated for the patient with severe respiratory distress or complete obstruction. In cases in which intubation is hampered by the injury

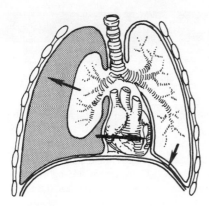

FIGURE 23-7 Closed pneumothorax. Simple pneumothorax is present in right lung with air in pleural cavity and collapse of right lung. (From Rosen P, Barkin RM, Hockberger RS et al: *Emergency medicine: concepts and clinical practice,* ed 4, St. Louis, 1998, Mosby.)

itself, tracheostomy is recommended.[1] Cricothyrotomy is usually performed in the emergency department (ED), with tracheostomy reserved for operative management.

Penetrating trauma to the larynx is readily apparent and requires immediate surgical intervention. Associated injuries to the carotid artery or jugular vein may occur. Penetrating missile injuries have been associated with extensive tissue destruction related to the blast effect.[1] Injury to the cervical spine must also be considered in any patient with injury to the neck.

Tracheal Injury

Trauma to the trachea may be blunt or penetrating; mechanisms of injury are often the same as for laryngeal injuries. Blunt injuries can be subtle or acute. Noisy breathing may be the only indication of partial obstruction, whereas absent breathing suggests complete obstruction. If the patient has an altered level of consciousness, diagnosis is more difficult. Diagnostic evaluation includes bronchoscopy, CT scan, and laryngoscopy. Treatment includes operative interventions for severe blunt or penetrating injuries. Less acute injuries may be managed with intubation or tracheostomy.

Bronchial Injury

Major bronchial injuries are unusual and often overlooked.[1] Blunt trauma to the chest that causes bronchial injury has a high mortality because of a delayed or missed diagnosis of the injury. Stab wounds or gunshot wounds of the bronchus are often identified during an operation performed for other reasons. Many patients die at the scene of the accident.[1] Most injuries occur within 1 inch of the carina. Signs and symptoms include hemoptysis, subcutaneous emphysema, mediastinal crunch (Hamman's sign), or tension pneumothorax with mediastinal shift. With bronchial disruption into both pleural spaces, bilateral tension pneumothoraces have occurred. The patient may present with dyspnea, tachycardia, and diminished or absent breath sounds. Persistent emphysema or air leak after chest tube insertion should increase the index of suspicion for this injury; bronchoscopy

confirms the diagnosis. Treatment may be limited to airway support until inflammation and edema resolve; however, surgical intervention is required for patients with a significant tear.

Pneumothorax

Pneumothorax refers to accumulation of air in the pleural space resulting in partial or complete collapse of the lung as intrapleural pressure is lost (Figure 23-7). Pneumothorax may be due to blunt or penetrating injuries. Laceration of lung tissue, often associated with rib fractures and subsequent air leak, is the most common cause of pneumothorax with blunt trauma.

A patient with a pneumothorax complains of chest pain and shortness of breath. Auscultation of the lung on the injured side shows decreased or absent breath sounds; percussion demonstrates hyperresonance. Normal breath sounds can occur as a result of resonance within the thoracic cavity. Tachycardia and tachypnea are usually present. If air accumulates in the mediastinum, a crunching sound called *Hamman's crunch* occurs. With each contraction the heart beats against air trapped between the heart and chest wall. Radiographs aid diagnosis of pneumothorax.

Pneumothorax is treated with chest tube placement in the fourth or fifth intercostal space, along the anterior axillary line.[1] The chest tube is connected to an underwater drainage system with suction attached to facilitate lung reexpansion. Box 23-4 identifies essential components for chest drainage systems and discusses general nursing implications. Figure 23-8 illustrates a typical chest drainage system. A radiograph taken after tube placement confirms tube placement and lung reexpansion. The patient is positioned upright after tube placement to prevent pressure forming from abdominal organs against the diaphragm. High-flow oxygen is continued.

Open Pneumothorax. Open pneumothorax, or sucking chest wound, occurs when an opening in the chest is more than two thirds the diameter of the trachea. Air preferentially moves into the chest through the chest wall rather than through the trachea. The injury is usually the result of penetrating trauma to the chest wall; however, blunt trauma may also cause an open chest wound. An open chest wound causes loss of intrathoracic pressure (Figure 23-9). The patient has chest pain, shortness of breath, and may be hypotensive. Breath sounds may be decreased or absent on the affected side, and a sucking sound may be heard with each breath. Bubbles often occur around the wound as air escapes through the blood. Immediate treatment consists of placing a sterile, nonporous, three-sided occlusive dressing over the injury. Taping three sides allows air to escape but prevents air from entering the wound. After placement of this dressing, the patient should be carefully monitored for development of tension pneumothorax. If a tension pneumothorax develops, the taped dressing must be removed immediately, with chest tube insertion to follow. Definitive treatment of the open chest wound is operative closure.

Tension Pneumothorax. Tension pneumothorax is a life-threatening condition that occurs when accumulation of air in one pleural space forces thoracic contents to the opposite side of the chest (Figure 23-10). Initial lung injury

Box 23-4 **CHEST DRAINAGE SYSTEMS—COMPONENTS AND MANAGEMENT**

FLUID COLLECTION CHAMBER

Fluid drains from the patient through a long tube to a collection chamber, marked for assessment of drainage.

WATER SEAL CHAMBER

Allows air to pass out via bubbles through the bottom of the chamber. Often calibrated for measuring intrathoracic pressure and may have float valve to protect patient from high negativity.

SUCTION CONTROL CHAMBER

Improves drainage and helps overcome the air leak. Keep suction control at -10 to -20 cm H_2O. Works by adding or removing water from the chamber with a regulator that adjusts to negative pressure changes, suction source or patient variations, and through a restrictive orifice mechanism that adjusts the opening to increase or decrease pressure.

NURSING RESPONSIBILITIES

Secure all connections. Monitor catheters to prevent kinking. Monitor drainage output. Assess for air leaks. Maintain unit in upright position. Monitor intrathoracic pressure.

ASSESSING FOR AIR LEAKS

Look at underwater seal. Leak may originate with the patient or the drainage system. For a patient receiving mechanical ventilation with positive end expiratory pressure, leaking causes continuous bubbling. Clamp chest tube at the dressing site with a toothless clamp. If bubbling stops, leak is from the lung. If bubbling continues, leak is distal to the clamp. Move clamp incrementally toward the drainage unit. If bubbling stops before the end of the tubing, leak is in the tube so tube must be replaced. If the unit is still bubbling when the very end of the tubing is clamped, the unit has the leak and should be changed.

INDICATIONS OF PATENCY

Water level in the water seal should fluctuate with breathing, rising with inspiration and falling with expiration, and is an indicator of chest tube patency. If the patient is on mechanical ventilation, this pattern is reversed because breaths are delivered under positive pressure. Fluctuations stop when the lung is fully reexpanded or when the tube is kinked or compressed.

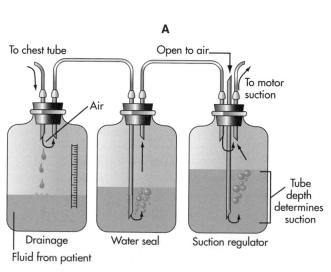

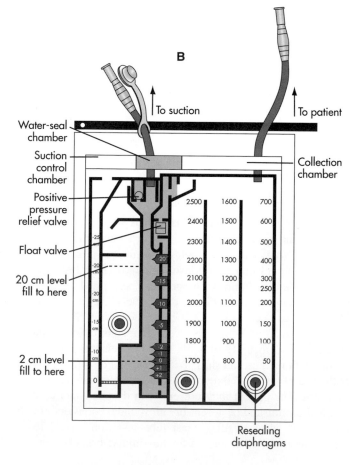

FIGURE 23-8 Chest tubes and chest tube drainage systems. **A,** Three-bottle water-seal suction. Bottle I is drainage bottle. Vertical piece of tape should be applied to outer surface of drainage bottle. Time and fluid level should be marked hourly on tape. Bottle II is water-seal bottle. Bottle III is suction control bottle. Length of glass tube below water surface determines amount of suction. **B,** Pleurevac disposable chest suction system. (From Lewis SM, Heitkemper MM, Dirkesn SR: *Medical-surgical nursing: assessment and management of clinical problems,* ed 5, St. Louis, 2000, Mosby.)

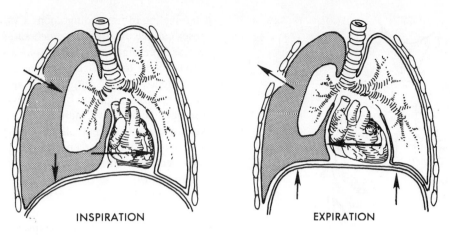

FIGURE 23-9   Open pneumothorax. Collapse of right lung and air in pleural cavity occurs with communication to outside through defect in chest wall. In sucking chest wound, lung volume is greater with expiration. (From Rosen P, Barkin RM, Hockberger RS et al: *Emergency medicine: concepts and clinical practice,* ed 4, St. Louis, 1998, Mosby.)

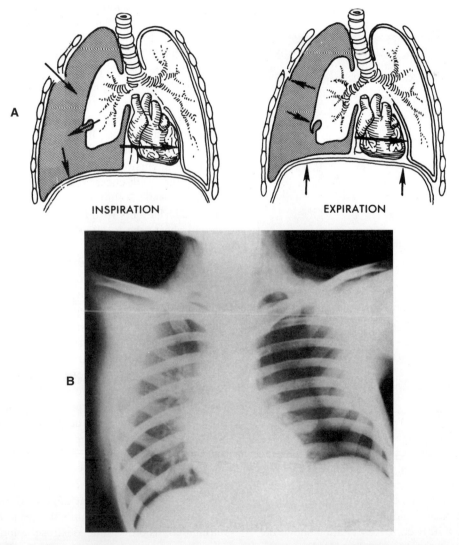

FIGURE 23-10   **A,** Tension pneumothorax. Right pneumothorax under tension, total collapse of right lung, and shift of mediastinal structures to left. **B,** Radiograph of left tension pneumothorax with shift of mediastinal structures to right. Note subcutaneous emphysema in soft tissues of neck. (From Rosen P, Barkin RM, Hockberger RS et al: *Emergency medicine: concepts and clinical practice,* ed 4, St. Louis, 1998, Mosby.)

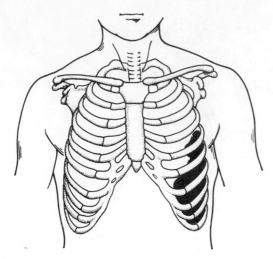

FIGURE **23-11** Hemothorax. (From Sheehy SB, Blansfield JS, Danis DM et al: *Manual of clinical trauma care: the first hour,* ed 3, St. Louis, 1999, Mosby.)

| Box 23-5 | **ADVANTAGES AND DISADVANTAGES OF AUTOTRANSFUSION**[2,12] |

ADVANTAGES

Blood is immediately available
Lower cost compared with banked blood
No risk of transfusion reaction
No risk of bloodborne pathogens
Potential psychologic comfort for the patient
Normothermic
Near-normal electrolytes and pH
Near-normal clotting factors
Greater oxygen-carrying capacity
Red blood cell half-life near normal

DISADVANTAGES

Depends on user competence with collection device
Potential for air embolism exists with reinfusion if air is not removed from collection bag
Sepsis possible if enteric contamination occurs
Coagulopathies may develop because of dilution of clotting factors when the amount of blood transfused is 25% to 50% of total blood volume
Citrate toxicity occurs with large doses of citrate
Blood trauma and hemolysis

allows air into the pleural space with inspiration; however, air cannot escape with expiration. Air continues to accumulate and intrathoracic pressure increases, forcing thoracic contents away from the injured side. Eventually the lung on the opposite side, the heart, and great vessels are compressed as mediastinal shift occurs. Auscultation shows decreased or absent breath sounds on the affected side and possibly decreased sounds on the unaffected side as the lung is compressed. If the patient is alert and able to speak, he or she may complain of chest pain, severe shortness of breath,

and a feeling of impending doom. Compression of the heart causes cardiac dysrhythmias, decreases diastolic filling, and decreases cardiac output. Vena cava compression impairs venous return to the heart, which worsens diastolic filling and decreases cardiac output. Neck vein distension occurs as venous return is impaired by compression of the heart; however, neck veins may remain flat if concurrent hypovolemia exists. The trachea eventually deviates to the unaffected side as mediastinal shift worsens.

Immediate needle decompression of the affected side is required. A 14- or 16-gauge catheter is inserted into the second intercostal space at the midclavicular line or fifth intercostal space at the anterior axillary line on the injured side. Definitive therapy is chest tube insertion.

Hemothorax

A hemothorax is free blood in the pleural space (Figure 23-11) resulting from bleeding from lung parenchyma, heart and major vessel injury, or injury to internal mammary arteries. The most common cause is an injury to the intercostal arteries that causes bleeding into the pleural space. In addition to chest pain, shortness of breath, and decreased or absent breath sounds on the affected side, the patient has dullness on chest percussion. Signs and symptoms of hypovolemic shock are often present. Treatment includes chest tube insertion, usually size 32F or 36F in an adult, high-flow oxygen by a nonrebreather mask, and large-bore intravenous lines for fluid replacement. Chest drainage should be carefully monitored to assess the need for autotransfusion and clots that occlude the tube. If blood return with chest tube insertion is 1000 to 1500 ml or blood loss is 200 to 300 ml/hr, surgical intervention is indicated.[6] Patients with a hemothorax may also require a second chest tube to allow the lung to maintain negative pressure.

Autotransfusion. Autotransfusion, collecting and reinfusing the patient's own blood, is a valuable tool during resuscitation of select hypovolemic trauma victims. Blood shed into the thoracic cavity can be easily collected and infused. Significant intrathoracic blood loss (more than 350 ml) and wounds that are less than 4 to 6 hours old are indications for potential autotransfusion.[1,3] Autotransfusion is also useful when homologous blood is not available or the patient's religious convictions forbid homologous transfusion. Box 23-5 highlights specific advantages and disadvantages of autotransfusion. Autotransfusion is not appropriate when enteric contamination has occurred (e.g., ruptured diaphragm).

Autotransfusion requires a chest drainage unit and autotransfusion device. An anticoagulant may be added before blood collection to prevent clotting during the collection phase and plugging of the blood filter and intravenous line during reinfusion. Citrate dextrose solution-A and citrate phosphate dextrose are the most common anticoagulants used. Serial assessment of laboratory values must be performed to monitor the patient response to autotransfusion and to the anticoagulants.

Pulmonary Contusion

Pulmonary contusion is the most common, potentially lethal chest injury seen in North America.[1] Almost 75% of patients with blunt chest trauma have a pulmonary contusion, with mortality about 40%. Contusion occurs when underlying lung parenchyma is damaged, causing edema and hemorrhage. Pulmonary laceration is usually not present. Concussive and compressive forces from blunt trauma are the most common cause of pulmonary contusion. Injury to lung parenchyma worsens progressively over time. Thoracic injuries associated with pulmonary contusion include rib fractures, flail chest, hemothorax, pneumothorax, and scapular fractures.[13]

Injury to the lung parenchyma causes rupture and hemorrhage into pulmonary tissue, alveoli, and small airways. As a result, airways collapse, followed by loss of ventilation, pulmonary shunting, and hypoxemia. The subsequent inflammatory response impairs gas exchange and worsens the clinical picture.[7] Diagnosis is based on the index of suspicion. Clinical evidence of dyspnea, hemoptysis, hypoxia, and possible chest wall abrasion or ecchymosis may be present. Fifty percent of patients with pulmonary contusion have no physical findings. Auscultation rarely detects abnormalities but a baseline arterial blood gas test may be helpful. The chest radiograph is usually not helpful during initial evaluation. CT may be used to quantify the contusion because it is a more sensitive indicator of tissue injury.[3]

Treatment consists of placing the patient in semi-Fowler's position to facilitate lung reexpansion, suctioning, and chest physiotherapy. Intubation and mechanical ventilation may be required if the patient has severe hypoxia or the contusion affects more than 28% of the lungs, as quantified by a CT scan. In general, intubation and mechanical ventilation are more likely with larger contusions. Intubation may also be required if the patient exhibits signs of shock, has fractured eight or more ribs, is elderly, or has underlying pulmonary disease. Fluids may be restricted when there is no evidence of hypovolemia.

Diaphragmatic Injury

Blunt or penetrating trauma may result in diaphragmatic injuries. Blunt injuries result in large radial tears that cause herniation of abdominal contents into the thorax. Herniation may develop slowly with penetrating injuries; sometimes years pass before this occurs.[1] Most injuries occur on the left side of the diaphragm because the right side is protected by the liver. The presence of hemothorax, pneumothorax, or intraabdominal hemorrhage suggests a possible ruptured diaphragm. A nasogastric tube is inserted before obtaining a chest x-ray; the tube is visible in the chest with diaphragmatic rupture. Other signs and symptoms include dyspnea, abdominal or epigastric pain that radiates to the left shoulder (Kehr's sign), bowel sounds in the lower chest, and decreased breath sounds on the affected side. Peritoneal lavage fluid may leak into the chest drainage system. Treatment is surgical repair.

Cardiac and Great Vessel Injuries

Cardiac Contusions

A cardiac contusion is a bruise of the heart, usually resulting from blunt trauma to the anterior chest. Common mechanisms of injury include steering wheel impact during a motor vehicle crash, falls, assaults, and direct blows from an object or large animal (e.g., kick from a horse). The myocardium may have a mild contusion or concussion injury or may have a severe injury that mimics acute myocardial infarction. An echocardiogram differentiates the extent of injury. A mild injury can cause cardiac dysrhythmia yet the echocardiogram is normal. Extensive myocardial contusion is characterized by dysrhythmia and some evidence of myocardial dysfunction on the echocardiogram.

Signs and symptoms of myocardial contusion and concussion are nonspecific and include chest pain, skin abrasions, or ecchymosis to the anterior chest. These signs occur with fractures or other chest wall injuries, so diagnosis is often difficult.[1] Not all patients have evidence of chest wall injury.[1,3] Chest pain associated with myocardial contusion mimics pain that occurs in angina. Unlike anginal pain, however, pain with myocardial contusion does not respond to coronary vasodilators.[3] Contusion is suggested by the patient's history of significant blunt trauma to the chest. Dysrhythmia seen with myocardial contusion includes sinus tachycardia, atrial fibrillation, atrial flutter, and premature ventricular contractions (PVCs). The most common dysrhythmia is PVCs, which increase with age of the victim.

Serial ECGs and continuous cardiac monitoring are essential. A two-dimensional echocardiography (2-D ECHO) is also recommended. Cardiac isoenzyme analysis has been abandoned because researchers have demonstrated lack of specificity and sensitivity for dysrhythmia development or injury with use of these enzyme values. Variable ECG findings occur in myocardial contusion. Specific findings include ST-segment and T-wave changes, prolonged QT interval, and right bundle branch block. Echocardiograms are useful for differentiating cardiac dysfunction from other pathologies such as myocardial contusion, pericardial tamponade, valve rupture, and pericardial effusion.[4]

Sequelae after injury include dysrhythmia, valve lesion, and rupture; thromboembolic events; and congestive heart failure. Treatment consists of cardiac monitoring of patients for at least 24 hours. Patients with abnormal ECGs or dysrhythmia should have a 2-D ECHO. Patients with an abnormal echocardiogram should be treated symptomatically. Patients with normal serial ECGs or those who remain asymptomatic for 24 hours require no further treatment.

Penetrating Cardiac Injuries

Person-against-person violence, usually seen in urban areas, is the leading cause of penetrating trauma in the United States. Most victims of penetrating cardiac injuries arrive in the ED in cardiac arrest or with significant hypotension secondary to cardiac tamponade or hemorrhage.[11] The right ventricle is the most frequently injured chamber because of

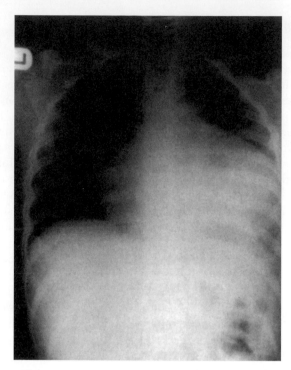

FIGURE **23-12**   Pericardial effusion. (From Barkin RM: *Pediatric emergency medicine: concepts and clinical practice,* ed 2, St. Louis, 1997, Mosby.)

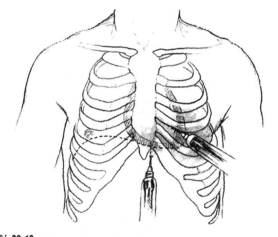

FIGURE **23-13**   Pericardiocentesis for acute cardiac tamponade can be performed via a left subxiphoid or parasternal approach. The subxiphoid route is generally preferred for acute trauma. (From Davis JH et al: *Essentials of clinical surgery,* St. Louis, 1991, Mosby.)

its anterior position. Other chambers injured are the left ventricle and right atrium. Gunshot wounds of the heart are significantly more lethal than stab wounds.[11] Penetrating injuries are associated with a high mortality (83%); only 20% to 25% of the victims reach the hospital alive.[5] Of those who arrive alive, only 20% are stable.[10] Patients who arrive with stable cardiac injuries have the best chance for survival with early diagnosis and treatment. Patients with injuries to the

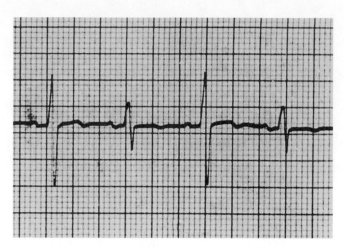

FIGURE **23-14**   Lewis-lead electrocardiogram shows total electrical alternation of amplitude and configuration of P and QRS complexes. (From Sotolongo RP, Horton JD: *Am Heart J* 101:853, 1981.)

chest between the midclavicular lines, clavicles, and costal margins should be aggressively evaluated for cardiac involvement.[10]

Immediate thoracotomy in the ED is indicated for patients in cardiac arrest.[11] Stabilization of the ABCs followed by echocardiography is recommended if the patient has cardiac activity. If the echocardiogram is negative, no further evaluation is indicated. Positive findings indicating tamponade suggest the need for a subxiphoid window. With positive subxiphoid exploration, cardiac surgery is indicated to repair the defect.[3,10,11]

Cardiac Tamponade

Cardiac tamponade occurs when rapid accumulation of blood in the pericardial sac decreases ventricular filling. As the pericardial sac fills, blood presses on the ventricles and impairs ventricular filling and the heart's pumping ability so cardiac output decreases. Figure 23-12 shows massive pericardial effusion with a "water bottle" appearance on radiograph. Classic signs of cardiac tamponade are a complex of symptoms called Beck's Triad: hypotension, muffled heart tones, and distended neck veins.[5]

Hypotension is secondary to myocardial compression and decreased cardiac output as more blood accumulates in the pericardium. Muffled heart sounds are caused by the insulating ability of blood in the pericardium, whereas neck vein distension occurs because the heart cannot expand normally to accommodate blood return to the heart. Classic symptoms may not always be evident because of associated injuries such as hypovolemia. As tamponade worsens, the patient exhibits air hunger, agitation, and deterioration in the level of consciousness. Knowing mechanisms of injury and location of the wounds is crucial for accurate assessment. Gunshot wounds and stab wounds to the chest are the most suggestive for this condition. Hemodynamically unstable patients with injuries to the chest should be immediately

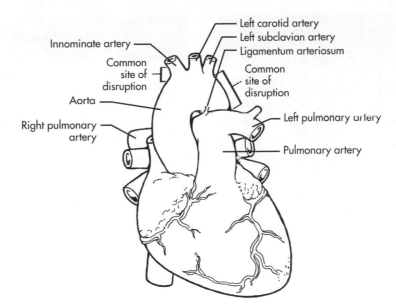

FIGURE 23-15   Common sites of aortic disruption.

evaluated for tamponade. In a stable patient an echocardio-gram and subxiphoid pericardial window are diagnostic tools of choice. Pericardiocentesis (Figure 23-13) may be life-saving for some patients with pericardial tamponade. However, it is not the best diagnostic tool for most patients because of significant false-positive rate and risks of sec-ondary injuries such as coronary vessel laceration and dys-rhythmia.[10] Pericardiocentesis may be a temporizing proce-dure performed to improve cardiac function while waiting for surgery. The ECG, chest radiograph, and central venous pressure readings are not reliable diagnostic tools because of inconsistent changes in assessment parameters for each.[9,10] Some patients exhibit an unusual rhythm known as electri-cal alternans (Figure 23-14). Early identification and prompt intervention are essential for patient survival.

Aortic Rupture

The majority of victims with aortic rupture caused by blunt trauma die at the scene of the crash; few survive transport to the hospital. Rapid diagnosis and surgical intervention are essential because half will die in the first 48 hours if left un-treated.[12] Traumatic aortic rupture is commonly associated with horizontal or vertical acceleration or deceleration in-juries such as high-speed motor vehicle crashes and falls from a great height. The most common site of injury in-volves the area of the aorta just distal to the left subclavian artery adjacent to the ligamentum arteriosum. The innomi-nate artery at the aortic arch and the aortic valve are also common sites of injury.[8,11] Figure 23-15 identifies common sites for aortic disruption.

The patient may complain of chest pain or pain between the scapulae, often described as unrelenting and severe. Other symptoms include dyspnea and hemoptysis. A loud systolic murmur may be heard over the precordium if aortic valve integrity has been lost. Signs of hemorrhagic shock may be present. A discrepancy between blood pressure val-ues in the right and left arms also occurs, depending on the level of the injury. Acute coarctation syndrome can occur as sympathetic fibers in the aorta respond to the stretch stimu-lus from a torn intima flap or hematoma. Blood pressure and pulse in the upper extremities are elevated, whereas pulses and blood pressure in the lower extremities are decreased or absent.[8]

The most common diagnostic test for aortic disruption is a chest radiograph; the most common finding is mediastinal widening (Figure 23-16). A supine chest radiograph may not adequately demonstrate mediastinal widening. Other chest radiograph findings include the presence of an "apical cap," a displaced esophagus (evidenced by visualization of the na-sogastric tube), trachea deviated to the right, obliteration of the aortic knob, fracture of the first or second ribs, depres-sion of the left mainstem bronchus, and massive left pleural effusion.[3,8,11] Radiographic findings are not specific or sensi-tive enough to pinpoint the injury; up to 28% of victims with aortic rupture have a normal chest radiograph.[11] The diag-nostic standard for identification of aortic injury is the aor-togram; however, this procedure is not without associated risks. Injection of radiopaque dye may worsen the tear in the aorta and cause complete disruption. Transesophageal echocardiography (TEE), used in some centers across the country, visualizes the aorta from the posterior aspect via the esophagus.

Definitive treatment for aortic disruption is immediate sur-gical repair. Management in the ED includes insertion of large-bore intravenous catheters and collection of blood for blood type and cross-match. Some patients require medical manage-ment with beta-blockers and antihypertensive agents when as-sociated injuries preclude the safe induction of anesthesia.[8]

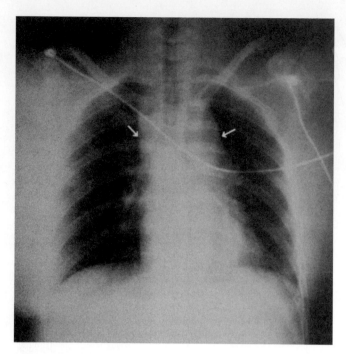

FIGURE 23-16   Radiograph of chest. Arrows demonstrate widened mediastinum.

Box 23-6   CHANGES IN MANAGEMENT OF THORACIC TRAUMA

Cardiac troponin 1 (cTn1) is a specific marker for myocardial necrosis. It is widely accepted for detecting myocardial necrosis after infarction but has not been sufficiently studied in the trauma patient for widespread use in evaluation of cardiac injury.[16]

Use of petroleum gauze for chest tube dressings has been abandoned in favor of bacteriostatic ointment, dry sterile dressing, and occlusive tape or dry sterile dressing and occlusive tape. Petroleum gauze macerates tissue and predisposes the patient to skin infection.[19]

Transesophageal echocardiography (TEE) may become the "gold standard" for diagnosis of ruptured aorta. It is less invasive, may be performed at the bedside, and is less costly than an aortogram. It is not widely accepted as a diagnostic tool, however, because of machine and user variability in interpretation of the test. Transthoracic echocardiography (TTE) may be used in place of subxiphoid exploration for identifying cardiac injuries in stable patients with penetrating traumas. The same issues apply to TTE as to TEE in terms of user expertise and interpretation.

Video-assisted thoracoscopy can reduce nontherapeutic laparotomies, patient morbidity, and costs. The diaphragm may be examined with a video camera through a small opening in the thoracic cavity, similar to laparoscopy.

Esophageal Injury

Injury to the esophagus usually results from penetrating trauma, but may be related to a severe blow to the lower abdomen. Esophageal injuries are rare and often lethal. Common causes of penetrating injury are iatrogenic events, such as instrumentation during certain procedures. Caustic ingestion, such as alkali or acid; crush injuries; and blast injuries also cause esophageal injury. Regardless of the mechanism, the final result is mediastinitis caused by contamination from saliva and gastric contents. The patient may experience pain or shock out of proportion to the apparent chest injury. Pneumothorax or hemothorax without rib fracture may be present. Chest tube drainage may have particulate matter. Diagnosis is confirmed by contrast studies or esophagoscopy. Urgent surgical repair is indicated.

SUMMARY

Thoracic injuries are challenging, chaotic to manage, and potentially life-threatening. Changes in technology such as TEE have made management easier. With more research, management of chest injuries may change significantly. Box 23-6 highlights some of these current and future changes.

The patient with a thoracic injury requires rapid assessment and intervention. The emergency nurse must anticipate potentially lethal thoracic injuries and rapidly intervene. Box 23-7 highlights nursing diagnoses for these patients.

Box 23-7   NURSING DIAGNOSIS FOR THORACIC TRAUMA

Airway clearance, Ineffective
Breathing pattern, Ineffective
Cardiac output, Decreased
Gas exchange, Impaired

References

1. American College of Surgeons: *Advanced trauma life support: course for physicians,* ed 5, Chicago, 1997, The College.
2. Atrium Medical Corporation: *Managing chest drainage and postoperative autotransfusion (study guide),* Hudson, NH, 1995, The Corporation.
3. Cohn SM et al: Exclusion of aortic tear in the unstable trauma patient: the utility of transesophageal echocardiography, *J Trauma Inj Infect Crit Care* 39:1087, 1995.
4. Doherty KA: Cardiovascular emergencies. In Jordan KS, editor: *Emergency nursing core curriculum,* ed 5, Philadelphia, 2000, WB Saunders.
5. Emergency Nurses Association: *Trauma nursing core course provider manual,* ed 5, Des Plaines, Ill, 2000, The Association.
6. Feliciano DV, Moore EE, Mattox KL: *Trauma,* ed 4, New York, 2001, McGraw-Hill.
7. James C: Respiratory emergencies. In Jordan KS, editor: *Emergency nursing core curriculum,* ed 5, Philadelphia, 2000, WB Saunders.

8. Kosmos CA: Multiple trauma. In Kitt S et al, editors: *Emergency nursing: a physiologic and clinical perspective,* Philadelphia, 1995, WB Saunders.

9. Meyer DM, Jessen ME, Grayburn PA: Use of echocardiography to detect occult cardiac injury after penetrating thoracic trauma: a prospective study, *J Trauma Inj Infect Crit Care* 39:902, 1995.

10. Nagy KK et al: Role of echocardiography in the diagnosis of occult penetrating cardiac injury, *J Trauma Inj Infect Crit Care* 38:859, 1995.

11. Rosenthal MA, Ellis JI: Cardiac and mediastinal trauma, *Emerg Med Clin North Am* 13(4):887, 1995.

12. Saletta S et al: Transesophageal echocardiography for the initial evaluation of the widened mediastinum in trauma patients, *J Trauma Inj Infect Crit Care* 39(1):137, 1995.

13. Tribble RW, Nolan SP: Pneumothorax. In Cameron JL, editor: *Current surgical therapy,* ed 5, St. Louis, 1995, Mosby.

14. Westaby S, Odell JA, editors: *Cardiothoracic trauma,* London, 1999, Arnold Publishing.

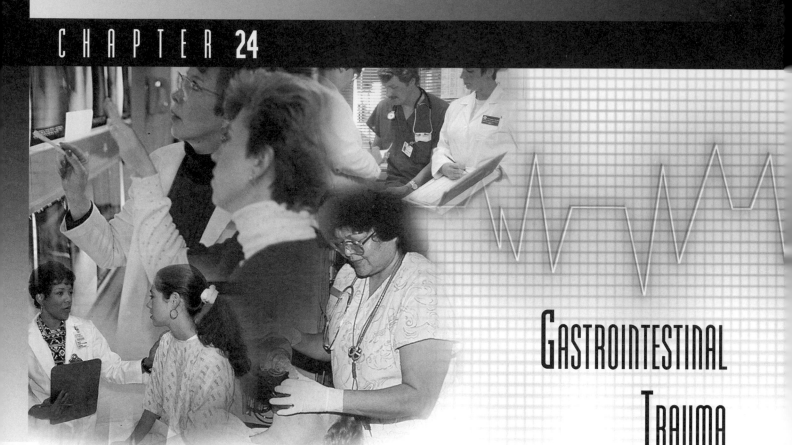

CHAPTER 24

Gastrointestinal Trauma

M. Lynn Herman

Abdominal trauma accounts for approximately 25% of all traumatic injuries and continues to be associated with high morbidity and mortality.[6a,10] It may occur as an isolated injury or in combination with other injuries, providing a wide range of symptoms from insignificant contusions, hypovolemic shock, and death. The need for recognition of life-threatening abdominal injuries and rapid surgical intervention cannot be overstated. Abdominal trauma is truly a surgical disease. The roles of the emergency nurse are assessment and intervention that focus on airway, breathing, and circulation (ABC) and rapid movement of the patient to the surgical area.

The incidence of abdominal trauma is directly associated with the geographic location of the patient. Abdominal trauma is further delineated by mechanism of injury (i.e., penetrating or blunt). The incidence of penetrating abdominal trauma is higher in urban centers but has increased in suburban areas as violence escalates across the country. Penetrating injuries are usually gunshot wounds (GSW) or stab wounds (SW). Foreign bodies such as wood, steel, or shrapnel from blasts or explosions are also considered penetrating injuries. Abdominal trauma secondary to blunt force is associated with motor vehicle crashes (MVC), assaults, and falls. Assaults and falls from heights are also more prevalent in urban areas compared with suburban areas. MVCs, the most common type of blunt trauma, has a higher incidence in the suburbs. Injury from blunt trauma occurs from diffuse energy over the abdomen that damages abdominal organs.

Preventing mortality and morbidity associated with abdominal trauma initially begins with understanding the mechanism of injury. Penetrating injuries are more straightforward in their presentation and their work-up is somewhat easier.[2] Blunt injuries carry a greater mortality than penetrating injuries because they are more difficult to diagnose— and are commonly associated with severe trauma to multiple intraperitoneal organs and extraabdominal systems.[6] Mortality varies with the organs injured, severity, associated extraabdominal injuries, promptness of definitive care, and the patient's preexisting health status. Missed or delayed diagnosis of abdominal injuries can be avoided if the trauma team is thorough and remains vigilant.

Life-threatening abdominal injuries can occur without outward sign of injury, so the emergency nurse must have a high index of suspicion for these injuries. Abdominal trauma is suggested when an energy source is applied to a person's trunk anywhere from the fourth rib to the hips. Inspiration lifts the diaphragm into the thoracic cavity, placing abdominal contents at risk for injury when the chest is injured below the fourth rib. It is also important to remember that infants and children, patients under the influence of mind-altering drugs or alcohol, those with an altered level of consciousness, or those with concurrent spinal injuries do not always exhibit abdominal pain, tenderness, or rigidity.

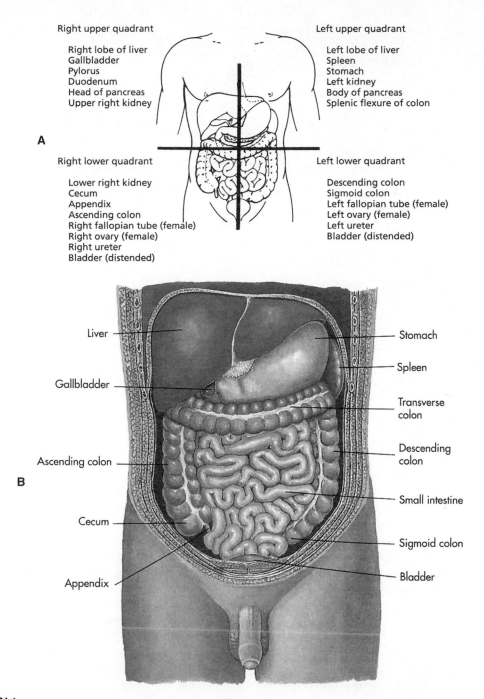

Right upper quadrant

Right lobe of liver
Gallbladder
Pylorus
Duodenum
Head of pancreas
Upper right kidney

Left upper quadrant

Left lobe of liver
Spleen
Stomach
Left kidney
Body of pancreas
Splenic flexure of colon

A

Right lower quadrant

Lower right kidney
Cecum
Appendix
Ascending colon
Right fallopian tube (female)
Right ovary (female)
Right ureter
Bladder (distended)

Left lower quadrant

Descending colon
Sigmoid colon
Left fallopian tube (female)
Left ovary (female)
Left ureter
Bladder (distended)

Liver — Stomach

Gallbladder — Spleen

— Transverse colon

— Descending colon

Ascending colon —

B

— Small intestine

Cecum — — Sigmoid colon

Appendix — — Bladder

FIGURE **24-1**   Gastrointestinal structures. (**A,** From Stillwell S: *Mosby's critical care nursing reference,* ed 2, St. Louis, 1996, Mosby. **B,** From Seidel HM et al: *Mosby's guide to physical examination,* ed 3, St. Louis, 1995, Mosby.)

The focus of this chapter is injury to the gastrointestinal (GI) system with brief discussion of abdominal vasculature. In the traditional sense abdominal trauma is viewed as an injury to the front of the patient (i.e., a blow to the abdomen). However, penetrating injury to the flank can also injure abdominal organs. In blunt trauma, injury to the flank usually damages the kidneys rather than abdominal organs. Chapter 25 discusses renal trauma in more detail. Trauma in the pregnant patient is discussed in Chapter 31, whereas pediatric trauma is discussed in Chapter 29.

ANATOMY AND PHYSIOLOGY

Organs in the abdominal cavity include the large and small intestines, liver, spleen, stomach, gallbladder, pancreas, and diaphragm. The spleen and liver are solid organs, whereas the stomach and intestines are hollow organs. Solid organs fracture when injured; hollow organs collapse or rupture. Vascular structures in the abdominal cavity include the aorta, vena cava, hepatic vein, iliac artery, and iliac vein. Most of these structures are located in the peritoneal space. Figures 24-1, *A* and *B,*

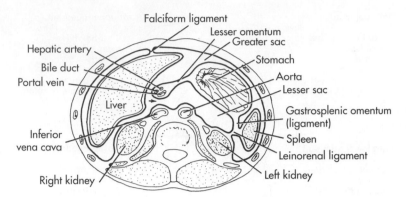

FIGURE 24-2   Retroperitoneal structures. (From Snell R, Smith M: *Clinical anatomy for emergency medicine,* St. Louis, 1993, Mosby.)

illustrates location of abdominal contents and gastrointestinal structures. Figure 24-2 delineates structures located in the retroperitoneal space.

Peritoneum

The peritoneum is the largest serous membrane in the body. The parietal peritoneum lines the abdominal wall, whereas the visceral peritoneum covers the abdominal organs. The peritoneal cavity is a potential space located between the parietal and visceral peritoneum. Closed in men, the peritoneal cavity in women communicates outside the body through the fallopian tubes, uterus, and vagina. The retroperitoneal space is that area posterior to the peritoneum containing the kidneys, parts of the colon, duodenum, pancreas, and female reproductive organs. The mesentery is a double layer of peritoneum that encloses an organ and connects it to the abdominal wall. Mesentery is found in most mobile parts of the intestine. Specific folds of the mesentery, the greater and lesser omentum, extend from the stomach to adjacent organs.

Organs

The stomach is a hollow organ located in the left upper quadrant that contains hydrochloric acid and other digestive agents. Gastric fluid has a pH of 1. The position of the stomach varies, moving with inspiration and expiration in and out of the thoracic cavity. Stomach size changes with consumption of food or liquids. The cardiac sphincter controls entry into the stomach with exit controlled by the pyloric sphincter. The stomach usually empties within 2 to 6 hours of food ingestion.

The small intestine connects to the pyloric sphincter and fills most of the abdominal cavity. Segments include the duodenum, jejunum, and ileum. The majority of digestion and absorption occurs here. The pH of the small intestines is between 6.5 and 7.5.

The large intestine interfaces with the ileum proximally and exits distally at the rectum. Divisions consist of the ascending colon, transverse colon, descending colon, and the sigmoid colon (Figure 24-3). Most absorption occurs in the proximal colon.

The liver, the largest gland in the body, accounts for almost 3% total body weight. It is specifically responsible for more than 500 separate metabolic functions, including secretion of bile, detoxification of poisons, and storage of glycogen. Box 24-1 lists just a few of the liver's functions.[3] Death occurs in less than 12 hours after complete destruction of the liver; however, only 10% to 20% of the liver is necessary to sustain life. The liver is extremely vascular. Blood flows through the portal vein at approximately 1000 ml/min and from the iliac artery at approximately 400 ml/min.

The gallbladder is a pear-shaped, hollow sac directly beneath the right lobe of the liver. Its principal function is storage and concentration of bile.

The pancreas, located behind the stomach, extends across the posterior abdomen from the duodenum to the spleen. The pancreas has both endocrine and exocrine functions. Exocrine cells produce lipase, amylase, trypsin, and other digestive enzymes. Endocrine cells produce insulin, glucagon, and somatostatin.

The spleen, a large vascular organ in the left upper quadrant behind the eighth to tenth ribs, is the largest single mass of lymphatic tissue in the body and is essential for defense against bacterial invasion. The spleen is extremely vascular with a blood flow of 200 ml/min, approximately 5% of the cardiac output.

Vascular Structures

Arterial blood supply for the abdominal cavity is the aorta (Figure 24-4). The abdominal aorta lies left of midline in the abdominal cavity and bifurcates into the iliac arteries just above the pelvic brim. Iliac arteries supply arterial blood to the lower extremities. Three unpaired arteries originating from the abdominal aorta supply abdominal organs: the celiac trunk, superior mesentery artery, and inferior mesentery artery. The celiac trunk branches into the hepatic, left gastric, and splenic arteries.

With the exception of the heart and lungs, venous blood returns from the body to the heart through the superior vena

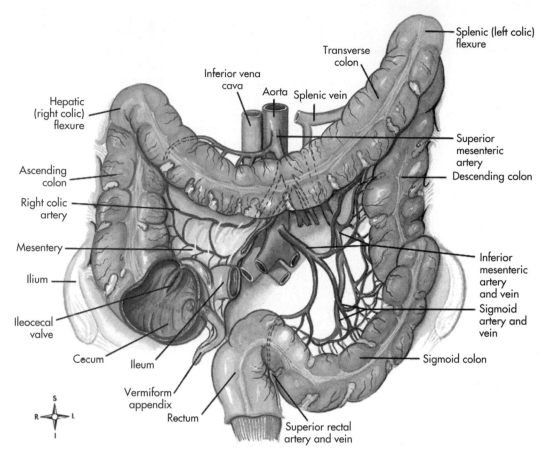

FIGURE **24-3** Anatomic locations of the large intestine. (From Thibodeau GA, Patton KT: *Anatomy and physiology,* ed 4, St. Louis, 1999, Mosby.)

Box 24-1 LIVER FUNCTIONS

Forms and excretes bile; metabolizes old red blood cells
Metabolizes carbohydrates, proteins, and fats
Helps maintain normal blood glucose and energy level
Stores glycogen to create energy reserve
Stores vitamins A, B12, D, E, K, copper, and iron
Detoxifies drugs and toxins
Acts as flood chamber for blood from the right heart
Inactivates and excretes aldosterone, glucocorticoids, estrogen, progesterone, and testosterone

cava or inferior vena cava. The inferior vena cava, formed by the union of the two common iliac veins, is the major vein in the abdomen. The superior vena cava is formed when the two brachiocephalic veins unite in the superior mediastinum.

PATIENT ASSESSMENT

Patient assessment remains the most important means of detecting abdominal trauma. The patient may come to the emergency department (ED) without specific signs of injury. Vascular organs such as the liver or spleen can lose blood rapidly or leak slowly over time. The nurse should assess the

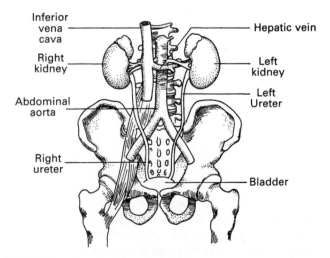

FIGURE **24-4** Vascular structures in the abdomen. (From Sheehy SB et al: *Manual of clinical trauma care: the first hour,* ed 3, St. Louis, 1999, Mosby.)

patient carefully and continually reassess hemodynamic status, level of consciousness, and level of pain. Initial assessment and stabilization begins with maintaining the ABCs. Critical interventions include oxygenation and intravenous (IV) access.

History

The patient with abdominal trauma may not have obvious injuries. The injury may also have happened days or weeks before onset of symptoms. Abdominal trauma should be suspected when the patient has a history of MVC or penetrating wounds to the torso or flank. It should also be considered in the patient with multisystem trauma or with a history of injury and unexplained hypotension or tachycardia. Alert patients may complain of abdominal or shoulder pain. Intraabdominal blood irritates the inferior surface of the diaphragm and phrenic nerve, causing referred pain to the shoulder. This finding, called *Kehr's sign,* should alert the emergency nurse to the possibility of peritoneal bleeding.

Mechanisms of Injury

To understand and help predict abdominal trauma, time and mode of injury are critical pieces of information. Injuries secondary to MVC are influenced by patient location in the vehicle; speed of the vehicle; use of a seat belt, shoulder harness, or air bag; and ejection from the vehicle. Use of seat belts has decreased mortality from injuries but has also led to identification of injuries caused by the seat belt. "Seat belt syndrome" refers to injuries in the plane of the body where the belt is located and includes injuries of the colon, small bowel, stomach, liver, spleen, vascular structures, and the spinal cord, usually the lumbar area.[1]

Motorcycle crashes can be placed in specific categories: frontal, lateral, angular, ejection, or "laying the bike down."[1] Details of the accident from bystanders or prehospital care providers facilitate better patient management.

Injuries secondary to falls vary with height of the fall, landing surface, and part of body that strikes the ground. Injuries are usually less severe if a person lands on a shock-absorbing surface such as mud. Surfaces such as concrete and steel do not absorb energy at impact so injuries are more severe. If the injury is due to assault with a blunt object, knowing what the object is and its size and weight is important.

With penetrating injuries the weapon must be identified. Knowing the type and caliber of guns, how close the assailant was when firing, and how many shots were fired is helpful. Length, width, and composition of the object that penetrated the abdomen can determine patient assessment and management. Injuries made with wood or other biologic material are more likely to cause infection and complications. Angle of entry suggests the path of the weapon, whereas length and width of the weapon can help estimate extent of injuries.[1]

Inspection

Bruising, abrasions, and lacerations are assessed. Bruising that mirrors location of the seat belt may be evident on admission to the ED, but usually does not occur for several hours after injury. Purplish discoloration of the flanks (Grey Turner's sign) or umbilicus (Cullen's sign) is associated with bleeding into the abdominal wall. Distension may be noted; however, it is not a reliable sign (2 L of fluid increases abdominal girth by only 0.75 inches). The nurse must note presence of GSWs or SWs. Inspection of the back for other wounds is essential with these injuries.

Old surgical scars should be noted because this may help narrow the search for organs that may be injured. For example, the patient with previous splenectomy has one less organ that may have been damaged. Previous surgical procedures can also cause adhesions that affect reliability of diagnostic peritoneal lavage (DPL).

Percussion/Auscultation

Percussion of the abdomen can provide helpful information; however, it is usually impossible to hear percussion sounds in the middle of trauma resuscitation. Auscultation can also provide helpful information about the presence or absence of bowel sounds. Absence of bowel sounds does not confirm intraabdominal injury; the absence may be due to shock or the presence of an ileus. A change in bowel sounds (i.e., diminishing or disappearing) is more diagnostic of abdominal trauma. Significantly decreased or absent bowel sounds have been reported in more than 50% of documented injuries.[8] On the other hand, absent bowel sounds occur in a significant number (20%) of patients with no injuries at laparotomy.[8] Bowel sounds in the chest, especially on the left side, are usually caused by diaphragmatic rupture.

Palpation

The abdomen is palpated carefully for pain, rigidity, tenderness, and guarding, examining all four quadrants. Abdominal masses suggest hematoma of the liver, spleen, or omentum. A sensation of popping bubbles when pressing down suggests injury of the duodenum or distal colon.

Initial Stabilization

Initial stabilization of the patient with abdominal trauma follows the same sequence as any patient with major trauma. After assessment of the patient's ABCs, the nurse inserts bilateral, large-bore intravenous (IV) catheters. Warm crystalloids such as lactated Ringer's solution or normal saline are infused at a rate adequate to maintain blood pressure. Baseline trauma lab tests including complete blood count, type and cross-match, and urinalysis are obtained. Coagulation studies, serum amylase, liver function tests, and blood chemistries may also be ordered for some patients. Serum pregnancy test should be performed on any woman of childbearing years. The MAST garment is no longer used to treat hypovolemic shock in the trauma patient; however, it may still be used to stabilize a fractured pelvis or femur. A nasogastric tube and urinary catheter should be inserted if the patient does not require immediate transport to surgery.

Diagnostic Evaluation

Diagnostic evaluation of a patient with abdominal trauma is based on the patient's hemodynamic stability. If the patient

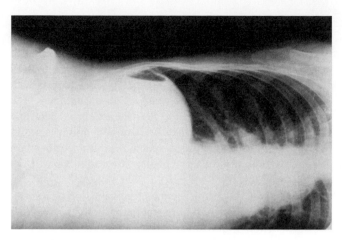

FIGURE **24-5**   Radiograph showing free intraperitoneal air. (Modified from Rosen P, Barkin RM, Hockberger RS et al: *Emergency medicine: concepts and clinical practice,* ed 4, St. Louis, 1998, Mosby.)

Table 24-1	POSITIVE DPL RESULTS
PARAMETER	**POSITIVE RESULTS**
Hematocrit	$2 ml/dl
Red blood cell count	$100,000 cells/mm^3
White blood cell count	$500 cells/mm^3
Amylase	$200 milliunits/ml
Bile	Present
Bacteria	Significant number present
Fecal material	Present
Food particles	Present

Modified from Ma OJ, Mateer JR, DeBehnke: Use of ultrasonography for the evaluation of pregnant trauma patients, *J Trauma* 40(4):665, 1996.
DPL, Diagnostic peritoneal lavage.

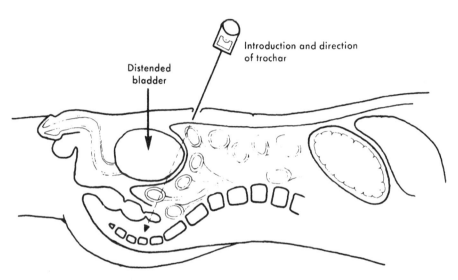

FIGURE **24-6**   Distended bladder may be perforated by trochar for peritoneal lavage. (From Sheehy SB, Lenehan GP: *Manual of emergency care,* ed 5, St. Louis, 1999, Mosby.)

is or becomes hemodynamically unstable secondary to intraperitoneal injury, transfusion with fluids or blood is begun and the patient is prepared for surgery. If the patient's condition permits, major diagnostic tools including diagnostic peritoneal lavage, high-speed computed tomography (CT) scanners, ultrasound, and laparoscopy may be used.

Initial radiographic evaluation of the patient with abdominal trauma includes an anteroposterior and lateral chest radiograph. Flat plate x-ray of the abdomen and pelvis may also be done; however, these tests are more effective in identifying bony abnormalities than life-threatening organ injuries. In some cases, free air (Figure 24-5), ileus, and ruptured diaphragm may be detected with these radiographs.

DPL, first developed in 1964, is used to determine the presence of intraabdominal blood and/or bile in the hemodynamically unstable patient. There are two widely used methods to introduce the peritoneal catheter: the cutdown method and the percutaneous method. In the cutdown method, an in-

cision is made through the entire abdominal wall below the umbilicus, and a catheter is introduced in a more controlled method. This technique is preferred if the patient has pelvic fractures or presents with advanced pregnancy. With the percutaneous method a catheter is introduced over a guidewire (Figure 24-6). Drawbacks to the percutaneous method include increased risk of injury to underlying organs and less accuracy. Insertion of a urinary catheter to empty the bladder and a gastric tube to decompress the stomach is essential to prevent injury to the organs during DPL. Immediate return of fluid or blood when the catheter is inserted is considered positive and the patient is prepared for surgery. If there is not immediate return of fluid, then 1 L normal saline or lactated Ringer's solution is instilled into the abdomen and allowed to drain back into the bag. Fifteen milliliters of blood are needed to cloud returning fluid. DPL is considered negative if newsprint can be read through the fluid; however, many institutions analyze specific components of the fluid. Table 24-1 gives parameters for a positive DPL test. It is important to note that in penetrating wounds DPL may be used on a limited basis to determine the presence of intraabdominal injury secondary to penetration through the peritoneum. A higher rate of false positives occurs in SWs. Most patients with GSWs usually require surgery, which obviates the need for DPL. Box 24-2 highlights the indications and contraindications for DPL.

CT is used to evaluate peritoneal and retroperitoneal injury in the stable patient. The high speed of newer helical or spiral CT scanners makes these studies safer for even the unstable patient, replacing DPL when available. The CT shows location of hemorrhage and skeletal injuries. Solid organ injuries are identified earlier than hollow organ injuries. Oral and IV contrast is used to evaluate abdominal structures. Noncontrast CT studies must be performed before contrast is given. Disadvantages of the CT scan include inability to differentiate fluid and blood in the peritoneal cavity; poor identification of injuries of the pancreas, diaphragm, small bowel, and mesentery; allergic reaction to contrast medium; and cost.

The primary goal of ultrasound in evaluating abdominal trauma is to determine the presence of free fluid in the abdominal cavity, thereby indicating the need for surgery.[4] Ultrasound is not widely used across the country but is gaining acceptance in larger centers and has been useful in evaluating the pregnant trauma patient. A minimum of 70 ml of blood is required for detection with ultrasound. Sensitivity in detecting as little as 100 ml of intraperitoneal fluid ranges from 60% to 95% in most recent studies.[7] Ultrasound advantages include portability (done at the bedside), speed (can be accomplished in less than 5 minutes), method (noninvasive), and cost. Ultrasound does not show retroperi-

toneal or diaphragmatic injuries and has limited use in the obese or agitated patient.

Laparoscopy is also making a comeback as a diagnostic tool for detecting abdominal trauma. Laparoscopy allows direct visualization of the abdominal cavity; however, as with all diagnostic tools, it too has its disadvantages. The retroperitoneum is difficult to view, the extent of liver and spleen injuries can not be clearly identified, and it is an invasive procedure. However, as techniques in this procedure improve, this tool may significantly affect diagnosis of abdominal injuries.

The range of diagnostic options for evaluation of abdominal trauma has increased with routine use of CT scans and the introduction of ultrasound. However, the basic principles of patient management have not noticeably changed. Immediate surgical intervention is indicated if the patient becomes hemodynamically unstable, has an enlarging abdominal mass without concomitant pelvic or vertebral fractures, or experiences a progressive drop in hemoglobin.

SPECIFIC INJURIES

Penetrating injuries can affect all abdominal structures. Assessment and treatment are usually straightforward. If the abdominal cavity is penetrated or the patient is in shock, surgery is indicated. With blunt trauma, assessment and treatment are more complex if accompanied by multisystem injuries. Abdominal organs injured most often by blunt trauma are the spleen and liver. The colon, vascular structures, stomach, pancreas, and diaphragm may also be injured, but the incidence is lower. The gallbladder is rarely injured by blunt trauma. Management of abdominal trauma in the ED focuses on stabilization of the patient's hemodynamic status, identification of potentially life-threatening injuries, and rapid transportation to the surgical suite when indicated. Specific injuries of the abdomen are described in the following section.

Spleen

The spleen is the organ injured most often by blunt trauma. Its small size makes it a difficult target, so it is injured less often with penetrating trauma. Because the spleen is encapsulated, injury may damage only the capsule or can actually fracture the spleen. Table 24-2 summarizes the types of splenic injuries that occur. Splenic injury is suggested when the patient has sustained blunt trauma to the left upper quadrant. When assessing for bruising or pain in the left upper quadrant, the presence of Kehr's sign suggests diaphragmatic irritation by peritoneal blood. Shock and hypotension are present in as few as 30% of patients with splenic trauma.

Not all patients with splenic injury require surgery. Operative management is reserved for unstable patients with splenic injury, GSWs of the spleen, or splenic injuries that violate all layers of the splenic capsule. SWs to the spleen and splenic hematoma are usually observed for changes in physical examination and hemoglobin and hematocrit lev-

Table 24-2	SPLENIC INJURIES	
GRADE	CATEGORY	DESCRIPTION
I	Hematoma	Subcapsular; involves less than 10% surface area; hematoma does not expand
	Laceration	Nonbleeding capsular tear; less than 1 cm deep
II	Hematoma	Subcapsular hematoma covering 10%-50% surface area
		Hematoma does not expand; intraparenchymal hematoma less than 2 cm wide
	Laceration	Capsular tear with active bleeding; intraparenchymal injury 1-3 cm deep
III	Hematoma	Subcapsular hematoma involving more than 50% surface area or one that is expanding; intraparenchymal hematoma less than 2 cm wide or expanding; ruptured subcapsular hematoma with active bleeding
	Laceration	More than 3 cm deep or involving intracellular vessels
IV	Hematoma	Ruptured intraparenchymal hematoma with active bleeding
	Laceration	Segmental laceration or one that involves hilar vessels
		Devascularization of more than 25% of spleen
V	Laceration	Shattered spleen
	Vascular	Hilar vascular injury; spleen is devascularized

From Pearl WS, Todd KH: Ultrasonography for the initial evaluation of blunt abdominal trauma, a review in prospective trials, *Ann Emerg Med* 27:353, 1996.

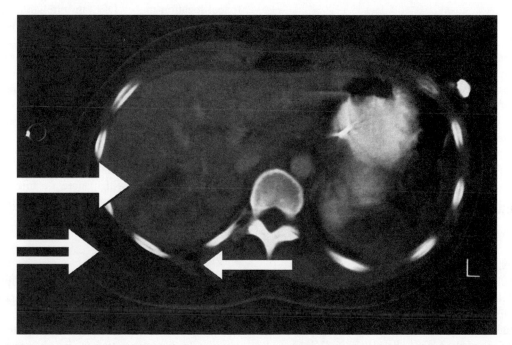

FIGURE 24-7   Computed tomography scan of the abdomen demonstrating a deep intrahepatic laceration *(large solid arrow)*, pneumothorax *(large hollow arrow)*, and retroperitoneal air *(small solid arrow)*. (From Rosen P, Barkin RM, Hockberger RS et al: *Emergency medicine: concepts and clinical practice*, ed 4, St. Louis, 1998, Mosby.)

els. The ultimate goal is to preserve the function of the spleen if at all possible.

Liver

The liver's size and anterior location make it an easy target for blunt and penetrating forces. Overall mortality for liver injuries is only 10%. MVCs still account for the majority of hepatic injuries. As with the spleen, the liver is encapsulated, so injuries can affect only the capsule or fracture the liver itself (Figure 24-7). Table 24-3 delineates types of liver in-

juries. Liver injuries are suggested when the patient has a direct blow to the right upper quadrant from the eighth rib to the central abdomen. Clinical indications include pain, bruising over the right upper quadrant, or referred pain to the right shoulder. Hemodynamic instability is almost always present when the liver sustains major damage. The trauma team should consider acute hepatic injury if the patient remains hypotensive despite aggressive IV fluid replacement. Surgical repair of liver injuries is determined by extent of injury to the liver and the patient's hemodynamic status. More than 50% of adults with liver injury are treated nonoperatively.

Table 24-3	LIVER INJURIES	
GRADE	CATEGORY	DESCRIPTION
I	Hematoma	Nonexpanding subcapsular hematoma less than 10% of liver surface
	Laceration	Nonbleeding capsular tear less than 1 cm deep
II	Hematoma	Nonexpanding subcapsular hematoma covering 10% to 50% surface area; less than 2 cm deep
	Laceration	Less than 3 cm parenchymal penetration; less than 10 cm long
III	Hematoma	Subcapsular hematoma more than 50% surface area or one that is expanding; ruptured subcapsular hematoma with active bleeding; intraparenchymal hematoma more than 2 cm
	Laceration	More than 3 cm deep
IV	Hematoma	Ruptured central hematoma
	Laceration	15% to 25% hepatic lobe destroyed
V	Laceration	More than 75% hepatic lobe destroyed
	Vascular	Major hepatic veins injured
VI	Vascular	Avulsed liver

From Pearl WS, Todd KH: Ultrasonography for the initial evaluation of blunt abdominal trauma, a review in prospective trials, *Ann Emerg Med* 27:353, 1996.

Stomach

The stomach is a hollow organ that can be easily displaced, so it is rarely injured with blunt trauma. Conversely, size and anterior location increase the risk of penetrating injury. Physical signs and symptoms associated with stomach injuries include left upper quadrant pain and tenderness. Diagnosis is based on patient assessment, aspiration of blood via the gastric tube, and presence of free air on the abdominal radiograph (see Figure 24-5). All patients with gastric injury require surgical exploration.

Large and Small Intestine

The intestines are hollow, highly vascular organs approximately 32 feet long that are fixed at various points in the peritoneal cavity. Their anterior location, relative lack of protection, vascularity, and fixed points of attachment make the intestines vulnerable to blunt and penetrating injuries. Penetrating trauma, particularly SWs, can eviscerate the bowel or omentum. Management includes covering the evisceration with saline-soaked pads, establishing IV access, and preparing the patient for surgery.

The intestines are frequently injured by inappropriately worn seat belts. Injury to the intestines usually causes rupture followed by spillage of chemical and bacterial contamination into the peritoneum. Initial signs and symptoms of intestinal injury include tenderness and rigidity. As time progresses and more peritoneal contamination occurs, fever, elevated white count, abdominal distension, and hypoactive bowel sounds occur.

Pancreas

The pancreas, a semisolid organ in the retroperitoneal space, is well-protected by the liver and stomach, so it is more likely to be injured by penetrating trauma. Pancreatic injury from blunt trauma is unusual, but does occur. Its retroperi-

toneal location makes DPL an unreliable indicator of pancreatic injury. Elevated serum amylase is also unreliable as an indicator of pancreatic injury—up to 40% of all patients with pancreatic injury initially have a normal serum amylase. Lipase is considered a better indicator of pancreatic injury. An assay for pancreatic fraction is proving more reliable; however, this test is not yet readily available. Endoscopic retrograde pancreatography has proven useful in identifying injury to the pancreatic duct. When surgery is required, every effort is made to preserve the pancreas because of its essential endocrine and exocrine functions. The majority of patients with pancreatic injury have other injuries, with associated hemorrhage being the major cause of death.

Diaphragm

Diaphragmatic rupture may be due to blunt or penetrating mechanisms. Rupture almost always occurs on the left side because the liver protects the right hemidiaphragm. Rupture should be suspected in all patients with thoracoabdominal injuries. In diaphragmatic rupture, abdominal contents spill into the thoracic cavity, causing respiratory compromise secondary to lung compression. Bowel sounds may be auscultated in the chest cavity. Loss of negative pressure in the chest and inability of the diaphragm to function normally further compromise respiratory function. Diagnosis is usually confirmed by a radiograph of the chest showing abdominal contents or the gastric tube in the left chest. These patients require immediate surgical repair. Mortality increases with delay in identification and treatment. (See Chapter 23 for additional discussion.)

Vascular Structures

Major vascular structures in the abdomen are the abdominal aorta, inferior vena cava, iliac artery, and hepatic veins. Vessels can be injured by blunt or penetrating mechanisms—

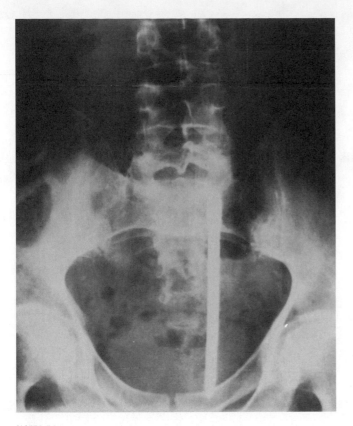

FIGURE 24-8 Radiograph of patient who inserted screwdriver into rectum. (From Rosen P, Barkin RM, Hockberger RS et al: *Emergency medicine: concepts and clinical practice,* ed 4, St. Louis, 1998, Mosby.)

injury of major abdominal vessels occurs in 5% to 10% of patients with blunt abdominal trauma. Disruption of vascular structures causes severe hemorrhage and death if the damage is not repaired. Identification of injuries is often made in the operating room, particularly in an unstable patient. A CT scan and arteriography may be used for the stable patient. ED management of patients with vascular injuries includes establishing IV access and providing rapid transport to the surgical suite.

Foreign Bodies

Another aspect of abdominal trauma is a foreign body in the stomach and rectum. This may be the result of ingestion, masturbation, autoeroticism, assault, confusion, mental retardation, or psychiatric illness. Many patients do not acknowledge the presence of a foreign body during initial evaluation. Complaints are often vague and relate to pain or discomfort. Diagnosis is usually made using a radiograph. Removal of the foreign body may be done in the ED or may require surgical intervention, depending on the size, shape, and location of the foreign body. Drug-filled condoms or plastic bags may also be swallowed or placed in the rectum. Other foreign bodies include vibrators, light bulbs, plastic bottles, screws (Figure 24-8), and live animals.

SUMMARY

A patient with abdominal trauma presents the caregiver with many unique challenges. The patient can have life-threatening injuries without any external evidence of injury. The emergency nurse must assume an injury is present until the possibility is ruled out. Consideration of how the patient was injured (i.e., mechanism of injury) can highlight potential injuries and enhance patient assessment. Ongoing assessment is critical for the patient with abdominal trauma; the patient's condition can change as the patient experiences continued blood loss or responds to bacterial contamination from a ruptured intestine. Box 24-3 summarizes nursing diagnoses for the patient with abdominal trauma.

References

1. Bennett BB, Hoyt KS: *Trauma nursing core course provider manual,* ed 5, Des Plaines, Ill, 2000, Emergency Nurses Association.
2. Fabian TC, Croce MA: Abdominal trauma, including indications for celiotomy. In *Management of specific injuries,* Stamford, Conn, 1996, Appleton & Lange.
3. Guyton AC, Hall JE: *Textbook of medical physiology,* ed 9, Philadelphia, 1996, WB Saunders.
4. Levin T: The use of ultrasound in blunt trauma, *J Emerg Nurs* 26:15, 2000.
5. Ma OJ, Mateer JR, DeBehnke DJ: Use of ultrasonography for the evaluation of pregnant trauma patients, *J Trauma* 40(4):665, 1996.
6. Marx JA: Peritoneal procedures. In Hedges JR, Roberts JR, editors, *Clinical procedures in emergency medicine,* ed 3, Philadelphia, 1997, WB Saunders.
6a. Mattox KL, Feliciano DV, Moore EE: *Trauma,* ed 4, New York, 2001, McGraw-Hill.
7. Pearl WS, Todd KH: Ultrasonography for the initial evaluation of blunt abdominal trauma, a review in prospective trials, *Ann Emerg Med* 27:353, 1996.
8. Rosen P, Barkin RM, Hockberger RS et al: *Emergency medicine: concepts and clinical practice,* ed 4, St. Louis, 1998, Mosby.
9. Rozycki GS, Shackford SR: Ultrasound, what every trauma surgeon should know, *J Trauma* 40(1):1, 1996.
10. Schwartz G, Hanke B, Mayer T et al: *Principles and practice of emergency medicine* ed 4, Baltimore, 1999, Williams & Wilkins.

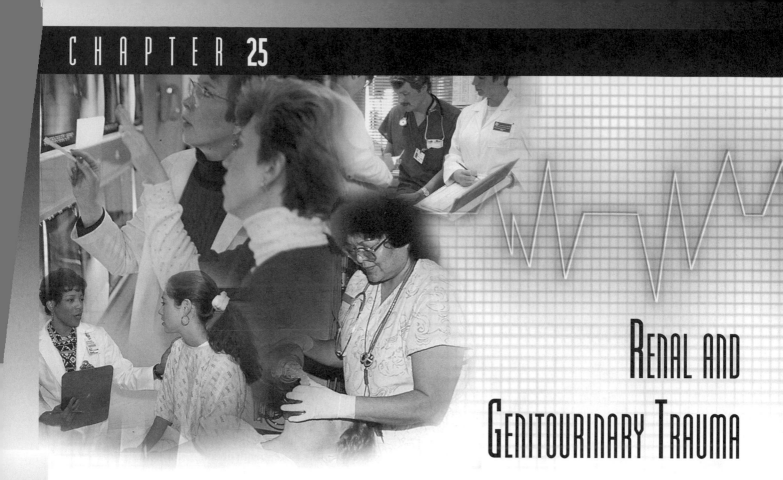

CHAPTER 25

RENAL AND GENITOURINARY TRAUMA

ELLEN E. RUJA

Genitourinary (GU) trauma occurs in approximately 8% to 10% of all trauma patients.[4] The kidney is the GU structure most commonly injured, followed by bladder, urethra, and ureter. Genitourinary injury is also common in children but rarely requires surgical management. Trauma to the GU system is divided into upper urinary tract, lower urinary tract, and genital injuries. Two basic injury mechanism categories exist: blunt and penetrating. Blunt urologic injury, the most common form of trauma, accounts for 70% to 80% of all urologic injuries.[2] Urologic injury should be considered in patients with severe lower abdominal blunt trauma and pelvic fracture. Urinary tract injury should be suspected for all patients with penetrating injuries to the abdomen, chest, or flank until proven otherwise. Prompt diagnosis and management are essential to minimize associated morbidity and mortality rates. This chapter reviews anatomy and physiology, mechanism of injury, presentation, investigation, and treatment of genitourinary injuries.

ANATOMY AND PHYSIOLOGY

The GU system consists of the kidneys, ureters, bladder, and urethra. Primary functions include control of body fluids, regulation of electrolyte concentration, and excretion of metabolic end products. Additional functions include prostaglandin production, renin production, insulin degradation, stimulation of red blood cell production through production of erythropoietin, and metabolic conversion of vitamin D to an active form.

Kidneys are retroperitoneal organs that lie high on the posterior abdominal wall (Figure 25-1). The right kidney, 1 to 2 cm lower than the left, lies inferior and posterior to the liver and posterior to the ascending colon and duodenum. The left kidney lies posterior to the descending colon and is associated with the tail of the pancreas medially and the spleen superiorly. Because of this relationship, major urinary tract trauma is associated with other intraabdominal injuries in approximately 73% of all penetrating trauma cases.[4] Kidneys are enclosed by a strong fibrous capsule and lie within a fatty tissue layer surrounded by Gerota's fascia. The perirenal space allows a large amount of blood to accumulate; however, the fascial layer can effectively tamponade renal bleeding in some cases. Normally, the kidneys are mobile within this area and can move vertically up or down three vertebral spaces (Figure 25-2). The kidney is well protected by the vertebral bodies and the back muscles posteriorly and abdominal viscera anteriorly.

The pediatric kidney is theoretically at greater risk for injury than the adult kidney because of its relatively larger size, increased lobulation, less thoracic cavity protection, less perirenal fat, and less-developed abdominal wall musculature. A child is more likely to undergo traumatic disruption of the ureteropelvic junction than an adult.

Ureters are small muscular tubes that are flexible and mobile. These hollow tubes drain urine from the kidneys to the bladder. Ureters do not contain valves or sphincters, so urine can reflux into the ureters from a distended bladder. The ureters are rarely injured in blunt abdominal trauma because

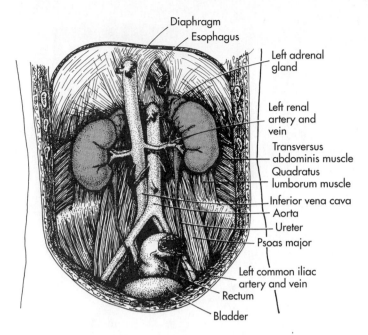

Diaphragm
Esophagus
Left adrenal gland
Left renal artery and vein
Transversus abdominis muscle
Quadratus lumborum muscle
Inferior vena cava
Aorta
Ureter
Psoas major
Left common iliac artery and vein
Rectum
Bladder

FIGURE 25-1   The genitourinary tract. (From Price SA, Wilson LM: *Pathophysiology: clinical concepts of disease processes,* ed 5, St. Louis, 1997, Mosby.)

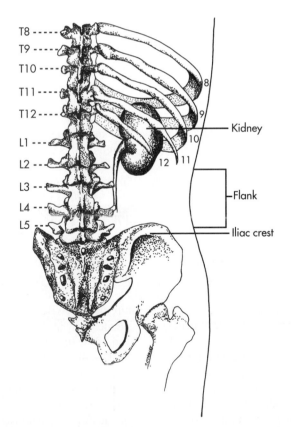

T8
T9
T10
T11
T12
L1
L2
L3
L4
L5
8
9
10
11
12
Kidney
Flank
Iliac crest

FIGURE 25-2   Anatomic relationship between kidneys and spine. (From Neff JA, Kidd PS, editors: *Trauma nursing: the art and science,* St. Louis, 1993, Mosby.)

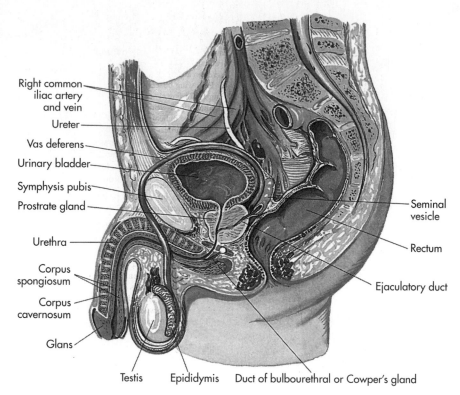

FIGURE 25-3 The male genital tract. (From Huether SE, McCance KL: *Understanding pathophysiology,* St. Louis, 1996, Mosby.)

Labels on figure:
Right common iliac artery and vein
Ureter
Vas deferens
Urinary bladder
Symphysis pubis
Prostrate gland
Urethra
Corpus spongiosum
Corpus cavernosum
Glans
Testis   Epididymis   Duct of bulbourethral or Cowper's gland
Seminal vesicle
Rectum
Ejaculatory duct

of their deep location in the retroperitoneal space and added protection from abdominal contents, spine, and surrounding muscles. The blood supply to the ureter comes from the renal artery, aorta, and iliac artery.

The bladder is an extraperitoneal hollow organ located in the pelvis that is well protected by pelvic bones laterally, urogenital diaphragm inferiorly, and the rectum posteriorly. Until age 6 years, the bladder is an intraperitoneal organ, lying just beneath the anterior abdominal wall, so it is more vulnerable to external trauma. In the adult the bladder is covered at the dome by a patch of peritoneum. Blood supply is abundant and mainly derived from branches of the internal iliac artery. In the male the prostate gland lies adjacent to the inferior margin and is fixed to the pubis anteriorly by ligaments and inferiorly by the urogenital diaphragm.

The female urethra is short and well protected by the symphysis pubis. In the male the urethra is approximately 20 cm long and lies outside the body. The urogenital diaphragm divides the urethra into posterior and anterior segments (Figure 25-3). The posterior urethra is composed of the prostatic and membranous urethra, extends from the inferior urogenital diaphragm to the bladder neck, and is approximately 3 to 4 cm long. The anterior urethra consists of the bulbous and pendulous urethra and extends from the external urinary meatus to the urogenital diaphragm.

The penis is composed of three vascular bodies: the paired corpora cavernosa and corpus spongiosum. These structures are surrounded by deep (Buck's fascia) and su-

perficial fasciae that allow mobility of the penile skin. The testis and epididymis reside in each scrotal compartment. Each testis receives blood via the spermatic cord and through the testicular artery, the artery to the vas deferens, and the cremasteric artery. Each testis is surrounded by a tough fibrous capsule. The scrotum is covered by a thin layer of skin and receives blood from branches of the femoral and internal pudendal arteries.

PATIENT ASSESSMENT

Rapid diagnosis and treatment of GU trauma can be very difficult because it seldom occurs independently and is often associated with abdominal injuries. For any trauma patient, the most immediate requirements are airway, breathing, and circulation (ABC). After basic life-support measures are implemented, immediate monitoring of their effectiveness should be instituted.

The first rule of urologic trauma management is to aggressively seek and diagnose urologic injury because many of these injuries are not obvious at the onset. Assessment of GU trauma begins with a brief history including allergies, medications, previous and current illnesses, and known anatomic abnormalities. Preexisting renal abnormalities can predispose the kidney to severe injury from even minor trauma. Abnormal kidneys occur in 0.1% to 23% of GU trauma cases.[4] Previous injuries to the GU tract may have caused chronic urologic infections and adhesions. Disorders such as chronic renal failure and renal artery stenosis profoundly influence initial treatment and long-term care of GU trauma.

Determining mechanism of injury, performing a detailed physical examination, and ensuring further diagnostic testing complete the clinical assessment of the injured patient. Certain mechanisms of injury carry a higher incidence of GU trauma (e.g., victim struck by a car, rapid deceleration incident, penetrating trauma). All clothing is removed for inspection. Several patterns of contusion and bruising are specific to GU injuries. Grey Turner's sign is bruising over the flank and lower back that occurs in retroperitoneal hematoma and is frequently present with pelvic fractures. An edematous and contused scrotum may be seen with straddle injuries, pelvic fractures, or dissecting retroperitoneal hematomas. Perineal bruising is a late sign in fracture of the symphysis pubis or pelvic rami. Fractures of the eleventh and twelfth ribs (Figure 25-2) have an increased potential of renal injury. Male genitalia are more easily examined than female genitalia. Laceration and avulsion injuries to the penis and scrotum are immediately apparent.

After observation the ED nurse auscultates the abdomen for bowel sounds. Absence of bowel sounds, abdominal rigidity, and guarding are not specific to GU injury but may be indicative of intraperitoneal urine extravasation or renal injuries. The abdomen is gently palpated for presence of a distended bladder—an empty bladder is not palpable. It is important to note that a full bladder may indicate the inability to void. If the patient cannot urinate, the urinary meatus should be checked carefully for blood. Blood at the meatus is a cardinal sign for anterior urethral injury. A digital rectal examination provides information on condition of the prostate gland and posterior urethra. A high-riding prostate or boggy mass indicates posterior rupture of the urethra. Extravasated urine and blood can dislocate the prostate. Percussion of the abdomen may reveal dullness, suggesting extravasated urine or blood.

Baseline hematologic, coagulation, and electrolyte panels should be obtained. Hematuria is a strong indication of GU trauma. Radiologic tests are discussed further in this chapter relative to specific injuries. If the patient's hemodynamic condition remains unstable despite control of external bleeding and fluid replacement, the patient should be prepared for exploratory surgery.

RENAL TRAUMA

Injuries to the kidneys may be limited to minor tissue damage or involve major vascular structures.

Blunt trauma accounts for 70% to 80% of renal injuries, whereas penetrating trauma accounts for only 6% to 14%. Blunt injuries are most commonly caused by a motor vehicle collision; sports injuries, occupational injuries, and assault are less common.[2] Injury from blunt trauma is due to three mechanisms—direct blow to the flank, laceration of renal parenchyma from a fractured rib or vertebrae, or sudden deceleration that causes shearing that leads to renal

Box 25-1	CLASSIFICATION OF RENAL INJURIES BY ORGAN INJURY SCALING COMMITTEE
Grade I	Contusion: microscopic or gross hematuria; normal urologic studies
	Subcapsular hematoma, nonexpanding; no laceration
Grade II	Laceration of renal parenchyma <1 cm; no extravasation
	Perinephric hematoma, nonexpanding
Grade III	Laceration of renal parenchyma >1
	No urinary extravasation; no collecting system involvement
Grade IV	Laceration involving collecting system
	Perinephric and paranephric extravasation
	Thrombosis of segmental renal artery
	Main renal artery or vein injury, hemorrhage controlled
Grade V	Fractured kidney
	Thrombosis of main renal artery
	Avulsion of main renal artery or vein

From Dixon MD, McAninch JW: *American Urological Association update series, traumatic renal injuries, part 1: assessment and management,* Houston, 1991, The Association.
*Grades I and II are minor; Grades III, IV, and V are major.

pedicle injury or parenchymal renal damage. Abdominal injuries resulting from seat belts include 11% that involve the urinary tract, half of which are renal injuries. Falls from heights are associated with ureteral avulsion at the ureteropelvic junction. Renal injuries are more common than splenic rupture, 4 times more common than hepatic and intestinal injuries, and 10 times more common than injuries to the lung, heart, pancreas, or major vessels. Boys sustain blunt renal injuries more often than girls; however, injuries in females are more severe. The majority of injuries caused by blunt trauma have limited severity and do not require exploration. Between 4% and 25% of blunt injuries are classified as major lacerations or vascular injuries as compared with 40% to 68% of penetrating injuries. Penetrating injuries are typically caused by gunshot or stab wounds, with gunshot wounds usually causing more complex injuries. A knife can readily cut the cortex of the kidney if the weapon is driven more than 3 inches into the victim. Damage to the kidney may be caused by a bullet, bullet fragment, or blast effect. The majority of penetrating injuries require surgical intervention. Iatrogenic injuries are an important subgroup of renal trauma. Percutaneous nephrostomy, renal biospy, and extracorporeal shock wave lithotripsy can produce a spectrum of renal injury, including hematomas and distal vascular lesions.

Classification of renal injuries has been established by the Organ Injury Scaling Committee of the American Association for the Surgery of Trauma (see Box 25-1 and Figure 25-4). A more practical staging system divides injuries into contusions, minor lacerations confined to the renal cortex,

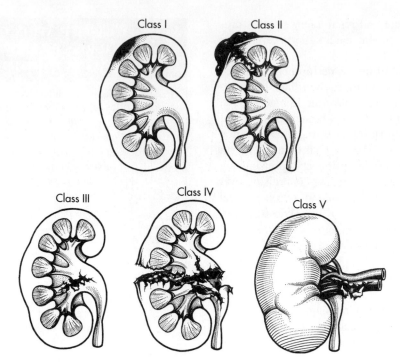

Class I Class II

Class III Class IV Class V

FIGURE 25-4 Classification of renal trauma. Class I, renal contusion; Class II, cortical laceration; Class III, caliceal laceration; Class IV, complete renal fracture; Class V, vascular pedicle injury. (From Rosen P, Barkin RM, Hockberger RS et al: *Emergency medicine: concepts and clinical practice,* ed 4, St. Louis, 1998, Mosby.)

major lacerations that involve the collecting system, and vascular injuries.

Clinical indicators of blunt renal injury include history of a direct blow to the flank, lower thoracic, or upper abdomen, and associated intraabdominal injuries. Signs of flank trauma include lower rib fractures, fracture of the lumbar transverse processes, bruising of the body wall, flank mass, and flank tenderness. Patients may develop microscopic or gross hematuria. Hematuria is the best indicator of renal injury; however, the degree of hematuria does not always correlate with degree of injury. Seven percent to 14% of patients with major lacerations or vascular injury and 6% to 10% of patients with minor lacerations after penetrating trauma do not have hematuria. Significant renal injury can occur with microhematuria in the absence of hypotension. Hypovolemic shock secondary to a major renal laceration can occur.

Initial radiographic evaluation of penetrating wounds consists of plain radiographs of the kidneys, ureters, and bladder (KUB) to determine path and appearance of the projectile. A flat plate radiograph of the abdomen may reveal loss of normal renal outline, loss of psoas muscle shadow on the affected side, scoliosis away from the kidney, and a flank mass. Fractures of transverse processes and lower ribs may also be clues that a renal injury has occurred. Indications for radiologic evaluation to stage renal trauma include penetrating injuries proximal to the GU system and blunt trauma with gross hematuria or microscopic hematuria associated with hypotension.

An intravenous pyelogram (IVP) is the initial examination of choice in patients with penetrating injury who are unstable and require immediate operative intervention. Usually, contrast is injected, then one view or radiograph is taken. However, an IVP has significant limitations in assessing associated intraabdominal injuries and staging renal injuries. An IVP should not be the initial study in patients with blunt trauma who are hemodynamically stable.

Color Doppler ultrasonography (US) can be limited by pain, ileus, or various wounds and is less sensitive than computed tomography (CT) for detecting parenchymal injury. The US study can show the presence of subcapsular and perirenal hematomas and detect vascular complications of the pedicle and intrarenal vasculature.

CT is the most accurate modality available for staging renal injuries, determining renal pedicle injuries, depicting size and extent of retroperitoneal hematoma, and evaluating associated intraabdominal injuries. Two types of CT scanners are currently available, conventional CT scanners and spiral CT scanners. The CT data set obtained during a spiral study is a continuous, nonoverlapping volume of data derived over 20 to 40 seconds.[5] These data create a volume of information that can be used for three-dimensional imaging. Spiral CT offers many advantages over conventional CT for evaluation of the retroperitoneum and specifically the kidneys. The kidneys are more completely imaged because of the single continuous x-ray exposure. The conventional CT images the kidney incompletely because of the discontinuous transverse sections acquired with separate breath holds.

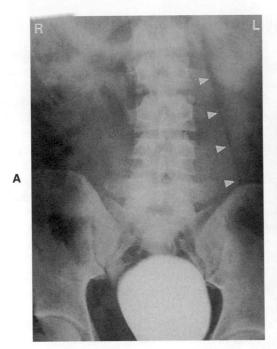

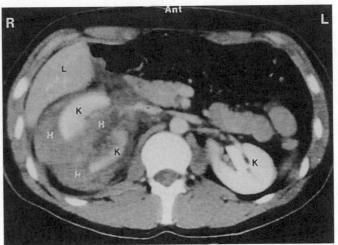

FIGURE 25-5 Renal laceration. A radiograph of the abdomen (**A**) in a young male involved in an automobile accident shows a well-defined left psoas margin *(arrowheads)*. The right psoas margin is not identified, and a contrast-enhanced computed tomography scan (**B**) at the level of the kidneys shows a fracture through the midportion of the right kidney. The kidney *(K)* can be seen in two separate pieces with intervening and surrounding hemorrhage *(H)*. *L* = liver. (From Mettler FA, Guiberteau MJ et al: *Primary care radiology*, Philadelphia, 2000, WB Saunders.)

Spiral CT findings in the acutely traumatized patient include renal parenchymal injuries such as contusions, lacerations, renal fractures, subcapsular hematomas, and renal pedicle injury (Figure 25-5). CT cannot differentiate various causes of traumatic vascular occlusion such as thrombosis, vascular tears, avulsions, intimal tears, and spasm.

Angiography is a sensitive modality for staging renal injuries and for ruling out vascular injuries. This invasive modality does not evaluate other abdominal injuries; therefore, angiography is reserved for high-risk patients with an indeterminate CT scan.

Magnetic resonance imaging (MRI) can complement a CT scan in patients with severe renal injury, preexisting renal abnormality, equivocal CT findings, or when a repeat radiographic follow-up is required. MRI is sensitive for detecting hematomas, edema, ischemia, and urinomas. MRI replaces CT in patients with an iodine allergy and may be used for initial staging when CT is not available.[3] A patient must be hemodynamically stable before MRI can be used.

Radionucleotide renal scans are particularly helpful in detecting arterial injury; however, minor extravasation is missed and lacerations are less likely to be seen than with other studies. US is appropriate for cases in which mild injury is present or suspicion of injury is low. This diagnostic modality cannot differentiate a hematoma, laceration, or urine; therefore, CT is more appropriate for a moderate-to-high suspicion of renal injury.

Significant progress in management of renal trauma during the last three decades has increased the rate of renal salvage. Surgical exploration is mandatory in patients with gunshot wounds. Vital renal structures are located toward the abdominal midline; therefore, penetration through the anterior abdomen has a greater chance for major injury. Management of stab wounds is different than management of gunshot wounds. Peripheral stab wounds such as flank wounds posterior to the anterior axillary line are more likely to injure nonvital structures.

Most blunt renal injuries can be treated nonoperatively with bed rest, frequent examinations, serial urinalyses, and analgesics. Controversy still exists about whether surgical or conservative management should be used in hemodynamically stable patients with severe renal injury. Unless immediate exploratory laparotomy is indicated for associated injuries or shock, most hemodynamically stable patients with major renal injuries, penetrating or blunt, can be managed by nonsurgical treatment with delayed intervention as needed. Hemodynamically unstable patients with renal pedicle or ureteral injuries, expanding retroperitoneal hematoma, falling hemoglobin levels, pulsatile hematoma, extensive extravasation, and nonviable tissue in more than 20% of the kidney may require immediate surgical management.

Early complications of renal injury include delayed bleeding, urinoma, abscess formation, renal insufficiency, urinary extravasation, and fistula formation. Late complications include arteriovenous fistulas, hydronephrosis, stone formation, chronic pyelonephritis, and pain. Hypertension can occur after renal artery injury or renal compression injury. Patients may become hypertensive within 24 hours of injury, or onset of hypertension can be delayed up to 10 years after injury. Patients with severe renal injuries require long-term follow-up to identify hypertension, perinephric cysts, arteriovenous fistulas, stones, renal failure, and retarded growth in the injured kidney.

Renal pedicle injuries usually occur in a seriously traumatized patient and represent 2% of all renal injuries. The majority of renal pedicle injuries occur in children and young adults with the left renal vein the most commonly injured vessel. The usual mechanism of renal artery occlusion is an intimal tear secondary to acceleration-deceleration injury. Renal vascular injuries include a vessel injury, renal artery thrombosis, and disruption of the renal artery intimal layer resulting in an aneurysm or thrombosis. No signs or symptoms are specific for renal pedicle injury. Hematuria is absent in one third of all cases. Despite immediate diagnosis by CT or IVP, most patients are not candidates for vascular repair because of the high incidence of severe associated injuries. Early diagnosis is essential. Surgical repair of pedicle injury within 12 hours is required to restore blood flow to the ischemic kidney and salvage renal function. Total avulsion of the renal pedicle is an indication for nephrectomy.

URETERAL INJURIES

Ureteral injuries from blunt trauma are rare. The most common mechanism of ureteral injury is penetrating trauma. A high index of suspicion is necessary to diagnose ureteral injury because early signs may not be evident on initial examination. Blunt trauma usually causes avulsion of the ureteropelvic junction subsequent to major hyperextension of upper lumbar and lower thoracic areas. A preponderance of the cases are children, with about one third of the cases involving adults. The right side is involved 3 times more often than the left side. Penetrating injury can cause partial or complete ureteral transection. With penetrating lower abdominal injury, careful examination of the wound with the ureter in mind is essential. Physical findings of ureteral injury are nonspecific and usually relate to an associated intraabdominal injury. Only when the ureter is obstructed and produces pain with classic radiation to the groin is diagnosis easy. Microhematuria is seen in 90% of cases.

Diagnosis of ureteral injury is made by IVP and retrograde ureteropyelography. Delayed spiral CT scanning of the kidney 5 to 8 minutes or longer after injection of contrast medium (during the excretory phase) should be added to visualize the ureters. Most patients with a ureteral injury require operative exploration for associated abdominal injuries. Dismembered pyeloplasty with ureteral stenting and nephrostomy tube is the treatment of choice. Untreated ureteral injury can lead to urinoma, abscess, or stricture.

BLADDER INJURIES

Major bladder trauma is relatively uncommon, accounting for less than 2% of abdominal injuries requiring surgical repair and occurring in only 5% to 10% of patients with pelvic fracture.[4] Rupture of the bladder does not usually occur as an isolated injury and rarely presents without fracture of the pelvis. The mechanism of injury in bladder rupture varies with patient population, amount of urine in the bladder at the time of injury, and location of injury within the bladder. Children are more susceptible to direct force and intraperitoneal rupture because of location. Injury to the bladder base and bladder neck may be caused by direct laceration from a fractured pelvic bone or shearing mechanism.

Bladder injuries are classified as contusions, extraperitoneal ruptures, intraperitoneal ruptures, and combined injuries. Nonpenetrating bladder injuries account for the majority of injuries. Twenty-five percent are intraperitoneal and usually not associated with pelvic fracture (Figure 25-6). Injuries are usually caused by a suprapubic blow in the presence of a full bladder. The bladder tends to rupture at the weakest point (i.e., dome or posterior wall of the bladder). Intraperitoneal ruptures involve extravasation of blood and urine into the peritoneal cavity. Fifty-six percent to 78% of bladder ruptures are extraperitoneal, secondary to a bony part rupture or shearing forces associated with pelvic fracture (Figure 25-7). Extraperitoneal bladder rupture involves perforation of the anterolateral bladder with extravasation of blood and urine into the retroperitoneal space. Seventy percent to 83% of blunt bladder injuries are associated with pelvic fracture; however, only 10% of patients with pelvic fractures have a ruptured bladder.[4] Combined intraperitoneal and extraperitoneal ruptures occur in up to 12% of cases, are associated with severe pelvic injury, and have a high mortality rate.[4]

Blunt lower abdominal trauma is suggested by patient history. Most patients with bladder perforation are unable to void and have suprapubic pain and hematuria. Associated leg fractures are often found. Hemodynamic instability is common because of extensive blood loss in the pelvis and associated injuries. Gross hematuria and pelvic fractures are present in more than 90% of bladder ruptures.[4] Extravasation of sterile urine may not initially lead to signs of peritoneal irritation. Late signs and symptoms are abdominal distension, acute abdomen, and increased blood urea nitrogen and serum creatinine levels.

Radiographic evaluation consists of retrograde urethrogram and cystogram in all male patients with pelvic fractures associated with gross hematuria, inability to urinate, blood at the meatus, perineal swelling, or nonpalpable prostate. Female patients with a pelvic fracture should undergo careful visual inspection of the urethra.

Retrograde or CT cystography with adequate bladder distention remains the primary method of detecting suspected bladder injuries. CT cystography over plain film cystography in patients undergoing CT evaluation for other blunt trauma related injuries is recommended. A plain film of the

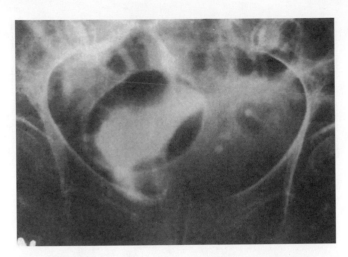

FIGURE 25-6 Bladder contusion secondary to a pelvic hematoma and pelvic fracture. (From Sandler CM et al: Radiology of the bladder and urethra in blunt pelvic trauma, *Radiol Clin North Am* 19:195, 1981.)

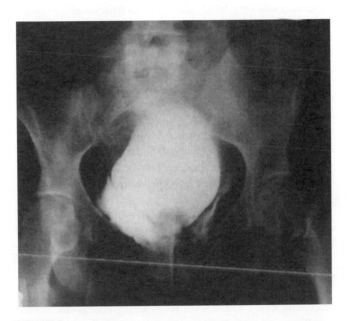

FIGURE 25-7 Extraperitoneal bladder rupture secondary to pelvic fracture. (From Gillenwater JY et al: *Adult and pediatric urology,* ed 3, vol 1, St. Louis, 1996, Mosby.)

pelvis should be obtained before cystography. Contrast infused into the bladder is seen as extravasate by CT. Only 15% of bladder injuries are identified with IVP.[4]

The usual treatment for bladder ruptures is surgical repair. Intraperitoneal ruptures do not close spontaneously, and most extraperitoneal ruptures are associated with bony injuries or other intraabdominal injuries that necessitate surgical exploration. Conservative therapy consisting of catheter drainage, antibiotics, and close clinical observation has been advocated for extraperitoneal tears in cases with minimal bleeding, no sepsis, and maintenance of adequate drainage.

Bladder injuries can lead to urinary ascites, abscess formation, and urinary fistula formation. Overall mortality of 9% reported for bladder rupture is clearly related to the high incidence of severe associated injuries.

URETHRAL INJURIES

A urethral injury should be suspected in any patient with a history of perineal or pelvic trauma. Urethral injuries rarely occur in females. When they do occur, they are usually associated with a pelvic fracture, obstetric injury, or anterior vaginal lacerations. Proximal urethral injuries almost invariably occur in men. Three percent to 25% of male patients sustaining a pelvic fracture suffer injury to the posterior urethra. Sixty-five percent experience complete urethral disruption, and 34% experience partial urethral tears. Urethral injuries are usually caused by shearing rather than direct laceration. If the injury is superior, the prostate can be forced upward by a developing hematoma. In addition, 10% to 20% of patients with bladder rupture caused by pelvic trauma have a concomitant urethral injury.[4] Injuries to the anterior urethra can occur as a result of straddle injury, blunt trauma, or sharp trauma to the penis caused by passage of a foreign body. Partial transection occurs most often. If Buck's fascia remains intact, urinary extravasation is confined to the penile shaft and perineum. With rupture of Buck's fascia, voiding can cause extensive extravasation along the abdominal wall.

Blunt trauma to the posterior urethra causes three general types of injuries, which may be incomplete or complete. With type I injuries, the urethra is stretched but does not rupture. Type II injuries are disruption of the urethra above the urogenital diaphragm; type III injuries are bulbomembranous injuries inferior to the urogenital diaphragm. Injuries to the anterior urethra are classified as contusions or partial or complete lacerations (Figure 25-8).

Clinical symptoms may be variable. Some patients have a classic triad of blood at the urethral meatus, inability to urinate, and a distended, palpable bladder. However, many patients with partial urethral tears can void. Other signs and symptoms include pain on micturition; perineal, scrotal, or penile hematoma or swelling; hematuria; and a "high-riding" prostate.

A digital rectal examination should be performed in all trauma patients to exclude associated rectal injury. Inability to palpate the prostate has been described as a classic sign of posterior urethral injury. A retrograde urethrogram is the study of choice for evaluation of urethral injuries. A urethral catheter should not be inserted if urethral injury is suspected. Such a procedure can convert a partial urethral disruption into a complete one, raise the risk of contamination, and increase the risk of further hemorrhage. Absence of blood at the meatus and a palpable prostate on rectal examination are sufficient evidence to allow passage of a urethral catheter. If resistance is encountered, the procedure should be stopped and urethrography performed. With minimal disruption of the urethra, gentle placement of a soft urinary

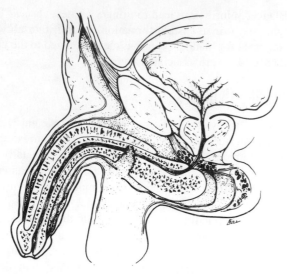

FIGURE 25-8   Depiction of anterior urethral injury. (From Neff JA, Kidd PS: *Trauma nursing: the art and science,* St. Louis, 1993, Mosby.)

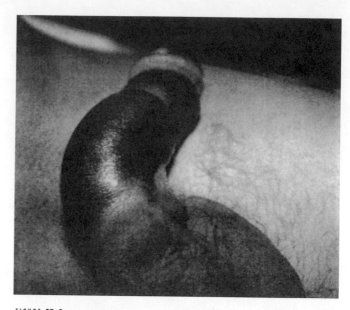

FIGURE 25-9   Fracture of the penis. Traumatic rupture of the corpus cavernosum, usually associated with sexual activity, results in a profound penile hematoma most often requiring operative repair. (From Rosen P, Barkin RM, Hockberger RS et al: *Emergency medicine: concepts and clinical practice,* ed 4, St. Louis, 1998, Mosby.)

catheter may be the only treatment required. With complete disruption, prompt suprapubic cystostomy drainage of the bladder is mandatory.

Impotence, stricture, and incontinence are the most severe complications of posterior urethral disruption. With anterior urethral injury, stricture formation is the most common complication. Impotence and incontinence are rare with anterior urethral injuries.

GENITAL INJURIES

Testicular and penile injuries are not common. The majority of injuries to the testes are secondary to blunt trauma. Patients with testicular contusions are treated with analgesics, elevation of the scrotum, ice compresses, and bed rest. Occasional lacerations of the scrotum and contents are seen. Penetrating and degloving injuries of the penis can occur in the workplace. Sexually related injuries involving strangulation or amputation of the penis have also been reported. Penetrating injuries mandate exploration and reconstruction. Traumatic amputation may be amenable to microsurgical reanastomosis.

Penile Trauma

Blunt trauma to the erect penis can rupture the tunica albuginea surrounding the corpora cavernosa, causing a penile fracture (Figure 25-9). The patient typically reports a "cracking or popping sound" during intercourse or sexual play, severe pain, and immediate detumescence. A hematoma with marked edema develops in the penile shaft. The fracture can sometimes be palpated and the defect detected. In 30% of patients, the urethra is lacerated, so urethrography should be considered.[4] MRI and cavernosography can be useful in evaluating atypical cases of penile fracture presentations.

In cases without urethral injury most patients can urinate normally. Occasionally, hematoma and edema cause exter-

nal urethral compression, leading to urinary retention. Management is controversial. Early surgical repair is associated with a lower risk of persistent penile angulation, shorter hospital stay, and more rapid functional return. Conservative treatment may be warranted in cases with minimal hematoma and no extravasation during a cavernosography. Treatment includes sedation, elevation of the penis, and ice packs.

Other penile injuries may be due to direct trauma from zippers, bites, machines, or knives. Treatment is determined by the severity of the injury.

Testicular Trauma

Traumatic injury to the testicles is an infrequent occurrence despite their exposed position in the male perineum. Injuries typically occur in young men, usually ages 15 to 40 years. Blunt trauma to the scrotum, which accounts for approximately 85% of cases, can cause testicular rupture. The patient with a scrotal injury may have acute pain, nausea, vomiting, syncope, and urinary retention. Patients can have large scrotal hematomas that make examination difficult; therefore, scrotal US imaging with Doppler studies is valuable. Nuclear imaging or MRI may be used to obtain additional information in equivocal cases. Minor cases are treated conservatively with scrotal support, nonsteroidal antiinflammatory medications, ice packs, and bed rest for 24 to 48 hours. Testicular rupture should be repaired immediately—reconstruction is possible in most cases. All penetrating testicular injuries should be explored and repaired. Orchiectomy is necessary in some cases but rarely indicated unless the entire testes is completely infarcted or shattered.

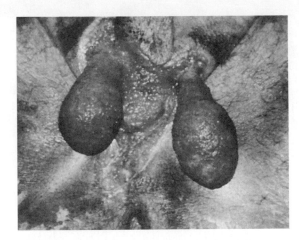

FIGURE 25-10 Scrotal avulsion injury. (From Neff JA, Kidd PS: *Trauma nursing: the art and science,* St. Louis, 1993, Mosby.

Avulsion injuries can cause loss of all or part of penile and scrotal skin (Figure 25-10). Industrial or farming accidents are often responsible for such injuries. The penile shaft can be covered with skin grafts; return of function is expected. Partial scrotal skin loss is managed by primary closure. The scrotum regenerates to accommodate the testicles and spermatic cords. Total skin loss leaves the testicles unprotected so the testicles are placed temporarily in thigh pouches when immediate grafting is not possible.

Straddle Injuries

Straddle injuries occur when a patient falls and takes the brunt of the fall on the perineum. These injuries commonly occur in young patients as they fall onto bicycle bars, motorcycles, and fences. On examination of a female patient, a vulvovaginal laceration with extensive ecchymosis of the perineum may be evident. Straddle injuries are often accompanied by vulvar hematomas that can extend into the retroperitoneal space. Associated urethral injuries and rectal tears should be ruled out. Treatment of straddle injuries involves repair of the laceration with evacuation and drainage of hematomas. The most common complication in the immediate postoperative period is infection. Sexual dysfunction may also occur.

Foreign Bodies

The medical literature contains numerous case reports of foreign bodies found in the urethra and bladder. Almost anything small and firm that can be passed into the urethra has been found there, including electric cable, tweezers, spaghetti, pebbles, paper clips, hairpins, and screws. In adults most foreign bodies are inserted for erotic stimulation. However, psychologic disorders and drug ingestion are other frequent reasons for such activity. It is unusual for children to present with foreign bodies in the urethra.

Patients may be too embarrassed to admit they inserted or applied any object and usually present when a complication or symptom occurs. The most common reason for consultation is dysuria. Other complaints are suprapubic or perineal pain, urethral discharge, hematuria, difficulty urinating, swelling, or abscess formation.

Clinical diagnosis is based on history and should always be considered in patients with chronic urinary tract infections. Radiographic studies, including plain radiographs, are usually helpful for radiopaque objects. Xeroradiography is effective for detecting nonmetallic foreign bodies traumatically or deliberately introduced into the genital tissues, including objects made of plastic, glass, rubber, cloth, or wood.

Foreign bodies below the urogenital diaphragm can usually be palpated and readily removed endoscopically, whereas foreign bodies above the urogenital diaphragm require greater endoscopic manipulation, perineal urethrostomy, or suprapubic cystotomy.

SUMMARY

Urinary trauma can be readily identified clinically and the extent of injury ascertained with radiographic imaging. An injured patient with potential urologic injury has a host of general surgical concerns, particularly in conjunction with pelvic fractures; however, life-threatening concerns related to airway control, ventilation, and hemodynamic status are still the first priority. After treatment of these concerns, organ-specific work-up can proceed. Close cooperation among the health care team is required for optimum outcome. Box 25-2 highlights nursing diagnoses for patients with GU trauma.

References

1. Carroll PR, McAninch JW: Staging of renal trauma, *Urol Clin North Am* 16:193, 1989.
2. Jordan KS: *Emergency nursing core curriculum,* ed 5, Philadelphia, 2000, WB Saunders.
3. Leppaniemi A et al: Comparison of high-field magnetic resonance imaging with computed tomography in the evaluation of blunt renal trauma, *J Trauma* 38(3):420, 1995.
4. Mattox KL, Feliciano DV, Moore EE: *Trauma,* ed 4, New York, 2001, McGraw-Hill.
5. Smith PA, Marshall FF, Fishman EK: Spiral computed tomography evaluation of the kidneys: state of the art, *Urology* 51(1):3, 1998.

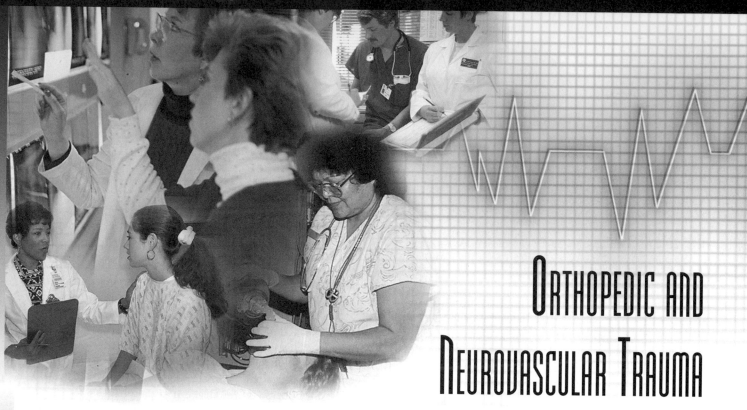

CHAPTER 26

ORTHOPEDIC AND NEUROVASCULAR TRAUMA

DEBORAH O'STEEN

Approximately 33 million musculoskeletal injuries occur annually, including 20 million fractures, dislocations, and sprains with approximately 8000 deaths. Primary mechanisms of injury are motor vehicle collisions (MVCs), assaults, falls, sports and recreation, and injuries sustained at work or home.

Musculoskeletal injury is one of the most common types of injury seen in the emergency department (ED) and a significant cause of disability. Bone, soft-tissue, and associated neurovascular injuries are rarely emergent unless accompanied by a life-threatening hemorrhage as in certain amputations and pelvic fractures. Fractures and soft-tissue injuries are primarily designated as urgent because of potential neurovascular injury with resultant limb disability and pain. Early intervention enhances preservation of limb and function. This chapter focuses on common orthopedic and neurovascular extremity injuries and appropriate therapeutic interventions. Related anatomy and physiology are briefly reviewed.

ANATOMY AND PHYSIOLOGY

The musculoskeletal system and related neurovascular structures consist of bones, joints, tendons, ligaments, muscles, vessels, and nerves. The skeletal system contains 206 bones, which provide support, strength, movement, and protection to the body and organs (Figure 26-1). Bones also store calcium and are involved in blood cell production.

Bones are characterized by shape as long, short, flat, or irregular with the shape of a particular bone suited for a unique function or purpose. The skeleton is composed of two types of bones: cancellous and cortical. Cancellous (spongy) bone is found in the skull, vertebrae, pelvis, and long-bone ends. Cortical (dense) bone is found in the long bones. Bones are supplied by blood vessels, nerves, and lymphatic vessels that nourish bone tissue and allow the bone to repair injuries. The periosteum covers the bones and provides an additional blood supply.

Bone is connected to other bone by stabilizing bands of elastic, fibrous connective tissue called *ligaments*. Nonelastic fibrous cords that connect muscle to bone are tendons. Dense connective tissue found between the ribs, in the nasal septum, ear, larynx, trachea, bronchi, between vertebrae, and on articulating surfaces is known as *cartilage*. Cartilage has a limited vascular supply, whereas bone tissue has abundant vascular structures.

Joints are classified as nonsynovial (immovable and slightly immovable) and synovial (freely movable). Synovial joints have two articulating surfaces covered with cartilage and surrounded by a two-layered synovial membrane sac. The entire joint is then encapsulated by dense, ligamentous material. Joints provide mobility and stability, flexion and extension, medial and lateral rotation, and abduction and adduction. Joint movement is enhanced by muscles and ligaments that overlie the joint.

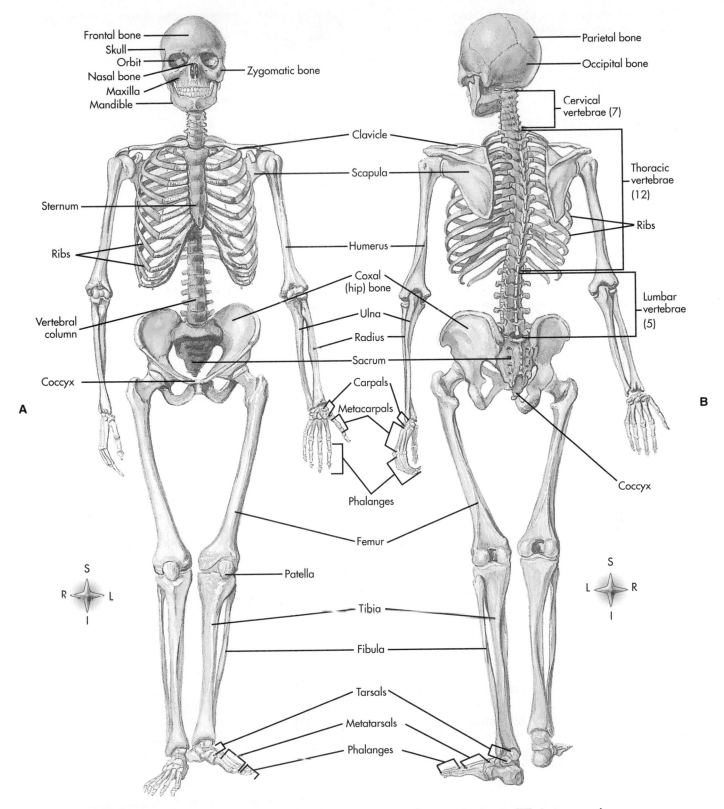

FIGURE 26-1 Skeleton. **A,** Anterior view. **B,** Posterior view. (From Thibodeau GA, Patton KT: *Anatomy and physiology,* ed 4, St. Louis, 1999, Mosby.)

Nerves and arteries lie in close proximity to bones and muscle groups, with arterioles distributed throughout the periosteum to provide nutrients. Nerves provide sensation and movement. The closeness of arteries and nerves to bone structures increases the risk for injury with trauma to soft tissue, muscle, bone, or joint.[2]

PATIENT ASSESSMENT

Assessment of orthopedic trauma begins with assessment of the airway, breathing, and circulation (ABCs). Rapid assessment identifies major injuries of head, cervical spine, chest, and abdomen, and prioritizes essential interventions. After ensuring that no life-threatening injury has been left unattended, the nurse assesses and stabilizes any extremity injuries. Box 26-1 highlights essential assessment parameters for orthopedic injuries.

Before immobilization, open fractures should be stabilized and bleeding controlled. Open fractures with obvious bone protrusion or deep laceration should be rinsed with sterile normal saline to remove gross contamination and covered with a dry sterile dressing.[4] Puncture wounds should not be irrigated over a fracture site because this can force bacteria deeper into the wound. Reduction of an open fracture also forces contaminants into the wound and should not be attempted in a prehospital setting.

To control bleeding apply pressure directly to the injury site, edges of the wound, or an adjacent pressure point. A tourniquet should not be used because of potential neurovascular compromise.

Immobilization

Immobilization should be accomplished as soon as possible to minimize further damage or complications secondary to bone fragments and to reduce pain in the injured limb. A splint should include the area above and below the injury. The neurovascular status should be checked before and after immobilization. If neurovascular status is initially compromised, gradual traction may be used to allow return of neurologic or vascular function before splinting. If neurovascular status is compromised after splinting or traction, the splint should be removed or traction decreased and the splint reapplied. Angulation should be corrected only if it prevents immobilization or if neurovascular compromise is present. Splinting is best accomplished with an assistant to support the limb while the padded splint is placed and wrapped with a noncompressive bandage. Neurovascular status is rechecked after splinting.

Four basic types of splints exist, including soft splints such as pillows; hard splints such as padded board, cardboard, aluminum, plaster (Table 26-1), fiberglass, or a ladder splint; inflatable air splints (Figure 26-2) or vacuum splints (Figure 26-3); and traction splints, which reduce angulation and provide support (Figure 26-4).[8]

Box 26-1	ASSESSMENT OF ORTHOPEDIC INJURIES

Swelling and deformity
Contusion, abrasion, laceration, puncture wound
Bruising
Crepitus
Point tenderness
Neurovascular assessment
   Pain
   Pulses
   Paralysis
   Paresthesia
   Pallor
   Tem*P*erature
   Ca*P*illary refill

Table 26-1	TYPES OF PLASTER SPLINTS AND THEIR INDICATIONS	
TYPE OF SPLINT	**INDICATIONS**	
Posterior short leg	Fracture or soft-tissue injury of the foot or ankle	
Forearm sugar tong	Fracture or soft-tissue injury of the forearm	
Humerus sugar tong	Immobilization of a humeral shaft fracture	
Thumb spica	Soft-tissue injury or metacarpal fracture of the navicular or scaphoid bone	
Volar forearm	Fracture or soft-tissue injury to wrist or carpal bone	
Ulnar gutter	Fracture or soft-tissue injury of the fourth or fifth metacarpal bone	
Radial gutter	Fracture or soft tissue injury of the first or second metacarpals	

Data from Proehl J: *Emergency nursing procedures,* ed 2, Philadelphia, 1999, WB Saunders.

Air splints were used extensively when first developed because they conformed well and provided visualization of the injured extremity. However, an air splint that is not open on the distal end does not allow neurovascular checks without deflating or unzipping the splint. An air splint should be inflated so that a finger can be slipped between the splint and the skin. Excessive pressure in the splint can compromise circulation. Air splints also stick to the skin, cause irritation, and are difficult to remove with excessive diaphoresis.

Several types of traction splints are available and are usually applied by prehospital providers. The Thomas ring splint, Sager splint, and Hare splint (see Figure 26-4) are used for fractures of the midshaft of the femur or upper third of the tibia but should not be used for the hip, lower tibia or fibula, ankle, or femur with associated tibial-fibular fractures.

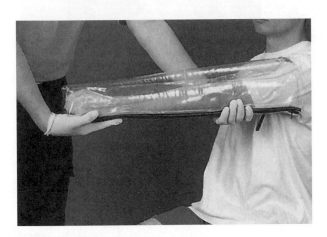

FIGURE **26-2**   Air splint. (From Stoy W: *Mosby's EMT: basic textbook,* St. Louis, 1996, Mosby.)

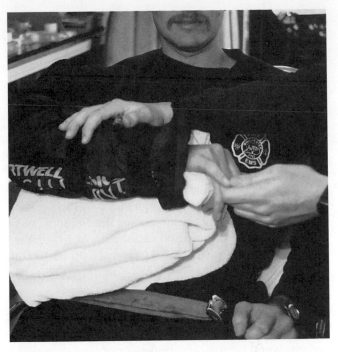

FIGURE **26-3**   Vacuum splint. (From Kidd PS, Sturt P: *Mosby's emergency nursing reference,* St. Louis, 1996, Mosby.)

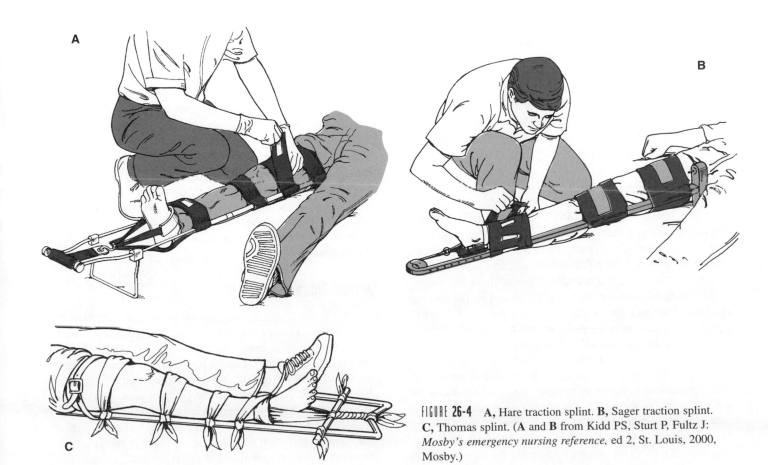

FIGURE **26-4**   **A,** Hare traction splint. **B,** Sager traction splint. **C,** Thomas splint. (**A** and **B** from Kidd PS, Sturt P, Fultz J: *Mosby's emergency nursing reference,* ed 2, St. Louis, 2000, Mosby.)

After immobilization the limb should be elevated and an ice pack applied to minimize swelling. Caution is advised because overzealous elevation may compromise arterial circulation and excessive, prolonged cold may damage tissues.

The patient should be completely disrobed and examined for anterior injuries, and then logrolled to identify posterior injuries while maintaining adequate cervical spine immobilization. Rings should be removed if the injury involves the hand, arm, foot, or toes. Elevation and cooling measures should be maintained, and neurovascular status should be checked periodically.

Careful history should include circumstances of the injury (time and mechanism) and significant medical history including acute and chronic alcohol use, medications, allergies, and tetanus immunization status. Time of last oral intake should be recorded and the patient should be NPO if surgical intervention is a possibility.

SOFT-TISSUE INJURIES

Soft-tissue injuries generally accompany orthopedic trauma; can involve skin, muscles, tendons, cartilage, ligaments, veins, arteries, and nerves; and can compromise circulation and function. Injuries to the skin include abrasions, avulsions, contusions, hematomas, lacerations, and puncture wounds (see Chapter 13).

Principles of nursing care are generally the same for various soft-tissue injuries. Inspection involves checking for wounds, swelling, hematomas, and bleeding, then assessing neurovascular status. A soft bulky dressing is applied and swelling is minimized with elevation and cooling measures. Radiographs are used to rule out foreign bodies and fractures. Analgesia is administered as prescribed for isolated injuries, and antibiotics are administered for significant, contaminated wounds. Written discharge instructions discuss elevation and cold therapy (e.g., apply a covered ice bag to the injury for 20 minutes every 2 to 3 hours for 24 to 48 hours).

Fingertip Injuries

Fingertip injuries are frequently seen in the ED, with the most common type being a crush injury to the distal phalanx that occurs when a heavy object falls on the finger or the digit is caught in a door. Crush injuries can also be associated with a fracture. If a hematoma forms under the fingernail (subungual hematoma), nail trephination by penetrating the fingernail over the hematoma with a nail drill, scalpel, pencil cautery, or superheated paper clip is done to release blood under the nail and relieve pressure.[4]

Fingertip injuries caused by a high-pressure paint or grease gun have increased in recent years. Reassessment after trephination is necessary because blood may not clot, so the hematoma reoccurs. This injury occurs when a person is cleaning the gun tip and a stream of paint or grease is released into the fingertip or hand under high pressure. Particular attention to history is crucial because the injury appears as a small pinhole in the fingertip but represents a serious,

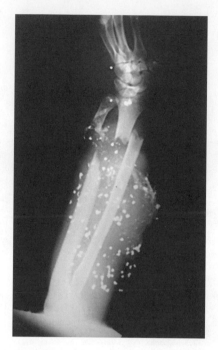

FIGURE 26-5   Gunshot wound fracture of radius and ulna with extensive soft tissue damage. (From Ballinger PW: *Merrill's atlas of radiographic positions and radiologic procedures,* ed 8, St. Louis, 1995, Mosby.)

limb-threatening surgical emergency. Therapeutic intervention requires debridement of the paint- or grease-infected limb under general anesthesia.

Impaling Injuries

Impaling injuries usually result from an industrial accident in which the victim falls onto a sharp, immobile object. Injuries with nails from a powered nail gun are also common. Nails used in these guns are coated with a special adhesive that can stick to tissue. Impaled objects are not immediately removed; surgical removal may be required. Complications from this type of injury include infection and problems specific to the structures in which the object is impaled. Biologic substances such as wood carry an increased risk of infection.

Gunshot Wounds

Gunshot wounds usually result from hunting or acts of violence. Tissue damage depends on the type of weapon and size of ammunition used, distance from the weapon, and part of the body injured (Figure 26-5). Tissue, bones, organs, and vessels away from the bullet's unpredictable path may also be injured. Appearance of the entrance wound does not always reflect destruction beneath. An extremity injury may be associated with a truncal injury because of a projectile path through the chest into the arm or through the arm into the chest or because of multiple bullet wounds. Careful assessment, including neurovascular assessment of all limbs,

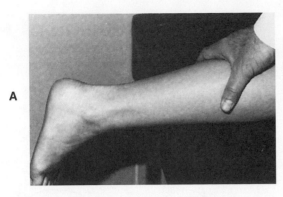 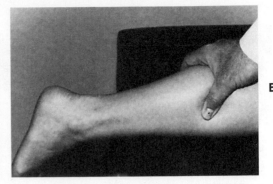

FIGURE 26-6   Thompson test. **A,** No pressure on gastrocnemius. **B,** Pressure on gastrocnemius and associated plantar flexion. If Achilles tendon is torn, plantar flexion does not accompany pressure. (From Nicholas JA, Hershman EB, editors: *The lower extremity and spine in sports medicine,* ed 2, vol 1, St. Louis, 1995, Mosby.)

is critical so that other wounds or tetanus immunization status are not overlooked. With gunshot wounds evidence surrounding the wound site or powder burns on the hand should be carefully protected until the police perform requisite testing. (See Chapter 3 for a discussion of evidence collection and preservation.)

Tendon and Muscle Rupture

Tendon and muscle ruptures are generally related to sports or recreation; however, metabolic disease and age may be a causative factor. Runners may experience a quadriceps tear, whereas a biceps tear can occur with minimal effort in middle-age or older individuals. Surgery may be required to restore function for complete tears. For incomplete injury, rest and application of ice for 24 to 48 hours followed by heat application may be prescribed.

An Achilles tendon rupture can occur in start-and-stop sports in which a person steps off abruptly on the forefoot with the knee forced in extension. This causes sharp pain extending from the heel into the back of the leg, sudden inability to use the foot, obvious deformity, and a positive Thompson's sign (Figure 26-6). The patient may also report hearing a loud crack or snap. A compression bandage should be applied and the patient prepared for surgery.

Crush Injuries

Crush injuries frequently occur in industrial settings (e.g., arm caught in the wringer of an industrial washing machine, press, or conveyor; limbs or trunk caught between equipment). Injury may involve only the distal end of a digit or large areas of the body. Depending on extent of damage, orthopedic, surgical, neurosurgical, or vascular-surgical intervention may be required.

Complications from crush injuries depend on the mechanism of injury and extent of tissue damage. With significant tissue necrosis (multicompartment), systemic crush syndrome characterized by myoglobinuria, extracellular fluid loss, acidosis, increased potassium, renal failure, shock, and cardiac disruption may occur.

Compartment Syndrome

Compartment syndrome occurs when swelling or compression-restriction causes pressure in the muscle compartment to rise to the point that microvascular circulation is interrupted. The resulting tissue ischemia threatens limb survival. Compression from severe soft-tissue injuries, fracture, casts, or a pneumatic antishock garment (PASG) can cause compartment syndrome resulting from pressure on the compartments from outside the compartment.[4] Prolonged pressure directly on a limb, frostbite, or snakebite can lead to compartment syndrome. Compartment syndrome usually occurs in compartments of the lower leg and forearm (Figure 26-7). Symptoms develop 6 to 8 hours after injury but may be delayed 48 to 96 hours.

Symptoms include deep, throbbing pain out of proportion to the original injury that is not relieved by narcotics; pain with passive flexion; decreased mobility of digits; paresthesia; decreased or absent pulses; coolness; pallor; and tenseness of overlying skin. Pulses may be absent, decreased, or palpable with compartment syndrome.

Irreversible tissue damage occurs within 4 to 6 hours of ischemia; therefore, prompt physician notification is essential. The limb is positioned level with the heart, then neurovascular function is assessed hourly or more often if indicated to identify changes. Diagnosis is made by measuring compartment pressure with a syringe or catheter device (Figures 26-8 and 26-9). Pressures greater than 30 to 60 mm Hg require fasciotomy.[7] A high index of suspicion is necessary when caring for injured comatose patients who cannot verbalize increasing pain or paresthesia.

Peripheral Nerve and Artery Injury

The most common causes of peripheral nerve and artery injuries are lacerations, penetrating wounds, fractures, and dislocations. Joints are well innervated and vascularized so they are especially prone to nerve or artery damage. Familiarity with major nerves and arteries is necessary for assessment of tissue injuries. Table 26-2 summarizes major vessels, associated injuries, and assessment findings.

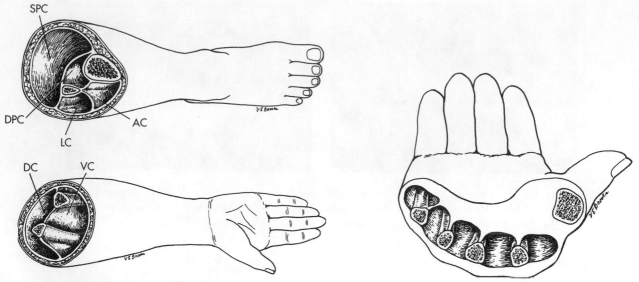

FIGURE 26-7   Cross-section anatomy of calf, forearm, and hand showing fibrosseous compartments. (From Matsen FA III: *Compartmental syndromes,* New York, 1980, Grune & Stratton.)

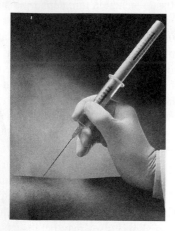

FIGURE 26-8   Intracompartmental pressure monitor. (Courtesy Millenium Medical Tech. Inc., Santa Fe, NM.)

Nerve injury may also occur from compression caused by prolonged PASG use or skeletal traction. Resolution of symptoms depends on the type of injury and length of time before compression is corrected. Partial nerve injury may be caused by a contusion that causes temporary paralysis and sensory deficit. Complete and total disruption of the nerve causes loss of all functions and usually requires surgical repair. Nerve evaluation and repair of an isolated injury may be done on an outpatient basis.

Axillary, brachial, radial, and ulnar arteries are the major arteries in the arms. Femoral, popliteal, anterior tibial, posterior tibial, and peroneal arteries are major arteries in the leg. High-impact and rapid-deceleration mechanisms are most likely to cause arterial injury. Assessment should evaluate pulse quality, skin color and temperature, capillary refill, bleeding, hematoma formation, and presence of bruits. Table 26-3 summarizes assessment for acute arterial is-

chemia. Arterial injuries may be difficult to discover; 10% to 15% of significant arterial disruptions can have detectable distal pulses. A Doppler ultrasonograph should be used for pulses that are difficult to palpate. Evaluation may require angiography; however, injury in association with an open fracture may be evaluated during surgery. Arterial injuries may not require repair if existing collateral circulation prevents ischemia. Complications of undiagnosed arterial disruptions include thrombosis, arteriovenous fistula, aneurysm, false aneurysm, and tissue ischemia with resultant limb dysfunction.

Strains

A strain is a weakening or overstretching of a muscle at the point of attachment to the tendon. Strains may occur as a result of almost any type of movement, from stepping off a curb and twisting the ankle to wrenching force caused by an MVC or violent muscle contraction. Strains are most often associated with athletic injuries.

A patient with a first-degree or mild strain complains of local pain, point tenderness, and slight muscle spasms. Therapeutic interventions include a compression bandage, intermittent elevation of the limb above heart level for 12 hours, application of a cold pack for the same period, and light weight-bearing on the injured part.

With a second-degree strain the patient has local pain, point tenderness, swelling, discoloration, and inability to use the limb for prolonged periods. Therapeutic interventions include a compression bandage, elevation and cold pack application for 24 hours; analgesia; and light weight-bearing.

Severe strains (third-degree) cause complete disruption of the muscle or tendon. This disruption can cause a small

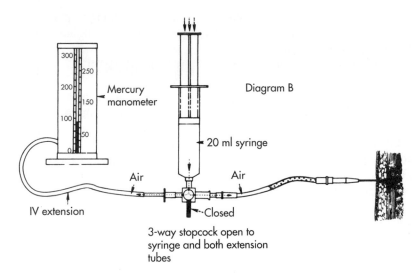

FIGURE 26-9 Whitesides' method for measuring intracompartmental pressure. (From Whitesides TE et al: Tissue pressure measurements as a determinant for the need of fasciotomy, *Clin Orthop Rel Res* 113:43, 1975.)

Table 26-2	ASSESSMENT OF COMMON PERIPHERAL NERVE INJURIES	
NERVE	FREQUENTLY ASSOCIATED INJURIES	ASSESSMENT FINDINGS
Radial	Fracture of humerus, especially middle and	Inability to extend thumb in "hitchhiker's sign"
Ulnar	distal thirds	Loss of pain perception in tip of little finger
Median	Fracture of medial humeral epicondyle	Loss of pain perception in tip of index finger
Peroneal	Elbow dislocation or wrist or forearm injury	Inability to extend great toe or foot; may also be associated with
	Tibia or fibula fracture; dislocation of knee	sciatic nerve injury
Sciatic and tibial	Infrequent with fractures or dislocations	Loss of pain perception in sole of foot

Table 26-3	THE "FIVE PS" OF ACUTE ARTERIAL ISCHEMIA	
NERVE	FREQUENTLY ASSOCIATED INJURIES	ASSESSMENT FINDINGS
Radial	Aching pain	Tenderness more proximal than numbness
Ulnar	Weakness or "giving out"	Weak extensors and flexors
Median	Numbness	Decreased to absent sensation, most dense distally
Peroneal	White and cold	Pallor (or dusky if has been dependent); coolness gradually decreasing proximally
Sciatic and tibial	Rarely appreciated by patient (pulselessness better replaced by coldness, such as in poikilothermia)	Better documented by segmental blood pressures or Doppler pulses being absent (pulselessness better replaced by "pressureless" or "Dopplerless" state)

From: Davis JH, Drucher WR et al: *Clinical surgery,* St. Louis, 1987, Mosby.

avulsion fracture that can be seen on x-rays. The patient complains of local pain, point tenderness, swelling, and discoloration. The patient describes a "snapping noise" at the time of injury. Therapeutic interventions include a compression bandage or splints, elevation, and cold pack application for 24 to 72 hours; analgesia; and no weight-bearing for 48 hours. Surgery may be required if a complete rupture occurs at the tendon-bone attachment site.

Sprains

Mechanism of injury for sprains may be the same as for strains, but a sprain is usually the result of more traumatic force. A sprain occurs when a joint exceeds its normal limit and damages ligaments. The patient may have a history of a popping or snapping sound. Sprains often occur in ankles, knees, and shoulders. In children, epiphyseal disruption is more common than ligamentous injury. A mild sprain (first-degree) produces slight pain and slight swelling. Therapeutic interventions include a compression bandage, elevation, cold pack application for 12 hours, and light weight-bearing. A moderate sprain (second-degree) causes pain, point tenderness, swelling, and inability to use the limb for more than a brief period. Therapeutic interventions include compression bandage, elevation, cold pack application for 24 hours, and light weight-bearing with crutches. A stirrup ankle brace applied to the ankle prevents inversion and eversion but allows flexion and extension. Figure 26-10 shows one brand of stirrup ankle brace.

A severe sprain (third-degree) involves torn ligaments, which cause pain, point tenderness, swelling, discoloration, and inability to use the limb. Therapeutic interventions include a splint or cast, elevation, and cold pack application for 48 hours, and light to no weight-bearing with crutches.

Knee Injuries

Knee injuries are a common form of soft-tissue injury in which rotational or extraflexion trauma strains or tears the medial meniscus, collateral ligament, or cruciate ligament. Symptoms include swelling, ecchymosis, effusion, pain, and tenderness. Therapeutic interventions include a compression bandage, knee immobilizer, or cylinder cast; elevation of the injured limb; intermittent cold pack application to the injured area for the first 24 hours; and non–weight-bearing

with crutch walking. If the injury is a ligament tear, surgical repair within 24 to 48 hours of injury is recommended.

TRAUMATIC AMPUTATIONS

Traumatic amputations occur among farm workers secondary to heavy farm machinery, in factory workers when a limb is caught by a heavy machine, and in motorcyclists when the motorcycle and driver collide with another vehicle. Other causes include snow blowers and lawn mowers. Body parts frequently amputated are digits (fingers, toes), distal half of the foot (transmetatarsal), leg (above, at, or below the knee), hand, forearm, arm, ears, nose, and penis.

Therapeutic interventions for amputations begin with stabilization of the ABCs including administration of high-flow oxygen, initiation of two large-bore intravenous (IV) lines, control of bleeding, and rapid transportation to a facility for definitive care. The limb should be supported and splinted in a position of anatomic function if the part is partially amputated. Figure 26-11 shows anatomic hand position. A completely amputated stump should be irrigated for gross contamination, dressed, and elevated. Antibiotics, a tetanus booster, and immune globulin as indicated should be initiated in the ED. Tourniquet application should be avoided.

Whenever possible the amputated part is preserved for reimplantation by wrapping it in saline gauze and placing in a plastic bag or container. The sealed container is then placed on top of crushed ice and water. This cools the part without causing direct damage to tissue. Placing the part directly on ice can cause cellular freezing and death. Cells are damaged by water moving across cellular membranes when the part is placed directly in water or ice. Distilled water is not used because of its deleterious effect on tissue.[4] Iodine should never be placed directly on the amputated part because of discoloration and effects on tissue viability. Maintain the limb in correct anatomic position.

Reimplantation

Occasionally reimplantation is possible. Limiting factors for successful reimplantation are availability of a reimplantation team, amount of damage to the attached and amputated parts, and time elapsed since the accident. Sharp cuts have a

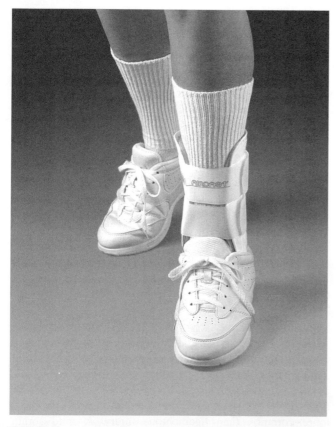

FIGURE **26-10** Stirrup splint. (Courtesy Aircast, Inc., Summit, NJ.)

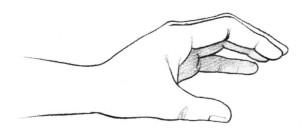

FIGURE **26-11** Anatomic position of the hand. (From Schwartz GR, editor: *Principles and practice of emergency medicine,* ed 4, Baltimore, 1999, Williams & Wilkins.)

better outcome than crush or avulsion-type injuries. Muscles can survive 12 hours of cold ischemia; bone, tendon, and skin can survive 24 hours. Warm survival time is much less. Predicted outcome of reimplantation is further determined by age, occupation, motivation, and general physical condition of the victim. Historically upper-extremity reimplantations are more successful than lower-extremity reimplantations, and children typically have a better outcome with this type of reimplantation.

FRACTURES

A fracture is a disruption or break in the bone. Patients arrive in the ED with angulation, deformity, pain, regional and point tenderness, swelling, immobility, and crepitus. Other findings include bony fragment protrusion, impaired neurovascular status, and occasionally shock.

Fractures are divided into two general categories. With closed or simple fractures, the bone is broken but the skin is intact. Open or compound fractures are characterized by bone protrusion or puncture wounds in which the bone punctures the skin or a foreign object penetrates the skin and bone, causing a fracture.

Open fractures are contaminated and require prophylactic antibiotic therapy. These fractures are graded by severity, then further categorized by wound size, amount of soft-tissue damage, injury to the periosteum, and vascular damage. Most open fractures require surgical debridement. Table 26-4 describes etiology for various types of fractures with illustrations for each type in Figure 26-12. A greater potential for shock exists with open fractures because of the potential for significant blood loss; closed injuries tamponade and limit blood loss. General nursing care includes IV access for fluid replacement, antibiotics, analgesia, and anesthesia. Wound

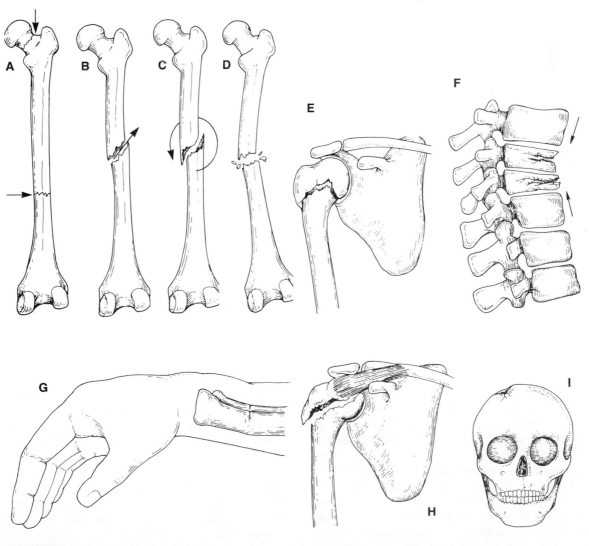

FIGURE 26-12 Types of fractures. **A,** Transverse fracture. **B,** Oblique fracture. **C,** Spiral fracture. **D,** Comminuted fracture. **E,** Impacted fracture. **F,** Compression fracture. **G,** Greenstick fracture. **H,** Avulsion fracture. **I,** Depression fracture.

Table 26-4 ETIOLOGY OF DIFFERENT TYPES OF FRACTURES	
TYPE	**ETIOLOGY**
Oblique fracture	Twisting force
Spiral fracture	Twisting force while foot is firmly planted
Comminuted fracture	Severe direct trauma causes more than two fragments
Impacted fracture	Severe trauma, causes fractured bone ends to jam together
Compression fracture	Severe force to top of head, sacrum, or os calsis (axial loading) forces vertebrae together
Greenstick fracture	Compression force; usually occurs in school-age children
Avulsion fracture	Forceful contraction of a muscle mass; causes a bone fragment to break away at the insertion point
Depressed fracture	Blunt trauma to a flat bone; usually associated with significant soft-tissue damage

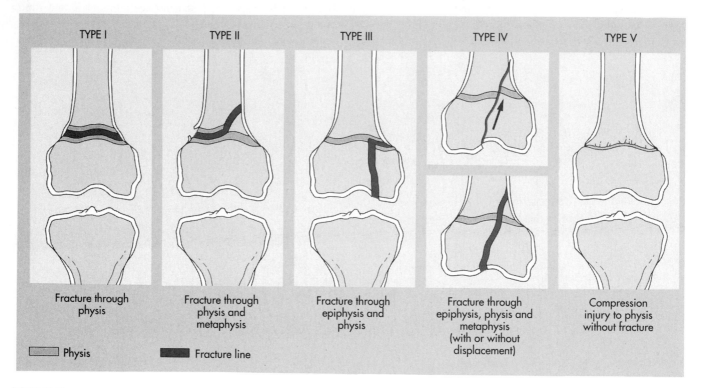

FIGURE 26-13 Salter Harris classification. (From Zittelli BJ, Davis HW: *Atlas of pediatric physical diagnosis,* ed 3, Philadelphia, 1997, WB Saunders.)

care includes irrigation with normal saline, covering with a dry sterile dressing, and verification of tetanus immunization status. Wound culture may be ordered before irrigation.

After evaluation of ABCs, specific limb injury assessment should be completed followed by immobilization, elevation, and ice packs. Repeated neurovascular assessments are essential to identify changes secondary to swelling. History should be obtained to determine mechanism of injury. The emergency nurse should also be alert for signs of abuse when the injury does not match the history. Understanding patterns of injury also facilitates assessment and identification of less obvious injuries. (Refer to Chapter 19 for discussion of mechanism of injury.)

When a limb suffers significant trauma, a fracture should be suspected until proven otherwise by radiologic studies. Radiography should include both anterior and lateral views because fractures may appear from only one angle.[1] Joints above and below the injury should be included in all radiographic evaluation.

Open fractures and certain closed fractures require surgical intervention. Ideally, patients with open fractures have surgery within 8 hours of injury. The patient should be kept NPO and prepared for surgery. IV lines are inserted, with consent obtained before narcotics are administered. Prophylactic broad-spectrum antibiotics are given as soon as possible for open fractures and vascular injuries.

Fractures are associated with numerous complications. Jagged bone ends may lacerate vital organs, arteries, and nerves, causing hemorrhage and neurovascular compromise. Open fractures can lead to serious infections that can lead to permanent limb dysfunction or limb loss. Long-term complications of fractures include nonunion, deformity, disability, avascular necrosis from decreased blood supply, and Volkman's contracture secondary to untreated compartment syndrome.

Fat embolism is a relatively uncommon, but life-threatening, sequela of bone injury, which presents 24 to 48 hours after injury. Seen most often with pelvic, femoral, or tibial fractures, this complication has a high mortality rate. Fracture causes release of fat particles into the bloodstream that embolize to end-organs, particularly pulmonary vasculature. The patient suddenly develops tachycardia accompanied by elevated temperature, altered level of consciousness, tachypnea, cough, shortness of breath, cyanosis, petechiae, and pulmonary edema leading to adult respiratory distress syndrome. Immediate therapeutic interventions include high-flow oxygen, support of ABCs, and possible administration of a corticosteroid and heparin (see Chapter 32).

Fractures occur frequently among children 6 to 16 years old and the elderly. Children's bones are softer and more porous, and therefore more likely to have a partial or greenstick fracture. Epiphyseal or growth plate (Salter-type) fractures may affect future bone growth because of early closure of the epiphyseal plate and resultant limb shortening (Figure 26-13). Angulation may occur with partial growth plate fractures because bone growth continues in the noninjured area. Epiphyseal fractures require close orthopedic follow-up for several months to monitor healing and identify growth abnormalities. Another concern with pediatric fractures is bleeding. A child with a femur fracture can lose 300 to 1000 ml of blood, a significant amount given the child's body size and circulating blood volume.

Elderly patients have brittle bones because of calcium loss associated with aging. This physiologic change combined with the problems the elderly have with balance increase the risk of falls and fractures. These patients may also have multiple medical problems that complicate recovery. Planning home care may be difficult for the elderly patient with a fracture who may be already challenged by normal activities of daily living. A cast and crutches cause greater loss of balance and impaired mobility.

Fracture Healing

Bone healing occurs over weeks or can take several months (Figure 26-14). Fracture healing is determined by the type of bone, type of fracture, degree of opposition, immobility, and general state of health. Infection and decreased neurovascular supply hamper healing, as does chronic hypoxia. Conversely, exercise promotes bone healing. Alterations in healing are described as delayed, malunion (residual deformity), and nonunion (failure to unite).

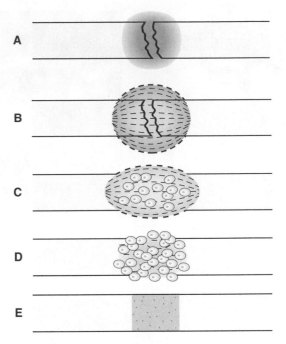

FIGURE 26-14   Bone healing (schematic representation). **A,** Bleeding at broken ends of the bone with subsequent hematoma formation. **B,** Organization of hematoma into fibrous network. **C,** Invasion of osteoblasts, lengthening of collagen strands, and deposition of calcium. **D,** Callus formation: new bone is built up as osteoclasts destroy dead bone. **E,** Remodeling accomplished as excess callus is reabsorbed and trabecular bone is laid down. (From Lewis SM, Collier IC, Heitkemper MM: *Medical-surgical nursing,* ed 4, St. Louis, 1996, Mosby.)

Upper Torso Fractures

Bones in the upper torso that communicate with the upper extremities include the clavicle and scapula.

Clavicular Fracture

Fracture of the clavicle occurs in all age-groups (Figure 26-15) but is particularly common in children and adolescents. A fall on an arm or shoulder, such as contact injury when athletes run into each other or with direct frontal impact, is a frequently reported mechanism of injury. Eighty percent of fractures occur in the middle third of the clavicle. Patients complain of pain in the clavicular area with point tenderness, swelling, deformity, and crepitus. The patient will not raise the affected arm and tilts the head toward the side of injury with the chin directed toward the opposite side. Neurovascular status of the arm is assessed, with the arm supported, and the shoulder placed in a figure eight support (Figure 26-16). A sling or sling and swathe may be used for an elderly patient. The patient should be instructed to apply a cold pack intermittently to the injured area for 12 to 24 hours and to take only tub or sponge baths. A referral should be given for orthopedic follow-up. Complications include

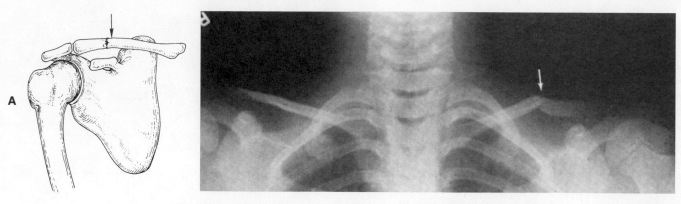

FIGURE 26-15 A, Clavicle fracture. B, Arrow on radiograph shows fracture.

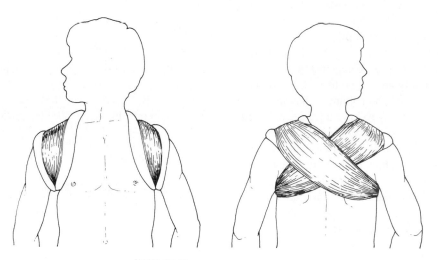

FIGURE 26-16 Figure-eight support.

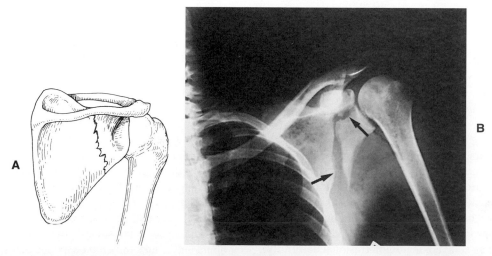

FIGURE 26-17 A, Scapular fracture. B, Radiograph. (B, From Ballinger PW: *Merrill's atlas of radiographic positions and radiologic procedures,* ed 8, St. Louis, 1995, Mosby.)

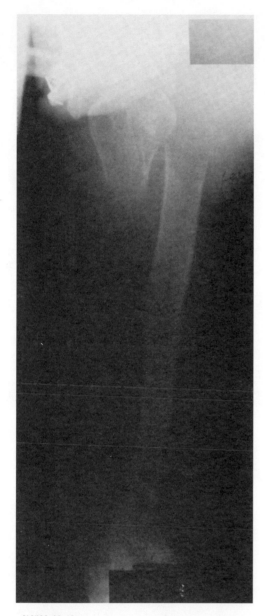

FIGURE 26-18 Radiograph of shoulder fracture.

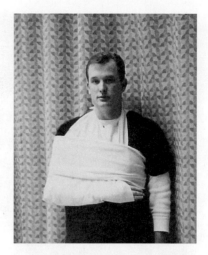

FIGURE 26-19 Sling and swath.

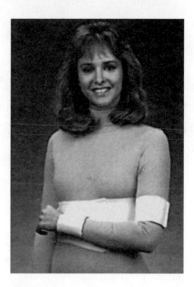

FIGURE 26-20 Example of shoulder immobilizer. (From Proehl JA: *Emergency nursing procedures,* ed 2, Philadelphia, 1999, WB Saunders.)

pneumothorax and hemothorax, particularly from the more serious frontal-impact injuries and brachial plexus injuries.[4]

Scapular Fracture

Scapular fractures occur in 1% of all fractures, primarily in young men (Figure 26-17). This injury is usually caused by violent, direct trauma but may be seen with severe muscle contraction. Associated injuries include pulmonary contusions and rib fractures. Common mechanisms of injury include MVCs, falls, and crush injuries. Patients complain of point tenderness and pain during shoulder movement. Bone displacement and swelling over the injured area may be evident. Therapeutic interventions include assessment of neurovascular status of the affected arm, placement of a compression bandage over the scapula if bone is not displaced, sling and swath bandage or shoulder immobilizer for 1 to 2 weeks, and application of a cold pack for the first 24 hours.

Complications include injuries to underlying ribs or viscera from the force required to cause the fracture.

Upper Extremity Fractures

Shoulder Fracture

A shoulder fracture is a fracture of the glenoid, humeral head, or humeral neck (Figure 26-18). Shoulder fractures occur frequently in elderly patients resulting from a fall on an outstretched arm or direct trauma to the shoulder. When this same mechanism of injury occurs in a younger person, shoulder dislocation usually occurs. Fracture occurs in an elderly person because of the weaker bone structure.

The patient arrives with pain in the shoulder area, point tenderness, immobility of the affected arm, gross swelling, and discoloration. The majority of injuries are impacted or nondisplaced and require only a sling and swath (Figure 26-19) or shoulder immobilizer (Figure 26-20). A Velpeau

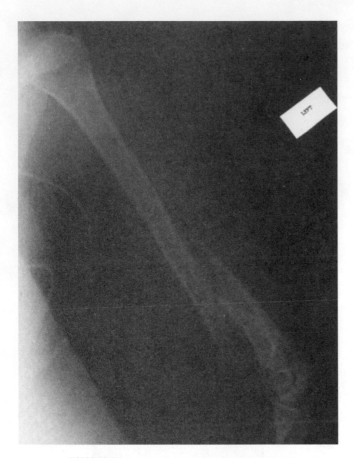

FIGURE **26-21**   Radiograph of humerus fracture.

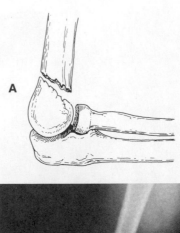

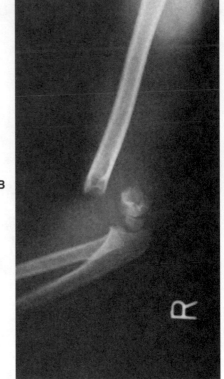

FIGURE **26-22**   **A,** Elbow fracture. **B,** Radiograph.

version of the sling and swath (with the affected hand pointing to the opposite shoulder) may be used. A significantly displaced fracture may require open reduction or skeletal traction but is generally reduced with closed traction. This injury truly complicates activities of daily living and requires extra planning for home care, particularly for an elderly patient living alone. Complications include neurovascular compromise (axillary nerve) and possible adhesive capsulitis or "frozen" (stiff) shoulder.

Upper Arm Fractures

Fractures of the upper arm (humeral shaft) are commonly seen in children and the elderly (Figure 26-21). This type of fracture results from a fall on the arm, direct trauma, or in association with dislocation of the shoulder and may also occur as a stress injury with lifting weights. The patient complains of point tenderness and significant discomfort. Swelling, inability or hesitancy to use the arm, severe deformity or angulation, and crepitus also occur. Therapeutic interventions include a sling and swath and assessment for other injuries (e.g., chest trauma). The fracture is usually reduced by closed reduction with mild, steady, downward traction. The arm is casted with a Y-shaped (sugar-tong) plaster splint applied from the axilla, around the elbow, and back to the shoulder (acromial process). The patient should

sit and lean forward during this procedure. The arm may be secured to the chest for additional stabilization. In addition to routine cast care instructions, the patient should be given instructions to exercise the wrist and fingers frequently. Radial nerve damage can accompany fracture of the middle or distal portion of the shaft. Hemorrhage is possible if bleeding is not controlled within moments of the injury.

Elbow Fractures

Elbow fractures (Figure 26-22) are seen most often in young children and athletes. These injuries occur with a fall on an extended arm or flexed elbow, such as a fall from a skateboard. Fractures of the elbow involve the distal humerus or head of the ulna or radius. Typically, supracondylar fractures of the humerus are extension injuries and are more likely to damage the brachial artery. Ulnar head fractures are generally the result of a direct blow and usually comminuted.

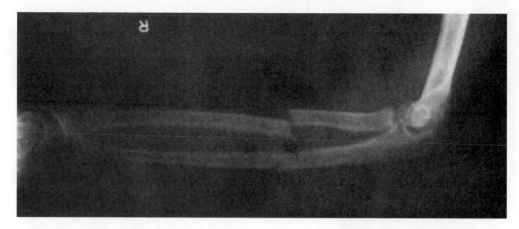

FIGURE **26-23** Radiograph of fracture of radius and ulna.

Elbow fractures are associated with considerable swelling and potential neurovascular compromise. Prompt initial assessment should be followed by serial assessment every 30 to 60 minutes. If compromise is present, the arm may be flexed at a greater angle. The arm should be splinted as found and a sling applied. When closed reduction is employed, the arm is casted and placed in a sling. Sling immobilization is usually sufficient for radial head fractures. Open reduction and fixation is required for comminuted or intra-articular fractures. Complications associated with elbow fractures include brachial artery laceration, nerve (median, radial, or ulnar) damage, and Volkmann's contracture.

Volkmann's contracture is due to ischemia of muscles and nerves from untreated compartment syndrome. The patient presents with inability to move his or her fingers, severe pain with manipulation, severe pain in forearm flexor muscles even after reduction, pulse deficit, swelling, extremity coolness, cyanosis, and decreased sensation. Temporary therapeutic intervention includes cast removal and extension of the forearm with possible cold pack application. Prompt orthopedic consultation is essential for further therapeutic intervention. Nonintervention leads to atrophy and a claw-like deformity.

Forearm Fractures

Forearm fractures include fractures of the radius and ulna. Common in adults and children, forearm fractures usually result from a fall on an extended arm or a direct blow (Figure 26-23). The patient has pain, point tenderness, swelling, deformity, angulation, and, occasionally, shortening of the extremity. Therapeutic interventions include a splint to immobilize the fracture and a sling. Many fractures can be manipulated by closed reduction, then casted with the elbow flexed 90 degrees. The shoulder and fingers should be free of the cast. If a sling is used the entire arm and hand should be supported. The hand should not become dependent or droop at the wrist. Complications of forearm fractures include neurovascular compromise leading to Volkmann's contracture.

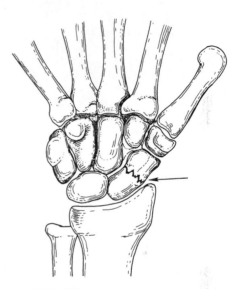

FIGURE **26-24** Wrist fracture (carpal).

Wrist and Hand Fractures

Carpal Fractures

The scaphoid is the carpal bone most prone to fracture (Figure 26-24). The patient complains of tenderness over the depression in the wrist on the thumb side of the hand (anatomic snuffbox). A specific navicular-view radiograph demonstrates scaphoid fractures best; however, fractures may not appear on radiographs for 2 to 4 weeks. If symptoms are present, a cast is placed regardless of negative radiographs. Complications include avascular necrosis or tissue death from loss of blood supply.

Wrist Fractures

Fractures of the wrist include the distal radius, distal ulna, and carpal bones of the hand (Figure 26-25). The most common mechanism is a fall onto an extended arm and open hand, causing swelling and deformity. Fractures of the distal radius and ulna are the most common fracture, typically

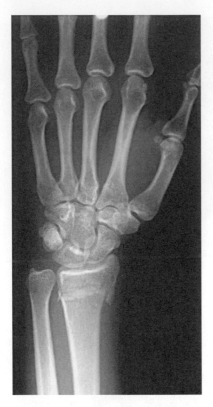

FIGURE **26-25** Wrist fracture (radius). (From Ballinger PW: *Merrill's atlas of radiographic positions and radiologic procedures,* ed 8, St. Louis, 1995, Mosby.)

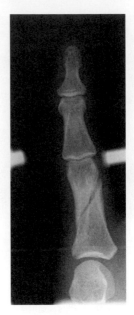

FIGURE **26-27** Fractured fifth digit. (From Ballinger PW: *Merrill's atlas of radiographic positions and radiologic procedures,* ed 8, St. Louis, 1995, Mosby.)

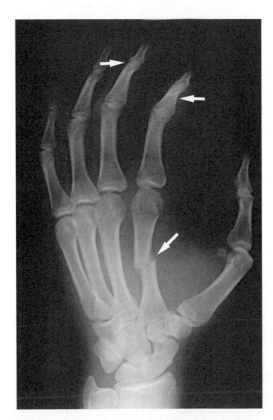

FIGURE **26-26** Metacarpal fracture. (From Ballinger PW: *Merrill's atlas of radiographic positions and radiologic procedures,* ed 8, St. Louis, 1995, Mosby.)

seen in the elderly. A Colles' fracture may also occur in association with a calcaneus and vertebral fracture sustained in a fall from a height. Wrist fractures are generally manipulated with closed reduction and then casted. Some physicians may not prescribe a sling because it can hinder elevation; some prefer a hanging apparatus, such as an IV pole for the first 2 days of elevation, even for home care.

Metacarpal Fractures

Fractures of the metacarpals (Figure 26-26) are common athletic injuries, particularly during contact sports. Striking a person or wall with a closed fist causes a boxer's fracture, a fracture of the fifth metacarpal. Throwing a baseball may cause the distal attachment of the extensor tendon to tear loose along with a segment of bone, causing an avulsion fracture. Industrial crush injuries to the hand can also fracture metacarpals. If an open fracture occurs, a compression bandage is used to control bleeding. Rings are removed before swelling increases and makes removal difficult. Metacarpal fractures are seldom displaced to any degree and are generally casted in the ED.

Phalanx Fractures

Fractured phalanges (fingers) are common in all age-groups (Figure 26-27). Symptoms are similar to those for carpal and metacarpal fractures with therapeutic interventions basically the same. Sometimes a phalanx fracture is associated with a hematoma beneath the fingernail (subungual hematoma) causing severe, throbbing pain. Therapeutic intervention for phalanx fractures is usually splinting the finger (Figure 26-28). Occasionally, surgical reduction is necessary to re-

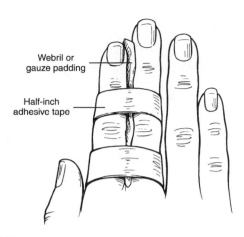

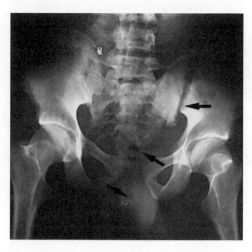

FIGURE 26-28 Buddy taping or dynamic splinting. (From Chudnofsky CR: Splinting techniques. In Roberts JR, Hedges JR, editors: *Clinical procedures in emergency medicine,* ed 3, Philadelphia, 1998, WB Saunders.)

FIGURE 26-29 Pelvis fracture. (From Ballinger PW: *Merrill's atlas of radiographic positions and radiologic procedures,* ed 8, St. Louis, 1995, Mosby.)

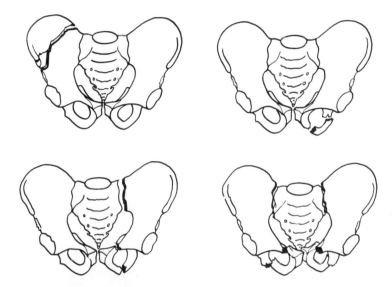

FIGURE 26-30 Types of pelvic fractures. (From Sheehy SB et al: *Manual of clinical trauma care,* ed 3, St. Louis, 1999, Mosby.)

align fractured segments. Subungual hematoma is treated with nail trephination.

Pelvic Fractures

Pelvic fractures (Figure 26-29) occur most frequently in middle-age and elderly adults with a mortality of 8% to 10%. Mortality is much greater when the patient has an open pelvic fracture. Open fractures into the rectum or vagina comprise approximately 3% of pelvic injuries but have a 40% to 60% mortality.[3] An estimated 65% of patients with pelvic fractures have other injuries, coexisting in nearly 30% of all multiple trauma injuries. Vehicular trauma, particularly in pedestrians, accounts for almost two thirds of pelvic fractures.[6] Other causes are direct trauma, falls from

a height, sudden contraction of a muscle against a resistance, and even doing splits while waterskiing. Pelvic fractures are classified as stable or unstable, depending on disruption of the pelvic ring (Figure 26-30). A particularly unstable fracture results from vertical-shear force, which causes significant bone and tissue damage. Specific neurovascular structures at risk for injury with pelvic fractures include the iliac artery, venous plexus, and sciatic nerve.

Compression of iliac wings causes tenderness over the pubis in the patient with a pelvic fracture. These patients also have paraspinous muscle spasm, sacroiliac joint tenderness, paresis or hemiparesis, pelvic ecchymosis, and hematuria. Hemorrhagic shock resulting from associated blood loss should be suspected in the patient with tachycardia and hypotension.

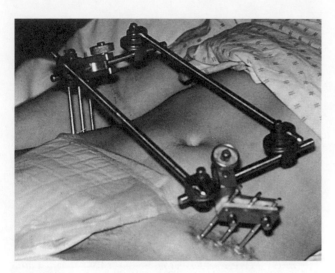

FIGURE 26-31 External fixator: pelvis. (From Maher AB, Salmond SW, Pellino TA: *Orthopedic nursing,* ed 2, Philadelphia, 1998, WB Saunders.)

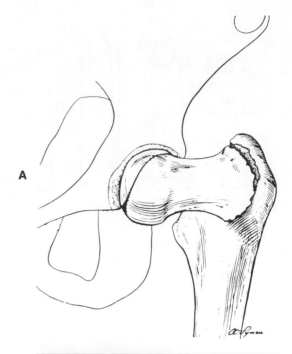

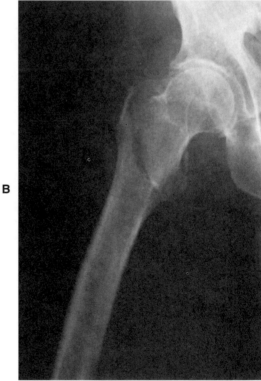

FIGURE 26-32 **A,** Hip fracture. **B,** Radiograph.

Therapeutic interventions include high-flow oxygen, serial vital signs, and two large-bore IV lines for volume replacement titrated to blood pressure and pulse rate. The spine and legs are immobilized with a long spine board. Flexing the knees may decrease pain. Patients with pelvic fractures bleed profusely, so blood should be typed and cross-matched for at least 4 to 5 units. Average blood loss is 2 units with potential loss of 4000 ml or more.[4] A urinary catheter should be inserted cautiously in the patient with pelvic trauma because of the potential for associated urethral injury. Never insert a urinary catheter when the patient has blood at the meatus or there is penile deformity in a male patient.

Definitive interventions depend on the severity of the fracture. Unstable, weight-bearing fractures are treated with external fixation devices or with open reduction using internal fixation devices. External fixation devices (Figure 26-31) may be applied in the ED for some patients. Less severe, non–weight-bearing injuries are treated with bed rest and traction.

Complications from pelvic fractures include bladder trauma, genital trauma, lumbosacral trauma, ruptured internal organs, sepsis, shock, and death. Long-term complications include thrombophlebitis, fat embolism, chronic pain, and loss of function.

Hip Fractures

Hip fractures are common in the elderly and are usually caused by falls or minor trauma (Figure 26-32). Conversely, major trauma accounts for most hip fracture in younger patients. Fractures can occur in the femoral head, femoral neck (intracapsular), and intertrochanteric region. Femoral head fractures are rare but generally are associated with a high-speed MVC. Symptoms associated with hip fractures include pain in the groin, hip, knee, severe pain with leg movement, and immobility. Patients with greater trochanteric fractures can be ambulatory. Extracapsular, trochanteric fractures are associated with pain in the lateral hip, increased shortening of the extremity, and a greater degree of external rotation.

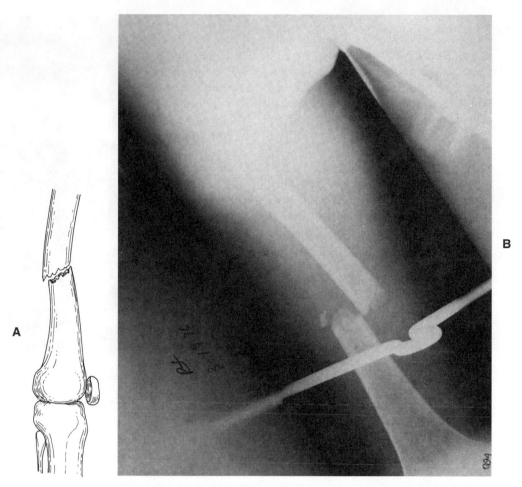

FIGURE 26-33 **A,** Femur fracture. **B,** Radiograph.

Immediate therapeutic interventions include splinting the hip to a long spine board or to the opposite leg. Monitoring serial vital signs is recommended because of the potential for blood loss. Early immobilization with Bucks traction or surgical intervention is often necessary. Complications of hip fracture include hypovolemia, shock, avascular necrosis with femoral head and neck fractures, and nonunion.

Lower Extremity Fractures

Femoral Fracture

Femoral fractures (Figure 26-33) occur in all age-groups, usually secondary to major trauma. The patient has severe pain, inability to bear weight on the injured leg, deformity, swelling, and angulation. Severe muscle spasms cause significant pain and also cause the limb to shorten. Crepitus occurs over the fracture site as bone pieces move.

Initial therapeutic intervention includes use of a Hare, Sager, or Thomas splint for traction. A long air splint with an enclosed foot or using the other leg as a splint is not recommended because these methods do not provide adequate stability. Associated injuries such as knee trauma are assessed. Intravenous access is established, ideally in two

sites, and vital signs are monitored frequently. Analgesia and volume replacement should be determined on an individual basis. The patient should be prepared for traction, pin placement in the ED, or surgery.

The greatest complication of femoral fracture is shock secondary to hypovolemia. Blood loss of more than 2 units into the thigh is not uncommon and can exceed 3000 ml. Severe muscle spasms can move bone ends, causing further soft-tissue injury, muscle damage, and pain. Neurovascular structures that can be damaged include the peroneal nerve, sciatic nerve, and popliteal artery.

Knee Fractures

Knee fractures may be supracondylar fractures of the femur or intraarticular fractures of the femur or tibia (Figure 26-34). This type of injury occurs in all age-groups and is usually the result of automobile, motorcycle, or automobile-pedestrian collisions that cause direct trauma to the knee.[5] Patients complain of knee pain, inability to bend or straighten the knee (depending on position of the knee at the time of injury), swelling, and tenderness. Therapeutic interventions include a long leg splint or securing one leg to the other. Depending on extent of injury, the patient may require

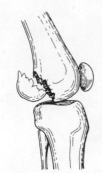

FIGURE 26-34 Knee fracture.

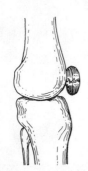

FIGURE 26-35 Patellar fracture.

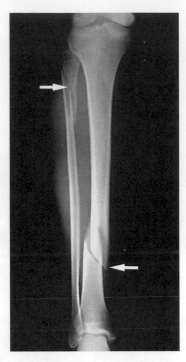

FIGURE 26-36 Tibia/fibula fracture. (From Ballinger PW: *Merrill's atlas of radiographic positions and radiologic procedures,* ed 8, vol 1, St. Louis, 1995, Mosby.)

surgical repair. The knee will most likely be casted. The most common complication of knee fractures is neurovascular compromise of the peroneal or tibial nerve or popliteal artery.

Patellar Fractures

Patellar fractures are seen in all age-groups (Figure 26-35), usually after direct trauma from a fall or impact with the dashboard. Indirect trauma such as a severe muscle pull can also cause fracture of the patella. The patient presents with knee pain and often has an obvious deformity of the patella. Open fractures also occur. Therapeutic interventions include covering the open wound and applying a long leg splint. Radiographs of the affected limb should be obtained to determine extent of the fracture. Treatment for a nondisplaced patellar fracture is use of a long leg cylinder cast. If the fracture is displaced, reduction is attempted to realign fractured parts with surgery if appropriate. The patella is an important part of the knee that aids in leverage and protects the knee joint. Complete disruption of extension warrants surgery.

Tibial and Fibular Fractures

Tibial and fibular fractures are seen in all age-groups (Figure 26-36) secondary to direct trauma, indirect trauma, or rotational force. The patient has pain in the leg, point tenderness, swelling, deformity, and crepitus. Many tibial and fibular fractures are open. Open and closed tibial injuries should be splinted as they are found; realignment should

not be attempted unless neurovascular compromise is present with an open fracture. Any open wounds should be covered with a dry sterile dressing. The patient with a stable, nondisplaced tibial fracture may be discharged in a long leg splint or cast. Open or closed reduction may be necessary when the fracture is unstable or displaced. Reduction of these fractures is followed by application of a splint or cast. Use of a cast or splint immediately after reduction is determined by the degree of edema and the potential for it to increase.[5]

An isolated fibular fracture is unusual. A walking cast is usually applied because the fibula is not a weight-bearing bone. Complications of tibial and fibular fractures include blood loss up to 2 L, infection, soft-tissue damage, neurovascular compromise, compartment syndrome, and Volkmann's contracture.[5]

Ankle Fractures

Fractures of the ankle involve the distal tibia, distal fibula, or talus and occur in all age-groups (Figure 26-37). Direct trauma, indirect trauma, or torsion can lead to open or closed ankle fractures. Fracture-dislocations also occur (Figure 26-38). The patient complains of pain in the injured area, inability to bear weight on the extremity, point tenderness, swelling, and deformity. After closed reduction the patient is placed in a walking cast. Depending on extent of injury, the patient may require open reduction and pinning. The most frequent complication is neurovascular compromise, particularly of the peroneal nerve.

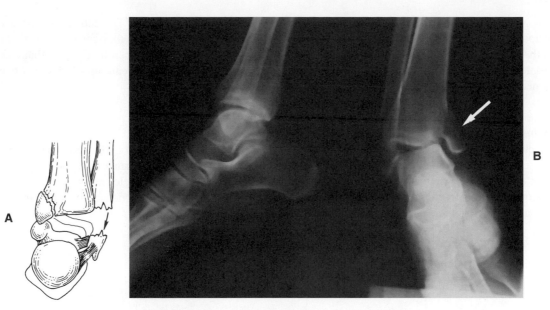

FIGURE 26-37 **A,** Ankle fracture. **B,** Radiograph.

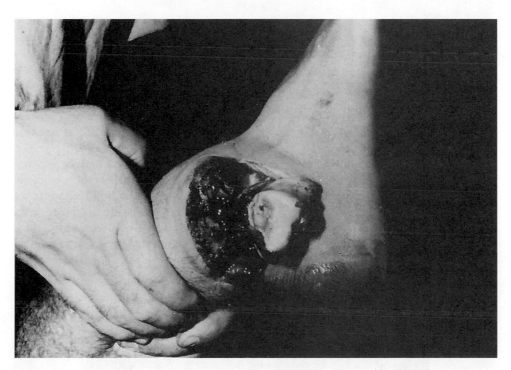

FIGURE 26-38 Open fracture dislocation of the talus. (From Davis et al: *Clinical surgery,* St. Louis, 1987, Mosby.)

Foot Fractures

Tarsal and Metatarsal Fractures. Fractures of the tarsals and metatarsals (Figure 26-39) occur in all age-groups, usually from MVCs, athletic injuries, crush injuries, or direct trauma. Fifth metatarsal fractures can occur with inversion injuries of the foot. The patient complains of pain in the foot and hesitates to bear weight. Therapeutic intervention includes a compression dressing and soft splint.

Minimally displaced fractures are treated with open-toed walking shoes or casts. With significant displacement, open reduction may be required. Crutches may be used to assist with weight-bearing or non–weight-bearing. Complications from this type of fracture are rare.

Calcaneus Fracture. Fractures of the calcaneus are usually seen in young adults secondary to a fall in which the victim lands on his or her feet (Figure 26-40). The patient complains of pain in the heel, point tenderness, and swelling. Dislocation may also occur. Management includes reduction of the fracture when necessary and application of a below-the-knee, weight-bearing cast. Open reduction is occasionally necessary. Associated injuries seen with calcaneus fractures include lumbosacral compression fracture and Colles' fracture.

Toe (Phalangeal) Fracture. Fractures of the toes (Figure 26-41) occur in all age-groups secondary to kicking a hard object or running into an immovable object. The patient has pain in the toe, swelling, and discoloration. Felt or cotton is placed between the fractured toe and adjacent toe, then both toes are taped together (buddy taped) so the unin-

jured toe acts as a splint. The patient may bear weight as tolerated and is instructed to wear hard-soled shoes, such as wooden or hard-soled open-toed shoes, that do not put pressure on the toes. Complications are rare, but nail injury may occur.

DISLOCATIONS

Dislocations occur when a joint exceeds its normal range of motion so that joint surfaces are no longer intact. Partial (subluxation) or complete separation of both articulating surfaces can occur. Soft-tissue injuries within the joint capsule and surrounding ligaments; severe swelling; and nerve,

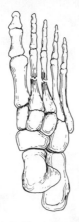

FIGURE **26-39**   Foot fracture.

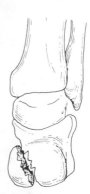

FIGURE **26-40**   Heel fracture.

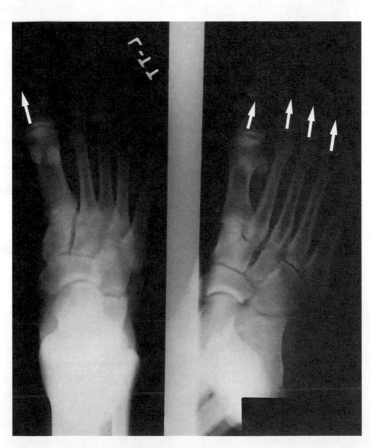

FIGURE **26-41**   Radiograph of toe fracture.

vein, and artery damage are observed with dislocations. Diagnosis can often be predicted before radiographs are taken by soliciting information about mechanisms of injury.

In general, dislocations produce severe pain, joint deformity, inability to move the joint, swelling, and point tenderness. Potential for vascular compromise also exists, so the pulse should be assessed carefully. Initial interventions include careful palpation of the joint and splinting the joint as it is found. Analgesia and sedation is given before reduction by the ED physician or orthopedist. Significant sedation (e.g., morphine, fentanyl, midazolan, methohexital, etomidate, propofol) may be required to reduce dislocations, so the patient should be carefully monitored.[7] Nitrous oxide is used in some institutions. Complications related to dislocations include ischemia, aseptic necrosis, and recurrent dislocations.

Acromioclavicular Dislocation

Acromioclavicular separations (Figure 26-42) are commonly seen in athletes secondary to a fall or direct force on the point of the shoulder. The patient complains of great pain in the joint area and cannot raise the affected arm or bring the arm across the chest. Deformity, point or area tenderness, swelling, and hematoma over the injury site are also noted. The separation is usually reduced, then the arm and shoulder is immobilized with a sling and swath. Occasionally, the patient requires surgery for open reduction and wiring. The patient may experience painful range of motion after reduction.

Shoulder Dislocation

Dislocations of the shoulder usually occur in children and athletes. Two general categories are anterior and posterior dislocations.

Anterior shoulder dislocations occur as an athletic injury when the athlete falls on an extended arm that is abducted and externally rotated. The force pushes the head of the humerus in front of the shoulder joint (Figure 26-43). Posterior dislocations are rare and usually occur in patients with seizures when the arm is abducted and internally rotated.

In all shoulder dislocations the patient complains of severe pain in the shoulder area, inability to move the arm, and deformity. Deformity is sometimes difficult to see in posterior dislocation. An estimated 55% to 60% of shoulder dislocations seen in the ED are recurrent.[9] The extremity is placed in the position of greatest comfort, then distal pulses are checked, followed by skin temperature and moisture evaluation, and neurologic status assessment. Radiographs are obtained before the joint is relocated unless neurovascular compromise has occurred. Figures 26-44 to 26-47 illustrate techniques for reducing shoulder dislocations. After the joint is relocated, it is immobilized with a sling and swath bandage or shoulder immobilizer. Postreduction radiographs are obtained to confirm placement. The patient should be re-

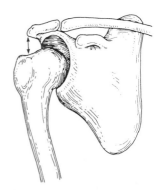

FIGURE 26-42 Acromioclavicular separation.

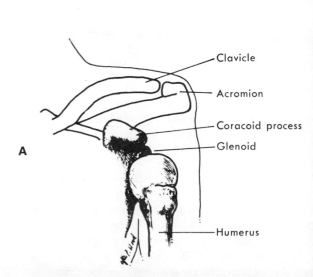

Clavicle
Acromion
Coracoid process
Glenoid
Humerus

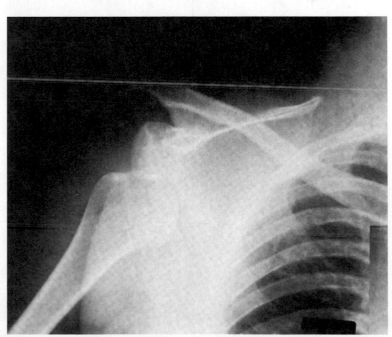

FIGURE 26-43 **A,** Anterior shoulder dislocation. **B,** Radiograph.

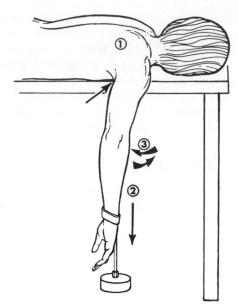

FIGURE **26-44** Stimson technique. *(1)* Patient lies prone on the edge of the stretcher with the shoulder at the edge. *(2)* Weights are attached to the arm, then the patient lies in this position for 20 to 30 minutes as needed. *(3)* Gentle external and internal rotation may also be used to aid reduction. (From Roberts J, Hedges J: *Clinical procedures in emergency medicine,* ed 3, Philadelphia, 1998, WB Saunders.)

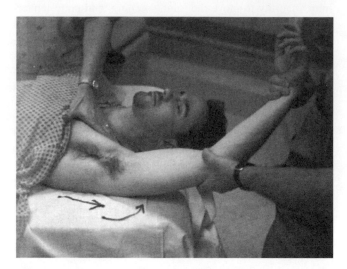

FIGURE **26-46** Milch technique. Apply slow steady abduction with overhead traction, external rotation (not shown), and direct pressure over the humeral head. (From Roberts J, Hedges J: *Clinical procedures in emergency medicine,* ed 3, Philadelphia, 1998, WB Saunders.)

A

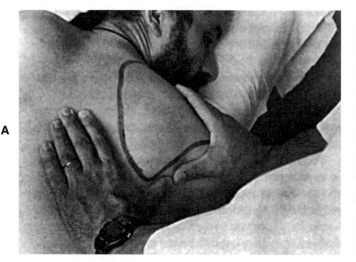

B

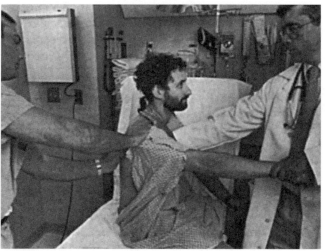

FIGURE **26-45** Scapular manipulation technique. **A.** Inferior tip of the scapula is pushed medially and dorsally with the thumbs while the superior aspect of the scapula is stabilized. Weights attached to the arm are used to apply hanging traction. **B.** With the patient seated, one hand applies traction and one hand applies countertraction while an assistant rotates the scapula in the same manner as A. (From Roberts J, Hedges J: *Clinical procedures in emergency medicine,* ed 3, Philadelphia, 1998, WB Saunders.)

ferred to an orthopedic surgeon. Complications from this type of injury are neurovascular compromise of the brachial plexus and axillary artery and associated fractures.

Elbow Dislocation

Dislocations of the elbow (Figure 26-48) are seen most often in children, teenagers, and young adults. Elbow dislocation is a common athletic injury caused from a fall on an externally rotated arm or when a young child is jerked or lifted by a single arm (known as nursemaid's elbow). The patient complains of pain in the joint, which may feel "locked." Any movement can produce severe pain. Swelling, deformity, and displacement are also noted. The arm is immobilized in the position of greatest comfort. The joint is relocated, then immobilized after radiographs are obtained. The most common complication of this injury is neurovascular compromise to the median nerve or brachial artery.

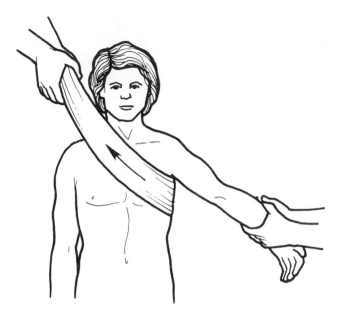

FIGURE 26-47   Traction-countertraction method for reducing anterior shoulder dislocations. (From Rosen P, Barkin RM, Hockberger RS et al: *Emergency medicine: concepts and clinical practice,* ed 4, St. Louis, 1998, Mosby.)

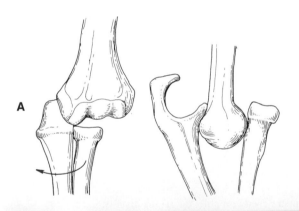

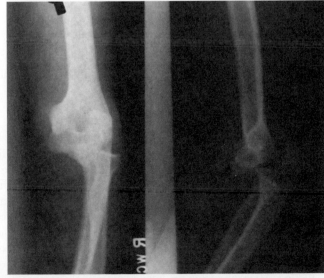

FIGURE 26-48   **A,** Elbow dislocation. **B,** Radiograph.

Radial head subluxation (nursemaid's elbow) accounts for about 20% of upper extremity injuries in children and is seen in children ages 6 months to 5 years, most often in 1- to 3-year-olds. History of a pull on the arm or a fall is reported. Figure 26-49 illustrates the process that leads to nursemaid's elbow. The child refuses to use the arm but does not seem in pain or distress. The injury does not require radiographic studies if the dislocation can be easily relocated with good return of function.

Wrist Dislocation

Dislocation of the wrist (Figure 26-50) is seen most frequently in athletes but does occur in all age-groups from a fall on an outstretched hand. The patient complains of severe pain in the wrist with swelling, deformity, and point tenderness. The wrist is placed in a splint in the position of comfort, then a cold pack is applied. Radiographic studies are obtained, the joint is relocated, and a cast is applied. Complications include neurovascular compromise, especially median nerve damage.

Hand or Finger Dislocation

Hand or finger dislocations (Figure 26-51) are usually seen in athletes secondary to a fall on an outstretched hand or finger and may also result from direct trauma to the tip of the finger. The patient presents with pain in area of the injury, inability to move the joint, deformity, and swelling. The injury is splinted in the position of comfort and a cold pack applied until radiographs are obtained and relocation is attempted. The injured area is usually splinted to immobilize the joint.

Hip Dislocation

Hip dislocations (Figure 26-52, p. 342) occur in all age-groups secondary to major trauma when the leg is extended before impact. The injury is common with head-on, frontal impact MVCs when the leg is extended with the foot on the brake pedal just before impact or when the knee jams into the dashboard (Figure 26-53, p. 343). Injury also occurs with falls and crush injuries. Dislocation may be anterior or posterior. The patient complains of pain in the hip and knee and arrives with the hip flexed, adducted, and internally rotated (posterior dislocation) or flexed, abducted, and externally rotated (anterior dislocation). The joint feels locked and the patient cannot move the leg.

The extremity is splinted in the presenting position or position of greatest comfort. Other injuries are assessed. Necrosis of the femoral head may occur if the joint is not relocated within 6 hours. Figures 26-54 and 26-55 on p. 343 show techniques for hip reduction. After the hip joint is relocated, the patient begins a period of bed rest with traction. Children may be placed in a spica cast. Complications from this type of injury are femoral artery and nerve damage.

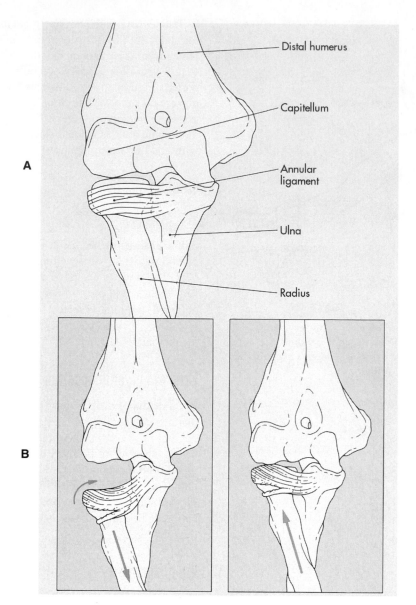

A

Distal humerus

Capitellum

Annular ligament

Ulna

Radius

B

FIGURE 26-49   Nursemaid's elbow. **A,** Sudden traction on the outstretched arm pulls the radius distally, causing it to slip partially through the annular ligament and tearing it in the process. **B,** When traction is released, the radial head recoils, trapping the proximal portion of the ligament between it and the capitellum. (From Zittelli B, Davis H: *Atlas of pediatric physical diagnosis,* ed 3, St. Louis, 1997, Mosby.)

Leg Dislocation

Knee Dislocation

Knee dislocations (Figure 26-56, p. 344) are common in all age-groups and are usually caused by major trauma. The patient complains of severe pain in the knee, inability to move the leg, swelling, and deformity. Immediate therapeutic intervention includes splinting the limb in position of comfort or presenting position. A fractured tibia is frequently associated with knee dislocation. Almost all people with dislocation of the knee joint have associated damage to the joint capsule.

After reduction the patient is admitted to the hospital for bed rest with the knee elevated and intermittent cold packs applied for 7 to 10 days. A cast is usually applied after this time. Complications include peroneal, popliteal, and tibial nerve damage.

Patellar Dislocation

Dislocation of the patella (Figure 26-57, p. 344) occurs in all age-groups, usually during athletic events secondary to direct trauma to the lateral aspect of the knee or rapid rotation on a planted foot. Patients usually have severe pain, keep the affected knee in a flexed position, and are unable to use the knee. Significant tenderness and swelling in the patellar area is evident. The leg is splinted in the presenting position and a cold pack applied. After radiographs the patella is reduced if spontaneous reduction does not occur with extension of the leg. After relocation the knee is placed in a compression bandage and knee immobilizer or cylinder cast.

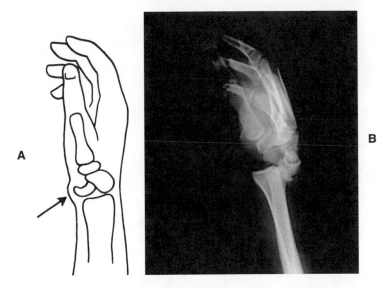

FIGURE **26-50**   **A,** Wrist dislocation. **B,** Radiograph. (**B,** From Ballinger PW: *Merrill's atlas of radiographic positions and radiologic procedures,* ed 8, St. Louis, 1995, Mosby.)

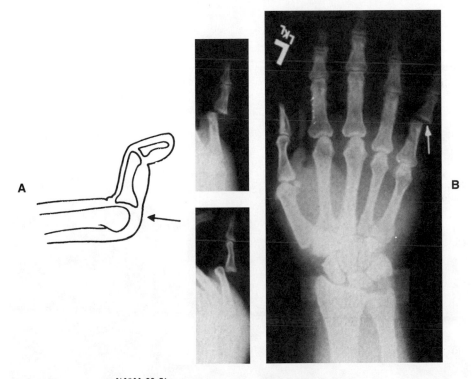

FIGURE **26-51**   **A,** Finger dislocation. **B,** Radiographs.

Ankle Dislocation

Ankle dislocation (Figure 26-58) is usually the result of athletic injury and is commonly associated with a fracture. Dislocation results from lateral stress motion when normal range of motion for the ankle is exceeded. Patients complain of severe pain in the ankle, inability to move the joint, swelling, and deformity. The ankle and foot are splinted in a position of comfort, and an ice pack is applied. The ankle may be relocated by a closed or open method, depending on the degree of injury and associated fractures. Primary com-

plication of this injury is neurovascular compromise including the tibial artery.

Foot Dislocation

Dislocations of the foot can occur in all age-groups but are rare. Injury is often the result of an automobile or motorcycle collision in which a combination of forces occur simultaneously. Foot dislocation is almost always associated with an open wound. The patient complains of severe pain in the foot with point tenderness and inability to use the foot.

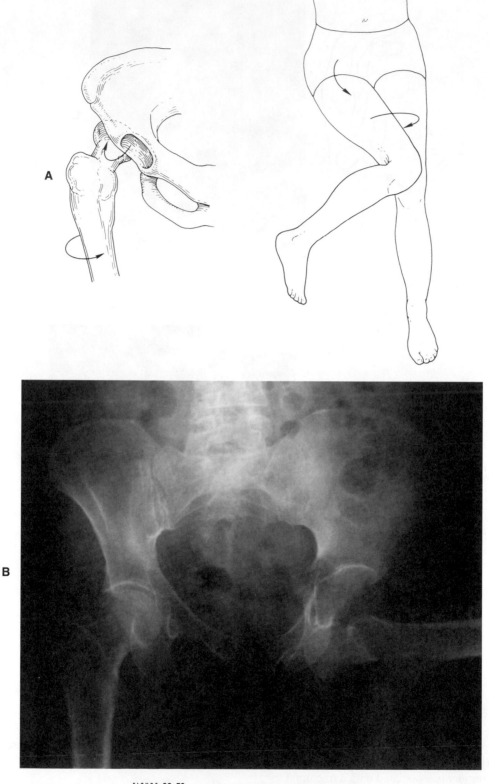

FIGURE 26-52   **A,** Hip dislocation. **B,** Radiograph.

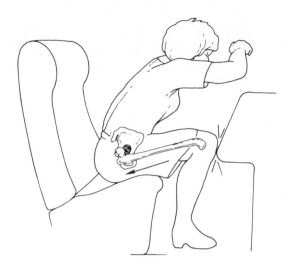

FIGURE **26-53**   Knee impact with dashboard.

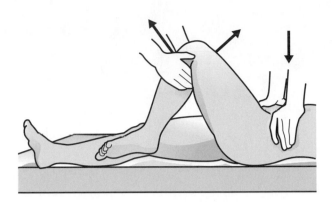

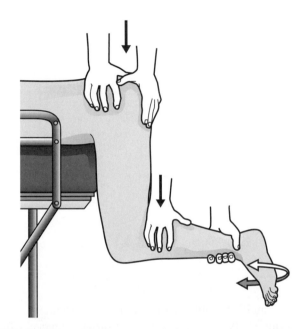

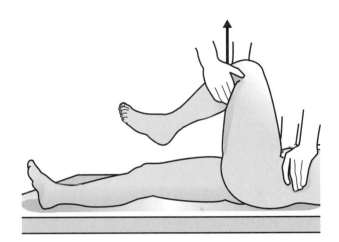

FIGURE **26-54**   Stimson method of reduction for posterior dislocation of the hip.

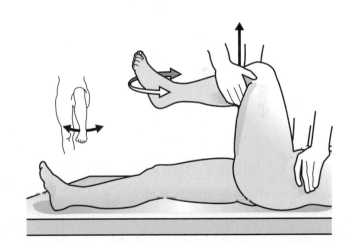

Significant swelling and deformity are evident. If present, an open wound is covered with a sterile dressing before a soft splint is applied. After the foot is relocated, a cast is applied. The patient is instructed to elevate the limb and apply cold packs for 24 hours. No weight-bearing is permitted.

Toe (Metatarsophalangeal) Dislocation

Dislocations of the metatarsophalangeal joints (toes) are rare (Figure 26-59). When they do occur they are often associated with open fractures, which should be reduced immediately because delay can result in an inability to perform closed reduction because of swelling. The patient complains of pain and point tenderness in the joint area with significant

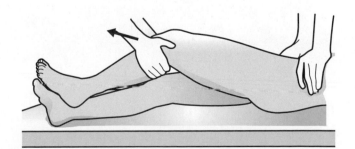

FIGURE **26-55**   Allis method of reducing posterior dislocation of the hip.

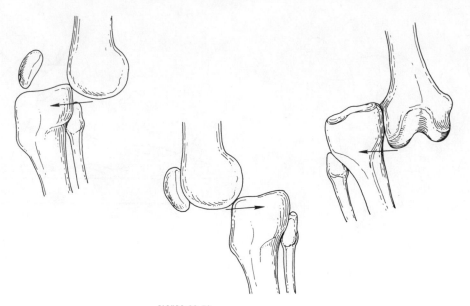

FIGURE **26-56** Knee dislocation.

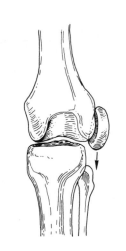

FIGURE **26-57** Patella dislocation.

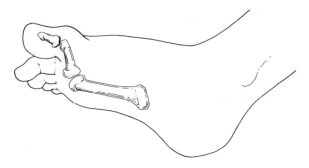

FIGURE **26-59** Metatarsophalangeal joint dislocation.

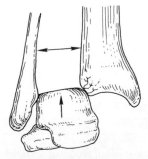

FIGURE **26-58** Ankle dislocation.

swelling and noticeable deformity. The area should be covered with a bulky dressing to prevent further damage. After radiographs have been obtained, the dislocation is reduced, then the foot and toes are immobilized.

REDUCTION ISSUES

The goal for reduction of fractures and dislocations is to restore anatomic alignment, allow bone healing, and preserve function. Fractures that do not require anatomic alignment for healing include an impacted fracture of the humeral neck, fractured clavicle (particularly in children), and pediatric nonangulated femur. Conversely, reduction is particularly important for intraarticular fractures, especially for weight-bearing bones.

Reduction methods are described as closed or open (surgical). Closed reduction uses traction-countertraction, angulation, and rotation (i.e., the reverse force of what caused the injury). A fingertrap and weights may be used for forearm reduction (Figure 26-60). Manipulation may require local

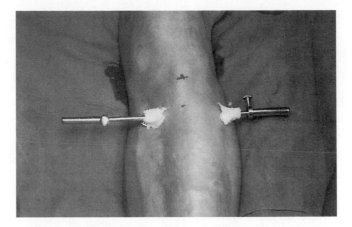

FIGURE **26-61** The pin is passed through the tibia to project equally medially and laterally. Points are protected with covers. (From Mills K, Morton R, Page G: *Color atlas and text of emergencies,* ed 2, London, 1995, Times Mirror International.)

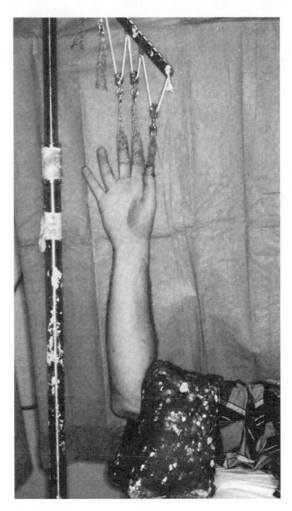

FIGURE **26-60** Finger traps and distal traction at the elbow to distract and reduce fracture dislocations. (From Rosen P, Barkin RM, Hockberger RS et al: *Emergency medicine: concepts and clinical practice,* ed 4, St. Louis, 1998, Mosby.)

anesthesia, conscious intravenous sedation, pain medications, or general anesthesia. Reduction should be accomplished as soon as possible after stabilization of other injuries because swelling can impede successful reduction. Postreduction radiographs are done after casting to verify acceptable bone alignment.

Open reduction is used for open fractures; multiple injuries; major fractures; and fractures involving intraarticular joints, epiphysis, or femoral neck. Surgical reduction is also used for soft-tissue entrapment; major nerve, arterial or ligament injuries; pathologic fractures; unsatisfactory or failed closed reduction; or delayed union. Open reduction employs internal fixation or external fixation devices.

TRACTION

Skin or skeletal traction may be initiated in the ED. A Hare traction splint can be used until more definitive stabilization is available. Bucks traction uses a wrapped dressing or boot to provide temporary immobilization before surgery for a hip or femur fracture and to reduce muscle spasm. Traction is set up on a hospital bed that is brought to the ED. This eliminates painful and possibly injurious removal of traction with transfer of the patient from the ED stretcher.

Steinman Pin

Skeletal traction may be applied in the ED with a Steinman pin (Figure 26-61). This provides temporary reduction of long-bone fractures until open reduction and internal fixation can be done. The pin is a round stainless steel rod drilled perpendicularly into the distal femur or proximal tibia for connection to a stirrup with traction (15 to 40 pounds). After pin placement, sterile dressings are placed around insertion sites. Osteomyelitis is a potential complication of pin insertion.

Casts

A brief overview of casting and care of casts is presented here. An orthopedic or medical-surgical text should be consulted for complete description of techniques and types of casts.

Before a cast is applied any particulate matter is removed and the skin completely dried. Any skin abnormalities are documented. Casting equipment includes plaster or fiberglass, stockinette and padding, a bucket of cool-to-warm water, gloves, and a gauze or elastic bandage if a splint is applied.

After the cast is applied, the patient should remain immobile with the limb placed on a plastic-coated pillow to avoid pressure and indentations for at least 20 minutes to allow the cast to set. A plaster cast generally requires 24 hours or more to dry thoroughly; a fiberglass cast dries in about an hour. Box 26-2 lists aftercare instructions for a patient with a cast.

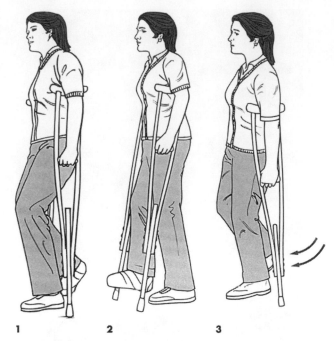

FIGURE 26-62 Three-point gait. *1,* Standing with crutches, all weight is on the good leg. *2,* Move crutches and injured leg forward simultaneously. *3,* Bearing weight on the palms of the hands, step forward onto the good leg. (From Proehl FA, Jones LM: *Mosby's emergency department patient teaching guides,* St. Louis, 1997, Mosby).

Compartment syndrome and pressure sores can occur with casts. Symptoms include elevated temperature and continuing pain after several days that keeps the patient awake. Interventions include immediate cast removal. Cast removal or a bivalve procedure is accomplished with an electric cast saw. The saw blade cuts by vibrating rapidly back and forth. The patient should be reassured that the blade does not cut the skin, but heat, vibration, or pressure may be felt. Burns secondary to the blade are rare. After the cast is cut, a cast spreader is used to widen the split and allow removal. Padding beneath the cast should be cut with bandage scissors.

ASSISTED AMBULATION: CRUTCH, CANE, AND WALKER

When fitting a patient for crutches, a cane, or a walker, measurement is ideally taken with the patient wearing shoes that will be worn for ambulating. The shoes should be sturdy, fit well, and fasten with a tie, buckle, or Velcro.

Axillary Crutches

Axillary crutches should fit so that each armpiece is 2 inches or two finger widths below the axilla with no weight on the axilla. Tips of the crutches should be placed 6 inches to the side and 6 inches to the front. Taller individuals require a broader base so crutches may be placed up to 12 inches to the side for these patients. Each handpiece should be fitted so that the elbow is flexed 30 degrees.

Cane

A cane should be fitted so that when it is held next to the heel, the elbow is at a 30-degree angle of flexion. A cane should be used for minimal support during ambulation and to assist with balance and stability.

Walker

A walker may be chosen for patients who are unsteady on crutches and those who can bear full weight on at least one leg. A walker is measured to fit with the arms bent at 30 degrees. Patients having difficulty ambulating with assist devices may require physical therapy for training, using a wheelchair temporarily until able to ambulate safely. A walker is not ideal for use on stairs.

Gait Training

A three-point gait is used when little or no weight-bearing is desired, making this gait ideal for ED patients. Figure 26-62 shows this gait. Figures 26-63 and 26-64 illustrate movement on stairs and changing from a sitting to standing position using crutches.

SUMMARY

Advances in surgical and orthopedic treatments have improved outcome for patients with soft-tissue injuries and fractures. However, the best outcome occurs if injury never occurs. Trauma prevention through education and legislation should be the primary goal of overall trauma management.

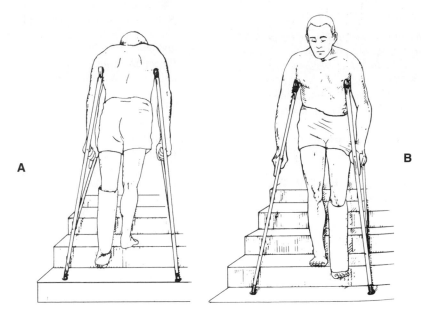

FIGURE 26-63 **A,** Going upstairs. **B,** Going downstairs with crutches. (From Barber J, Stokes L, Billings D: *Adult and child care,* ed 2, St. Louis, 1977, Mosby.)

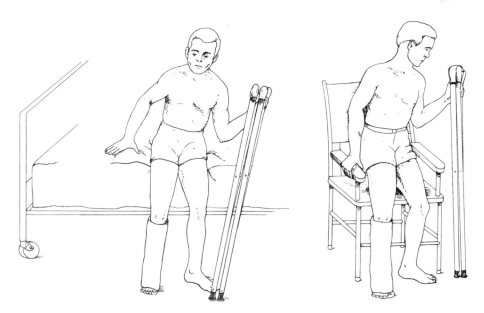

FIGURE 26-64 Transferring from sitting to standing with crutches. (From Barber J, Stokes L, Billings D: *Adult and child care,* ed 2, St. Louis, 1977, Mosby.)

The main objective for nursing care of the patient with an orthopedic or soft-tissue injury is to preserve or restore normal neurovascular status and motor function. Attention to these injuries is a secondary priority to ABCs. The emergency nurse must assess and intervene as soon as possible and monitor for developing complications to prevent further harm to the extremity. Box 26-3 summarizes nursing diagnoses for these patients.

Box 26-3	**NURSING DIAGNOSES FOR ORTHOPEDIC OR SOFT-TISSUE INJURY**

Fluid volume, Deficient
Infection, Risk for
Pain
Physical mobility, Impaired
Skin integrity, Impaired
Tissue perfusion, Ineffective

References

1. Ballinger PW et al: *Merrill's atlas of radiographic positions and radiologic procedures,* ed 9, vol 1, St. Louis, 1999, Mosby.
2. Butler AB, Salmond SW, Pellino TA: *Orthopedic nursing,* ed 2, Philadelphia, 1998, WB Saunders.
3. Cwinn AA: Pelvis and hip. In Rosen P et al, editors: *Emergency medicine: concepts and clinical practice,* vol 1, St. Louis, 1998, Mosby.
4. Emergency Nurses Association: *Musculoskeletal trauma: trauma nursing core course provider manual,* ed 5, 2000, Des Plaines, Ill, The Association.
5. Fultz J: Extremity trauma. In Kidd PS, Sturt P, editors: *Mosby's emergency nursing reference,* St. Louis, ed 2, 2000, Mosby.
6. Geiderman JM: Orthopedic injuries: management principles. In Rosen P, Barkin RM, Hockberger RS et al, editors: *Emergency medicine concepts and clinical practice,* ed 4, St. Louis, 1998, Mosby.
7. Harwood-Nuss A et al: *The clinical practice of emergency medicine,* ed 3, Philadelphia, 2000, JB Lippincott.
8. Nolan BG, Sturt P: Splint application. In Kidd PS, Sturt P, editors: *Mosby's emergency nursing reference,* ed 2, St. Louis, 2000, Mosby.
9. Proehl JA: *Emergency nursing procedures,* ed 2, Philadelphia, 1999, WB Saunders.

Additional Reading

1. del Piñal F, Herrero F, Jado E et al: Acute thumb ischemia secondary to high-pressure injection injury: salvage by emergency decompression, radical debridement, and free hallux hemipulp transfer, *J Trauma* 50:571, 2001.
2. Lewis SM, Heitkemper MM, Dirksen SR: *Medical-surgical nursing: assessment and management of clinical problems,* ed 5, St. Louis, 2000, Mosby.
3. Mattox KL, Feliciano DV, Moore EE: *Trauma,* ed 4, New York, 2000, McGraw-Hill.
4. Walker J: Orthopedic emergencies. In Jordan KS, editor: *Emergency nursing core curriculum,* ed 5, Philadelphia, 2000, WB Saunders.

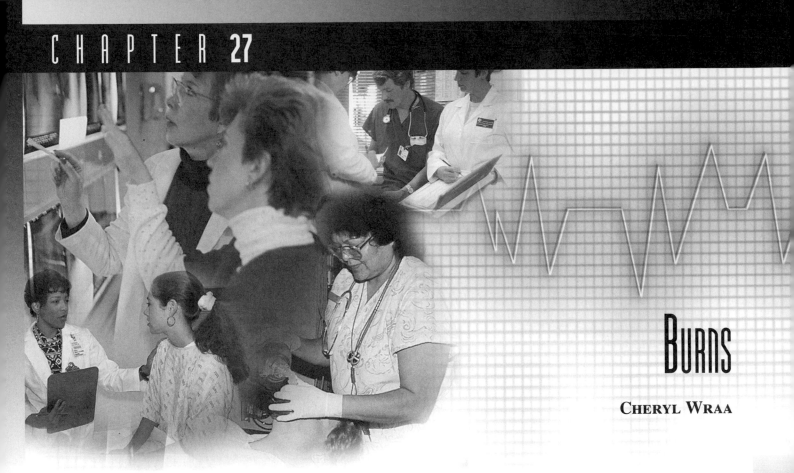

CHAPTER 27

BURNS

CHERYL WRAA

Burn trauma continues to be an immense challenge to caregivers. In the United States close to 1.2 million people annually are treated for burn injuries. Of these, approximately 6000 die and 60,000 require hospitalization. The recent decline in mortality is attributed to early excision and closure of the burn wound. Other factors contributing to the decline are improved resuscitation, control of infection, and support of the hypermetabolic response. A significant portion of morbidity and mortality associated with burn injuries is due to associated injuries. Pulmonary pathology from inhalation injury is the major cause of burn trauma death with the majority of deaths at the extremes of age. Burn injury and deaths associated with fires are the third leading cause of accidental death in children between the ages of 1 and 14 years [6-8,11]

More than 90% of all burns are considered preventable. Education, particularly in the school-age population, combined with legislative efforts is helping decrease the number of burn injuries. The American Burn Association has developed effective public education programs. Legislation has been enacted that requires smoke alarms and sprinkler systems in public buildings, hotels, apartments, and new homes. For the caregiver an accurate classification of injury, timely intervention, and rapid transport to an appropriate burn facility significantly reduces burn injury mortality and morbidity.[9,10]

ETIOLOGY

Not all burns are caused by fire. Tissue damage may be secondary to chemicals, tar, electricity, lightning, or frostbite.

The location and duration of exposure to the source affects outcome, regardless of the specific source of burn injury. Specific mechanisms of burn injury are described in the following sections.

Thermal Burns

Thermal injuries represent 60% of all burns. They may result from flame, flash, steam, or scalding liquid.[2,10] Figure 27-1 is an example of one cause of burn injury.

Scald Burns

Scalds from hot liquids are the most common cause of all burns. Exposure to water at 140° F (60° C) for 3 seconds can cause a deep partial-thickness or full-thickness burn. If water is 156° F (69° C), the same burn occurs in 1 second. As a comparison, fresh brewed coffee is about 180° F (82° C). Soups and sauces, which are a thicker consistency, remain in contact longer with the skin and cause deeper burns. Immersion burns are usually deep and severe because of prolonged contact with a scalding liquid.

Other liquids that cause scalds are cooking oil and grease. When used for cooking, oil and grease may reach 400° F (204° C).

Flame Burns

Burns from flames are the next most common cause of burns. Fortunately, the number of house fires has decreased with increased use of smoke detectors. Most flame burns are caused by careless smoking, motor vehicle crashes, and clothing ignited from stoves or space heaters. Flame burns that occur outdoors are usually secondary to misuse of cooking stoves fueled by white gasoline, lanterns in tents, smoking in a sleeping bag, and gasoline or kerosene in a charcoal fire.[2]

Flash Burns

Explosions of natural gas, propane, gasoline, or other flammable liquids cause flash burns—the third most common type of thermal burn. The explosion causes intense heat for a very brief time. Flash burns are usually partial thickness, although depth is dependent on amount and kind of fuel that explodes. Flash burns can be large and are often associated with significant thermal upper airway damage.[2]

Contact Burns

Contact with a hot object such as metal, plastic, glass, or hot coals results in contact burns. The burns are usually not extensive but tend to be deep. People involved in industrial accidents often have contact burns associated with crush injuries from machine presses or hot, heavy objects. An increase has been seen in toddlers with contact burns secondary to the increased use of wood-burning stoves. The most common injury is to the palm when a child falls against the stove with hands outstretched.[2]

Electrical Burns

As electricity passes through the body and meets resistance from body tissues, it is converted to heat in direct proportion to amperage and the body's electrical resistance. It initially passes through the skin, causing an external burn at the entry and exit sites, with extensive damage internally between these sites. Nerves, blood vessels, and muscle are less resistant and more easily damaged than bone or fat. The heart, lungs, and brain can sustain immediate damage. The nervous system is particularly sensitive to electrical burns. Damage to the brain, spinal cord, and myelin-producing cells causes devastating transverse myelitis. The smaller the body part through which the electricity passes, the more in-

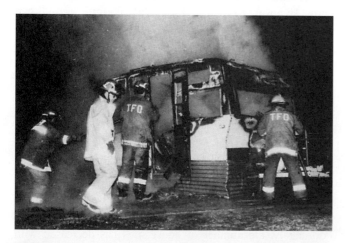

FIGURE 27-1   Burn injuries occur as a result of exposure to flame and smoke. (Courtesy Tacoma Fire Department, Tacoma, Wash.)

tense the heat and the less it is dissipated. Consequently, extensive damage can occur in the fingers, hands, forearms, toes, feet, and lower legs. If the path is near or through the heart, damage to the heart's electrical conduction system can cause spontaneous ventricular fibrillation or other dysrhythmias. Papillary muscle damage may lead to sudden valvular incompetence and cardiac failure. Alternating current is more likely to induce fibrillation than direct current.

Most lightning injuries do not traverse the body but flow around it, creating a shock wave capable of causing fractures and dislocations. About 70% of patients who survive a lightning strike complain of paresthesia or paralysis. Fortunately, both conditions are usually temporary.[2]

Chemical Burns

Chemicals cause a denaturing of protein within the tissues or a desiccation of cells. Chemical concentration and time of exposure determine extent of the burn. Alkali products cause more tissue damage than acids. A wet chemical should be removed as soon as possible by flushing with copious amounts of water. Dry substances should be brushed off the skin before the area is flushed. Care must be taken not to expose the caregiver to the chemical during this procedure. All fluids used to decontaminate the patient should be contained; the fluid should not be allowed to drain into the general drainage system. Chemical burns can be deceiving as to depth; appearances can be similar in surface discoloration until tissue begins to slough days later. Consequently, all chemical burns should be considered deep partial thickness or full thickness until proven otherwise. After chemical removal, wounds are managed in the same manner as thermal burns.[2,10]

Frostbite

Frostbite is actual freezing of tissue from exposure to freezing or below-freezing temperatures. In a cold environment the body attempts to maintain heat by vasoconstriction of peripheral blood vessels to reduce heat exchange. The longer the period of exposure, the more peripheral blood flow is reduced. When extremities are left unprotected, intracellular and extracellular fluids can freeze, forming crystals that damage local tissues. Blood clots may form and impair circulation to the area.

Signs, symptoms, and classification of frostbite are the same as thermal burns. The affected extremity should be rapidly rewarmed using warm water. Use of excessive heat such as steam is dangerous and can cause unnecessary damage. Dress the rewarmed extremity and immobilize it with a padded splint. As with flame burns, frostbite can be very painful, so pain management is needed.[4,7]

BURN ASSESSMENT

Burn depth and extent are assessed to determine severity of burn injury. In many cases final determination is not made for several days.

Depth of Burn

Burns are described as partial thickness or full thickness. Identification of the depth of injury may be difficult initially because depth may actually increase over time as edema forms and circulation to the area of injury is compromised. This process usually peaks at 48 hours; therefore, a more accurate determination of depth can be made between 48 and 72 hours. Depth determination is not a priority during initial resuscitation.

Extent of Burn

Extent of injury for thermal and chemical injuries is assessed by using formulas such as the Rule of Nines (Figure 27-2), Berkow formula, or Lund and Browder table (Figures 27-3 and 27-4).[10] The caregiver should remember that the Rule of Nines must be modified for children. As noted in Figure 27-2, *B,* the head and neck of an infant represent 18% of body surface area (BSA), whereas legs represent 13% for each lower extremity. To correct for age 1% is subtracted from the head for each year of age through 10 years, and 0.5% is added to each lower extremity. To estimate scatter burns, the size of the patient's palm (excluding fingers) is used to represent 1% of total BSA (TBSA). The palm is visualized over the burned areas. To obtain a more accurate estimate of the extent of burns, both burned and unburned areas are calculated. The two estimates should then be compared. If the total is more or less than 100%, the areas should be reestimated. Assessing extent of injury in electrical burns is more difficult because surface damage is minimal when compared with underlying damage. When discussing an electrical injury, describing the injury anatomically is more important than calculating percentage of BSA burned.

Severity of Burn

The severity of burn injury is based on assessment of extent and depth of injury, patient age, presence of concomitant injuries, smoke inhalation, or preexisting diseases. The American Burn Association's guidelines for classification of severity for burn injuries are listed in Table 27-1.

Care of patients with burns of different severity is determined by availability of specialized care facilities. Initial stabilization of the burn patient should be available in any community hospital with 24-hour emergency capabilities. Patients with minor burns may be treated as outpatients or admitted to the community hospital. Patients with moderate burns may be treated in a community hospital with appropriate staff and facilities to deliver burn care or transferred to a specialized burn care facility. Patients with major burns require care in a specialized burn care facility. Transfer agreements with special-care units should be developed in advance to facilitate timely and uneventful transfer. Box 27-1 summarizes criteria for transfer to a burn center. Any patient with concomitant trauma that poses increased risk for morbidity or mortality should be treated in a trauma cen-

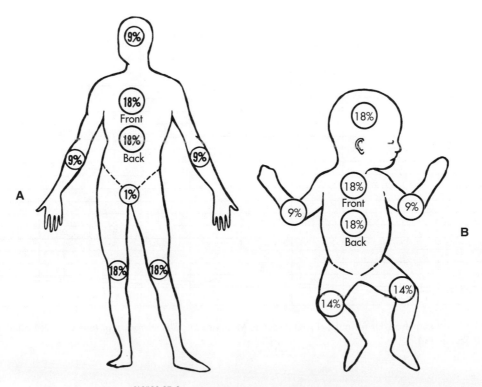

FIGURE 27-2   Rule of Nines. **A,** Adult. **B,** Child.

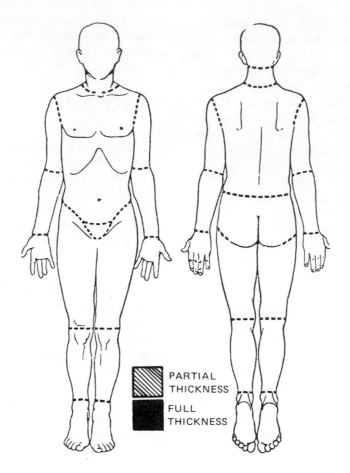

Percent Surface Area Burned

AREA	1 YEAR	1-4 YEARS	5-9 YEARS	10-14 YEARS	Y 15 YEARS	ADULT	2°	3°
Head	19	17	13	11	9	7		
Neck	2	2	2	2	2	2		
Ant. Trunk	13	13	13	13	13	13		
Post Trunk	13	13	13	13	13	13		
R. Buttock	2½	2½	2½	2½	2½	2½		
L. Buttock	2½	2½	2½	2½	2½	2½		
Genitalia	1	1	1	1	1	1		
R. U. Arm	4	4	4	4	4	4		
L. U. Arm	4	4	4	4	4	4		
R. L. Arm	3	3	3	3	3	3		
L. L. Arm	3	3	3	3	3	3		
R. Hand	2½	2½	2½	2½	2½	2½		
L. Hand	2½	2½	2½	2½	2½	2½		
R. Thigh	5½	6½	8	8½	9	9½		
L. Thigh	5½	6½	8	8½	9	9½		
R. Leg	5	5	5½	6	6½	7		
L. Leg	5	5	5½	6	6½	7		
R. Foot	3½	3½	3½	3½	3½	3½		
L. Foot	3½	3½	3½	3½	3½	3½		
TOTAL								

FIGURE 27-3   Lund and Browder formula. (From Artz CP, Moncrief JA: *The treatment of burns,* ed 2, Philadelphia, 1979, WB Saunders.)

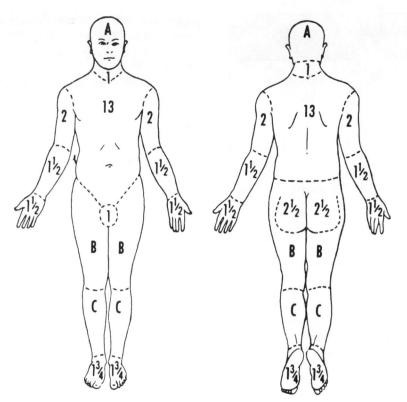

Relative Percentage of Areas Affected by Growth

	Age in Years					
	0	1	5	10	15	Adult
A—½ of head	9½	8½	6½	5½	4½	3½
B—½ of one thigh	2¾	3¼	4	4¼	4½	4¾
C—½ of one leg	2½	2½	2¾	3	3¼	3½

FIGURE 27-4   Lund and Browder formula. (From Artz CP, Moncrief JA: *The treatment of burns,* ed 2, Philadelphia, 1979, WB Saunders.)

Table 27-1 AMERICAN BURN ASSOCIATION'S CLASSIFICATION OF SEVERITY OF INJURY		
CLASSIFICATION	**CHARACTERISTICS**	**TREATMENT FACILITY**
Minor	SPT DPT, <15% TBSA adult DPT, <10% TBSA child or older adult FT, <2% TBSA adult, child (not involving face, hands, feet, or perineum)	Outpatient or inpatient (for 24 hr)
Moderate	DPT 15% to 25% TBSA adult DPT 10% to 20% TBSA child or older adult FT 2% to 10% TBSA adult, child (not involving face, hands, feet, or perineum)	Community hospital

Major	DPT, >25% TBSA adult
	DPT, >20% child <10 years of age or adult >50 years of age
	FT, >10% TBSA adult, child
	Burns of face, hands, feet, and perineum
	Burns complicated by:
	    Inhalation injury
	    Major associated trauma
	    Preexisting illness
	    All major electrical injuries
	    Burns caused by caustic chemical agent
		Burn center

Data from Edlich R, Moghtader J: Thermal burns. In Rosen, P, Barkin RM, Hockberger RS et al, editors: *Emergency medicine: concepts and clinical practice,* ed 4, St. Louis, 1998, Mosby.
SPT, Shallow partial thickness; *DPT,* deep partial thickness; *TBSA,* total body surface area; *FT,* full thickness.

1. Partial thickness burns greater than 10% total body surface area (TBSA)
2. Burns that involve the face, hands, feet, genitalia, perineum, or major joints
3. Third-degree burns in any age-group
4. Electrical burns, including lightning injury
5. Chemical burns
6. Inhalation injury
7. Burn injury in patients with preexisting medical disorders that could complicate management, prolong recovery, or effect mortality
8. Any patient with burns and concomitant trauma (such as fractures) in which the burn injury poses the greatest risk of morbidity or mortality, In such cases, if the trauma poses the greater immediate risk, the patient may be initially stabilized in a trauma center before being transferred to a burn unit. Physician judgement will be necessary in such situations and should be in concert with the regional medical control plan and triage protocols.
9. Burned children in hospitals without qualified personnel or equipment for the care of children
10. Burn injury in patients who will require special social, emotional, or long-term rehabilitative intervention

Data from American College of Surgeons: *Resources for optimal care of the injured patient: 1999,* Chicago, 1998, The College.

ter until he or she is stable and then transferred to a burn center as appropriate.

PATHOPHYSIOLOGY

Burn injury occurs when skin is exposed to more energy than it can absorb. The cause of the burn may vary but local and systemic responses are generally similar. To understand the pathophysiology of burns, one must first understand the functions of the skin, which consists of two layers: the epidermis and the dermis. The epidermis, the outer layer of the basement layer of cells, consists of cells that migrate upward to become surface keratin. The dermis, or inner layer, consists of collagen and elastic fibers and contains hair follicles, sweat and sebaceous glands, nerve endings, and blood vessels. The skin is the largest organ of the body and acts as an infection barrier, vapor barrier, and a heat regulator.[6,9]

Three zones of tissue damage occur at the burn site. First is the central zone of coagulation, an area of irreversible damage. Concentrically surrounding this area is the zone of stasis where capillary and small vessel stasis occurs. The ultimate fate of the burn wound depends on resolution or progression of the zone of stasis. Edema formation and prolonged compromise of blood flow to this area cause a deeper, more extensive wound; therefore, depth and severity of burn wounds may not be known for 2 or more days after the initial injury.

The third zone of damage is the zone of hyperemia, an area of superficial damage that heals quickly on its own.[2,10]

The body responds to the burn injury with varying degrees of tissue damage, cellular impairment, and fluid shifts. A brief decrease in blood flow to the affected area is followed by a marked increase in arteriolar vasodilation. Damaged tissues release mediators that initiate an inflammatory response. Histamine, serotonin, prostaglandin derivatives, and the complement cascade are all activated. Release of proinflammatory mediators combined with vasodilation causes increased capillary permeability, then intravascular fluid loss and wound edema. For burn injuries less than 20% TBSA, these actions are usually limited to the burn site. As the affected TBSA goes beyond 20%, local response becomes systemic. Hypoproteinemia resulting from increased capillary permeability aggravates edema in nonburned tissue. Basal metabolic rate increases from insensible fluid loss, which along with fluid shift produces hypovolemia. Capillary permeability increases for 2 to 3 weeks with the most significant changes occurring in the first 24 to 36 hours.[2,6,10,11]

Initially blood viscosity increases when hematocrit rises secondary to vascular fluid shifts into the interstitium. Because of a marked increase in peripheral resistance, decreased intravascular fluid volume, and increased blood viscosity, cardiac output falls. Capillary leak and depressed cardiac output can depress central nervous system function, causing restlessness, followed by lethargy, and finally coma. Decreased cardiac output, blood volume, and intense sympathetic response decrease perfusion to the skin, viscera, and renal perfusion. Levels of thromboxane A2, a potent vasoconstrictor, have been shown to be significantly increased in burned patients and contribute to mesenteric vasoconstriction and decreased splanchnic blood flow. Decreased flow can convert a zone of stasis to zone of coagulation, which increases depth of the burn. Decreased circulating plasma with increased hematocrit can cause hemoglobinuria, which can lead to renal failure. Immediate hemolysis of red cells occurs, with the life span of remaining red cells reduced by approximately 30% of normal. Platelet count and platelet survival time initially drop drastically then continue to decrease for 5 days after injury. This period is followed by a rebound increase in platelets over the next 2 to 3 weeks.[2,6,10,11]

Cardiovascular changes begin immediately after a burn; their extent varies with burn size and presence of additional injuries. Patients with an uncomplicated burn less than 15% TBSA can usually be treated with oral fluid resuscitation. Burns that surpass 20% TBSA have massive shifts of fluid and electrolytes from the intravascular to extravascular space. This shift begins to resolve in 18 to 36 hours; however, normal extracellular volume is not completely restored until 7 to 10 days after the burn. If intravascular volume is not replenished, hypovolemic shock occurs. If untreated the patient dies of cardiovascular collapse. Inadequate treatment also leads to renal failure from acute tubular necrosis.

The hypermetabolic response after burn trauma is huge and far exceeds the response seen in other forms of trauma.

The patient's metabolic rate can increase as much as 2 to 3 times the normal rate. Release of catabolic hormones, including catecholamines, cortisol, and glucagon, initiates a persistent hypermetabolic response. This response causes accelerated breakdown of skeletal muscle, decreased protein synthesis, increased peripheral lipolysis, and increased utilization of glucose, which rapidly depletes glycogen stores. This response manifests clinically as severe muscle wasting, decreased muscle strength, and increased liver fat with hepatomegaly and functional impairment. The hypermetabolic response is commensurate with size of the burn. The adverse effects of the response are managed through nutritional and pharmacologic intervention to improve net nitrogen balance, preserve lean body mass, decrease cardiac work, and decrease hepatic fatty infiltration.[11]

Burn injuries can affect every organ system in the body, causing cerebral perfusion abnormalities, impaired coronary blood supply, renal insufficiency, and acid-base imbalance.[2,9] Realization of these broad effects can enhance management of the burn patient.

Pulmonary Response to Smoke Inhalation

Inhalation injury or smoke inhalation is a syndrome comprising three distinct problems: carbon monoxide intoxication, upper airway obstruction, and chemical injury to the lower airways and lung parenchyma.

Carbon monoxide intoxication is the most common killer of victims of fire. Most people who die in a fire have been overcome by carbon monoxide before they sustain a burn injury. In the body, carbon monoxide has a 200-times greater affinity for hemoglobin than oxygen, which causes inadequate tissue-oxygen delivery. Carbon monoxide combines with myoglobin in muscle cells, causing muscle weakness. Tissue hypoxia and the resultant confusion and muscle weakness may be the major reasons for most fire fatalities. Combining carbon monoxide with the cytochrome oxidase system of the brain may account for prolonged coma in some fire victims.

Carbon monoxide poisoning is characterized by pink-to-cherry-red skin, tachypnea, tachycardia, headache, dizziness, and nausea. An arterial blood gas sample is drawn to measure carboxyhemoglobin level. Levels up to 15% are rarely associated with symptoms of carbon monoxide poisoning and can be normal for a heavy smoker. Levels of 15% to 40% are associated with varying disturbances such as headache and confusion. Levels greater than 40% are associated with coma. All patients with suspected carbon monoxide poisoning should be placed on 100% oxygen.[6,10]

Upper airway obstruction is the result of intrinsic or extrinsic edema that may lead to airway occlusion at or above the vocal cords (Figure 27-5). This injury is primarily a thermal injury resulting in tissue damage in the posterior pharynx. Figure 27-6 shows radiographic evidence of epiglottis secondary to thermal/chemical injury. Actual thermal injury below the vocal cords is rare because the posterior pharynx

is such an efficient heat exchange system. True thermal injury below the vocal cords is usually the result of superheated steam in which water vapor carries heat into the lungs. Injuries that occur in an oxygen-enriched atmosphere or one in which the person was inhaling explosive gases (e.g., during inhalation anesthesia) also cause true thermal injury below the vocal cords. True thermal injury to the lungs is almost always fatal. Thermal injury to the upper airway is usually associated with facial burns. Edema progresses rapidly, totally occluding the airway in minutes to hours. Management for airway edema is early intubation or tracheostomy if intubation is not possible.

Chemical injury to the lower airway is a common problem with inhalation of smoke. Chemical injury from acids and aldehydes in the smoke may damage the lung parenchyma. These chemicals, attached to carbon particles in the smoke, are heavier than air, so they are readily inhaled and find their way down the bronchi into alveoli. This chemical injury causes hemorrhagic tracheobronchitis, increased edema formation, decreased surfactant levels, and decreased pulmonary macrophage function. This condition leads to rapid development of adult respiratory distress syndrome (ARDS) over 24 to 48 hours. Severe inhalation injury may increase the patient's fluid needs in the first 24 hours by as much as 50% of calculated values.

PATIENT MANAGEMENT

The burn patient may have other injuries in addition to the burn; therefore, the patient should be initially evaluated using the ABCD survey for trauma.[1] The cervical spine is stabilized while assessing for an adequate airway. Assessment of specific burn injuries should then be done. A history is obtained as time and patient condition permit. How did the injury occur? What caused the injury—flame, scald, etc? Was smoke involved? Did injury occur in a confined space? What was the patient doing before the injury? Did the patient have a stroke or myocardial infarction before the injury? Does the patient have any medical problems or allergies? General assessment and interventions for the burn patient are described in this section.

Airway

A high index of suspicion for smoke inhalation is essential for these patients. Burns that occur in small spaces are often associated with smoke inhalation. The oropharynx and vocal cords should be inspected for redness, blisters, and carbonaceous particles. The patient is observed for increasing restlessness, dyspnea, difficulty swallowing, increasing hoarseness, and rapid, shallow respirations. The patient may have increasing difficulty managing secretions with a significant risk for impending airway obstruction. Early intubation is recommended before complete obstruction occurs. Tracheostomies should be avoided initially because edema of the neck makes this procedure difficult.

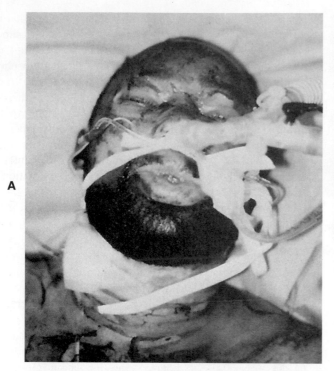

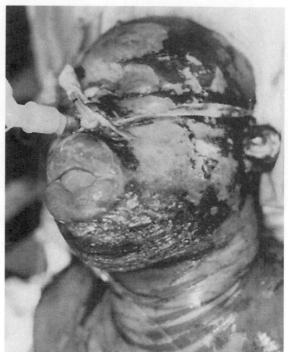

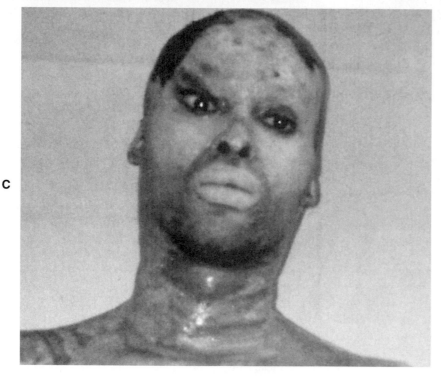

FIGURE 27-5 Facial edema.
A, Four to 5 hours after burn.
B, Thirty hours after burn, showing distortion of facial features and necessity of intubation before the full extent of burn edema development. **C,** Facial contour 3 months after burn. (Courtesy Anne E. Missavage, MD, UC Davis Regional Burn Center, Sacramento, Calif.)

Breathing

Circumferential full-thickness burns of the chest can impair breathing by limiting chest wall excursion and preventing adequate gas exchange. The chest should be visually inspected for tight, leathery eschar that circles the chest. Evidence of breathing compromise includes inadequate chest expansion, restlessness, confusion, decreased oxygenation, decreased tidal volume, and rapid, shallow respirations.

Escharotomy is indicated for circumferential burns that compromise breathing. Surgical incisions are made in burned tissue on the chest to release eschar and expose underlying subcutaneous tissue. Improvement in chest wall expansion should occur immediately after incisions are made. General anesthesia is not required because the incisions are made in a full-thickness burn. Intravenous narcotic analgesia is usually adequate to relieve any pain associated with escharotomy.

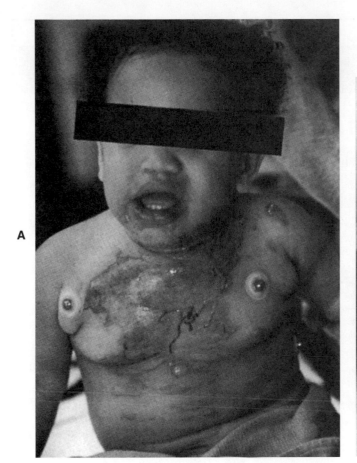

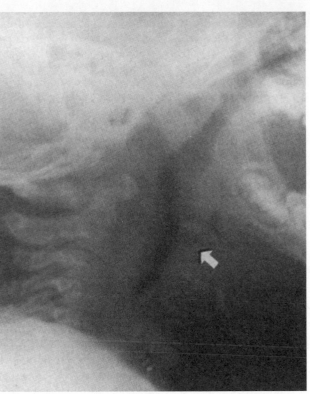

FIGURE 27-6   **A,** Photograph of 22-month-old child showing burn primarily to the anterior chest wall. **B,** Lateral airway radiograph of the same child demonstrating effects of thermal or chemical epiglottis. (From Barkin RM: *Pediatric emergency medicine: concepts and clinical practice,* ed 2, St. Louis, 1997, Mosby.)

The patient with a burn injury is also at risk for carbon monoxide poisoning. Altered breathing patterns such as decreased respirations or apnea may be evident, as may the characteristic cherry-red skin, or it can appear slightly cyanotic. Confusion, irritability, or coma may be present. Carboxyhemoglobin level and chest radiograph are obtained to assess for carbon monoxide poisoning and the presence of pulmonary damage or associated injuries. High-flow oxygen with a nonrebreather mask or bag-valve mask is administered as appropriate. If the patient does not respond after 1 to 1.5 hours of regular oxygen therapy, hyperbaric oxygen therapy may be used.

ARDS occurs in patients with CO poisoning but is usually not a problem until approximately 18 hours after injury. Clinical findings associated with ARDS include decreased oxygenation, increased secretions, rapid respirations, confusion, and increasing patchy infiltrates on the radiograph. Treatment includes intubation and ventilation with positive end expiratory pressure. Bronchodilators may be indicated; however, corticosteroids are not. Giving corticosteroids to patients with burns and smoke inhalation can increase morbidity and mortality. Refer to Chapter 32 for additional information on ARDS.

The burn patient should be assessed for other injuries that can affect breathing, such as pneumothorax, hemothorax, tension pneumothorax, and flail chest. These problems occur with a burn injury from a motor vehicle crash or explosion. Additional injuries may be present when a patient has jumped to escape the fire. Preexisting health problems that may affect respiratory functions (e.g., chronic obstructive pulmonary disease, asthma) should be noted.

Circulation

The patient with a burn injury is at significant risk for hypovolemia from actual fluid loss and fluid movement from increased capillary permeability and vasodilation. Assess the patient for increased respirations, increased pulse, decreased blood pressure, decreased urine output, diminished capillary refill, restlessness, confusion, nausea, and vomiting. Additional indications of volume compromise include central venous pressure less than 3 cm H_2O, hematocrit greater than 50 mg/dl, presence of an ileus, and urine output less than 0.5 ml/kg/hr.

One or two large-bore intravenous (IV) catheters should be started. A single IV catheter is adequate for a burn less

Table 27-2 FLUID REPLACEMENT FORMULAS

FORMULA	ELECTROLYTE SOLUTION	COLLOID	WATER	RATE	EXAMPLE: 70 KG/45% TBSA (PER 24 HR)
Evans	1 ml/kg/% TBSA NS	1 ml/kg/%	2000 ml	½, 1st 8 hr; ½, next 16 hr	3150 ml NS 3150 ml colloid 2000 ml water 8300 ml TOTAL
Brooke	1.5 ml/kg/% TBSA LR	0.5 ml/kg/%	2000 ml	½, 1st 8 hr; ½, next 16 hr	4725 ml LR 1575 ml colloid 2000 ml water 8300 ml TOTAL
Modified Brooke	2-3 ml/kg/% TBSA LR	None	None	½, 1st 8 hr; ½, next 16 hr	6300-9450 ml LR
Parkland (Baxter)	4 ml/kg/% TBSA LR	None	None	½, 1st 8 hr; ½, next 16 hr	12,600 ml LR
Hypertonic formula	Rate based on urine output of 30 ml/hr with hypertonic LR (sodium, 250 mEq/L)	None	None	To maintain urine output	Unknown

From Neff JA, Kidd PS: *Trauma nursing,: the art and science,* St. Louis, 1992, Mosby.
TBSA, Total body surface area; *NS,* normal saline; *LR,* lactated Ringer's solution.

than 40% TBSA. Two are begun if the burn is greater than 40% TBSA or the patient will be transferred. Leg veins are avoided because of increased risk of thrombophlebitis. The IV catheter can be inserted into burned tissue if no other access is available, but this should be considered a last resort. Fluid volume requirements are calculated using an accepted formula such as the Parkland or Baxter formula (Table 27-2). These formulas are guidelines for fluid replacement type and volume and should be adjusted to the patient's response to the fluid. Ideally, fluid resuscitation is adequate if pulse and blood pressure are within normal limits for age and urine output is 0.5 ml/kg/hr for adults and 1 to 1.5 ml/kg/hr for infants.

No formula exists for calculating fluid resuscitation in electrical injuries. An infusion of lactated Ringer's solution is administered at 1 to 2 L/hr in the average adult until he or she shows signs of adequate resuscitation. Urine output should be maintained at 2 to 3 times the normal volume to facilitate excretion of myoglobin. After urine output is established, mannitol may be given to increase urine flow and aid excretion of myoglobin. Significant acidosis can occur; so repeated administration of sodium bicarbonate may be required to prevent dysrhythmias. After fluid therapy corrects acidosis, repeated administration may not be necessary.

Infection

The patient with a burn injury has lost the greatest protection against invasion by various pathogens and must be protected with scrupulous aseptic technique. Gloves, masks, caps, and gowns must be worn. Sterile technique is necessary for all procedures. Wounds are kept covered with clean sheets while other care is provided. If the patient is transferred, sterile sheets are used to cover the patient. If treatment is followed

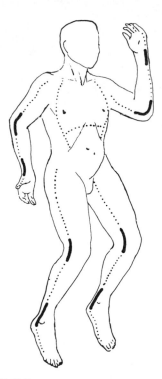

FIGURE 27-7 Placement of escharotomies.

by discharge, the nurse should debride the burn, apply a topical antibiotic, and cover the wound with a fluffy dressing. Systemic antibiotics are rarely indicated even in severe burns until infection is confirmed by culture. Exceptions to this guideline include young children, elderly patients, diabetic patients, or those with immune system compromise.

For minor or moderate burns, tetanus immunization is given if the patient has not been immunized within the past 10 years. In major burns or grossly contaminated burns,

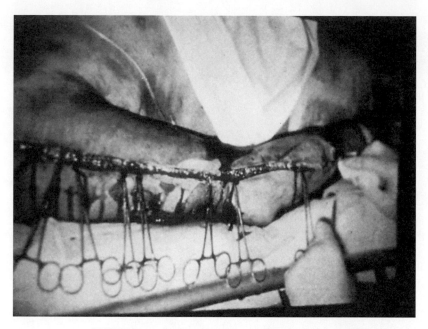

FIGURE 27-8   Control of bleeding from escharotomy.

tetanus immunization is given if previous immunization has occurred within 5 years. If the patient has never been immunized or no clear history of immunization exists, tetanus hyperimmune globulin (Hypertet) and tetanus immunization is given.

Pain Management

Burn wounds are exquisitely painful and deserve special consideration. The pain of primary tissue damage and nerve damage may be worsened by primary and secondary hyperalgesia. Studies have shown that opioid administration should be the prime treatment for burn pain.[4] During initial resuscitation, analgesics or anesthetics should be titrated to effect. After 24 hours, decreased plasma protein levels increase bioavailability of free drugs, especially those that are protein bound. Giving pain medication as needed may increase the patient's awareness of pain and other symptoms. Administering opioids on a schedule, based on drug half-life or by continuous infusion, can facilitate the patient's ability to cope with the pain. The opioid of choice has been IV morphine, 25 to 50 μg/kg/hr, titrating to avoid respiratory depression. Fentanyl may also be used for some patients. Studies have shown that unfortunately, there is a low correlation between pain assessment by the nurse and the patient's self-assessment of pain severity.[5]

For the burn victim, pain can be made worse by fear of pain or disfigurement, anxiety related to loss of control, and distress over losing family members or material possessions at the time of injury. Anxiety decreases pain tolerance. Reducing anxiety minimizes interplay between acute pain and sympathetic arousal. For the burn patient, anxiolytics may help decrease anxiety and improve pain tolerance. They are especially helpful during painful procedures. The most commonly used anxiolytics are benzodiazipine drugs. Diazepam has a long half-life and high lipid solubility. After repeated use in the burn patient, prolonged mental impairment may occur when the drug is stopped. Therefore short-term administration of lorazepam and midazolam are preferred.[4,5]

Patients with burn-induced or traumatic nerve injury may develop neuropathic pain. Pain is usually described as tingling, burning, shooting, or numbing. When a postburn patient comes to the emergency department (ED) with this type of pain, it is because the pain did not respond to opiate analgesics. Drugs that decrease neuronal excitability by mechanisms other than opiate receptors are useful for this type of pain. Tricyclic antidepressants in low doses are often successful in relieving neuropathic pain. Sodium channel-blocking drugs such as IV lidocaine, carbamazepine, phenytoin, and mexiletine have also produced successful analgesia.[5]

Wound Care

Wound care should be delayed until the patient's condition is stabilized; however, initial management must include removal of jewelry and constrictive clothing. Wounds must be kept covered with clean sheets until more definitive care can be provided. All patients with full-thickness burns are assessed for circulatory problems. Capillary refill and the presence of paresthesia are evaluated with distal pulses checked by Doppler ultrasonography. Burn tissue does not stretch, so swelling beneath burned tissue compromises circulation because of lack of elasticity. If the patient has signs of compromise, escharotomy is indicated. Figure 27-7 illustrates placement of these surgical incisions. Significant bleeding that occurs with escharotomy can be controlled with an electrocautery unit or small hemostats (Figure 27-8). After the procedure is completed a topical antibacterial agent is applied

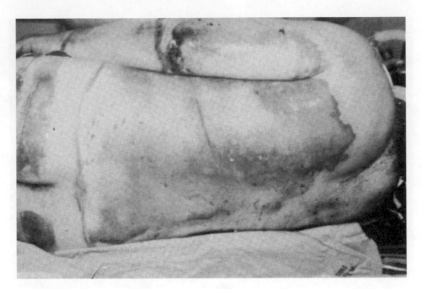

FIGURE 27-9   Flame burns to back.

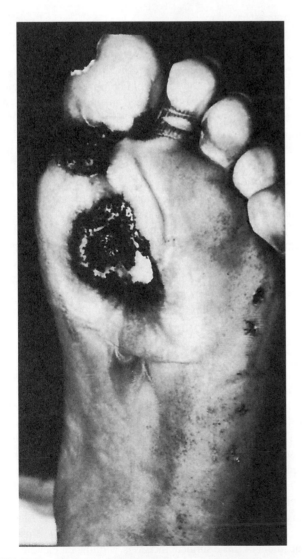

FIGURE 27-10   Exit wound from direct current. (From National Flight Nurses Association: *Flight nursing,* ed 2, St. Louis, 1996, Mosby.)

to the open wound, a light pressure dressing is applied, and the extremity is slightly elevated.

Thermal burns may be secondary to flame, flash, scalds, or hot objects. Figure 27-9 shows an example of a thermal burn. Thermal burns are cleaned with sterile saline or commercially available products containing polaxamer 188. The outer covering of blisters larger than a half dollar are broken and removed, except for those on the palms and soles of the feet. Hair is shaved from burns and surrounding areas. The wound is covered immediately with a topical antibacterial agent such as silvadene or bacitracin. Burns of the face should be left open and covered by bacitracin ointment, which is reapplied every 6 hours after gently washing the skin.

Chemical burns should be immediately irrigated with tap water or saline for at least 5 to 10 minutes to remove the chemical. Clothing and jewelry is removed, and unburned areas adjacent to the burned areas are rinsed. These areas can be injured but may not hurt, blister, or turn red immediately. If the chemical is dry, it can be brushed from the patient before irrigating. After the wound is thoroughly irrigated, it is treated like a thermal burn. Chemical burns of the eye are an ophthalmologic emergency. The eye must be irrigated thoroughly with copious amounts of water or saline. (Refer to Chapter 48 for additional discussion of chemical eye injuries.)

Electrical injuries are different from thermal and chemical burns. These wounds may have little superficial tissue loss; however, massive muscle injury may be present beneath normal-looking skin or minor to severe exit wounds (Figures 27-10 and 27-11). Wounds should be cleaned gently with water or saline and 0.25 strength povidone iodine (Betadine); they rarely need immediate debridement. Topical agents such as mafenide acetate (Sulfamylon) that deeply penetrate tissue are used to cover the wound. Light dressings may be applied to cover these often grotesque wounds; however, dressings

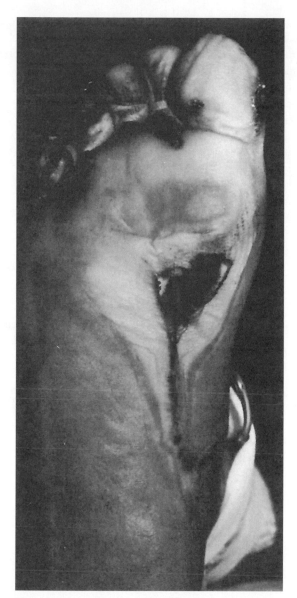

FIGURE 27-11 Exit wound from alternating current. (From National Flight Nurses Association: *Flight nursing,* ed 2, St. Louis, 1996, Mosby.)

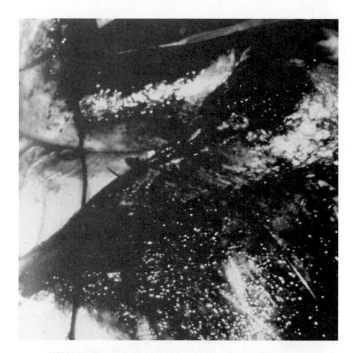

FIGURE 27-12 Tar burns of chest before removal of tar.

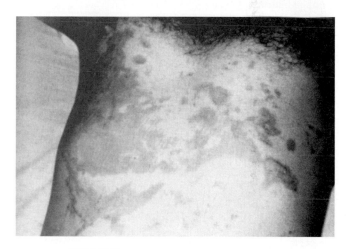

FIGURE 27-13 Tar burns after removal of tar.

must not interfere with assessment for circulatory compromise and possible compartment syndrome. High voltage injuries are associated with severe muscle contractions, so radiographs of the cervical spine may be indicated.

Electrical injuries of the extremities cause significant damage that leads to tissue swelling. Consequently, these patients are at risk for compartment syndrome. Symptoms associated with this condition include pain, pallor, paresthesia, pulselessness, and paralysis. Fasciotomies are used to relieve compartment syndrome.

Tar or asphalt burns may be deep or superficial depending on temperature of the tar, which may range from 150° F to more than 600° F. Figure 27-12 shows a tar burn before tar removal. Figure 27-13 shows the same burn after tar has been removed. Immediate treatment of a tar burn is to cool the tar, but do not try to peel it off the patient's skin. Using mineral oil, petroleum jelly, or a solvent such as Medi-Sol loosens the tar. In areas where the burn is not circumferential, oil or ointment is applied and the burn is covered with a light dressing. Dressings are removed in 4 to 12 hours, oil or ointment reapplied, and a new dressing applied. For areas with circumferential tar, oil or ointment can be applied with light dressings and changed every 20 to 30 minutes until tar is removed. After the tar is removed, the burn is treated as a thermal injury.

Temperature Regulation

The patient with a burn injury has lost a major control mechanism for temperature regulation. This heat loss is worsened by administration of IV fluids, irrigation of burned tissue, and environmental coolness often encountered in the ED. The patient's temperature should be documented as soon as possible after arrival in the ED and rechecked within 1 hour. Keeping the patient covered, using warmed IV fluids, and increasing room temperature minimizes heat loss.

SUMMARY

Burn injury can be devastating to the patient and family; for the caregiver, it can also be visually disturbing. Regardless of how severe the burn may be, a primary survey should be performed for potentially life-threatening injuries. Resuscitation of the burn patient includes evaluation of the burn, replacement of fluid losses, wound care, protection against contamination, maintenance of body temperature, and pain

control. Box 27-2 summarizes nursing diagnoses appropriate for the burn patient. A multidisciplinary approach to burn care can reduce mortality and morbidity. Appropriate application of burn center transfer criteria ensures the best outcome for the patient with a major burn injury.

References

1. American College of Surgeons: *Advanced trauma life support student manual,* Chicago, 1997, The College.
2. Auerbach P: *Wilderness medicine,* ed 4, St. Louis, 2001, Mosby.
3. Edlich R, Moghtader J: Thermal burns. In Rosen P, Barkin RM, Hockberger RS et al, editors: *Emergency medicine: concepts and clinical practice,* ed 4, St. Louis, 1998, Mosby.
4. Hedderich R, Ness T: Analgesia for trauma and burns, *Crit Care Clin* 15:1, 1999.
5. Kowalske K, Tanelian D: Burn pain, *Anesth Clin N Amer* 15:2, 1997.
6. McCloskey K, Orr R: *Pediatric transport medicine,* St. Louis, 1995, Mosby.
7. National Association of Emergency Medical Technicians: *Pre-hospital trauma life support,* ed 4, St. Louis, 2001, Mosby.
8. National Flight Nurses Association: *Flight nurse advanced trauma course student manual,* Park Ridge, Ill, 1995, The Association.
9. National Flight Nurses Association: *Flight nursing: principles and practice,* ed 2, St. Louis, 1996, Mosby.
10. Neff J, Kidd P: *Trauma nursing: the art and science,* St. Louis, 1992, Mosby.
11. Ramzy P, Barret J, Nerndon D: Thermal injury, *Crit Care Clin* 15:2, 1999.

Box 27-2	NURSING DIAGNOSES FOR BURN INJURY

Body image, Disturbed
Fluid volume, Deficient
Gas exchange, Impaired
Hypothermia, Risk for
Infection, Risk for
Pain
Tissue perfusion, Ineffective

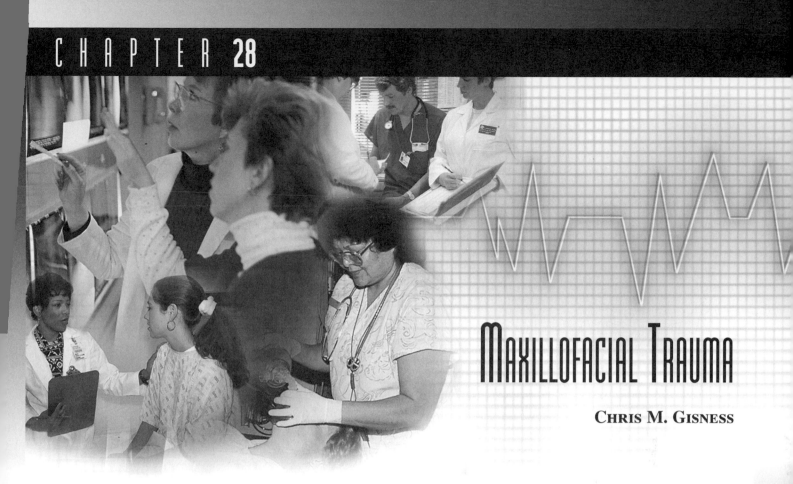

CHAPTER 28

MAXILLOFACIAL TRAUMA

CHRIS M. GISNESS

Maxillofacial trauma involving injury of the facial bones, neurovascular structures, skin, subcutaneous tissue, muscles, and glands is a common injury in patients treated in the emergency department (ED). Facial trauma is a complicating factor in management of patients with multisystem injuries. Studies document a 20% to 50% incidence of closed head injury with significant facial trauma.

Motor vehicle collisions (MVCs) are the most common cause of facial injury in the United States; however, facial trauma from assaults and personal altercations is increasing. Domestic violence is reported as the cause in 25% of all facial fractures.[9] Handguns also cause facial injury. With bullet trajectory above the mandible, intracranial injury should also be considered. Facial injury from falls is common among the elderly and children. In children, skull and facial bone flexibility absorb energy associated with deceleration injuries such as MVCs and falls. Significant energy is required to fracture the maxilla or midface—100 times the force of gravity; consequently patients with midface fractures often have multisystem injuries.[10] Figure 28-1 illustrates the relative strength of facial bones, whereas Table 28-1 identifies gravitational forces required to fracture various facial bones.

Thorough assessment of the eyes is a priority after life-threatening injuries have been addressed. Globe disruption and blindness can occur with injuries involving the eyes. Damage to the optic nerve or retina may also occur.

Use of air bags and seat belt restraints in vehicles save lives but not without some risk.[3] Facial injuries involving lacerations, abrasions, and chemical burns have been documented. Pediatric occupants are at significant risk for life-threatening injuries when seated in the front seat if an airbag deploys.[2] Infants weighing less than 40 pounds should be placed in the rear seat, with those less than 20 lbs or 1 year of age placed in a rear-facing car seat. Children should also be placed in the rear seat with a size- and weight-appropriate car seat.[10]

Assessment and treatment of facial injuries—regardless of severity—does not take priority over recognition and treatment of life-threatening injuries. Rapid, thorough assessment using a systematic approach with emphasis on airway, breathing, circulation (ABCs), and cervical spine stabilization is essential.

ANATOMY AND PHYSIOLOGY

Principal facial bones include the frontal, nasal, maxilla, zygoma, and mandible (Figure 28-2). The frontal bone articulates with the frontal process of the maxilla and nasal bone and laterally with the zygoma. The orbital complex is composed of the frontal bone superiorly, zygoma laterally, maxilla inferiorly, and processes of the maxilla and frontal bone medially. Paired nasal bones that form the bridge of the nose articulate with the frontal bone above and maxilla below (Figure 28-3). The nasal cavity is divided by the nasal septum (Figure 28-4); the lateral wall has ridges or concha that affect phonation (Figure 28-5).

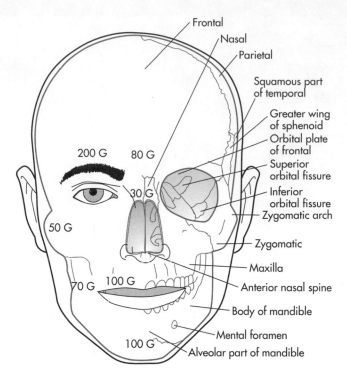

FIGURE 28-1 Relative strength of facial bones. (From Shepard S, Reyes I: Maxillofacial injury. In Norwood-Nass A, Wolfson A, editors: *The clinical practice of emergency medicine,* Philadelphia, 2001, Lippincott Williams & Wilkins.)

Table 28-1	FORCE OF GRAVITY IMPACT REQUIRED FOR FACIAL FRACTURE	
BONE	**FORCE OF GRAVITY (G)**
Nasal bones	30
Zygoma	50
Angle of mandible	70
Frontal-glabellar region	80
Midline maxilla	100
Midline mandible (symphysis)	100
Supraorbital rim	200

From Rosen P et al: *Emergency medicine,* ed 4, vol I, St. Louis, 1998, Mosby.

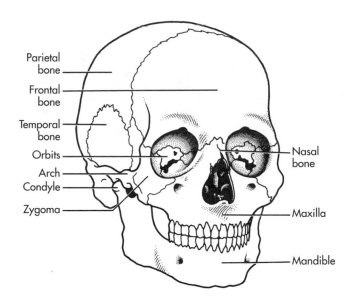

FIGURE 28-2 Facial skeleton. (From Rosen P et al: *Emergency medicine,* ed 4, St. Louis, 1998, Mosby.)

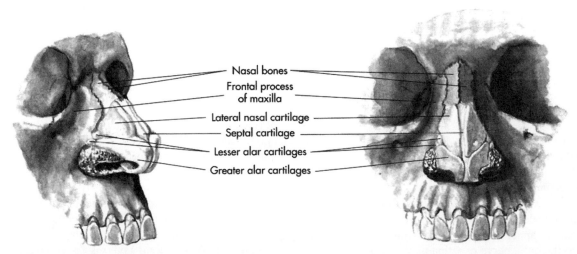

FIGURE 28-3 Nasal structures. (From *Mosby's medical, nursing, and allied health dictionary,* ed 5, St. Louis, 1998, Mosby.)

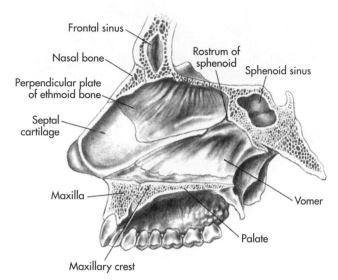

FIGURE **28-4** Nasal septum, medial view of sagittal section. (From Agur A, Lee M: *Grant's atlas of anatomy,* ed 10, Philadelphia, 1999, Lippincott Williams & Wilkins.)

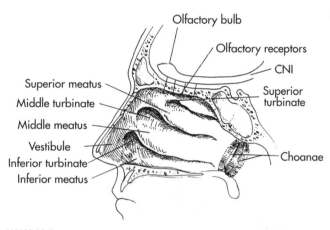

FIGURE **28-5** Lateral view of the left nasal cavity. (Modified from Barkauskas VH et al: *Health and physical assessment,* ed 2, St. Louis, 1998, Mosby.)

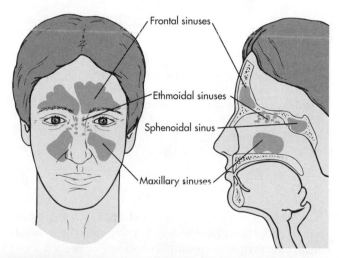

FIGURE **28-6** Paranasal sinuses. (From Agur A, Lee M: *Grant's atlas of anatomy,* ed 10, Philadelphia, 1999, Lippincott Williams & Wilkins.)

The midface, or maxilla, forms the upper jaw, anterior hard palate, part of the lateral wall of the nasal cavity, and part of the orbital floor. Below the orbit the maxilla is perforated by the infraorbital foramen to allow passage of the infraorbital vessels and nerves. Projecting downward, the alveolar process joins the opposite side to form the alveolar arch, which houses the upper teeth. Sinus cavities in the midface decrease weight and act as resonating chambers (Figure 28-6).

The zygoma forms the cheek and the lateral wall and floor of the orbital cavity. Articulations with the maxilla, frontal bone, and zygomatic process of the temporal bone form the zygomatic arch.

The mandible is a horizontal horseshoe body with two rami, anterior coronoid processes, and posterior condyloid processes.[11] The mandibular notch lies medial to the zygomatic arch and separates the two processes. The mandible articulates with the temporal bone to form the temporomandibular joint, whereas the upper body of the mandible, called the *alveolar part,* contains lower teeth.

The facial nerve (Cranial nerve VII) provides sensory and motor innervation to the side of the face. It originates in the brainstem, then divides into six branches to innervate the scalp, forehead, eyelids, facial muscles for expression, cheeks, and jaw (Figure 28-7). Specific functions for each branch are listed in Table 28-2. Other cranial nerves that may be affected by facial trauma are the oculomotor, trochlear, and trigeminal. Function and testing for each are described in Table 28-3.

The parotid gland located adjacent to the anterior ear drains into the oral cavity through the parotid duct (Figure 28-8). These structures are located adjacent to branches of the facial nerve on top of the masseter muscle.[1]

PATIENT ASSESSMENT

An organized approach to patient assessment is essential for identification and stabilization of facial injuries (Table 28-4). Regardless of injury or mechanism for injury, the first priority is a clear, secure airway. Damaged facial structures can cause airway obstruction. If the mandible is displaced, the tongue loses anatomic support and occludes the airway. Foreign objects (e.g., dentures or avulsed teeth) can obstruct the airway, whereas fractures of the naso-orbital complex compromise the airway secondary to hemorrhage. Gunshot wounds to the face cause significant swelling and hematoma formation, which obstruct the airway. When airway compromise is recognized, the chin lift–head tilt method should be used unless cervical spine injury is possible, in which case the jaw-thrust maneuver is indicated. Altered mental status from alcohol, drugs, or head injury can diminish the patient's gag reflex and leave the airway unprotected. Frequent suctioning of the oropharynx or nasopharynx is required when bleeding or excessive secretions are present. A tonsil tip suction catheter can be provided for an alert patient to self-suction. Allow the patient to sit upright or elevate the head of bed to promote drainage

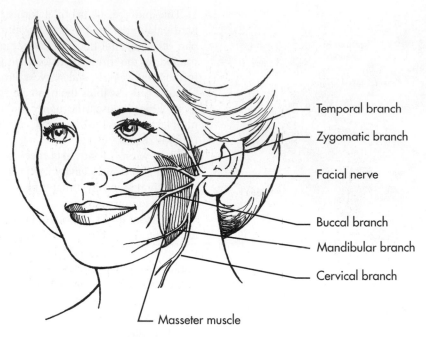

FIGURE 28-7   Anatomy of the facial nerve.

Table 28-2	FACIAL NERVE BRANCH FUNCTIONS	
BRANCH	**FUNCTION**	
Buccal	Wrinkle nose	
Cervical	Wrinkle skin of neck	
Mandibular	Purse and depress lips	
Temporal	Raise eyebrows, wrinkle forehead	
Zygomatic	Close eyelids	

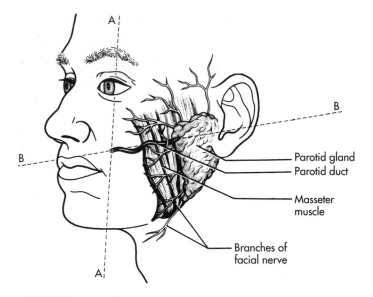

FIGURE 28-8   Parotid gland and parotid duct with nearby branches of facial nerve. Line B demonstrates approximate course of parotid duct from parotid gland, entering mouth at junction of lines *A* and *B*. (From Rosen P et al: *Emergency medicine,* ed 4, St. Louis, 1998, Mosby.)

if cervical spine injury is not a consideration or the cervical spine has been cleared.

Excessive bleeding and swelling of the mouth and facial structures, coupled with inability to clear the airway, requires aggressive airway control. Supplemental oxygen and assisted ventilations can be accomplished with a bag-valve-mask; however, swelling and facial fractures can make use of a bag-valve-mask difficult with some patients. An oropharyngeal airway can be used in an unconscious patient with obstruction from the tongue. A nasopharyngeal airway can be used in the conscious patient with no nasal or midface fractures.

Orotracheal intubation is preferred in patients with facial injuries; however, nasotracheal intubation should be avoided. Cribriform plate fractures increase the risk for cerebral penetration by an endotracheal tube. Rapid-sequence induction facilitates intubation and has the added benefit of protecting the patient from increases in intracra-

nial pressure.[6] If rapid-sequence induction is used, equipment to perform surgical airway opening must be available should cricothyroidotomy or tracheostomy be needed. Pulse oximetry is an essential adjunct for monitoring the airway. Cervical spine injury should be considered in all facial

Table 28-3	CRANIAL NERVES INVOLVED IN FACIAL TRAUMA			
NERVE	NAME	FUNCTION	DESCRIPTION	ASSESSMENT
III	Oculomotor	Motor	Eyeball movement; supplies 5 of 7 ocular muscles	Pupil response; ocular movement to four quadrants
IV	Trochlear	Motor	Eyeball movement (superior oblique)	Same as above
V	Trigeminal	Motor and sensory	Facial sensation; jaw movement	Assessing pain, touch, hot and cold sensations, bite, opening mouth against resistance
VII	Facial	Motor and sensory	Facial expression; taste from anterior two thirds of tongue	Zygomatic branch: have patient close eyes tightly; temporal branch: have patient elevate brows, wrinkle forehead; buccal branch: have patient elevate upper lip, wrinkle nose, whistle

Table 28-4	SYSTEMATIC ASSESSMENT FOR FACIAL TRAUMA
COMPONENT	DESCRIPTION
Airway	Assess for open airway; avoid using head-tilt method; consider airway adjuncts; nasopharyngeal airway adjunct is particularly useful with significant edema unless nasal or midface fractures are present
Breathing	Ensure adequate breathing; consider supplemental oxygen; noisy breathing suggests obstructed breathing
Circulation	Ensure adequate pulse rate and blood pressure
Cervical spine	Protect cervical spine; assume injury until proven otherwise by cross-table lateral radiograph of cervical spine; 10% of patients with severe head trauma have concurrent cervical spine trauma
Control hemorrhage	Use direct pressure whenever possible; protect airway when hemorrhage is present
Neurologic examination	Perform brief neurologic examination; assess for level of consciousness; pupillary response, and accommodation; rate, rhythm, and depth of respiration; and extraocular movement
Eyes	Evaluate eyes for visual acuity, loss of vision, diplopia (double vision), lid laceration, foreign bodies, penetrating bodies, and hemorrhage
Face	Check for malocclusion, tenderness, asymmetry of infraorbital rim; assess zygomatic arch, anterior wall of antrum, angles of jaw, and lower borders of mandible; check for cerebrospinal fluid leak from nose or face; anesthesia of lip, mouth, tongue; intraoral lacerations, ecchymosis, and loose or broken teeth

trauma patients with plain radiographs or computed tomography (CT) scan used to rule out injury.

After a patent airway is established, the next priority is hemorrhage control. Adult patients with facial injury rarely develop shock from facial bleeding, so hypotension is usually caused by associated injuries in the chest, abdomen, retroperitoneal space, or bones. Facial bleeding can be quickly controlled with direct pressure. An external compression dressing, such as a Barton bandage, wrapped circumferentially, can be used to temporarily control bleeding. Bleeding vessels on the face should be carefully assessed before ligation to prevent accidental clamping of facial nerve branches. A large cotton-tip swab can be used to apply direct pressure to bleeding vessels; ice packs and direct nasal pressure usually stop bleeding from the nose. A nasal tampon may be inserted to control anterior bleeding; a nasal catheter can be used to control posterior bleeding. Severe fa-

cial trauma such as LeFort II or III fractures requires manual reduction of the face to control bleeding. With closed fractures, bleeding from lacerated arteries and veins in sinus cavities can cause significant posterior pharyngeal bleeding; ligation of arteries and veins is necessary to control blood loss.

Palpate facial structures before edema and hematomas obscure bony landmarks (Figure 28-9). Use both hands simultaneously to palpate for step-off irregularities and crepitus of supraorbital ridge and zygoma. Take a bird's-eye view by looking down on the face from the eyebrows to compare height of malar eminences, then take a worm's-eye view and look up from below the chin. Gently palpate nasal bones and look intranasally for septal hematoma. Palpate laterally for depressions in the zygomatic arch, then visualize the mouth for gross dental malocclusion. Ask the patient if teeth close and fit together properly, then check the patient's ability to

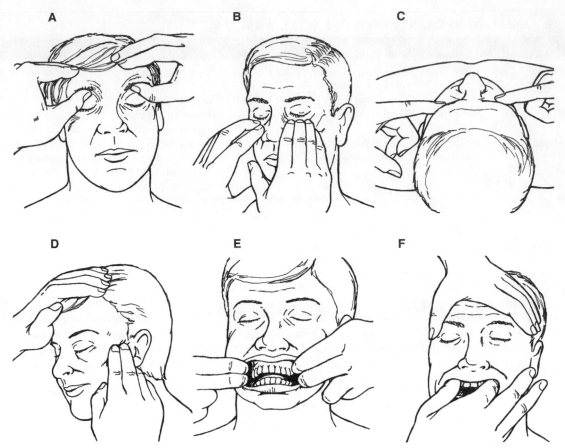

FIGURE 28-9 Palpation examination techniques for facial injuries. **A,** Palpation for irregularities of supraorbital ridge. **B,** Palpation for irregularities of infraorbital ridge and zygoma. **C,** Comparing height of malar eminences. **D,** Palpation for depression of zygomatic arch. **E,** Visualization of gross dental occlusion. **F,** Maneuver to ascertain motion in maxilla.

completely open the jaw. Upper and lower jaws should be carefully palpated intraorally (wearing gloves). Check midface stability by attempting to move the upper teeth and hard palate.

Evaluate the facial nerve and branches. Loss of sensation over the lower lip may indicate injury to the inferior alveolar nerve and possible mandibular fracture. Numbness over the upper lip occurs with fracture in the maxilla and injury to the infraorbital nerve. Assessment of the eye should be done early, before increasing lid edema makes it more difficult. Visual acuity is determined with use of the Snellen chart, hand-held card, or standard chart. If the patient is unable to count fingers, check for light perception and document findings before other testing is done.[3] Assess eyes for loss of vision, visual acuity, pupillary reactivity and symmetry, and extraocular movements. Ensure that pupils are on the same facial plane and observe closely for enophthalmos and proptosis. A teardrop-shaped pupil suggests a ruptured globe. Hyphema and subconjunctival hemorrhage often indicate a serious eye injury. In some patients with periorbital injuries, widening of the distance between the medial canthus (called telecanthus) may indicate serious orbital injury. Raccoon eyes or periorbital ecchymosis suggests anterior basilar skull fracture, LeFort fracture, or nasoethmoid injury, whereas nasal or ear drainage positive for cerebrospinal fluid (CSF) occurs with cribriform plate fracture or basilar skull fracture. Appearance of a bull's eye or halo when bloody drainage from the nose or ear is placed on white paper indicates the presence of CSF (Figure 28-10). Clear fluid positive for glucose or clear fluid that does not crust also indicates CSF. A ruptured tympanic membrane or laceration of the external ear canal can occur with mandible fractures. Deep lacerations of the cheek should be carefully evaluated for injury to the parotid gland, parotid (Stenson's) duct, and branches of the facial nerve. Diagnostic evaluation for maxillofacial injury includes radiographs, CT, and magnetic resonance imaging. Table 28-5 describes various diagnostic tests used to evaluate facial injuries.

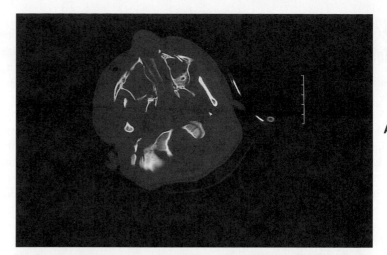

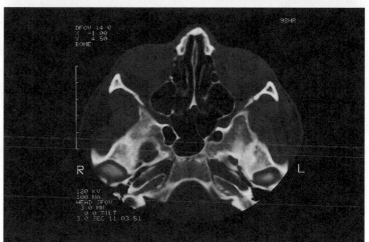

FIGURE 28-10   LeFort III fracture. This 10-year-old girl was hit by a car while sled riding. Clinically she had bilateral raccoon eyes, severe facial edema with a mobile maxilla, and bleeding from the nose, mouth, and eyes. She had the constellation of fractures that constitutes a LeFort III fracture and numerous other facial and skull fractures. **A,** In this cut, multiple fractures involving the anterior, posterior, and medial walls of the maxillary sinuses are shown. **B,** Bilateral zygoma fractures are evident in another cut. (From Zittelli B, Davis H: *Atlas of pediatric physical diagnosis,* ed 3, St. Louis, 1997, Mosby.)

Table 28-5	**RADIOGRAPHIC EXAMINATION FOR MAXIOLLOFACIAL INJURY**
TEST	**DESCRIPTION**
Water's view (posteroanterior)	Single most useful x-ray in maxillofacial injury
	Delineates orbital rim and floor
	Detects blood in maxillary sinus
Towne's view	Mandible condyles-subcondylar regions of orbital floor
Anterior, posterior, and lateral	Skull
	Sinus, roof of orbit
Submental vertex (jughandle)	Zygomatic arch
	Details base of skull
AP and lateral oblique mandible	Condylar, coronoid, body, and symphysis
Occlusal and apical	Palate, symphysis, roots of teeth
CT scan	Provides definitive diagnosis in C-spine injury
	Standard for assessing soft tissue injuries
	Complex facial fractures
MRI	Useful for identifying soft tissue injuries in optic nerve
	Muscle herniation, infraocular and intraocular hematomas, entrapment

AP, Anteroposterior; *CT,* computed tomography; *MRI,* magnetic resonance imaging.

SPECIFIC MAXILLOFACIAL INJURIES

Soft-Tissue Trauma

For cosmetic purposes, repair of facial lacerations should occur as quickly as possible. Simple lacerations can be cleaned, debrided, and sutured by primary intention within 24 hours of injury. Deeper lacerations and lacerations associated with fractures are conservatively debrided, irrigated, and closed after reduction. Degloving injuries usually involve subcutaneous tissues and underlying skeletal structures.[7] Tissue is considered viable, so excessive debridement should be avoided. Repair of facial lacerations in uncooperative patients is extremely difficult and may injure other important structures. Delaying repair until the patient is more cooperative usually results in better outcome. Figure 28-11 shows contusions, abrasions, and lacerations of the face.

Lacerations caused by animal or human bites are highly contaminated because of the bacteria and debris in the mouth. Human bites should be meticulously cleaned and irrigated; however, controversy surrounds wound closure.[3] Extensive or gaping wounds on the face present cosmetic problems, so consultation with a plastic surgeon is recommended. Treatment of animal bites is also controversial. Most experts recommend closing the wound after meticulous irrigation and debridement. Both human and animal

bites should be inspected for tooth fragments. Extensive animal bites, usually caused by large dogs, frequently require surgical exploration and repair. A helpful mnemonic for dealing with animal bites is RATS (rabies, antibiotics, tetanus, and soap). Patients with animal and human bites receive prophylactic antibiotics and are immunized for tetanus as appropriate.

Road rash or friction injuries present a unique problem because of potential tattooing or epidermal staining. Debridement should be done within 12 hours to avoid accidental but permanent tattooing from grease and asphalt. Skin should be vigorously scrubbed with mild soap after the area has been injected with local anesthetic. Gunpowder can cause permanent discoloration of skin with subsequent cosmetic disfigurement; therefore, black powder fragments embedded in facial skin should be removed by using a local anesthetic and scrubbing with a hard brush or hard bristle toothbrush in the first hour whenever possible. Gunpowder penetrating the skin is very hot and continues to burn epithelial and collagen layers. Removal after 72 hours increases risk for permanent discoloration, so dermabrasion may be performed after the fifth to seventh day.[8] When glass fragments are visible, tape applied to the face helps pick up the glass.

Air bags usually cause minor abrasions of the face, neck, and upper chest.[5] Corneal or scleral injury may also occur but is not a common event. Lacerations of eyebrows and eyelids should be repaired before swelling occurs so borders can be matched. Eyebrows should never be shaved because landmarks are eliminated and the brow is unlikely to grow back. When suturing the brow, hairs are aligned so they slant in a downward and outward direction.

Vermilion-cutaneous and vermilion-mucosal margins are important anatomic landmarks in repair of lip lacerations. Borders must be perfectly aligned to prevent development of step-off deformity of the lip. Figure 28-12 illustrates closure

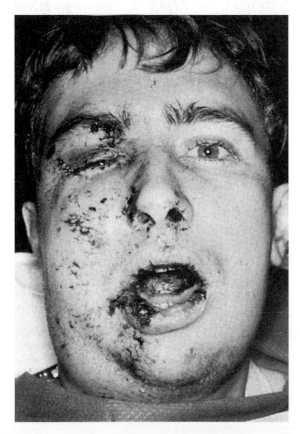

FIGURE 28-11 Facial injuries. (From Sheehy SB, Jimmerson CL: *Manual of clinical trauma care,* ed 2, St. Louis, 1994, Mosby.)

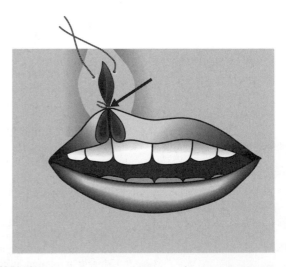

FIGURE 28-12 Lip laceration through the vermillion border. Closure requires proper alignment with the first suture placed at the vermillion-cutaneous border.

of this type of laceration. Tissue loss from the lip requires reconstruction by a plastic surgeon.

Intraoral injuries should be carefully inspected for debris, crushed tissue, and tooth fragments. Injuries should be meticulously cleaned and irrigated. Gaping intraoral lacerations tend to develop ulcerations and become infected, so they should be closed. Antibiotics are usually prescribed.

When the tongue is lacerated, inspect the mouth carefully for other lacerations from teeth. Gaping or bleeding lacerations are sutured and antibiotic therapy is indicated. Children are prone to hard and soft palate lacerations, usually from falling with a sharp object in the mouth.

Ear injuries are categorized into three groups: hematomas, lacerations, and avulsions. Hematomas must be properly drained and dressed to prevent a scar deformity that resembles a cauliflower (Figure 28-13). Lacerations may involve skin or skin and cartilage. Wounds require minimal debridement and are usually closed in two layers; however, avulsion injuries of the ear require skin preservation; otherwise grafts from other body sites are required. Anesthetics containing epinephrine should not be used on the ear because of the deleterious effects of vasoconstriction. Antibiotics are prescribed to prevent cartilage infection. Cartilage necrosis can occur if bandages are left unpadded or unchecked for long periods.

Deep cheek lacerations can damage the parotid gland, parotid duct, and branches of the facial nerve, a motor nerve that governs muscles of facial expression. Injury to the temporal branch causes forehead asymmetry because the patient cannot wrinkle the forehead on the affected side. With injury to the temporal or zygomatic branch, the patient is unable to fully close the eyelids on the affected side. Buccal branch injury keeps the patient from pursing the lips to whistle, and injury to the mandibular branch causes inability to lower or depress the lower lip. At rest, elevation of the lower lip occurs on the affected side. Injury to the facial nerve can be easily missed if the patient is unconscious or

has numerous facial dressings. Facial paralysis after blunt facial trauma has a good prognosis for complete recovery if minimal soft-tissue damage occurs. Lacerations of the parotid duct or the parotid gland are an infrequent occurrence. Duct cannulization is used to determine patency when injury is suspected.

Nasal Fractures

Nasal fractures are the most common facial fracture because the nose offers the least resistance. The mechanism of injury is usually blunt trauma. Overlooked nasal injury can lead to permanent deformity and airway obstruction. Clinical findings include swelling, deformity, bleeding, and crepitus. Table 28-6 provides a detailed look at the clinical and radiographic aspects of these and other facial fractures. In children the nose is more elastic and resistant to fractures; however, dislocations are common. Unrecognized or untreated nasal fractures can lead to abnormal nasal bone growth that affects nasal contour.

Nasal bones are lined with mucoperiosteum, which becomes an open fracture when overlying skin is lacerated. Fractures caused by a frontal blow damage ethmoid and frontal sinuses, lacrimal duct, and orbital margins. If the cribriform plate is affected and the dura torn, cerebrospinal fluid rhinorrhea occurs. Careful examination of each naris can identify septal hematomas, lacerations, and ability of the patient to breathe through his or her nose.[3] A septal hematoma appears as a bulging tense bluish mass that feels doughy when palpated. Septal hematomas should be emergently drained to prevent airway obstruction and necrosis of septal cartilage. Untreated septal hematoma causes a permanent nasal deformity called *saddle deformity*.[10]

Initial interventions focus on controlling bleeding with direct pressure. Bleeding may be intranasal and in the pharynx. Ice compresses applied to the bridge of the nose aid hemostasis and help relieve pain. Anterior or posterior nasal packing may be required to control bleeding. Splinting maintains position, ensures alignment, and prevents further edema and injury. In some cases the physician may not set the fracture until the swelling subsides. When the fracture involves the nasal mucosa of the lacrimal system, blowing the nose causes intracranial air or subcutaneous emphysema that can later cause localized infection or meningitis.

Maxillary Fractures

Maxillary, or midface fractures, caused by significant force, are usually a combination of fractures involving several facial structures. Maxillary fractures are classified as LeFort I, II, and III (i.e., lower third, middle third, and orbital complex). Plain radiographs of the face with emphasis on Water's view are used to confirm diagnosis (Figure 28-14), with CT scan used to substantiate extent of fractures. Maxillary fractures are rarely seen in children because of the flexibility and pliable nature of their maxillofacial structures.

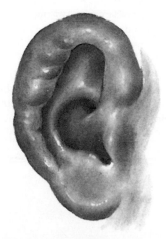

FIGURE 28-13 Cauliflower ear. (Modified from Seidel HM et al: *Mosby's guide to physical examination*, ed 3, St. Louis, 1995, Mosby.)

Table 28-6   FACIAL FRACTURES: CLINICAL AND RADIOGRAPHIC FINDINGS, AND COMPLICATIONS FOR SPECIFIC FACIAL FRACTURES

FRACTURE	CLINICAL PRESENTATION	RADIOGRAPHIC	COMPLICATIONS
Naso-orbital	Symptoms: pain, visual abnormalities Signs: massive periorbital and upper facial edema and ecchymosis, epistaxis, traumatic telecanthus, foreshortening of nose with telescoping; associated intracranial injuries	Views: CT scan Findings: disruption of interorbital space and comminution of nasal pyramid; frontal, zygomatic, orbital, maxillary fractures common	Residual upper midface deformity ("dish face"); telecanthus; frontal sinus-nasolacrimal system pathology with mucocele, mucopyocele, dacryocystitis
Zygoma			
Arch	Symptoms: pain in lateral cheek, inability to close jaw Signs: swelling, crepitus over arch, obvious asymmetry	Views: Water's submentovertex Findings: depression of arch, comminution	Contour irregularities of arch area, flattening of arch
Body "tripod fracture"	Symptoms: pain, trismus, diplopia, numb upper lip, lower lid, bilateral nasal area Signs: swelling, ecchymosis of malar and periorbital areas; palpable infraorbital rim "step-off"; entrapment of extraocular muscles with disconjugate gaze; scleral ecchymosis, displacement of lateral canthal ligament	Views: Water's submentovertex, CT scan Findings: clouding, air/fluid level maxillary sinus, separation of zygomaticomaxillary, zygomaticofrontal, and zygomaticotemporal suture lines	Residual malar deformity, enophthalmos, diplopia, infraorbital nerve anesthesia, chronic maxillary sinusitis
Orbital floor	Symptoms: diplopia, orbital pain Signs: periorbital edema, ecchymosis, enophthalmos, extraocular muscle entrapment, disconjugate gaze; hyphema, subluxation of lens, retinal detachment, rupture of globe with direct eye trauma	Views: Water's, CT scan, tomograms Findings: air/fluid level maxillary sinus, herniated adnexa and/or orbital floor fragments in maxillary sinus	Enophthalmos, diplopia; recurrent orbital cellulitis with implant (alloplastic) extrusion
Mandible			
Condyle	Symptoms: pain at fracture site, referred pain to ear Signs: crepitus, excessive salivation, swelling of condylar region, deviation of jaw toward fracture, cross-bite or open-bite deformity	Views: AP, oblique, Water's, Panorex Findings: nondisplaced, or displaced anteriorly and medially	Ankylosis of TMJ; chronic TMJ
Angle	Symptoms: pain at fracture site, inability to close mouth Signs: swelling at angle of jaw, ecchymosis, crepitus, malocclusion	Views: Panorex, mandibular series Findings: nondisplaced (favorable) or posterior fragment displaced upward and medially (nonfavorable)	Nonunion, malunion, osteomyelitis
Body	Symptoms: pain at fracture site, limitation of movement Signs: swelling, ecchymosis, crepitus, malocclusion	Views: Panorex, mandibular series Findings: nondisplaced (favorable), or posterior fragment displaced upward and medially, anterior fragments rotated lingually (nonfavorable)	Osteomyelitis, infection (tooth in fracture line)
Symphysis	Symptoms: pain Signs: malocclusion, frequent association with soft tissue wounds of lower lip, tongue	Views: mandibular series, submentovertex Findings: nondisplaced or lingual rotation or anterior fragments, may be associated with angle or condyle fractures	Residual malocclusion, loss of chin projection, asymmetry; osteomyelitis

Modified from Trunkey DD, Lewis FR: *Current therapy of trauma,* ed 2, Toronto, 1986, BC Decker.
CT, Computed tomography; *AP,* anteroposterior; *TMJ,* temporomandibular joint.

Table 28-6	FACIAL FRACTURES: CLINICAL AND RADIOGRAPHIC FINDINGS, AND COMPLICATIONS FOR SPECIFIC FACIAL FRACTURES—cont'd		
FRACTURE	**CLINICAL PRESENTATION**	**RADIOGRAPHIC**	**COMPLICATIONS**
Maxilla			
LeFort I (transverse)	Symptoms: pain upper jaw, numb upper teeth Signs: midfacial edema and ecchymosis, epistaxis, malocclusion, mobility of maxillary dentition	Views: Water's, Panorex, CT scan Findings: opaque maxillary sinus, displacement of fragments of alveolus if comminuted; fracture through maxillary sinus and pterygoid plates	Loss of teeth, infection, malocclusion
LeFort II (pyramidal)	Symptoms: pain midface, numb upper lip, lower lid, lateral nasal area Signs: midfacial edema and ecchymosis, epistaxis, malocclusion, mobility of midface, nasal flattening, anesthesia infraorbital nerve territory	Views: Water's, CT scan Findings: opaque maxillary sinuses, separation through frontal process, lacrimal bones, floor of orbits, zygomaticomaxillary suture line, lateral wall of maxillary sinus, and pterygoid plates	Nonunion, malunion lacrimal system obstruction, infraorbital nerve anesthesia, diplopia, malocclusion
LeFort III (craniofacial dysjunction)	Symptoms: pain face, difficulty breathing Signs: "donkey-face" deformity, malocclusion, mobile face, marked facial edema and ecchymosis, epistaxis, CSF rhinorrhea	Views: Water's, CT scan Findings: separation of midthird of face at zygomaticofrontal, zygomaticotemporal, and nasofrontal sutures, and across orbital floors; opaque maxillary sinuses	Nonunion, malunion, malocclusion, lengthening of midface, lacrimal system obstruction

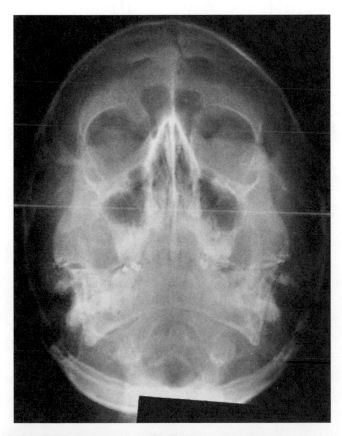

FIGURE 28-14 Posteroanterior (Water's) radiograph of the paranasal sinuses of a 9-year-old girl. (From Snell R, Smith M: *Clinical anatomy for emergency medicine,* St. Louis, 1993, Mosby.)

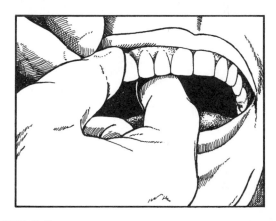

FIGURE 28-15 Clinical examination for fracture of maxilla.

Patients with maxillary fractures complain of severe facial pain, anesthesia or paresthesia of the upper lip, and some visual disturbances (see Table 28-6). Clinically, the patient has severe facial swelling, ecchymosis, periorbital or orbital swelling, subconjunctival hemorrhage, elongation of the face, facial asymmetry, epistaxis, and malocclusion, and may occasionally exhibit complete airway obstruction.[4] CSF may leak from the nose. Figure 28-15 shows a technique used to assess for maxillary mobility.

LeFort I, or lower third fracture (Figure 28-16, *A*) is a horizontal fracture in which the body of the maxilla is separated from the base of the skull above the palate but below the zygomatic process attachment. Separation may be unilateral or bilateral. There is a free-floating segment of the upper teeth and lower maxilla; however, the fracture may not be displaced. The hard palate and upper teeth are mobile when moved by grasping the alveolar process and anterior teeth.

Lateral view   Frontal view

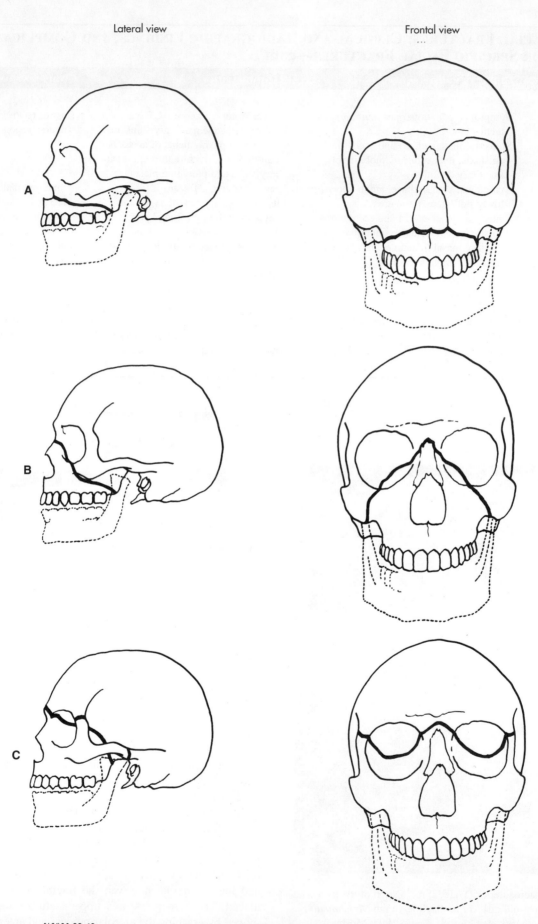

FIGURE 28-16   **A,** LeFort I facial fracture. **B,** LeFort II facial fracture. **C,** LeFort III facial fracture.

LeFort II, or middle third fracture (Figure 28-16, *B*), involves the pyramidal area including the central maxilla, nasal area, and ethmoid bones. This portion of the face is a tripod shape with the apex at the nose. Grasping the front teeth and palate causes movement of the nose and upper lip with no movement of the orbital complex. Significant force is required to fracture this area so the patient should be carefully evaluated for other injuries. The nose, lips, and eyes are usually edematous with subconjunctival hemorrhage and epistaxis frequently noted. The presence of CSF rhinorrhea suggests an open skull fracture.

LeFort III, or orbital complex fracture (Figure 28-16, *C*), causes total cranial facial separation. The nose and dental arch move without frontal bone involvement. Massive edema, ecchymosis, epistaxis, and malocclusion are present with a spoonlike appearance of the face noted in side profile. Early ocular examination is necessary to prevent unrecognized ocular injuries secondary to extensive swelling. Fractures of the cribriform plate and bleeding from the middle meningeal artery threaten airway patency; cervical spine fracture-dislocation can also occur.[3]

Management of maxillary fractures includes aggressive airway control. Endotracheal intubation may be difficult because of edema and loss of normal anatomic contour, so anticipate cricothyroidotomy or tracheotomy. Excessive secretions and bleeding require frequent suctioning, so allow the patient to use a Yankauer suction when appropriate.[5] Position the patient upright and leaning forward (as soon as the cervical spine is cleared) to promote drainage and decrease swelling. Apply ice compresses for pain relief and to decrease swelling and administer prophylactic antibiotics and tetanus immunization as appropriate.

Zygoma Fractures

Fractures of the zygoma usually occur in two patterns: zygomatic arch fracture and tripod fracture. Fracture of the orbital floor may also be present with zygomatic fractures. Injury is usually caused by blunt trauma to the front and side of the face. With a tripod fracture, the zygoma fractures in three places: zygomatic arch, posterior half of the infraorbital rim, and frontozygomatic suture. A step deformity is palpated at the infraorbital rim and frontozygomatic suture area with flattening or asymmetry of the cheek, periorbital edema, circumorbital or subconjunctival ecchymosis, and pain exacerbated by jaw motion (see Table 28-6).

Entrapment of the inferior rectus muscle causes double vision and asymmetry of ocular levels and anesthesia of the upper lip, cheek, teeth, and gums. The mnemonic TIDES is helpful in determination of zygomatic fractures (Box 28-1). Interventions focus on pain control and decreasing swelling. Plain radiographs with a "jughandle" view demonstrate zygomatic arch fracture (Figure 28-17), whereas CT scans are often needed to demonstrate extent of a tripod fracture.

Orbital Blowout Fractures

Zygoma fractures and orbital blowout fractures can occur independently but are often found in combination. Plain radiographs with Water's view can help distinguish these injuries. Orbital blowout fracture occurs when blunt trauma to the globe causes abrupt rise in orbital pressure. The orbital floor is the weakest part of the bony orbit, so increased pressure causes orbital contents to prolapse into the maxillary sinus (Figure 28-18).[4] Inferior rectus muscle, inferior oblique muscle, infraorbital nerve, orbital fat, and connective tissue become entrapped in the orbital floor, so extraocular movements should be carefully evaluated. The globe may also become entrapped. This fracture frequently results from sports, such as a baseball thrown at the eye, and altercations such as fist fights. Golf balls can extend past the protective orbital rim and rupture the globe. If the globe is perforated, manipulating the eyes or noseblowing can lead to intraorbital air.

Subcutaneous orbital emphysema suggests fracture in the sinus arch. Noseblowing, coughing, sneezing, vomiting, and straining can force air from sinuses through the fracture into the orbital space. Proptosis or bulging of the eye and limitation of extraocular motion suggest orbital involvement (Figure 28-19). Double vision, pupil asymmetry, enophthalmos (sunken appearance), anesthesia of the cheek and upper lip, ptosis or drooping of the lid, and a sunken appearance are clinical manifestations of blowout fracture (see Table 28-6). Globe injuries may occur concurrently with blowout fractures. Ruptures usually occur at the weakest area of the globe or opposite the side of impact.[4] If a ruptured globe is

Box 28-1	TIDES MNEMONIC FOR ZYGOMATIC FRACTURES	
T	Trismus	Tonic contracture of muscles of mastication
I	Infraorbital	Hypoesthesia or anesthesia
D	Diplopia	Double vision
E	Epistaxis	Nosebleed
S	Symmetry absence	Flatness or depression of cheek

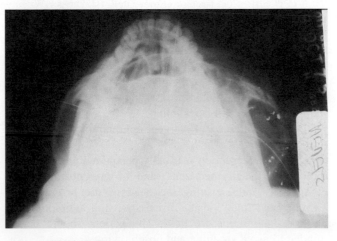

FIGURE 28-17 Radiograph of zygomatic fracture.

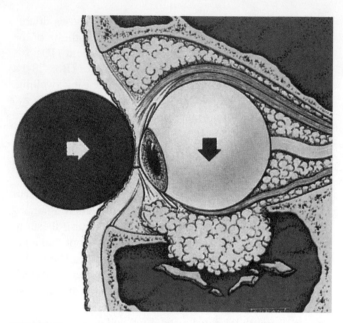

FIGURE 28-18 Mechanism of a blowout fracture caused by the impact of a ball. The periorbital fat is forced through the floor of the orbit. (From Ragge N: *Immediate eye care,* London, 1990, Wolfe Medical Publications.)

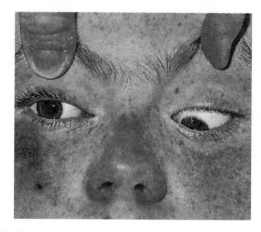

FIGURE 28-19 Blow-out fracture. (From Zitelli BJ, Davis HW: *Atlas of pediatric physical diagnosis,* ed 2, London, 1992, Gower Medical.)

suspected, an eye shield or plastic cup should be used over the eye to prevent further injury. The globe is ruptured in 3.5% of blunt trauma.[9] Emergent ophthalmologic consultation is indicated.

Surgical intervention is usually postponed until swelling diminishes, usually between 7 and 14 days postinjury. Ice compresses and elevating the head of the bed decrease swelling and relieve pain. Broad spectrum antibiotics and nasal decongestants are used. The patient should be reminded to avoid straining and noseblowing.[7]

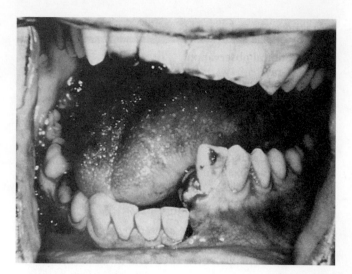

FIGURE 28-20 Malocclusion caused by fracture. (From Sheehy SB, Jimmerson CL: *Manual of clinical trauma care,* ed 2, St. Louis, 1994, Mosby. Courtesy Dr. Daniel Cheney.)

Mandibular Fractures

Mandibular fractures are the second most common facial fracture. Blunt force, such as a severe blow to the face during contact sports, altercations, and MVCs, is the usual mechanism of injury. Mandible fractures can be a significant life-threatening injury if loss of bony support displaces the tongue posteriorly and obstructs the airway. Malocclusion is a cardinal indication of mandible fracture (Figure 28-20). Signs and symptoms vary with fracture site; however, point tenderness and crepitus may be palpated and step-off deformity found. Trismus and decreased range of motion are usually noted. The face may be asymmetric with swelling and ecchymosis. Paresthesia in the lower lip and chin imply injury to the inferior alveolar nerve (see Table 28-6). The oral cavity should be assessed for broken or loose teeth, lacerations, or ecchymosis. Sublingual hematoma can compromise the airway. Inspect ears for tears in the external canal and tympanic membrane.

Mandibular fractures are classified according to the region of the jaw injured. The most common sites for fracture are the angle of the mandible, condyle, and molar and mental regions, with the symphysis the least common injury site (Figure 28-21). Reciprocal fractures can occur on the side opposite the point of impact. A panoramic radiograph is best for radiographic imaging of the mandible (Figure 28-22). Treatment consists of surgical intervention with open reduction and internal fixation or wiring jaws, depending on location of the fracture. Nursing care in the ED includes allowing the patient to sit upright as soon as the cervical spine is cleared and applying ice compresses to the face to minimize swelling and relieve pain. Oral saline rinses for the mouth may also be used. Intravenous antibiotics are indicated for open fractures, and repair of lacerations should occur as soon as possible.

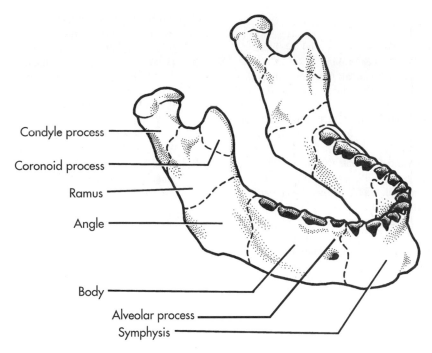

Condyle process
Coronoid process
Ramus
Angle
Body
Alveolar process
Symphysis

FIGURE 28-21 Fracture sites of mandible. (Modified from Rosen P et al: *Emergency medicine,* ed 3, St. Louis, 1992, Mosby.)

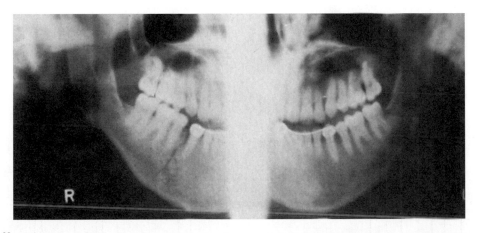

FIGURE 28-22 Panoramic radiograph of mandible. Note fractures in left angle and right body. (Dental retainer appliance is in place on lower incisors.) (From Rosen P et al: *Emergency medicine,* ed 4, St. Louis, 1998, Mosby.)

SUMMARY

Maxillofacial injuries are a common occurrence in the ED. Special attention should be given to stabilizing the cervical spine, maintaining a patent airway, and controlling hemorrhage. The goal of treatment is life, function, and aesthetics. Box 28-2 identifies priority nursing diagnoses for facial injuries.

Box 28-2 NURSING DIAGNOSES FOR FACIAL INJURIES

Airway clearance, Ineffective
Infection, Risk for
Pain
Skin integrity, Impaired

References

1. Agur A, Lee M: *Grant's atlas of anatomy,* ed 10, Philadelphia, 1999, Lippincott Williams & Wilkins.
2. Bailey H, Perez N, Blank-Reid C et al: Atlanto-occiptal dislocation: an unusual lethal airbag injury, *J Emerg Med* 18(2):215, 2000.
3. Colucciello S: Maxillofacial trauma. In Tintinall J: *Emergency medicine: a comprehensive study guide,* ed 5, New York, 2000, McGraw–Hill.
4. Ellis E, Scott K: Assessment of patients with facial fractures. In Rutkauskas J, Reddings S, Mulliken R, editors: *Emergency medicine clinics of North America: oral facial emergencies,* Philadelphia, 2001, WB Saunders.
5. Emergency Nurses Association: *Emergency nursing core curriculum,* ed 5, Philadelphia, 2000, WB Saunders.
6. Howes D, Dowling P: Triage & initial evaluation of oral facial emergency, *Emerg Med Clin N Am Oral Facial Emerg* 18(3):371, 2000.
7. Kitt S, Selfredge-Thomas J, Proehl J et al: *Emergency nursing: a physiologic and clinical perspective,* ed 2, Philadelphia, 1995, WB Saunders.
8. Mayor T, Constant E: Trauma to the face. In Schwartz G, editor: *Principles & practice of emergency medicine,* Baltimore, 1999, Williams & Wilkins.
9. Moore S, Reyes I: Maxillofacial injuries. In Harwood-Nuss A, Wolfson A, editors: *The clinical practice of emergency medicine,* ed 3, Philadelphia, 2001, Lippincott Williams & Wilkins.
10. Paige K, Barlett S: Facial trauma and plastic surgical emergencies. In Fleisher O, Ludwig S, editors: *Textbook of pediatric emergency medicine,* ed 4, Philadelphia, 2000, Lippincott Williams & Wilkins.
11. Snell R, Smith M: *Clinical anatomy for emergency medicine,* St Louis, 1993, Mosby.

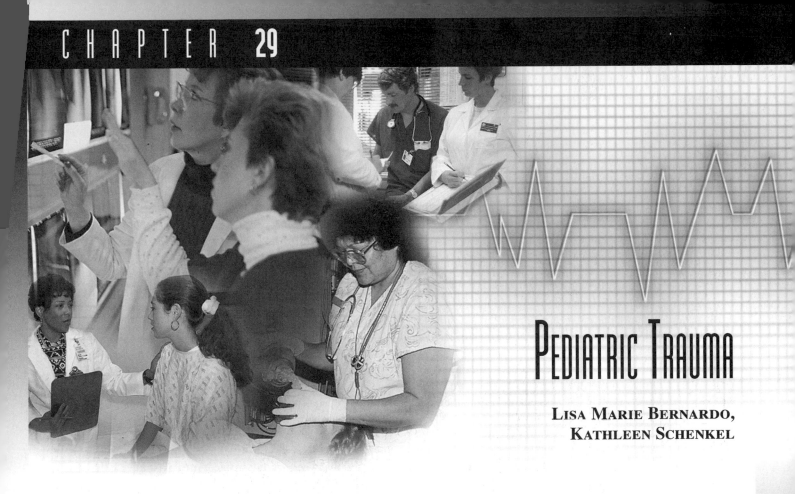

CHAPTER 29

PEDIATRIC TRAUMA

LISA MARIE BERNARDO,
KATHLEEN SCHENKEL

Despite scientific advances in injury prevention and treatment, traumatic injury continues to be the leading cause of death in children older than 1 year of age. Approximately 22 million children are injured in the United States each year.[34] There are 10,000 children who die annually from trauma, and more than 100,000 have permanent disabilities.[38] Among ethnic groups in the United States, Alaska Native and Native American Indian children have the highest rates of injury-related morbidity and mortality.[16]

Of the estimated 31,447,000 annual emergency department (ED) visits made by children and adolescents in the United States, 13,562,000 (43%) are injury-related (17.8 visits per 100 people).[50] These injury-related visits peak in the 0- to 2-year and 18- to 20-year age-groups. Males accounted for almost 59% of injury-related ED visits, with the rate of visits between Caucasian and minority pediatric and adolescent patients similar.[50] The home was the most frequently reported injury location (5,984,000, 44%). The majority of patients (84%) had an Injury Severity Score (ISS) less than 3. Only 4% of these ED patients were admitted, transferred, or pronounced dead on arrival.[50] An estimated $4 billion is paid annually for all injury-related ED visits by children and adolescents, of which $2.4 billion (60%) is paid for males.[50]

The frequency of childhood injuries compels the emergency nurse to participate in primary, secondary, and tertiary prevention of pediatric injuries. This chapter highlights anatomic and physiologic differences in pediatric patients, describes patient assessment, reviews essential interventions, discusses treatment of selected traumatic injuries, and identifies specific injury prevention strategies.

HISTORICAL PERSPECTIVE

Dr. William E. Ladd is considered the pioneer of pediatric surgery.[29] In 1917 he was a medical volunteer who treated thousands of people injured in the collision of two ships in Halifax, Nova Scotia. The burned and injured children had a profound effect on him. He returned to Boston and devoted himself exclusively to surgical care of children.[29] Ladd is credited with being the first pediatric surgeon and the originator of pediatric surgery as a specialty.

During the World Wars, surgeons exposed to new techniques in trauma care were not interested in care of pediatric trauma patients. However, pediatric trauma care could not have advanced without their efforts.[45] In the 1960s pediatric trauma gained recognition as the number of children injured and killed from "accidents" increased. During the late 1980s and early 1990s, pediatric trauma care gathered even more interest. The American Pediatric Surgical Association's Trauma Committee developed guidelines for care of injured children, and *Emergency Medical Services for Children* grants were implemented. Community groups such as the *National Safe Kids Campaign* became popular, promoting pediatric injury prevention to the public. Interest in pediatric trauma care— from the prehospital arena through rehabilitation into the prevention phase—continued to grow through ongoing clinical, education, and research endeavors.

EPIDEMIOLOGY

Blunt force trauma is the most common mechanism of pediatric morbidity and mortality,[38] including motor vehicle crashes (MVCs), falls, pedestrian incidents, and bicycle crashes. MVCs are the leading cause of death from blunt force trauma,[35] with most fatalities resulting from head injuries.[38] In 1999 MVCs killed 1135 child occupants between 0 and 10 years of age and injured approximately 182,000 children in the United States alone. This represents approximately 3 deaths and 500 injuries to American children every day.[47] Frontal collisions (43%) are the most common crash pattern among fatal crashes, followed by side impact collisions (34%), first-event rollovers (13%), and rear end collisions (10%).[47] Most children who die in MVCs are not restrained in child safety seats or seat belts.[47] Although only 8% of all children younger than 5 years of age traveled as unrestrained motor vehicle passengers in 1998, they accounted for more than half of child passenger fatalities.[47] In one study of 5751 children injured in MVCs, more than 40% were unrestrained.[3] Restraint systems minimize the risk for vehicular ejection and contact with the vehicle's interior structures and passengers, allow the passenger to "ride down" the vehicle's velocity during a crash, and spread energy from impact over large body areas.[52] As unrestrained passengers, young children are thrown about the vehicle, suffering injuries to the head, chest, abdomen, and extremities. They can be pinned beneath the dashboard, impaled on the gearshift, and bounced against doors, seats, and other passengers. Children held on the lap of an adult can be crushed between the adult and point of impact; for example, the dashboard, steering column, or front seat. Unrestrained children have a greater chance of ejection through the windshield, side windows, or rear windows.

Safety seats are the most effective protection against fatal injury to child motor vehicle passengers. Rear-facing infant safety seats reduce the risk of death in an MVC by 71%, forward-facing seats for toddlers reduce risk of death by 54%, and safety belts reduce risk of death by 45%.[47] However, parents must know how to correctly install and use child safety seats to achieve the most protection for their children. Infants are placed in rear-facing seats until they are at least 1 year of age and weigh at least 9 kg because they have large heads, proportionally, and weak neck muscles place them at risk for cervical distraction and dislocation during frontal crashes.[52] Children ages 4 to 9 years restrained with lap belt and shoulder harness are susceptible to certain injuries. Young children have a shorter sitting height than adults, with a higher center of gravity above the lap belt. Greater proportion of body mass is located above the safety belt, which may cause more forward motion and increase the risk for head and neck injury. Children can jackknife over restraints, causing an airway or hanging injury. Similarly, a child can "submarine" under the restraint system, leading to neck and airway injuries. The lap belt itself can also cause injuries. During sudden deceleration children are thrown forward with their full body weight going into the lap belt. Resulting injuries include lumbar spine fractures, small bowel injuries, and abdominal bruising.

Sitting in the rear seat of a car offers significant protection during an MVC. Restraint use enhances this effect[3]; therefore, parents must be encouraged to restrain children with proper child safety devices in the vehicle's rear seat for optimal protection in the event of an MVC.

Children riding in the back of pickup trucks are at risk for serious injury or death. In 1997, 161 deaths of occupants riding in the back of pickup trucks were reported; 77 (48%) were children and adolescents.[48] Passengers riding in the back of pickup trucks are more likely to sustain multiple injuries, sustain injuries of greater severity, and are more likely to die compared with occupants riding in the cab portion of the truck.[14] The danger of riding in the back area is passenger ejection during a crash or noncrash event, such as a sudden stop, turn, swerve with loss of balance, intentional jumps or falls, and unintentional jumps and falls.[14]

Children and adolescents sustain injuries as passengers or operators of off-road vehicles (two-, three-, and four-wheel unlicensed motor vehicles). Most injuries occur from disruptions in the driving surface, such as bumps, holes, and uneven terrain.[13] Young children riding as passengers can be crushed by the adult driver on impact with a stationary or moving object. Older children who are not the appropriate size or weight to operate such vehicles can flip vehicles onto themselves and sustain serious multisystem injuries.

Falls are the most common mechanism of injury in children, accounting for 3,125,000 (23%) of all ED injury-related visits.[50] Young children are most frequently injured during falls in the home. Children fall from varying heights, such as from furniture or out windows. They also fall while running, playing, and participating in sports. Injuries sustained from falls vary from mild to severe single-system or multisystem trauma.

Baby walkers are the most common nursery products that cause injury.[18] Baby walkers were implicated in 14,300 ED visits made by children younger than 15 months in 1997; most children sustained injuries from falls down stairs while in the walker.[19] Shopping carts also have the potential for injuring children younger than 5 years of age. In 1996 an average of 22,200 children younger than 5 years of age were treated in EDs for shopping cart-related injuries; an average of 12,800 were treated for falls from carts.[22] An almost even percentage of children fell from the seat portion (51%) compared with the basket portion[22] (49%) of the cart. Eleven thousand (66%) children were treated for head injuries.[22]

Pedestrian injuries are a common cause of morbidity and mortality in the pediatric population. As pedestrians, children are struck by moving vehicles while playing, walking, running, crossing the street, or entering or exiting a school bus. Rates of childhood pedestrian injuries have been reported as 2.5 times higher on one-way streets compared to two-way streets.[49] Most injuries occur in the afternoon and early evening hours on urban streets. Lower socioeconomic status and urban domicile have also been implicated in pedestrian incidents, with a rate 3 times higher for children from poorer neighborhoods compared with wealthier neighborhoods.[49]

Young children struck by motor vehicles in driveways sustain a tenfold increase in mortality as compared to all other pedestrian incidents.[39] Among 527 children younger than 18 years of age injured as pedestrians, 51 (10%) were struck in their own driveway. Children younger than 5 years of age struck in their driveway had a higher ISS, were more likely to sustain a closed-head injury, and were more likely to die compared with children older than 5 years of age struck in their driveway.[39] If the child's shoes are knocked from the body, the vehicle's speed is estimated at 40 mph.[46]

Bicycle crashes result in fatal and nonfatal injuries. Approximately 300 children are killed and more than 400,000 receive ED treatment for bicycle-related injuries each year in the United States.[20] Children ages 5 to 14 years have the highest rate of bicycle-related injuries.[20] Head injuries are the most frequent, with most fatal injuries associated with bicycle-related crashes. Other injuries associated with bicycle crashes are long bone fractures and abdominal, thoracic, and facial injuries. Wearing a bicycle helmet can reduce the likelihood of head injuries by 85% or more.[20] A national survey of children ages 8 to 13 years reported that they were aware of the serious head injuries that could result from not wearing a helmet while bicycling; however, most respondents reported not wearing a bicycle helmet because helmets "make you look like a nerd . . . make you sweat and are tight."[18] Ways to make helmets more appealing include commercials with role models wearing helmets, adding decals and bills, and designing helmets for girls with ponytails.[18] Helmet use significantly reduces morbidity and mortality associated with bicycle-related head injuries.

Children can sustain injuries from skateboards and scooters. Children have a high center of gravity, which limits their ability to break a fall. The Committee on Injury and Poison Prevention[15] recommends that children younger than 5 years of age not use skateboards because these children do not have a well-developed neuromuscular system, do not have good judgment, and cannot protect themselves from injury. Skateboards should not be ridden in traffic. Proper protective wear, including helmets, elbow pads, and knee pads, should be worn. For the calendar year 2000, there were approximately 39,800 ED visits for scooter-related injuries.[21] Approximately 85% of these injuries were sustained by children less than 15 years of age, with two thirds of those injured males.[21] Five scooter-related deaths have been reported; three (60%) were in children younger than 12 years of age.[21] Proper protective gear for scooter safety includes a helmet, knee pads, and elbow pads; wrist guards are not recommended because they make it difficult to grip the handle and steer the scooter. Children less than 8 years of age should use scooters, skates, and skate boards under close adult supervision.[21]

ANATOMY AND PHYSIOLOGY

Children differ from adults developmentally, anatomically, and physiologically. Recognizing differences and implementing appropriate interventions to support these differences can result in increased survivability of the pediatric trauma patient.

Respiratory System

Crucial anatomic and physiologic differences exist between the adult and pediatric airway. The child's oropharynx is relatively small; therefore, the airway is easily obstructed by the large tongue. The U-shaped epiglottis protrudes into the pharynx, with the tonsils and adenoids often enlarged. Vocal cords are short and concave, with the larynx relatively cephaloid and easily collapsible if the head is hyperflexed or extended. In a child younger than 10 years of age, the narrowest portion of the airway is the cricoid cartilage.[10] Lower airways are smaller and supporting cartilage less developed in infants and small children, so airways are easily obstructed by mucus and edema.[10]

Ribs are pliable and do not provide adequate support for the lungs; therefore, blunt trauma to the chest causes pulmonary contusions rather than rib fractures. If rib fractures are present, a high index of suspicion for severe internal trauma should be raised. The mediastinum is more mobile, causing greater susceptibility to great-vessel damage. Retractions are more likely when the child is in respiratory distress. These can be suprasternal, supraclavicular, infraclavicular, intercostal, or substernal. Breathing is primarily diaphragmatic or abdominal in children younger than 7 or 8 years of age. Crying children are more prone to swallowing air, which causes gastric distention and hampers respiratory excursion. A thin chest wall transmits breath sounds easily, so accurate respiratory assessment may be difficult. Respiratory rates are higher in children because of higher metabolic rates. Oxygen consumption in infants is 6 to 8 ml/kg/min compared with 3 to 4 ml/kg/min in adults, so hypoxemia can occur rapidly.[10]

Cardiovascular System

The child's estimated blood volume is 80 milliliter per kilogram. Although this absolute blood volume is small, it is larger than an adult's on a milliliter per kilogram basis. Seemingly small amounts of blood loss can impair perfusion and decrease circulating blood volume. Because of their large cardiac reserve and catecholamine response, children can maintain a high to normal blood pressure even with significant blood loss. Hypotension is not observed until the child has lost 20% to 25% of circulating blood volume.[10] Falling blood pressure is a late sign of hypovolemia in children and signals imminent cardiac arrest. The best assessment for cardiac perfusion is capillary refill—normal is less than 2 seconds. Other assessment factors are presence of bradycardia or tachycardia with decreased urinary output.

Children have a higher metabolic rate and oxygen requirements that require higher cardiac output per kilogram.[10] Tachycardia is the first response to decreased oxygenation. When tachycardia fails to increase oxygen delivery, tissue hypoxia and hypercapnia occur, followed by bradycardia.[10] Bradycardia is a late sign of cardiac decompensation.

Children can have a variety of congenital heart defects that may impair circulatory status (tetralogy of Fallot, truncus arteriosus, and large ventricular septal defects). If a child has had a Blalock-Taussig shunt, blood pressure readings are unattainable in the arm from which the subclavian artery was used (that arm is perfused by collateral circulation). Children may also have functional or nonfunctional heart murmurs. Finally, dextrocardia (heart on the right side) or situs inversus (transposition of all thoracic and abdominal organs) may be present.

Neurologic System

An infant's head is larger in proportion to the rest of the body than an adult's. The skull is more malleable, providing less protection to the brain. The posterior fontanelle closes at age 4 months; the anterior fontanelle is normally closed by age 18 months. Although open fontanelles allow for release of increased intracranial pressure (ICP), they may allow direct injury to the brain or cause extensive bleeding. Infants bleed significantly from a scalp laceration because of the large surface area and increased vascularity. Finally, a young child has a higher center of gravity, which, together with the larger head, makes the child prone to head injuries.

Children's cerebral tissues are thin, soft, and flexible compared with that of adults. Sulci are still deepening during childhood, and myelinization is still occurring. These differences make brain tissues more easily damaged, especially from shearing injuries. Several features make the cervical spine vulnerable to injury in children younger than 9 years of age[27]:

- The head is disproportionately large, making the child vulnerable to flexion-extension injury.
- The neck muscles are underdeveloped.
- The vertebral bodies are wedge shaped.
- The articulating facets are angled horizontally, resulting in subluxation from minimal force.
- The end plates are cartilaginous.
- The interspinous ligaments are elastic and lax, leading to increased spinal mobility.

Gastrointestinal and Genitourinary Systems

Young children have protuberant abdomens as a result of underdeveloped abdominal musculature trauma.[41] Because solid abdominal organs are relatively larger in children compared with adults, there is an increased risk of direct organ injury following blunt and penetrating kinetic forces.[41] A pliable rib cage does not afford adequate protection to abdominal organs and can predispose children to further internal injuries. Though partially protected by the flexible rib cage, the liver is still vulnerable to injury because of its large size and fragility. The transverse diameter of the abdomen is small, and lower abdominal organs are not well protected by the pelvis.[37] Renal injuries occur because the relatively large kidneys are not protected by the small amount of perinephric fat, weak abdominal muscles, and elastic rib cage. The kidneys also retain fetal lobulations, which may predispose these organs to separation and fracture.[41] Congenital abnormalities such as hydronephrosis, horseshoe kidneys, and ectopic kidneys make the child more susceptible to renal trauma. Many congenital anomalies are not diagnosed until abdominal trauma has occurred. Greater elasticity makes ureteral tearing rare. Ureteral injuries are suspected with penetrating trauma to the abdomen or flank area. The bladder is an abdominal organ and not well protected. In girls the bladder neck is also less protected. Tissues of a prepubescent girl are more rigid because of a lack of estrogen; they do not become more pliable until adolescence, when estrogen is released.

Musculoskeletal System

The periosteum in a growing child is stronger, thicker, and more osteogenic compared with periosteum in an adult, which results in decreased fracture displacement and fewer open fractures, as compared with adults.[24] Consequently, four unique bone fracture patterns are found in children: plastic deformity (the bone is deformed but not broken); torus (buckle) fracture (compression forces applied at the metaphysis and diaphysis causes bone to buckle rather than break due to its porous nature); Greenstick fracture (an incomplete fracture where the compressed side's cortex and periosteum are intact); and physis fractures (injury to the growth plate, which can lead to angulation deformities if not diagnosed and treated properly).[24] Bone osteogenicity allows rapid callus formation, permitting bones to heal quickly. Even though bone is strong, fractures occur more frequently than muscle sprains or ligament tears because these structures are stronger than the bones themselves.

Another unique feature of the pediatric musculoskeletal system is presence of a physis or growth plate. This area of bone, which is responsible for longitudinal bone growth, is found between the epiphysis and metaphysis. The physis is cartilaginous and does not ossify until puberty; therefore, treatment to attain proper anatomic alignment is critical to optimize bone growth and reduce the risk of deformity.[24]

Integumentary System

Children have a larger ratio of body surface area to weight, which makes them prone to convective and conductive heat loss. Infants younger than 6 months of age do not have the fine-motor coordination to shiver and are unable to keep themselves warm. Nonshivering thermogenesis occurs, in which brown fat is broken down to produce warmth. Shivering is a high-energy consuming, nonproductive muscular activity initiated for thermogenesis.[6] Shivering may not be possible in injured children receiving sedation or neuromuscular blocking agents.[6] Children have less subcutaneous fat for insulation and can lose heat through radiation, convection, conduction, and evaporation.

PATIENT ASSESSMENT

Each ED should be equipped with personnel and supplies necessary to treat an injured child effectively and efficiently. Equipment should be readily available and prepared before arrival. Table 29-1 provides a quick reference to emergency equipment for the pediatric patient.

Initial assessment and stabilization of the pediatric trauma patient requires knowledge of developmental and physiologic differences among infants, children, and adolescents. Injured children are frightened—strange, painful things are happening. The patient may feel he or she is being punished for a real or imagined wrongdoing. Talking with the child in language he or she understands is essential for relieving anxiety and developing trust.

Initial assessment consists of primary and secondary assessment. During primary assessment, airway/cervical spine, breathing, circulation, and disability (neurologic status) are assessed. Life-threatening injuries are identified and treated. Table 29-2 describes primary survey in the preferred order. During secondary assessment, all other body systems are assessed and other injuries are treated. Table 29-3 details the secondary survey. Throughout initial assessment and stabilization, airway, breathing, and circulation are continually reassessed.

Initial Stabilization

Airway/Cervical Spine

The tongue is the most common cause of airway obstruction in the child. Opening the airway with the jaw-thrust technique to prevent hyperextension of the cervical spine is the initial step in relieving airway obstruction. Suction the oropharynx with a tonsil suction device if vomitus, blood, or loose teeth are present.

Place an oropharyngeal airway to help maintain airway patency in the child with altered level of consciousness who does not have an intact gag reflex. Oropharyngeal airways are measured from the corner of the mouth to the tragus of the ear. An oropharyngeal airway that is too small or too large will obstruct the airway, so correct size is critical. Use a tongue depressor to insert the airway directly. Do not rotate 90 degrees as in the adult patient because a child's oropharyngeal tissues can be damaged and the tongue inadvertently pushed posteriorly, causing obstruction. A nasopharyngeal airway may be used for airway patency if there is no evidence of head trauma. This airway is measured from the naris to the tragus of the ear.

In a child who requires continuous airway maintenance, rapid-sequence endotracheal intubation (RSI) is necessary. RSI is "a technique in which a potent sedative or induction agent is administered virtually simultaneously with a paralyzing dose of a neuromuscular blocking agent to facilitate rapid tracheal intubation."[12] This procedure must be undertaken by a health care professional skilled in pediatric intubation. The orotracheal route is preferred because the nasotracheal route can be difficult or contraindicated in severe facial trauma or basilar skull fracture.

Before the intubation attempt, cardiac and pulse oximetry monitoring devices are placed on the child. Sedating medications followed by paralyzing agents are administered while the child's lungs are ventilated with 100% oxygen. After the trachea is intubated, auscultate breath sounds over the epigastrium, then the trachea and bilateral anterior aspect of the chest. Listen high in the axilla because breath sounds are easily transmittable across the thin chest wall. Correct endotracheal tube placement is determined through auscultation of equal, bilateral breath sounds in all fields, observation of condensation in the endotracheal tube, and assessment of end tidal carbon dioxide measurements. Final confirmation is made by chest radiograph.

Right mainstem bronchus intubations are a common complication with pediatric intubation; therefore, bilateral chest wall movement should be observed during ventilation with a bag-valve-mask device. Movement is best assessed by standing at the foot of the bed watching chest rise and fall during ventilation. After endotracheal tube placement is confirmed by auscultation, a chest radiograph must be obtained. In the meantime the tube must be securely taped with benzoin and adhesive tape. The tube should not press on the corner of the mouth (nares with nasotracheal intubation) because of the potential for tissue breakdown. Frequent suctioning may be necessary if aspiration is suspected or injury to the airway or lung tissue has occurred.

Children are diaphragmatic breathers so compression on the diaphragm impedes lung expansion. A gastric tube is inserted to relieve gastric distension. The tube is inserted nasally if the child has no obvious facial trauma or signs of a basilar skull fracture. After the tube is inserted it is taped to the child's face and connected to low intermittent suction.

Cricothyrotomy and tracheostomy are reserved for severe cases of airway instability from facial, head, and neck trauma. Fortunately, these procedures are rarely required in children.

Spinal precautions are initiated in the multiply-injured child, including application of a rigid collar, cervical immobilization device, and immobilization board. Care must be taken to prevent cervical spine flexion from the cervical collar or backboard (Figure 29-1). Movement can worsen spinal cord injury and compromise the airway. Immobilization devices remain intact until radiographic and clinical evidence demonstrate that spinal cord injury is not present.

Use of the appropriately sized cervical collar is essential to prevent spinal cord injury and airway compromise. A collar that is too large pushes the jaw backward, causes airway obstruction, and allows the child to move the head from side to side, which prevents cervical spine control. A collar that is too small does not provide appropriate alignment and may cause airway compromise from constriction. A cervical col-

Table 29-1 QUICK REFERENCE TO PEDIATRIC EMERGENCY EQUIPMENT

EQUIPMENT	PREMATURE	NEONATE	6 MOS	1Y	2Y	3Y	4Y	5Y	6Y	7Y	8Y	9Y	10Y	11-18Y
Airway														
Oral airway[b] (size)	Infant	Infant/small	Small	Small	Small	Small	Med	Med	Med	Med	Med/Lg	Med/Lg	Med/Lg	Large
Endotracheal tube[c] (mm) C = cuffed	2.5-3.0	3.0-3.5	3.5-4.0	4.0-4.5	4.0-4.5	4.0-4.5	4.0-5.5	5.0-5.5	5.5-6.0	5.5-6.0	6.0 C 6.5 C	6.0 C 6.5 C	6.0 C 6.5 C	7.0 C 8.0 C
Laryngoscope blade[b] s = straight c = curved	0 s	1 s	1 s	1 s	1 s	1 s	2 s/c	2 s/c	2 s/c	2 s/c	2-3 s/c	2-3 s/c	2-3 s/c	3 s/c
Suction catheter[c] (French)	5	6	6	8	8	8	10	10	10	10	10	10	10	12
Breathing														
Face mask[b] (size)	Premie NB	NB	NB	Ped	Ped	Ped	Ped	Ped	Ped	Ped	Ad	Ad	Ad	Ad
Bag-valve device[b] (size)	Inf	Inf	Inf	Ped	Ped	Ped	Ped	Ped	Ped	Ped/Ad	Ad	Ad	Ad	Ad
Chest tube[b] (French)	10-14	12-18	14-20	14-24	14-24	14-24	20-32	20-32	20-32	20-32	28-38	28-38	28-38	28-38
Circulation	22-24	22-24	22-24	20-22	20-22	20-22	20-22	18-22	18-20	18-20	16-20	16-20	16-20	14-18
Over-the-needle catheter[d] (gauge)														
Intraosseous device (gauge)	18	15	15	15	15	15	15	15	—	—	—	—	—	—
Gastrointestinal/ Genitourinary														
Nasogastric tube[e] (French)	5	5	8	8	10	10	10	10	10	12	12	12	12	14-16
Urinary catheter[b] (French)	5 feeding tube	5-8 feeding tube	8	10	10	10	10-12	10-12	10-12	10-12	12	12	12	12-18

From Bernardo L, Bove M: *Pediatric emergency nursing procedures*, Boston, 1993, Jones & Bartlett.

[a]This reference demonstrates suggested sizes only. Always consider each child's size and health condition when selecting appropriate equipment for procedures.

[b]Committee on Trauma: *Advanced trauma life support student manual*, Chicago, 1989, American College of Surgeons.

[c]Motoyama E: Endotracheal intubation. In Motoyama E, Davis P, editors: *Smith's anesthesia for infants and children*, St. Louis, 1990, Mosby.

[d]Chameides L, editor: *Textbook of pediatric advanced life support*, Dallas, 1988, American Heart Association, Academy of Pediatrics.

[e]Skale N: *Manual of pediatric nursing procedures*, Philadelphia, 1992, JB Lippincott.

Table 29-2   PRIMARY SURVEY OF THE PEDIATRIC TRAUMA PATIENT

COMPONENT	ACTIONS
Airway	Assess for patency; look for loose teeth, vomitus, or other obstruction; note position of head.
	Suspect cervical spine injury with multiple trauma; maintain neutral alignment during assessment; evaluate effectiveness of cervical collar, cervical immobilization device, or other equipment used to immobilize the spine.
	Open cervical collar to evaluate neck for jugular vein distention and tracheal deviation.
Breathing	Auscultate breath sounds in the axillae for presence and equality.
	Assess chest for contusions, penetrating wounds, abrasions, or paradoxic movement.
Circulation	Assess apical pulse for rate, rhythm, and quality; compare apical and peripheral pulses for quality and equality.
	Evaluate capillary refill; normal is less than 2 seconds.
	Check skin color and temperature.
	Assess level of consciousness; check for orientation to person, place, and time in the older child.
Disability	In a younger child, assess alertness, ability to interact with environment, and ability to follow commands. Is the child easily consoled and interested in the environment? Does the child recognize a familiar object and respond when you speak to him or her?
	Check pupils for size, shape, reactivity, and equality.
	Note open wounds or uncontrolled bleeding.
Expose	Remove clothing to allow visual inspection of entire body.

Table 29-3   SECONDARY SURVEY OF THE PEDIATRIC TRAUMA PATIENT

COMPONENT	ACTIONS
Head, eye, ear, nose	Assess scalp for lacerations or open wounds; palpate for stepoff defects, depressions, hematomas, and pain.
	Reassess pupils for size, reactivity, equality, and extraocular movements; ask the child if he or she can see.
	Assess ears and nose for rhinorrhea or otorrhea.
	Observe for raccoon eyes (bruising around the eyes) or Battle's sign (bruising over the mastoid process).
	Palpate forehead, orbits, maxilla, and mandible for crepitus, deformities, stepoff defect, pain, and stability; evaluate malocclusion by asking child to open and close mouth; note open wounds.
	Inspect for loose, broken, or chipped teeth as well as oral lacerations.
	Check orthodontic appliances for stability.
	Evaluate facial symmetry by asking child to smile, grimace, and open and close mouth.
	Do not remove impaled objects or foreign objects.
Neck	Open cervical collar and reassess anterior neck for jugular vein distention and tracheal deviation; note bruising, edema, open wounds, pain, and crepitus.
	Check for hoarseness or changes in voice by asking child to speak.
Chest	Obtain respiratory rate; reassess breath sounds in anterior lobes for equality.
	Palpate chest wall and sternum for pain, tenderness, and crepitus.
	Observe inspiration and expiration for symmetry or paradoxic movement; note use of accessory muscles.
	Reassess apical heart rate for rate, rhythm, and clarity.
Abdomen/pelvis/ genitourinary	Observe abdomen for bruising and distention; auscultate bowel sounds briefly in all four quadrants; palpate abdomen gently for tenderness; assess pelvis for tenderness and stability.
	Palpate bladder for distention and tenderness; check urinary meatus for signs of injury or bleeding; note priapism and genital trauma such as lacerations or foreign body.
	Have rectal sphincter tone assessed, usually by physician.
Musculoskeletal	Assess extremities for deformities, swelling, lacerations, or other injuries.
	Palpate distal pulses for equality, rate, and rhythm; compare to central pulses.
	Ask child to wiggle toes and fingers; evaluate strength through hand grips and foot flexion/extension.
Back	Logroll as a unit to inspect back; maintain spinal alignment during examination; observe for bruising and open wounds; palpate each vertebral body for tenderness, pain, deformity, and stability; assess flank area for bruising and tenderness.

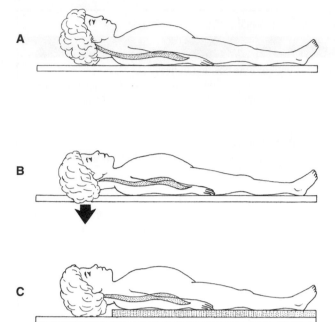

FIGURE 29-1 **A,** Young child immobilized on a standard backboard; note how the large head forces the neck into flexion. Backboards can be modified by an occiput cutout (**B**) or a double mattress pad (**C**) to raise the chest. (From Roberts J, Hedges J: *Clinical procedures in emergency medicine,* ed 3, Philadelphia, 1998, WB Saunders.)

lar fits properly if the chin rests securely in the chin holder, the collar is beneath the ears, and the upper part of the sternum is not covered. Figure 29-2 illustrates the procedure for sizing cervical collars.

Infants and young children may arrive in the ED secured in their car safety seat. Children can initially remain in their car seats if there are no signs of distress and the car seat is intact.[25] Cervical immobilization with a collar, if possible, and towel rolls should be completed.[25] Although no evidence-based guidelines indicate that car seat immobilization is effective, it may be an option for emergency medical services personnel to transport stable, injured children.[25]

Cervical spine radiographs from C1 through T1 are obtained in the anterior-posterior and lateral views to evaluate for vertebral fractures. The radiograph is assessed for vertebral symmetry, alignment, and spacing. Spinal immobilization can be removed if there is no radiographic evidence of cervical spine injury and the child has normal neurologic findings.

Breathing

Supplemental oxygen is administered to any child with multiple trauma. The child breathing spontaneously with effective air exchange can receive humidified oxygen via nasal cannula, partial nonrebreather face mask, or nonrebreather face mask.

Flow rate for a nasal cannula should be no more than 6 L/min of oxygen; higher flow rates irritate the nasopharynx. A cannula is used in children with minimal oxygen requirements. With infants and young children, secure the cannula in the nares, then start oxygen flow. (Remember that oxygen flow may frighten the child.) A partial rebreathing mask set at a flow rate of 10 to 12 L/min delivers an inspired oxygen concentration of 50% to 60%. Blowby oxygen can be used for those who do not tolerate the cannula or mask.

Nonrebreather oxygen masks are used for a child with greater oxygen requirements; flow rate is set at 10 to 12 L/min. A properly fitting face mask fits snugly on the face, covering nose and mouth without covering eyes or cheeks. In the child who is not breathing spontaneously or effectively, ventilations are assisted with a bag-valve-mask set at 15 L/min, which allows oxygen delivery up to 90%.[10] A bag-valve-mask must have a minimum volume of 450 ml, be self-refilling, and available in both pediatric and adult sizes.[10] Bag-valve devices are equipped with pop-off valves, which can be used when great resistance is met during ventilation attempts. When assisting ventilations with a bag-valve-mask device, the bag is squeezed until enough air volume is delivered to allow easy rise and fall of the chest. Care must be taken not to ventilate with extreme force because pneumothorax can occur.

A pulse oximeter is applied to the child's finger, earlobe, or toe to determine oxygen saturation. Pulse oximetry readings should be 95% or more.

Chest tubes are inserted if there is evidence of hemothorax, pneumothorax, or hemopneumothorax. Local anesthetic (and preferably sedatives) should be administered before insertion of chest tubes.

Circulation

Continuous cardiopulmonary and blood pressure monitoring devices are connected to the child. Vital signs are measured every 5 minutes until the child's condition stabilizes. Blood pressure readings should be evaluated against other vital signs. A properly fitting blood pressure cuff fits two thirds of the upper arm. A cuff that is too small gives false high readings, whereas a cuff that is too large gives false low readings.

Apply direct pressure to open, bleeding wounds. Tourniquets are not recommended because direct tissue damage may occur.

Two large-bore intravenous catheters are inserted, preferably in the antecubital fossae, for venous access and fluid replacement. Catheter size is determined by the size of the child's veins. After the catheter is secured, obtain blood for laboratory analyses, then initiate crystalloid fluid replacement.

If peripheral venous access is not established after three attempts, alternate methods of access are employed. Intraosseous route should be considered in children younger than 6 years of age, although this age limit is gradually increasing. Calcifying bones in older children can make intraosseous access difficult, so access through the jugular,

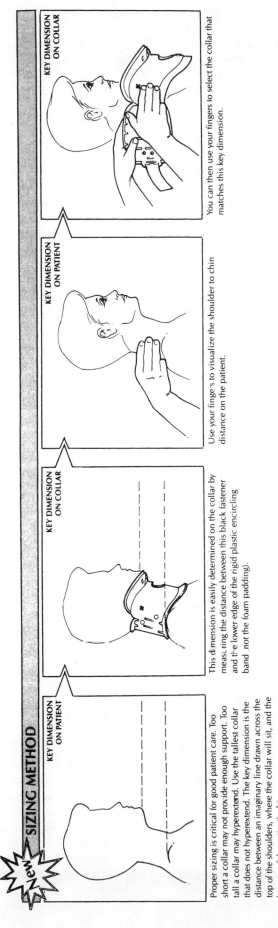

SIZING METHOD

New

KEY DIMENSION ON PATIENT

Proper sizing is critical for good patient care. Too short a collar may not provide enough support. Too tall a collar may hyperextend. Use the tallest collar that does not hyperextend. The key dimension is the distance between an imaginary line drawn across the top of the shoulders, where the collar will sit, and the bottom of the patient's chin.

KEY DIMENSION ON COLLAR

This dimension is easily determined on the collar by measuring the distance between this black fastener and the lower edge of the rigid plastic encircling band (not the foam padding).

KEY DIMENSION ON PATIENT

Use your fingers to visualize the shoulder to chin distance on the patient.

KEY DIMENSION ON COLLAR

You can then use your fingers to select the collar that matches this key dimension.

FIGURE **29-2** Method for predetermining the correct size for an extrication collar. (Courtesy of Laerdal Medical Corporation, Wappingers Falls, NY.)

subclavian, or femoral vein by an experienced physician is the next possibility. Venous cutdown in the saphenous or brachial vein is the last choice. Central venous pressure monitoring or arterial pressure monitoring is reserved for severely injured children and should be performed only under controlled circumstances by experienced personnel.

Crystalloid fluid replacement is initiated with lactated Ringer's solution, which should be warmed when large volumes will be administered. Stopcocks connected to intravenous (IV) tubing allow easy administration of fluid boluses. Crystalloids are infused at a maintenance rate based on estimated weight. If the child is hemodynamically stable or has a head injury, infusion rate may be decreased, usually to two thirds of the maintenance rate. Excessive fluid administration in the child with a head injury may increase ICP.

Hypovolemic shock is suspected in the child with tachypnea, tachycardia, decreased level of consciousness, decreased urinary output, and prolonged capillary refill. Fluid bolus of 20 ml/kg lactated Ringer's solution is rapidly administered, with effectiveness observed almost immediately. If there is no improvement, another bolus can be administered followed by a third bolus. Warm O-negative blood may be given at 10 ml/kg if there is no improvement after the third fluid bolus.[10]

Children may arrive in the ED in traumatic arrest and require cardiopulmonary resuscitation (CPR). In one study of 957 pediatric trauma patients requiring CPR, only 225 (24%) survived to hospital discharge.[33] Children receiving CPR at the scene had a higher survival rate (26%) than those who did not receive CPR until ED arrival (19%).[33] Children arriving at the ED with CPR en route for traumatic arrest may require ED thoracotomy (EDT). Injured children likely to benefit from EDT are those with a single penetrating injury to the left side of the chest who have or had vital signs and pupillary response within 5 minutes of EDT.[11] The technique for performing an EDT is reported by Clemence.[11] Despite CPR and EDT, the outcome after traumatic arrest in the pediatric population is bleak.

Routine blood tests include complete blood count (CBC) and differential, electrolytes, blood urea nitrogen (BUN), creatinine, glucose, and type and screen. If abdominal trauma is suspected, amylase, lipase, and liver enzymes may be obtained. In suspected cardiac or muscle damage, creatine phosphokinase levels are also obtained. Other blood tests include prothrombin time, partial thromboplastin times, toxicology screening, and arterial blood gases. Urine may be sent for complete urinalysis and toxicology testing. Pregnancy testing should be considered in the postmenarcheal female.

Pneumatic antishock garments are not routinely used in pediatric trauma but can be used as a splint for pelvic fractures or femur fractures when other forms of splinting are not available.

An indwelling urinary catheter is placed if there is no sign of genitourinary trauma (i.e., no blood at the meatus). A urimeter on the urine collection bag allows careful monitoring of urinary output. Decreased output can indicate hypovolemic shock. Hematuria suggests genitourinary trauma; however, the first urine specimen may test negative for blood because of urine in the bladder before injury. Therefore a subsequent urine specimen may be necessary. Normal urinary output for children younger than 1 year of age should approach 2 ml/kg/hr; for children older than 1 year of age, 1 ml/kg/hr is optimal.[10]

Disability

Serial neurologic assessments are necessary to identify changes in mental status. Changes in level of consciousness can indicate hypovolemia or increased ICP. Early signs of increased ICP are vomiting and irritability. In infants a bulging fontanelle is a late sign of increasing ICP.

In older children the first sign of increased ICP is disorientation to time, place, and familiar people, then to self. This description is not applicable to the younger child, who has no concept of time or place. The Glasgow Coma Scale (GCS), although appropriate for adults and older children, is not appropriate for infants and preverbal children. The Pediatric Coma Scale is a more reliable measurement of neurologic status in these age-groups (Figure 29-3). Children as young as 3 months old should recognize their parents, and those as young as 6 months should recognize siblings and may know the names of their pets. They may also recognize popular cartoon or television characters or favorite toys.

In a child with severe head trauma, hyperventilation with 100% oxygen is initiated to keep arterial carbon dioxide pressure ($PaCO_2$) between 30 and 35 mm Hg.[30] Mannitol may be administered at 0.5g to 1 g/kg to decrease cerebral swelling.[30]

Exposure/Environmental Control

The child's temperature is recorded initially and monitored throughout initial stabilization to detect and treat hypothermia. Common temperature measurement routes are tympanic, oral, rectal, and bladder. In one study comparing rectal and tympanic membrane temperatures in injured children, an 85% correlation was found, with rectal temperatures an average 0.3° C higher.[4] Factors to consider when selecting route for temperature measurement in pediatric trauma patients include safety, accuracy, and compliance. Refer to Bernardo, Henker, and O'Connor[8] for discussion of advantages and disadvantages of selected temperature measurement routes.

Numerous factors during the child's initial ED care increase the risk of hypothermia, including transfusion of large amounts of unwarmed IV fluids or blood products[38]; clothing removal during assessment and treatment; large, open wounds; neurologic or multisystem injuries; administration of paralytic or sedative agents; treatment in cold trauma rooms; and transport and transfer in unheated ambulances, helicopters, and hospital diagnostic suites.[6] Therefore measures to prevent heat loss and promote thermoregulation should be initiated. Passive warming measures include increasing ambient temperature by using overhead

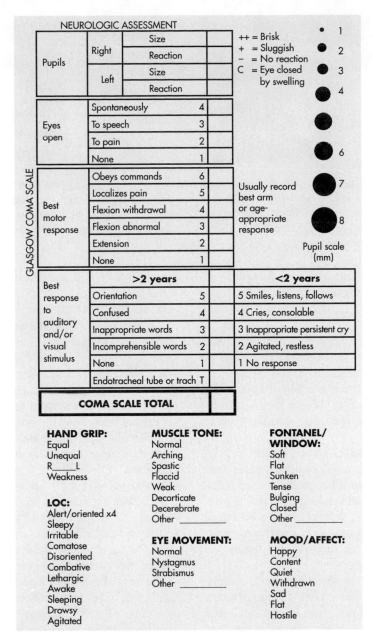

FIGURE 29-3 Pediatric coma scale. (From Wong D et al: *Wong's essentials of pediatric nursing,* ed 6, St. Louis, 2001, Mosby.)

lights and applying warm blankets. Active warming measures include administering warm IV fluids and blood products. In one study of 30 injured children randomized to receive either room temperature or warmed IV fluids during initial ED treatment, there was a trend toward increased body temperature in those children receiving warmed IV fluid. However, this trend was not statistically significant.[7] In another study of eight injured children randomized to receive either warmed IV fluids or a convective warming blanket, there was no statistically significant difference in temperatures for both groups on ED discharge—all maintained body temperature in the normothermic range.[5] No evidence-based practice is defined for nursing interventions to prevent heat loss in injured children during initial ED

treatment. Further, measures effective in adults cannot be extrapolated for application in injured children.[9] Clinical trials are needed to identify effective interventions for preventing heat loss and maintaining normothermia in injured children.

Full Set of Vital Signs

Vital signs (temperature, heart rate, respiratory rate, blood pressure) are measured on ED arrival and throughout initial ED treatment. Vital signs are measured continuously and recorded every 5 minutes in unstable patients and every 15 minutes in stable patients. Documenting patient care on a trauma flowsheet allows visual inspection of trends in patient vital signs and permits rapid interventions as needed.

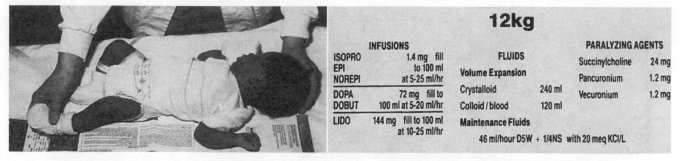

12kg

INFUSIONS			FLUIDS		PARALYZING AGENTS	
ISOPRO	1.4 mg fill		Volume Expansion		Succinylcholine	24 mg
EPI	to 100 ml				Pancuronium	1.2 mg
NOREPI	at 5-25 ml/hr		Crystalloid	240 ml	Vecuronium	1.2 mg
DOPA	72 mg fill to		Colloid / blood	120 ml		
DOBUT	100 ml at 5-20 ml/hr		Maintenance Fluids			
LIDO	144 mg fill to 100 ml		46 ml/hour D5W + 1/4NS with 20 meq KCl/L			
	at 10-25 ml/hr					

FIGURE 29-4   The Broselow tape can be used as a rapid method for generating drug and fluid doses, as well as endotracheal tube, and suction catheter sizes. The tape uses the principle that length correlates with body surface area and weight. The patient is measured with the tape in the supine position and the line on which the foot of the patient reaches contains the precalculated drug doses and equipment sizes appropriate for the patient. (From Barkin R et al: *Pediatric emergency nursing,* ed 2, St. Louis, 1997, Mosby.)

Weight should be determined through actual measurement or by estimation with a Broselow tape (Figure 29-4).

Family Presence

The presence of a supportive parent does wonders for a frightened child. Allow parents to see the child as soon as possible after stabilization is complete. Explain to the parents beforehand what they will see and why. Explanations prevent any surprises. Parents may believe they need permission to touch or talk to their child, so encourage them to do so.

Controversy exists as to whether parents should be present during resuscitation. If parents are present, a nurse must stay with them and explain what is happening to their child. The Emergency Nurses Association advocates parental presence during resuscitation. Such presence may be beneficial to the child and the family members. A designated emergency nurse or social worker can stay with the family and explain treatment that is taking place.

While parents are waiting to see their child, a social worker, emergency nurse, or designated patient advocate should keep them apprised of the situation and serve as a support person. If the decision is made to transfer the child to another facility, parents should see their child before departure. If the child dies before parents arrive at the accepting institution, they may feel guilty because they were not able to see the child or agreed to have their child transferred elsewhere. When the child leaves, say "Mommy will see you later" rather than "goodbye" because "goodbye" implies that they may never see each other again. Most flight programs have policies in place for transport of a family member with a patient. Many factors influence the decision to have a parent or other family member accompany a child in a helicopter, so the decision to do so ultimately rests with the pilot and flight crew and should be respected.[28]

Give Comfort Measures

The injured child has a number of fears—mutilation, losing control, getting in trouble with his or her parents for engaging in a forbidden activity, death, disfigurement, and pain. It is the responsibility of the emergency nurse to help the child cope effectively with these fears during trauma resuscita-

tion. Children who are hearing impaired or require a translator should have an interpreter other than a family member present during the examination.

Assign one nurse as the child's support person. When the child has cervical and spinal immobilization, the nurse should stand at the child's side and down from his or her face, about chest level, so the child is able to see the person. Standing directly over the child's face is frightening, especially when different faces keep appearing and reappearing. Hold the child's hand or stroke his or her hair to provide tactile comfort. Talk softly and slowly, using words he or she can understand (e.g., "The doctor is going to listen to your heartbeat," "You will feel a pinch in your right arm. You can scream, but you must keep your right arm still."). Avoid words such as "take" or "cut out" because they imply mutilation. Use words such as "make it better." If the child requires general anesthesia, avoid telling the child he or she will "be put to sleep." If the child had a pet that was "put to sleep," this statement may create death fears. Instead, tell the child he or she will get "special medicine to help you take a short nap." The child understands "nap" is a short time. Tell the child what will happen before it happens. Children do not like surprises any more than adults do. Prepare them by using feeling terms, that is, "This will feel cold; this will feel heavy; this will smell sweet." If a procedure will hurt, tell the child. Lying will only cause him or her to mistrust you.

Children cope in a variety of ways. Because young children are mobile, crying and kicking are ways for them to cope. To them, being restrained may mean not being alive. School-age children and adolescents cope by seeking information; they may ask the same questions over and over again. Be patient. Scolding or threatening the child is fruitless and will only increase fear and resistance.

Severe injuries should be shielded from the child's visual field. Refrain from discussing the magnitude of an injury in the child's presence. It is not known if unconscious children remember discussions in their presence, so it is best to avoid talking about other family members or the child's condition in his or her presence. Talk to the child who is comatose or unresponsive just as if he or she were awake.

Pain management is of utmost importance when treating the injured child; however, it may be neglected. Recent re-

Table 29-4	HISTORY BASED ON MECHANISM OF INJURY
MECHANISM OF INJURY	HISTORY
Pedestrian MVC	Speed of vehicle; distance child thrown; run over or struck by vehicle; where child was struck (right or left side)
Passenger MVC	Restrained or unrestrained; position in vehicle; ejection from vehicle; extrication time; scene fatalities; site of impact (rear, head on; side impact); crash scene (stationary or moving vehicle); vehicle speed at impact
Bicycle crash	Speed of bicycle; helmet use; crash into stationary object or moving vehicle
Fall	Height of fall; landing surface; body area striking ground first
Gunshot wound	Bullet size (caliber/millimeter); number of shots fired; type of firearm; range; suicide or homicide (i.e., presence of a suicide note or death threats; entrance or exit wounds)
Stab wound	Penetrating object (i.e., knife; entrance or exit wounds; object still in place)

MVC, Motor vehicle crash.

Box 29-1	AMPLE MNEMONIC
A	Allergies
M	Medications
P	Past health history
L	Last meal eaten
E	Events leading to the injury

quirements from the Joint Commission on the Accreditation of Health Care Organizations require that all patients receive pain assessment and appropriate pain relief measures. Various pain scales are available to measure pain in preverbal and verbal children. Analgesics may be administered after all injuries are identified and the child is determined to be physiologically and neurologically intact. Pharmacologic management of pain includes narcotic and nonnarcotic analgesics. Nonpharmacologic management of pain includes comfort measures such as distraction techniques, progressive relaxation, positive self-talk, and deep breathing exercises. Allowing an infant to suck a pacifier promotes comfort, whereas allowing a toddler to hold a transitional object such as a blanket or toy promotes security. The awake child may be able to use a pain scale to rate the pain. Reevaluation is necessary after any pain relief measures are initiated.

Head-to-Toe-Assessment

The secondary survey is outlined in Table 29-3. In addition, frequent monitoring of the neurovascular status of an injured extremity is necessary to identify impairment of circulation or possible compartment syndrome. An injured extremity can be splinted for protection and comfort until definitive care is provided. After the extremity is splinted or casted, frequent reevaluation is necessary because edema may develop and impede circulation.

Inspect the Posterior Surface

The child is logrolled as a unit to inspect the posterior surface for contusions, abrasions, open wounds, and impaled objects; the spine and flank are palpated for tenderness and pain. The child is logrolled back into the supine position with spinal immobilization resumed or removed at that time.

History

History allows the trauma team to prepare for the patient and anticipate interventions that may be required. However, this information is not always available because the injury may not have been witnessed. The awake, nonverbal child cannot relate circumstances surrounding the injury. Such situations require special attention, because child neglect or abuse may be involved (see Chapter 49). Information related to mechanism of injury is found in Table 29-4. In all injuries it is important to ascertain if loss of consciousness occurred.

The AMPLE mnemonic (Box 29-1) is helpful for organizing and obtaining an adequate patient history. This information may be obtained from the parent, family member, or awake older child or adolescent. In addition to this information, it is important to determine the need for vision or hearing aids, such as eyeglasses, contact lenses, or hearing aids. These may or may not be with the child on arrival.

Additional Interventions

Additional interventions undertaken during emergency treatment of the injured child include radiologic testing, medication administration, management of pain, and provision of emotional support.

Radiologic Testing. Along with cervical spine radiographs, other radiographic testing may be undertaken relative to suspected injuries. An abdominal series may be indicated in a child with abdominal trauma, whereas chest and spine films may be indicated for the child with multiple injuries. Intravenous pyelogram may be performed if renal trauma is suspected. Specific radiographs with views of injured extremities before definitive treatment is administered may also be performed. Radiographs may be obtained in the trauma room or the child may be transported to the radiology department. A nurse should remain with the child to explain procedures and monitor the child's condition.

Usefulness of sonography to detect fluid and organ injury in children with abdominal trauma is uncertain. Benya, Lim-Dunham, Landrum, and Statter[2] performed an abdominal sonogram on 51 injured children before the children underwent abdominal computed tomography (CT) scan. Both tests were reviewed independently by two radiologists for the presence of fluid and organ injury. Agreement between the observers was excellent for sonographic identification of fluid ($\kappa = 0.82$) but poor for detection of organ injury ($\kappa = 0.34$). In contrast, Corbett, Andrews, Baker and colleagues[23] performed bedside ultrasound during secondary survey of 47 injured children. A CT scan of the abdomen and pelvis or laparotomy were performed as indicated and served as the "gold standard" to verify presence or absence of free fluid in the abdomen. The agreement between an ED physician and radiologist blinded to interpretations of test results had a moderate level of agreement ($\kappa = 0.56$) for presence of free fluid in the abdomen. Although detection of free fluid in the abdomen may be possible using sonography, additional research is needed to validate usefulness of this diagnostic tool in the initial care of children with abdominal injuries.

A CT scan is indicated in children with head, chest, spinal, or abdominal trauma. Xenon testing may be used in the child with severe head injury. Again, a nurse must accompany the child for continuous monitoring. Appropriate equipment should be readily available in case there is a change in the child's status. Sedation may be required for stable children undergoing a CT scan of the head after head injury. Sedation practices vary widely among health care providers. Survey results from 304 pediatric emergency medicine physicians found that 74% followed published guidelines for sedation.[17] In three clinical scenarios midazolam was the most frequently chosen sedative.[17] Emergency nurses should follow hospital policies for sedation of these and all trauma patients undergoing diagnostic procedures.

Medications. Antibiotics may be administered in the child with large, open contaminated wounds, open fractures, or arterial injury. Determine the child's immunization status to ensure appropriate tetanus prophylaxis. Children bitten by domestic or wild animals may require rabies prophylaxis, in which case local health department guidelines should be followed.

SPECIFIC CONDITIONS

TRAUMATIC BRAIN INJURIES

Traumatic brain injury (TBI) is the leading cause of trauma-related death in children. Three percent (419,000) of all child and adolescent injury-related ED visits are for TBI.[50] Falls were the mechanism of injury in 49% (206,000) of these visits.[50] Thirteen percent (54,000) of these patients were hospitalized.[50] TBI often results from blunt trauma from MVCs, bicycle crashes, falls, and maltreatment. Children are susceptible to brain injury because of their larger head-to-body ratio, thin cranial bones, and less-myelinated brain. These factors leave the brain relatively unprotected and vulnerable to injury.[30] The thinner cranium allows injury forces to be transmitted directly to the brain itself.[30] Unmyelinated brain tissue in infants and young children appears to be more susceptible to shearing forces when compared to older children and adults.[30] Furthermore, cranial sutures remain open in early infancy, with the anterior fontanelle open until 18 months. These features increase the child's susceptibility to head injury but also serve as an outlet for swollen cerebral tissues, allowing greater tolerance for increases in intracranial pressures.

Mild to moderate TBI (Glasgow Coma Scale [GCS] 13 to 15) are more common than severe head injuries.[30] Brain injuries are divided into primary and secondary phases. Primary injury results from mechanical damage from traumatic forces applied to the brain where the brain contacts the interior skull or foreign bodies that cause direct brain injury.[30] Diffuse axonal injury, skull fractures, contusions, and hemorrhage result (Figure 29-5). Secondary injury occurs from the resultant changes in the brain caused by the initial injury; for example, cerebral edema, hypoxia, ICP, and decreased cerebral blood flow.[30]

Mild to Moderate TBI

Mild to moderate TBI may cause persistent vomiting, posttraumatic seizure, and loss of consciousness. Persistent vomiting (over a few hours) warrants further observation and evaluation with possible hospital admission.[51] Children who experience posttraumatic seizures require a CT scan and hospital admission, especially in children older than 5 years of age when seizures occur late after the injury, reoccur, persist, or if other symptoms suggest severe injury.[51] Loss of consciousness immediately after injury may not be known because no witnesses may have been present. The child may arrive in the ED awake and alert or unconscious. In either situation, further assessment and evaluation are warranted.

Children with mild to moderate TBI must receive serial neurologic evaluations to determine if ICP is increasing. Serial evaluations include measurement of level of consciousness, pupillary response, motor and sensory response, and vital signs. Making a game of assessment may elicit cooperation from the young, awake, and frightened child. Having the awake child touch the nose and move the heels down the shins tests cerebellar function, whereas having the child squeeze the nurse's fingers and "push on the gas pedal" tests motor strength. The awake infant and toddler should be able to focus on and reach for a toy or object. This child should recognize the parent and be easily consoled. Any changes in the child's level of consciousness should be reported immediately to avoid subsequent deterioration and possible brainstem herniation from increased ICP. The child should be evaluated for clinical signs of TBI including hemotympanum, cerebrospinal fluid (CSF) otorrhea, CSF rhinorrhea, orbital bruising (raccoon eyes), or mastoid bruising (Battle's sign) that may indicate a basilar skull fracture.[51] Other clinical findings that may be evident are altered level of consciousness, pupillary responses, speech deficits, and sensory motor deficits.

A CT scan without contrast may be obtained if intracranial pathology is suspected. Skull radiographs are obtained to detect location and extent of skull fractures in infants and young children. Toxicology screening is considered in children with altered level of consciousness. In general, children with mild to moderate TBI are admitted to the hospital for observation if they have any neurologic deficits, seizures,

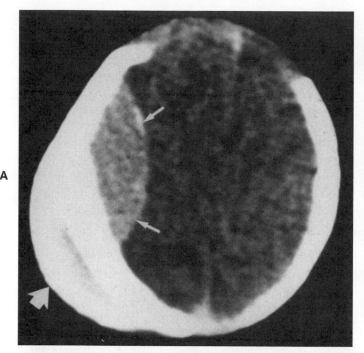

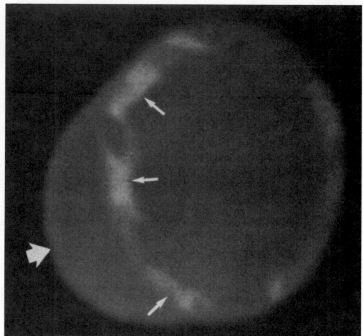

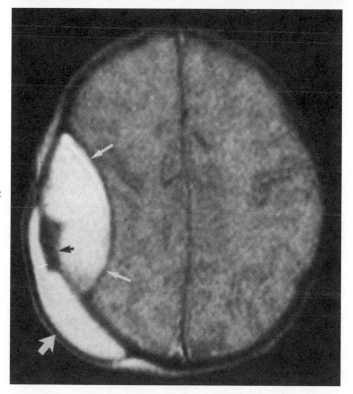

FIGURE 29-5   **A,** Axial unenhanced CT scan demonstrating acute epidural hematoma *(small white arrows)* and right subgaleal hematoma *(large white arrow).* **B,** Axial unenhanced CT scan (bone settings) in the same patient as **A** demonstrates multiple linear and depressed fractures *(small arrows)* of the right parietal bone and a subgaleal hematoma *(large arrow).* **C,** Axial MR T2-weighted image of the same patient as in **A** and **B** demonstrates subacute epidural hematoma *(small white arrows)* of the right-convexity parietal region of the brain, a subgaleal hematoma *(large white arrow)* of the scalp, and depressed bone fracture *(black arrow).* (From Silverman FN, Kuhn JP, Berdon WE et al: *Caffey's pediatric x-ray diagnosis: an integrated approach,* ed 9, St. Louis, 1997, Mosby.)

vomiting, severe headache, fever, prolonged loss of consciousness, skull fracture, altered level of consciousness, or suspected child maltreatment.[30]

Children with mild TBI may be discharged home if parents or guardians understand the required home care. Survey results of 765 pediatricians, emergency physicians, and family physicians answering clinical vignettes about children with minor head trauma showed that for children with minor head trauma without complications, observation at home was the most common initial management

choice.[1] Parents should be instructed to return to the ED if the child has persistent vomiting, changes in vision, unequal pupil size, persistent headache or drowsiness, changes in level of consciousness, unequal strength or gait, or seizures. Over the next 10 to 12 hours, parents should awaken the child every few hours to evaluate for changes in level of consciousness. Be sure parents understand the child may sleep and that sleeping is not an indication of a problem. They should be instructed to observe for nose or ear drainage on the pillow and to contact the ED if this is observed. Acetaminophen may be administered for headache.

Infants with skull fractures may be admitted for 24-hour observation. Among 101 infants hospitalized with an isolated skull fracture, the median length of hospital stay was 1 day, with 88% (89) staying less than 24 hours.[31] Among this series of infants, neurologic symptoms and signs of head injury, such as loss of consciousness, vomiting, lethargy, irritability, focal neurologic abnormalities, and seizures, were not sensitive predictors of isolated skull fractures. However, physical examination revealed that the majority of these infants had local signs of injury at the fracture site location.[31] Infants with isolated skull fractures may not require hospitalization if they can be cared for by reliable parents, child maltreatment is not suspected, and neurologic symptomatology is not present.[31]

Skull fractures that occur in one of the suture lines should create a high index of suspicion for epidural hematomas. A complication of these fractures is growth of the fracture. This expansion of the fracture is usually observed in infants and young children younger than 3 years of age and is thought to result from cerebral tissue or arachnoid membrane herniation through a dural laceration[30] causing a pulsatile mass. Surgery may be indicated for these situations; therefore, infants and young children with this fracture must receive follow-up treatment. Infants can sustain significant blood loss from scalp lacerations, so they require close observation for development of hypovolemic shock.

Severe TBI

Severe TBI is characterized by decreased level of consciousness, posturing, combative behavior, and abnormal neurologic findings. This catastrophic injury can be caused by severe shaking, falls, or motor vehicle collisions. Severe shaken impact syndrome is characterized by retinal hemorrhaging, seizures, and decreased level of consciousness (see Chapter 49).

In severe TBI the airway is secured using RSI and is followed by hyperventilation. A quick neurologic assessment should be completed before administering paralytic and sedative agents. Because carbon dioxide is a potent vasodilator, $PaCO_2$ should be maintained between 30 to 35 mm Hg to allow adequate cerebral blood flow.[30] Arterial oxygen saturation should be maintained at greater than 90% with mean arterial pressure slightly higher than age-appropriate norms. IV fluids such as normal saline or lactated Ringer's solution are administered, preferably at one half to two thirds of maintenance requirements. Glucose-containing fluids are avoided because of potential for cerebral edema. Mannitol 0.5 g to 1 g/kg may be infused to remove fluid from interstitial spaces. Phenobarbital or phenytoin is administered to prevent seizures for patients with increased risk resulting from injury; however, administration is usually limited to 7 days.

Babinski's reflex may be present with severe brain injury. Laboratory analyses, including type and cross-match, toxicologic testing, and clotting times (prothrombin time/partial thromboplastin time) should be performed in the event surgery is required. A CT scan without contrast is usually performed to determine location and extent of the injury. Operative management may be indicated followed by admission to an intensive care unit for ongoing nursing and medical care.

Generally children have better outcomes than do adults after TBI, although the reasons are not clear. Neurologic deficits are the most common complications of TBI and are relative to the area of brain injury. For example, frontal brain injury results in cognitive deficits. Children may require rehabilitation for speech, motor, and cognitive improvements.

Maxillofacial Injuries

The incidence of maxillofacial injuries in children older than 5 years and younger than 16 years is estimated at 1% to 14% and 0.87% to 1% for children younger than 5 years of age.[34] MVCs account for the largest proportion of maxillofacial injuries.[34] The most frequently fractured facial area is the mandible, followed by the midface and upper face.[34] One concern in the young pediatric population is damage to growing facial structures, such as incomplete calcification of bone, developing dentition, and cartilaginous and soft tissue. Facial injuries are diagnosed by clinical assessment and confirmed by diagnostic tests such as CT scan; plain or panoramic radiographs are not effective in detecting facial injuries[34] because of the aforementioned composition of facial structures.

Dental injuries are the most common orofacial injuries sustained during sports activities.[43] More than 5 million teeth are avulsed annually.[43] Avulsed primary teeth should not be replaced, but avulsed adult (permanent) teeth should be reimplanted within 2 hours (preferably 30 minutes).[34] The avulsed tooth is handled by the crown and placed in milk, saline, or tooth preservative solution; tissues attached to the teeth are left in place and not scrubbed away.[43] Consultation with a maxillofacial surgeon should be considered for children with severe facial injuries; attention to airway maintenance is critical.

Spinal Cord Injuries

Spinal cord injuries are relatively uncommon in the pediatric population. When these injuries do occur, rapid acceleration-deceleration forces and hyperflexion-hyperextension forces are suspected. Children younger than 9 years of age are susceptible to cervical spine injuries because of their larger head size, weaker neck muscles and ligaments, and horizontal facets.[27] Laxity of the pediatric spine contributes to spinal cord injury without bony abnormality. This phenomenon, known as spinal cord injury without radiographic abnormalities (SCIWORA), occurs because of inherent elasticity of the pediatric spine, which allows transient displacement of the cerebral column by flexion-extension or acceleration-deceleration forces.[40] Hyperflexion or hyperextension of the spinal cord leads to injury or transection. The spinal cord then returns to normal length and the vertebrae to normal alignment. The child may exhibit signs of spinal cord injury, such as numbness, tingling, or weakness; however, subsequent radiographs show no evidence of bony abnormality. Although SCIWORA is most often diagnosed at the cervical level, thoracic SCIWORA is also possible. One review of reported literature demonstrates an approximate 35% incidence of SCIWORA in children with traumatic myelopathy.[40] Most children younger than 8 years of age experience SCIWORA at a higher spinal level with greater severity of injury as compared with older children.[40]

Signs and symptoms of spinal cord injury are the same in children as in adults. Numbness, tingling, weakness, and spasticity or flaccidity may be observed. Priapism and perianal wink may also be demonstrated. The child may complain of pain in the back or neck with tenderness on palpation. The awake child with a spinal cord injury may feel helpless and afraid, so continuous reassurance is essential.

Spinal injuries should always be suspected in children with multiple injuries. Complete spinal immobilization is maintained until it is clinically determined that spinal cord injury is not present. Endotracheal intubation and mechanical ventilation are indicated in children with high spinal cord injuries. Children with lower cervical injuries require close observation for changes in their respiratory status. IV fluids should be administered at one half to two thirds of maintenance requirements. High-dose steroids are administered within 8 hours of injury. Methylprednisolone 30 mg/kg is administered over 15 minutes followed by normal saline over the next 45 minutes. A continuous infusion of 5.4 mg/kg/hr is then run for 23 hours if the injury occurred within 8 hours.[53] There is limited research in children younger than 13 years of age; however, they may benefit from this protocol.[53] Lateral, anterior-posterior, and open mouth (odontoid) radiographic views of the cervical spine are obtained. Anterior-posterior views of the thoracic or lumbar spine are obtained as needed. Serial neurologic assessments are performed to identify changes in neurologic function such as increasing cord swelling.

Unconscious children with suspected spinal cord injury should remain immobilized until they are awake and able to complete a neurologic examination. Advanced diagnostic tests, such as MRI and somatosensory evoked potentials, may be indicated to determine the presence or extent of spinal cord injury. Operative management may be needed for children with unstable vertebral fractures or dislocations.

Complications or sequelae of spinal cord injury range from mild neurologic deficits to complete hemiplegia, paraplegia, or quadriplegia. Autonomic areflexia, bowel and bladder incontinence, and ventilator dependence occur relative to the level of the cord lesion. Rehabilitation assists the child to maximize his or her potential for recovery.

Thoracic Injuries

Most thoracic injuries are caused by blunt trauma. With infants and young children these injuries are usually caused by falls, whereas older children sustain these injuries as pedestrians or passengers in motor vehicles. Penetrating chest trauma is seen in adolescents as a result of violence—intentional or self-inflicted. Common thoracic injuries in the pediatric population are pulmonary contusion, cardiac contusion, and pneumothorax.

Children are susceptible to transmission of blunt forces to underlying thoracic structures (heart, lungs, great vessels) because soft cartilage and developing bones make the thorax pliable.[36] Rib fractures should raise a high index of suspicion for severe blunt forces. Similarly, when flail segments are present, severe parenchymal pulmonary injury should be suspected.[36] The mediastinum is easily displaced by air or fluid. As the mediastinum shifts, venous return, cardiac output, and lung volume are severely compromised.[36]

Rib Fractures

Rib fractures are associated with chest pain, tenderness on palpation, and respiratory distress. Flail segments lead to paradoxic chest wall movement during respiration. Changes in pulse oximetry and respiratory rate and effort may occur. Children should receive oxygen via face mask and analgesics for pain relief. A chest radiograph is obtained to determine location and extent of fractures. Evaluate carefully for spleen or liver injury with lower rib fractures.

Pneumothorax/Hemothorax

Pneumothorax may be open, closed, or tension. Clinical signs and symptoms vary with severity of injury but can include respiratory distress, air hunger, decreased or absent breath sounds on the affected side, and anxiety. In a tension pneumothorax, tracheal deviation away from the affected side and jugular vein distention are often observed. Hemothorax from severe blunt or penetrating chest trauma is characterized by hypovolemic shock, decreased or absent breath sounds on the affected side, and respiratory distress.

Pneumothoraces are treated relative to severity. Chest radiographs confirm the presence of air in the pleural space but should not delay treatment in a symptomatic child. Children in no acute distress with a small pneumothorax receive supplemental oxygen and are observed for worsening of the pneumothorax. Large pneumothoraces require needle decompression followed by chest tube placement. The needle is inserted at the fourth intercostal space at midaxillary line, followed by chest tube placement with water seal suction. In tension pneumothoraces, needle insertion precedes chest radiograph because this situation is an immediate threat to life. After needle decompression, chest tubes are inserted and a chest radiograph is obtained. Similarly, in hemothoraces chest radiographs may be delayed until chest tubes are inserted. Autotransfusion should be considered for these patients when there are no contraindications; for example, enteric contamination or wound greater than 6 hours old. Surgical intervention is indicated with ongoing blood loss into the chest drainage system greater than 100 ml/hr or immediate blood loss greater than 20% of the child's estimated circulating blood volume.[36]

Pulmonary Contusion

Pulmonary contusions should be suspected in children with respiratory distress after blunt chest trauma without abnormal radiographic findings. Pulmonary contusion is usually not diagnosed until after hospital admission. Signs and symptoms include increasing respiratory distress, hemoptysis, and decreased pulmonary function. Chest radiographs show changes from the initial film. Management of these patients in the ED begins with supplemental oxygen. Endotracheal intubation and subsequent ventilation with positive end-expiratory pressure is usually reserved for severe injuries. Fluids may be limited if the child is not hypovolemic.

Tracheobronchial Injury

Tracheobronchial rupture, although rare, can occur with blunt or penetrating forces to the neck and chest. The child may have respiratory distress, subcutaneous emphysema, and cyanosis. Severe tracheobronchial rupture causes massive subcutaneous emphysema, persistent air leak, mediastinal air, tension pneumothorax, and failure of the lung to expand after chest tube insertion. Airway management with endotracheal intubation or tracheostomy is imperative. Chest tubes may also be required. Fibroscopy may be helpful in identifying the area of injury.[44]

Diaphragmatic Injury

Diaphragmatic rupture usually occurs after blunt trauma. In this case diminished breath sounds are auscultated (usually on the left side), bowel sounds are heard within the chest cavity, or a scaphoid abdomen (Gibson's sign) is present.[42] Diaphragmatic rupture requires early identification, operative management, and repair—mortality increases with delayed identification and treatment.

Cardiac Injury

In general, cardiac injuries are suspected in children with chest bruising, upper body cyanosis, unexplained hypotension, and dysrhythmias. Injuries include cardiac tamponade, myocardial contusion, and great vessel injuries. Management of cardiac injuries includes initial and ongoing evaluations of electrocardiograms, cardiac enzymes, and echocardiographic studies.

Abdominal Injuries

Blunt force is the most common cause of abdominal trauma in children, with subsequent hemorrhaging a common cause of traumatic death. Because of the child's smaller abdomen, injuries can occur to multiple organs. The spleen followed by the liver are the most commonly injured abdominal organs in blunt trauma[42]; the stomach and intestines are the most commonly injured abdominal organs in penetrating trauma.[41] Trauma can result from pedestrian motor vehicle crashes, MVCs, falls or forces applied to the abdomen, bicycles, and child maltreatment. Penetrating abdominal trauma usually results from acts of violence. The lap belt complex—small bowel contusion/laceration, lumbar flexion distraction injury (Chance fracture), and cutaneous bruising—occurs in restrained passengers in an MVC.

The alert child who sustains abdominal trauma may complain of tenderness with palpation. Deep palpation should be avoided to prevent guarding.[37] For young infants and toddlers, placing a warm hand on the abdomen for a few seconds before palpation may avoid startling or frightening the patient.[37] Abdominal distention, abrasions, or contusions may be noted. Hypovolemic shock indicates internal hemorrhaging. CT can identify injury to solid abdominal organs.

Children with blunt abdominal trauma are treated according to their hemodynamic stability. A nasogastric tube (or orogastric tube in the child with TBI) is inserted to decompress the stomach and avoid aspiration. Serial CBCs are obtained to monitor for ongoing blood loss. A CT scan with contrast is used to determine extent of the injuries in the hemodynamically stable child. This is preferred over diagnostic peritoneal lavage because of accuracy in detecting specific abdominal injuries. Many injuries are treated conservatively with serial reevaluation; however, surgical intervention is indicated for persistent hemorrhaging or peritonitis. The hemodynamically unstable child who does not respond to fluid and blood boluses must be prepared for immediate surgery.

Splenic injury is suspected in children with tenderness in the left upper quadrant. Pain in the left shoulder may be elicited with abdominal palpation (Kehr's sign). Splenic injury is suspected in children with altered level of consciousness, altered vital signs, low blood count, left lower rib fractures, abdominal pain, or grunting.[42] Children with splenic injuries who are hemodynamically stable are admitted to the hospital and managed with bed rest and serial reevaluation. Hemodynamically unstable patients (those who are hypotensive even with fluid and blood administration) require operative management.

Liver injuries are suspected in children who sustain any blunt force trauma to the abdomen. Right upper quadrant pain, tenderness, or diffuse pain are symptoms of liver injury.[42] Serum asparate aminotransferase and serum alanine aminotransferase are obtained and evaluated, with a threshold of 200 for each test indicative of hepatic injury.[37] Large liver lacerations cause significant blood loss and require immediate surgical repair, whereas smaller lacerations without signs of hypovolemia can be managed conservatively. In one review of 328 children sustaining liver injuries, 72% were hemodynamically stable and managed nonoperatively.[32]

Pancreatic injuries cause abdominal pain that radiates to the back and persistent epigastric tenderness or vomiting; however, these injuries may not be noted until several days postinjury.[37] Serum amylase and lipase levels are obtained and the patient is hospitalized for further evaluation.

Intestinal injury is suspected in MVC passengers with abdominal bruising from the seat belt, bicycle riders who strike the handlebars, and those sustaining penetrating trauma.[42] Pain can be the only symptom, but free air may be noted on radiographs in some patients. These patients require a CT scan, hospitalization, and observation for possible intestinal perforation and subsequent surgical repair.[42] Intestinal perforation should be suspected in children with lap-belt injuries. Symptoms include fever, increasing pain, hypotension, and peritoneal signs.[42]

All children who sustain high-velocity abdominal trauma (e.g., gunshot wounds) should undergo surgical exploration.[42] Children sustaining low-velocity injuries (e.g., stab wound to the anterior torso) and who are hemodynamicaly stable are hospitalized and observed.

Genitourinary Injuries

Genitourinary injuries result from pedestrian or passenger MVCs, sledding, sports activities, falls, and altercations. Bladder and urethral injuries result mostly from blunt trauma and are often associated with pelvic fractures. Blunt and penetrating injuries of the kidneys and ureters also occur. Renal injuries may be minor or so severe that surgical intervention is necessary.

Renal Injury

Renal injury should be considered in children who sustain fractures to the lower ribs or the transverse process of the vertebrae. In such cases, there may be direct flank trauma or rapid deceleration forces that crush the kidney against the rib cage or vertebral column.[42] Symptoms of renal trauma include abdominal, back, or flank tenderness. The awake, stable child may be able to provide a urine specimen by voiding spontaneously, or an indwelling bladder catheter can be inserted to measure urine output and obtain urine specimens for testing. A catheter is not passed in suspected urethral trauma. Physical signs include localized abrasions or lacerations and hematuria. Hematuria is an important indicator of both severe and nonsevere renal injury, with the degree of hematuria correlating to a higher risk of abdominal injury.[41] Hematuria may also occur without substantial renal injury resulting from capillary disruption after blunt force trauma.[41] In the presence of gross hematuria, CT scan of the abdomen is indicated because there is an association between gross hematuria and severe intraabdominal injury.[41] Bedside urine screening may be performed to identify blood in the urine. Urinalysis testing with a threshold of more than 50 red blood cells (RBCs) per high-power field indicates the need for further genitourinary tract evaluation; a threshold of more than 10 RBCs/hpf is used in children with high-risk injuries such as pelvic or proximal lower extremity fractures.[37]

A CT scan with contrast dye is usually obtained. Treatment is specialized relative to the type of injury and may range from observation and bed rest to surgical exploration for patients with pedical injuries or renal pelvis rupture.[42]

Ureteral Injury

Ureteral injuries are rare, so recognition may be delayed unless the possibility for this injury is entertained. Hematuria or urinary leak may be present with flank mass and iliac pain

present. Symptoms may not be noted until 7 to 10 days after the initial injury. Urine may appear at entrance or exit wounds or on a surgical dressing. If no wound is present, signs of retroperitoneal abscess such as chills, fever, lower abdominal pain, palpable mass, pyuria, and frequency may ocur. Surgical repair is indicated for ureteral injuries, with a ureteral stent required in some patients.

Bladder Injury

Symptoms of bladder injuries vary with sustained injury. Suprapubic tenderness, urgency to void, inability to void, hematuria, and palpable abdominal mass may be observed with a ruptured bladder. Children with an extraperitoneal rupture may be able to pass small amounts of sanguineous urine but with significant discomfort. If severe hemorrhaging is present, signs of shock are observed. Most bladder contusions are minor and managed conservatively with observation and reevaluation. Large extraperitoneal injuries and intraperitoneal bladder ruptures with pelvic fractures necessitate surgical intervention for most patients.[42]

Urethral Injury

Urethral injury should be suspected in patients with vaginal bleeding; penile, scrotal, perineal, and prostate trauma; and the inability to advance an indwelling bladder catheter.[41] No attempt should be made to insert a urinary bladder catheter when there is blood at the meatus because the child may have a partial urethral tear. Inserting a catheter may convert a partial tear to a complete tear. Urthrography is indicated with cystography and CT cystography/CT scan of the abdomen and pelvis may be performed for some patients.[41] Partial urethral tears are managed conservatively with a suprapubic catheter or indwelling urethral catheter inserted under fluoroscopy. Complete urethral tears require surgical repair.

Genital Injuries

Injuries to female genitalia can result from falls, straddle-type injuries (e.g., falls on monkey bars, picket fences, or diving boards), and sexual abuse or assault. Testicular trauma can also result from straddle-type injuries. The most common cause of penile injuries is direct forces such as zipper injuries and trauma from toilet seats. Infants can sustain a tourniquet injury from threads, bands, rings, or human hair lodged in the coronal groove, which forms a constricting ring and lacerates the penile shaft. Sexual abuse must be considered in any child with genital trauma, particularly when injuries are inconsistent with the history. In children with suspected sexual abuse or assault, proper evidence collection is critical (see Chapter 49).

Musculoskeletal Injuries

Musculoskeletal injuries are common occurrences in the pediatric population. Long-bone fractures occur from falls, sports activities, and motor vehicle and pedestrian crashes. Strong ligaments account for the prevalence of fractures rather than ligamentous injury.

Table 29-5	SALTER-HARRIS CLASSIFICATION, FRACTURE DESCRIPTIONS, AND OUTCOME	
TYPE	**DESCRIPTION OF FRACTURES**	**TREATMENT AND OUTCOME**
Type I	Horizontal separation of epiphysis and metaphysis; point tenderness; radiographs may be normal; mild soft-tissue swelling produced by shearing forces	No disturbance in growth if properly diagnosed; favorable prognosis; treated with closed reduction and casting
Type II	Separation of epiphysis and metaphysis with some avulsion of the metaphysis produced by shearing forces	No disturbance in growth if properly diagnosed; favorable prognosis; treated with closed reduction and casting
Type III	Produced by intraarticular shearing forces; intraarticular fracture; fracture extends through epiphyseal plate into the metaphysis	Angular deformities may occur; requires good reduction; variable-poor prognosis
Type IV	Fracture starts at the articular surface and extends through the epiphysis, epiphyseal plate, and metaphysis; intraarticular fracture produced by shearing forces	Open reduction and external fixation is needed; variable-poor prognosis; angular deformity may result
Type V	Epiphyseal plate is crushed without fracture or displacement; radiographic diagnosis virtually impossible, produced by crushing forces	Poor prognosis, even when correctly identified and treated

From Bernardo LM, Trunzo R: Pediatric trauma. In Kitt S, Selfridge-Thomas J, Proehl J et al, editors: *Emergency nursing: a physiologic and clinical perspective,* ed 2, Philadelphia, 1995, WB Saunders.

The most unique feature of the child's musculoskeletal system is the epiphyseal growth plate (physis) located at the articulating ends of bones between the epiphysis and metaphysis. The epiphyseal growth plate is responsible for longitudinal bone growth; therefore, injury can cause growth disturbance or arrest. In general, growth is completed in boys by age 16 years and in girls by 14 years of age. Children sustaining injuries near the physis should have appropriate follow-up to detect limb-length discrepancies and angular deformities.[24] Growth plate fractures are categorized with the Salter-Harris classification (Table 29-5).

Signs of musculoskeletal trauma include point tenderness, soft-tissue swelling, discoloration, limitations in range of motion, loss of function, altered sensory perception, and changes in pulses, temperature, or capillary refill distal to the injury.[24] An obvious deformity may be noted or an actual open fracture may be observed. The child may complain of pain and splint the injured extremity by holding the broken arm with the other hand, for example.

Musculoskeletal trauma is rarely life threatening, so the child's airway, breathing, circulation, and neurologic status are usually intact. The injured extremity is elevated and ice is applied. A splint or sling and swath can be applied, provided neurovascular status is assessed before and after splint application. A sterile dressing is applied to any open fracture. Prophylactic antibiotics are given for open fractures, and tetanus prophylaxis is administered. Analgesia is required during splinting and during any reduction measures.

Radiographs of the anteroposterior and lateral views of the injured extremity are obtained, including the joint above and below the injury.[24] Comparative views of the injured and uninjured extremities may be obtained. Such radiographs allow for detection of previous fractures that may not have been reported by the family. Child maltreatment should be investigated in nonambulatory children with spiral fractures in the lower extremities or upper arms, toddlers with femur fractures, young children with multiple fractures, or in circumstances in which the injury does not match the history.

Most children require a simple cast when the fracture is nondisplaced. After cast application, the child is discharged from the ED. Parents or guardians are given discharge instructions to observe for swelling of the toes or fingers, odor from the cast, and changes in skin color and temperature. Parents should contact the ED with any of these complaints or if the child complains of sharp pain or numbness. Severe swelling can prohibit application of a cast, so some children are discharged with a splint with the cast applied after swelling subsides.

Displaced fractures require manipulation to realign the fractured bone(s). In such situations the ED physician or orthopedic surgeon may attempt closed reduction in the ED. Conscious sedation is administered using analgesics and sedatives such as midazolam, fentanyl, or ketamine. The nurse must carefully monitor the child throughout the procedure for adverse effects to the sedation. After the fracture is reduced, sedatives are stopped, the cast is applied, and postreduction radiographs are obtained. If reduction is not successful, the child may require open reduction and internal fixation in the operating room.

Treatment for femoral fractures varies with age. Infants are placed in spica casts, often in the ED. Reamed and non-reamed intramedullary rodding used in older children allows early mobilization. Tibial skeletal traction, external fixation, and plating techniques are also used depending on the type of fracture and the child's age. Children with pelvic fractures require admission to the hospital and subsequent bed rest. Unstable pelvic fractures may require application of an external fixation device.

SUMMARY

Pediatric trauma patients provide a unique challenge for the emergency nurse. The ability to identify potentially life-

Box 29-2 **NURSING DIAGNOSES FOR THE PEDIATRIC TRAUMA PATIENT**

Airway clearance, Ineffective
Anxiety
Breathing pattern, Ineffective
Cardiac output, Decreased
Family processes, Interrupted
Fear
Fluid volume, Deficient
Gas exchange, Impaired
Pain

threatening conditions is essential. Box 29-2 highlights nursing diagnoses appropriate for these patients. Emergency nurses are in a unique position to offer anticipatory guidance to families concerning primary injury prevention. Becoming actively involved in trauma prevention and safety education is another way for emergency nurses to promote safety through education, engineering, and enforcement strategies. Educating parents and children during ED visits using posters, pamphlets, one-on-one discussions, and videos provides families with opportunities for discussion with nurses and with each other regarding their safety practices. Volunteer to speak with students and parent-teacher groups about safety on such topics as wearing bicycle helmets, firearm safety, or wearing safety belts. Engineering efforts include becoming a car seat safety inspector with the National Safe Kids Campaign to check proper installation and security of car safety seats. Write to manufacturers to express concerns about product safety. Report unsafe products or patients injured by products to the Consumer Product Safety Commission. Enforcement includes promoting safety laws in one's community. Become politically aware and support legislators who favor legislation aimed at reducing injuries (e.g., mandatory bicycle, motorcycle, and skateboard helmet use). Educate legislators and government officials about unsafe road conditions, traffic problems, and other community hazards that cause injuries in children.

Emergency nurses can become involved in organizations such as the *National Safe Kids Campaign* and *Emergency Nurses Cancel Alcohol Related Emergencies*. The Emergency Nurses Association has resources related to injury control and prevention. Emergency nurses can minimize the effects of pediatric trauma by providing quality patient care to injured children and their families. Participating in injury prevention activities helps reduce the incidence of pediatric trauma and enhances the professional image of nursing.

References

1. Aitken M, Herrerias C, Davis R et al: Minor head injury in children: current management practices of pediatricians, emergency physicians, and family physicians, *Arch Pediat Adolesc Med* 152:1176, 1998.
2. Benya E, Lim-Dunham J, Landrum O et al: Abdominal sonography in examination of children with blunt abdominal trauma, *Am J Roentgenol* 174:1613, 2000.
3. Berg M, Cook L, Corneli H et al: Effect of seating position and restraint use on injuries to children in motor vehicle crashes, *Pediatrics* 105:831, 2000.
4. Bernardo L, Clemence B, Henker R et al: A comparison of aural and rectal temperature measurements in children with moderate and severe injuries, *J Emerg Nurs* 22:403, 1996.
5. Bernardo L, Gardner M, Lucke J et al: The effects of core and peripheral warming methods on temperature and physiologic variables in injured children, *Pediatr Emerg Care* 12(2):138, 2001.
6. Bernardo L, Henker R: Thermoregulation in pediatric trauma: an overview, *Int J Trauma Nurs* 5:101, 1999.
7. Bernardo L, Henker R, Bove M et al: The effect of administered crystalloid fluid temperature on aural temperature of moderately and severely injured children, *J Emerg Nurs* 23:105, 1997.
8. Bernardo L, Henker R, O'Connor J: Temperature measurement in pediatric trauma patients: a comparison of thermometry and measurement routes, *J Emerg Nurs* 25:327, 1999.
9. Bernardo L, Henker R, O'Connor J: Treatment of trauma-associated hypothermia in children: evidence-based practice, *Am J Crit Care* 9:227, 2000.
10. Chameides L, Hazinski M: *Textbook of pediatric advanced life support*, Dallas, 1997, American Heart Association, American Academy of Pediatrics
11. Clemence B: Emergency department thoracotomy: nursing implications for pediatric cases, *Int J Trauma Nurs* 6:123, 2000.
12. Clinical Policies Committee: Rapid-sequence intubation, *Ann Emerg Med* 29:573, 1997.
13. Committee on Injury and Poison Prevention: All-terrain vehicle injury prevention: two-, three-, and four-wheeled unlicensed motor vehicles, *Pediatrics* 105:1352, 2000.
14. Committee on Injury and Poison Prevention: Children in pickup trucks, *Pediatrics* 106:857, 2000.
15. Committee on Injury and Poison Prevention: Skateboard and scooter injuries, *Pediatrics* 109(3):542, 1995.
16. Committee on Native American Child Health and Committee on Injury and Poison Prevention: The prevention of unintentional injury among American Indian and Alaska Native children: a subject review, *Pediatrics* 104:1397, 1999.
17. Conners G, Sacks W, Leahey N: Variations in sedating uncooperative, stable children for post-traumatic head CT, *Pediatr Emerg Care* 15:241, 1999.
18. Consumer Product Safety Commission: *CPSC, AAA release study on kids and bike helmets,* 2001. Retrieved February 2, 2001 from the World Wide Web: http:www.cpsc.gov/cpscpub/prerel/prhtml95/95127.html.
19. Consumer Product Safety Commission: *CPSC gets new, safer baby walkers on the market,* CPSC document #5086, 2001. Retrieved February 2, 2001 from the World Wide Web: http://www.cpsc.gov/cpscpub/pubs/5086html.
20. Consumer Product Safety Commission: *CPSC study shows more kids wear bicycle helmets, but deaths and injuries still common,* 2001: Retrieved February 2, 2001 from the World Wide Web: http://www.cpsc.gov/cpscpub/prerel/prhtml96/96072.html.
21. Consumer Product Safety Commission: *More scooter information,* 2001. Retrieved February 2, 2001 from the World Wide Web: http://www.cpsc.gov/pr/prscoot.html.
22. Consumer Product Safety Commission: *Shopping cart injuries: victims 5 years old and younger,* 2001. Retrieved February 2, 2001 from the World Wide Web: http://www.cpsc.gov/library/shopcart.html.

23. Corbett S, Andrews H, Baker E et al: ED evaluation of the pediatric trauma patient by ultrasonography, *Am J Emerg Med* 18:244, 2000.

24. Della-Giustina K, Della-Giustina D: Emergency department evaluation and treatment of pediatric orthopedic injuries, *Emerg Med Clin North Am* 17:895, 1999.

25. Dietrich A, Shaner S: *Pediatric basic trauma life support,* Oakbrook Terrace, Ill, 1995, Basic Trauma Life Support International.

26. Durkin M, Laraque D, Lubman I et al: Epidemiology and prevention of traffic injuries to urban children and adolescents, *Pediatrics* 103(6):e74, 1999.

27. Eleraky M, Theodore N, Adams M et al: Pediatric cervical spin injuries: report of 102 cases and review of the literature, *J Neurosurg Spine* 92:12, 2000.

28. Fultz J: Tips for helping the families of patients transported by helicopter, *J Emerg Nurs* 25:132, 1999.

29. Goldbloom R: Halifax and the precipitate birth of pediatric surgery, *Pediatrics* 77:764, 1986.

30. Greenes D, Madsen J: Neurotrauma. In Fleisher G, Ludwig S, editors: *Textbook of pediatric emergency medicine,* ed 4, Philadelphia, 2000, Lippincott Williams & Wilkins.

31. Greenes D, Schutzman S: Infants with isolated skull fracture: what are their clinical characteristics, and do they require hospitalization? *Ann Emerg Med* 30:253, 1997.

32. Gross M, Lynch F, Canty T et al: Management of pediatric liver injuries: a 13-year experience at a pediatric trauma center, *J Pediatr Surg* 14:816, 1999.

33. Guohua L, Tang N, DiScala C et al: Cardiopulmonary resuscitation in pediatric trauma patients: survival and functional outcome, *J Trauma* 47:1, 1999.

34. Haug R, Foss J: Maxillofacial injuries in the pediatric patient, *Oral Surg Oral Med Oral Pathol Oral Radiol Endodontics* 90:126, 2000.

35. Hogert D, Kochunek K, Murphy P: *Deaths: final data for 1997,* Hyattsville, Md, 1999, National Center for Health Statistics.

36. Kadish H: Thoracic trauma. In Fleisher G, Ludwig S, editors: *Textbook of pediatric emergency medicine,* ed 4, Philadelphia, 2000, Lippincott Williams & Wilkins.

37. Meyer M, Burd R: The top 10 things to evaluate in children with suspected blunt abdominal injuries, *J Trauma Nurs* 7:98, 2000.

38. Moulton S: Early management of the child with multiple injuries, *Clin Orthop Related Res* 376:6, 2000.

39. Partrick D, Bensard D, Moore E et al: Driveway crush injuries in young children: a highly lethal, devastating, and potentially preventable event, *J Pediatr Surg* 33:1712, 1998.

40. Pollack I, Pang D: Spinal cord injury without radiographic abnormality (SCIWORA). In Pang D, editor: *Disorders of the pediatric spine,* New York, 1995, Raven Press.

41. Rothrock S, Green S, Morgan R: Abdominal trauma in infants and children: prompt identification and early management of serious and life-threatening injuries. Part 1: injury patterns and initial assessment, *Pediatr Emerg Care* 16:106, 2000.

42. Rothrock S, Green S, Morgan R: Abdominal trauma in infants and children: prompt identification and early management of serious and life-threatening injuries. Part II: specific injuries and ED management, *Pediatr Emerg Care* 16: 189, 2000.

43. Rudy C: Dental trauma, *School Nurse News* 18: 33, 2001.

44. Slimane M, Becmeur F, Aubert D: Tracheobronchial ruptures from blunt thoracic trauma in children, *J Pediatr Surg,* 34:1847, 1999.

45. Stylianos S, Harris B: The history of pediatric trauma care. In Buntain W, editor: *Management of pediatric trauma care,* Philadelphia, 1995, WB Saunders.

46. Templeton J: Mechanisms of injury. In Eichelberger M, editor: *Pediatric trauma,* St Louis, 1993, Mosby.

47. U.S. Department of Transportation, National Highway Traffic Safety Administration: *Child restraint systems safety plan (draft),* Washington, D.C., 2000, U.S. Department of Transportation.

48. U.S. Department of Transportation, National Highway Traffic Safety Administration, National Center for Statistics and Analysis: *Fatality analysis reporting system,* Washington, D.C., 1998, U.S. Department of Transportation.

49. Wazana A, Rynard V, Raina P: Are child pedestrians at increased risk of injury on one-way compared to two-way streets? *Can J Public Health* 91:201, 2000.

50. Weiss H, Mathers L, Forjuoh S: *Child and adolescent emergency department visit databook,* Pittsburgh, Pa, 1997, Center for Violence and Injury Control, Allegheny University of the Health Sciences.

51. Wiley P: Paediatric head injuries: a literature review, *Aust Emerg Nurs J* 1:20, 1997.

52. Winston F, Durbin D: Buckle up! Is not enough: enhancing protection of the restrained child, *JAMA* 281:2070, 1999.

53. Woodward G: Neck trauma. In Fleisher G, Ludwig S, editors: *Textbook of pediatric emergency medicine,* ed 4, Philadelphia, 2000, Lippincott Williams & Wilkins.

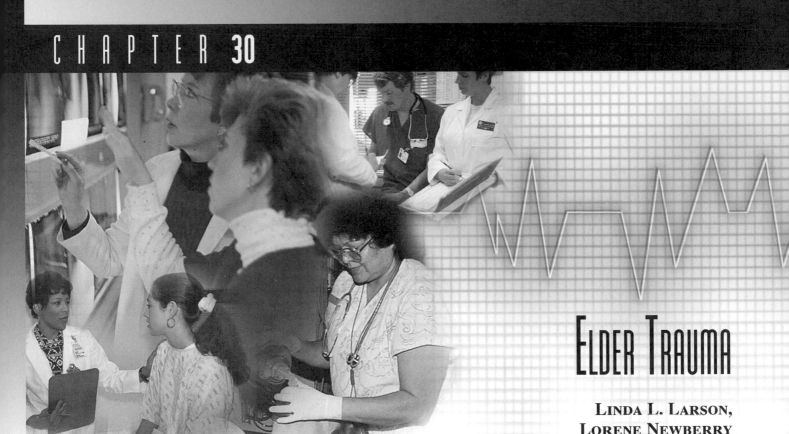

CHAPTER 30

ELDER TRAUMA

LINDA L. LARSON,
LORENE NEWBERRY

Elders, or geriatrics, are individuals older than age 65,[10] a definition that follows government statistics and matches when Medicare benefits begin. By the year 2000, 13% of the U.S. population were older than age 65.[3] Factors that contribute to the expanding elder population include increasing life expectancy and improved health care.

More individuals live past age 65 years; the number of individuals between ages 75 and 84 years is currently 13 times greater than it was in the year 1900. The number of individuals age 85 years and older is 24 times greater than it was in the year 1900 and is the fastest-growing segment of the population today. Birthday celebrations for centenarians are increasingly common. Women in every age-group have a lower probability of dying than men. Three quarters of men older than age 65 are still married, whereas more than half of older women are widows.

Although geriatric patients comprise 13% of the population, they consume one third of all trauma resources.[7] There is a higher mortality rate in the geriatric population despite greater use of resources. This is likely the result of the aging process that diminishes this population's physiologic reserves.

PHYSIOLOGIC CHANGES

Aging is progressive, predictable, and inevitable—it is the evolution of life from birth until death. Progressive deterioration of homeostatic control mechanisms causes slower reactions to stimuli and longer recovery periods. Organ reserves diminish to the point that any stress causes more extensive injury with less ability to compensate.

Nervous System

The brain shrinks with age, whereas the dura adheres tightly to the skull.[9] Progressive loss of brain volume occurs as the brain shrinks, and cerebrospinal fluid production decreases. Consequently, space around the brain increases, which may decrease incidence of contusions. However, stretching of dural connections increases the risk of bleeding.[8] The brain is also at greater risk for ricochet or coup-contrecoup injuries because of increased freedom of movement within the cranial vault.

Age-related changes in the autonomic nervous system, primarily the baroreflex, affect the elder person's ability to respond to injury. The problem may lie in the baroreceptor or α-adrenergic or β-adrenergic response. Normally the baroreflex increases peripheral vascular resistance, heart rate, blood pressure, and ultimately, cardiac output. In elders, heart rate and blood pressure do not always increase with stimulation of the baroreflex.

Thermoregulation decreases in elders, which increases their risk for hypothermia and hyperthermia. Decrease in lean body mass, decreased muscle activity, less efficient shivering, and 50% reduction in glucose-induced thermogenesis make maintaining normal body temperature difficult. Problems in thermoregulation are associated with inability to regulate body fluid. Vasopressin secretion may be inhibited by inadequate release of stimulating hormones. The elderly also experience less thirst with water deprivation, so water consumption may not be adequate.

Other age-related changes that may affect assessment of the elderly patient include chronic dementia, previous strokes, decreased visual acuity, and decreased hearing. Table 30-1 summarizes variances in assessment of the nervous system in older patients.

Respiratory System

Healthy elderly patients also experience increased calcification of the trachea, decreased elasticity, and stiffening of the rib cage, which decrease pulmonary function.[9] Increased

residual lung volume and decreased alveolar surface area lead to slightly elevated carbon dioxide pressure levels. The work of breathing is complicated by structural changes in the chest that decrease overall pulmonary reserve and may cause more complications in the injured elder; for example, atelectasis, aspiration, pneumonia, or adult respiratory distress syndrome. Table 30-2 identifies age-related differences in assessment of the respiratory system.

Cardiovascular System

Changes in the peripheral vascular system decrease arterial compliance,[5] increase blood pressure, and decrease ventricular filling.[9] Ventricular filling decreases by 50% between

Table 30-1 GERONTOLOGIC DIFFERENCES IN ASSESSMENT: NERVOUS SYSTEM		
COMPONENT	**CHANGES**	**DIFFERENCES IN ASSESSMENT FINDINGS**
CENTRAL NERVOUS SYSTEM		
Brain	Reduction in cerebral blood flow and metabolism	Alterations in selected mental functioning
	Decrease in efficiency of temperature-regulating mechanism	Decrease in body temperature, impairment of ability to adapt to environmental temperature
	Decrease in neurotransmitter content, disruption in integration as result of loss of neurons	Repetitive movements, tremors
	Decrease in oxygen supply, changes in basal ganglia caused by vascular changes	Changes in gait and ambulation (e.g., extrapyramidal, parkinson-like gait); diminished kinesthetic sense
PERIPHERAL NERVOUS SYSTEM		
Cranial and spinal nerves	Loss of myelin and decrease in conduction time in some nerves	Decrease in reaction time in specific nerves
	Cellular degeneration, death of neurons	Decrease in speed and intensity of neuronal reflexes
FUNCTIONAL DIVISIONS		
Motor	Decrease in muscle bulk	Diminished strength and agility
	Decrease in electrical activity	Decrease in reactions and movement time
Sensory	Decrease in sensory receptors caused by degenerative changes and involution of fine corpuscles of nerve endings	Diminished sense of touch; inability to localize stimuli; decrease in appreciation of touch, temperature, and peripheral vibrations
	Decrease in electrical activity	Slowing of or alteration in sensory reception
	Atrophy of taste buds	Signs of malnutrition, weight loss
	Degeneration and loss of fibers in olfactory bulb	Diminished sense of smell
	Degenerative changes in nerve cells in vestibular system of inner ear, cerebellum, and proprioceptive pathways in nervous system	Poor ability to maintain balance, widened gait
Reflexes	Possible decrease in deep tendon reflexes	Below-average reflex score
	Decrease in sensory conduction velocity as result of myelin sheath degeneration	Sluggish reflexes, slowing of reaction time
RETICULAR FORMATION		
Reticular activating system	Modification of hypothalamic function, reduction in stage IV sleep	Increase in frequency of spontaneous awakening together with tiredness, interrupted sleep, insomnia
AUTONOMIC NERVOUS SYSTEM		
SNS and PSNS	Morphologic features of ganglia, slowing of ANS responses	Orthostatic hypotension, systolic hypertension

From Lewis SM, Heitkemper MM, Dirksen SR: *Medical-surgical nursing: assessment and management of clinical problems,* ed 5, St. Louis, 2000, Mosby.
ANS, Autonomic nervous system; *PSNS,* parasympathetic nervous system; *SNS,* sympathetic nervous system.

ages 20 and 80 years. Peripheral vascular resistance increases 1% per year. Intracellular calcium levels remain higher for a longer period in the elderly, which changes the action potential and electrical activity of the heart in relation to mechanical activity. Inotropic response to catecholamines and cardiac glycosides decreases, and refractoriness to electrical stimulation increases. Other age-related changes that affect assessment may include ischemic myocardial disease and conduction abnormalities. Gerontologic differences in cardiovascular assessment are summarized in Table 30-3.

Renal System

Renal perfusion decreases by 50% and renal mass decreases 25% to 30%, mostly in the renal cortex.[9] As the number of nephrons with long Henle's loops into the cor-

---

Table 30-2   GERONTOLOGIC DIFFERENCES IN ASSESSMENT: RESPIRATORY SYSTEM

CHANGES	DIFFERENCES IN ASSESSMENT FINDINGS
STRUCTURE	
↓ Elastic recoil ↓ Chest wall compliance ↑ Anteroposterior diameter ↓ Functioning alveoli	Barrel chest appearance; ↓ chest wall movement; ↓ respiratory excursion; ↓ vital capacity; ↑ functional residual capacity; diminished breath sounds particularly at lung bases; ↓ PaO_2 and SaO_2; normal pH and $PaCO_2$
DEFENSE MECHANISMS	
↓ Cell-mediated immunity ↓ Specific antibodies ↓ Cilia function ↓ Cough force ↓ Alveolar macrophage function	↓ Cough effectiveness; ↓ secretion clearance; ↑ risk of upper respiratory infection, influenza, or pneumonia; respiratory infections may be more severe and last longer
RESPIRATORY CONTROL	
↓ Response to hypoxemia ↓ Response to hypercapnia	Greater ↓ in PaO_2 and ↑ in $PaCO_2$ before respiratory rate changes. Significant hypoxemia or hypercapnia may develop from relatively small incidents. Retained secretions, excessive sedation, or positioning that impairs chest expansion may substantially alter PaO_2.

Modified from Lewis SM, Heitkemper MM, Dirksen SR: *Medical-surgical nursing: asssment and management of clinical problems,* ed 5, St. Louis, 2000, Mosby.
SaO₂, Arterial oxygen saturation; *PaO₂,* arterial oxygen pressure; *PaCO₂,* arterial carbon dioxide pressure.

Table 30-3   GERONTOLOGIC DIFFERENCES IN ASSESSMENT: CARDIOVASCULAR SYSTEM

CHANGES	DIFFERENCES IN ASSESSMENT FINDINGS
CHEST WALL	
Senile kyphosis	Altered chest landmarks for palpation, percussion, and auscultation; distant heart sounds
HEART	
Myocardial hypertrophy, increase in collagen and scarring, decrease in elasticity	Decrease in cardiac reserve, slight decrease in HR
Downward displacement	Difficulty in isolating apical pulse
Decrease in CO, HR, SV in response to exercise or stress	Slowed, decreased response to stress; slowed recovery from activity
Cellular aging changes and fibrosis of conduction system	Decrease in amplitude of QRS complex and lengthening of PR, QRS, and QT intervals; left axis deviation; irregular cardiac rhythms
Valvular rigidity from calcification, sclerosis, or fibrosis, impeding complete closure of valves	Systolic murmur (aortic or mitral) possible without indication of cardiovascular pathology
BLOOD VESSELS	
Arterial stiffening caused by loss of elastin in arterial walls, thickening of intima of arteries, and progressive fibrosis of media	Elevation in systolic and possibly diastolic BP (e.g., 160/90) possible widened pulse pressures; more pronounced arterial pulses; pedal pulses often not detectable; color and temperature changes in extremities; loss of hair on lower legs
Increase in tortuosity and varicosities of veins	Ulcerated, inflamed, painful, or cordlike varicosities

From Lewis SM, Collier IC, Heitkemper MM: *Medical-surgical nursing: assessment and management of clinical problems,* ed 4, St. Louis, 1996, Mosby.
BP, Blood pressure; *CO,* cardiac output; *HR,* heart rate; *SV,* stroke volume.

tex decreases, glomerular filtration rate decreases, whereas blood urea nitrogen and creatinine levels increase. Elderly people also have decreased renin, angiotensin, and aldosterone levels, a condition which ultimately leads to inability to regulate fluid and electrolyte balance. Table 30-4 describes age-related differences in the assessment of the urinary system.

Musculoskeletal System

Muscle weight relative to total body weight decreases with aging. Bone reabsorption increases with decreased bone remodeling and decreased bone density. Bone loss occurs more rapidly in women than in men, leading to osteoporosis and increased risk of fractures. Loss of water content makes

Table 30-4 GERONTOLOGIC DIFFERENCES IN ASSESSMENT: URINARY SYSTEM

CHANGES	DIFFERENCES IN ASSESSMENT FINDINGS
KIDNEY	
Decrease in amount of renal tissue	Less palpable
Decrease in number of nephrons and renal vascular bed; thickened basement membrane of Bowman's capsule and glomeruli	Decrease in creatinine clearance, increase in BUN level
Decrease in function of loop of Henle and tubules	Alterations in drug excretion; nocturia; loss of normal diurnal excretory pattern because of decreased ability to concentrate urine; less concentrated urine
URETER, BLADDER, AND URETHRA	
Decrease in elasticity and muscle tone	Palpable bladder after urination because of retention
Weakening of urinary sphincter	Stress incontinence (especially during Valsalva maneuver), dribbling of urine after urination
Decrease in bladder capacity and sensory receptors	Frequency, urgency, nocturia, overflow incontinence
Estrogen deficiency leading to thin, dry vaginal tissue	Stress or urge incontinence, dysuria, positive urine culture
Uninhibited bladder contractions	Urge incontinence
Prostatic enlargement	Hesitancy, frequency, urgency, nocturia, straining to urinate, retention, dribbling

From Lewis SM, Heitkemper MM, Dirksen SR: *Medical-surgical nursing: assessment and management of clinical problems,* ed 5, St. Louis, 2000, Mosby. *BUN,* Blood urea nitrogen.

Table 30-5 GERONTOLOGIC DIFFERENCES IN ASSESSMENT: MUSCULOSKELETAL SYSTEM

CHANGES	DIFFERENCES IN ASSESSMENT FINDINGS
MUSCLE	
Decreased number and diameter of muscle cells, replacement of muscle cells by fibrous connective tissue	Decreased muscle strength and bulk, abdominal protrusion, muscle flabbiness
Loss of elasticity in ligaments and cartilage	Decreased fine motor activity, decreased agility
Reduced ability to store glycogen; decreased ability to release glycogen as quick energy in times of stress	Slowed reaction times, slowing of most muscle neuronal reflexes, slowing of impulse conduction along motor units, easy fatigability
JOINTS	
Erosion of articular cartilage, possible direct contact between bone ends	Manifestations of osteoarthritis, joint stiffness, possible crepitation on movement of joints, pain with range-of-motion movements
Overgrowth of bone around joint margins (osteophytes)	Heberden's nodes in fingers (especially in women), limited mobility in affected joints
Loss of water from disks between vertebrae, narrowing of joint vertebral spaces	Loss of height, back pain, joint subluxation
BONE	
Decrease in bone mass	Dowager's hump (kyphosis) caused by compression of vertebral bodies Decreased height

From Lewis SM, Heitkemper MM, Dirksen SR: *Medical-surgical nursing: assessment and management of clinical problems,* ed 5, St. Louis, 2000, Mosby.

cartilaginous structures stiffer and more susceptible to injury. Assessment of the musculoskeletal system in older patients is addressed in Table 30-5.

Gastrointestinal System

Peristalsis decreases significantly with aging, so elders are prone to constipation.[1] Decreased blood flow to the rectum contributes to this problem and may affect healing of rectal injuries. Diminished intestinal enzymes affect digestion and electrolyte balance. Changes in appetite can lead to poor eating habits and malnutrition, which also affect wound healing. Assessment findings related to aging and the gastrointestinal system are listed in Table 30-6.

Integumentary System

Dermal thickness decreases as much as 20% with age,[4] with significant loss of vascularity and proliferative ability. Dermatologic changes affect wound healing and thermoregulation while decreasing the barrier against bacterial invasion.

Additional information on age-related changes in the integumentary system is presented in Table 30-7.

Other Systems

Aging affects every cell and every body system. These physiologic changes affect the elder's ability to survive trauma. For example, changes in the clotting cascade (Table 30-8) may place the elder at risk for bleeding disorders, whereas changes in the endocrine system decrease the elder's response to stress (Table 30-9).

EPIDEMIOLOGY OF TRAUMA

"Trauma is the seventh leading cause of death in persons over 65 years of age . . ."[8] Etiology includes motor vehicle collisions, falls, burns, and penetrating trauma. The most common cause of injury in the geriatric population is falls. Factors that predispose the elderly to falls include impaired sensation, visual disturbances, weakness of musculature, unsteady gait and balance, degenerative joint disease,

---

Table 30-6 GERONTOLOGIC DIFFERENCES IN ASSESSMENT: GASTROINTESTINAL SYSTEM

CHANGES	DIFFERENCES IN ASSESSMENT FINDINGS
MOUTH	
Loss of teeth	Presence of dentures, difficulty chewing
Decreased taste buds, decreased sense of smell	Diminished sense of taste (especially salty and sweet)
Decreased volume of saliva	Dry oral mucosa
Atrophy of gingival tissue	Poor-fitting dentures
ESOPHAGUS	
Decreased tone and motility	Complaints of pyrosis (heartburn), dysphagia, eructation
ABDOMINAL WALL	
Thinner and less taut	More visible peristalsis, easier palpation of organs
Decrease in number and sensitivity of sensory receptors	Less sensitivity to surface pain
STOMACH	
Decreased acid secretion, atrophy of gastric mucosa, hypochlorhydria	Food intolerances, signs of anemia as result of vitamin B_{12} malabsorption
SMALL INTESTINES	
Decreased secretion of most digestive enzymes, decreased motility	Complaints of indigestion
LIVER	
Increased size and lowered position	Easier palpation
LARGE INTESTINE, ANUS, RECTUM	
Decreased anal sphincter tone and nerve supply to rectal area	Fecal incontinence
Decreased muscular tone, decreased motility	Flatulence, abdominal distention, relaxed perineal musculature
Decrease in transit time	Constipation, fecal impaction

From Lewis SM, Heitkemper MM, Dirksen SR: *Medical-surgical nursing: assessment and management of clinical problems,* ed 5, St. Louis, 2000, Mosby.

Table 30-7	GERONTOLOGIC DIFFERENCES IN ASSESSMENT: INTEGUMENTARY SYSTEM
CHANGES	**DIFFERENCES IN ASSESSMENT FINDINGS**
SKIN	
Decreased subcutaneous fat, muscle laxity, degeneration of elastic fibers, collagen stiffening	Increased wrinkling, sagging breasts and abdomen, redundant flesh around eyes, slowness of skin to flatten when pinched together (tenting)
Decreased extracellular water, surface lipids, and sebaceous gland activity	Dry, flaking skin with possible signs of excoriation caused by pruritus
Less active apocrine and sebaceous gland activity	Dry skin with minimal to no perspiration
Increased capillary fragility and permeability	Evidence of bruising
Increased melanocytes in basal layer with pigment accumulation	Senile lentigines on face and back of hands
Diminished blood supply	Decrease in rosy appearance of skin and mucous membranes; cool to touch; diminished awareness of pain, touch, temperature, and peripheral vibration
Decrease in proliferative capacity	Diminished rate of wound healing
HAIR	
Decreased melanin and melanocytes	Graying hair
Decreased oil	Dry, coarse hair; scaly scalp
Decrease in density of hair follicles	Thinning and loss of hair; loss of hair in outer one half or one third of eyebrow
Cumulative androgen effect; decreasing estrogen levels	Facial hirsutism; baldness
NAILS	
Decreased peripheral blood supply	Thick, brittle nails with diminished growth
Increased keratin	Ridging
Decreased circulation	Prolonged return of blood to nails on blanching

Lewis SM, Heitkemper MM, Dirksen SR: *Medical-surgical nursing: assessment and management of clinical problems,* ed 5, St. Louis, 2000, Mosby.

Table 30-8	EFFECTS OF AGING ON HEMATOLOGIC STUDIES
STUDY	**CHANGES**
CBC STUDIES	
Hb	Decreased
MCV	Increased
MCHC	Decreased
WBC count	Diminished response to infection
Platelets	Unchanged
CLOTTING STUDIES	
Partial thromboplastin time	Reduced
Fibrinogen	May be elevated
Factors V, VII, VIII, IX	May be elevated
ESR IRON STUDIES	Increased significantly
Serum iron	Reduced
Total iron-binding capacity	Reduced

From Lewis SM, Heitkemper MM, Dirksen SR: *Medical-surgical nursing: assessment and management of clinical problems,* ed 5, St. Louis, 2000, Mosby.
CBC, Complete blood count; *ESR,* erythrocyte sedimentation rate; *Hb,* hemoglobin; *MCHC,* mean corpuscular hemoglobin concentration; *MCV,* mean corpuscular volume; *WBC,* white blood cell.

dementia, neuromuscular disorders, and predisposition to syncope and near-syncope. The challenge in caring for elderly patients with trauma from a fall is to determine not only the injuries but also the cause of the fall.

The second leading cause of trauma in the elderly is motor vehicle collisions. Motor vehicle collisions involving the elderly are more likely to occur when split-second decisions or reactions to specific hazards are required: for example, at intersections, rights of way, or traffic signs. Box 30-1 identifies factors that may play a role in these crashes.

Elderly people have one of the highest rates of pedestrian accidents, representing 46% of all pedestrian fatalities.[2] Auto-pedestrian collisions may result from decreased mobility, diminished vision, hearing loss, and slowed reaction times. Skeletal changes caused by osteoporosis limit upward gaze and can make visualization of traffic lights or signs difficult.[8] In the United States crossing time for intersection lights is set at a standard 4 ft/sec.

Mobility may be one of the most significant problems facing the elderly. Limited mobility is a major factor in increased incidence of falls and injury. One in three elderly people falls each year.[3,6] Five percent of falls in institutionalized or community-dwelling adults cause fractures and an additional 5% to 10% cause restricted activity for days or weeks because of hematomas, sprains, or dislocations. Up to

Table 30-9 EFFECTS OF AGING ON THE ENDOCRINE SYSTEM

HORMONE	BASAL LEVEL	SECRETION	MCR	TARGET ORGAN RESPONSE	CLINICAL SIGNIFICANCE
POSTERIOR PITUITARY					
ADH	↑	↑	—	↓ (renal)	Sodium imbalance, syndrome of inappropriate ADH, hyponatremia
ANTERIOR PITUITARY					
GH	↓	↓	—	—	Unknown significance
TSH	—	—	—	—	Unknown significance
ACTH	—	—	—	—	
Prolactin	—	—	?	?	
LH and FSH	↑	↑	?	↓	
THYROID					
T$_4$	—	↓	↓	↓	Atypical presentation of hyperthyroidism
T$_3$	—	—	↓	↓	Increased hypothyroidism
PARATHYROIDS					
PTH	↑	↑	?	↓ (renal)	Hypercalcemia, hypercalciuria, increased bone resorption
ADRENAL CORTEX					
Cortisol	—	↓	↓	↓	
Androgens	↓	↓	?	?	
Aldosterone	↓	↓	↓	?	Decreased response to sodium restriction and upright posture
ADRENAL MEDULLA					
Epinephrine	—	—	—	↓	Decreased response to β-blockers (e.g., less of a decrease in heart rate and cardiac output)
Norepinephrine	↑	↑	↑	↓	Increased sympathetic nervous system activity, possible increase in hypertension
PANCREAS					
Insulin	↑	↓	—	↓	Impaired glucose tolerance
GONADS					
Estrogen	↓	↓	—	?	Increased hot flashes, decreased vaginal secretions, increased risk for atherosclerosis, osteoporosis
Testosterone	↓	↓	?	?	Decreased ejaculatory force
KIDNEYS					
Renin	↓	↓	?	?	Decreased response to sodium restriction, upright posture
Vitamin D	↓	N/A	?	↓	Decreased intestinal absorption of calcium

From Lewis SM, Heitkemper MM, Dirksen SR: *Medical-surgical nursing: assessment and management of clinical problems,* ed 5, St. Louis, 2000, Mosby.
↑, increased; ↓, decreased; —, no change; ?, no data or conflicting data.
ACTH, Adrenocorticotropic hormone; *ADH,* antidiuretic hormone; *FSH,* follicle-stimulating hormone; *GH,* growth hormone; *LH,* luteinizing hormone; *MCR,* metabolic clearance rate; *N/A,* not applicable; *TSH,* thyroid stimulating hormone.

25% of all elders who have previously fallen admit to restricting their activities because of fear of additional falls and injury. Factors leading to falls in the elderly may be environmental or physiologic (Box 30-2). The elderly also have an increased risk for head injury, fractured mandibles, and ruptured globes. Loss of teeth leads to mandibular instability and increased incidence of fractures. Thinning of the limbus increases the risk for globe rupture.

Decreased reaction time, preexisting health problems, and altered sense of hearing, vision, and smell place elders at greater risk for burn injuries. Elderly people do not tolerate burn injuries as well as younger patients because of diminished cardiac, pulmonary, and metabolic reserves. Mortality is reported between 33% and 40%, depending on the percent of body surface involved. A rule of thumb in elderly burn patients is that the percent of body surface area burned is roughly equivalent to mortality.

Other causes of injury in the elderly are penetrating trauma and abuse. Mortality from penetrating injuries is higher in the elderly patient than in younger age groups, 17.3% compared with 4.7%.[11] Increased mortality is the result of diminished patient reserves and increased incidence of complication. Elderly suicide patients tend to use guns more often than substance ingestion, so they are usually more successful in their attempts. Increased violence across the country may lead to an increased number of elderly patients with penetrating trauma. Elder abuse has also increased over the past decade. Refer to Chapter 51 for more discussion of this disturbing health problem.

Box 30-1	POTENTIAL FACTORS IN MOTOR VEHICLE CRASHES INVOLVING ELDERLY PEOPLE

Slowed reaction time
Diminished visual acuity
Decreased peripheral vision
Impaired hearing
Loss of motor strength
Arthritis
Dementia
Attention deficits
Concurrent medical conditions
Prescription drugs
Severe sensory stimulation

Box 30-2	FACTORS THAT CONTRIBUTE TO FALLS IN THE ELDERLY

ENVIRONMENTAL	PHYSIOLOGIC
Throw rugs	Musculoskeletal weakness
Staircases	Arthritis
Changes in floor surface	Poor balance
Furniture out of place	Impaired proprioception
Animals	Syncope
Lack of assist devices	Dizziness
(e.g., handrails,	Vertigo
walkers, canes)	Hypoglycemia
Small children	Postural hypotension
Doorway transitions not level	Anemia
Poor lighting	Medications
	Decreased vision

INJURIES

Injuries in the elderly are similar to injuries in younger patients. Differences relate to frequency of specific injuries and absence of significant hemodynamic changes in response to blood loss. Physiologic changes of aging and medications such as beta blockers affect elders' ability to respond to blood loss. Elder trauma patients can be in profound cardiogenic shock with minimal changes in vital signs. Some centers suggest early, invasive hemodynamic monitoring for the severely injured elder. Fluid should be administered cautiously because of potential fluid overload and decreased cardiac reserve, which can lead to pulmonary edema.

The most common injury in the elderly patient is fracture. With decreased bone density, less stress is required to break bones. Older patients are particularly prone to long-bone fractures secondary to osteoporosis. Early stabilization is recommended to decrease potential pulmonary complications. Significant retroperitoneal bleeding can occur with minor pelvic or hip fractures. Approximately half of elderly patients with hip fractures will die within 1 year. Rib fractures in the elderly also increase mortality because of decreased lung expansion and other complications. Careful assessment and monitoring are essential to minimize associated complications.

Delayed wound healing is a problem in elderly patients with lacerations, surgical incisions, or burn injuries. Geriatric patients are at risk for infectious complications resulting from changes in skin and the immune system. Tetanus prophylaxis is not always adequate in the elderly. Elderly women in rural areas, particularly those who never worked outside the home, may have never received or completed tetanus immunization. Elderly men are more likely to have served in the military, where they would have received tetanus immunization.

SUMMARY

The elderly trauma patient presents an assessment challenge for the emergency nurse. Knowledge of physiologic changes of aging is essential for management of these patients. Geriatric patients also require awareness of their worth as individuals and their right to make their own health care decisions. Box 30-3 summarizes potential nursing diagnoses for the elderly trauma patient.

Box 30-3	NURSING DIAGNOSES FOR THE ELDERLY TRAUMA PATIENT

Anxiety
Breathing pattern, Ineffective
Cardiac output, Decreased
Fear
Fluid volume, Deficient
Fluid volume, Excessive
Gas exchange, Impaired

References

1. Beck JC, editor: *Geriatric review syllabus: a core curriculum in geriatric medicine,* New York, 1991, American Geriatrics Society.
2. Ciccone A, Allegra JR, Cochrane DG et al: Age-related differences in diagnoses within the elderly population, *Am J Emerg Med* 16(1):43, 1998.
3. Eachempati SR, Reed RL II, St. Louis JE et al: "The demographics of trauma in 1995" revisited: an assessment of the accuracy and utility of trauma preditions, *J Trauma* 45(2):208, 1998.
4. Kaminer MS, Gilchrest BA: Aging of the skin. In Hazzard WR et al, editors: *Principles of geriatric medicine and gerontology,* New York, 1994, McGraw-Hill.
5. Lewis SM, Heitkemper MM, Dirksen SR: *Medical-surgical nursing: assessment and management of clinical problems,* ed 5, St. Louis, 2000, Mosby.
6. Ludwick R, Dieckman B, Snelson CM: Assessment of the geriatric orthopaedic trauma patient, *Orthop Nurs* 18(6):13, 1999.
7. Mandavia D, Newton K: Geriatric trauma, *Emerg Med Clin North Am* 16(1):257, 1998.
8. Mattox KL, Feliciano DV, Moore EE: *Trauma,* ed 4, New York, 2001, McGraw-Hill.
9. McCance KL, Huether SE: *Pathophysiology: the biologic basis for disease in adults and children,* ed 4, St. Louis, 2001, Mosby.
10. Reuben DB, Yoshikawa TT, Besdine RW, editors: *Geriatric review syllabus supplement: a core curriculum in geriatric medicine,* New York, 1993, American Geriatrics Society.
11. Yoshikawa TT, Norma DC, editors: *Acute emergencies and critical care of the geriatric patient,* New York, 2000, Mercel Dekker.

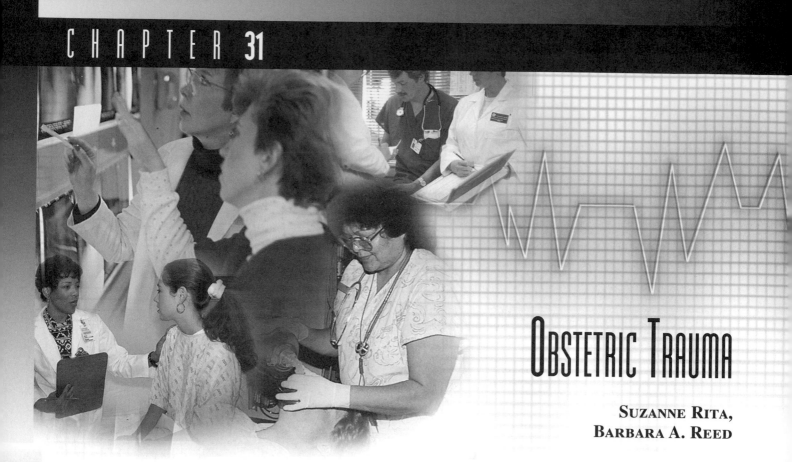

CHAPTER 31

OBSTETRIC TRAUMA

SUZANNE RITA,
BARBARA A. REED

The actual incidence of obstetric trauma is unknown, but it has been estimated that it occurs in 7% of all pregnancies.[3] Most obstetric trauma involves minor injury, although significant injuries related to trauma can occur. Head injury and hemorrhagic shock account for most maternal deaths from trauma.

Abruptio placentae and maternal shock are other common causes of fetal demise. Mechanisms for obstetric trauma are blunt and penetrating injuries. Blunt injuries occur secondary to motor vehicle collisions (MVCs), falls, and assaults. Penetrating injuries includes gunshot wounds and stab wounds.

ANATOMY AND PHYSIOLOGY

Initial assessment and management of the pregnant trauma patient is often provided by prehospital and emergency personnel. Optimal outcome for mother and fetus is based on sound knowledge of maternal anatomy and physiology and implications for interventions.

Uterine

The uterus grows from 7-cm and 70-g to a 36-cm and 1100-g walled organ. As the uterus grows, its wall becomes thinner. Until 12 weeks of pregnancy the uterus remains a small, self-contained intrapelvic organ protected from abdominal injury by the bony pelvis. The uterus becomes an intraabdominal organ as it enlarges and ascends, encroaching on the peritoneal cavity and confining the intestines to the upper abdomen. Figure 31-1 shows uterine size for various gestation periods. During the second trimester the uterus is susceptible to abdominal injury, although the fetus remains small and relatively cushioned by large amounts of amniotic fluid. By the third trimester the uterus is large and thin walled. During the last 2 to 8 weeks of gestation, the fetus descends and the fetal head engages in the pelvis. The fetus occupies most of the space when the head becomes fixed in the pelvis. Maternal pelvic fractures during this trimester are frequently associated with fetal skull fractures and intracranial hemorrhage.

Uterine blood flow increases from a baseline of 60 ml/min to 600 ml/min during the third trimester. Uterine blood flow has no autoregulation and depends solely on maternal perfusion pressure; therefore, uterine injury may be a major source of blood loss.

By the third trimester the uterus and placenta have reached maximum vasodilatation and cannot increase blood flow in response to decreased perfusion. During maternal stress or injury, catecholamines released by the sympathetic nervous system cause marked uteroplacental constriction and decreased perfusion, which lead to fetal distress.

Cardiovascular

Anatomically, the heart is elevated and rotated forward by the ascending diaphragm pushed up by the enlarging uterus. This cardiac displacement causes a 15-degree left axis deviation

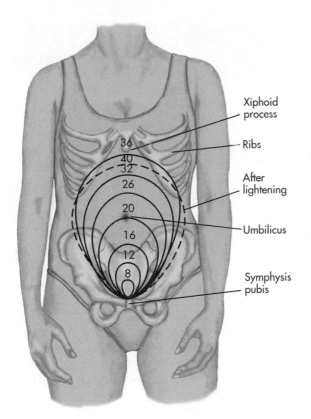

Xiphoid
process

Ribs

After
lightening

Umbilicus

Symphysis
pubis

FIGURE 31-1 Uterine growth pattern during pregnancy. (From Gorrie TM, McKinney ES, Murray SS: *Foundations of maternal-newborn nursing,* ed 2, Philadelphia, 1998, WB Saunders.)

that is considered a normal change of pregnancy. An electrocardiogram may also show a flattened or inverted T wave in lead III and Q waves in III and aVF. Ectopic beats are also common during pregnancy.

Cardiovascular physiology is profoundly altered during pregnancy. Maternal blood volume increases by the tenth week of gestation and increases 40% to 50% by the twenty-eighth week, remaining at that level until delivery. Uterine blood flow increases to 600 ml/min by the end of pregnancy. Increased blood flow and volume increase maternal cardiac output by 1 to 1.5 L/min.[3] After approximately 20 weeks' gestation, cardiac output can decrease through compression of the vena cava and aorta by the fetus when the mother is in a supine position. This event is called *inferior vena cava syndrome* or *supine hypotensive syndrome.* Because the uterus at 20 weeks has grown and risen to the level of the inferior vena cava, compression of the vena cava by the uterus may decrease cardiac output by 28% and systolic blood pressure by 30 mm Hg. Sequestering blood in the venous system may decrease perfusion to the uterus. Displacing the gravid uterus to the left by placing the pregnant patient in the left lateral decubitus position reverses aortocaval compression. When spinal injury is suspected, maintain spinal immobilization and tilt the backboard 15 degrees or manually displace the uterus to the left.

Resting heart rate increases until the second trimester and remains 10 to 20 beats per minute above baseline for the du-

ration of the pregnancy. Systolic and diastolic blood pressures decrease in the first trimester, then level off during the second trimester. A decrease of 15 mm Hg for systolic and diastolic pressure is normal. A gradual increase to prepregnant levels occurs at the end of the third trimester.

Hemodynamic measures may be misleading. Signs of shock such as tachycardia and hypotension may be normal physiologic changes of pregnancy. Conversely, normal findings may mask an underlying shock state. Hypervolemia of pregnancy enables a woman to tolerate acute blood loss of 10% to 15% or gradual loss of 30% (1500 ml) without a change in vital signs.[3]

Catecholamine release caused by maternal hypovolemia vasoconstricts peripheral and uterine vascular beds, shunting blood to vital maternal organs. A 15% to 30% reduction of uterine blood flow can occur without obvious change in maternal blood pressure. Uterine hypoperfusion and fetal hypoxia can occur before evidence of maternal shock. Signs of fetal distress include fetal bradycardia, fetal tachycardia, and decreased fetal movement.

Gravid women in shock may not have the cool, clammy skin typical of shock because of maternal vasodilatation in the first and second trimester. Vasoconstriction in response to stress occurs predominately in the third trimester.

Adequate and appropriate fluid replacement is necessary to restore maternal and uteroplacental perfusion. Lactated Ringer's solution is the recommended fluid. Blood transfusions should be given with Rh-compatible blood. In cases of impending shock, only O-negative or type-specific blood is acceptable. Vasopressors are not indicated for initial management of hypovolemic shock but may be used early in management of cardiogenic shock secondary to cardiac contusion or distributive shock resulting from spinal cord injury.

Hematologic

Dilutional anemia in pregnancy is caused by the disproportionate increase of plasma volume relative to erythrocyte volume. Dilutional states can reduce the hematocrit level from 31% to 34% and hemoglobin to 11.0 g. These changes are referred to clinically as "physiologic anemia of pregnancy."[1]

Platelet levels may be normal or slightly decreased. Physiologic leukocytosis occurs during the second and third trimesters. An increase in white blood cells of 15,000 may occur by term and rise even higher during stress or labor. Sedimentation rate also increases during pregnancy. Cautious interpretation of lab values is required; increased levels may mask or falsely indicate an infectious process.

Fibrinogen levels start to rise in the third month and double by term. An increase in clotting factors VII, VIII, IX, and X produces hypercoagulability and increased thromboembolic risk. Deep vein thrombosis and pulmonary embolism are a significant risk, especially when the gravid woman is inactive. The pregnant woman that sustains trauma is at a high risk for disseminated intravascular coagulopathy if abruptio placentae or amniotic fluid embolism occur.

Pulmonary

Significant anatomic and physiologic alterations occur in the pulmonary system during pregnancy. Capillary engorgement of the mucosal lining of the respiratory tract predisposes gravid women to nosebleeds and airway obstruction. Gentle suction and gentle intubation may be necessary to control epistaxis and prevent airway compromise.

The diaphragm elevates as the uterus enlarges, up to 4 cm with associated flaring of the ribs. During the third trimester, chest tubes, when needed, should be inserted in the third or fourth intercostal space to avoid diaphragm injury.

Diaphragm elevation reduces pulmonary functional reserve capacity by 20% at the end of pregnancy. Reduction is associated with increased maternal oxygen consumption and diminished oxygen reserve. Maternal tidal volume and minute ventilations decrease to 40% by late pregnancy. Respiratory rates will increase. Arterial carbon dioxide pressure ($PaCO_2$) decreases to approximately 30 mm Hg by the end of the second trimester and remains at this level until delivery. Arterial oxygen pressure levels increase to 101 to 104 mm Hg.[1]

The maternal respiratory center is especially sensitive to minute changes in $PaCO_2$ levels. Partially compensated respiratory alkalosis occurs during pregnancy, although normal arterial and venous pH are maintained by increased renal excretion of bicarbonate. Diminished maternal oxygen reserve makes the gravid uterus vulnerable to hypoxia. Maternal hypoxia affects fetal oxygenation, so fetal compromise may occur. Fetal heart rate changes are frequently the first indicator of maternal hypoxia. Maternal trauma requires measurement of arterial blood gas (ABG) levels to determine hypoxia and acidosis. Supplemental oxygen at 100% is essential until maternal and fetal hypoxia are ruled out or resolved.

Gastrointestinal

Various anatomic and physiologic gastrointestinal (GI) changes occur during pregnancy. The small bowel is pushed up by the uterus into the upper abdomen, and the large bowel moves posteriorly. Diminished bowel sounds may be a normal finding in pregnancy or indicate intraperitoneal injury. Stretching of the abdominal wall by uterine growth can impair maternal sensitivity to peritoneal irritation, so muscle guarding, rigidity, or rebound tenderness may be dulled or absent.

Progesterone has a smooth-muscle effect on the GI tract, reducing motility and tone and relaxing the gastric sphincter. Gastric emptying is delayed and gastroesophageal reflux occurs frequently, increasing the risk of aspiration. Assume all gravid trauma patients have a full stomach; therefore, a nasogastric tube should be promptly inserted to minimize risk of aspiration.

Genitourinary

Maternal susceptibility to traumatic bladder injury increases as the bladder moves from a pelvic organ to an intra-abdominal position by 12 weeks' gestation. Urinary frequency increases in the third trimester from bladder compression by the uterus. Dilation of the ureters (right greater than left), renal calyces, and pelvis from compression by the ovarian plexus can result in urinary stasis. Glomerular filtration rate increases; therefore, blood urea nitrogen and creatinine decrease.

Musculoskeletal

The pelvis becomes more flexible during pregnancy in preparation for fetal delivery. Hormonal changes loosen ligaments of the symphysis pubis and sacroiliac joints. By 7 months' gestation, there is considerable widening of the pelvis. An unsteady gait caused by the widening pelvis and heavy abdomen predisposes the gravid female to falls.

Neurologic

Changes in the central nervous system (CNS) related to pregnancy are abnormal findings. Preeclampsia occurs after 20 to 24 weeks' gestation and is characterized by hypertension, proteinuria, and edema. CNS irritability can lead to eclampsia, which is marked by seizure activity. Hypoxia from seizure activity places the mother and fetus at risk. Altered mentation, seizures, and hypertension may also indicate head injury; therefore, meticulous neurologic assessment of the pregnant trauma patient is essential.

Endocrine

The pituitary gland doubles in size and weight by term, requiring a greater blood supply. Hypoperfusion causes ischemia and can lead to pituitary necrosis. Hemorrhage within the gland can occur with reperfusion. Sheehan's syndrome, which is necrosis of the anterior pituitary gland, produces long-term complications related to decreased hormone levels. Aggressive and rapid treatment of shock are required to prevent these serious complications.

PATIENT ASSESSMENT

Anatomic and physiologic changes during pregnancy can obscure the mother's response to trauma. Maternal compensatory mechanisms preserve vital maternal functions at the expense of the fetus. Fetal survival depends on adequate gas exchange and uterine perfusion. Rapid and efficient assessment and correct intervention for specific abnormalities provide optimal maternal-fetal outcome.

Maintenance of cervical spine immobilization is necessary when neck injury is suspected until the neck is clinically and radiographically cleared. A lateral backboard tilt of 15 degrees maintains immobilization and deflects the uterus from the vena cava. Repositioning the airway by chin-tilt or jaw-thrust maneuvers may be enough to establish patency and should not interfere with cervical immobilization. Use oral or nasal airways; the mother may be predisposed to nasopharyngeal bleeding that can lead to further obstruction. Early orotracheal or nasotracheal intubation prevents further trauma or obstruction.

All trauma patients need supplemental oxygen. Injury can exacerbate existing pulmonary alterations related to pregnancy, such as decreased pulmonary reserve and increased maternal oxygen consumption, compromising the mother and fetus. Oxygen is critical for fetal survival because of fetal inability to tolerate hypoxia.

Assessment and intervention for external and internal hemorrhage is necessary to ensure maternal-fetal survival. Apply direct pressure to sites of uncontrolled external bleeding. The mother can lose 1500 ml of blood before signs of shock are evident. Retroperitoneal and uteroplacental injury can be sources of occult blood loss. Venous access with two large-bore catheters and aggressive fluid volume replacement optimize maternal blood volume and oxygen-carrying capacity. Initiate blood replacement with Rh-compatible blood if crystalloids do not stabilize circulatory status. Aortocaval compression can occur by 20 weeks' gestation; therefore, displacing the uterus to the left can increase cardiac output by 20%.

Insertion of an arterial line or central venous line provides accurate monitoring of circulation and response to treatment and may be used in some centers. Assessment of neurologic defects should include consideration of eclampsia.

Secondary assessment involves identification of other injuries. Thorough history includes standard trauma history and obstetric history—last menstrual period (LMP), expected date of confinement, parity, problems and complications of current or past pregnancies, presence of uterine contractions, and current fetal activity. Specific obstetric assessment in the secondary survey includes the abdomen, uterus, and fetus.

Abdomen

The abdomen may be difficult to assess because of blunted signs of intraperitoneal irritation. Severe occult intraabdominal hemorrhage may occur without signs of impending shock. Liver and splenic injuries are a common injury encountered in MVCs. The most common cause of intraperitoneal hemorrhage in gestational trauma is splenic rupture.

Inspect the abdomen for signs of injury, including ecchymosis, abrasions, and contusions. Note the shape and contour of abdomen. Irregularity or deformity may indicate uterine rupture. Inspect for fetal movement. Palpate for masses and abdominal tenderness. Remember abdominal rigidity, guarding, and rebound tenderness may be blunted by the stretched abdominal wall.

Diagnostic peritoneal lavage (DPL) has been safely and accurately used to detect intraperitoneal hemorrhage in obstetric trauma. Abdominal computed tomography (CT) is used to determine abdominal injuries in the stable trauma patient. Ultrasonography (US) is also beneficial in determining intraabdominal injury and fetal status.

Fetus and Uterus

Simultaneous assessment of the fetus and uterus should occur early in the secondary survey. Signs of abdominal pain, uterine tenderness, or contractions may indicate uteroplacental injury and potential for maternal-fetal compromise.

Determining gestational age is critical because this guides fetal assessment and intervention. The best indicator of gestational age is LMP. If the woman is unsure or unresponsive, she is assumed pregnant until a negative human chorionic gonadotropin (HCG) is documented. Normal gestation is 40 weeks, with the uterus usually palpable by 12 to 14 weeks' gestation. The fundus generally reaches the umbilicus by 20 weeks' gestation. Fundal height just below the xiphoid indicates a term fetus. Fetal gestational age should be determined by US. If emergency US is not available, an estimate of gestational age of a single fetus can be accomplished by measuring fundal height. A measurement midline from the symphysis pubis to the top of the uterus correlates gestational age with the height of the fundus in centimeters. A fundal height of 25 cm corresponds to gestational age of 25 weeks. Fetal viability is generally considered 24 to 25 weeks' gestation, although viability has occurred earlier with advanced neonate resuscitation and treatment in a neonatal intensive care unit. Serial fundal measurements are beneficial because increased fundal height may indicate occult intrauterine bleeding or uterine injury.

Evaluation of fetal well-being begins with a baseline fetal heart tone (FHT) on arrival at the emergency department (ED). Fetal heart tones are audible by Doppler testing by 10 to 12 weeks' gestation. Normal FHTs range from 120 to 160 beats/min. Fetal bradycardia is defined as FHT less than 110 beats/min and indicates serious fetal stress and decompensation. Sustained fetal tachycardia greater than 160 beats/min also indicates fetal distress. Significant FHT patterns such as variability or late deceleration are ominous signs of fetal distress. Early continuous monitoring should be initiated for the fetus. Monitoring fetal heart rate and contractions should be continued for 4 to 6 hours in the absence of uterine tenderness, vaginal bleeding, fetal distress, or serious maternal injury.[2] A competent staff member should interpret fetal monitoring.

Another indicator of fetal well being is fetal movement. US can determine fetal cardiac activity, body movement, placental location, estimated gestational age, and volume of amniotic fluid. Fetal death may also be diagnosed by US.

Uterine and fetal assessment includes inspection of the perineum for blood or amniotic fluid. The presence of amniotic fluid is most accurately identified by a microscopic procedure. A fern pattern appears on the slide if the specimen contains amniotic fluid. In the absence of blood or urine, nitrazine paper can be used to differentiate amniotic fluid from vaginal fluid. Normal vaginal fluid has a pH of 4.5 to 5.5. Amniotic fluid has a pH of 7.0 to 7.5, which turns nitrazine paper blue. Kleihauer-Betke staining is used to determine the presence of fetal blood in maternal circulation.

A general pelvic examination identifies crowning, fetal presentation, blood, and fluids. The necessity for speculum examination is determined by the trauma physician and may be deferred to the attending obstetrician. Direct visualization allows assessment of cervical dilation, locates source of blood or fluids, and identifies uterine or fetal injury. Bimanual examination is avoided unless delivery is imminent or genital tract injury is present. Urinary catheter placement is indicated to empty the bladder. Return of blood or hematuria suggests genitourinary (GU) injury.

Diagnostics

Cardiotocography

Fetal monitoring should begin immediately but should not interfere with maternal resuscitation and stabilization. Initial FHT may be determined by intermittent doptone; however, the obstetric trauma patient requires continuous fetal monitoring. Cardiotocography consists of continuous electronic monitoring of FHT, patterns, and uterine contractions. An external transducer registers motion of fetal heart valves, and a second transducer monitors uterine contraction. Signals interpreted as electrical impulses are recorded as fetal heart tracings. Figure 31-2 shows a normal tracing for fetal heart rate. Box 31-1 summarizes FHT changes that indicate fetal distress, whereas Figure 31-3 shows types of deceleration in fetal heart rate. A minimum of 4 hours of fetal monitoring is recommended in the absence of FHT abnormalities or maternal complications, with 24-hour monitoring with FHT abnormalities until fetal well-being is established. Fetal monitoring should be performed by a clinician skilled in use of equipment, interpretation of data, and requisite intervention.

Laboratory

Laboratory studies include standard trauma profiles; however, results should be interpreted cautiously because of hematologic changes with pregnancy. Standard lab studies include complete blood count, serum electrolytes, amylase, coagulation profile, arterial blood gas, type and screen or type and cross, toxicology screen, and urinalysis. Hospital policy and the attending physician determine the need for hepatitis B and human immunodeficiency virus screening. HCG levels should be obtained for all women of childbearing age if LMP is unknown or greater than 4½ weeks before admission. Special attention to antibody screening is needed for Rh immune status because maternal Rh sensitization can occur when an Rh-negative mother carries an Rh-positive fetus. Administration of Rh (D) immune globulin (RhoGam) can prevent maternal sensitization.

Radiographic Evaluation

Radiodiagnostic procedures necessary for trauma evaluation should not be omitted in the presence of a gravid uterus. Studies should be performed with a vigilant attempt to minimize fetal irradiation and limit radiation risks to decrease potential fetal injury. Radiographic studies are determined by clinical examination and physician suspicion of injury.

Box 31-1	**FETAL MONITORING INDICATORS OF FETAL DISTRESS**

Decreased variability in rate
Rate decelerations
Tachycardia greater than 160 beats/min
Bradycardia less than 110 beats/min
Uterine activity greater than eight contractions per hour

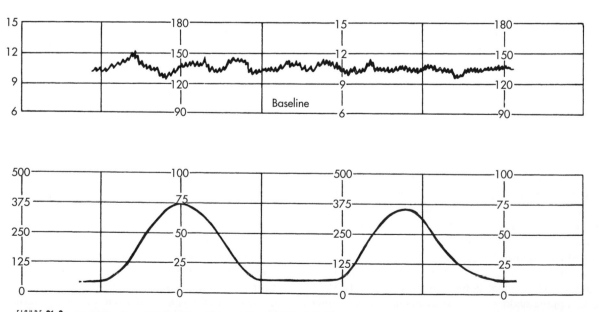

FIGURE 31-2   Tracing of normal fetal heart rate. (From AJN: *AJN/Mosby nursing boards review for the NCLEX-RN examination,* ed 10, St. Louis, 1997, Mosby.)

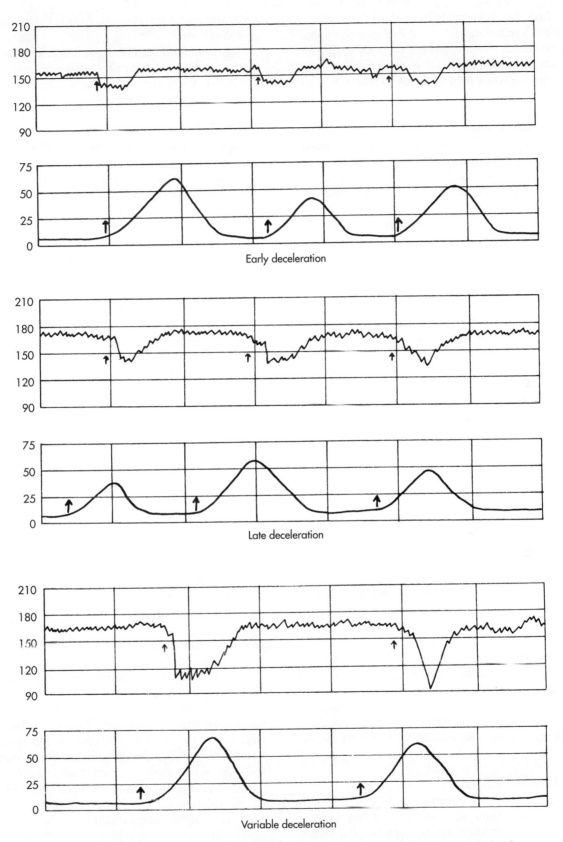

FIGURE 31-3 Types of deceleration in fetal heart rate. (From AJN: *AJN/Mosby nursing boards review for the NCLEX-RN examination,* ed 10, St. Louis, 1997, Mosby.)

Every effort should be made to minimize fetal risk. An expert radiology technician can avoid duplicate films, shield the uterus whenever possible, and perform only essential radiodiagnostics. Counseling with an obstetrician or geneticist may be beneficial when fetal radiation exposure is a concern.

Diagnostic Peritoneal Lavage

DPL can effectively assess abdominal injury for hemoperitoneum and is considered safe and accurate for the gravid trauma patient. DPL does not assess retroperitoneal or intrauterine injury. Indications for DPL after blunt trauma are abdominal signs and symptoms, altered level of consciousness, unexplained shock, severe thoracic injuries, and multiple or major orthopedic injuries. Before the procedure, insert an in-dwelling urinary catheter to decompress the bladder and decrease the risk of perforation. Insertion of an orogastric or nasogastric tube serves the same purpose but also decreases the risk of aspiration. The peritoneal catheter is inserted with direct visualization using the open technique to avoid the gravid uterus. An intraumbilical incision may be used during the first trimester; however, the supraumbilical route is performed in later trimesters. Further diagnostics are required to locate source and extent of injury. Immediate, delayed, or deferred laparotomy is determined by maternal and fetal condition.

INJURIES

Blunt Trauma

Blunt abdominal trauma can cause minor or severe life-threatening trauma to mother and fetus. The most common causes of abdominal trauma are MVCs, falls, and assaults, with falls the most common cause of minor injury. Hormonal changes soften joints and relax pelvic ligaments, which produces increasing instability in balance and gait. These changes in combination with the protruding abdomen and easy fatigue increase the mother's susceptibility to falls. Many falls occur during the third trimester.

Injury to the abdomen can result from direct force as the abdomen impacts the dashboard or steering wheel or secondary to organ displacement and hemorrhage from a coup-contrecoup event. Injury to the uterus can cause severe complications for the fetus, including premature labor, abruptio placentae, uterine rupture, fetal head injury, and fetal-maternal hemorrhage.

Premature Uterine Contractions

A frequently occurring complication of obstetric trauma is uterine contractions. Damage to myometrial and decidual cells releases prostaglandins, which stimulate the uterus. The extent of uterine damage, release of prostaglandins, and fetal age determine labor progression. Usually contractions are self-limiting and tocolysis is not indicated. Tocolysis, pharmacologic suppression of contractions, may be effective in halting preterm labor of the injured but hemodynamically stable gravida. Pharmacology is determined by physician discretion.

Adequate fluid volume replacement and positioning the mother in the left lateral tilt position can minimize uterine irritability. Cardiotocographic monitoring should be initiated early to assess uterine activity and fetal response.

Abruptio Placentae

Abruptio placentae is premature separation of the normally implanted placenta from the uterine wall. Abruptio placentae is divided into two main types: (1) those in which hemorrhage is concealed and (2) those in which hemorrhage is apparent (Figure 31-4). In both types, placental abruption can be complete or partial. Partial detachment occurs with placental detachment from the uterine wall at the center of the placenta. This results in hidden hemorrhage. Abruptio placentae can also occur at the rim or outer portions, causing vaginal bleeding and subsequent hemorrhage. Blood trapped behind the separating placenta is old blood and appears dark. Fresh bleeding is usually bright red, whereas a port-wine color is seen when blood is mixed with amniotic fluid. Predisposing factors for abruptio placentae are related to hypertension, part of the preeclampsia-eclampsia syndrome, glomerulonephritis, diabetes, increased maternal age, cigarette smoking, drinking alcohol during pregnancy, or possible dietary deficiencies.[4]

Abdominal trauma is a direct force that can trigger abruptio placenta. Energy from blunt force is dissipated to the elastic uterus, causing the placenta, which is relatively inelastic, to shear away from the uterine lining. Risk for abruptio placentae is usually immediately after injury. Bleeding can be severe enough to cause immediate maternal circulatory shock. Lack of oxygenation from impaired maternal-fetal gas exchange can lead to infant mortality resulting from hypoxia or intracranial hemorrhage.

Classic signs of abruption include vaginal bleeding, uterine tenderness, abdominal pain, back pain, and uterine hyperactivity with poor relaxation between contractions. Presentation may be vague or severe. Other indications of abruption include preterm labor, maternal shock, increasing fundal height, and fetal distress. Vaginal bleeding may be absent, with concealed retroplacental bleeding. Fetal distress may be the first indication of uteroplacental injury and potential abruption. Rapid deterioration can occur in both mother and fetus, so intensive monitoring is indicated. Two large-bore intravenous IV catheters should be started with lactated Ringer's solution. A complete blood count and type and cross-match should be immediately sent to the lab. Fetal monitoring is essential. A small abruption may be compatible with fetal survival; however, a viable fetus in distress requires immediate surgical delivery.

Uterine Rupture

Rupture of the uterus is an uncommon catastrophic injury resulting from blunt abdominal trauma. Previous cesarean section is a predisposing factor because rupture can occur at the healed incision site. Rupture of the posterior aspect of

Direct Fetal Injury

Blunt trauma infrequently results in direct fetal injury, with fetal skull fractures and intracranial hemorrhage the most common injuries noted. Injuries usually occur in association with maternal pelvic fractures. Later in pregnancy when the head is engaged in the pelvis, the fetal skull can become trapped and injured by the fractured pelvis. Compression of the fetal skull may occur between the maternal spine and re-straining lap belt or a striking object. Other fetal fractures include clavicle and long-bone injury.

Penetrating Injury

Increasing size and position make the gravid uterus suscep-tible to penetrating trauma. Fetal injury is a frequent occur-rence with a high rate of fetal mortality. Gunshot wounds to the abdomen are more common than stab wounds. Degree of injury depends on type, caliber, and range of the weapon. Upper abdominal wounds involve bowel perforation or retroperitoneal injuries caused by compartmentalization by the gravid uterus. Lower abdominal entry wounds cause di-rect injury to the fetus. Indirect injury to the fetus may be caused by trauma to the cord, placenta, or membrane. All gunshot wounds require exploratory laparotomy.

Stab wounds have a better prognosis for the mother and fetus. Visceral organs can slide away from the penetrating object, so fewer organs are injured. Surgical exploration is usually required in cases of upper abdominal trauma from a bullet or stab wound. Conservative management of lower abdominal injuries is indicated if the patient is stable or there is no evidence of GI or GU trauma. Diagnostic options include local exploration of wounds, DPL, US, and CT of the abdomen. Emergency exploratory laparotomy is indi-cated for the pregnant patient with penetrating trauma and unstable vital signs or fetal distress. The decision to deliver the fetus depends on (1) gestational age, (2) evidence of penetration of the amniotic sac, (3) evidence of fetal death or distress, and (4) maternal injuries requiring abdominal exploration. Otherwise, vaginal delivery can be anticipated as the fetus continues to grow and mature in utero.[4]

Seat Belts

MVCs are one of the most common causes of maternal in-jury or mortality. Ejection from the vehicle with resulting head trauma accounts for most deaths. Fetal death rates are also high when the mother is ejected. Combined lap and shoulder restraints (i.e., three-point restraints) reduce mater-nal ejection and risk of fetal injury. Lap belts without shoul-der harnesses also decrease ejection from the vehicle; how-ever, the lap restraint alone can cause intraabdominal injuries. Elevation of the small bowel during pregnancy ex-poses the protuberant uterus and increases the risk for uter-ine or fetal injury from the lap belt. The two-point shoulder harness without lap restraint does not prevent ejection. Proper use of three-point restraints is advocated to reduce maternal mortality and fetal risk. The lap belt should be

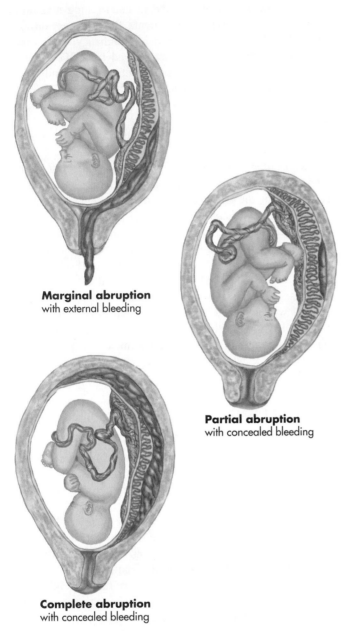

Marginal abruption
with external bleeding

Partial abruption
with concealed bleeding

Complete abruption
with concealed bleeding

FIGURE 31-4 Types of abruptio placentae. (Gorrie TM, McKinney ES, Murray SS: *Foundations of maternal-newborn nursing,* ed 2, Philadelphia, 1998, WB Saunders.)

the uterus usually occurs in an unscarred uterus and is likely to involve bladder injury. Increased maternal blood volume and perfusion increases the risk for maternal hypovolemic shock with uterine rupture. Fetal limbs can be easily pal-pated outside the uterine borders with uterine rupture. Fetal mortality is almost 100%. Rarely can the uterus be repaired, so hysterectomy is indicated for almost all patients with uterine rupture.

worn snugly across the pelvis below the abdomen and uterus; the shoulder harness should be worn in the normal position across the chest and between the breasts.

Burns

Most burn injuries in pregnant women occur in the home, with extremities, face, and neck burned most often. Fortunately the majority of burn injuries are minor. Pregnancy does not appear to affect maternal outcome; however, fetal outcome is affected by maternal condition. Total body surface area involved and severity of burn affect maternal outcome, premature delivery, and fetal death. A severely burned pregnant woman develops contractions a few days to a week postburn.[4] Fetal mortality results from hypoxia, hyponatremia, sepsis, and prematurity. Spontaneous abortion usually occurs within the first week after the burn event. Occasionally, delivery of a healthy term infant is possible.

Immediate care of the burned pregnant woman is the same as that of the nonpregnant patient. Severe burns require treatment at a burn center. Aggressive and appropriate fluid resuscitation, electrolyte therapy, supplemental oxygen, ventilation, and prevention of infection are critical. Sterile, dry dressings should be applied. Avoid wet or cool dressings. Antibiotics should be used if necessary; however, silver sulfadiazine cream should be avoided because of possible development of fetal kernicterus.

Electrical Injury

Few cases of electrical injury during pregnancy are reported; however, fetal mortality has been associated with even minor electrical shock. Most electrical accidents occur at home. Alternating current found in the home follows a hand-to-foot route. Consequently, the fetus lies in the direct path of the current. Fetal injury can result from cardiac conduction changes or uteroplacental lesions. If the fetus survives, oligohydramnios or growth retardation can develop. Pregnant women should report all incidents of electrical shock to the obstetrician. Baseline fetal monitoring and close, frequent follow-ups are necessary to evaluate fetal well-being.

SPECIAL CONSIDERATIONS
Cardiac Arrest

Objectives for cardiopulmonary resuscitation during pregnancy are to sustain circulation and perfusion for both patients—the mother and fetus. Basic and advanced life support should be initiated early and performed with slight variations. The maternal heart is located cephalad and laterally rotated; therefore, compressions are slightly higher on the sternum. Prompt, gentle intubation may reduce risk of nasoesophageal or oroesophageal bleeding and aspiration. In the presence of maternal hypoxia and acidemia, vasocon-

striction occurs in the uteroplacental vascular bed. Monitoring ABGs and serum pH is vital to determining maternal acidosis and response to treatment. Renal excretion of sodium bicarbonate increases during pregnancy; therefore, bicarbonate administration is determined by ABG results. Aggressive ventilation with supplemental oxygen and fluid loading are necessary for resuscitation. Vasopressors should be used with caution because of uteroplacental vasoconstriction and deleterious effects on the fetus. There are no contraindications to external defibrillation during pregnancy.

Later in pregnancy, supine hypotension can occur from compression of the inferior vena cava, abdominal aorta, and pelvic veins by the gravid uterus. Cardiac output and venous return may be significantly reduced. Displacing the uterus to the left during chest compressions minimizes this effect and increases cardiac output. At gestation greater than 26 weeks, fetal viability and survival must be considered. Perimortem cesarean section (PMCS) promotes survival of the mother and fetus. There are minimal documented cases of maternal recovery with return to the preresuscitation state after cesarean delivery. After the need for perimortem cesarean section is determined, the procedure must be performed quickly, with a neonatal resuscitation team immediately available.

Perimortem Cesarean Section

The injured mother may require emergency delivery of a viable fetus. Indications for cesarean delivery include fetal distress, placental abruption, uterine rupture, unstable pelvic or lumbosacral fracture during labor, or impending maternal death.

A PMCS is delivery of the neonate before maternal death. Fetal survival depends on the interval between maternal arrest and fetal delivery, gestational age, fetal condition, and cause of maternal arrest. Gestational age is best determined by LMP; however, measurement of fundal height can be used to estimate fetal age. A fundus above the umbilicus suggests a viable fetus greater than 26 weeks' gestation.

The interval between maternal arrest and fetal delivery is the most important factor predictive of fetal survival. Most infants that survive are delivered within 5 minutes of maternal arrest.[3] As the interval increases, neonatal survival decreases. PMCS should be initiated while maternal cardiopulmonary resuscitation (CPR) is performed to ensure uteroplacental perfusion. The "4-minute rule" (that is, PMCS should be initiated within 4 minutes after maternal cardiac arrest and the infant delivered by the fifth minute) promotes best maternal and fetal outcome. Maternal recovery may occur after cesarean section secondary to release of aortocaval compression, increased cardiac output, and increased tissue perfusion.

Fetal condition should be determined early during maternal arrest. Evidence of FHT is a primary indication for PMCS, with PMCS recommended regardless of fetal viability resulting from potential neonatal or maternal survival.

Neonatal Resuscitation

Emergency delivery of a neonate is performed because of maternal or fetal stress or both. Compromised fetal condition secondary to maternal arrest or other stressors may necessitate aggressive resuscitation. A neonatal team skilled in assessment and treatment of the newborn should be prepared with equipment necessary to resuscitate fetus. Assessment and resuscitation should be performed simultaneously in a stepwise fashion. Drying, warming, suction, and tactile stimulation are the first interventions. Oxygen is needed by a compromised neonate when minimal respiratory effort is made with an adequate heart rate. The neonate requires only bag-valve-mask ventilation with 100% oxygen. Chest compressions should be initiated when heart rate is absent or the neonate has a heart rate less than 60 beats/min after 30 seconds of adequate assisted ventilation. Intubation and med-ications are the final steps of neonate resuscitation. APGAR scoring is calculated at 1 minute after delivery and repeated in 5 minutes to determine success of resuscitative efforts; however, determining the APGAR score should not interfere with neonatal resuscitation. Box 31-2 summarizes neonatal resuscitation.

Patient Transport

Prehospital care and transport of the pregnant woman are influenced by several factors. As with any trauma patient, the initial focus is on spinal integrity, basic life support assessment, and emergency interventions. Supplemental oxygen benefits the mother and fetus because the pregnant woman is at higher risk for respiratory compromise than a nonpregnant woman and the fetus cannot tolerate hypoxia. Application of supplemental oxygen throughout transport is

---

Box 31-2 NEONATAL RESUSCITATION

Dry baby as soon as born. Keep infant warm!

AIRWAY

Clear the airway
Position baby supine or on side with head in neutral or slightly extended position
If meconium-stained amniotic fluid present and infant displays: absent or depressed respirations, heart rate less than 100 beats/min or poor muscle tone, direct tracheal suctioning is recommended

BREATHING

Begin ventilations if respirations are absent or if heart rate is less than 60 beats/min and cyanosis persists despite 100% oxygen

Oxygen

Preferred method: Simple facemask held firmly on face using 5 to 10 L/min flow
May use standard oxygen tubing and a flow rate of 5 to 10 L/min to direct blow-by oxygen toward the neonate's nares
Endotracheal intubation if needed

Bag-valve-mask ventilation

Rate: 40 to 60 breaths/min
Adequate ventilation is assessed by chest wall movement, auscultation of bilateral breath sounds and use of an exhaled carbon dioxide indicator
Bag-valve volume for full-term neonate: at least 450 to 750 ml

COMPRESSIONS

Begin compressions if heart rate is absent, heart rate remains less than 60 beats/min after 30 seconds of adequate assisted ventilation

Acceptable methods in newborns

Thumb technique (preferred method): Two thumbs on the lower third of the sternum with hands encircling the body and fingers supporting the back
Two-finger technique: Two fingers, using the tips of the fingers to compress the lower third of the sternum and the other hand to support the back (unless on a firm surface)

Compression: Ventilation ratio

3:1 ratio (three compressions to one ventilation)
Results in 90 compressions and 30 ventilations per minute
Important to allow for adequate ventilation between compressions

Compression depth: Depress the sternum $\frac{1}{2}$ to $\frac{3}{4}$ inch

Modified from American Heart Association: Guidelines 2000 for cardiopulmonary resuscitation and emergency cardiac care, *Circulation*, 102(suppl I):I-1, 2000.

required until respiratory status is evaluated. IV access is needed for fluid replacement to treat maternal hypovolemia and ensure uterine perfusion. To avoid serious maternal-fetal complications, appropriate maternal positioning during transport is vital. The left lateral decubitus position is advocated to avoid aortocaval compression in gestation greater than 20 weeks. If spinal immobilization is needed, a cervical collar and backboard with a left lateral tilt of 15 degrees should maintain immobilization and minimize compression.

SUMMARY

Obstetric trauma, although rare, can be a catastrophic event. Two patients, the mother and the fetus, must be considered during assessment and treatment of the obstetric patient. Clinical management requires a team approach. The emergency physician, emergency nurse, trauma surgeon, obstetrician, perinatologist, labor and delivery nurse, and neonatal nurse may be key members of the trauma team during resuscitation of an obstetric trauma patient.

Optimal fetal outcomes are the result of maternal survival. Aggressive resuscitation and stabilization of the mother promotes the best maternal and fetal outcomes. Box 31-3 highlights nursing diagnoses for the obstetric trauma patient. Concern for maternal and fetal condition produces elevated stress levels in the patient and family, so emotional care should not be forgotten. Reassurance is indispensable during trauma intervention.

Prevention efforts can decrease the incidence and severity of obstetric trauma. Public and private education about proper use of seat belts can reduce maternal and fetal injury. Violence, especially domestic violence, should be assessed in the ED. Appropriate intervention may prevent a repeat attack and avoid maternal injury. Education that fetal condition basically depends on maternal condition may help the mother choose actions that promote fetal well-being.

Box 31-3	NURSING DIAGNOSES FOR THE PREGNANT TRAUMA PATIENT

Anxiety
Aspiration, Risk for
Fear
Fluid volume, Deficient
Gas exchange, Risk for impaired
Infection, Risk for
Tissue perfusion, Ineffective

References

1. Bennett BB, Hoyt KS: Trauma and pregnancy. In Emergency Nurses Assocation: *Trauma nursing core course provider manual,* ed 5, Park Ridge, Ill, 2000, The Association.
2. Emergency Nurses Association: *The obstetrical patient in the ED: position statement,* Park Ridge, Ill, 1993, The Association.
3. Knudsen M, Rozycki GS, Strear CM: Reproductive system trauma. In Mattox KL, Feleciano DV, Moore EE, editors: *Trauma,* ed 4, New York, 2001, McGraw-Hill.
4. Pearlman MD, Tintinalli JE: *Emergency care of the woman,* New York, 1998, McGraw-Hill.

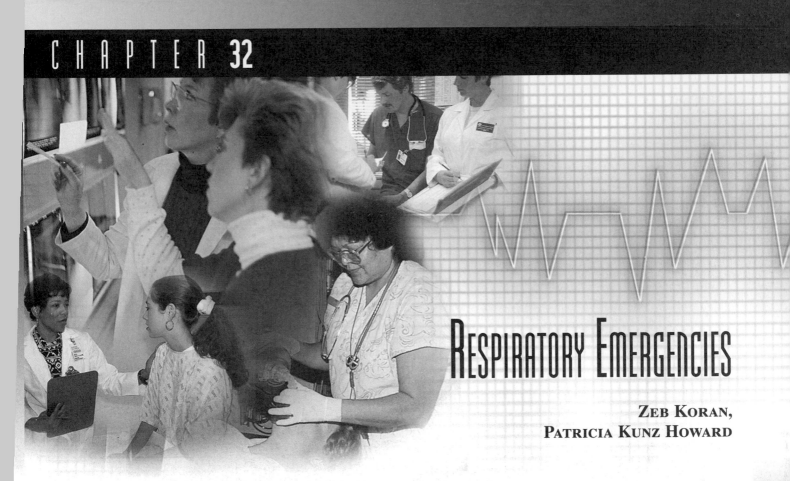

CHAPTER 32

RESPIRATORY EMERGENCIES

ZEB KORAN,
PATRICIA KUNZ HOWARD

Respiratory emergencies may present as a minor problem, such as upper respiratory infection, or impending respiratory arrest caused by epiglottitis. Rapid assessment and intervention are essential to prevent escalation of respiratory compromise. Because respiratory distress is caused by impaired oxygenation or ventilation, it is an emergent condition, regardless of etiology.

This chapter focuses on common respiratory emergencies including asthma, bronchitis, emphysema, pulmonary edema, pulmonary embolus, near-drowning, and spontaneous pneumothorax. Respiratory emergencies that occur more often in the pediatric population (i.e., croup, epiglottitis, bronchiolitis) are addressed in the chapter on pediatric emergencies (see Chapter 48), whereas tuberculosis is included in the discussion of infectious diseases (see Chapter 40). Anatomy and physiology of the respiratory system are included to facilitate understanding of these potentially life-threatening conditions.

ANATOMY AND PHYSIOLOGY

Anatomic structures of the pulmonary system include the oral cavity, epiglottis, trachea, bronchi, and lungs (Figure 32-1). Ciliated epithelium located from the proximal trachea to the terminal bronchioles trap dust particles and other debris, preventing contamination of the lower airways. Goblet cells secrete mucus, which keeps airways moist and traps debris that might otherwise enter alveoli. The airway distal to the larynx is considered sterile because of these and other protective mechanisms such as coughing and alveolar macrophages. Upper airways have C-shaped cartilaginous rings that prevent airway collapse. Rings gradually disappear in the lower branches and are replaced by smooth muscle in the bronchioles. The functional unit of the pulmonary system is the alveolus, which interacts with adjacent capillaries to ensure oxygen transport from alveolus into blood (Figure 32-2). Alveoli remain open because of the presence of surfactant, a detergent-like substance that reduces surface tension within the alveoli.

Respiration is divided into pulmonary ventilation, diffusion of oxygen and carbon dioxide across the alveolar capillary membrane, transport of oxygen and carbon dioxide to and from cells, and regulation of ventilation. Pulmonary ventilation refers to flow of air between the atmosphere and alveoli. Figure 32-3 illustrates movement of the chest wall during respiration. Negative intrathoracic pressure is the impetus for movement of air into the lungs, whereas flow out of the lungs occurs passively.

Normal gas exchange in the lung depends on adequate ventilation and perfusion (Figure 32-4). Imbalance in either area creates a ventilation/perfusion ($\dot{V}/\dot{Q}$) mismatch.[4] Figure 32-5 illustrates the effect of inadequate ventilation and the consequences of poor perfusion. Extreme imbalance between ventilation and perfusion shunts blood to the arterial system without benefit of oxygenation (Figure 32-6, p. 425). Congenital heart conditions such as patent ductus arteriosus are a common cause of shunts. Consolidated pneumonia and pulmonary embolus also lead to shunting.

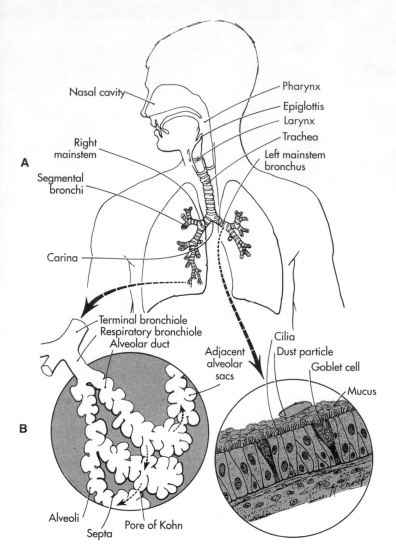

FIGURE **32-1** Structures of the respiratory tract. **A,** Pulmonary functional unit. **B,** Ciliated mucous membrane. (From Price SA, Wilson LM: *Pathophysiology: clinical concepts of disease processes,* ed 5, St. Louis, 1997, Mosby.)

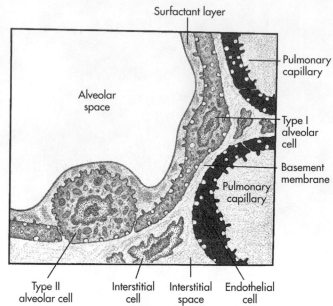

FIGURE **32-2** Alveolar wall and space. (From Thompson JM et al: *Mosby's clinical nursing,* ed 5, St. Louis, 2001, Mosby.)

Cellular oxygenation depends on transport of adequate oxygen to cells, affinity of hemoglobin for oxygen, and the ease with which hemoglobin releases oxygen to cells. Hemoglobin's affinity for oxygen is described by the oxygen-hemoglobin dissociation curve (Figure 32-7, p. 426). If the curve shifts to the left, hemoglobin picks up oxygen more easily in the lungs but does not easily release oxygen to tissues. When the curve shifts to the right, oxygen uptake by hemoglobin is less rapid, but oxygen delivery to cells is easier. Conditions that affect oxygen dissociation are temperature, acid-base balance, and carbon dioxide pressure (pCO_2) levels.

PATIENT ASSESSMENT

Assessment of the patient with a respiratory emergency begins with evaluation of airway, breathing, and circulation (ABCs). After ABCs are ensured, assess for objective findings such as flaring of nostrils, cyanosis, pallor, decreasing level of consciousness, and dyspnea. Assess level of consciousness, vital signs, use of accessory muscles, and breath sounds. Presence of barrel chest and clubbed fingers suggests chronic obstructive pulmonary disease (COPD), cardiovascular abnormalities, valvular heart disease, or congenital defects; however, these can be normal findings in patients living at high altitudes or those who are elderly. Physical examination of the chest varies with condition. Table 32-1 on p. 426 lists these assessment findings for various pulmonary emergencies.

Obtain historical information related to onset of symptoms, preexisting conditions, smoking, and presence of orthopnea or nocturnal dyspnea. Tobacco smoke decreases efficacy of pulmonary mucosa, cilia, and alveolar macrophages. Table 32-2 on p. 427 highlights tobacco's effects on the respiratory system. Determining the patient's occupation can provide helpful information because certain occupations have an increased incidence of pulmonary diseases (Table 32-3, p. 427).

Nursing interventions include frequent assessment of oxygen saturation, vital signs, and cardiac rhythm. Early identification and treatment of hypoxia can prevent ventricular dysrhythmias related to myocardial ischemia. Oxygen saturation is monitored using noninvasive pulse oximetry (Figure 32-8, p. 428). Patients with respiratory emergencies frequently have decreased oxygen saturation. Administer oxygen in cases of decreased oxygen saturation. Chest radiograph, complete blood count (CBC), and measurement of arterial blood gases should also be obtained. Table 32-4 provides normal arterial and venous blood gas values; abnormal arterial blood gas values are listed in Table 32-5.

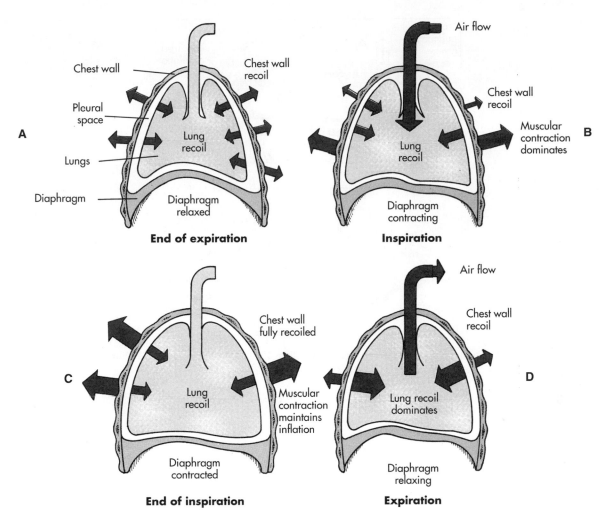

FIGURE 32-3 Interaction of forces during inspiration and expiration. **A,** Outward recoil of the chest wall equals inward recoil of the lungs at the end of expiration. **B,** During inspiration, contraction of respiratory muscles, assisted by chest wall recoil, overcomes tendency of lungs to recoil. **C,** At the end of inspiration, respiratory muscle contraction maintains lung expansion. **D,** During expiration, respiratory muscles relax, allowing elastic recoil of the lungs to deflate the lungs. (From Huether SE, McCance KL: *Understanding pathophysiology,* ed 2, St. Louis, 2000, Mosby.)

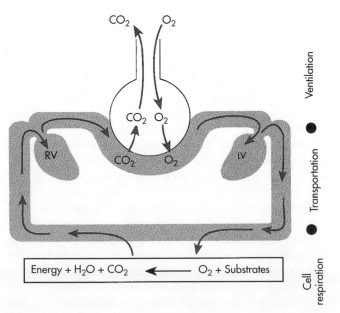

FIGURE 32-4 Normal gas exchange in the respiratory process. *RV,* Right ventricle; *LV,* left ventricle. (From Price SA, Wilson LM: *Pathophysiology: clinical concepts of disease processes,* ed 5, St. Louis, 1997, Mosby.)

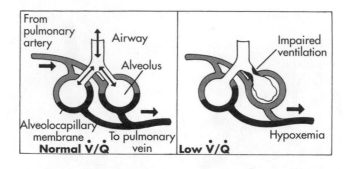

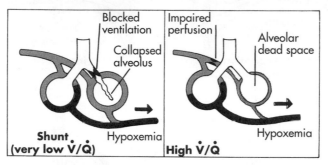

FIGURE 32-5   Ventilation-perfusion abnormalities. (From Huether SE, McCance KL: *Understanding pathophysiology,* ed, 2, St. Louis, 2000, Mosby.)

Acute Bronchitis

Acute bronchitis occurs in all age groups and is more common during cold and flu seasons. Acute inflammation from infectious agents such as influenza, parainfluenza, adenovirus, and rhinovirus is the most common cause. Secondary infection with *Mycoplasma pneumoniae, Haemophilus influenzae,* and pneumococci and streptococci organisms also occurs. Acute bronchitis usually clears independently except in patients with COPD, the elderly and debilitated, or patients with other chronic disorders.

Clinical manifestations include recent upper respiratory infection such as sore throat, stuffy nose, and cough. Cough is initially dry, hacky, and nonproductive and most troublesome at night, usually interrupting sleep. Exposure to cold, deep breathing, talking, and laughing may also cause coughing. Within days, sputum production is evident with a retrosternal, scratchy feeling present. Dyspnea is not present unless there is underlying cardiopulmonary disease. Inflammation and hypersensitivity may occur.

Chest radiographs may be normal or show signs of inflammation. Scattered wheezing and a mild or elevated fever may also be present. Management includes bed rest, humidification, cough preparations to allow sleep, antibiotic for secondary infection—especially with underlying pulmonary disease, and increasing oral fluid intake. Prognosis is good with self-limiting acute bronchitis but can progress to pneumonia with underlying pulmonary disease.

Chronic Bronchitis

Chronic bronchitis occurs more frequently in middle-age men, is uncommon in nonsmokers, and involves excessive, chronic production of mucus.[3] Direct correlation exists between the amount and duration of cigarette smoking and severity of the bronchitis. The size and work of goblet and mucous gland cells increase, causing peripheral mucus plugs, inflammation of bronchiole walls, and loss of cilia without decrease in peak expiratory flow rates. Resistance in smaller (less than 2 mm) airways causes a mismatch of $\dot{V}/\dot{Q}$ ratio and hypoxemia. In advanced stages, emphysema, increased pulmonary vascular resistance, right ventricular failure, increased airway obstruction, and polycythemia predispose the patient to thrombi and emboli. Table 32-6 on p. 429 highlights clinical differences between chronic bronchitis and emphysema.

Chronic bronchitis is diagnosed when cough with increased sputum production occurs at least 3 consecutive months each year for 2 successive years.[5] The cough may become purulent. Dyspnea indicates obstruction but has slow onset unless there is acute exacerbation. In advanced stages, prolonged expiration with wheezing and dyspnea at rest resembles emphysema. A chest radiograph is insignificant in uncomplicated chronic bronchitis but in the late stages reveals hyperinflation. Pulmonary function tests are normal in the early stages, but chronic obstructive changes increase residual volume, indicating small airway obstruction.

Management for chronic bronchitis, as with COPD in late stages, includes bronchodilators, nebulized inhalers, and

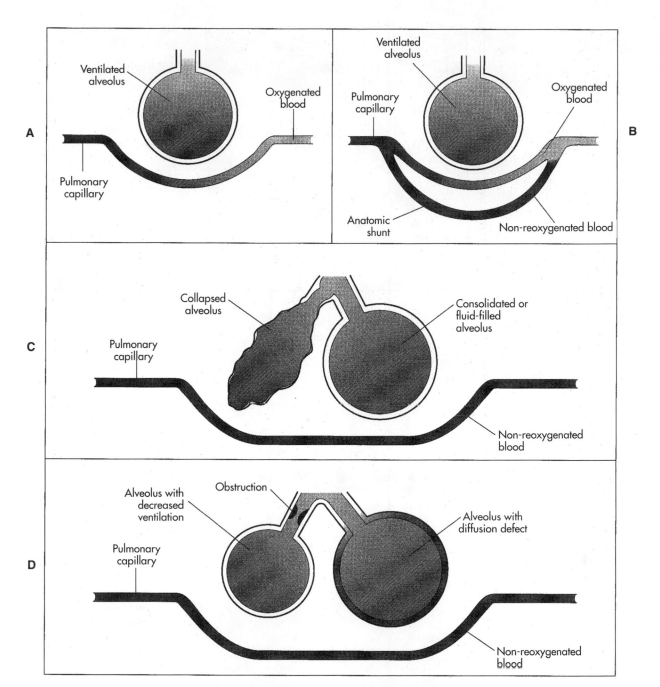

FIGURE 32-6   Pulmonary shunting. **A,** Normal alveolar-capillary unit. **B,** Anatomic shunt. **C,** Types of capillary shunts. **D,** Types of shuntlike effects. (From NFNA: *Flight nursing,* ed 2, St. Louis, 1996, Mosby.)

usually steroids. Antibiotics are not used unless obvious infection is present. Unless these patients stop smoking, the majority will progress to COPD. The course of chronic bronchitis is cough with expectoration for years.

Pneumonia

Pneumonia results from an acute bacterial, viral, or fungal infection and may be preceded by upper respiratory tract infection, ear infection, or eye infection, or can occur as the primary illness without precipitating causes. Pneumonia occurs primarily in young children and debilitated individuals and is the leading cause of death among the elderly.[3]

Figure 32-9 on p. 430 illustrates types of pneumonia. Patients who are bedridden, have rib fractures, or have underlying cardiac or pulmonary disorder have an increased risk for pneumonia. Pneumonia is more likely to occur in those with a previous episode of pneumonia. Other causes include smoking, diabetes mellitus, exposure to extreme changes in environmental temperature, steroids, or immunosuppressive

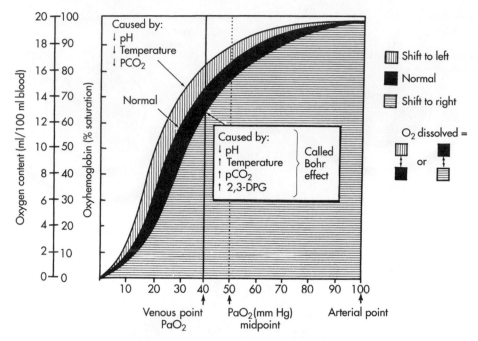

FIGURE 32-7 Oxygen-hemoglobin dissociation curve. Effects of acidity and temperature changes are shown. (From Thompson JM et al: *Mosby's clinical nursing,* ed 5, St. Louis, 2001, Mosby.)

Table 32-1   CHEST EXAMINATION FINDINGS IN COMMON PULMONARY PROBLEMS

PROBLEM	INSPECTION	PALPATION	PERCUSSION	AUSCULTATION
Chronic bronchitis	Barrel chest; cyanosis	↑Movement ↓Fremitus	Hyperresonant or dull if consolidation	Crackles; rhonchi; wheezes
Emphysema	Barrel chest; tripod position; use of accessory muscles	↓Movement	Hyperresonant or dull if consolidation	Crackles; rhonchi; diminished if no exacerbation
Asthma: In exacerbation	Prolonged expiration; tripod position; pursed lips	↓Movement ↓Fremitus if hyperinflation	Hyperresonance sounds	Wheezes; ↓ breath sounds ominous sign if no improvement (severely diminished air movement)
Not in exacerbation	Normal	Normal	Normal	Normal
Pneumonia	Tachypnea; use of accessory muscles; duskiness or cyanosis	Unequal movement if lobar involvement; ↑fremitus over affected area	Dull over affected areas	Early: bronchial sounds lower in chest Later: crackles; rhonchi
Atelectasis	No change unless involves entire segment, lobe	If small, no change; if large, ↓movement; ↑fremitus	Dull over affected areas	Crackles (may disappear with deep breaths); absent sounds if large
Pulmonary edema	Tachypnea; labored respirations; cyanosis	↓Or normal movement	Dull or normal depending on amount of fluid	Fine or coarse crackles
Pleural effusion	Tachypnea; use of accessory muscles	↓Movement ↑Fremitus above effusion; absent fremitus over effusion	Dull	Diminished or absent over effusion; egophony over effusion
Pulmonary fibrosis	Tachypnea	↓Movement	Normal	Crackles

From Lewis SM, Heitkemper MM, Dirksen SR: *Medical-surgical nursing: assessment and management of clinical problems,* ed 5, St. Louis, 2000, Mosby.

Table 32-2 EFFECTS OF TOBACCO SMOKE ON THE RESPIRATORY SYSTEM

AREA OF DEFECT	ACUTE EFFECTS	LONG-TERM EFFECTS
Respiratory mucosa		
Nasopharyngeal	↓Sense of smell	Cancer
Tongue	↓Sense of taste	Cancer
Vocal cords	Hoarseness	Chronic cough, cancer
Bronchus and bronchioles	Bronchospasm, cough	Chronic bronchitis, asthma, cancer
Cilia	Paralysis, sputum accumulation, cough	Chronic bronchitis, cancer
Mucous glands	↑Secretions, ↑cough	Hyperplasia and hypertrophy of glands, chronic bronchitis
Alveolar macrophages	↓Function	Increased incidence of infection
Elastin and collagen fibers	↑Destruction by proteases, ↓function of antiproteases (α-1-antitrypsin), ↓synthesis and repair of elastin	Emphysema

From Lewis SM, Heitkemper MM, Dirksen SR: *Medical-surgical nursing: assessment and management of clinical problems,* ed 5, St. Louis, 2000, Mosby.

Table 32-3 OCCUPATIONAL LUNG DISEASES

DISEASE	AGENTS/INDUSTRIES	DESCRIPTION	COMPLICATIONS
Asbestosis	Asbestos fibers present in insulation, construction material (roof tiling, cement products), shipyards, textiles (for fireproofing), automobile clutch and brake linings	Disease appears 15-35 yr after first exposure; interstitial fibrosis develops; pleural plaques, which are calcified lesions, develop on pleura; dyspnea, basal crackles, and decreased vital capacity are early manifestations	Diffuse interstitial pulmonary fibrosis; lung cancer, especially in cigarette smokers; mesothelioma (rare type of cancer affecting pleura and peritoneal membrane)
Berylliosis	Beryllium dust present in aircraft manufacturing, metallurgy, rocket fuels	Noncaseating granulomas form; acute pneumonitis occurs after heavy exposure; interstitial fibrosis can also occur	Progress of disease possible after removal of stimulating inhalant
Bird fancier's, breeder's, or handler's lung	Bird droppings or feathers	Hypersensitivity pneumonitis is present	Progressive fibrosis of lung
Byssinosis	Cotton, flax, and hemp dust (textile industry)	Airway obstruction is caused by contraction of smooth muscles; chronic disease results from severe airway obstruction and decreased elastic recoil	Progression of chronic disease after cessation of dust exposure
Coal worker's pneumoconiosis (black lung)	Coal dust	Incidence is high (20%-30%) in coal workers; deposits of carbon dust cause lesions to develop along respiratory bronchioles; bronchioles dilate because of loss of wall structure; chronic airway obstruction and bronchitis develop; dyspnea and cough are common early symptoms	Progressive, massive lung fibrosis; increased risk of chronic bronchitis and emphysema with smoking
Farmer's lung	Inhalation of airborne material from moldy hay or similar matter	Hypersensitivity pneumonitis occurs; *acute* form is similar to pneumonia, with manifestations of chills, fever, and malaise; *chronic,* insidious form is type of pulmonary fibrosis	Progressive fibrosis of lung
Siderosis	Iron oxide present in welding materials, foundries, iron ore mining	Dust deposits are found in lung	
Silicosis	Silica dust present in quartz rock in mining of gold, copper, tin, coal, lead; also present in sandblasting, foundries, quarries, pottery making, masonry	In *chronic* disease, dust is engulfed by macrophages and may be destroyed, resulting in fibrotic nodules; *acute* disease results from intense exposure in short time; within 5 yr, it progresses to severe disability from lung fibrosis	Increased susceptibility to tuberculosis; progressive, massive fibrosis; high incidence of chronic bronchitis
Silo filler's disease	Nitrogen oxides from fermentation of vegetation in freshly filled silo	Chemical pneumonitis occurs	Progressive bronchiolitis obliterans

From Lewis SM, Heitkemper MM, Dirksen SR: *Medical-surgical nursing: assessment and management of clinical problems,* ed 5, St. Louis, 2000, Mosby.

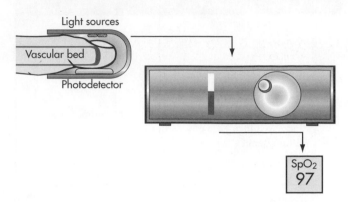

FIGURE 32-8 A pulse oximeter passes light from a light-emitting diode through a vascular bed to a photodetector. The oximeter compares the amount of light emitted with the amount absorbed and calculates the SpO_2. The oximeter displays the SpO_2 as a digital reading. SpO_2, Arterial oxyhemoglobin saturation. (From Lewis SM, Heitkemper MM, Dirksen SR: *Medical-surgical nursing: assessment and management of clinical problems,* ed 5, St. Louis, 2000, Mosby.)

therapy. Those who abuse alcohol or drugs have a tendency to aspirate, so pneumonia is seen more often in these individuals.[9] Box 32-1 highlights factors that predispose people to pneumonia.

Patients who have an elevated temperature (39° C to 40° C) exhibit diaphoresis and may complain of chest pain, which is often referred diaphragmatically and mistaken for gastrointestinal disorders. Productive cough, tachypnea, tachycardia, cyanosis, and apprehension may occur. Pleuritic chest pain is frequently noted. Breath sounds are present but are diminished over the area of pneumonia. Rales also occur. Abdominal distention, vomiting, and headache have also been reported. Table 32-7 on p. 432 compares symptoms and characteristics for types of pneumonia.

Therapeutic interventions for emergency department (ED) patients with pneumonia include administering humidified oxygen and antibiotics, and controlling fluid and electrolyte balance. Diagnostic assessment includes sputum culture and gram stain, chest radiograph, and CBC. Pulse oximetry is obtained initially and monitored over time to

Table 32-4 NORMAL ARTERIAL AND VENOUS BLOOD GAS VALUES*

	ARTERIAL BLOOD GASES			
LABORATORY VALUE	**SEA LEVEL BP 760 MM HG**	**1 MILE ABOVE SEA LEVEL (5280 FT) BP 629 MM HG**	**MIXED VENOUS BLOOD GASES**	
pH	7.35-7.45	7.35-7.45	pH	7.34-7.37
PaO_2	80-100 mm Hg	65-75 mm Hg	PVO_2	38-42 mm Hg
SaO_2	>95%†	>95%†	SVO_2	60-80%†
$PaCO_2$	35-45 mm Hg	35-45 mm Hg	$PVCO_2$	44-46 mm Hg
HCO_3^-	22-26 mEq/L	22-26 mEq/L	HCO_3^-	24-30 mEq/L

From Lewis SM, Heitkemper MM, Dirksen SR: *Medical-surgical nursing: assessment and management of clinical problems,* ed 5, St. Louis, 2000, Mosby.
BP, Barometric pressure; *PaO_2,* arterial oxygen pressure; *PVO_2,* partial pressure of oxygen in venous blood; *SaO_2,* arterial oxygen saturation; *SVO_2,* venous oxygen saturation; *$PaCO_2$,* arterial carbon dioxide pressure; *$PVCO_2$,* partial pressure of carbon dioxide in venous blood; *HCO_3^-,* bicarbonate.
*Assumes patient is ≤60 years of age and breathing room air.
†The same normal values apply when SaO_2 and SVO_2 are obtained by oximetry.

Table 32-5 ARTERIAL BLOOD GASES WITH VARIOUS STAGES OF COMPENSATION

	CAUSE	pCO_2	UNCOMPENSATED		PARTIALLY COMPENSATED		FULLY COMPENSATED	
VALUES			pH	HCO_3^-	pH	HCO_3^-	pH	HCO_3^-
Respiratory alkalosis	Hyperventilation	↓	↑	Normal	↑	↓	Normal	↓
Respiratory acidosis	Drug ingestion (hypoventilation)	↑	↓	Normal	↓	↑	Normal	↑

	CAUSE	HCO_3^-	UNCOMPENSATED		PARTIALLY COMPENSATED		FULLY COMPENSATED	
VALUES			pH	pCO_2	pH	pCO_2	pH	pCO_2
Metabolic alkalosis	Severe vomiting	↑	↑	Normal	↑	↑	*	↑
Metabolic acidosis	Diabetic ketoacidosis	↓	↓	Normal	↓	↓	*	↓

*Metabolic cannot be fully compensated to a normal pH by the respiratory system.
HCO_3^-, Bicarbonate; *pCO_2,* carbon dioxide pressure.

Table 32-6 COMPARISON OF EMPHYSEMA AND CHRONIC BRONCHITIS*		
	EMPHYSEMA	**CHRONIC BRONCHITIS**
CLINICAL FEATURES		
Age	30-40 yr (onset)	20-30 yr (onset)
	60-70 yr (disabling)	40-50 yr (disabling)
Body build	Thin	Tendency toward obesity
Health history	Generally healthy, occasional insidious dyspnea, smoking	Recurrent respiratory tract infections, smoking
Weight loss	Often marked	Absent or slight
Dyspnea	Slowly progressive and eventually disabling	Variable, relatively late
Sputum	Scanty, mucoid	Copious, mucopurulent
Cough	Negligible	Considerable
Chest examination	Marked increase in AP diameter, quiet or diminished breath sounds, limited diaphragmatic excursion	Slight to marked increase in AP diameter, scattered crackles, rhonchi, wheezing
Cor pulmonale	Rare except terminally	Frequent with many episodes
DIAGNOSTIC STUDY RESULTS		
ABGs	Near normal, mild $\downarrow PaO_2$, normal or $\uparrow PaCO_2$	$\downarrow PaO_2$, $\uparrow PaCO_2$
Chest x-ray	Hyperinflation, flat diaphragm, attenuated peripheral vessels, small or normal heart, widened intercostal margins	Cardiac enlargement, normal or flattened diaphragm, evidence of chronic inflammation, congested lung fields
LUNG VOLUMES		
Total lung capacity	Increased	Normal or slightly increased
Residual volume	Increased	Increased
Vital capacity	Decreased	Decreased
FEV1	Decreased	Decreased
FEV1/FVC	Decreased (<70%)	Decreased (<70%)
Hematocrit and hemoglobin	Normal until late in disease	Increased
PATHOLOGY		
	Panlobular emphysema	Centrilobular emphysema

From Lewis SM, Heitkemper MM, Dirksen SR: *Medical-surgical nursing: assessment and management of clinical problems,* ed 5, St. Louis, 2000, Mosby.

ABGs, Arterial blood gases; *AP,* anteroposterior; *FEV1,* forced expiratory volume in 1 second; *FVC,* forced vital capacity; *PaO₂,* arterial oxygen pressure; *PaCO₂,* arterial carbon dioxide pressure.

*Most people with chronic obstructive pulmonary disease have features of both pulmonary emphysema and chronic bronchitis.

determine changes in the patient's respiratory status. Arterial blood gas values are usually obtained for these patients.

Asthma

Asthma, as defined in *Guidelines for the diagnosis and management of asthma,*[7] is "a chronic inflammatory disorder of the airways in which many cells and cellular elements play a role . . .". Three to four percent of the U.S. population are affected by asthma.[3] Asthma can be controlled, not cured, and has an unpredictable course with increasing prevalence and hospitalization. Onset occurs before age 10 in 50% of patients and there is positive family history in more than one third of asthmatic patients. Thirty percent of those diagnosed with asthma during childhood will have it as adults.

Those having symptoms into the second decade of their life will usually have asthma throughout their life.[1]

Development of airway inflammation and hyperresponsiveness occur in response to immunologic or nonimmunologic stimuli or triggers (Box 32-2). Immunologic triggers cause a humoral immune response with complex multicell activation, including mast cells, eosinophils, and immunoglobulin E (IgE) antibodies (Figure 32-10, p. 434). Inflammatory mediators cause smooth muscle contraction, vasodilation, mucosal edema, increased mucus secretion, and macrophage eosinophil infiltration. Acetylcholine directly increases airway resistance and bronchial secretions. This cholinergic response further stimulates histamine and inflammatory mediator release, excluding IgE antibodies.

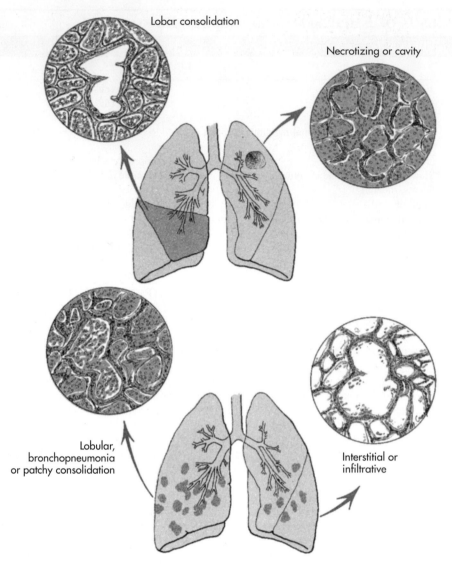

FIGURE 32-9 Types of pneumonia. Lobar: entire lobe consolidated, exudate chiefly intraalveolar, pneumococcus and *Klebsiella* organisms are common infecting organisms. Necrotizing: granuloma may undergo caseous necrosis and form cavity; fungi and tubercle bacillus infections are common causes. Lobular: patchy distribution, fibrinous exudate chiefly in bronchioles, *Staphylococcus* and *Streptococcus* species are common infecting organisms. Interstitial: perivascular exudate and edema between alveoli caused by virus or mycoplasmal infection. (From Price SA, Wilson LM: *Pathophysiology: clinical concepts of disease processes,* ed 5, St. Louis, 1997, Mosby.)

Nonimmunologic triggers stimulate the autonomic nervous system and cause mast cell and inflammatory mediator response. The pathway of emotional triggers is through the parasympathetic nervous system and stimulation of the hypothalamus. Aspirin sensitivity causes asthma through reaction to prostaglandin synthesis. Exercise-induced asthma occurs after 10 to 20 minutes of vigorous exercise through airway cooling secondary to decreased warming, reduced humidification, and increased respiratory rates. Exercise may be the only trigger for some patients and is usually limited to the early phase. Gastroesophageal (GE) reflux, a common condition associated with asthma, involves esophageal spasm with reflux of gastric acid causing spasm of nearby bronchial and esophageal structures.

Immunologic and nonimmunologic triggers cause increased mucus production, airway hyperresponsiveness, airway narrowing, and chronic inflammatory airway changes. Reaction phases in response to asthma triggers are early and late. Early-phase reaction involves rapid bronchospasm; late-phase reaction involves inflammatory epithelial lesions, increased mucosal edema, and increased secretions. Complex interactions among cells in the lungs cause a chronic inflammatory process that irritates airways. Acute exacerbation involves airway obstruction from spasm, inflammation, and mucus plugging.

<table>
<tr><td>

Box 32-1 FACTORS PREDISPOSING TO PNEUMONIA

Smoking
Air pollution
Altered consciousness: Alcoholism, head injury, seizures, anesthesia, drug overdose
Tracheal intubation (endotracheal intubation, tracheostomy)
Upper respiratory tract infection
Chronic diseases: Chronic lung disease, diabetes mellitus, heart disease, uremia, cancer
Immunosuppression drugs (corticosteroids, cancer chemotherapy, immunosuppressive therapy after organ transplant)
HIV
Malnutrition
Inhalation or aspiration of noxious substances
Debilitating illness
Bed rest and prolonged immobility
Altered oropharyngeal flora

</td></tr>
</table>

From Lewis SM, Heitkemper MM, Dirksen SR: *Medical-surgical nursing: assessment and management of clinical problems,* ed 5, St. Louis, 2000, Mosby.
HIV, Human immunodeficiency virus.

Morphologic changes of lung tissue from asthma include bronchial infiltration with inflammatory cells; vascular dilation, edema, and epithelial damage and detachment; smooth muscle hypertrophy; subepithelial fibrosis; and mucous gland hypertrophy. Radiographs of patients dying from asthma show air trapping caused by mucous plugs containing detached epithelium and eosinophils, with thickened bronchial walls infiltrated by inflammatory cells.

Diagnosis is based on careful history, examination, and lab studies. History includes symptoms, patterns, usual triggers, family history, and allergic background. Physical examination may reveal upper airway rhinitis, sinusitis, or nasal polyps. Wheezes and prolonged expiratory phase may be noted, with flexural eczema a common finding.[9] CBC with differential may reveal increased eosinophils. Nasal smears or sputum specimens should also be obtained. Chest radiograph may show increased hilar or basilar infiltrates or areas of atelectasis secondary to mucus plugging and alveolar collapse.

Seventy-five percent to 85% of asthmatic patients have positive skin reaction, so allergy testing is indicated.[2] Inhaled allergens are important triggers, particularly for patients younger than age 30 years. However, food allergens are not common triggers for most patients. Sinusitis and allergic rhinitis with postnasal drip are common triggers and may necessitate sinus radiographs. Polyps are associated with asthma in patients older than age 40 years. Nasal polyps, asthma, and allergy to aspirin are components of what is known as Triad disease.

Viral, occupational exposures, and GE reflux are more common triggers in older adults and can be identified by careful history. GE reflux is associated with nocturnal exacerbations that respond poorly to nebulized therapy.[6] Gastrointestinal workup is indicated when GE reflux is suspected.

Occupational asthma initially presents with rhinitis or eye irritation along with evening or nocturnal cough. Coughing, wheezing, and dyspnea progress with continued exposure but symptoms decrease on days off work. Smokers have a higher incidence of occupational asthma than nonsmokers, secondary to increased airway irritation. More than 240 occupational triggers have been identified. Occupations and agents associated with asthma are listed in Box 32-3 on p. 435.

The hallmark of asthma diagnosis is spirometry before and after bronchodilator therapy to document reversibility of airway narrowing, usually by peak expiratory flow rates (PEFR). PEFR is the greatest flow velocity produced during forced expiration after fully expanding lungs during inspiration. Peak expiratory flow measurement is simple, portable, and quantitative; however, lung volumes are not measured and measurement is effort dependent. Bronchoprovocation may be used with histamine, methacholine, or exercise. The lower the dose that causes a 20% fall in forced expiratory volume, the more severe the disease.

Clinical manifestations include cough, wheezing, prolonged expiratory time, and reduced peak expiratory flow. Increased work of breathing and use of accessory muscles may also be present. Arterial blood gas values initially have reduced arterial oxygen pressure (PaO_2) and arterial carbon dioxide pressure ($PaCO_2$) from hyperventilation. $PaCO_2$ eventually rises, which indicates further $\dot{V}/\dot{Q}$ mismatching. Fine crackles may be heard with opening and closing of distal air sacs in response to mucous plugging and atelectasis. Breath sounds may be diminished in lower lobes. Decreased air sounds, decreased oxygen saturation, decreased respiratory effort, and decreased level of consciousness are signs of impending failure that require immediate intervention. Asthma is classified according to severity; however, asthma is a chronic state, with exacerbations ranging from mild to severe (Table 32-8). Severity can be assessed by examining medications required to control symptoms, need for prednisone, prior intubation, recent hospitalizations, spirometric indices of air flow obstruction, occurrence of night symptoms, and number of ED visits.

Management goals are to maintain near-normal pulmonary function and exercise levels, prevent chronic symptoms and acute exacerbations, and avoid adverse effects of medications. Therapy includes objective measurement of lung function, environmental control, avoidance of triggers, select drugs, and comprehensive patient education.

PEFR provides objective data for management, documents personal best and daily variations, detects impending exacerbation, guides medicine therapy, and helps identify triggers. To correctly obtain peak expiratory flow measurements the patient should stand, if able, take a deep breath, and forcefully blow out all inspired air. The highest of three readings is recorded. A diary of peak expiratory flow measurements, along with documentation of viral infections,

Table 32-7 COMPARISON OF TYPES OF PNEUMONIA

CAUSATIVE AGENT	CHARACTERISTICS	CLINICAL MANIFESTATIONS AND COMPLICATIONS
GRAM-POSITIVE BACTERIAL PNEUMONIAS		
Pneumococcal pneumonia (*Streptococcus pneumoniae*)	URI usually preceding; usual involvement of 1 or more lobes; incubation period of 1-3 days; peak incidence in winter and spring; damage to host by overwhelming growth of organism; necrosis of lung tissue (unusual); chest x-ray shows lobar infiltration; nasopharyngeal carriers; frequent finding of herpes labialis in association with pneumonia; risk factors of chronic heart or lung disease, diabetes mellitus, cirrhosis	Abrupt onset, elevated temperature, tachypnea, chills and rigor, productive cough (often bloody, rusty, or green), nausea, vomiting, malaise, myalgia, weakness, pleuritic chest pain, atelectasis, lung abscess (rare), pleural effusions (25%-50%), empyema, metastatic infection (meninges, joints, heart valves), bacteremia (25%)
Staphylococcal pneumonia (*Staphylococcus aureus*)	Acquisition via hematogenous route or via aspiration into lungs; nasopharyngeal carriers (35%-50% of population); necrotizing infection causing destruction of lung tissue; chest x-ray shows bronchopneumonia; risk factors of chronic lung disease, leukemia, other debilitating diseases; influenza infection (10-14 days earlier) often preceding; drug abusers, diabetics, patients on long-term hemodialysis at risk as carriers; occurrence more frequent in hospitalized patients than in persons in community; prolonged antibiotic therapy usually necessary; high mortality rate in chronically debilitated patients, newborns	Abrupt onset, chills, high fever, productive cough with sputum (often bloody and purulent), tachypnea, progressive dyspnea, pleuritic chest pain, empyema, pleural effusions, lung abscess
Streptococcal pneumonia (*Streptococcus pyogenes*)	Occurrence in military populations after influenza epidemics and sporadically in community; often associated with strep throat; occurrence most frequent in winter; transmission to lung by inhalation or aspiration; destruction of lung tissue; chest x-ray shows bronchopneumonia	Fever (usually >102.2° F [39° C]), chills, cough, pharyngitis, hemoptysis, pleuritic chest pain, dyspnea, myalgia, empyema (common), pleural effusions, bacteremia, mediastinitis, pneumothorax, bronchiectasis
Anthrax pneumonia (*Bacillus anthracis*)	Association with agricultural or industrial exposure (e.g., individuals working with animal hair or contaminated animal hides or bones); transmission to lung via inhalation; formation of spores; ingestion and transport of spores to hilar lymph nodes (site of multiplication of bacteria) by alveolar macrophages; hemorrhagic pneumonitis possible	Early manifestations: insidious onset (2-4 days), mild fever, myalgia, malaise, fatigue, nonproductive cough Later manifestations: dyspnea, profuse diaphoresis, cyanosis
GRAM-NEGATIVE BACTERIAL PNEUMONIAS		
Friedländer's pneumonia (*Klebsiella pneumoniae*)	Most common gram-negative pneumonia acquired outside hospital; alcoholics, diabetics, people with chronic lung disease, and postoperative patients at risk; transmission to lungs via aspiration of oropharyngeal organisms; chest x-ray shows lobar consolidation; rapid progression to lung abscess possible; high mortality and morbidity rates	Sudden onset, fever, cough, purulent sputum, hemoptysis, malaise, pleuritic chest pain, extensive lung necrosis, lung abscess, empyema, pericarditis, meningitis
Pseudomonas pneumonia (*Pseudomonas aeruginosa*)	Most common gram-negative hospital-acquired pneumonia; predisposition from endotracheal intubation, intermittent positive-pressure breathing treatments, suctioning, respiratory therapy equipment; high mortality rate in critically ill patients; chest x-ray shows nodular bronchopneumonia; persons with chronic lung disease, debilitating diseases, tracheostomies, cancer, and kidney transplants or those taking immunosuppressive drugs or broad-spectrum antibiotics at risk; high mortality rate (50%-90%)	High fever, cough, copious sputum, hypoxia, cyanosis, lung abscess

From Lewis SM, Heitkemper MM, Dirksen SR: *Medical-surgical nursing: assessment and management of clinical problems,* ed 5, St. Louis, 2000, Mosby.
GI, Gastrointestinal; *GU,* genitourinary; *HIV,* human immunodeficiency virus; *URI,* upper respiratory tract infection.
*Organism has characteristics of both bacteria and viruses.

Table 32-7 COMPARISON OF TYPES OF PNEUMONIA—cont'd

CAUSATIVE AGENT	CHARACTERISTICS	CLINICAL MANIFESTATIONS AND COMPLICATIONS
GRAM-NEGATIVE BACTERIAL PNEUMONIAS–cont'd		
Influenza pneumonia (*Haemophilus influenzae*)	Increase in incidence; transmission to lung by endogenous aspiration; chest x-ray shows bronchopneumonia in multiple lobes or lobar consolidation; alcoholics and persons with chronic lung disease, recent viral infections, and immune deficiencies at risk; high mortality rate, especially in older adult patients	Usually gradual onset, sometimes abrupt; fever; chills; cough; purulent sputum; hemoptysis; sore throat; dyspnea; nausea and vomiting; pleuritic chest pain; pleural effusions; lung abscess (common); empyema (common)
Legionnaires' disease *Legionella pneumophila*)	Occurrence in outbreaks or sporadic; transmission to lung from airborne organisms; proliferation of organisms in water reservoirs (e.g., air-conditioning cooling towers); cigarette smokers and persons with serious underlying diseases (e.g., chronic lung or heart conditions) at increased risk; erythromycin effective	Myalgia (initially), headache (initially), fever, chills, nonproductive cough, pleuritic chest pain, nausea and vomiting, diarrhea, mental confusion, respiratory failure (major complication), healing with fibrosis common
ANAEROBIC BACTERIAL PNEUMONIAS		
Anaerobic streptococci Fusobacteria *Bacteroides* species	Transmission to lung usually by aspiration of oropharyngeal secretions but occasionally via blood from GI or GU tract or wound infections; three or four anaerobes usually causing infections; persons with poor dental hygiene, periodontal disease, and history of altered consciousness at risk; chest x-ray often shows lung abscess, empyema, necrotizing pneumonia	Similar to pneumococcal pneumonia, except for insidious onset; foul-smelling sputum; necrotizing pneumonitis (aspiration induced); lung abscess; empyema
MYCOPLASMA PNEUMONIA		
Mycoplasma pneumonia (*Mycoplasma pneumoniae*)*	Transmission from person to person by respiratory droplets; incubation period of 9-21 days; involvement of epithelial lining of respiratory system; common in children, military populations, college-age groups; increase in cold agglutinin titer in serum or complement fixation with negative bacterial culture; chest x-ray shows interstitial pneumonia, often bilaterally	Gradual onset; URI, including fever (low-grade), nasal congestion; pharyngitis; lower respiratory tract involvement (e.g., bronchitis, bronchiolitis); headache; malaise; cough (initially usually nonproductive); maculopapular rashes
VIRAL PNEUMONIAS		
Influenza viruses Adenovirus Parainfluenza viruses Respiratory syncytial virus	Influenza A most common in civilian adults; responsible for about one half of all pneumonias; peak incidence in winter; transmission from person to person by respiratory droplets; usually self-limiting; symptomatic treatment; adverse effect on many respiratory defense mechanisms, predisposing patients to secondary bacterial pneumonia; chest x-ray shows interstitial pneumonia	Fever, chills, headache, myalgia, anorexia, sneezing, nasal congestion, cough (initially nonproductive)
PROTOZOAN PNEUMONIA		
Interstitial plasma cell pneumonia (*Pneumocytis carinii*)	Opportunistic infection; persons with immunosuppression (e.g., recipients of organ transplants, patients with HIV infection, and those with hematologic malignancies) at highest risk; presentation similar to other atypical pneumonias	Cough (usually nonproductive), fever, night sweats, dyspnea (may be only with exertion)

weather, medicine changes, environments, and other possible triggers aid in management of asthma.

Avoidance and environmental control of allergens such as dust mite antigen, animal dander, pollens, and molds can greatly reduce symptoms. Encasing pillows and mattresses in vinyl and washing bedding every week in water temperatures greater than 130° F, along with carpet removal or anti-mite treatment, reduces dust mite allergen. Keeping cats and dogs outside the house reduces dander allergen and outdoor pollens and mold. Asthma patients should remain inside with air conditioning during early morning and midday hours to further reduce exposure.

Allergen inhalation
  Animal danders
  House dust mite
  Pollens
  Molds
Air pollutants
  Exhaust fumes
  Perfumes
  Oxidants
  Sulfur dioxides
  Cigarette smoke
  Aerosol sprays
Viral upper respiratory
  infection
Paranasal sinusitis
Exercise and cold, dry air
Drugs
  Aspirin
  Nonsteroidal antiinflam-
    matory drugs
  β-adrenergic blockers

Occupational exposure
  Metal salts
  Wood and vegetable dusts
  Industrial chemicals and plastics
  Pharmaceutical agents
Food additives
Sulfites (bisulfites and metabi-
  sulfites)
Tartrazine
Menses
Gastroesophageal reflux
Emotional stress

From Lewis SM, Heitkemper MM, Dirksen SR: *Medical-surgical nursing: assessment and management of clinical problems,* ed 5, St. Louis, 2000, Mosby.

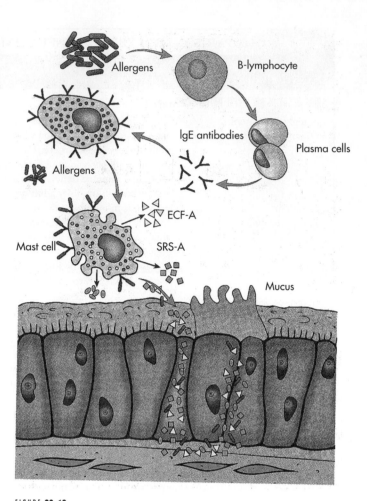

FIGURE 32-10 Early-phase response in asthma is triggered when an allergen or irritant cross-links immunoglobulin E receptors on mast cells, which are then activated to release histamine and other inflammatory mediators. (From Lewis SM, Heitkemper MM, Dirksen SR: *Medical-surgical nursing: assessment and management of clinical problems,* ed 5, St. Louis, 2000, Mosby.)

Drugs for asthma reduce contraction and spasm of bronchial smooth muscle, airway inflammation, mucosal edema, and airway hyperreactivity. Medications are given orally, intravenously, subcutaneously, and via inhalation (Table 32-9 and Box 32-4, p. 439). Several forms of aerosolized therapy are used (Table 32-10). Advantages of aerosol therapy include smaller drug amounts, rapid onset of action, direct delivery to respiratory system, fewer side effects, and painless, convenient administration.[8] Table 32-11 on p. 439 highlights over-the-counter drugs used for managing asthma.

Asthma education and clinician-patient communication are primary concerns when treating and controlling asthma. Asthma education should convey clinician-patient partnership, the concept of asthma as a chronic but controllable disease, role of environmental control and use of medication, the importance of objective PEFR measurements, individualized guidelines for managing acute exacerbations, and when to call for help. Action, indication for use, and side effects of each medication should be provided orally and in written form in easy-to-understand language. More in-depth information can be added for individuals with specific learning needs. Detailed, written instructions are given to outline a plan for continuing care that is individualized to each patient's capability. Correct use of spacers, inhalers, and PEFR meters must be assessed (Figure 32-11, p. 440). The emergency nurse should take every opportunity to dispel common misconceptions about asthma (Box 32-5, p. 441).

Heliox is being used more often with asthma; however, literature regarding this treatment is minimal. Ongoing research is evaluating magnesium sulfate for treatment of acute bronchospasm in asthma. Research is based on the theory that magnesium acts as a calcium channel antagonist, blocks uptake of calcium in bronchial smooth muscle, and causes bronchial relaxation. Recent studies suggest magnesium may be beneficial for patients with acute, severe asthma when conventional therapy does not control exacerbation.

Emphysema

Emphysema refers to permanent abnormal enlargement of air spaces distal to terminal bronchioles and associated destructive changes of the alveolar wall. In contrast, asthma is characterized by simple overdistention without alveolar destruction. Three types of emphysema are categorized according to area of lung tissue involved. There are 25,000

Box 32-3	OCCUPATIONS AND AGENTS ASSOCIATED WITH ASTHMA

OCCUPATION	AGENT
Veterinarians, animal lab workers, animal handlers, shepherds, grooms, jockeys, veterinarians, and kennel workers	Dander, urine, mites, small insects, bacterial or protein dusts
Bakers, millers, food processors	Flour, wheat, rye, fungal amylases
Beauticians, hair dressers, stylists	Henna, persulphage
Coffee roasters	Green coffee bean
Farmers	Storage mites, grain mites, egg protein
Health care workers	Latex, formaldehyde, gluteraldehyde
Oil industry, dock workers	Castor bean
Painters, insulation installers	Isocyanates, anydrides
Pharmaceutical workers	Pancreatin, papain, pepsin, gums, latex, penicillin and other anti-biotics, cimetidine, psyllium, others
Photographers	Amines
Printers, carpet makers, textile workers	Gum, latex, rubber, dyes, cotton, flax, hemp dust
Saw mill workers, joiners, cabinet makers, carpenters	Wood dust and bark
Welders, platinum refinery workers, hard metal grinders, aluminum refinery workers	Platinum salts, cobalt, aluminum emissions, stainless steel fumes, nickel salts

Table 32-8	ASTHMA SEVERITY CLASSIFICATION

VARIABLES	MILD	MODERATE	SEVERE
Symptom frequency	<1 hr, 1-2 times/wk	>1-2 times/wk lasting several days, occasional ED visits	Daily signs and symptoms
Activity intolerance	<½ hr of wheezing or cough with activity	Moderate activity intolerance	Marked limitation
Nocturnal asthma	<1-2 times/month	2-3 times/wk	Almost every night
School-work	Attendance rarely affected	Attendance affected	Poor attendance
PEFR	>80% best	60%-80% best	<60% best
	<20% daily variations	20%-30% daily variations	>30% daily variations

ED, Emergency department; *PEFR,* peak expiratory flow rate.

acini, or airways distal to the terminal bronchiole or conducting airway, and 3 million alveoli. Centrilobular emphysema occurs in the center of lobules and corresponds to enlargement of respiratory bronchioles, is associated with chronic bronchitis, rarely occurs in nonsmokers, and involves upper lung fields. Panlobular emphysema is less common, occurs throughout the lung but primarily in lower and anterior fields, has less correlation with smoking, and is more associated with familial α-1 antiprotease deficiency.[9] Entire acini and many bullae (airspaces less than 1 mm in diameter in distended state) are involved. Bullous emphysema is characterized by isolated emphysemic changes in bullae with absence of generalized emphysema.

There is a definite relationship between smoking, chronic bronchitis, and emphysema; however, all smokers do not develop emphysema, so some genetic or familial trait may predispose patients. A small minority of patients have a genetic deficiency of serum α-1 antiprotease, otherwise known as antitrypsin, which inhibits protease that digests proteins such as elastic and collagen fibers of the lung. Protease is present in macrophages and polymorphonuclear leukocytes

released during inflammatory processes. Protease-antiprotease imbalance infection or respiratory irritants such as smoke and pollutants inactivate inhibitors.

The end result is destruction of elastic properties of the lung and loss of natural recoil and support. During expiration, increased intrathoracic pressure causes collapse with premature closure of airways, whereas decreased support of the lung causes large residual volumes and decreased flow rates. Inspiratory rates are normal unless there is airway obstruction from chronic bronchitis, air trapping, and overdistended airspaces. Eventually the area for gas exchange at the alveolar capillary membrane decreases because of destruction of alveolar wall, so $\dot{V}/\dot{Q}$ mismatch occurs with patchy emphysemic changes, increased physiologic dead space, and abnormal arterial blood gases.

Early manifestations include signs of chronic bronchitis but may not be otherwise specific. Dyspnea on exertion occurs first and progresses to dyspnea at rest. Primary emphysema presents with dyspnea without cough or expectoration. The severity of dyspnea does not correlate with severity of destructive changes in the lung. Increasing dyspnea indicates

Table 32-9 COMMON PULMONARY DRUGS

MEDICATION	ACTIONS	STRENGTH/DOSAGE	SIDE EFFECTS/COMMENTS/PRECAUTIONS
BRONCHODILATORS			
Sympathomimetics Epinephrine (Adrenalin)	Stimulates β-receptors for bronchodilation	Epi: 1:100 (1%) neb 0.25-0.5 ml QID or q 20-30 min for 3 doses (0.3 mg/max)	Unwanted SE: tremor, palpitations, increased blood pressure, headache, nervousness, dizziness, and nausea because both α and β are stimulated
Racemic epi (Micronefrin, Asthma nefrin)		Racemic: 2.25% neb; 0.25-0.5 ml	Racemic has ½ cardiac effects of epinephrine. Rapid onset, short duration of action. Monitor for rebound effect 2-4 hours after treatment
Terbutaline (Brethaire, Brethine)	As above	Brethaire MDI 0.2 mg/puff, 2 puffs q 4-6 hr. Brethine SQ 1 mg/ml, 0.1 mg/kg/q 2-6 hr, 0.3 mg max	4-6 hour duration. β-2 specific so less cardiac effects. Peak 30-60 min. Onset 5-15 min
Albuterol (Proventil, Ventolin)	As above	Neb: 0.5%, 2.5-5.0 ml TID/QID. MDI: 90 μg/puff, 2 puff TID/QID. Tab: 2 and 4 mg tabs, 2-4 mg TID/QID. Extended release tabs (Repetabs): 4 mg/tab, q 12 hr. Spinhaler: 200 μg/cap, 1 cap q 4-6 hr	As above
Isoetharine (Bronkosol, Bronkometer)	As above	Neb: 1.0% 0.25-0.5 ml QID. MDI: 340 μg/spray, 1-2 puffs QID	β-2 specific. Short duration of action. Rapid onset. Minimal β-1 or cardiac stimulation
Salmeterol zinafoate (Serevent)	As above	MDI: 35 μg/puff, 1-3 puffs q 12 hr	Not for use in acute bronchospasm and asthma attacks because of long onset of action. Onset 20-30 min. Peak 2-3 hr. Duration 8-12 hr. SE are cough with administration and same as albuterol, especially when given with albuterol for control of acute symptoms
Zanthines	Smooth muscle dilation, CNS stimulation, and cerebral vasoconstriction, vasodilation of periphery and cardiac vessels, cardiac stimulation, and diuresis	Dosage depends on age, previous theophylline therapy, acute or chronic situation. Dosage altered with: *increased serum levels*—barbiturates, calcium channel blockers, cimetidine, zantac, corticosteroids, ephedrine, viral infections, pneumonia; *decreased serum levels*—barbiturates, β-agonist, rifampin, phenytoin, cigarette smoking	Levels: <5 μg/ml—no effects. 10-20 μg/ml—therapeutic range. >20 μg/ml—nausea. >30 μg/ml—cardiac dysrhythmias. >40-45 μg/ml—seizures. Dosages decreased with children, liver failure, and CHF
Theophylline anhydrous (100% theophylline—Theodur, Respbid, Solphyllin, Bronkodyne)	As above	Oral or IV rapid onset load: 5-6 mg/kg. Each 0.5 mg/kg increase will increase serum level by 1 μg/ml	SE: CNS—headache, anxiety, restlessness, dizziness, insomnia, tremor, seizures. GI—abdominal pain, nausea/vomiting, anorexia, diarrhea, GE reflux. Resp—increased respiratory rate

QID, 4 Times a day; *SE*, side effects; *MDI*, metered-dose inhaler; *TID*, 2 times a day; *CNS*, central nervous system; *CHF*, chronic heart failure; *IV*, intravenous; *GI*, gastrointestinal; *CV*, cardiovascular; *SVT*, supraventricular tachycardia; *WBC*, white blood cells; *HPA*, hypothalmic-pituitary-adrenal.

Table 32-9 COMMON PULMONARY DRUGS—cont'd

MEDICATION	ACTIONS	STRENGTH/DOSAGE	SIDE EFFECTS/ COMMENTS/PRECAUTIONS
BRONCHODILATORS—cont'd			
Aminophyline (79% theophylline)		Chronic therapy load: 16 mg/kg per 24 hr or 400 mg/24 hr, whichever is less	CV—palpitations, SVT, ventricular dysrhythmias, hypotension Renal—diuresis (increase hydration to prevent thick secretions) Food/drug interactions: Increased levels with caffeine (tea, cola, chocolate), and char-broiled foods, increased protein and decreased carbohydrate diets
PARASYMPATHOLYTICS/ANTICHOLINERGICS			
Atropine Ipratropium (Atrovent)	Antimuscarinic action: blocks acetylcholine by occupying receptor site and blocks PSNS bronchoconstriction effect, inhibits mast cell release (decreased mucus and chemotaxis), blocks cough receptors	Neb: 0.2% (1 mg/0.5 ml), 0.025 mg/kg TID/QID MDI: 18 μg/puff, 2 puff QID	SE: 0.5 mg—dryness of mouth and eyes 2.0 mg—pupil dilation, increased heart rate, blurred vision 5.0 mg—slurred speech, impaired swallowing and urination, flushed skin >5.0 mg—CNS excitement Onset 15 min Peak ½ to 1 hr for atropine and 1-2 hr for ipratropium Duration 3-4 hr for atropine and 4-6 hr for ipratropium
CORTICOSTEROIDS			
	Decreased inflammation of inflamed epithelial cells in asthma		Systemic SE are related to dose and minimal compared to systemic administration but can occur with >800 μg/day, >400 μg/day in children SE topical under 800 μg/day: oropharyngeal fungal infections, hoarseness, cough, and can be eliminated or reduced with use of spacers and rinsing mouth after each puff Can be used intranasally to prevent allergic rhinitis or decrease signs and symptoms; must be figured into overall total daily dose

Continued

increasing airway obstruction. In advanced stages the patient may have increased anteroposterior (A-P) diameter of the chest, dorsal kyphosis, elevated ribs, flare at the costal margin, and widening of the costal angle; that is, barrel chest. Breath sounds are decreased with expiratory wheezes. Chest radiographs may show depression and flattening of the diaphragm, indicating hyperinflation of lungs.[9] Decreased vascular markings, hyperlucency, deeper space between sternum and heart, and increased A-P diameter may also be present. Pulmonary function tests reveal hyperinflation, increased residual volume, reduced vital capacity, and increased total lung capacity with decreased expiratory flow

rates.[8] Reduction in diffusion capacity differentiates emphysema from asthma or bronchitis. Arterial blood gases are normal in mild cases, with decreased PaO_2 being the most common change; in advanced stages or acute exacerbation $PaCO_2$ is elevated. Chest auscultation usually finds hyperresonance in all fields.

The cause of emphysema is variable and may include annual decline in expiratory flow rates. Progression varies, but increased obstruction correlates with increased severity. ED management includes pulse oximetry, oxygen therapy, bronchodilators, and steroids. Decreased oxygen saturation should be addressed immediately.

Table 32-9 COMMON PULMONARY DRUGS—cont'd

MEDICATION	ACTIONS	STRENGTH/DOSAGE	SIDE EFFECTS/ COMMENTS/PRECAUTIONS
CORTICOSTEROIDS—cont'd			
Inhaled corticosteroids			
Dexamethasone (Decadron Respinhaler)	As above	MDI (μg/puff) AND dose Dexamethasone (84) 3 puffs TID/QID	As above
Beclomethasone (Beclovent, Vanceril)		Beclomethasone, etc—(42) 2 puffs TID/QID	
Triamcinolone (Azmacort)		Triamcinolone (100) 2 puffs TID/QID	
Flunisolide (Aerobid)		Flunisolide (250) 2 puffs TID/QID	
Oral corticosteroids Outpatient: prednisone	As above	Short bursts for 3 days may be all that is needed, >5 days need to taper reduction of doses, 1-2 mg/kg/day in single or divided doses	SE: Increased appetite, mood swings, fluid retention, increased WBC, hypertension (fluid retention), ulcer, gastritis, increased serum glucose
Inpatient: methyl-prednisone		1-2 mg/kg/dose q 6 hr, length depends on severity, dose tapered off	Long-term SE: Osteoporosis, myopathy of striated muscle, cataract formation, immunosuppression, suppression of HPA axis
Antiasthmatics Cromolyn (Intal) Nedocromil (Tilade)	Inhibition of mast cell degranulation—blocks release of chemical mediators of inflammation (can prevent late phase reaction of asthma)	MDI: Cromolyn: 0.8 mg/puff, 2 puffs QID Nedocromil: 1.75 mg/puff, 2 puffs QID Neb: Cromolyn: 20 mg/amp, 1 amp QID	Comes in intranasal, ophthalmic, and oral preparations SE: Minimal, seen mostly with inhaled powder form—cough, bronchospasm **Does not treat acute attacks of bronchospasm** Peak 5-30 min Duration 4-6 hr

Table 32-10 FORMS OF AEROSOLIZED THERAPY[7]

TYPES	DESCRIPTION	INDICATIONS
Nebulizers (ultrasonic, small particle, and small volume)	Drug solution in liquid reservoir chamber is shattered into suspension by aerosol or acoustic energy with varying particle size	Unable to cooperate or is disoriented Incapable of inspiratory hold Reduced tidal volume Tachypneic or unstable respiratory pattern Achieves better distribution of drug to lower airways
MDI	Suspension of drug (micronized powder or liquid) in chlorofluorocarbon liquid propellant (freon)	Able to follow instructions Capable of inspiratory hold Stable respiratory pattern Needs drug available in MDI form Requires timing and coordination of inspiration and delivery of drug
Auxiliary devices	Spacers: Increase vaporization of particles and increase lung penetration, decrease loss of drug in air or mouth, simplify coordination (puff then inhale versus puff and inhale during midpuff with MDI)	Spacers: Increase delivery of drug Decrease coordination requirements with MDI
	Breath actuated devices: Aimed at reducing coordination and grip strength problems (elderly, arthritic)	Breath actuated devices: Reduce coordination and grip strength requirements for use with MDI
Dry powder inhalers	Powdered drug to be inhaled to cause aerosolization of solid particles	Poor MDI coordination Sensitive to CFC propellents in MDI Capable of high inspiratory volumes May cause bronchospasm in hyperreactive airways

MDI, Metered-dose inhaler; *CFC,* chlorofluorocarbon.

Box 32-4 COMMON COUGH AND COLD AGENTS USED WITH ASTHMA MEDICATIONS

ADRENERGIC NASAL DECONGESTANTS

Oral: Phenylephrine (Neosynephrine, Coricidin), pseudoephedrine (Sudafed)
Topical: Oxymetazoline (Afrin)
Cause vasoconstriction
Side effects include increased blood pressure and heart rate, especially with oral preparation
Side effects with topical administration include necrosis of nasal septum with prolonged use—use only during acute episodes and no more than 3 days BID per month

ANTIHISTAMINE DRYING AGENTS

Diphenhydramine (Benadryl)
Clemastine (Tavist)
Promthazine (Phenergan)
Terfenadine (Seldane)
Axtemizole (Hismanal)
Block H1 receptors of bronchopulmonary smooth muscle and blood vessels
Sedative and anticholinergic effects: drowsiness and dryness of mouth and eyes

EXPECTORANTS

Guaifenesin (e.g., Robitussin)
Iodinated glycerol (Organidin)
SSKI (potassium iodide)
Aid in mucus clearing by mucolytic or stimulant action; major use in bronchitis
Iodides associated with hypersensitivity reactions

ANTITUSSIVES

Codeine (e.g., Robitussin AC)
Hydrocodone (Tussionex, Triaminic Expectorant DH)
Dextromethorphan (e.g., Vicks Formula 44D, Robitussin DM)
Control cough; use only with dry hacking cough; do not use with productive cough
Use of products that have cough suppression with expectorant and antihistamine with expectorant is questionable

Table 32-11 NONPRESCRIPTION COMBINATION ASTHMA DRUGS

| | INGREDIENTS | | |
DRUG PRODUCT	SYMPATHOMIMETIC	XANTHINE	OTHER
Amodrine	Ephedrine	Aminophylline	Phenobarbital
Asthma Nefrin inhalant	Epinephrine	—	Chlorobutanol
Bronkaid tablets	Ephedrine	Theophylline	Guaifenesin
Bronkaid mist	Epinephrine	—	Ascorbic acid, alcohol
Bronkotabs	Ephedrine	Theophylline	Guaifenesin, phenobarbital
Primatene M tablets	Ephedrine	Theophylline	Pyrilamine
Primatene P tablets	Ephedrine	Theophylline	Phenobarbital
Primatene Mist	Epinephrine	—	Ascorbic acid, alcohol
Tedral	Ephedrine	Theophylline	Phenobarbital
Vaponefrin inhalant	Epinephrine	—	Chlorobutanol
Verquad	Ephedrine	Theophylline	Guaifenesin, phenobarbital

From Lewis SM, Heitkemper MM, Dirksen SR: *Medical-surgical nursing: assessment and management of clinical problems,* ed 5, St Louis, 2000, Mosby.

COPD

Chronic obstructive pulmonary disease (COPD) is a disease process that is a combination of three other diseases: emphysema, chronic bronchitis, and asthma. Most patients have a combination of emphysema and bronchitis, with asthma involved less in frequency and less in severity. The blends of the two disease processes vary from patient to patient with two types more frequently observed, the "blue bloater" and the "pink puffer."

With the "blue bloater," chronic bronchitis is the more dominant disease process. These patients have increased mucous production and inflammation from bronchitis and

How To Use Your Metered-Dose Inhaler the Right Way

Using an inhaler seems simple, but most patients do not use it the right way. When you use your inhaler the wrong way, less medicine gets to your lungs. (Your doctor may give you other types of inhalers.)

For the next 2 weeks, read these steps aloud as you do them or ask someone to read them to you. Ask your doctor or nurse to check how well you are using your inhaler.

Use your inhaler in one of the three ways pictured below (**A** or **B** is best, but **C** can be used if you have trouble with **A** and **B**).

Steps for Using Your Inhaler

Getting ready
1. Take off the cap and shake the inhaler.
2. Breathe out all the way.
3. Hold your inhaler the way your doctor said (A, B, or C below).

Breathe in slowly
4. As you start breathing in **slowly** through your mouth, press down on the inhaler **one** time. (If you use a holding chamber, first press down on the inhaler. Within 5 sec, begin to breathe in slowly.)
5. Keep breathing in **slowly**, as deeply as you can.

Hold your breath
6. Hold your breath as you count to 10 slowly, if you can.
7. For inhaled quick-relief medicine (β_2-agonists), wait about 1 min between puffs. There is no need to wait between puffs for other medicines.

A. Hold inhaler 1 to 2 in in front of your mouth (about the width of two fingers).

B. Use a spacer/holding chamber. These come in many shapes and can be useful to any patient.

C. Put the inhaler in your mouth. Do not use for steroids.

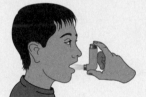 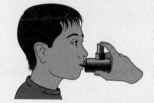 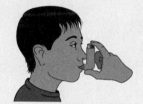

Clean Your Inhaler as Needed

Look at the hole where the medicine sprays out from your inhaler. If you see "powder" in or around the hole, clean the inhaler. Remove the metal canister from the L-shaped plastic mouthpiece. Rinse only the mouthpiece and cap in warm water. Let them dry overnight. In the morning, put the canister back inside. Put the cap on.

Know When to Replace Your Inhaler

For medicines you take each day (an example):
Say your new canister has 200 puffs (number of puffs is listed on canister) and you are told to take 8 puffs per day.

$$8 \text{ puffs per day} \overline{)200 \text{ puffs in canister}} \begin{array}{c} 25 \text{ days} \end{array}$$

So this canister will last 25 days. If you started using this inhaler on May 1, replace it on or before May 25.
You can write the date on your canister.

For quick-relief medicine take as needed and count each puff.

Do not put your canister in water to see if it is empty. This does not work.

FIGURE **32-11** Correct use of a metered-dose inhaler. (From Lewis SM, Heitkemper MM, Dirksen SR: *Medical-surgical nursing: assessment and management of clinical problems,* ed 5, St. Louis, 2000, Mosby.)

---

panlobular emphysema. Decrease in ventilation and increase in cardiac output causes a ventilation perfusion mismatch, which leads to polycythemia and hypoxemia.

Emphysema is the lead disease with the "pink puffer." Alveolar cell destruction decreases oxygen exchange; however, the body compensates with hyperventilation and decreased cardiac output. Unlike the "blue bloater," the end result is highly oxygenated blood with decreased cardiac output. Table 32-12 compares characteristics of these COPD categories.

COPD is the fourth leading cause of death in the United States, with an estimated 32 million people affected by the disease.[3] Cessation of smoking may prevent development of COPD in smokers. Early changes with chronic bronchitis are reversible when limited to small airways. Structural changes with emphysema are not reversible, so further in-

Box 32-5 COMMON MISCONCEPTIONS AND THE REALITY ABOUT ASTHMA

MYTHS AND MISCONCEPTIONS	REALITY
Asthma is an emotional problem, not a physiologic problem.	Asthma is caused by exposure to various triggers.
People with asthma should never exercise.	Activity and exercise is part of the overall plan of care for a patient with asthma.
You can get addicted to asthma medicine.	Asthma medication is *not* addictive.
I don't want to take those steroids because it will make me look like a man.	Inhaled, oral, or IV corticosteroids are *not* the same as anabolic steroids.
The more I use my medicine the less likely it is to work when I need it.	Medication *does not* lose effectiveness with increased or continuous use.
An asthma attack happens without warning.	Episodes can be predicted by identifying triggers and PEFR measurements.

IV, Intravenous; *PEFR,* peak expiratory flow rate.

Table 32-12 CHRONIC OBSTRUCTIVE PULMONARY DISEASE

PINK PUFFER	BLUE BLOATER
PROMINENT DISEASE	
Emphysema	Chronic bronchitis
HISTORY	
Dyspnea for a long period	Productive cough
Cough at late onset	Eventual dyspnea
Minimal to no sputum production	
PHYSICAL ASSESSMENT	
Pursed lip breathing; distant heart sounds; barrel chest; sitting in tripod position; accessory muscle use; wheezing	Cyanotic; symptoms of right heart failure; rhonchi; obese; use of accessory muscles
COURSE OF DISEASE	
Progressive dyspnea	Frequent, recurrent, pulmonary infections
Eventual cachexia	Worsening cough
Respiratory failure	Cardiac or respiratory failure

sults must be avoided. Outpatient management includes avoiding irritants, good bronchial hygiene (adequate hydration, humidification, and postural drainage), bronchodilators, expectorants, and mucolytics. Nebulized therapy is as effective as intermittant positive pressure breathing (IPPB) treatments, whereas anticholinergic bronchodilators may have better results. Corticosteroids are used sparingly, although infections should be treated aggressively. Viral and bacterial infections play a major role in exacerbations of COPD and contribute to disability. Preventive measures include pneumococcal and viral immunizations. Antibacterial prophylaxis may be used for bacteria-prone patients, although resistant organisms have made this practice questionable. Changes in cough and sputum production and characteristics require prompt antibiotic therapy. Proper education, patient compliance, adequate nutrition, and exercise are important parts of therapy. In advanced disease chronic respiratory failure with severe hypoxemia and hypercapnia are present, so serum carbon dioxide levels no longer provide the drive for respiration. Hypoxia, or low serum oxygen, is the drive for respiration. Chronic oxygen delivery is necessary if PaO_2 falls below 55. High-flow oxygen should not be withheld when the patient is in respiratory failure. ED management includes oxygen therapy, nebulized inhalers, bronchodilators, and steroids. Low-flow oxygen may be administered with nasal cannula or venturi mask, which uses entrained air to provide a specific percent of oxygen.

Pulmonary Embolus

Signs and symptoms of pulmonary embolus are frequently confused with those of myocardial infarction, pneumothorax, rib fracture, or other phenomena with the chief complaint of chest pain. Consequently, pulmonary embolus is extremely difficult to diagnose in the emergency setting. Pulmonary embolus is the third leading cause of death in the United States and the most common form of death among hospitalized patients. Each year approximately 400,000 people in the United States have a pulmonary embolus that is not diagnosed.[3]

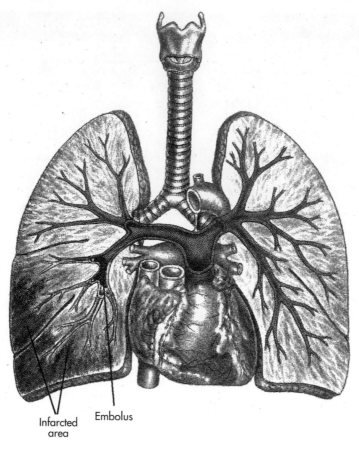

Infarcted   Embolus
area

FIGURE 32-12   Pulmonary embolism. (From Wilson SF, Thompson JM: *Mosby's clinical nursing series: respiratory disorders,* St. Louis, 1990, Mosby.)

Pulmonary embolus commonly results from trauma to the lower extremities or pelvis, surgery, long-bone fractures, or immobility but is seen occasionally with obesity, decreased peripheral circulation, congestive heart failure, or thrombophlebitis. Cardiac diseases such as congestive heart failure or myocardial infarction may cause pulmonary emboli. Pulmonary emboli may also appear in conjunction with acute infections, blood dyscrasias, childbirth (amniotic fluid emboli), scuba diving (air emboli), oral contraceptives, cigarette smoking, neoplasms, and central venous catheter insertion. Administration of IV fluids and blood (particularly autotransfusion) under pressure can lead to air embolus if air is not removed before administration.

The most common source of pulmonary embolism is deep leg veins. Stasis of blood, damage to epithelium of the vessel wall, or alterations in coagulation lead to formation of venous thrombi. The clot is dislodged and travels through the venous system and right side of the heart, finally lodging in a pulmonary vessel, obstructing blood flow and decreasing perfusion to a portion of the lungs (Figure 32-12). Lack of perfusion to an area of the lung with continued respirations leads to a disproportionate amount of blood when compared with oxygen in the bloodstream (i.e., $\dot{V}/\dot{Q}$ mismatch). If the embolism lodges in a large pulmonary vessel, pulmonary vascular resistance increases and cardiac output is decreased. The embolism causes the body to react microscopically by releasing serotonin, histamines, prostaglandins, and catecholamines that trigger bronchospasms and vasoconstriction. The production of surfactant ceases and alveoli collapse.

Pulmonary embolus is usually underdiagnosed. Signs and symptoms of pulmonary embolus can be nonspecific and lead the emergency nurse to think of other reasons for the signs and symptoms. Common signs and symptoms include shortness of breath, tachypnea, tachycardia, and sudden-onset pleuritic chest pain that increases with respirations. The patient may have a cough, hemoptysis (from alveolar damage), diaphoresis, syncope, fever, and crackles. Petechiae (most often seen on the chest) also occur, but are more common with fat emboli. If the embolism occludes a large vessel, symptoms may be more severe and include anxiety, hypotension, and signs of right ventricular failure.

Diagnosis of pulmonary embolism is primarily made from arterial blood gas values and lung scan, high-resolution helical computed tomographic angiography, or pulmonary angiogram. Figure 32-13 shows a lung scan positive for pulmonary embolism. Decreased oxygen pressure and decreased pCO_2 are highly suggestive of pulmonary emboli in the presence of other symptoms. Chest radiographs are obtained but are usually normal. Baseline laboratory studies are com-

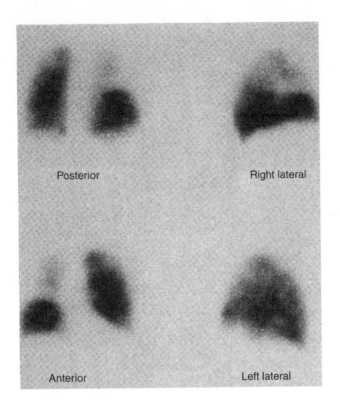

Box 32-6	CARDIOGENIC PULMONARY EDEMA

Inefficient pumping of left ventricle
Fluid pressure increases in left ventricle
Left atrium inhibited from pumping efficiently
Increased alveolar-capillary membrane pressure
Fluid in alveoli

pleted to rule out other sources of respiratory distress. Electrocardiogram changes significant for a pulmonary embolism include new-onset right bundle branch block and right axis deviation with peaked P waves in limb leads and depressed T waves in right precordial leads (V1-3).

Management of the patient with pulmonary embolism includes variable oxygen administration, from low-flow oxygen by nasal cannula to intubation, depending on patient needs. Analgesics may be administered intravenously if the patient is extremely uncomfortable. Intravenous fluids and vasopressors should be used to maintain pressure. Intravenous anticoagulants are initiated to prevent further clot formation. Weight-based heparin protocols are the preferred anticoagulant for these patients. Oral anticoagulants are usually not started in the ED. Fibrinolytic therapy should be started immediately in the unstable patient and should be considered in the ED for any patient with a diagnosed pulmonary embolus. Administration is dependent on the fibrinolytic used.

Pulmonary Edema

Pulmonary edema is not a primary disease process, but rather the result of an acute event. Pulmonary edema may be cardiogenic or noncardiogenic. Cardiogenic pulmonary edema occurs with inadequate left ventricular pumping that leads to increased fluid pressure (Box 32-6). Increased left ventricular pressure inhibits left atrial emptying, so that blood backs up into alveolar-capillary membranes and pulmonary capillary filtration increases. Fluid from the pulmonary circulation floods the alveolar-capillary membrane and fills alveolar spaces normally containing air. The end result is increased fluid in the lungs. Potential causes of cardiogenic pulmonary edema include myocardial infarction and congestive heart failure.

Excessive extracellular fluid volume can result in pulmonary edema as increased pressure at the arterial capillary membranes pushes fluid into surrounding tissues. Fluid shifts across the alveolar-capillary membrane into the alveoli, resulting in pulmonary edema.

Fluid overload inhibits left ventricular pumping so excess fluid backs up into the left atrium with the same effect as cardiogenic pulmonary edema (Figure 32-14). Excessive fluid volume may be caused by increased sodium intake, such as with packaged foods, abuse of tap water enemas, or overload of intravenous fluids high in sodium. Renal disorders and cirrhosis also cause fluid overload.

Noncardiogenic pulmonary edema, or acute respiratory distress syndrome (ARDS), is the result of primary damage to the alveolar-capillary membrane. Loss of integrity increases membrane permeability, which causes fluid and protein accumulation in interstitial spaces that eventually floods the alveoli, causing significant fluid accumulation in the lungs. Figure 32-15 illustrates pathophysiology of ARDS. A multitude of conditions (e.g., trauma, sepsis, fluid overload) predispose patients to ARDS (Box 32-7, p. 446).

Patients with pulmonary edema exhibit cardiovascular and respiratory symptoms. Cardiovascular symptoms result from generalized fluid overload. Poor left ventricular functioning is generally followed by poor right ventricular functioning, which leads to heart failure with engorged neck veins, sacral edema when the patient is sitting with legs not in a dependent position, lower extremity pitting edema, weight gain, rapid, bounding pulse, and S3-S4 heart sounds. If the pulmonary edema is untreated, the pulse eventually becomes weak and thready as the condition worsens. The skin is cool, pale, and moist and may appear cyanotic or mottled in some patients. Blood pressure initially increases in an attempt to pump extra fluid but decreases as the condition worsens.

Respiratory symptoms occur as increased alveolar fluid impairs oxygen exchange across the alveolar-capillary membrane. The patient develops dyspnea, and respiratory rate increases in an effort to increase oxygenation. Increased respiratory rate decreases pCO_2, causing respiratory alkalo-

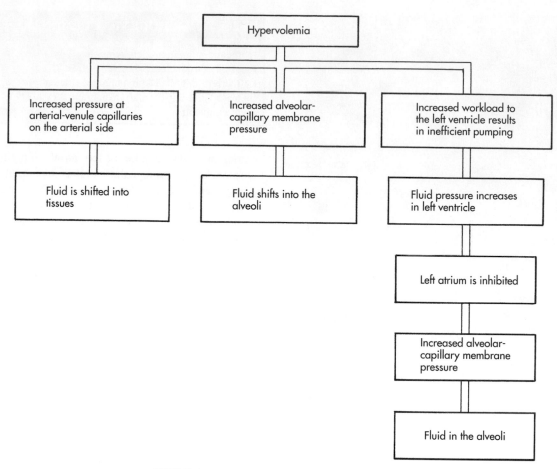

FIGURE 32-14 Hypervolemia and pulmonary edema.

sis. As the condition worsens, metabolic acidosis occurs in an effort to rid the body of metabolic waste products. Respiratory effort becomes labored as the patient tires from the effort of breathing. Fluid causes crackles and productive cough with frothy, white sputum. Sputum has a pink tinge in fulminant pulmonary edema. Cyanosis may be present, and oxygen saturation decreases as hypoxia increases. Bronchospasms may develop, causing wheezing, rales, and rhonchi. Chest radiographs usually show bilateral interstitial and alveolar infiltrates (Figure 32-16). The left ventricular wall is usually enlarged, which gives the heart a water-bottle shape.

Treatment focuses on improving oxygenation through administration of high-flow oxygen (nonrebreather mask or intubation), improving cardiac function, and decreasing cardiac workload. Bronchodilators may be given through aerosol inhalation treatments to decrease bronchospasms. Positive end-expiratory pressure is indicated when hypoxia continues despite aggressive oxygen therapy. Most patients with hypoxemia refractory to maximum ventilation have a poor prognosis because of secondary multiple system organ failure.

Heart rate increases in an attempt to manage excess fluid; however, this leads to decreased filling time and decreased contractility. Digoxin is given via intravenous push to increase contractility and decrease heart rate. Dobutamine is given intravenously to increase contractility and reduce peripheral vascular resistance. Dopamine is indicated for hemodynamically significant hypotension, whereas Nitroprusside is used to decrease afterload by vasodilation. Cardiac workload is also decreased through diuretic therapy (e.g., furosemide, bumetanide) and positioning the patient in high-Fowler's position with legs dependent. Dependent-leg position results in venous distention in lower extremities or pooling of blood, which decreases circulatory volume. Intravenous morphine causes vasodilation, which increases venous pooling and decreases preload—pressure in the left ventricle at end of diastole. Preload is the result of blood volume in the left ventricle. In pulmonary edema, treatment is given to decrease volume so backflow into the atria is decreased and to increase strength of contraction by preventing overstretch of muscle fibers (Starling's law). Nitroglycerin may be administered to increase venous distention and venous pooling, which decrease blood return to the heart.

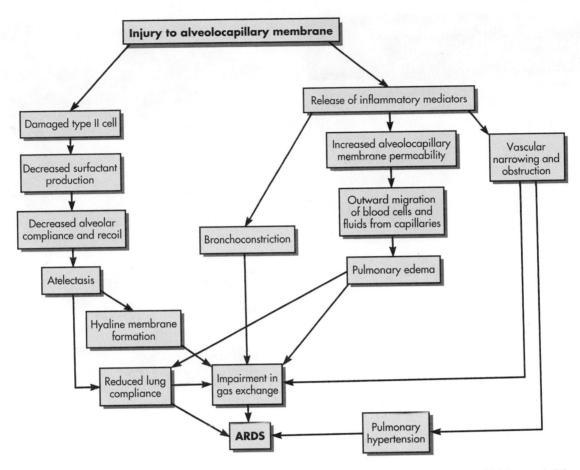

FIGURE 32-15 Pathophysiology of acute respiratory distress syndrome (ARDS). (From Lewis SM, Heitkemper MM, Dirksen SR: *Medical-surgical nursing: assessment and management of clinical problems,* ed 5, St. Louis, 2000, Mosby.)

Other interventions include using a urinary catheter to monitor urine output and effects of diuretics.

Lung Transplants

Lung transplant patients now have longer survival rates, so emergency nurses must have a level of knowledge regarding health problems these patients may experience. The most common complications that drive a lung transplant patient to seek emergency care fall into four categories: pleural space complications, pulmonary parenchymal complications, opportunistic infections, and immunosuppresion-induced complications. Table 32-13 discusses the categories with more specific information. One of the most important facts for a nurse to consider in the ED is that these patients are immunocompromised because of the medications they routinely take. Precautions should be taken to protect these patients from exposure to other disease processes while they are in the ED, including the waiting room.

Nontraumatic Pneumothorax

Primary spontaneous pneumothorax occurs in individuals without underlying pulmonary disease, whereas a secondary spontaneous pneumothorax occurs in those individuals with a history of underlying pulmonary conditions, such as COPD or pulmonary fibrosis. Most frequently, primary spontaneous pneumothorax occurs in males 20 to 40 years of age, but occurring most commonly in men in their twenties. Secondary spontaneous pneumothoraces occur more frequently in older males.[3] Typically, a spontaneous pneumothorax will occur during rest. There is an increased risk for spontaneous pneumothorax in tall individuals and in smokers. With spontaneous pneumothorax the cause is usually rupture of an apical, subpleural emphysematous bleb. An iatrogenic pneumothorax is the result of an invasive procedure such as insertion of a subclavian catheter or transthoracic needle aspiration. However, iatrogenic pneumothorax can also be the result of mechanical ventilation and cardiopulmonary resuscitation.

Patients with a pneumothorax have dyspnea and chest pain on the affected side. Subcutaneous emphysema may be present with cyanosis, hypotension, and severe dyspnea if the pneumothorax is large. Oxygen saturation should be carefully monitored. Interventions are determined by clinical presentation and the degree of collapse. Asymptomatic patients with less than 15% pneumothorax may be observed on an inpatient or outpatient basis. Other treatment options

Box 32-7 CONDITIONS PREDISPOSING TO ACUTE RESPIRATORY DISTRESS SYNDROME

INFECTIOUS CAUSES

Gram-negative sepsis
Bacterial pneumonia
Viral pneumonia
Pneumocystis carinii
Tuberculosis

ASPIRATION

Gastric
Fresh and salt water (drowning)
Ethylene glycol
Hydrocarbon fluids

SHOCK

Septic
Traumatic
Hemorrhagic

TRAUMA

Generalized
Fat embolism
Lung contusion
Multiple major fractures
Head injury
Burns

METABOLIC DISORDERS

Pancreatitis
Uremia
Diabetic ketoacidosis

INHALED TOXIC AGENTS

Oxygen
Smoke
Toxic gases

HEMATOLOGIC DISORDERS

Massive blood transfusion
Disseminated intravascular coagulation
Transfusion reaction
Postcardiopulmonary bypass or resuscitation

IMMUNOLOGIC REACTIONS

Drug allergy
Anaphylaxis

DRUG-RELATED

Dextran 40
Heroin
Methadone
Salicylates
Thiazides
Propoxyphene
Colchicine

OTHER

Radiation pneumonitis
Amniotic fluid emboli
Increased intracranial pressure
High altitude
Fluid overload
Eclampsia
Goodpasture's syndrome
Drug overdose
Bowel infarction
Dead fetus

From Lewis SM, Heitkemper MM, Dirksen SR: *Medical-surgical nursing: assessment and management of clinical problems,* ed 5, St. Louis, 2000, Mosby.

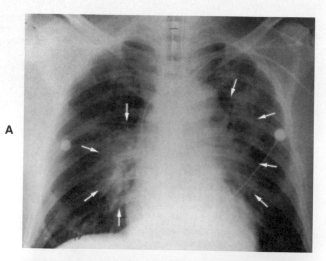

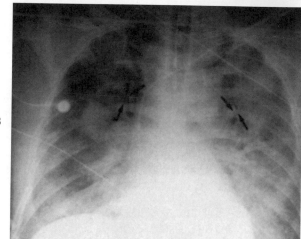

FIGURE 32-16   Pulmonary edema. Pulmonary edema, or fluid overload, can be manifested by indistinctness of the pulmonary vessels as they radiate from the hilum **(A).** This is sometimes termed a "bat wing" infiltrate. As pulmonary edema worsens **(B),** fluid fills the alveoli, and "air bronchograms" *(arrows)* become apparent. (From Mettler FA et al: *Primary care radiology,* Philadelphia, 2000, WB Saunders.)

include needle aspiration and tube thoracostomy. It is important to remember that these individuals are more likely to experience another spontaneous pneumothorax.

Inhalation Injury

Three factors to consider when evaluating a patient with inhalation injury are exposure to asphyxiants (or asphyxiation), thermal or heat injury, and smoke poisoning (or pulmonary irritation). Exposure to asphyxiants is the most frequent cause of early mortality, with carbon monoxide (CO) the most frequent asphyxiant from a fire.

Carbon Monoxide Poisoning

CO affinity for hemoglobin is 200 times greater than for oxygen, resulting in oxygen being displaced from hemoglobin. Without a mechanism for oxygen transport, tissue becomes hypoxic. Carboxyhemoglobin (COHb) levels greater than 10% indicate smoke inhalation; however, smokers or individuals exposed to automobile exhaust can have baseline COHb levels of 10% to 15%. Fetal hemoglobin binds even more quickly with CO, so the fetus is at greater risk for injury from smoke inhalation. As COHb levels increase, symptoms worsen (Table 32-14). Refer to Chapter 41 for additional discussion of CO poisoning.

An additional consideration with CO poisoning is the potential for exposure to other asphyxiants. For example, cyanide can be produced with combustion of wool, silk, paper products, rubber, plastics, and polyurethane. Cyanide

Table 32-13 LUNG TRANSPLANT COMPLICATIONS

COMPLICATION CATEGORY	SPECIFIC COMPLICATION	MOST COMMON TIME FOR OCCURRENCE	SPECIAL CONSIDERATIONS	EMERGENCY DEPARTMENT TREATMENT
Pleural Space	Pneumothorax—may be tension or simple	Early postoperative period		Standard treatment for pneumothorax
	Hemothorax	Early postoperative period	Dependent upon amount of blood loss, may be hypoxic or hypovolemic	Chest tube for drainage and fluid replacement
	Chylothorax	Early postoperative period	Symptoms resemble pleural effusion	Thoracentesis
	Empyema	Middle to late postoperative	May also occur on the nontransplanted side	Thoracentesis with possible chest tube; antibiotics
Pulmonary parenchymal	Acute rejection		May be acute or chronic; may be difficult to identify if in the presence of a superimposed infection	Immunosuppressive therapy should be started immediately
	Pulmonary embolism	Any postoperative phase		Initiate heparin
Opportunistic infections	Bacterial		May be intrapulmonary, such as pneumonia or extrapulmonary with the genitourinary tract being the most common; generally gram-negative rods or gram-positive cocci	Initiation of antibiotics
	Viral-CMV	3 weeks to 4 months postoperatively	Usually mild; can result in pneumonitis or hepatitis	Ganciclovir
	Viral-RSV		Generally more serious than CMV but less frequent occurrence; results in pneumonia	Ribavirin
	Mycotic		Common because of immunosuppression; most common in pulmonary and gastrointestinal systems	Antifungals
	Parasitic		*Pneumocystitis carinii* most common; typically affects the transplanted lung	Antibiotics
Immunosuppression-induced complications	Azathioprine		Depression bone marrow; may present with signs of infection or pancreatitis	
	Corticosteroids		May result in infections or pancreatitis from toxicity	
	Cyclosporine		Nephrotoxic and hepatotoxic	

CMV, Cytomegalovirus; *RSV,* respiratory syncytial virus.

impedes cellular metabolism, causing anaerobic metabolism that in turn causes lactic acidosis and decreased oxygen consumption. Inhalation of cyanide affects the central nervous, respiratory, and cardiovascular systems so clinical presentation is characterized by symptoms related to each system. Treatment in the ED utilizes a cyanide antidote kit containing amyl nitrate, sodium nitrate, and thiosulfate.

Thermal or Heat Injury
Unless the cause of heat injury is from steam, explosive or volatile gases, or hot liquid aspiration, it is rare to have heat injury below the oropharyngeal airway. The respiratory tract's ability to efficiently exchange heat, combined with closure of the glottis, protects lower airways from extreme heat. Extreme heat on the upper airway initially causes erythema, edema, and blisters of the mucosa. Within the first 24 to 48 hours after injury, the airway can become obstructed from increasing mucosal edema.

Smoke Poisoning
Smoke poisoning refers to inhalation of toxic gases, such as hydrogen chloride, phosgene, ammonia, and sulfur dioxide.

Table 32-14	COHB LEVELS AND SYMPTOMS
COHB LEVELS	**SYMPTOMS**
5%-10%	Can be asymptomatic or have mild headache, vertigo
10%-20%	Headache, nausea, vomiting, loss of coordination, may appear flushed, dyspnea
20%-30%	Confusion, lethargy, ST depression, visual disturbances
40%-60%	Coma, seizures, ectopy
60%	Death

Table 32-15	AGE-RELATED RISK FACTORS IN DROWNING AND NEAR-DROWNING
AGE-GROUP	**RISK FACTORS**
Children	Lack of supervision, abuse, neglect, inability to swim, no recognition of dangers of rivers and lakes
Adolescents	Risk-taking, peer pressure, poor swimming skills, alcohol consumption, no recognition of dangers of rivers and lakes, underlying medical conditions such as seizures
Adults	Risk-taking, alcohol consumption, poor swimming skills, underlying medical conditions

These toxins damage pulmonary endothelial cells and destroy epithelial cilia, leading to mucosal edema. Surfactant production decreases, followed by atelectasis. Clinically the patient develops pulmonary edema, usually within 24 to 48 hours of the initial injury. Clinical interventions focus on presenting symptoms and include humidified oxygen, vigorous pulmonary toilet, and bronchodilators. Intubation and mechanical ventilation are indicated if severe pulmonary edema occurs.

Obtaining a careful history is essential when caring for the patient with potential inhalation injury. It is important to know if the fire occurred in an enclosed space, how long the patient was exposed, and the elements in the environment. The patient's medical history is also important because mortality increases with physical and cognitive disabilities and with age. Patients with carbonaceous sputum, singed facial or nasal hair, or burns of the neck or face should be carefully evaluated for inhalation injury. Hoarseness, wheezing, dyspnea, and restlessness may also be present. Early ventilation is recommended.

Initial interventions are directed toward protecting and maintaining a patent airway and supporting the patient's hemodynamic status. A secure airway and oxygen administration are important in all patients with an inhalation injury or the possibility of an inhalation injury. COHb half-life is 320 minutes with room air but can be decreased to 90 minutes with administration of 100% oxygen and 23 minutes in a hyperbaric chamber. Studies exist that investigate the use of surfactant instillation and aerosolized deferoxamine with inhalation injury.

Submersion Injury

Submersion-related injuries are the third leading cause of accidental death in the United States; approximately 8000 people die from drowning each year. The highest incidence occurs in toddlers younger than 4 years of age and young adults 15 to 24 years of age.[3] Risk factors associated with drowning and near-drowning include alcohol, poor swimming skills, and hypothermia. Table 32-15 identifies risk factors associated with various age groups.

The significant physiologic effect of drowning is hypoxemia from laryngospasm. In some individuals the state of asphyxiation results in relaxation of the airway allowing water to enter the lungs. This is referred to as wet drowning. In approximately 10% to 20% of patients, the airway does not relax but remains in laryngospasm until cardiac arrest and cessation of respiratory attempts. This prohibits aspiration of water and is referred to as dry drowning.

Freshwater and salt water drowning both lead to profound hypoxia, the cause of death in all drowning victims. Aspiration of water floods alveoli and impairs gas exchange because of a loss of surfactant. Pulmonary injury is worsened by contaminants such as chlorine, algae, sand, and mud.

Clinically, patients can have respiratory distress, bronchospasm, loss of consciousness, pulmonary edema (cardiogenic and noncardiogenic), hypothermia, poor perfusion, hypotension, dysrhythmias, metabolic acidosis, electrolyte abnormalities, and associated injuries such as spinal cord damage. Spinal cord injuries are more common in adolescents and young adults injured when diving or falling head first into water. Outcome is determined by age, length of submersion, type of fluid, fluid temperature, and associated injuries. Submersion injury in cold, icy waters is associated with better neurologic recovery. In young children cold water submersion creates a response known as the mammalian diving reflex. Bradycardia, apnea, and vasoconstriction occur when cold submersion causes shunting of blood and oxygen to the coronary and cerebral vasculature. With submersion injuries the earlier the victim regains consciousness, the greater the likelihood of return to prior level of function. Most patients who are alert and conscious on arrival survive without neurologic deficits.

ED management involves maintaining a patent airway and stabilizing the cervical spine. Supplemental oxygen should be administered and oxygenation and ventilatory status assessed. Intubation and mechanical ventilation are indicated when supplemental oxygen cannot maintain adequate oxygen saturation. Hypothermic patients should be warmed slowly. Fluid resuscitation with isotonic solutions may be indicated for noncardiogenic pulmonary edema. Diagnostic studies include CBC, electrolyte measurements, arterial blood gas values, and chest radiographs. A nasogastric tube is inserted to decompress the stomach and minimize risk of aspiration; a urinary catheter is used to monitor output and volume status. Diuretic therapy, intracranial pressure monitoring, and neuromuscular paralyzing agents may be indicated for some patients. Prophylactic antibiotics and steroids are not recommended. Refer to Chapter 41 for additional discussion of submersion injuries.

SUMMARY

Respiratory emergencies may be subtle or obvious. The ability to manage obvious cases of respiratory distress and to identify subtle cases of impending respiratory crisis is a hallmark of an effective emergency nurse. Without essential interventions, respiratory emergencies can progress to respiratory arrest and death. Box 32-8 identifies nursing diagnoses applicable to patients with a respiratory emergency.

Box 32-8	NURSING DIAGNOSES FOR RESPIRATORY EMERGENCIES

Airway clearance, Ineffective
Fluid volume, Excessive
Gas exchange, Impaired
Tissue perfusion, Altered

References

1. Black JM, Matassarin-Jacobe E, editors: *Medical-surgical nursing: clinical management for continuity of care,* ed 5, Philadelphia, 1997, WB Saunders.
2. Davis MA, Votey SR, Greenough PG, editors: *Signs & symptoms in emergency medicine,* St. Louis, 1999, Mosby.
3. Emedicine: *Instant access to the minds of medicine,* (Retrieved February 13, 2002 from the World Wide Web: http://www.emedicine.com.
4. Guyton AC, Hall GE: *Textbook of medical physiology,* ed 10, Philadelphia, 2000, WB Saunders.
5. Jordan KS, editor: *Emergency nursing core curriculum,* ed 5, Philadelphia, 2000, WB Saunders.
6. Lewis SM, Heitkemper MM, Dirksen SR: *Medical-surgical nursing: assessment and management of clinical problems,* ed 5, St. Louis, 2000, Mosby.
7. National Asthma Education and Prevention Program: *Guidelines for the diagnosis and management of asthma: expert panel report 2,* Bethesda, 1997, National Institutes of Health.
8. *Nursing 2000 drug handbook,* ed 20, Springhouse, Pa, 2000, Springhouse Publications.
9. Siberry GK, Iannone R, editors: *The Harriet Lane handbook,* ed 15, St. Louis, 2000, Mosby.

Suggested Reading

Demling RH: Smoke inhalation injury. In Shoemaker W, Ayres S, Grenvik A et al: *Textbook of critical care,* ed 4, Philadelphia, 2000, WB Saunders.

Goodwin S, Boysen P, Modell J: Near drowning: adults and children. In Shoemaker W, Ayres S, Grenvik A et al: *Textbook of critical care,* ed 4, Philadelphia, 2000, WB Saunders.

Scanlon C et al: *Egan's fundamentals of respiratory care,* ed 7, St. Louis, 1999, Mosby.

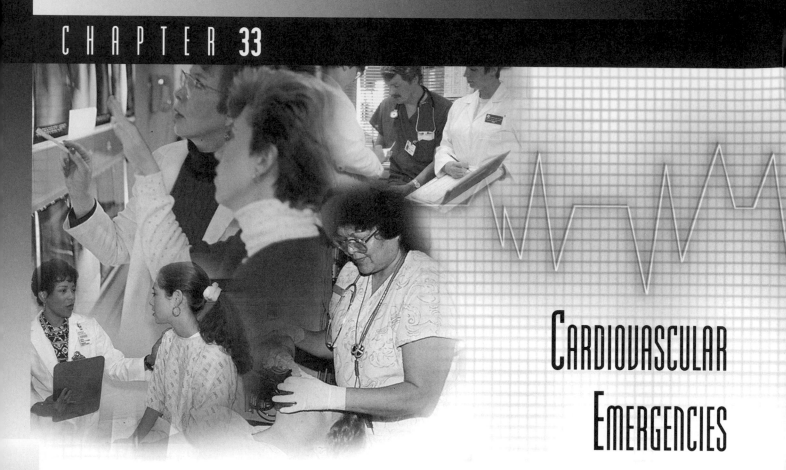

CHAPTER 33

CARDIOVASCULAR EMERGENCIES

SUSAN BARNASON

Cardiovascular emergencies affect the heart and great vessels. The event may be subtle or obvious, caused by progressive disease development or a sudden traumatic event. Emergencies secondary to trauma are described in Chapter 23. Cardiovascular emergencies in children are discussed in Chapter 48. This chapter describes cardiovascular emergencies caused by progressive disease development or a sudden nontraumatic cardiac event.

CARDIAC ANATOMY AND PHYSIOLOGY

The heart is a four-chambered, muscular structure with valves between each chamber to prevent back flow with pumping action of the heart (Figure 33-1). The heart works in synchrony as a two-pump system. Deoxygenated blood from the venous system enters the right atrium through the inferior and superior vena cavae. Blood is pumped from the right ventricle into the pulmonary vasculature. After oxygenation, blood returns to the left atrium via the pulmonary veins. The left ventricle then pumps blood to the body via the arterial system. Figure 33-2 illustrates blood flow through the heart. The left side of the heart is the stronger side, with the ability to pump 4 to 8 L of blood per minute. Oxygenation of the heart muscle is provided by blood from the right and left coronary arteries. Arteries arise from the right and left sinuses of Valsalva of the aortic valve. Coronary arteries lie on the surface of the heart and fill during ventricular diastole.[21]

The heart is surrounded by a fibrous, fluid-filled sac called the pericardium. Pericardial fluid lubricates the heart and prevents friction with contraction. The heart is divided into three distinct layers, the epicardium, myocardium, and endocardium. Epicardium serves as the visceral surface of the pericardium. Myocardium, the thickest portion of the heart, is composed of concentric rings of muscle fibers. Contraction of concentric rings facilitates blood flow up and out of the ventricles. The endocardial layer is a smooth tissue that is the inner layer of the atria and ventricles. Endocardium also functions as the surface of the heart valves.

One of the unique characteristics of cardiac tissue is automaticity or intrinsic ability to initiate electrical activity. Figure 33-3 shows the heart's electrical conduction system. The sinoatrial (SA) node has the highest rate of automaticity, spontaneously depolarizing 60 to 100 times per minute. Impulses generated by the SA node are carried to the atrioventricular (AV) node by intraatrial tracts; that is, Bachmann, Bundle, Wenckebach's, and Thorel's tracts. Electrical stimulation of heart muscle at the level of the atria causes the mechanical event of atrial contraction. At the AV node, slight delay in impulse transmission allows completion of atrial contraction before ventricular stimulation. From the AV node, the electrical impulse is carried to the ventricles by the right and left bundle branches of the His bundle. Bundles terminate with Purkinje fibers, which deliver the impulse to the ventricular muscle, causing ventricular contraction.[27]

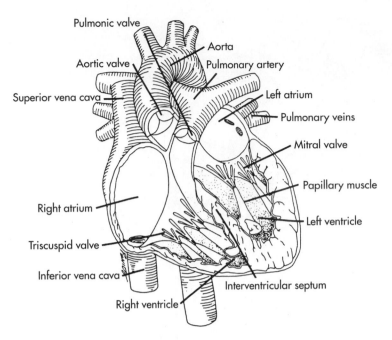

FIGURE 33-1 Anatomy of the heart. (From Lounsberry P, Frye SJ: *Cardiac rhythm disorders: a nursing process approach*, ed 2, St. Louis, 1992, Mosby.)

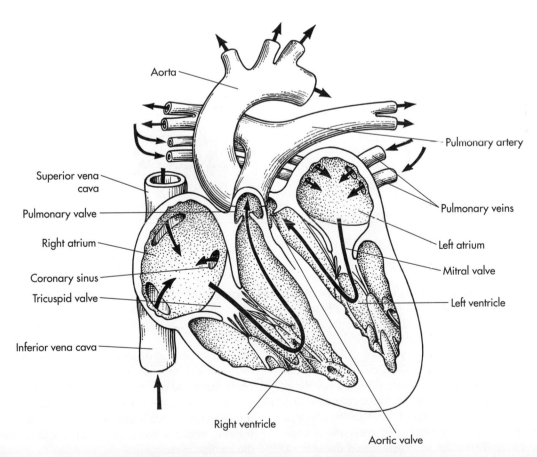

FIGURE 33-2 Circulation of blood through the heart. Arrows indicate direction of flow. (From Atkinson LJ, Fortunato NM: *Berry & Kohn's operating room technique*, ed 8, St. Louis, 1996, Mosby.)

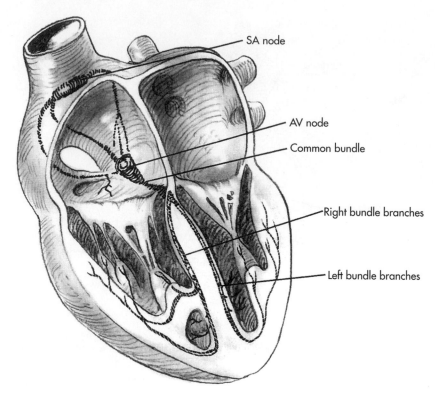

FIGURE **33-3** Conduction system of the heart. (From Davis JH, Drucker WR et al: *Clinical surgery,* vol 1, St. Louis, 1987, Mosby.)

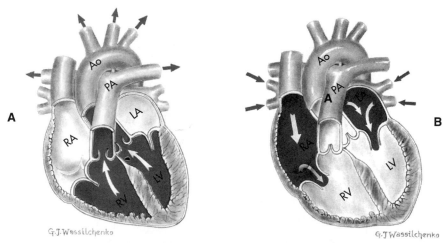

FIGURE **33-4** Blood flow during (**A**) systole, and (**B**) diastole. (From Canobbio MM: *Mosby's clinical nursing series, cardiovascular disorders,* vol 1, St. Louis, 1990, Mosby.)

Mechanical events of the cardiac cycle are called diastole and systole. Approximately 60% of the cardiac cycle is diastole, the time when the ventricles are filling. Diastole is also the time when aortic and pulmonic valves close. Mitral and tricuspid valves open during this time. Electrically, this corresponds to electrical stimulation and mechanical contraction of the atria. With atrial contraction and opening of AV valves, pressure in the atria is higher than pressure in the ventricles.[9] Therefore blood flows from an area of greater pressure to an area of lesser pressure (Figure 33-4). The systolic phase of the cardiac cycle corresponds with ventricular contraction and opening of pulmonic and aortic valves. During contraction, AV valves close and chordae tendineae contract to prevent regurgitation. Figure 33-5 depicts the relationship between electrical and mechanical components of the cardiac cycle.

Pressures within the cardiovascular system affect cardiac output because of the effect on preload and afterload. After-

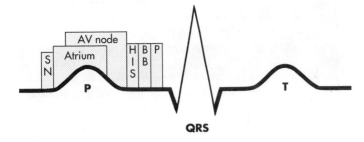

QRS

FIGURE 33-5 Schematic drawing of cardiac activation related to the surface ECG. The timing of activation of the components of the conduction system is superimposed on the surface ECG. *SN,* Sinus node; *HIS,* common bundle of HIS; *BB,* bundle branches; *P,* Purkinje network; *ECG,* electrocardiogram. (From Lounsberry P, Frye SJ: *Cardiac rhythm disorders; a nursing process approach,* ed 2, St. Louis, 1992, Mosby.)

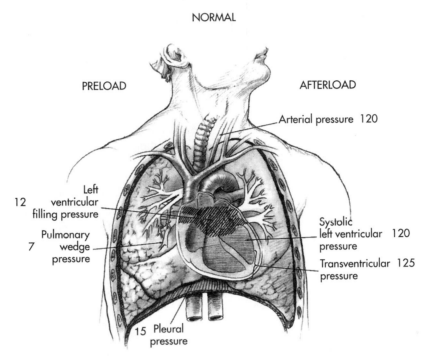

FIGURE 33-6 The effects of normal pleural pressure on cardiac filling pressure. (From Davis JH, Drucker WR et al: *Clinical surgery,* vol 1, St. Louis, 1987, Mosby.)

load refers to pressure in the arterial system, which opposes blood flow from the left ventricle. Preload refers to blood volume coming into the right side of the heart [21] Figure 33-6 illustrates the effect of these pressures on cardiac filling.

Cardiac activity is regulated by branches of the autonomic nervous system. Specific effects of each branch are described in Table 33-1. Receptors in the heart and great vessels respond to signals from the sympathetic nervous system (Table 33-2). Stimulation affects heart rate, contractility, automaticity, conduction, and vascular smooth muscle. These receptors prepare the body to fight or flee perceived threats, including loss of blood volume.

SPECIFIC CARDIOVASCULAR EMERGENCIES

Specific emergencies discussed are cardiac arrest, acute coronary syndromes, dysrhythmias, heart failure, acute pericarditis, abdominal aortic aneurysm, and hypertensive crisis.

Cardiac Arrest

Sudden cardiac arrest can be defined as nontraumatic death resulting from cardiac causes that occurs within 1 hour of onset of acute symptoms.[16,36] More than 600 people experience sudden cardiac death daily, or an annual rate of approximately 365,000, which represents more than 50% of all cardiovascular deaths.[3,16] Common causes of sudden cardiac arrest are ventricular tachycardia (VT) and ventricular fibrillation (VF). These lethal dysrhythmias are usually a late complication of myocardial infarction, but they may also be associated with aneurysm rupture, cardiomyopathies, rheumatic heart disease, mitral valve prolapse, and cardiac surgery. Sudden cardiac arrest can also be associated with other conditions or events. Table 33-3 presents etiologic factors associated with other causes of cardiopulmonary arrest.

In patients ages 18 to 35 years, approximately 23% of sudden cardiac deaths are related to coronary artery disease.[23]

Table 33-1 PARASYMPATHETIC AND SYMPATHETIC STIMULATION OF THE HEART		
NERVE ACTIVATION	**CARDIAC EFFECT**	**CLINICAL MANIFESTATIONS**
Parasympathetic	Slows SA node discharge	Symptomatic bradycardia
	Slows AV node conduction and increases refractoriness	Transient heart block
Sympathetic	Heart rate increases	Tachycardia
	Enhances AV node function	Hypertension
	Shortens His-Purkinje and ventricular muscle refractoriness	Increased cardiac output
	Increased ventricular contraction	
	Increased peripheral vascular resistance	

SA, Sinoatrial; *AV,* atrioventricular.

Table 33-2 SYMPATHETIC NERVOUS SYSTEM RECEPTORS		
SYMPATHETIC RECEPTOR	**LOCATION**	**CLINICAL RESPONSE**
α	Vascular smooth muscle	Vasoconstriction
β-1	Myocardium	Increased heart rate, contraction, automaticity, and conduction
β-2	Peripheral vasculature and lungs	Vasodilation of peripheral vasculature and bronchodilation
Dopaminergic	Renal, mesenteric, cerebral, and coronary arteries	Vasodilation

Another condition associated with death among young adults is hypertrophic cardiomyopathy, which causes left ventricular outflow obstruction or myocardial ischemia secondary to small intramural vessels, and may potentiate lethal dysrhythmias. Other etiologic factors associated with sudden cardiac arrest[6] in the young include congenital coronary artery anomalies, myocarditis, idiopathic concentric left ventricular hypertrophy, Marfan's syndrome, mitral valve prolapse, aortic stenosis, idiopathic long QT syndrome, and miscellaneous causes (e.g., Wolff-Parkinson-White syndrome, high-risk behaviors inclusive of alcohol and drug use—cocaine, tricyclic agents, heroin, anabolic steroids).

Among people 30 years of age and older, an estimated 20% to 30% of sudden cardiac deaths are secondary to acute myocardial infarction causing pump failure.[16] Immediate interventions include establishing an airway, supporting oxygenation, and providing circulation with chest compressions. Airway management and oxygenation are discussed in greater detail in Chapter 32. Circulation for the pulseless patient is produced with chest compressions. Properly performed chest compressions can produce 30% of the patient's normal cardiac output, which is enough blood flow through the heart and brain to sustain tissue viability for a short time. Cerebral blood flow must be at least 50% of normal volume to maintain consciousness.[6]

Chest compressions are best accomplished with the victim on a firm surface to allow even compression of the thoracic cavity. Compressions should be forceful enough to generate a carotid or femoral pulse. Mechanical chest compression devices should be an adjunct to manual chest compressions and used only by trained personnel in limited situations, for example, reducing rescuer fatigue in prolonged resuscitation efforts. The most common mechanical compression device is the compressed gas-powered plunger mounted on a backboard. During use of such devices, remember to place the plunger in the correct location over the sternum to provide maximum cardiac output and minimize adverse events, for example, fractured ribs. Another mechanical device reported in the literature is a cardiopulmonary resuscitation (CPR) vest; however, use of this device is still considered investigational.[4,10]

Open thoracotomy and cardiac massage may be required in cases of penetrating wounds to the heart, penetrating abdominal trauma with deterioration and arrest, pericardial tamponade, tension pneumothorax, or crushing chest injuries. This technique may also be used for patients with chronic lung disease who have a barrel chest when other more conservative measures for chest compression have failed. Studies have demonstrated that direct cardiac chest massage provides better hemodynamics than closed chest compressions; however, this procedure must be performed within 15 minutes of arrest to be effective.

Defibrillation

Advanced cardiac life support measures implemented in the emergency department (ED) augment basic life support measures with administration of drugs, fluids, and defibrillation. Restoring normal circulation for the patient who has experienced sudden cardiac arrest or cardiopulmonary arrest requires vigilance to restore or stabilize cardiac rhythm. If the patient has VF or pulseless VT, the intervention of choice is immediate defibrillation. For defibrillation to be effective, an electric current sufficient to depolarize a critical portion of the left ventricle must pass through the heart. When treating VF and pulseless VT in adults, up to three countershocks should be rapidly delivered, the first at 200 joule (J), the second at 200 to 300 J, and the third at 360 J. Check the pulse and ECG rhythm between shocks to determine if defibrillation has been effective.

Table 33-3	DIFFERENTIAL DIAGNOSIS OF CARDIOPULMONARY ARREST*			
CAUSES	SPECIFIC CAUSE	SIGNS AND SYMPTOMS	THERAPEUTIC INTERVENTION	NOTES
Metabolic	Hypoglycemia	Physical signs of insulin or oral hypoglycemic agent usage; tachydysrhythmias; seizures; aspiration	Dextrose, 50%	Consider hypoglycemia a strong possibility in patients who have a history of diabetes
	Hyperkalemia	ECG Prolonged QT interval; peaked T waves; loss of P waves; wide QRS complexes	Calcium chloride; sodium bicarbonate	Often seen in hemodialysis and renal failure patients; also seen in patients taking spironolactone (Aldactone)
Drug-induced	Tricyclic antidepressants amitriptyline (Elavil), amitriptyline and perphenazine (Etrafon, Triavil), imipramine (Tofranil), doxepin (Sinequan), protriptyline (Vivactil)	Tachydysrhythmias	Sodium bicarbonate; physostigmine (however, efficacy has been questioned)	Causes direct cardiac toxicity; often delayed toxicity in adults
	Narcotics	Bradydysrhythmias; heart blocks	Naloxone (Narcan)	There is a question of direct cardiac toxicity
	Propranolol	Cardiac Heart blocks; bradydysrhythmias; PVCs	Atropine	PVCs may be caused by slow rate
		Respiratory Bronchospasm	Aminophylline	
		Metabolic Hypoglycemia	Dextrose, 50%	
Pulmonary (any disease causing severe hypoxia)	Asthma	Severe bronchospasm causing hypoxia and respiratory acidosis ECG Tachydysrhythmias (especially ventricular fibrillation)	Endotracheal intubation and ventilatory support	Abuse of sympathomimetic inhalants
	Pulmonary embolus	Pleuritic chest pain; shortness of breath in high-risk patients (postoperative, those taking birth control pills); syncope (recent study shows 60% have syncope as part of initial complaint; tachydysrhythmias	Good ventilatory support; consider fibrinolytic agents	Pathophysiology; acute hypoxia and cor pulmonale leading to tachydysrhythmias
	Tension pneumothorax	Distended neck veins; tracheal deviation; asymmetric chest expansion ECG Often electrical mechanical dissociation	Needle thoracotomy; chest tube	Often seen in patients with blunt chest trauma; often occurs during CPR because of chest compressions (especially in patients with COPD)

ECG, Electrocardiogram; *PVC,* premature ventricular contraction; *COPD,* chronic obstructive pulmonary disease; *IV,* intravenous; *CPR,* cardiopulmonary resuscitation.

*Many causes of cardiopulmonary arrest exist other than primary cardiac abnormalities. It is important for the nurse or rescuer to be familiar with these causes and to be alert to their signs and symptoms, as identification of these may modify the type of therapeutic intervention given. This table lists some of the conditions that may lead to cardiopulmonary arrest but are not primary cardiac abnormalities. All therapeutic interventions listed are in addition to basic and advanced cardiac life support measures.

SPECIAL NOTE FOR PREHOSPITAL CARE: Consider early transport for young patients in cardiac arrest, since definitive therapeutic intervention will most likely include procedures not performed in the field.

Continued

Table 33-3	DIFFERENTIAL DIAGNOSIS OF CARDIOPULMONARY ARREST—cont'd			
CAUSES	SPECIFIC CAUSE	SIGNS AND SYMPTOMS	THERAPEUTIC INTERVENTION	NOTES
Neurogenic	Increased intracranial pressure from any cause (e.g., subarachnoid hemorrhage; subdural hematoma)	Central neurogenic breathing; dilated pupil(s); decerebrate/decorticate posturing ECG Wide range of dysrhythmias, especially heart blocks	Central neurogenic hyperventilation (causes respiratory alkalosis, which results in cerebral vasoconstriction); steroids; diuretic agents; surgery	Damage to brainstem and autonomic centers
Hypovolemic	Anything that causes volume loss such as gastrointestinal bleeding, severe trauma with organ damage, ruptured ectopic pregnancy, dissecting or leading aneurysm	Tachycardia; decreasing blood pressure; skin cool, clammy, pale; obvious signs of external blood loss	IV fluids; shock position; surgery	A major cause of cardiopulmonary arrest that may be unrecognized
Other cardiac causes	Pericardial tamponade	Distended neck veins; decreasing blood pressure; distant heart sounds, widening pulse pressure ECG Electromechanical dissociation of bradydysrhythmias	IV fluids: Atropine; isoproterenol; pericardiocentesis; thoracotomy	Look for it, especially in patients with blunt chest trauma or prolonged CPR efforts

When preparing to defibrillate, make sure the machine has a charged battery or is plugged into an electrical outlet. Turn the machine on and select "defib" or "unsynchronized" mode. Select the energy level and prepare defibrillation paddle electrodes by applying conducting gel or by placing defibrillation pregelled patches on the patient's chest. Saline-soaked gauze pads may be used if other conductive media are not available, but these are not ideal conductors. Most commonly, anterolateral paddle placement (Figure 33-7) is used; however, anteroposterior paddle placement may also be used. To defibrillate, apply firm pressure, ensure the area around the patient is clear of personnel and electrical equipment, then discharge the paddles by depressing discharge buttons simultaneously.

An alternative to manually defibrillating the patient is automated external defibrillation (AED). The AED uses two large adhesive patches placed on the patient's chest in the anterolateral position. These patches serve as electrodes to monitor the rhythm and to deliver countershocks. Some AEDs are considered fully automated because they analyze the electrocardiogram (ECG) rhythm, determine rhythm lethality (e.g., VF, VT), charge, and deliver countershocks as appropriate. These AEDs are found in public areas for use by lay people in the event of an emergency. Other AEDs are considered semiautomated or shock-advisory defibrillators. These devices monitor the rhythm, but require the user to interpret the rhythm, charge the defibrillator, and discharge the countershock. Both types provide "hands-free" defibrillation. All personnel should be clear of the patient when the countershock is delivered; however, a bag-valve-mask can

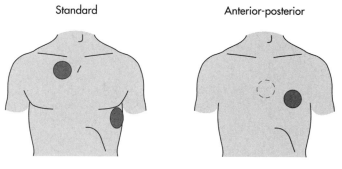

Defibrillator electrode placement

Standard   Anterior-posterior

FIGURE 33-7   Standard and anterior-posterior electrode placement for defibrillation. (From Rosen R, Barkin R: *Emergency medicine: concepts and clinical practice,* ed 4, St. Louis, 1998, Mosby.)

be safely used during defibrillation, as long as the rescuer touches only the bag. Compressions are stopped while the patient is defibrillated. Some AEDs have a minimum energy level of 200 J. This level of energy is contraindicated in patients who weigh less than 90 lb. Other AEDs allow the user to program the energy level appropriate for the size of the patient. When transporting a patient, the AED should be in the semiautomatic mode so that inappropriate discharge of energy does not occur if the AED interprets motion artifact as VF or VT.[10]

Internal defibrillation during open cardiac massage requires internal paddles. Follow the same set-up procedure as

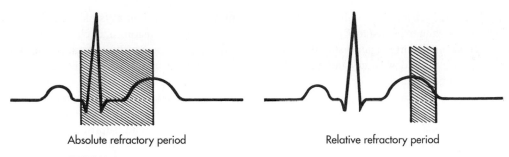

FIGURE 33-8   Absolute and relative refractory periods on the electrocardiogram.

external defibrillation. Apply sterile saline solution to sterile gauze sponges placed over internal defibrillation paddles. The energy level for defibrillation is usually 10 to 50 J for adults.

Successful defibrillation depends on the metabolic state of the heart and decreasing resistance (thoracic impedance) to the countershock.[10] Improved effectiveness of defibrillation can be accomplished with appropriately sized defibrillator paddle or patch electrodes (8 to 12 cm for adults), appropriate placement of defibrillator paddles or patches, and good interface between the defibrillator paddle or patches and the patient's chest wall. In addition, if using paddles, the amount of electrode-chest contact pressure (minimum of 11 kg or 25 pounds of pressure recommended) when using defibrillator paddles improves defibrillation effectiveness.

Cardioversion

Synchronized cardioversion is used when the patient becomes hemodynamically unstable or pharmacologic intervention has been unsuccessful in management of sustained ventricular tachycardia, paroxysmal supraventricular tachycardia, and atrial fibrillation or atrial flutter. In synchronized cardioversion, energy is delivered to the heart during the absolute refractory period, which occurs a fraction of a second after the QRS (ventricular depolarization). Synchronized cardioversion decreases potential energy delivery during the vulnerable period of repolarization; that is, the T wave of the ECG (Figure 33-8).

The procedure for cardioversion is the same as defibrillation with two specific exceptions. The machine must be set on synchronous mode and sedation may be given for the conscious patient. Sedatives such as diazepam (Valium) or midazolam (Versed) are administered slowly via intravenous (IV) push in small, incremental doses. Explain the procedure to the patient and obtain informed consent when possible. Check serum potassium; hypokalemia predisposes the heart to ventricular fibrillation. If the procedure is elective, ask the patient to empty his or her bladder and remove dentures before the procedure. A baseline 12-lead ECG is obtained before the procedure. After cardioversion, monitor vital signs, level of consciousness, and cardiac rhythm frequently until the patient is hemodynamically stable and returns to the preintervention level of consciousness. Complications of cardioversion include asystole, junctional rhythms, premature ventricular contractions, ventricular

tachycardia, ventricular fibrillation, embolization, and return to atrial fibrillation or atrial flutter.

Another method to cardiovert a patient's rhythm is through manual stimulation of the vagus nerve by a Valsalva maneuver, retching or emesis, or carotid sinus massage. Ocular pressure and application of ice water to the patient's face are no longer recommended for vagal stimulation.

Carotid sinus massage is accomplished by placing pressure on the carotid bodies, which stimulates the baroreceptors and therefore the parasympathetic branch of the autonomic nervous system. Stimulation decreases blood pressure and heart rate. The patient should be supine with oxygen supplied at 4 to 6 L/min via nasal cannula. A patent IV line and ECG monitor should be present before the procedure. The physician auscultates the carotid arteries for bruits. Bruits are produced by turbulent flow through the carotid arteries and suggest presence of atherosclerotic plaque, which could break off if manipulated and cause a stroke. If a bruit is auscultated, carotid massage is not performed on that artery.

Start carotid massage with the right carotid sinus. In more than 75% of the population, preferential massage of the right carotid body affects the SA node, whereas left carotid body massage affects the AV node. Even when the SA node is completely shut down, the AV node can provide pacemaker activity. If the left side is massaged first, complete block of the AV node may occur and lead to slow ventricular rate. Pressure is applied gently to the carotid artery just below the mandible in small, circular motions, rotating the fingers backward and medially. Carotid massage should not exceed 5 to 10 seconds and should be discontinued sooner if the rhythm changes. Even when properly performed, carotid massage may cause asystole for 15 to 30 seconds, followed by a few idioventricular complexes before a new pacemaker site becomes active. Emergency equipment and medications should always be available whenever carotid massage is performed. If carotid massage is successful, monitor the patient continuously for several hours after the procedure. Complications of carotid massage include further dysrhythmias (e.g., ventricular tachycardia, ventricular fibrillation, asystole), cerebral occlusion that leads to stroke, cerebral anoxia, and seizures.[6]

Fluids

Use of IV fluids in sudden cardiac arrest or cardiopulmonary arrest must be guided by suspected etiology of arrest and patient response to fluids. Expansion of circulating volume is needed when there has been unexpected loss of blood volume (e.g., ruptured abdominal aortic aneurysm, trauma). Volume expansion is accomplished with crystalloids (e.g., normal saline, lactated Ringer's solution) or colloids (e.g., albumin). Fluid therapy is also beneficial in circumstances in which the patient has decreased cardiac output (e.g., secondary to acute myocardial infarction).

Because of adverse effects on cerebral tissue, dextrose solutions are not recommended during CPR. Recommended fluids in cardiac arrest are normal saline or lactated Ringer's solution. Dextrose solutions are reserved for patients with actual or suspected hypoglycemia. All emergency drugs routinely administered for cardiac arrest are stable in 0.9% normal saline solution.[10]

Drug Therapy

Emergency drug therapy is dependent on ECG rhythm and hemodynamic stability. Table 33-4 provides an overview of commonly used emergency medications. Epinephrine is the first-line drug in management of cardiac arrest, specifically asystole, pulseless electrical activity (PEA), VF, and pulseless VT. Vasopressin can be used for VF and pulseless VT followed by epinephrine if the rhythm does not convert. It is important to remember that management of VF and pulseless VT is immediate defibrillation before any medications are administered.

Patients with ventricular dysrhythmias associated with cardiac-cardiopulmonary arrest benefit from amiodarone (cordarone) administration. Other antidysrhythmic agents considered for management of patients with VF or pulseless VT include lidocaine (xylocaine), magnesium, and procainamide (pronestyl). After the ventricular dysrhythmia is controlled, an infusion of the medication is necessary to sustain therapeutic drug levels. These pharmacologic agents should not be given to patients with third-degree AV block and with an escape rhythm or patients with bradycardia and premature ventricular contractions (PVCs). Ectopic beats may contribute to the patient's cardiac output; therefore, lidocaine could effectively reduce output and cause further decompensation or asystole.

Bradycardia dysrhythmias are initially managed with atropine, which blocks stimulation of the vagus nerve. Atropine may not be effective for high-degree AV block dysrhythmias. Atropine can also be used for asystole and PEA. Isoproterenol (Isuprel) is a β-adrenergic agonist and may be used to increase cardiac output in bradydysrhythmias in some cases. Routine use of isoproterenol is not recommended because of effects on ventricular irritability; however, it is considered a first-line drug for the heart transplant patient with symptomatic bradycardia. Bradycardic rhythms that affect hemodynamic stability may ultimately require cardiac pacing.

Supraventricular rhythms can impair effective cardiac output (because of decreased filling time) and hemodynamic stability. Adenosine (Adenocard) is an extremely fast-acting agent (half-life <10 seconds) for reentry dysrhythmias. The drug must be given rapidly and followed with a 20-ml saline bolus to maximize effects. Side effects include transient bradycardia, transient asystole, ventricular ectopy, flushing, dyspnea, hypotension, and chest pain. Symptoms usually terminate spontaneously without further intervention. Other pharmacologic agents such as Ibutilide, β-adrenergic blocking drugs (e.g., metoprolol [Lopressor]) and calcium channel blocking agents (e.g., verapamil [Calan] and diltiazem [Cardizem]) can be used for controlling ventricular response rate in patients with supraventricular tachycardias (e.g., atrial fibrillation, atrial flutter, paroxysmal supraventricular tachychardia, atrial tachycardia). Monitor for bradycardia and hypotension when administering these drugs. Drugs should be used only for narrow complex supraventricular tachycardia (SVT), because of the potential to induce or worsen reentry ventricular dysrhythmias.[10]

Other miscellaneous drugs that may be used during cardiac arrest include sodium bicarbonate, calcium, and magnesium sulfate. Sodium bicarbonate is reserved for specific clinical situations, including hyperkalemia, preexisting bicarbonate-responsive acidosis, and tricyclic antidepressant overdose. Magnesium is considered useful in treatment of torsades de pointe, suspected hypomagnesemia, and refractory VF. Calcium, an ion essential to myocardial contraction and impulse formation, is recommended for hyperkalemia, hypocalcemia, and calcium channel–blocker toxicity.

During cardiopulmonary arrest, hemodynamic status is unstable and requires intervention to stabilize not only the patient's cardiac rhythm but also the cardiovascular system. Table 33-5 reviews vasoactive drugs more commonly used during cardiac arrest.[4,17,22,34] Refer to Table 33-6 for overview of cardiovascular drugs that can be given via endotracheal tube or interosseous route when IV access cannot be established.[10,38]

Acute Coronary Syndromes

The broader terminology of acute coronary syndromes is inclusive of Q wave myocardial infarction (full-thickness myocardial necrosis), non–Q wave myocardial infarction, now called non–ST elevation MI or non–STEMI (subendocardial or intramural wall damage), and unstable angina (myocardial ischemia without necrosis). Approximately 1.5 million people experience acute myocardial infarction (AMI) annually in the United States; 40% die before reaching the hospital. The majority of patients die in the first 2 hours after onset of infarction. Mortality from infarction can be reduced significantly if the patient receives proper medical care in the early phases of infarction. All these syndromes evolve from rupture or erosion of atheromatous plaque. An estimated 5.5 million people over age 18 years in the United States have atherosclerosis. Pathogenesis of atherosclerosis includes accumulation of lipids on intimal lining of the arteries, calcific sclerosis of the medial layer of arteries, and thickening of the walls of the arteries (Figure 33-9 on p. 465). Generally, atherosclerosis affects the aorta and the coronary, cerebral, femoral, and other large or middle-size arteries. Risk factors for atherosclerosis include smoking, hyperlipidemia, hypertension, diabetes mellitus, stress, lack of exercise, aging, diet high

Table 33-4 DRUGS COMMONLY USED IN CARDIOPULMONARY RESUSCITATION

DRUG	CATEGORY	ACTIONS	INDICATIONS	DOSE	COMMENTS
Adenocard (Adenosine)	Unclassified anti-dysrhythmic	Slows conduction through the AV node; also can interrupt the reentry pathways through the AV node to decrease the heart rate	PSVT	**SVT:** 6 mg rapid IV push over 1 to 3 seconds; may give additional 12 mg rapid IV push if first dose not effective, may repeat 12 mg after 1 to 2 min It is helpful to rapidly bolus 10 ml normal saline after giving adenocard to clear IV tubing completely	May cause brief heart block or transient asystole; may cause other dysrhythmias (e.g., PVC, PAC, sinus bradycardia, sinus tachycardia) during time of conversion from PSVT These symptoms are usually brief because of the short half-life of the drug (i.e., <10 seconds) Contraindications include: Second- or third-degree AV block, or sick sinus syndrome
Amiodarone (Cordarone)	Combined β-adrenergic blocker and calcium channel blocker	Prolongs myocardial cell action potential duration and refractory period; decrease AV conduction and sinus node function	Recurring ventricular fibrillation and unstable ventricular tachycardia	**Arrest:** 300 mg IV push followed by 150 mg IVP if no response **Nonarrest:** Initial infusion: 150 mg over 10 min; can repeat every 10-15 min as needed Early maintenance: 1 mg/min for 6 hours Late maintenance: 0.5 mg/min Do not exceed 2.2 g in 24 hours, including initial dose	May cause hypotension, nausea, bradycardia
Atropine	Parasympatholytic; anticholinergic	Increases the rate of SA node firing; increases conduction through AV node; decreases vagal tone	Hemodynamically significant bradycardia; asystole; high-degree AV blocks	**Bradycardia and AV blocks:** 0.5 to 1.0 mg (IV push) or intratracheally every 5 min to maximum dose of 0.04 mg/kg **Asystole:** 1.0 mg IV push or intratracheally; repeat every 3-5 min up to a total of 0.04 mg/kg	May cause paradoxic slowing of heart rate when given slowly or in doses of less than 0.5 mg

PSVT, Paroxysmal supraventricular tachycardia; *SVT,* supraventricular tachycardia; *IV,* intravenous; *PVC,* premature ventricular contraction; *PAC,* premature atrial contraction; *AV,* atrioventricular; *SA,* sinoatrial; *VF,* ventricular fibrillation; *VT,* ventricular tachycardia; D$_5$W, 5% dextrose in water; *gtt,* drops.

Continued

in fat and cholesterol, gender, and family history. Multiple existing risk factors increase a person's chance of developing acute coronary syndromes.[4,11,31]

Overview of Acute Coronary Syndromes

The major cause of the final event leading to AMI is thrombosis formation in a narrowed coronary artery from ruptured or fissured atherosclerotic plaque. Subsequent vessel occlusion and thrombosis cause myocardial hypoxia and necrosis. Myocardial hypoxia may also be caused by coronary artery spasm and dissecting aortic aneurysm. Complete necrosis occurs in 4 to 6 hours. The area surrounding the zone of necrosis is ischemic. Damage to the myocardium predisposes the patient to pump failure and various dysrhythmias secondary to conduction defects and irritability of myocardial tissue. Location and size of the infarct depend on which coronary artery is affected and where the occlusion occurs (Table 33-7, p. 466). Most

Text continued on p. 464

Table 33-4 **DRUGS COMMONLY USED IN CARDIOPULMONARY RESUSCITATION—cont'd**

DRUG	CATEGORY	ACTIONS	INDICATIONS	DOSE	COMMENTS
Epinephrine (Adrenalin)	Sympathomimetic	Both α- and β-adrenergic effects; increases mean arterial pressure; decreases fibrillatory threshold; stimulates heart in asystole and idioventricular rhythms	Allergic reaction; cardiac arrest; bronchoconstriction or bronchospasm	**Cardiac arrest**: 1 mg IV push or intratracheally; repeat every 5 min when needed	Available as 1:10,000 solution (1 mg in 10 ml) May cause tachycardia, palpitations, PVCs, angina
Isoproterenol (Isuprel)	Sympathomimetic	Nonspecific β-adrenergic stimulation	Hemodynamically significant bradycardia refractory to Atropine	**Bradycardia**: 1 mg in 250 ml D_5W (4 μg/ml); 2-20 μg/min IV (30-300 μ-gtts/min); titrate to achieve heart rate of >60 beats/min	Causes an increased workload on the heart; use with extreme caution: exacerbates ischemia and extends infarct
Lidocaine (Xylocaine)	Category IB antidysrhythmic	Decreases automaticity; suppresses ventricular ectopy; depresses conduction through reentry pathways; elevates VF threshold	PVCs, VT, VF, preintubation for patients with suspected increased intracranial pressure or laryngospasm	**VF and VT with collapse**: 1.5 mg/kg IV push or intratracheally; repeat in 3-5 min; not to exceed 3 mg/kg **PVC's and VT**: 1 mg/kg IV push or intratracheally; repeat at 0.5 mg/kg every 8-10 min not to exceed 3 mg/kg **IV infusion**: 1 g in 250 ml D_5W (4 mg/ml) at 2-4 mg/min (30-60 μgtts/min) **Preintubation**: 1.5 mg/kg IV push, wait 90 seconds then intubate	May cause central nervous system depression, drowsiness, dizziness, confusion, anxiety Contraindications include: Bradycardia-related PVCs, bradycardia, idioventricular rhythm; if given too rapidly, may cause seizures
Procainamide (Pronestyl)	Category IA antidysrhythmic	Suppresses PVCs; suppresses reentry dysrhythmias; may elevate VF threshold; negative chronotrope and dromotrope; mild negative inotrope; potent peripheral vasodilator	PVCs and VT refractory to lidocaine; hemodynamically significant SVT	**IV push**: 100 mg IV (slow IV push—20 mg/min) repeat every 5 min; dose not to exceed 1 g **IV infusion**: 1 g in 250 ml D_5W (4 mg/ml) at 1 to 4 mg/min (15-60 μgtt/min)	May cause hypotension, bradycardia Contraindications: Third-degree AV block, digoxin toxicity
Sodium bicarbonate	Alkalotic agent	Buffers or neutralizes metabolic acidosis	Suspected acidosis in cases of cardiac arrest	1 mEq/kg IV push; repeat 0.5 mEq/kg every 10 to 15 min when required	May inactivate catecholamines when given together in the same IV line; when possible use arterial blood gases to guide administration
Verapamil (Calan, Isoptin)	Category IV antidysrhythmic	Blocks entry of Ca++ into cells; negative dromotrope and depresses atrial automaticity; negative chronotrope; negative inotrope; vasodilator	SVT	**IV push**: 0.075 to 0.15 mg/kg IV (slow IV push) Elderly patients: give 2 mg over 3 to 4 min Maximum dose 10 mg	May cause hypotension

Table 33-5	COMMONLY USED PARENTERAL VASOACTIVE DRUGS FOR CARDIOVASCULAR EMERGENCIES				
DRUG	**CATEGORY**	**ACTIONS**	**INDICATIONS**	**DOSE**	**COMMENTS**
Brevibloc (Esmolol)	β-adrenergic blocker Class II antiarrhythmic	Depresses AV conduction and myocardial automaticity, especially in the SA node; prolongs the refractory period	SVT (e.g., PAT, atrial fibrillation/ flutter, sinus tachycardia)	**IV push**: Initial loading dose of 500 mcg/kg given over 1 min, followed by 50 mcg/kg over 4 min May repeat initial loading dose followed by the 4 min. infusion increased at increments of 50 mcg/kg/min Do not give over 200 mcg/kg/min **IV infusion**: Follow loading dose with an infusion of 100 mcg/kg/min	May cause significant bradycardia, hypotension, bronchospasm, heart failure Contraindications: Heart block, CHF, severe asthma Has an immediate onset of action Duration of action approx 30 min after end of infusion
Calcium chloride	Electrolyte replacement	Improves vascular tone and myocardial contractility	Rapid electrolyte replacement In seriously hypotensive patients who respond poorly to fluid/ vasopressors when hypocalcemia suspected	**IV push**: For Ca++ Replacement: 500 mg to 1 g (i.e., 7 to 14 mEq) For hyperkalemic ECG changes: 100 mg to 1 g For hypocalcemic tetany: 300 mg to 1.2 g For hypotension associated with Ca++ channel blockers: 500 mg to 2 g Administer slowly at a rate not to exceed 0.7 to 1.4 mEq/min **IV infusion**: Administer diluted solution over 30-60 min (i.e., dilute calcium chloride in 50-100 ml D_5W, LR, or 0.9% NS)	May cause hypotension, bradycardia, dysrhythmias Contraindications: Hypercalcemia, ventricular fibrillation
Diazoxide (Hyperstat)	Antihypertensive vasodilator	Direct relaxation of arteriolar smooth muscle Inhibits release of pancreatic insulin	Significant hypertension	**IV push**: 1-3 mg/kg (e.g., approx. 50-150 mg) May repeat every 5-15 min as needed Maintenance Dose = 50-150 mg every 4-24 hours	Inject drug rapidly as slow administration reduces hypotensive effects Onset of action <1 min, with peak in 2-5 min May cause hypotension CHF, dysrhythmias, myocardial and cerebral ischemia, and hyperglycemia

PAT, Paroxysmal atrial tachycardia; *CHF,* congestive heart failure; *ECG,* electrocardiogram; *HCL,* hydrochloride; *BP,* blood pressure; *AMI,* acute myocardial infarction; *PVC,* polyvinyl chloride; *ICP,* intracranial pressure; see Table 33-4 for other definitions.

Continued

Table 33-5   COMMONLY USED PARENTERAL VASOACTIVE DRUGS FOR CARDIOVASCULAR EMERGENCIES—cont'd

DRUG	CATEGORY	ACTIONS	INDICATIONS	DOSE	COMMENTS
Diltiazem HCL (Cardizem)	Calcium channel blocker	SA node automaticity decreased; AV conduction prolonged; increased refractoriness of AV node; and vasodilation including coronary arteries	SVT (e.g., atrial fibrillation/flutter, PSVT)	**IV push:** 0.25 mg/kg to be administered over 2 min May give additional dose in 15 min of 0.35 mg/kg if initial dose inadequate to control HR **IV infusion:** 5-15 mg/hr	May cause hypotension, bradycardia, AV heart block Has an immediate onset when given IV, with peak effect in 15 min Contraindications: Heart block, accessory conduction pathways or preexcitation syndromes
Dobutamine HCL (Dobutrex)	Sympathomimetic, β-1 adrenergic receptor agonist	Positive inotropic effects (e.g., increases force of myocardial contraction); increases heart rate at higher doses	To optimize cardiac output; may be used as concurrent therapy with afterload-reducing agents to also increase cardiac output	**IV infusion:** Initially 2.5 mcg/kg/min; continue titration to maintain effective cardiac output Maintenance dose usually 2.5-10 mcg/kg/min Maximum dose = 40 mcg/kg/min	May cause tachycardia, dysrhythmias (e.g. ventricular) Consider dose reduction of dobutamine if heart rate >10% above baseline
Dopamine HCL (Intropin, Dopastat)	Sympathomimetic, β-1 and α-adrenergic agent; also a dopaminergic stimulator	At low doses: Vasodilates mesenteric and cerebral blood flow At intermediate doses: Increase myocardial contractility and peripheral vasodilation At high doses: Increased peripheral/renal vascular resistance and increased myocardial contractility	At low doses: To increase urinary output At intermediate doses: To increase cardiac output At high doses: To increase BP in nonhypovolemic shock	**IV infusion:** *low* dose: 0.5-2 mcg/kg/min *intermediate* dose: 2-10 mcg/kg/min *high* dose: >10 mcg/kg/min Maximum dose = 20 mcg/kg/min	May cause dysrhythmias Extravasation of the drug may cause tissue sloughing and necrosis
Enalaprilat (Vasotec)	Angiotensin-converting enzyme (ACE) inhibitor	Reduces vascular tone	Significant hypertension Adjunct to digitalis and diuretics for acute CHF	**IV push:** Initial dose 0.625 mg IVP; may repeat in 1 hour Maintenance dose=1.25 mg every 6 hours IVP	May cause hypotension, pulmonary edema
Ibutilide (Corvert)	Class III antiarrhythmic	Slows conduction; delays repolarization by activation of slow, inward current (mostly sodium) resulting in prolongation of atrial and ventricular action potentials	Recent onset atrial fibrillation or atrial flutter	**IV:** ≥60 kg: 1 mg administered over 10 min, may repeat dose in 10 min if not effective in converting rhythm <60 kg: 0.01mg/kg over 10 min, may repeat dose in 10 min if needed	May have proarrhythmic effects—monitor closely for torsades de pointes or polymorphic ventricular tachycardia; especially within 4-6 hours after administration

PAT, Paroxysmal atrial tachycardia; *CHF,* congestive heart failure; *ECG,* electrocardiogram; *HCL,* hydrochloride; *BP,* blood pressure; *AMI,* acute myocardial infarction; *PVC,* polyvinyl chloride; *ICP,* intracranial pressure; see Table 33-4 for other definitions.

Table 33-5	COMMONLY USED PARENTERAL VASOACTIVE DRUGS FOR CARDIOVASCULAR EMERGENCIES—cont'd				
DRUG	**CATEGORY**	**ACTIONS**	**INDICATIONS**	**DOSE**	**COMMENTS**
Labetalol (Normodyne, Trandate)	Selective α-adrenergic blocker and nonselective β-adrenergic blocker	Blocks sympathetic stimulation, thereby causing vasodilation	Hypertension	**IV push**: 20 mg (0.25 mg/kg) IV to be administered over 2 min. Additional doses of 40-80 mg of the drug can be given at 10-min intervals up to maximum dose of 300 mg total	May cause hypotension, bradycardia, heart block, bronchospasm
Magnesium sulfate	Electrolyte replacement	Adequate Mg++ is needed for normal cardiac automaticity, excitability, conduction and contractility	Supraventricular and ventricular dysrhythmias	**IV push**: 1-3 g of magnesium sulfate (concentration of magnesium should *not* exceed 200 mg/ml. Also Mg++ should not be administered faster than 150 mg/min) **IV infusion**: Follow initial IV dose with 1-2 g of Mg++ per hour	Rapid injection may cause hypotension, heart block, cardiac/respiratory arrest. Onset of action is immediate when given IV. Observe for hypermagnesemia: Flushing, hypotension, bradycardia, confusion, weakness, depressed deep tendon reflexes, respiratory depression
Metaprolol tartrate (Lopressor)	β-adrenergic blocker	Selectively blocks β-1 adrenergic receptors, which slows sinus heart rate, decreases cardiac output, decreases BP	Hypertension; AMI in hemodynamically stable patient	**IV push**: 5 mg IVP for hypertension **Treatment for AMI**: 3 IV injections of 5 mg; give 50 mg metaprolol "orally" every 6 hours after last dose IV metaprolol	May cause bradycardia, hypotension, bronchospasm
Nicardipine (Cardene)	Calcium channel blocker	Significantly decreases peripheral vascular resistance	Hypertensive emergency	**IV infusion**: 5 mg/hr to be titrated to desired effect—up to 15 mg/hr	May cause tachycardia, angina, hypotension
Nitroglycerin (Tridil)	Vasodilator	Relaxation of vascular smooth muscle, promoting venous and coronary artery vasodilation; reduces venous return	Angina, hypertension	**IV infusion**: Initiate infusion at 5-10 mcg/min. Increase infusion by 5-10 mcg/min every 5-10 min. Maximum dose: 200 mcg/min	May cause hypotension, headache, dizziness. Nitroglycerin is absorbed by many soft plastics; therefore dilute the concentrate in a glass bottle and consider using non-absorbing, non-PVC tubing or flush tubing with 20-25 mls before starting infusion
Nitroprusside, sodium (Nipride)	Vasodilator	Relaxes vascular smooth muscle—lowering both arterial and venous BP	Significant hypertension	**IV infusion**: Initiate infusion at 0.3-0.5 mcg/kg/min. Increase infusion by 1-2 mcg/kg/min to attain desired hemodynamic effects. Maximum infusion rate = 10 mcg/kg/min	May cause hypotension, angina, increased ICP, seizures. The IV solution needs to be protected from the light by using a light-resistant covering (e.g., aluminum foil, opaque plastic). Onset of action immediate, with peak action of 1-2 min

Continued

Table 33-5	COMMONLY USED PARENTERAL VASOACTIVE DRUGS FOR CARDIOVASCULAR EMERGENCIES—cont'd				
DRUG	**CATEGORY**	**ACTIONS**	**INDICATIONS**	**DOSE**	**COMMENTS**
Norepinephrine bitartrate (Levophed)	Vasopressor	Peripheral venous/arterial vasoconstriction; cardiac stimulation	Short-term use for hypotension or shock	**IV infusion**: Initiate infusion at 2 mcg/min and titrate to desired BP Usual range = 2-12 mcg/min	May cause ventricular tachycardia/ fibrillation (i.e., secondary to increased myocardial oxygen consumption) Extravasation of the drug may cause tissue sloughing and necrosis
Phenylephrine (Neo-Synephrine)	Vasopressor	Potent postsynaptic α-adrenergic agonist	Short-term use for hypotension/ shock	**IV push**: 0.1-0.5 mg to be given over 1 min **IV infusion**: Dilute to yield solution of 0.1/ml and titrate gtt every 10-15 min to achieve and to maintain BP >90 mm Hg	May cause hypertension, dysrhythmias, reflex bradycardia, cerebral hemorrhage Extravasation of the drug may cause tissue sloughing and necrosis
Propranolol HCL (Inderal)	Nonselective β-adrenergic blocker and class II antidysrhythmic	Blocks sympathetic stimulation of β-1 adrenergic receptors	Control of hypertension and suppression of rapid-rate cardiac dysrhythmias	**IV push**: 0.5 to 3 mg Give slowly 1 mg/min; may repeat dose after 2 min	May cause bronchospasm, hypotension, heart block, angina
Vasopressin (Pitressin)	Vasopressor	Directly stimulates contraction of smooth muscles; causes vasoconstriction wih reduced blood flow to coronary, peripheral, cerebral, and pulmonary vessels	Short-term use for hypotension or shock Alternative to epinephrine in cardiac arrest d/t VF or pulseless VT in patients without CV disease	**IV infusion**: Dilute with 5% dextrose in water or 0.9% NaCl to a concentration of 0.1 to 1.0 U/ml titrate gtt every 10-15 min to achieve and to maintain BP >90 mm Hg **Cardiac arrest**: 40 units IV push	May cause hypertension, dysrhythmias Contraindicated in preexisting CV disease; IV dose same as IO and ET dose

AMIs are caused by blockage of the left anterior descending coronary artery, which causes involvement of the anterior wall of the myocardium.[11]

Non–STEMI is usually related to intermittent occlusive thrombosis causing distal myocyte necrosis of the region supplied by the related coronary artery. As the clot enlarges around the thrombus, it may embolize and eventually occlude coronary microvasculature, which results in small elevations of cardiac enzymes. Underlying pathology for unstable angina is partial occlusion by thrombus of atherosclerotic plaque. Patients with either non–STEMI or unstable angina are at high risk for progression to transmural myocardial infarction.[2,29,32,33]

When the coronary artery(s) becomes narrowed or occluded, myocardium becomes hypoxic, often resulting in classic retrosternal chest discomfort or angina pectoris. Pain is described as crushing, burning, sharp, heavy, or a variety of other descriptors. The pain lasts several minutes to several weeks and may vary in location. Local hypoxia, lactate buildup, and sensory response of the hypoxic myocardium contribute to pain. Pain may localize in the substernal area or radiate to the jaw and down the left arm. Associated symptoms include nausea, vomiting, diaphoresis, and hiccups if the phrenic nerve is stimulated.

Blood pressure decreases with AMI because poor pump action decreases cardiac output. Sodium and water retention may occur as a result of decreased cardiac output and increased venous pressure. When AMI occurs, ventricular failure occurs. With severe ventricular failure, stroke volume decreases and ventricular diastolic pressure increases, whereas the sympathetic response decreases blood flow to the periphery. Decreased blood flow and pressure to the kidneys slows glomerular filtration rate (GFR). Decreased GFR stimulates renal cells to produce renin so angiotensin levels rise and aldosterone is secreted. Increased aldosterone and decreased GFR cause sodium and water retention and formation of interstitial edema.[11]

Table 33-6 ALTERNATE ROUTES FOR DRUG ADMINISTRATION IN CARDIOVASCULAR EMERGENCIES

ROUTE	NURSING MANAGEMENT
ENDOTRACHEAL (ET)	
When IV access not available, can administer selected emergency drugs: Epinephrine Atropine Lidocaine Naloxone	Dilute drug in sterile saline or sterile water (i.e., 10 ml for adults and 1 to 2 ml for children) Administer medications as far down ET tube as possible; consider inserting intracatheter in ET tube and advancing to give medication
Consider dose 2.0 to 2.5 times recommended IV dose (for above medications) Vasopressin (ET dose same as IV dose)	Administer drug quickly down ET tube, follow with three to four rapid insufflations of ambu-bag to aerosolize medication in tracheobronchial tree
INTRAOSSEOUS (IO)	
Used most often in children age 6 years or younger Intraosseous needle placed in proximal tibia Can be placed in any portion of the tibia excluding the epiphyseal plates (e.g., distal tibia, midanterior distal one third of the femur, iliac crest, humerus); the sternum can be used as a site in patients age 3 years or older Use for medications, fluids, and blood and blood products	Use sterile technique to insert an intraosseous needle; alternative methods include using #16 or #18 gauge hypodermic, spinal, or bone marrow needle Confirm placement by aspiration of bone marrow, and freely flowing IV without evidence of infiltration Secure firmly with sterile dressing and tape to prevent dislodgement Monitor for extravasation and patency Flush with dilute saline or heparin to maintain patency Dilute hypertonic-alkaline solutions before administration

IV, Intravenous.

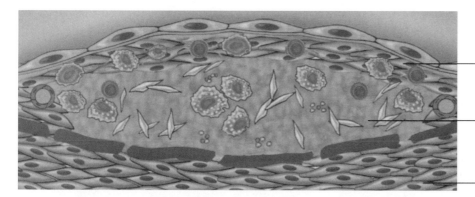

FIBROUS CAP
(smooth muscle cells, macrophages, foam cells, lymphocytes, collagen, elastin, proteoglycans, neovascularization)

NECROTIC CENTER
(cell debris, cholesterol crystals, foam cells, calcium)

MEDIA

FIGURE 33-9 Major components of well-developed atheromatous plaque. From Cotran R, Kumar V, Collins T: *Pathologic basis of disease,* ed 6, Philadelphia, 1999, WB Saunders.)

Patient Assessment for Acute Coronary Syndrome

Prompt assessment of the patient with acute coronary syndromes is crucial because the incidence of ventricular fibrillation is 15 times greater during the first hour after onset of AMI symptoms. On average, patients delay 2 or more hours before seeking medical care for AMI symptoms.[40] Most patients are resting or engaged in only moderate activity when symptoms begin. Chest pain indicative of AMI is usually severe, lasts longer than 30 minutes, and is not relieved with rest or vasodilators such as nitroglycerin. Ironically, up to 20% of patients with AMI do not experience chest pain. Patients with diabetes mellitus are more prone to neuropathy and may not experience pain. Among patients older than 85 years, the classic symptom of AMI is shortness of breath.

Heart transplant patients do not experience chest pain because pain receptors are disconnected during transplant.

Obtaining a concise, brief history of chest pain is crucial; the PQRST mnemonic is particularly useful for these patients (Table 33-8). Patients who have chest pain must have a differential diagnosis made between angina pectoris and AMI.[8,19] There are two types of angina—stable and unstable (Table 33-9). Stable angina, known as typical angina, occurs as a predictable event after activities such as exercise or body strain. Two categories of unstable angina are typical unstable angina and Prinzmetal's angina. Attacks of typical unstable angina, also called preinfarction angina, are prolonged, occur more frequently, and worsen with each episode. Typical unstable angina is associated with higher incidence of left main and proximal left anterior descending coronary artery disease. Half the patients with typical unstable angina have total or near-total occlusion (70% to 100% stenosis) of a coronary artery (Figure 33-10). Prinzmetal's angina, or variant angina, occurs when the patient is at rest, usually at the same time each day. Prognosis with Prinzmetal's angina is poor, with 50% mortality during the first year.

In addition to assessing pain, assess for associated symptoms and pertinent medical history. Associated symptoms include diaphoresis, nausea, vomiting, indigestion, dyspnea, palpitations, dizziness, or lightheadedness. Evaluate risk factors for cardiac disease; for example, smoking, hypertension, hyperlipidemia, diabetes, and related medical history (i.e., previous angina, previous AMI or cardiac surgery, peripheral vascular disease, and immediate family history of AMI). Medication history may include antianginals, antidysrhythmics, antihypertensives, anticoagulants, and digitalis preparations. Such drugs as H_2 blockers, antacids, sucralfate, and nonsteroidal antiinflammatory drugs may assist in differentiating gastrointestinal problems and/or musculoskeletal discomfort.

In addition to cardiac disease, other etiologies may be associated with chest pain (Table 33-10, p. 469). Hyperventilation, a common condition in the ED, may occur as a result of anxiety disorder or may be a response to disease processes such as AMI, salicylate overdose, or intracerebral hemorrhage. Treat these patients with extreme caution and assess carefully for signs and symptoms of an underlying disorder.

A patient with hyperventilation is a difficult diagnostic problem. Hyperventilation may be a response to an organic process in which having the patient breathe into a paper bag may be detrimental. Hyperventilation is a sign of many illnesses and conditions, including anxiety, pregnancy, fever, liver disease, trauma, hypovolemia, pulmonary embolus, stress, ketoacidosis, high altitude, thyrotoxicosis, pulmonary hypertension, pulmonary edema, anemia, stroke, central nervous system lesion, and fibrotic lung disease. Hyperventilation causes partial arterial carbon dioxide pressure to drop and cerebral vasculature to constrict, resulting in respiratory alkalosis and tetany. Signs and symptoms include anxiety; panic; shortness of breath; paresthe-

Table 33-7	CORONARY ARTERIES IN MI	
RIGHT CORONARY ARTERY		**LEFT CORONARY ARTERY**

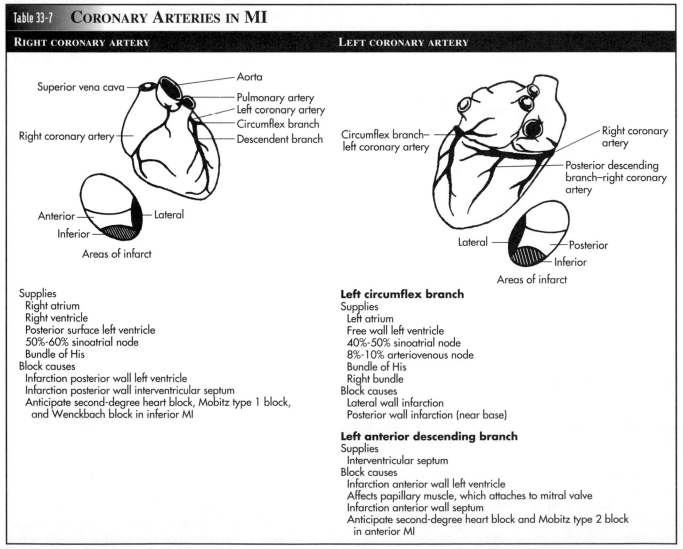

Right coronary artery

Supplies
  Right atrium
  Right ventricle
  Posterior surface left ventricle
  50%-60% sinoatrial node
  Bundle of His
Block causes
  Infarction posterior wall left ventricle
  Infarction posterior wall interventricular septum
  Anticipate second-degree heart block, Mobitz type 1 block, and Wenckbach block in inferior MI

Left circumflex branch
Supplies
  Left atrium
  Free wall left ventricle
  40%-50% sinoatrial node
  8%-10% arteriovenous node
  Bundle of His
  Right bundle
Block causes
  Lateral wall infarction
  Posterior wall infarction (near base)

Left anterior descending branch
Supplies
  Interventricular septum
Block causes
  Infarction anterior wall left ventricle
  Affects papillary muscle, which attaches to mitral valve
  Infarction anterior wall septum
  Anticipate second-degree heart block and Mobitz type 2 block in anterior MI

MI, Myocardial infarction.

sia of the fingers, toes, and periorbital area; carpopedal spasms; confusion; syncope; and, occasionally, chest pain. Therapeutic intervention includes calming and reassuring the patient. Have the patient talk; it is difficult to hyperventilate when speaking. As a last therapeutic intervention, have the patient breathe into a paper bag to facilitate carbon dioxide rebreathing.

Chest pain may also be caused by abdominal illnesses such as hiatal hernia, gastric or peptic ulcer, pancreatitis, esophageal spasms, Mallory-Weiss syndrome, or Boerhaave's syndrome. Other problems that cause chest pain are musculoskeletal disorders involving trauma, degenerative disk disease, xiphoidalgia, costochondritis, Mondor's disease, and postherpetic syndrome.

Physical findings associated with AMI are usually consistent with a patient who is acutely ill. Because of hemodynamic effects of AMI, the patient may have a variety of heart rates and heart dysrhythmias. The patient may be hypertensive secondary to low cardiac output and sympathetic stimulation or hypotensive from pump failure. The first heart sound may be decreased because of decreased myocardial contractility, whereas the second heart sound may be increased because of increased pulmonary artery pressure. An S3 sound (gallop) may be present as the result of ventricular dilation and increased ventricular fluid pressure. The presence of a new systolic murmur indicates ischemic mitral regurgitation or ventricular septal defect.

A transient pericardial friction rub occurs secondary to the inflammatory response to necrosis. There also may be an alternating pulse rate caused by left-sided heart failure. Increased pressure from congestion causes backflow of blood into jugular veins so jugular vein distention occurs when the patient is sitting at a 45-degree angle. There may also be a prominent V wave with rapid Y wave descent. The patient may also have an elevated temperature caused by inflammation and necrosis of myocardial tissue.

The patient is often diaphoretic and anxious. Diaphoresis is related to the autonomic nervous system response, whereas anxiety may be due to pain and fever. Cyanosis may be caused by decreased oxyhemoglobin concentration and decreased blood supply to the peripheral vascular system.

ECG

Changes in the ECG provide information about the site of coronary artery occlusion, myocardial ischemia, and the presence of tissue necrosis. Lead placement of an ECG determines which area of the heart the ECG signal is representing (Figures 33-11 and 33-12, p. 471). Changes in the ECG occur because of changes in electrical current flow when there is myocardial damage or ischemia (Figure 33-13, p. 471). When current flows toward a lead (arrowhead, positive electrode), an upward ECG deflection occurs. When current flows away from a lead (arrowhead, positive electrode), downward deflection occurs. When current flows perpendicular to a lead

Table 33-8	PQRST MNEMONIC FOR CHEST PAIN ASSESSMENT	
FACTOR	DESCRIPTION QUESTIONS
P Provokes, palliates, precipitating factors	What provoked the pain? What makes the pain better? What makes the pain worse? Have you had this type of pain before? What were you doing when the pain occurred?
Q Quality	What does the pain feel like? Is it burning? Crushing? Tearing? Sharp?
R Region, radiation	Show me where the pain is. How large an area is involved? Does the pain radiate? If so, where?
S Severity, associated symptoms	How severe is the pain? If you were to rate the pain on a scale from 0 to 10 with 10 being the most severe pain you can imagine, how would you rate your pain? What else did you feel besides the pain?
T Time, temporal relations	When did the pain start? How long did it last? Does it come and go? Were you awakened by the pain? Is the pain always present?

Table 33-9	DIFFERENTIAL DIAGNOSIS OF ANGINA	
CHARACTERISTIC	STABLE ANGINA	UNSTABLE (PREINFARCTION) ANGINA
Location of pain	Substernal; may radiate to jaws, neck, and down arms and back	Substernal; may radiate to jaws, neck, and down arms and back
Duration of pain	1-5 min	5 min; occurring more frequently
Characteristic of pain	Aching, squeezing, choking, heavy burning	Same as stable angina but more intense
Other symptoms	Usually none	Diaphoresis; weakness
Pain worsened by	Exercise; activity; eating; cold weather; reclining	Exercise; activity; eating; cold weather; reclining
Paine relieved by	Rest; nitroglycerin; isosorbide	Nitroglycerin, isosorbide may give only partial relief
ECG findings	Transient ST depression; disappears with pain relief	ST segment depression; often T wave inversion; ECG may be normal

ECG, Electrocardiogram.

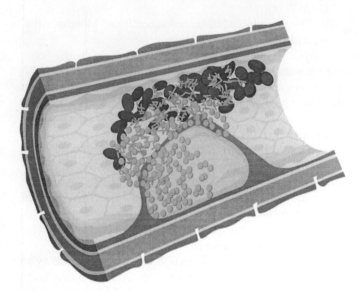

FIGURE **33-10** Thrombus formation. (From Roetting M, Tanabe P: Emergency Management of acute coronary-syndromes, *J Emerg Nurs* (suppl) 26(6):S1, 2000.)

(arrowhead), biphasic ECG deflection occurs.[20] Figures 33-14 through 33-17 on p. 472 illustrate ECG changes with myocardial infarction. Serial ECGs are used in conjunction with patient assessment, history, and other diagnostic measures to confirm the diagnosis of AMI. A single ECG cannot be used exclusively. ECG findings are sensitive only 50% of the time, and ECG changes occur with other conditions. Patients with stable angina can have ST segment depression, and ST segment elevation can occur with unstable angina and Prinzmetal's angina. Pericarditis may cause ST segment elevation in many leads, hemorrhagic stroke is associated with T wave inversion, and ventricular aneurysms may be associated with ST elevation.[12,14,28]

Elevation of the segment between the end of the S wave and the beginning of the T wave (ST segment) is indicative of myocardial injury and occurs minutes after occlusion of a coronary artery. The ST segment can remain elevated for 24 hours. T wave inversion occurs 6 to 24 hours after occlusion, may persist months to years, and is due to ischemia. (Hypoxia should also be considered with T wave inversion.) Pathologic Q waves, measuring more than 0.04 seconds in width and at least 25% or more of overall QRS height, occur within 24 hours and indicate irreversible myocardial cell death. ST segment depression may also be associated with AMI. Reciprocal changes (ST segment depression and peaked T wave) may be seen in ECG leads that view regions opposite the damaged area. Hyperkalemia should be eliminated as a cause of tall, peaked T waves. Changes in ECG[20] have an overall 79% sensitivity and 44% specificity in detecting an AMI (Box 33-1, p. 473).

A Q wave has been associated with transmural AMI; however, studies now demonstrate both Q wave and non–Q wave (non–STEMI) infarcts can be transmural or subendocardial. In general, Q wave infarctions are associated with a larger region of myocardial necrosis, higher enzyme levels,

fresh coronary thrombosis, frequent vomiting, congestive heart failure, conduction defects, dysrhythmias, and less collateral circulation. When ST segment depression occurs in the inferior (II, III, aVF), lateral (I, aVL, V5, V6), or anterior (V1 through V6) leads and cardiac enzymes are elevated, diagnosis of non–STEMI is supported. ST elevation is most frequently associated with Q wave infarctions and almost 50% of non–STEMIs.[12,14,28]

All patients with suspected inferior or lateral AMI should be evaluated for right ventricular infarction. Right ventricular infarct is present in up to 40% of patients with inferior myocardial infarctions resulting from occlusion of the right coronary artery. Changes noted on the ECG may include isolated ST segment elevation in V1 or ST elevation in V1 to V4. A more reliable method of determining right ventricular infarct is use of right ventricular leads (V3R to V6R). Figure 33-18 and Box 33-2 on p. 473 illustrate right ventricular lead placement. Use of lead V4R has 92% sensitivity for right coronary artery occlusion.[35]

ECG changes in posterior infarct (ST depression in V1 to V4) represent reciprocal changes of the anterior wall, the portion of the heart opposite the posterior portion. Other changes include R waves longer than 0.04 seconds in V1 and V2 and R wave to S wave ratio larger in V1 and V2.[35] Further evaluation may include posterior ECG leads (V7 to V9) (Figures 33-19 and 33-20, p. 474 and Box 33-2, p. 473).

Continuous ECG monitoring in one or more leads is essential for the AMI patient. Dual lead or continuous ST segment monitoring is available to detect changes in the ECG and identify dysrhythmias. The best lead to use for diagnosing wide complex QRS rhythms is MCL-1 and MCL-6 (see Figure 33-19). This combination of a limb lead and precordial lead is valuable in detecting both ST segment changes associated with further blockage of coronary arteries and for dysrhythmia detection. If bedside monitoring permits, the combination of leads V1, I, and aVF allows quick evaluation of ECG axis. Figure 33-20 on p. 474 provides an overview of axis based on leads I and aVF. Evaluation of axis during wide-complex QRS rhythms or dysrhythmias assists in differentiating supraventricular from ventricular dysrhythmias. In one study, three lead combinations were 100% sensitive for ischemic changes in the major coronary vessels. Leads III, V2, and V5 reflect the coronary artery and left circumflex artery. Leads III, V3, and V5 reflect left anterior descending artery. As technology evolves, multilead ECG monitoring and continuous ST segment monitoring may become increasingly common in the ED.[13]

Cardiac Markers

In addition to ECG monitoring, cardiac markers are measured as part of the diagnostic workup for acute coronary syndromes.* Myoglobin is a nonspecific protein associated with muscle oxygen transport. Myoglobin levels elevate about 1 hour sooner than creatine kinase (CK) after myocardial injury and peak in 2 to 4 hours, and are therefore considered an early cardiac biomarker. Myoglobin is found in striated muscle of the heart and skeletal muscle; thus, el-

---

*1,18,26,30,31,33,39

Table 33-10	ETIOLOGIC FACTORS TO BE CONSIDERED IN THE DIFFERENTIAL DIAGNOSIS OF CHEST PAIN				
ETIOLOGIC FACTORS	**P** PRECIPITATING/ PALLIATING	**Q** QUALITY	**R** RADIATING/REGION	**S** SEVERITY/SYMPTOMS	**T** TIME/ TEMPORAL
Ischemic/ Anginal	Precipitating factors: Effort-related activity, large meals, emotional stress Palliation: Ceases with activity abatement, relief with nitroglycerin, relief with rest	Tightness, burning, deep, constrictive	Retrosternal, area affected the size of the palm of the hand Pain may radiate to left shoulder, left hand (e.g., especially the 4th and 5th fingers), epigastrium, trachea, larynx Never involves region above the level of the eye	Associated symptoms: Profuse diaphoresis, weakness, shortness of breath, nausea, vomiting	Gradual onset of pain builds up to maximum pain intensity; usually anginal pain lasts 1-5 minutes
Myocardial infarction	Precipitating factors: Effort-related activity, large meals, emotional stress	Severe chest pain	Chest pain; may have radiation of pain to back, jaw, or left arm	Associated symptoms: Palpitations, dyspnea, diaphoresis, nausea, vomiting, dizziness, weakness, sense of impending doom	Usually pain has lasted 30 minutes or more
Acute pericarditis	Precipitating factors: May occur after AMI, may also be related to viral, collagen, or vascular disorders	Chest pain may be dull to severe and crushing type pain	Anterior chest pain with radiation to the neck, arms, or shoulders; pain may be intensified by deep inspiration	Associated symptoms: Fever (i.e., between 101-102° F or 38.3-38.9° C); pericardial friction rub; ECG: ST segment elevation in all leads except V1 and aVR	May be hours to days
Dissecting aortic aneurysm	Sudden onset	Severe, ripping, tearing type pain	Anterior and posterior chest Often radiates from anterior chest to intrascapular region or to abdomen Pain may move with progression of aortic dissection	Associated symptoms: Dyspnea, tachypnea, CHF (i.e., secondary to aortic regurgitation caused by dissection); also, CVA, syncope, paraplegia and pulse loss associated with dissecting aneurysm	Sudden onset
Esophageal disorders (esophageal reflux, esophageal spasm)	Precipitating factors: Often triggered by exercise, or by food (large meal, spicy foods, acidic foods, cold foods) or ethanol intake	Burning or pressure-like pain May be severe	May radiate to neck, ear, jaw or lower abdomen	Associated symptoms: Dysphagia, aspiration	Minutes to days
Cocaine induced	Precipitating factors: Cocaine use Palliation: Relieved with nitroglycerin	Sharp, heaviness, pressure of the chest Severe type pain	Substernal location, with radiation to both arms	Associated symptoms: Tachycardia, palpitations, diaphoresis, nausea, dizziness, syncope, dyspnea	Occurs from 1-6 hours after cocaine use

AMI, Acute myocardial infarction; *ECG,* electrocardiogram; *CHF,* congestive heart failure; *CVA,* Cerebrovascular accident; *COPD,* chronic obstructive pulmonary disease.

Continued

Table 33-10   ETIOLOGIC FACTORS TO BE CONSIDERED IN THE DIFFERENTIAL DIAGNOSIS OF CHEST PAIN—cont'd

ETIOLOGIC FACTORS	**P** PRECIPITATING/ PALLIATING	**Q** QUALITY	**R** RADIATING/REGION	**S** SEVERITY/SYMPTOMS	**T** TIME/ TEMPORAL
Postoperative coronary artery bypass graft (CABG) due to harvest of internal mammary artery (IMA)	Precipitating factors: Use of IMA for graft of CABG patient	Mild to severe chest pain, burning, prickling, and dull-type sensations	Anterior chest, may radiate over entire chest wall and particularly over the site of the graft, may radiate to neck or axilla	Associated symptoms: Numbness, tenderness on palpation of the sternum, hyperesthesia along the incisional line, delayed healing of the sternum	Persistent type of pain Shooting type pain may last for several seconds and occur several times per day
Mitral valve prolapse	Palliation: Relief in recumbent position, no relief with nitroglycerin	Dull and aching; although may also be sharp	Nonretrosternal chest pain	Associated symptoms: Systolic murmur, unexplained dyspnea, weakness, midsystolic (apical) click	Onset may be sudden or recurrent May last for a few seconds, or be persistent for days
5-Fluorouracil (FU) therapy	Precipitating factors: Following infusion of 5-FU Palliation: relief with nitroglycerin	Mild to severe pain	Central chest pain; radiates to left shoulder and left arm	Associated symptoms: Nausea, vomiting, tachycardia, hypertension	Occurs several hours after IV bolus or infusion of 5-FU No chest pain between treatment
Spontaneous pneumothorax	COPD, chronic asthma	Sharp or stabbing; described as moderate to severe	Usually pain of entire lung region (hemithorax), may rediate to back and neck	Associated symptoms: Decreased or absent breath sounds; pneumothorax per chest radiograph	Continuous pain until treated
Tachydysrhythmias	Precipitating factors: anxiety, digitalis toxicity, exercise, organic heart disease Palliation: terminated by antiarrhythmics, direct current shock, vagal maneuvers	Sharp, stabbing type of chest pain May have palpitations, "skipped beats"	Precordial chest pain	Associated symptoms: Weakness, fatigue, lethargy, palpitations, dizziness, vertigo	Paroxysmal in onset Lasts briefly to hours
Anxiety disorders	May have history of depression or anxiety	Pain may be vague, diffuse; may be further described as disabling	Anterior chest and abdomen	Associated symptoms: Dyspnea, fatigue, anorexia	Variable; often continuous for hours to days
Monosodium glutamate	Occurs with food ingestion high in monosodium glutamate	Burning type of chest pain	Retrosternal chest pain	Associated symptoms: Facial pain, nausea, vomiting	Occurs shortly after meals or up to several hours after meal
Musculoskeletal	Precipitating factors: pain with inspiration or with musculoskeletal movement	Generalized aching, stiffness with point tenderness, swelling	Tenderness of the anterior chest wall	Persistent chest pain without relief with rest	

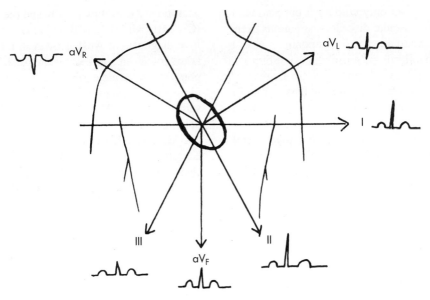

FIGURE 33-11   Six-limb lead (leads I, II, III, aV$_R$, aV$_L$, and aV$_F$) normally appear as shown.

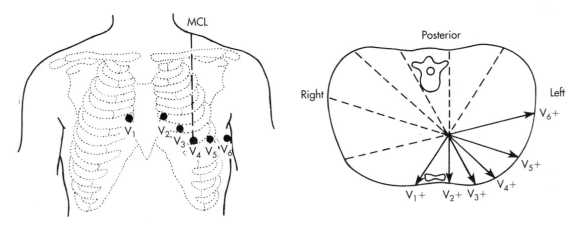

FIGURE 33-12   Precordial or chest (V$_{1-6}$) leads.

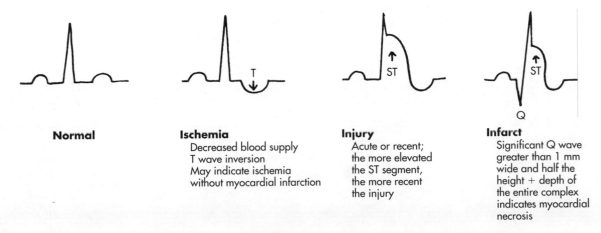

Normal

Ischemia
Decreased blood supply
T wave inversion
May indicate ischemia
without myocardial infarction

Injury
Acute or recent;
the more elevated
the ST segment,
the more recent
the injury

Infarct
Significant Q wave
greater than 1 mm
wide and half the
height + depth of
the entire complex
indicates myocardial
necrosis

FIGURE 33-13   ECG changes.

evations can be associated not only with AMI but also with conditions such as neuromuscular disorders, strenuous exercise, and renal failure. Cardiac-specific troponin is also a protein found in the myofibrils of muscle. Two subforms, cardiac-specific troponin T (cTn T) and troponin I, are very specific for the cardiac muscle because they have a role in contraction of myocardial muscle. Some studies have found not only that troponin elevations occur with AMI, but some studies have reported cTn T is released from myocardial cells in unstable angina. Troponin is detectable 4 to 6 hours after AMI, peaks at 10 to 24 hours, and remains elevated 5 to 7 days. Other primary cardiac markers released from

necrotic myocardium are CK and the MB fraction of the CK (CK-MB); with CK-MB once the "gold" standard for definitive diagnosis of AMI. However, CK-MB may take 4 to 6 hours to elevate, so biomarkers such as myoglobin and troponins that elevate earlier can be useful to the clinician for a more timely diagnosis. In addition, there are isoforms or subforms of CK-MB: CK-MB1 and CK-MB2. Studies have demonstrated that CK-MB2 of more than 1 U/L or a ratio of CK-MB2 to CK-MB1 of 1.5 is also indicative of AMI.[5,31] Lactate dehydrogenase (LDH), which is released by ischemic heart muscle, is elevated after AMI. Examine especially the isoforms LDH-1 and LDH-2; normally, LDH-2 is

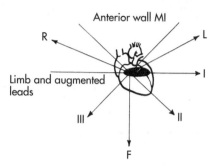
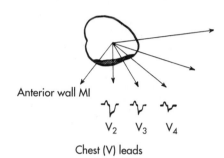

FIGURE 33-14 Anterior myocardial infarction (V$_2$, V$_3$, and V$_4$)

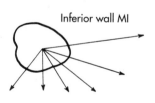
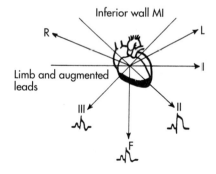

FIGURE 33-15 Inferior myocardial infarction (II, III, and aV$_F$).

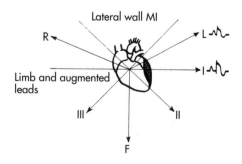
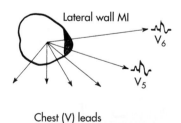

FIGURE 33-16 Lateral myocardial infarction (I, aV$_L$, V$_5$, and V$_6$).

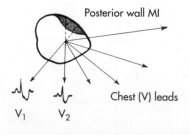
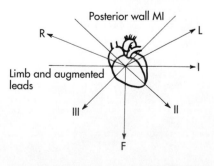

FIGURE 33-17 Posterior myocardial infarction (V$_1$ and V$_2$).

higher but with AMI the ratio "flips" and the LDH-1 level will be higher than LDH-2. Because of its lengthy time of elevation, LDH can be useful for prolonged retrospective diagnosis of myocardial infarction. Table 33-11 on p. 475 describes markers released with myocardial tissue necrosis.

Further evaluation of the patient with acute coronary syndromes includes a chest radiograph to rule out other causes of chest pain such as pneumonia, pneumothorax, trauma, and malignancy. A chest radiograph is also valuable in determining the presence of cardiomegaly and pulmonary congestion. In some situations, an echocardiogram may be used to evaluate myocardial wall motion, valve abnormalities, and septal wall defect. Although not diagnostic of AMI, an echocardiogram is useful in determining the extent of damage to the myocardium. Extensive myocardial damage puts the patient at risk for complications such as heart failure and cardiogenic shock.

Patient Management

While obtaining the history and assessing the patient's status, the emergency nurse should convey a calm and reassuring manner. Any patient with AMI or suspected AMI should have low-flow oxygen (2 to 6 L/min) and the head of the bed should be elevated. Maintain oxygen saturation greater than 95%. If oxygenation cannot be maintained or the patient is acidotic, intubation and mechanical ventilation are indicated.

After oxygen therapy is initiated, establish IV access for medications and fluid therapy. Insert at least two large-bore (18-gauge) catheters and infuse normal saline as needed. Ongoing assessment includes frequent determination of blood pressure, continuous ECG monitoring, and continuous pulse oximetry monitoring. Assessment of pain intensity, location, radiation of pain, and applicable descriptors establishes baseline. Assessment parameters should be reassessed after any intervention for chest pain. Nitroglycerin is the initial drug of choice for treatment of chest pain related to angina pectoris and AMI. Nitroglycerin can be administered sublingually in 0.3- or 0.4-mg tablets or in a spray. One tablet or spray is administered every 5 minutes, up to three doses. Nitroglycerin dilates coronary arteries, reduces afterload by dilating peripheral venous circulation, and reduces preload; that is, decreases venous return to the heart. Nitroglycerin is not usually given unless systolic blood pressure (SBP) is at least 100 mm Hg because of potential decreased blood pressure that can occur. If sublingual nitroglycerin is not effective, IV nitroglycerin (Tridil) can be used. Initiate nitroglycerin infusion at 10 to 20 mcg/min and titrate in increments of 5 to 10 mcg/min up to 50 to 180 mcg/min.[4,31]

If nitroglycerin fails to relieve chest pain, the next drug of choice is morphine sulfate. This narcotic analgesic relieves

---

Box 33-1   CRITERIA FOR SIGNIFICANT ECG CHANGES

PROBABLE NEW TRANSMURAL AMI

$\geq$ 1 mm ST segment elevation in $\geq$ two leads
OR
Abnormal Q waves in $\geq$ two leads

NEW STRAIN OR ISCHEMIA

$\geq$1 mm ST segment depression in $\geq$ two leads

NEW ST OR T WAVE CHANGES OF ISCHEMIA OR STRAIN

ST depression <1 mm and T wave inversions (can represent ischemia or strain)

ECG, Electrocardiogram.

Box 33-2   LEAD PLACEMENT FOR RIGHT VENTRICULAR AND POSTERIOR LEADS

RIGHT VENTRICULAR LEADS

V_{3R} = Between V_1 and V_{4R}
V_{4R} = Fifth intercostal space right midclavicular line
V_{5R} = Fifth intercostal space right anterior axillary line
V_{6R} = Fifth intercostal space right midaxillary line

POSTERIOR LEADS

V_7 = Fifth intercostal space posterior axillary line
V_8 = Fifth intercostal space between V_7 and V_9
V_9 = Fifth intercostal space next to vertebral column

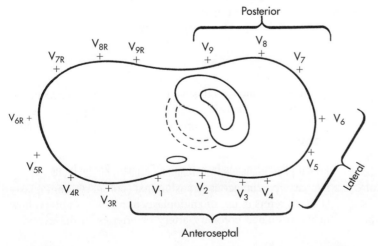

FIGURE 33-18   Right ventricular and posterior wall electrocardiogram lead placement. (Modified from Hearns PA: Differentiating ischemia, injury, infarction: expanding the 12-lead electrocardiogram, *Dimen Crit Care Nurs* 13(4):176, 1994.)

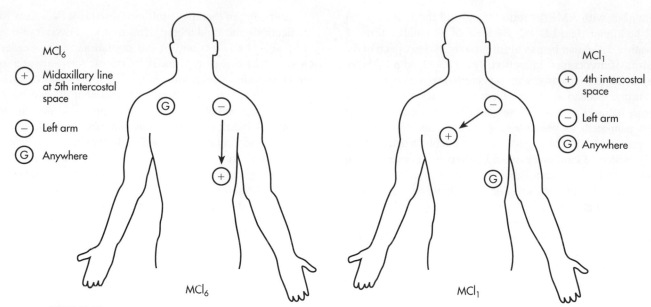

FIGURE 33-19 Monitoring on three-lead electrocardiogram monitor. Leads MCl$_6$ and MCl$_1$ are the best leads for monitoring dysrhythmias.

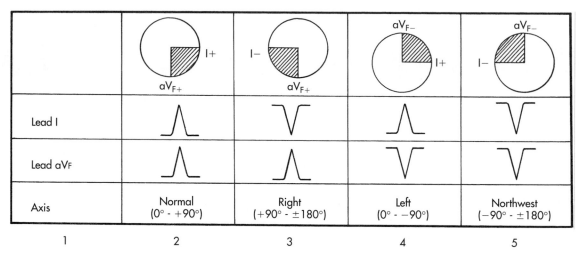

FIGURE 33-20 Determination of QRS axis. *(1)* Note predominant QRS polarity in leads I and aV$_F$. *(2)* If QRS during tachycardia is primarily positive in I and aV$_F$, axis falls within normal quadrant from 0 degrees to 90 degrees. *(3)* If complex is primarily negative in I and positive in aV$_F$, right axis deviation is present. *(4)* If complex is predominantly positive in I and negative in aV$_F$, left axis deviation is present. *(5)* If QRS is primarily negative in both I and aV$_F$, markedly abnormal "northwest" axis is present that is diagnostic of ventricular tachycardia. (Modified from Drew BJ: Bedside electrocardiographic monitoring, *Heart Lung* 20(6):610, 1991.)

chest pain and anxiety, which decreases myocardial oxygen consumption.[25] If SBP is greater than 100 mm Hg, administer morphine 2 to 4 mg IV every 5 to 10 minutes until pain is relieved. Monitor respiratory status and hemodynamic response carefully after morphine administration.

After the patient is initially evaluated, aspirin should be given orally (to be chewed) unless contraindicated (e.g., allergy, active gastrointestinal [GI] bleeding). If the patient is unable to tolerate oral aspirin, one rectal suppository can be given. Recommended dosage ranges from 160 to 325 mg. If the patient is "allergic" to aspirin, other antiplatelet agents such as dipyridamol, ticlopidine, or clopidogrel can be considered.[4,31]

Primary Percutaneous Transluminal Coronary Angioplasty

Primary percutaneous transluminal coronary angioplasty (PTCA) refers to use of angioplasty to reestablish blood flow in the occluded coronary artery or arteries in the evolving

Table 33-11	CARDIAC MARKERS FOR ACUTE MYOCARDIAL INFARCTION		
CARDIAC MARKER	**INITIAL ELEVATION AFTER ACUTE MYOCARDIAL INFARCTION**	**MEAN PEAK TIME**	**TIME TO RETURN TO BASELINE**
Myoglobin	1-4 hours	6-7 hours	18-24 hours
Troponin-I (cTn I) (cardiac specific)	3-12 hours	10-24 hours	3-7 days
Troponin-T (cTn T) (cardiac specific)	3-12 hours	12-48 hours	10-14 days
Creatine kinase-MB (CK-MB)	4-12 hours	10-24 hours	48-72 hours
CK-MB subforms: MB1 & MB2	1-6 hours	18 hours	Unknown
Lactate dehydrogenase (LDH)	8-12 hours	24-48 hours	10-14 days
*LDH-1/LDH-2 ratio >0.76 is significantly associated with acute myocardial infarction			

AMI process and is considered potentially superior to fibrinolytic therapy.[4,31] Current standards indicate that primary angioplasty should be performed in tertiary care centers with qualified clinicians. Targeted times from door to balloon should be 90 ± 30 minutes for patients with diagnosed AMI. Thus early diagnosis and decision-making regarding optimal treatment are necessary to facilitate primary PTCA.

Fibrinolytic Therapy

Fibrinolytic therapy for the patient with AMI is a crucial component of overall therapy to reduce patient mortality and morbidity. Patients benefit from therapy if the fibrinolytic agent is initiated within 12 hours of onset of chest pain. The goal of fibrinolytic therapy is to lyse coronary thrombi, restore blood flow to a hypoperfused myocardium, and abort or prevent complete evolution of the infarction process. When treatment begins within 3 hours of new symptoms, the incidence of successful reperfusion is 60% to 70% for all fibrinolytic agents.

Fibrinolytic therapy targets elements of the clotting process to cause fibrinolysis, the process of clot degradation. Lysis of the clot begins with activation of plasminogen, which converts to plasmin. Plasmin degrades or breaks down fibrin in the clot, circulating fibrinogen, factor V, and factor VIII. Fibrinolytic agents are an exogenous source of plasminogen. Refer to Table 33-12 for a comparison of fibrinolytic agents.[31]

Fibrinolytic agents have a significant potential for bleeding complications. Absolute contraindications for fibrinolytic therapy include recent internal bleeding (less than 1 month before arrival), known bleeding diathesis, history of cerebrovascular accident (CVA), recent surgery (e.g., intracranial, intraspinal, intraocular), intracranial AV malformations, uncontrolled hypertension (SBP greater than 180 mm Hg, diastolic blood pressure [DBP] greater than 110 mm Hg), recent trauma (in the past 10 days), and CPR. Relative contraindications include minor trauma, diabetic retinopathy, pregnancy, concurrent anticoagulation, severe trauma (e.g., in the past 6 months), any previous central nervous system event, and unsuccessful central venous puncture. If the patient will receive streptokinase or anistreplase, the patient should be screened for recent history of a streptococcal infection (less than 6 months ago) or prior treatment with streptokinase or anistreplase. Additional lab data

such as a complete blood cell count, prothrombin time, partial thromboplastin time (PTT), fibrinogen, and platelet count can assist with determining potential bleeding problems and serve as baseline data.

Additional nursing management for the patient receiving fibrinolytic therapy focuses on assessing for potential complications, monitoring for reperfusion, and minimizing tissue trauma. The major complication for the patient receiving fibrinolytic therapy is bleeding and hemorrhage. Bleeding occurs most often at cut-down sites, arterial puncture sites, and injection sites. Systemic bleeding, that is, GI, urinary, vaginal, cerebral, or retroperitoneal, and neurologic impairment (e.g., CVA) may also occur. Monitor for hypotension, decreased hemoglobin and hematocrit, and tachycardia. The other major complication that occurs is an allergic reaction, particularly with use of streptokinase or anistreplase. Monitor for respiratory distress, rash, or urticaria. Minimize tissue trauma by keeping the patient on bed rest, limiting arterial and venous punctures, and limiting use of noninvasive blood pressure cuffs. Reperfusion cannot be absolutely determined without benefit of cardiac angiography; however, markers of reperfusion that can be assessed by the emergency nurse include resolution of chest pain, normalizing of ST changes, and occurrence of reperfusion dysrhythmias such as accelerated idioventricular rhythms.

A heparin infusion is recommended in conjunction with fibrinolytic therapy to prevent formation of a new clot and reocclusion of the coronary vessel. The recommended dose is 60 U/kg as a bolus at the same time as initiating fibrinolytic therapy. A maintenance infusion of 12 U/kg per hour is titrated to maintain the patient's PTT at 1.5 to 2 times the control levels. Heparin is also recommended for patients who receive nonselective fibrinolytic agents (e.g., streptokinase, anistreplase); however, heparin should be withheld 6 hours and activated PTT (aPTT) checked before initiation of heparin to ensure aPTT is less than 2 times the control.

Heparin is also indicated for use in patients with non-ST elevation acute coronary syndromes. Options for heparin include IV heparin, subcutaneous unfractionated heparin (7500 U twice daily), or low molecular weight heparin (e.g., enoxaparin [Lovenox], dalteparin [Fragmin]) at 1 mg/kg twice daily.[31]

Table 33-12   COMPARISON OF FIBRINOLYTIC AGENTS

AGENT	ACTION	DOSE	COMMENTS
Streptokinase (Steptase, Kabikinase)	Exogenous plasminogen activator; not clot specific	**IV:** 1.5 million units IV over 1 hr **Intracoronary:** 10,000 to 30,000 U; followed by maintenance infusion of 2,000 to 4,000 U/min until thrombolysis occurs (e.g., 150,000 to 500,000 U total)	Half-life in plasma is 18 min; has a prolonged effect on coagulaiton because of depletion of fibrinogen, which persists for 18-24 hr; antibodies to the drug may be present in persons who have been exposed to *Streptococcus* infection resulting in: allergic reactions (e.g., rash, fever, chills); patients should not be retreated with streptokinase for a period of 2 wk to 1 yr after initial administration because of secondary resistance to development of antibodies
Anistreplase (Eminase)	Inactivated derivative of thrombolytic enzyme synthesized from streptokinase and lysoplasminogen; promotes thrombolysis after activation within the body	**IV:** 30 U over 2-5 min; dilute only with 5 ml sterile water	Do not give to patients who are allergic to streptokinase; may not be as effective as usual when administered more than 5 days after the previous dose or after streptokinase therapy or streptococcal infection; discard if not used within 30 min of mixing
Alteplase (Activase, Activase rt-PA)	Proteolytic enzyme; direct activator of plasminogen; high degree of clot specificity	**IV:** 15 mg IV bolus over 1-2 min; then 50 mg over 30 min, then 35 mg over 60 min	Half-life in plasma is 5-7 min; may cause sudden hypotension; inline IV filters can remove as much as 47% of the drug
Reteplase (Retavase)	Activates the conversion of plasminogen to plasmin; high degree of clot specificity	**IV:** 10 U over 2 min; then repeat 10 U in 30 min after initiation of first bolus	Give normal saline fluid before and after administraiton of Reteplase (Retevase) Reconstitute just before administration and use within 4 hr after reconstituting
TNK-tissue plasminogen activator (TNKase)	Activates clot-bound plasminogen to plasmin	**IV:** 30-50 mg bolus over 5 sec Dosing based on patient weight: <60 kg=30 mg TNK ≥60 to <70 kg = 35 mg TNK ≥70 to <80 kg = 40 mg TNK ≥80 to <90 kg = 45 mg TNK ≥90 mg = 50 mg TNK	More fibrin specificity and less incidence of bleeding than rt-PA

IV, Intravenous; *rt-PA,* recombinant prurokinase.

Additional Pharmacologic Therapy

Nitroglycerin IV infusions are recommended for the first 24 to 48 hours after AMI, especially anterior AMI. Nitroglycerin dilates coronary arteries, increases collateral blood flow, and decreases preload and afterload. Recent studies recommend additional pharmacologic agents to provide further protection for the AMI patient from mortality and morbidity. β-Blocker therapy should be initiated within 12 hours after AMI or for non-ST elevation acute coronary syndromes if there are no absolute contraindications, such as severe left ventricular failure and pulmonary edema, bradycardia (heart rate less than 60 bpm), hypotension (SBP lower than 100 mm), signs of poor peripheral perfusion, and second or third degree heart block. β-Blockers have proven especially useful in AMI patients with recurrent symptoms of ischemia, hypertension, sinus tachycardia, and in patients younger than 65 years of age. Additional therapy that may be initiated in the ED includes angiotensin-converting enzyme (ACE) inhibitor agents for those patients with AMI (e.g., enalapril, captopril, lisinopril). These agents should be started within 24 hours of AMI. Use of ACE inhibitors has been associated with reduced mortality. Known contraindications to ACE inhibitor therapy include allergies, Killip class III and IV (classification system for cardiac severity), history of renal failure, or bilateral renal artery stenosis.[4,31]

Table 33-13	OVERVIEW OF GLYCOPROTEIN IIB/IIIA INHIBITORS	
GLYCOPROTEIN IIB/IIIA INHIBITOR	**DOSAGE**	**POTENTIAL SIDE EFFECTS**
Abciximab (ReoPro)	0.25 mg/kg over 10-60 min 0.125mg/kg/min for 12 hr	Potential for increased bleeding, hypotension, bradycardia, nausea and vomiting, diarrhea
Eptifibatide (Integrilin)	180 mcg/kg over 1 to 2 min 2 mcg/kg/min for up to 72 hr	Potential for increased bleeding, hypotension
Tirofiban HCL (Aggrastat)	0.4 mcg/kg/min for 30 min 0.1 mcg/kg/min for 12-24 hr	Potential for increased bleeding, nausea, bradycardia

Another aspect of management of non-ST elevation acute coronary syndromes is the use of glycoprotein IIB/IIIA inhibitors. Platelet adhesion, activation, and aggregation play major roles in development of thrombus, which can potentiate evolution of these acute coronary syndromes into an AMI. Glycoprotein IIB/IIIA inhibitors antagonize or inhibit the receptor sites, which inhibits platelet aggregation. It has been demonstrated that these reduce risk for development of thrombus independent of aspirin and heparin therapies. Refer to Table 33-13 for an overview of these agents.[4,17,22,31,34]

Dysrhythmias

Blood flow deprivation to the myocardium as a result of AMI can affect the heart's electrical conduction system, causing various dysrhythmias. Table 33-14 summarizes dysrhythmias and categories of antidysrhythmics according to modified Vaughan-Williams classification schema. By understanding drug classifications, the emergency nurse can anticipate expected action of the drug and nursing implications for drug administration and patient assessment.[17,22,34]

PVCs are the most common dysrhythmia associated with cardiac ischemia and AMI, occurring in approximately 85% of patients with AMI. After initiation of oxygen therapy, lidocaine is the drug of choice for symptomatic PVCs. Lidocaine may be used prophylactically for AMI patients, even without PVCs, because of the high incidence of ventricular tachycardia and ventricular fibrillation that occurs without warning dysrhythmias. Some studies suggest that prophylactic use of lidocaine in patients with AMI may increase mortality; therefore, lidocaine use must be considered with respect to potential adverse effects. PVCs may also be caused by hypoxemia, acidosis, alkalosis, electrolyte imbalances, digoxin toxicity, and bradycardia.[6] The underlying mechanism responsible for the patient's PVCs should be evaluated and treated.

Bradycardia is defined as a heart rate less than 60 beats per minute and occurs in approximately 65% of AMI patients, particularly those with inferior wall infarction. Bradycardic dysrhythmias include AV blocks. Four different types occur, depending on area and degree of damage to the conduction system. These AV blocks are referred to as first-degree, second-degree Mobitz I (Wenckebach), second-degree Mobitz II, and third-degree or complete heart block. Blocks in conduction may be caused by myocardial infarc-

---

Box 33-3   SYSTEMATIC EVALUATION OF CARDIAC RHYTHMS

RATE

Bradycardia: <60 beats/min
Normal rate: 60 to 100 beats/min
Tachycardia: >100 beats/min

RHYTHM

Is the rhythm regular or irregular?

P WAVES

Are P waves present? Does one P wave appear before each QRS? Is P wave deflection normal?

QRS COMPLEX

Normal is 0.06 to 0.12 second. Are the QRS complexes normal shape and configuration?

P/QRS RELATIONSHIP

Does QRS complex follow every P wave?

PR INTERVAL

Normal is 0.12 to 0.2 second. Is the interval prolonged? Shortened?

---

tion, infection, degenerative changes in the conduction system, rheumatic heart disease, and medications such as beta blockers, calcium channel blockers, and cardiac glycosides. Management of symptomatic bradycardias and heart blocks includes drugs such as atropine and epinephrine. An external pacemaker or transvenous pacemaker may also be used. Second-degree Mobitz I heart block, associated with a conduction defect through the AV node, is usually benign and transient. This rhythm is commonly associated with inferior infarction because the right coronary artery supplies this area and the AV node. Second-degree Mobitz II AV block occurs when conduction through the bundle branches is impaired, usually because of blockage of the left coronary artery, which supplies the anterior wall and bundle branches.[6] This form of second-degree block is more likely than the other form to progress to third-degree block.

Other dysrhythmias that commonly occur are supraventricular tachycardias, which may be indicative of

Table 33-14	ANTIDYSRHYTHMIC PHARMACOLOGIC AGENTS AS CLASSIFIED BY MODIFIED VAUGHAN-WILLIAMS CLASSIFICATION SCHEMA				
CLASS	PHARMACOLOGIC ACTION	ELECTROPHYSIOLOGIC EFFECTS	INDICATIONS	DRUG EXAMPLARS	COMMENTS
I	Sodium channel blockade (stabilizes cell membrane)	Decreases conduction velocity; prolongs PR and QRS intervals	Ventricular dysrhythmias	Moricizine (Ethmozine)	Risk of proarrhythmia potential
IA		Blocks and delays repolarization, thereby lengthening the action potential duration and the effective refractory period	Atrial and ventricular dysrhythmias	Quinidine sulfate (Quinidex) Procainamide HCL (Pronestyl) Disopyramide (Norpace)	Observe for heart block, hypotension, prolonged PR/QRS/QT intervals
IB		Shortens the action of potential duration	Ventricular dysrhythmias	Lidocaine HCL (Xylocaine) Tocainide HCL (Tonocard) Mexilitene HCL (Mexitil)	Potential toxicity: Dizziness, vertigo, confusion, seizures
IC		Slows conduction of electrical impulses in atria, AV node, and ventricular/His—Purkinje fibers	Ventricular dysrhythmias	Flecainide acetate (Tambocar) Propafenone (Rhythmol)	Risk of proarrhythmia potential
II	β-adrenergic blockade	Inhibition of the sympathetic stimulation—reducing heart rate and decreasing myocardial irritability and shortens action potential	Supraventricular & ventricular dysrhythmias	Propranolol HCL (Inderal) Esmolol HCL (Brevibloc) Acebutolol (Sectral)	Observe for hypotension, bradycardia, heart block
III	Potassium channel blockade	Delayed repolarization and prolongation of the action potential, thus decreasing myocardial irritability	Ventricular tachycardia and ventricular fibrillation	Amiodarone HCL (Cordarone) Dofetilide (Tikosyn) Ibutilide fumarate (Corvert)	Observe for exacerbation of dysrhythmias, hypotension Pulmonary fibrosis may occur with amiodarone use
IV	Calcium channel blockade	Slows conduction of electrical impulses and decreases rate of impulse initiation	SVT and atrial dysrhythmias	Verapamil (Calan) Diltiazem (Cardizem) Nifedipine (Procardia)	Observe for hypotension, bradycardia, heart block
Unclassified	Potassium channel opener	Slows conduction through AV node and increases refractory period in AV node	SVT	Adenosine (Adenocard)	Has very rapid effect, short half-life

HCL, Hydrochloride; *AV,* atrioventricular; *SVT,* supraventricular tachycardia.

myocardial ischemia or anterior wall infarct. Often associated with chest pain, tachycardias are dangerous because they increase myocardial oxygen consumption and may extend the infarct. Treatment depends on clinical findings. For hemodynamically unstable patients, therapy may include pharmacologic agents such as adenosine, ve-rapamil, and procainamide, and vagal maneuvers or synchronized cardioversion.

Evaluation of dysrhythmias requires a systematic approach (Box 33-3). An overview of each rhythm is presented, including rhythm strip in lead II, significance of the rhythm, and therapeutic interventions for adults.

Pulseless Electrical Activity (PEA)

Rate	Varies
Rhythm	No characteristic pattern
P waves	None
QRS complex	Relatively normal or wide and bizarre
P/QRS relationship	None
PR interval	None

NOTE: By definition a patient is having pulseless electrical activity (PEA) when current rhythm should be perfusing but the patient has no pulse. Idioventricular rhythm at rate of 20 beats/min without a pulse is *not* PEA, but normal sinus rhythm at 72 beats/min in a patient who is unconscious, pulseless, and apneic is PEA.

Significance: Electrical complexes are present without mechanical contraction of the heart. The most common causes of this dysrhythmia are hypoxemia, hypovolemia, tension pneumothorax, acidosis, cardiac tamponade, and pulmonary embolism.

Intervention: Perform CPR and treat the underlying cause. Intubate, establish IV access, and give epinephrine every 3 to 5 minutes. If the electrical rate is less than 60 beats/min, atropine is given.

Dysrhythmias originating in the sinus node
Normal sinus rhythm

Rate	60 to 100 beats/min
Rhythm	Regular
P waves	Present
QRS complex	Present; normal duration
P/QRS relationship	P wave preceding each QRS complex
PR interval	Normal

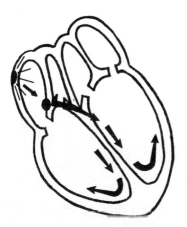

Impulse travels from
SA to AV node
through His bundle
to Purkinje fibers

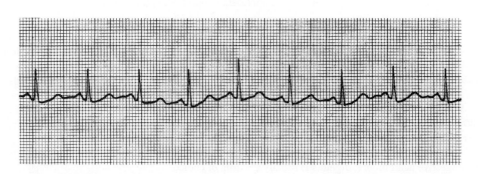

Significance: The sinoatrial (SA) node is the normal pacemaker of the heart and is influenced by parasympathetic and sympathetic branches of the autonomic nervous system.

Intervention: None required.

Sinus tachycardia

Rate	>100 beats/min; seldom >160 beats/min
Rhythm	Regular
P waves	Normal; present; with rapid rates, P waves may be buried in previous T wave
QRS complex	Present; normal duration
P/QRS relationship	P wave precedes each QRS complex
PR interval	Normal

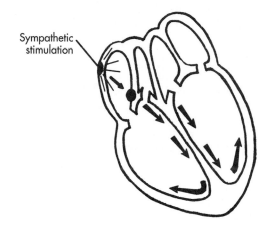

Sympathetic stimulation

SA node originates impulses at regular rate of greater than 100/minute

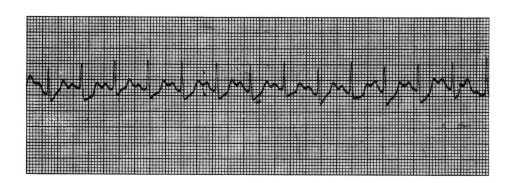

NOTE: If rate is exactly 150, consider possibility that rhythm is atrial flutter with a 2:1 conduction.

Significance: The normal pacemaker of the heart is firing at an increased rate because of anxiety, fever, pain, exercise, smoking, hyperthyroidism, heart failure, volume loss, specific drugs, or other reasons that cause increased tissue oxygen demands. Decreased vagal tone (parasympathetic stimulation) allows the sinus node to increase rate. Cardiac output may decrease with rates greater than 180 beats/min because of inadequate ventricular filling. Very rapid rates during AMI can lead to further ischemia and tissue damage.

Intervention: Treat the underlying cause. No specific drug is given for sinus tachycardia except in congestive heart failure; digitalis is usually the drug of choice.

Sinus bradycardia

Rate	<60 beats/min; seldom <30 beats/min
Rhythm	Regular or slightly irregular
P waves	Present; normal
QRS complex	Present; normal duration
P/QRS relationship	P wave precedes each QRS complex
PR interval	Normal

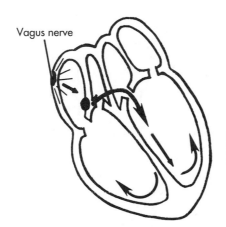

Vagus nerve

SA node originates impulses at a regular rate of less than 60/minute

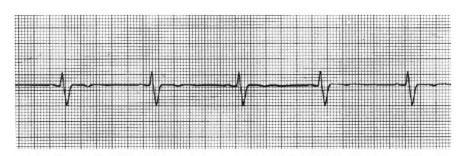

Significance: The normal pacemaker (SA node) is slowed by increased vagal tone (parasympathetic stimulation). Causes include rest, normal athletic heart, anoxia, hypothyroidism, increased intracranial pressure, acute myocardial infarction, vagal stimulation (such as vomiting, straining at stool, carotid sinus massage, or ocular pressure), and specific drugs.

Intervention: With heart rate less than 50 beats/min, cardiac output, coronary perfusion, and electrical stability may be reduced, causing PVCs. No treatment is needed if the patient is alert, has normal blood pressure, and no PVCs. Hypotension and PVCs should be treated. Symptomatic PVCs should be treated with oxygen and atropine, not lidocaine. Increasing the heart rate can eradicate the PVCs, whereas eliminating PVCs can decrease cardiac output.

Sinus arrhythmia

Rate	60 to 100 beats/min, but rate increases with inspiration and decreases with expiration
Rhythm	Regularly irregular
P waves	Present
QRS complex	Present; normal duration
P/QRS relationship	P wave precedes each QRS complex
PR interval	Normal

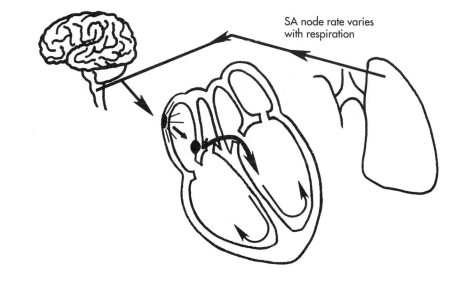

SA node rate varies with respiration

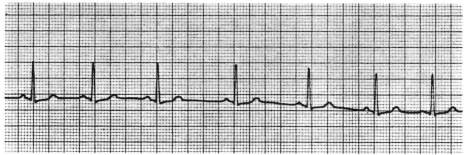

Significance: Normal finding in children and young adults with variation of vagal tone in response to respirations. As an abnormal finding, may occur in patients with mitral or aortic valve problems or as a response to increased intracranial pressure or specific drugs. To be considered a dysrhythmia, variation must exceed 0.12 seconds between the longest and shortest cycles.

Intervention: Observe the patient and document findings. If not related to respiratory problems, treat the underlying cause.

Dysrhythmias originating in the atria

Premature atrial contractions (extrasystoles)

Rate	Usually 60 to 100 beats/min
Rhythm	Usually regularly irregular; may be regular
P waves	Present, but premature P wave may appear different in configuration because it did not originate in the SA node
QRS complex	Present; normal duration
P/QRS relationship	P wave precedes each QRS complex
PR interval	Normal in regular beats, variable in premature atrial contractions (PACs)

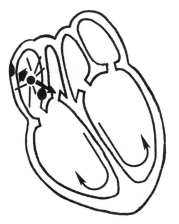

Atrial origin of abnormal impulse

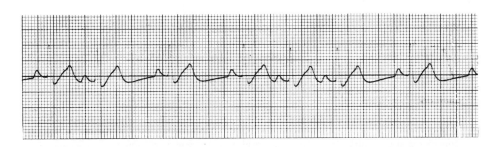

NOTE: Always describe underlying rhythm. For example, "Sinus tachycardia with approximately two PACs per minute."

Significance: PACs are the result of an irritable ectopic focus that may be caused by fatigue, alcohol, coffee, smoking, digoxin, congestive heart failure, or ischemia; sometimes the cause is unknown. PACs may be a prelude to atrial fibrillation, atrial flutter, or paroxysmal atrial tachycardia.

Intervention: Treatment is usually unnecessary. If the patient has symptoms, tranquilizers, quinidine, procainamide, verapamil, β-adrenergic blockers, and diltiazem may be tried. Encourage the patient to limit alcohol, coffee consumption, and smoking.

Supraventricular tachycardia

Rate	140 to 220 beats/min; atrial rate usually 160 to 240 beats/min
Rhythm	Atrial rhythm regular; ventricular rhythm usually regular, may be 2:1 AV block
P waves	Absent or abnormal; may be difficult to identify if P waves buried in preceding T wave; differ from normal sinus P waves
QRS complex	Normal or prolonged because of bundle branch block or aberrant conduction
P/QRS relationship	May be a block
PR interval	Normal or prolonged

Impulse travels from
site above ventricles
through HIS bundle to
Purkinje fibers

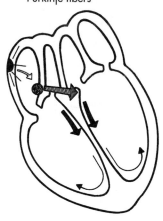

NOTE: Rhythm that is regular, greater than 150 beats/min, and associated with narrow QRS complex is considered supraventricular tachycardia. A part of the atria or AV junction, is serving as the pacemaker for the heart. Called paroxysmal supraventricular tachycardia when it begins and ends abruptly.

Significance: In elderly individuals and those with heart disease, rapid heart rates may precipitate myocardial ischemia, infarction, or pulmonary edema. May also be caused by digoxin overdose.

Intervention: Treatment should be initiated promptly when the patient has chest pain, hypotension, pulmonary edema, or signs of AMI. Determine whether the rhythm is paroxysmal supraventricular tachycardia or ventricular tachycardia. Vagal maneuvers, verapamil, adenosine, digoxin, overdrive pacing, and synchronized cardioversion are used to treat this rhythm.

Wandering atrial pacemaker

Rate	Usually 60 to 100 beats/min
Rhythm	Irregular
P waves	Present; configuration varies
QRS complex	Present; normal duration
P/QRS relationship	P wave preceding each QRS
PR interval	Normal, although may vary from beat to beat

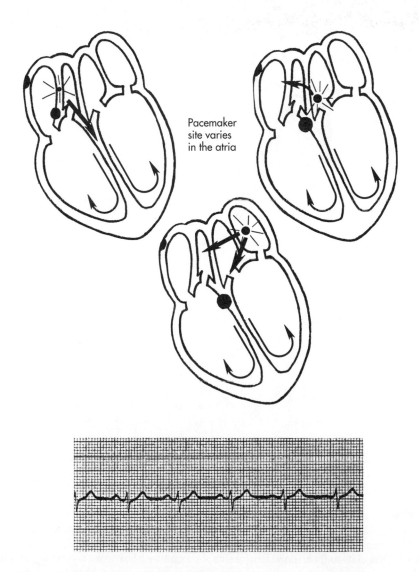

Pacemaker site varies in the atria

Significance: SA node is suppressed or other atrial foci become excited and take over pacemaker function of the heart. This dysrhythmia may be caused by specific drugs, inflammation, or chronic obstructive pulmonary disease.

Intervention: Treatment is usually unnecessary. Consider withholding digoxin until serum level confirmed. When necessary, treat the underlying cause.

Atrial flutter

Rate	Atrial rate of 240 to 360 beats/min
Rhythm	Regular or irregular
P waves	Saw-toothed pattern (F waves, or flutter waves)
QRS complex	Present; normal duration
P/QRS relationship	Ventricular response varies; because of rapid atrial rate, there may be regular or irregular ventricular response
PR interval	Not measurable

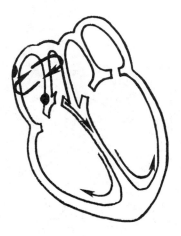

Circus movement in atria; variable degree of block

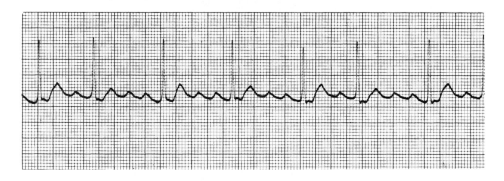

Significance: Irritable focus in the atria is responsible for this dysrhythmia. Usually a 2:1 AV block with ventricular rate approximately 150 beats/min. Ventricular response may be regular or irregular. New-onset atrial flutter is a dangerous dysrhythmia because ineffective atrial contractions may cause mural clots to form in the atria, which subsequently break loose and form pulmonary or cerebral emboli. Atrial flutter may occur with coronary artery disease, rheumatic heart disease, chronic obstructive pulmonary disease, shock, anoxia, electrolyte imbalance, hyperthyroidism, and in response to various drugs.

Intervention: Ventricular rate may be slowed with digitalis, verapamil, adenosine, diltiazem, or β-blocking agents. If pharmacologic therapy is unsuccessful, synchronized cardioversion is indicated. Verapamil and β-blockers may exacerbate bradycardia, congestive heart failure, or both.

Atrial fibrillation

Rate	Atrial rate 350 to 600 beats/min; ventricular rate 60 to 160 beats/min
Rhythm	Irregularly irregular
P waves	No P waves; F waves (fibrillatory) appear
QRS complex	Irregular rhythm; normal duration
P/QRS relationship	Indistinguishable P waves; irregular ventricular response
PR interval	Indistinguishable

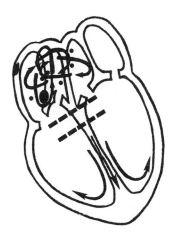

Chaotic impulses from atria; variable degree of block

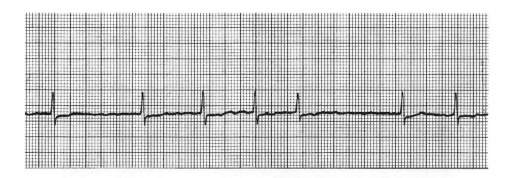

Significance: Multiple atrial pacemakers fire chaotically in rapid succession. Atria never firmly contract. Ventricles respond irregularly. Poor atrial emptying causes danger of mural clot formation and embolism. Cardiac output drops because there is no "atrial kick" (15% to 20% decrease in cardiac output). Patients who have chronic atrial fibrillation controlled with digitalis whose ventricular rate is less than 100 beats/min do not need treatment. Dysrhythmia frequently occurs in coronary artery disease, rheumatic heart disease, hyperthyroidism, and, most commonly, digitalis toxicity.

Intervention: Cardioversion is recommended for patients with ischemic heart disease. For asymptomatic patients, heart rate may be controlled with digitalis, calcium channel–blockers, or β-adrenergic blockers. Use of the latter two drugs in the undigitalized patient may not be effective and can cause congestive heart failure.

Dysrhythmias originating in the AV node
Nodal (junctional) rhythm

Rate	Usually 40 to 60 beats/min
Rhythm	Regular
P waves	May appear inverted before or after the QRS complex, or may be absent
QRS complex	Regular; normal duration
P/QRS relationship	Variable
PR interval	<0.12 second when the P wave precedes the QRS complex

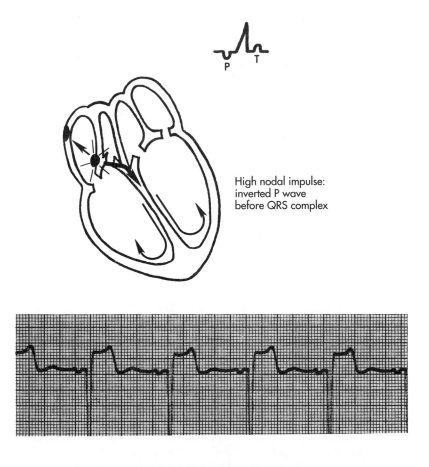

High nodal impulse:
inverted P wave
before QRS complex

Significance: AV junction has assumed pacing function for the heart. There is retrograde depolarization of the atrium, which may or may not result in detectable P waves.

Intervention: If the patient has been receiving digitalis therapy, withhold digitalis and obtain serum digoxin level to check for toxicity. There is no specific therapy for this dysrhythmia. If the patient becomes symptomatic from decreased heart rate, atropine may be administered. If no response to the atropine, pacing is indicated.

Nodal (junctional) rhythm—cont'd

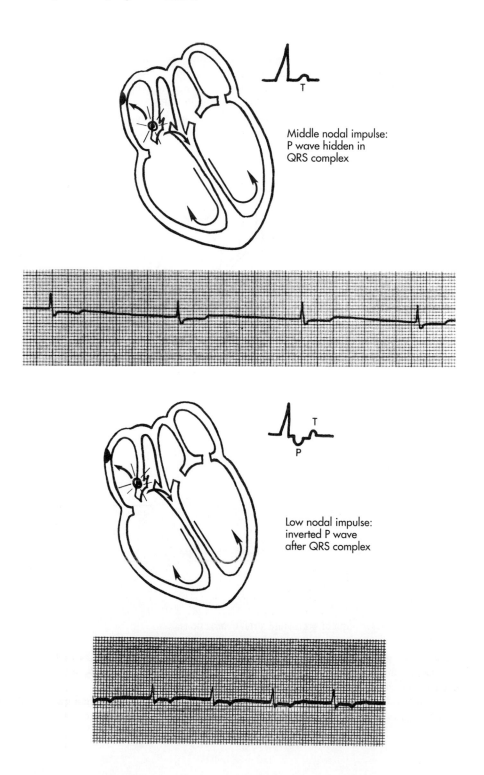

Middle nodal impulse:
P wave hidden in
QRS complex

Low nodal impulse:
inverted P wave
after QRS complex

Premature nodal contractions and premature junctional contractions

Rate	Usually normal or bradycardic
Rhythm	Irregularly irregular
P waves	May appear inverted or may be absent
QRS complexes	Regular; normal duration
P/QRS relationship	P waves may appear inverted, may be absent, and may occur before, during, and after the QRS complex
PR interval	<0.12 second when the P wave is seen in a premature beat

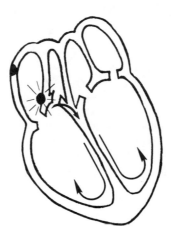

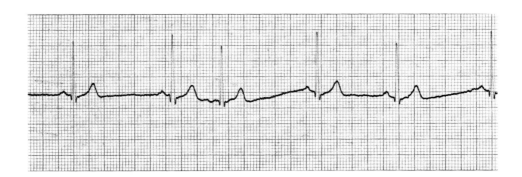

NOTE: See the description of premature atrial contractions.

Significance: AV junction serves episodically as pacemaker for the heart. Dysrhythmia is seen less frequently than premature atrial contractions or PVCs; may precede first-, second-, or third-degree heart block.

Intervention: Premature nodal contractions and premature junctional contractions are usually benign. If therapy is indicated, treatment is similar to that for premature atrial contractions.

Nodal tachycardia (junctional tachycardia)

Rate	100 to 800 beats/min
Rhythm	Regular
P waves	May appear inverted or may be absent
QRS complex	Regular; normal duration
P/QRS relationship	P waves may appear inverted before or after the QRS complex or may be absent
PR interval	<0.12 second when the P wave is present

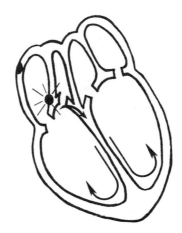

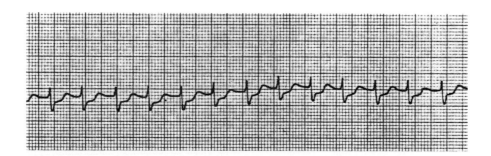

NOTE: Accelerated junctional rhythm is a junctional rhythm with increased sympathetic stimulation. Rate is 60 to 100 beats/min.

Significance: An irritable focus takes over as the heart's pacemaker. Nodal tachycardia may be caused by heart disease, electrolyte imbalance, chronic obstructive pulmonary disease, anoxia, or specific drugs.

Intervention: Dysrhythmia generally considered a variant of supraventricular tachycardia and is treated accordingly. In cases of nonparoxysmal episodes caused by digitalis intoxication, digitalis should be withheld and serum level checked. Serum potassium level should also be obtained.

First-degree AV block

Rate	Usually 60 to 100 beats/min
Rhythm	Usually regular
P waves	Present; normal configuration
QRS complex	Regular; normal duration
P/QRS relationship	P wave precedes each QRS complex
PR interval	>0.20 second

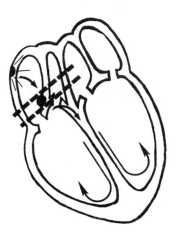

SA node originates impulse; partial block at AV node.

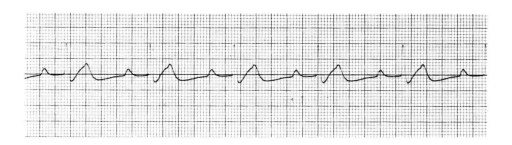

Significance: Conduction of impulse generated by the SA node is delayed through the atrioventricular node. Causes are varied and include anoxia, ischemia, atrioventricular node malfunction, edema after open-heart surgery, digitalis toxicity, myocarditis, thyrotoxicosis, rheumatic fever, clonidine, and tricyclic antidepressants.

Intervention: Usually no treatment is required. Observe the patient, noting level of consciousness and vital signs. If the patient becomes symptomatic (rarely), atropine is the drug of choice. If the patient is on a regimen of digitalis, withhold it and obtain serum digitalis and potassium levels.

Second-degree AV block (Mobitz I, Wenckebach)

Rate	Usually normal
Rhythm	Regularly irregular
P waves	One P wave preceding each QRS complex, except during regular dropped ventricular conduction at periodic intervals
QRS complex	Cyclic missed conduction; when QRS complex is present, duration normal
P/QRS relationship	P wave before each QRS complex, except during regular dropped ventricular conduction at periodic intervals
PR interval	Lengthens with each cycle until one QRS complex is dropped, then cycle is repeated

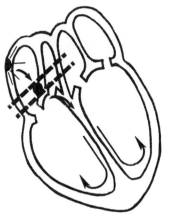

SA node originates impulse; partial block at AV node

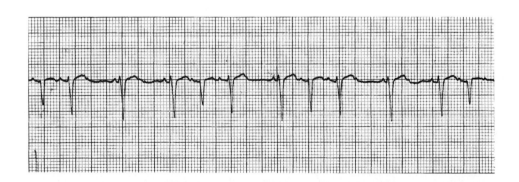

Significance: Each atrial impulse takes progressively longer to travel through the AV node until a beat is dropped, then the cycle begins again. Dysrhythmia is the less serious form of second-degree heart block; usually transient and reversible. In rare instances, dysrhythmia may progress to complete heart block. Commonly occurs after inferior wall infarct.

Intervention: Treatment needed when heart rate is <50 beats/min or if the patient becomes symptomatic. Therapy includes atropine and temporary pacing.

Second-degree AV block (Mobitz II)

Rate	Atrial rate usually 60 to 100 beats/min; ventricular rate slower
Rhythm	Usually regularly irregular
P waves	Two or more P waves for every QRS complex; normal configuration; regular interval
QRS complex	Normal duration, when present
P/QRS relationship	One or more nonconducted impulses appearing as P waves not followed by QRS complexes
PR interval	Normal or delayed on the conducted beat but regular throughout the dysrhythmia

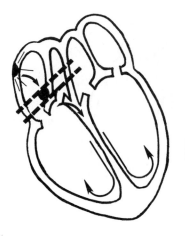

Partial intermittant block at AV node.

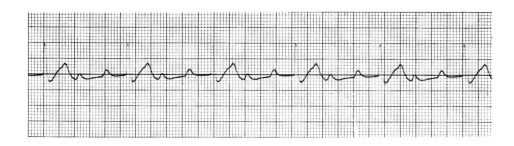

Significance: One or more atrial impulses are not conducted through the AV node to the ventricles. May occur in anterior myocardial infarction and progress rapidly to complete heart block. Other causes are anoxia, digitalis toxicity, and hyperkalemia.

Intervention: If the patient is asymptomatic, immediate treatment is not required. As with other heart block, atropine and pacing measures are used. If the patient is taking digitalis, withhold medication and obtain serum level.

Third-degree AV block (complete heart block)

Rate	Atrial rate 60 to 100 beats/min; ventricular rate usually <60 beats/min
Rhythm	Usually normal for atria and ventricles when examined separately
P waves	Occur regularly
QRS complex	Slow; usually wide (>0.10 second)
P/QRS relationship	Completely independent of each other
PR interval	No PR interval because there is no consistent relationship between P wave and QRS complex

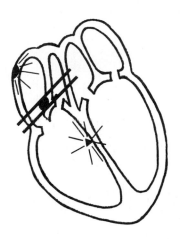

Complete block at AV node; may have nodal or ventricular independent pacemaker

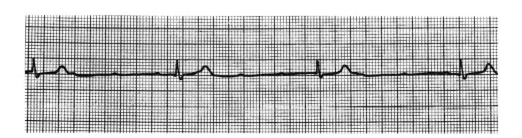

Significance: No SA impulses conducted through AV node. AV node or ventricle initiates impulse; the atria and ventricles beat independently. Bradycardia reduces myocardial perfusion and may lead to ventricular tachycardia or ventricular fibrillation.

Intervention: Pacemaker insertion is required. Transcutaneous pacing may be used until a transvenous pacer can be inserted. Atropine can be used until pacing unit is available. Be prepared to perform CPR and advanced life support. Do not give lidocaine to a patient with complete heart block, even when wide, bizarre QRS complexes are present.

Dysrhythmias originating in the ventricles

Premature ventricular contractions (premature ectopic beats, extrasystoles, premature ventricular beats, ventricular premature beats)

Rate	Usually 60 to 100 beats/min
Rhythm	Irregular
P waves	Present with each sinus beat; do not precede premature ventricular contractions (PVCs)
QRS complex	Sinus-initiated QRS complex normal; QRS complex of PVC wide and bizarre: >0.10 second; full compensatory pause
P/QRS relationship	P wave before each QRS complex in normal sinus beats; no P wave preceding PVC; compensatory pause following PVC
PR interval	Normal in sinus beat; none in PVC

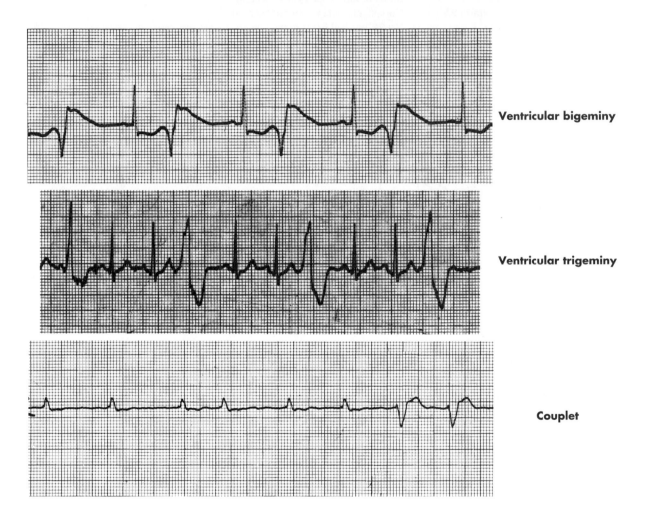

Ventricular bigeminy

Ventricular trigeminy

Couplet

Significance: PVCs indicate ventricular irritability. Impulse is initiated by ventricular pacemaker cell. PVCs may occur as a result of hypoxia, hypovolemia, ischemia, infarction, hypocalcemia, hyperkalemia, acidosis, or from alcohol, tobacco, coffee, or other stimulants. PVCs may originate from the same focus (unifocal) or from various foci (multifocal). Multifocal PVCs have various morphologies. PVCs may occur in repetitive patterns, every other beat (bigeminy), every third beat (trigeminy), in pairs (couplet), three contractions together (triplet). Four or more consecutive PVCs is referred to as a short run of ventricular tachycardia.

Intervention: Administer oxygen. If possible, treat the underlying cause. If treating the cause is not possible, pharmacologic therapy is indicated. First try lidocaine as a bolus. If this treatment is not successful, procainamide and amiodarone may be used. After ectopy is resolved, IV drip of effective antidysrhythmic drug should be instituted. When the PVCs are related to a slow heart rate, atropine is the drug of choice.

Ventricular tachycardia

Rate	150 to 250 beats/min
Rhythm	May be slightly irregular
P waves	Not seen
QRS complex	Wide and bizarre; width is >0.12 second
P/QRS relationship	None
PR interval	None

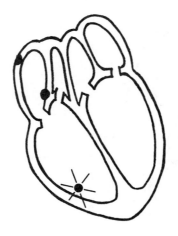

One ventricular
pacemaker fires
rapidly

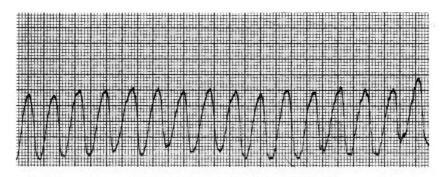

Significance: Rhythm cannot be tolerated for long periods because cardiac output is significantly reduced. If the rhythm persists, will deteriorate into ventricular fibrillation and asystole.

Intervention: Pulseless ventricular tachycardia should be treated as ventricular fibrillation. If a pulse is present and the patient is stable, give an antidysrhythmic agent (amiodarone, lidocaine, or procainamide). If the patient becomes unstable, cardioversion is the treatment of choice. Be prepared to begin CPR and initiate advanced life support measures.

Ventricular fibrillation

Rate	Rapid, disorganized
Rhythm	Irregular
P waves	Not seen
QRS complex	Absent; fibrillatory waves of varying size, shape, and duration occur
P/QRS relationship	None
PR interval	None

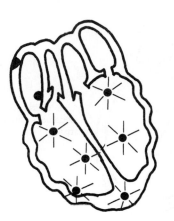

Ventricular ectopic
sites firing so fast that
quivering results

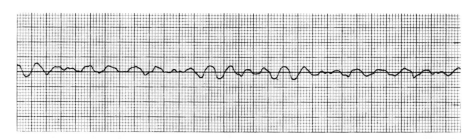

Significance: Dysrhythmia is the most common cause of sudden cardiac death. Ventricular fibrillation produces no cardiac output; cerebral death results when dysrhythmia persists more than 4 to 6 minutes. Ventricular fibrillation may be preceded by ventricular tachycardia.

Intervention: Begin CPR until a defibrillator is available. Check the rhythm, differentiating between asystole and fine ventricular fibrillation. Defibrillate, start with 200 J, continue with 200 to 300 J, and increase as high as 360 J if no response. If no pulse is present, continue CPR while establishing IV access, intubating the patient, or both. Next, administer epinephrine (or vasopressin if there is no history of CV disease), defibrillate up to 360 J, administer amiodarone then defibrillate at 360 J. Continue administration of antidysrhythmics alternated with countershocks.

Remember to check pulse and rhythm between each countershock. If ventricular fibrillation reoccurs after conversion, begin defibrillation at whatever energy level was previously successful.

Idioventricular rhythm

Rate	Usually <40 beats/min
Rhythm	Regular or irregular
P waves	None
QRS complex	Wide and bizarre (>0.10 second)
P/QRS relationship	None
PR interval	None

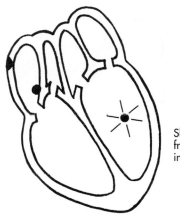

Slow impulses
from ectopic site
in ventricle

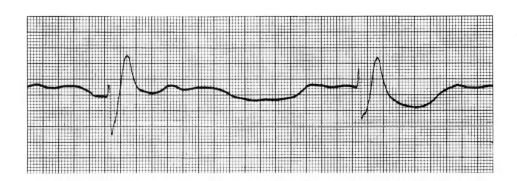

Significance: Rhythm is escape rhythm of ventricular origin. Effective cardiac contractions and pulses may or may not be present. May be caused by complete heart block, AMI, cardiac tamponade, or exsanguinating hemorrhage. Outcome is usually poor.

Intervention: Administer atropine; consider pacing. Treat the underlying cause.

Asystole (ventricular standstill)

Rate	None
Rhythm	None
P waves	May or may not appear
QRS complex	Absent or rare with bizarre configuration
P/QRS relationship	None
PR interval	None

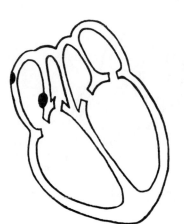

No electrical activity

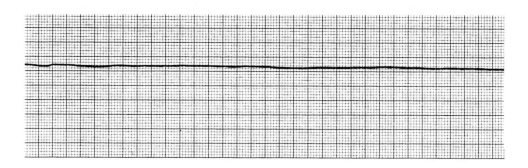

Significance: Mortality greater than 95%. Asystole often implies the patient's heart has been in arrest for a prolonged period. Confirm presence of asystole in two limb leads.

Intervention: Begin CPR. Differentiate between asystole and ventricular fibrillation. Intubate and establish IV access. Administer epinephrine; repeat every 3 to 5 minutes as needed. Next, give atropine (repeat once in 3 to 5 minutes) and use external pacemaker.

Pacemakers

Temporary pacing is used when a patient's condition deteriorates secondary to a bradycardic or tachycardic dysrhythmia unresponsive to other therapy. Indications for pacing include severe bradycardia, high-degree AV blocks, atrial tachycardia, atrial flutter, and recurrent ventricular tachycardia.

Three methods can be used for pacing—transthoracic, transvenous, and external (transcutaneous) methods. The transthoracic approach is not used in the ED because of associated risks, time required to complete the procedure, and interference with chest compressions. The transvenous method involves inserting a catheter electrode percutaneously into the right atrium or ventricle via the subclavian, internal jugular, brachial, or femoral vein. The procedure is guided by the changes in the ECG or fluoroscopy. Atrial pacing is used to suppress atrial tachycardia, whereas ventricular pacing suppresses ventricular ectopy by overdrive pacing.

Transcutaneous or external pacing is used more often in the ED. A negative electrode is placed posteriorly at midthoracic level of the spine with a positive electrode placed anteriorly at the chest lead V3 position. This position provides a lower pacing threshold and is away from large skeletal muscles, thus decreasing muscle stimulation. Electrode placement should not interfere with defibrillation. The rate of pacing impulses may be "fixed" (asynchronous, competitive, or nondemand) or set to fire on demand. A fixed rate delivers electrical current at regular intervals and is usually used when patients have bradycardia causing hemodynamic instability; for example, complete heart block. The demand pacing mode senses the patient's own QRS complexes and generates an impulse only if the patient does not have an intrinsic QRS generated during a set time frame. Fixed-rate pacing is rarely used because of potential competition with the patient's own rhythm or ventricular fibrillation if the pacer discharges on the T wave (relative refractory period) of the patient's own cardiac cycle.[6]

Successful pacing depends on condition of the myocardium. Patients with severe bradycardia, heart block, or idioventricular rhythm who can generate a pulse with each QRS complex usually respond to cardiac pacing and have a better outcome. Patients in asystole are less likely to respond to pacing.

Factors that indicate successful pacemaker capture—that is, successful electrical stimulation followed by mechanical response—include combined pacing spike and QRS complex 0.14 seconds in duration and resolution of the dysrhythmia being treated. Mechanical capture occurs when the heart responds to pacing with effective contractions. Mechanical capture is evaluated by the presence of a pulse consistent with paced beats. Both types of capture (electrical and mechanical) must be present for effective pacing. Assess the patient's hemodynamic and neurologic response by palpating the carotid or femoral pulse, obtaining vital signs, and evaluating the level of consciousness.

Two major reasons for lack of capture are acidosis and hypoxemia. Evaluate the patient's oxygen saturation and acid-base levels to determine appropriate interventions for such disorders. Another reason for lack of capture is related to the external pacing device and pacing electrodes. Check all connections. Consider repositioning the posterior electrode to the fifth intercostal space, midaxillary line (V6 chest lead position). Replace dry pacing electrodes. Make sure contact between external pacing electrodes and skin surface is adequate. Skin should be clean and dry before electrode application; benzoin may be used to improve adherence to the skin.

Implanted Cardioverter Defibrillator Therapy

The implanted cardioverter defibrillator (ICD) is a device that may be used as a treatment modality to reduce the incidence of sudden death from AMI. Approved in 1985, the ICD monitors the patient's cardiac rhythm and provides pacing or defibrillation to the patient depending on programming. Newer models can deliver multiple or tiered therapies, antitachycardia pacing (fast pacing), single-chamber ventricular demand pacing for bradycardia (slow pacing), cardioversion, or defibrillation shocks.

ICD generators are implanted under skin and subcutaneous tissue. Depending on device, the ICD generator may be implanted in the abdomen or upper chest. Older ICD devices require a surgical approach for applying electrodes to the epicardial surface of the heart. Newer devices allow subcutaneous or submuscular insertion of the ICD patch along the left anterior axillary line, left midaxillary area, or left posterior area. The lead is then tunneled along the left anterior chest wall and connected to the ICD generator.

If the patient requires defibrillation, external defibrillation can still be performed. Defibrillator paddles should not be placed over the ICD generator. If defibrillation attempts are unsuccessful, consider anterior-posterior placement of paddles to improve conduction of electrical current around ICD electrodes on the chest wall. Anyone in physical contact with the patient when the ICD device fires may experience a harmless, slight tingling sensation. If the ICD fires inappropriately, the physician can deactivate the device by placing a magnet over the ICD generator.[6]

Acute Ischemic Heart Failure

Heart failure (HF) occurs when the myocardium fails to function adequately as a pump. This inadequacy results in venous congestion, decreased stroke volume, decreased cardiac output, and increased peripheral systemic pressure. Onset may be gradual or sudden. The primary precipitating event for HF is some type of myocardial damage that activates many compensatory mechanisms. Over time, compensatory mechanisms are exhausted and cause adverse events. HF rarely occurs at the same time as AMI. Development is generally more insidious, occurring over time. HF may be seen alone or in conjunction with pulmonary edema. The onset of HF is a symptom of an underlying problem such as AMI, hypertension, fluid overload, intracranial injury, valvular heart disease, dysrhythmias, cardiomyopathy, hyperthyroidism, fever, and adult respiratory distress syndrome.[6] HF may also occur with oxygen toxicity syndrome, pneumothorax, uremic pneumonia, intracranial tumors, and drugs such as methotrexate (Rheumatrex), busulfan (Myleran), and nitrofurantoin (Furadantin).

HF is characterized by severe dyspnea, orthopnea, fatigue, weakness, abdominal discomfort (secondary to ascites or hepatic engorgement), dependent edema, distended neck veins, bilateral rales, third heart sound (gallop), laterally displaced apical pulse, and hepatomegaly. Assess patient and ensure adequate airway, breathing, and circulation (ABCs), then check vital signs, monitor ECG rhythm and oxygenation, auscultate lungs and heart, and observe for distended neck veins and peripheral edema.

Therapeutic interventions include maintaining the patient on bed rest in high-Fowler's position; administering oxygen, digitalis, and diuretics; maintaining an IV line at keep-open rate or use of a saline or intermittent needle therapy; monitoring intake and output; and weighing the patient daily. Additional therapy may include vasodilators to dilate arteries, ACE inhibitors to decrease systemic vascular resistance, and digitalis or other pharmacologic agents (e.g., dobutamine [Dobutrex]) to increase cardiac output. [9,21] Left ventricular assistive devices are also used in these patients as a temporary measure.

Acute Pericarditis

Acute pericarditis is inflammation of the pericardial sac caused by AMI, trauma, infection, or neoplasms. Among younger patients, infectious processes such as coxsackie virus, streptococci, staphylococci, tuberculosis, and *Haemophilus influenzae* can cause pericarditis. Early pericardial friction rub may occur with pericarditis in conjunction with AMI. Friction rub occurs when an inflamed area over a transmural infarction causes the pericardial surface to lose lubricating fluid. Pericarditis is most evident 2 to 3 days after an AMI.

Patients with pericarditis have severe chest pain that increases during inspiration and increased activity, fever, chills, and dyspnea. Tachycardia or other dysrhythmias may also be present. Pericardial friction rub increases in intensity when the patient leans forward. The patient has general malaise with ST segment elevation 1 to 3 mm in all ECG leads except aVR and V1. Therapeutic intervention includes oxygen by nasal cannula 4 to 6 L/min, sedation, analgesia, and bed rest. Antiinflammatory agents and steroids may also be indicated.[6,9,21]

Aortic Aneurysm

An aneurysm is "irreversible dilatation of an artery secondary to a localized weakness of the arterial wall that may predispose the artery to thrombosis, distal embolization, or rupture." Aneurysms can occur anywhere along the aorta; however, 80% occur in the abdominal aorta

rather than the thoracic aorta. Abdominal aortic aneurysms (AAA) are more common in individuals ages 50 to 70 years, and account for 10,000 deaths per year.[15] One postmortem study suggested 5% of men ages 65 to 74 years had AAA.

The primary etiology of aortic aneurysms is atherosclerosis and related factors; that is, hyperlipidemia, smoking, diabetes, and hereditary factors. Other causes include arteritis, congenital abnormalities, trauma, infection, and syphilis. The atherosclerotic process contributes to weakening and eventual destruction of the medial wall of the artery. Over time hemodynamic forces of blood flow cause thickening of the wall and replacement of muscle fibers with fibrous tissue and calcium deposits. The aneurysm enlarges over time and the wall tension of the aneurysm increases. Dilation of the aneurysm allows development of a thrombus, which may be dislodged and cause thromboembolism distally in the patient's circulation, for example, lower extremities.[9,21]

Three types of aneurysms are fusiform, saccular, and dissecting. Fusiform aneurysms are characterized by a segment of artery dilated around the entire circumference of the artery, whereas a saccular aneurysm dilates only a portion of the artery. A dissecting aneurysm actually results in a tear of the artery's intimal layer, which allows blood to flow between the intimal and medial layers (Figure 33-21). Dissecting aneurysms are further classified by the extent of the tear and location. Type 1 dissection occurs in the ascending aorta and extends beyond the aortic arch. Type 2 dissection occurs only in the ascending aorta. Type 3 dissection begins distal to the left subclavian artery.[6]

As the aorta dissects, major vessels that branch off the aorta may be occluded. Occluded vessels include myocardial, cerebral, mesenteric, and renal vessels. Rupture of the dissection can cause pericardial tamponade or hemorrhage into the thoracic cavity, resulting in exsanguination, shock, and imminent death.

Patient Assessment

Fifty percent of patients with aortic aneurysms are asymptomatic. AAA may be discovered on physical examination suggested by widened midline pulsation proximal to the umbilicus. Patients who present to the ED with a leaking or rupturing AAA have a classic presentation characterized by extreme back pain accompanied by abdominal pain and tenderness with palpation. Back pain may radiate to legs, groin, or lower back secondary to stretching of the anterior spinal ligament. Patients with a thoracic aneurysm may complain of excruciating substernal chest pain felt through to the posterior cavity. Rupture of the aneurysm compromises hemodynamic stability and blood flow distal to the aneurysm. Signs and symptoms include dyspnea, orthopnea, diaphoresis, pallor, apprehension, syncope, tachycardia, unilateral absence of major pulses, bilateral blood pressure differences, hypertension, pulsation at the sternoclavicular joint, murmur of aortic insufficiency (in ascending aortic aneurysm), hemiplegia or paraplegia, and shock.

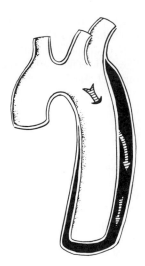

FIGURE 33-21   Dissecting aortic aneurysm.

Patient Management

The most common diagnostic test for aortic aneurysm is the chest radiograph. Patients must be in an upright position to validate the widened mediastinum. Extremely large aneurysms may appear as soft masses, displace other organs, or cause abnormal gas patterns. Other diagnostic tests that may be used if the patient is hemodynamically stable include ultrasound and computed tomography scan.

Therapeutic intervention includes placing the patient in a high-Fowler's position, administering high-flow oxygen, and inserting two large-bore IV catheters with lactated Ringer's solution. Maintaining blood pressure control is critical. If hypertension is present such drugs as nitroprusside sodium (Nipride) are used to decrease blood pressure. If the patient has hypovolemic shock, intervention focuses on maintaining ABCs, fluid resuscitation, and preparing for emergency surgery.

Hypertensive Crisis

Hypertension can be defined as a systolic blood pressure ≥140 mm Hg and/or a diastolic pressure ≥90 mm Hg. When blood pressure becomes abruptly elevated to extreme levels, the patient has a life-threatening situation. An estimated 50 million people in the United States have hypertension. The actual incidence of hypertensive crisis is relatively rare, occurring in approximately 1% of the hypertensive population.[24]

Hypertensive crisis is categorized by the degree of acute-target end-organ damage and the rapidity with which the blood pressure must be lowered. Hypertensive crisis has been further categorized into hypertensive emergencies and hypertensive urgencies. Hypertensive emergencies are those clinical situations in which excessively high blood pressure must be lowered quickly, within minutes to hours, to prevent new or worsening organ damage. Hypertensive urgencies develop over days to weeks and generally demonstrate an elevated diastolic blood pressure without signs of end organ damage. Determination of end-organ damage is made by clinical presentation.

Regardless of underlying mechanism of hypertension, elevated blood pressure increases systemic or peripheral vascular resistance and cardiac output. These increases perpetuate the cycle by stimulating release of catecholamines, which increases a sympathetic activity and activates the renin-angiotensin system. The net result is continued increases in blood pressure. Hypertensive crisis usually occurs in patients with a history of hypertension. Other conditions that may cause or precipitate hypertensive crisis include renal parenchymal disease (e.g., acute glomerulonephitis, vasculitis), endocrine problems (e.g., pheochromocytoma, Cushing's syndrome), use of sympathomimetic drugs (cocaine, amphetamines, phencyclidine, lysergic acid diethylamide, diet pills) and food-drug interactions (e.g., monoamine oxidase and tyramine interaction).[37]

Patient Assessment

Patients with hypertensive crisis usually have DBP higher than 120 mm Hg. Primary symptoms are consistent with new or evolving end-organ damage. Increase in systemic peripheral vascular resistance and sympathetic stimulation imposed by the significant hypertension increase myocardial workload and myocardial oxygen consumption. Symptoms associated with cardiovascular manifestations include congestive heart failure, chest pain, angina, and AMI. Neurologic changes include headache, nausea, vomiting, dizziness, visual disturbances (e.g., blurred vision, temporary visual loss, decreased visual acuity, photophobia), altered mental states (e.g., agitation, confusion, lethargy, coma), and seizures.[6] Other neurologic symptoms include focal cranial nerve palsy, sensory deficits, motor deficits, aphasia, and hemiparesis. Fundoscopic evaluation may reveal papilledema from effects of hypertension on retina[7].

Patient Management

In addition to cardiac and vital sign monitoring, IV access should be established. An arterial line provides the most accurate blood pressure readings; however, a noninvasive blood pressure device can also be used for continuous BP monitoring. The goal of management is to lower SBP to 100 to 110 mm Hg. Intravenous pharmacologic agents such as nitroprusside sodium (Nipride), nitroglycerin (Tridil), fenoldopam mesylate (Corlopam), enalaprilat (Vasotec), labetalol hydrochloride (Normodyne), nicardipine hydrochloride (Cardene), esmolol hydrochloride (Brevibloc), phentolamine mesylate (Regitine), and propranolol (Inderal) are used so they can be titrated for safe, effective reduction of SBP. Assess the patient's response to these agents (i.e., presenting symptoms improved or new symptoms not present).

SUMMARY

Cardiovascular attacks are frequent and challenging aspects of emergency nursing. Box 33-4 lists a few nursing diagnoses

Box 33-4	**NURSING DIAGNOSES FOR CARDIOVASCULAR EMERGENCIES**

Anxiety
Breathing pattern, Ineffective
Cardiac output, Decreased
Coping, Ineffective
Fear
Fluid volume, Deficient
Fluid volume, Excessive
Gas exchange, Impaired
Pain
Tissue perfusion, Ineffective
Ventilation, Impaired spontaneous

pertinent for patients with cardiovascular emergencies. Recent changes in management of these patients include new drugs, new doses for old drugs, and new diagnostic modalities. The emergency nurse is challenged to maintain an effective knowledge base as new technologies emerge.

References

1. Adams JE: Cardiac biomarkers: past, present, and future, *Am J Crit Care* 7(6):418, 1998.
2. Albert NM: Inflammation and infection in acute coronary syndromes, *J Cardiovasc Nurs* 15(1):13, 2000.
3. American Heart Association: *2001: heart and stroke statistical update,* Dallas, Tex, 2001, The Association.
4. American Heart Association: Guidelines 2000 for cardiopulmonary resuscitation and emergency cardiovascular care, *Circulation* 102(8)(suppl I):I-1, 2000.
5. Antman EM, Braunwald E: Acute myocardial infarction. In Braunwald E, editor: *Heart disease: a textbook in cardiovascular medicine,* ed 5, Philadelphia, 1997, WB Saunders.
6. Barnason S: Cardiovascular emergencies. In Newberry L, editor: *Sheehy's emergency nursing principles and practice,* ed 4, St. Louis, 1998, Mosby.
7. Capriotti T: New recommendations: intensify control of patient blood pressure, *Medsurg Nurs* 8(3):207, 1999.
8. Carpenter DO, editor: *Professional guide to signs and symptoms,* ed 3, Springhouse, Penn, Springhouse.
9. Clochesy JM, Breu C, Cardin S et al: *Critical care nursing,* ed 2, Philadelphia, 1996, WB Saunders.
10. Cummins RO, editor: *Advanced cardiac life support,* Dallas, Tex, American Heart Association.
11. Doering LV: Pathophysiology of acute coronary syndromes leading to acute myocardial infarction, *J Cardiovasc Nurs* 13(3):1, 1999.
12. Drew BJ, Ide B: EKG puzzles & pearls: use of the EKG in risk stratification, *Progr Cardiovasc Nurs* 13(2):32, 1998.
13. Drew BJ, Krucoff MW: Multilead ST-segment monitoring in patients with acute coronary syndromes: a consensus statement for healthcare professionals, *Am J Crit Care* 8(6):372, 1999.
14. Drew BJ, Pelter MM, Adams MG et al: 12-lead ST-segment monitoring vs. single-lead maximum ST-segment monitoring for detecting ongoing ischemia in patients with unstable coronary syndromes, *Am J Crit Care* 7(5):355, 1998.
15. Fink HA, Lederle FA, Roth CS et al: The accuracy of physical examination to detect abdominal aortic aneurysm, *Arch Int Med* 160:833, 2000.
16. Flutterman LG, Lemberg L: Sudden cardiac death— preventable— reversible, *Am J Crit Care* 6(6):472, 1997.
17. Gutierrez K, editor: *Pharmacotherapeutics: clinical decision-making in nursing,* Philadelphia, 1999, WB Saunders.
18. Harrison H: Troponin I, *Am J Nurs* 99(5):24TT, 1999.
19. Hill B, Geraci SA: A diagnostic approach to chest pain based on history and ancillary evaluation, *Nurse Pract* 23(4):20, 1998.
20. Jacobson C: Bedside cardiac monitoring, *Crit Care Nurse* 18(3):82, 1998.
21. Kinney MR, Dunbar SB, Brooks-Brunn J et al, editors: *AACN clinical reference for critical care nurses,* ed 4, St. Louis, 1998, Mosby.
22. Kuhn MA, editor: *Pharmacotherapeutics: a nursing approach,* ed 4, Philadelphia, 1998, FA Davis.
23. Liberthson RR: Sudden death from cardiac causes in children and young adults, *New Engl J Med* 334(16):1039, 1996.
24. Mansfield J, Daley K: Hypertensive emergencies, *Am J Nurs* September (suppl):20, 2000.
25. Moore JM, Wilson EM: Treatment of acute myocardial infarction emergencies in a community hospital setting, *Am J Nurs* September (suppl):15, 2000.
26. Murphy MJ, Berding CB: Use of measurements of myoglobin and cardiac troponins in the diagnosis of acute myocardial infarction, *Crit Care Nurse* 19(1):58, 1999.
27. Paul S, Hebra JD: *The nurse's guide to cardiac rhythm interpretation,* Philadelphia, 1998, WB Saunders.
28. Pelter MM, Adams MG, Wung S et al: Peak time of occurrence of myocardial ischemia in the coronary care unit, *Am J Crit Care* 7(6):411, 1998.
29. Roettig ML, Tanabe P: Emergency management of acute coronary syndromes, *J Emerg Nurs* 26(6):S1, 2000.
30. Ryan TJ, Anderson JL, Antman EM et al: ACC/AHA guidelines of the management of patients with acute myocardial infarction, *J Am Coll Cardiol* 28(5):1328, 1996.
31. Ryan TJ, Antman EM, Brooks NH et al: 1999 update: ACC/AHA guidelines for the management of patients with acute myocardial infarction, *J Am Coll Cardiol* 34(3):890, 1999.
32. Schoenhagen P, McErlean ES, Nissen SE: The vulnerable coronary plaque, *J Cardiovasc Nurs* 15(1):1-12, 2000.
33. Siomko AJ: Demystifying cardiac markers, *Am J Nurs* 100(1):36, 2000.
34. Spratto GR, Woods AL: *PDR nurse's drug handbook,* Montvale, NJ, 2000, Delmar Publishers
35. Stewart S, Haste M: Prediction of right ventricular and posterior wall ST elevation by coronary care nurses: the 12-lead electrocardiograph versus the 18-lead electrocardiograph, *Heart Lung* 25(1):14, 1996.
36. Tedesco C, Reigle J, Bergin J: Sudden cardiac death in heart failure, *J Cardiovasc Nurs* 14(4):38, 2000.
37. Vaughan CJ, Delanty N: Hypertensive emergencies, *Lancet* 356:411, 2000.
38. West VL: Alternative routes of administration, *J Intravenous Nurs* 21(4):221, 1998.
39. Wu AHB, Apple FS, Gibler B et al: National academy of clinical biochemistry standards of laboratory practice: recommendations for the use of cardiac markers in coronary artery disease, *Clin Chem* 45(7):1104, 1999.
40. Zerwic JJ: Patient delay in seeking treatment for acute myocardial infarction symptoms, *J Cardiovasc Nurs* 13(3):21, 1999.

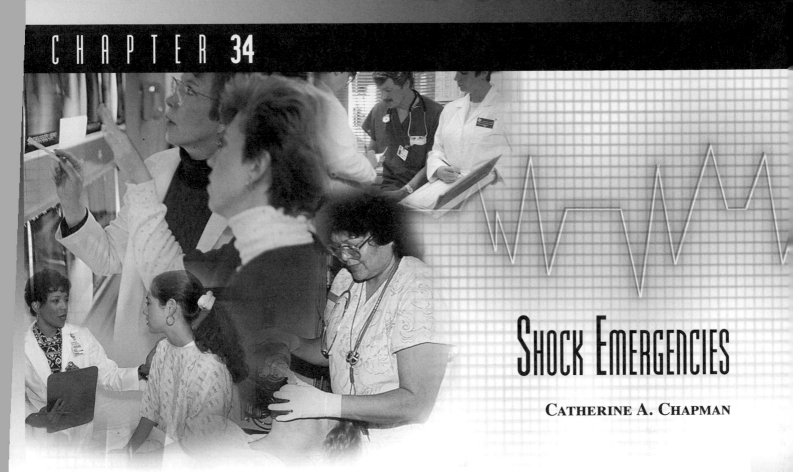

CHAPTER 34

SHOCK EMERGENCIES

CATHERINE A. CHAPMAN

Shock has been superficially described as low blood pressure. The reality is much more complex. Low blood pressure may be the last thing to occur in shock. Blood pressure is not the determinant for deciding someone is in shock but rather whether he or she is in compensated or decompensated shock. Identifying the patient in shock requires astute assessment skills based on a strong clinical foundation. Shock is a potentially fatal condition that occurs when cells become hypoxic as a result of decreased perfusion. Clinically, shock is found in patients of all ages as the result of blood loss, infection, myocardial infarction, and other conditions that alter cellular perfusion. This chapter reviews the pathophysiology of shock, describes four categories of shock, and discusses patient assessment, evaluation, and treatment for each type of shock.

CATEGORIES OF SHOCK

Normal circulation and cellular perfusion are products of adequate circulating volume, cardiac output, and peripheral vascular resistance. Blood pressure is a product of systemic vascular resistance (SVR) and cardiac output (CO). Change or damage to any of these components alters cellular perfusion and oxygenation. Shock is categorized by which essential component is affected. Specific categories of shock are hypovolemic shock, cardiogenic shock, distributive shock, and obstructive shock. Box 34-1 lists categories of shock by causative agent.

Hypovolemic shock results from loss or redistribution of blood, plasma, or other body fluids, which ultimately leads to overall reduction in intravascular volume (preload). Hypovolemic shock is primarily an alteration in circulating volume. Volume loss can occur from traumatic injury, gastrointestinal bleeding, ruptured ectopic pregnancy, vaginal bleeding, posterior nasal bleed, osmotic diuresis associated with diabetic ketoacidosis (DKA), gastric suctioning, or excessive vomiting or diarrhea. Redistribution of body fluids is most often caused by thermal injuries.

Cardiogenic shock occurs when loss of ventricular effectiveness (contractility) decreases cardiac output. Cardiac pump failure can result from myocardial infarction, myocardial contusion, cardiomyopathies, ruptured papillary muscle, dysrhythmias, valvular disease, or ruptured ventricular septum.

Distributive shock, or vasogenic shock, is caused by overall reduction in SVR and vasodilation. Blood volume is normal; however, the circulating blood volume is decreased by massive vasodilation and decreased SVR. Distributive shock is categorized by etiology into neurogenic, septic, and anaphylactic shock.

Obstructive shock occurs when an obstruction decreases circulating volume by preventing the myocardium from mechanically emptying during systole or filling during diastole. Causes include pulmonary embolism, air embolism, tension pneumothorax, pericardial tamponade, intracardiac clot, vena cava obstruction, aortic stenosis, or aortic aneurysm.

Box 34-1	CAUSES OF SHOCK
Hypovolemic shock	Massive external bleeding, hemothorax, hemoperitoneum, fractures, gastrointestinal bleeding, massive vomiting, massive diarrhea, massive diaphoresis, diabetes mellitus, diabetes insipidus, excessive diuretic use, burns, ascites
Cardiogenic shock	Myocardial infarction, cardiomyopathy, cardiac contusion, dysrhythmias, heart valve disease
Distributive shock	Sepsis, anaphylaxis, spinal cord injury, overdose, anoxia
Obstructive shock	Tension pneumothorax, pericardial tamponade, pulmonary embolus, intracardiac clot, vena cava clot, aortic aneurysm, aortic stenosis, valvular disease, gravid uterus

Box 34-2	CELLULAR EFFECTS OF SHOCK
Decreased ATP production
Excess lactic acid production
Mitochondrial death
Cellular edema
Deterioration of the sodium-potassium pump
Hyperkalemia

ATP, Adenosine triphosphate.

Obstructive shock decreases filling or obstructs outflow, which results in decreased cardiac output.

PATHOPHYSIOLOGY

Shock is defined as an alteration in tissue perfusion that occurs at the cellular level. Conditions that result in hypoxia or poor cellular perfusion precipitate a complex clinical syndrome known as shock. In the presence of hypoxia and inadequate tissue perfusion, cells do not receive oxygen and nutrients or remove waste products. Cellular damage or death ensues when cellular oxygen demands exceed the tissue's oxygen supply.

Normal cell metabolism requires an aerobic environment to break down glucose and oxidize substrates. Enzyme-mediated chemical reactions transfer energy from this process into adenosine triphosphate (ATP). Oxidative energy synthesis of ATP is necessary for cell survival and is a fundamental characteristic of life. This process is also referred to as cellular respiration.

Cellular respiration occurs within organelles known as mitochondria, which are located in the cell's cytoplasm. Mitochondria are the site of ATP synthesis and energy production. Lysosomes in the cytoplasm store hydrolytic or digestive enzymes that mediate chemical reactions within the cell.

The production of cellular energy and synthesis of ATP is dependent on a continuous oxygen supply. Availability of oxygen is influenced by blood flow, oxygen saturation, and cardiac output. Oxygen consumption is the amount of oxygen removed by the tissues for metabolism. Oxygen debt refers to the difference between cellular demand for oxygen and cellular consumption of available oxygen. A continuous oxygen debt related to tissue hypoxia creates an anaerobic environment that adversely affects cellular metabolism.

In abnormal cell metabolism the synthesis of ATP is altered, so pyruvic acid is reduced to lactic acid. Concurrently, the sodium-potassium pump deteriorates, so redistribution of ions and fluid occurs. Sodium and fluid move into the cell, displacing potassium extracellularly, causing hyperkalemia and cellular engorgement. Altered calcium ions within the mitochondria cause constriction of the mitochondria and eventually damage the mitochondrial membrane. Damage to the membrane exacerbates cellular engorgement and leads to organelle death. In addition, changes within the cell damage lysosomal membranes, leading to release of enzymes followed by further cell devastation. Lactic acid produced from the initial abnormal cellular metabolism precipitates metabolic acidosis. Box 34-2 summarizes adverse cellular effects of shock.

COMPENSATORY BODY RESPONSES

Regardless of the type of shock, the body mobilizes a series of responses to compensate for the evolving shock state. Compensatory responses are stimulated by decreasing tissue perfusion. Ideally, the outcome of these compensatory mechanisms is restoration of cardiac output and tissue perfusion. To accomplish this, blood is shunted from the kidneys, gastrointestinal tract, liver, and skin to vital organs; that is, the heart, lungs, and brain. Key compensatory responses include the baroreceptors, sympathetic nervous system, fluid shifts, and endocrine system. Without these compensatory mechanisms, shock progresses and ultimately death occurs. Box 34-3 summarizes the progression of the shock state.

Baroreceptors

Baroreceptors are a collection of specialized neural tissues located in the aortic arch and bifurcation of the common carotid arteries. Baroreceptor reflexes respond to small changes in vascular tone or pressure. Inhibition of baroreceptors by the vasomotor center of the brain in response to decreasing cardiac output results in sympathetic stimulation followed by peripheral vasoconstriction in an effort to increase circulating volume and to maintain blood pressure. Similarly the resulting decrease in vagal tone decreases coronary resistance in an attempt to improve myocardial oxygen supply.[5]

Box 34-3 **SHOCK PROGRESSION**

Compensatory shock	Body responses initiated to increase cardiac output, tissue (cellular perfusion), and vital organ perfusion
Progressive shock	Body responses become inadequate to maintain perfusion and multisystem failure ensues
Irreversible shock	Pervasive cellular destruction; death is imminent

Sympathetic Nervous System

Stimulation of the sympathetic nervous system by decreases in circulating volume and cardiac output results in release of epinephrine, norepinephrine, and other catecholamines that stimulate α- and β-receptors.

Stimulation of α-receptors is followed by arteriole and venous vasoconstriction, which shunts blood to organs. Other effects include stimulation of the adrenal glands, which ultimately leads to fluid retention by the kidneys. The chronotropic effect is tachycardia. β-Receptor stimulation has a positive inotropic effect, increasing myocardial contractility and improving coronary artery blood flow. The α- and β-adrenergic affects augment venous return, increasing ventricular filling or preload, heart rate, and myocardial contractility, which facilitates ventricular emptying and improves cardiac output and blood pressure.

Fluid Shifts

Normal distribution of body fluid is 75% intracellular and 25% extracellular. Of the extracellular fluid one third is located intravascularly; the remainder is interstitial. Hydrostatic pressure and plasma colloid oncotic pressure (COP) are forces that maintain normal fluid distribution between the intravascular and interstitial compartments. Hydrostatic pressure pushes fluid from the arterial end of the capillary bed into the interstitial space. COP pulls fluid into the venous capillary bed because of plasma proteins such as albumin.

Alterations in circulating volume or cardiac output that reduce hydrostatic pressure cause less fluid to be distributed interstitially. However, the pressure gradient continues to push fluid into the intravascular space.

Endocrine Response

The endocrine system response to decreased circulating volume or decreased cardiac output is a product of the adrenal glands, the kidneys, the pituitary gland, and the lungs. Components are the renin-angiotensin-aldosterone system and antidiuretic hormone (ADH).

Renin-angiotensin-aldosterone System

Renal hypoperfusion and mediation of β-receptors by the sympathetic nervous system secondary to shock causes release of renin. Renin activates conversion of angiotensinogen to angiotensin I, which is then converted by the lungs into angiotensin II, which causes release of aldosterone and produces vasoconstriction. Aldosterone promotes sodium reabsorption within the renal tubule. Water follows reabsorption of sodium, so the net effect is water movement from the interstitial space into the intravascular space. Ideally, circulating volume and cardiac output increase. There is a corresponding decrease in urinary output as a result of this response.

Antidiuretic Hormone

ADH is released by the posterior pituitary gland in response to increased plasma osmolarity, altered circulating volume, and in response to angiotensin. ADH causes sodium and water reabsorption from the distal renal tubules in an attempt to increase circulating volume and cardiac output. Urine output decreases and urine specific gravity increases as a result of this process.

PATIENT ASSESSMENT

Assessment, stabilization, and reassessment of the patient with actual or potential shock is critical for a positive patient outcome. Astute assessment and observation reveal subtle changes in clinical variables that indicate improvement or deterioration in the patient's status.

The initial approach to patient assessment is the primary assessment, which addresses airway, breathing, circulation, and level of consciousness.[2] Priority is given to controlling and maintaining the airway, effective breathing, and adequate oxygenation. Augmentation of circulating volume and cardiac output may also be required to support circulation. Secondary assessment follows the primary assessment and includes temperature, blood pressure, pulse, respiratory rate, history, and head-to-toe inspection, auscultation, and palpation of the patient. Attention is directed to focused assessment, which is a detailed assessment of the patient's problem. It is guided by findings of the primary and secondary assessment. In most cases of shock, all systems require a focused assessment after the priority sequencing of the primary and secondary assessment.

History

History is an important part of the secondary assessment and may provide important information about the patient's clinical presentation, precipitating events, and preexisting health status. History may be determined by interviewing the patient, significant others, or prehospital personnel and can also be acquired during physical assessment. Box 34-4 highlights pertinent historical data.

Common Clinical Manifestations

Although shock occurs at the cellular level, manifestations of the shock state are evident at the systemic level. Clinical

Box 34-4	PERTINENT HISTORICAL DATA
Chief complaint	Vomiting, hematemesis
Pain, pressure (PQRST)	Diarrhea, melena
Provocation	Vaginal bleeding
Quality	Fever, chills
Radiation/region	Rash, urticaria
Severity (scale 0-10)	Polyuria, thirst
Time (time of onset)	Injury, location, mechanism,
Level of consciousness	force, protective device
Dizziness, syncope	Bleeding, site, estimated blood
Weakness, fatigue	loss
Difficulty breathing	Medical-surgical history
Edema: Location and type	Allergies

changes are noted in the respiratory and circulatory systems and in "nonessential" organs such as the kidneys and skin. Astute assessment depends on recognition of these common clinical manifestations of shock.

Respiratory

During shock, respiratory effectiveness is affected by hypoxia (which also decreases the level of consciousness), injury, or pulmonary congestion. Evaluation of respiratory rate, rhythm, and depth may reveal air hunger, accessory muscle use, and tachypnea. Tachypnea is an effort to decrease carbon dioxide and compensate for cellular acidosis. Adequate oxygenation may be indicated by pulse oximetry but inadequate circulating volume perpetuates cellular hypoxia and anerobic cellular metabolism. Therefore a gradual increase in depth and rate of respiration may be early signs of impending shock. Breath sounds may also be absent, unequal, or diminished. Wheezes, crackles, or coarse breath sounds indicating pulmonary congestion occur with cardiogenic shock.

Circulatory

Cardiac output is determined by preload, afterload, contractility, and heart rate. Preload is the volume in the right and left ventricles at the end of diastole. It is affected by circulating volume, right arterial pressure, and intrathoracic pressure.[5] Preload affects myocardial stretch and the force of myocardial contractility. Afterload is the arterial pressure or resistance the ventricles must overcome with each contraction; that is, the amount of pressure necessary for the left ventricle to contract. Afterload is affected by aortic pressure, pulmonary arterial pressure, and systemic vascular resistance. An increase in afterload decreases stroke volume and subsequently decreases cardiac output. Contractility refers to the heart's contractile force.

Pulse rate increases when the sympathetic nervous system responds to decreased cardiac output in shock. A corresponding decrease in stroke volume results in weak, thready

pulses. Evaluate and compare peripheral pulses to central pulses for presence, rate, equality, and quality.

A drop in systolic blood pressure occurs from decreased cardiac output or decreased venous return. In early shock the diastolic blood pressure rises from sympathetic effect on peripheral vascular resistance, which causes vasoconstriction. Consequently, pulse pressure narrows in the presence of decreased systolic blood pressure. As shock progresses, sympathetic activity becomes less effective and diastolic blood pressure begins to fall.

A reduction in arterial distention caused by decreased cardiac output and a proportionate decrease in stroke volume causes flattened jugular veins when the patient is supine. However, the patient in obstructive shock and cardiogenic shock can have neck veins that appear full as a result of right-sided ventricular failure or increased pulmonary pressures. Assessment of neck veins may help determine the presence and cause of shock.

Auscultate heart sounds to evaluate rate, quality, and the presence of abnormal sounds such as S3 or S4 and identify irregularities such as murmurs, friction rubs, or a gallop. Cardiac dysrhythmias develop frequently as a result of zonal lesions resulting from myocardial hypoxia, which can interfere with the normal electrical conduction patterns. Stimulation of the sympathetic nervous system causes tachycardia. Progression of shock and depletion of epinephrine stores lead to bradycardia, heart blocks, and ventricular dysrhythmia including ventricular fibrillation.

Level of consciousness is a sensitive assessment measurement of shock and its progression. Decreased cerebral perfusion and hypoxia are initially manifested by restlessness, anxiety, or confusion. Continued progression of shock with significant cerebral hypoperfusion and hypoxia leads to an obtunded, unresponsive patient.

Nonessential Organs

When tissue perfusion decreases, the body considers only three organs essential—the brain, heart, and lungs. All others (the kidneys, intestines, and skin) are nonessential for self-preservation. Blood is shunted away from these nonessential organs in an attempt to maintain cardiac output and cerebral perfusion. Sympathetic nervous system activity and peripheral vasoconstriction shunt blood from the skin, causing cool skin, pallor (especially around the lips), cyanosis, and diaphoresis. Children develop mottled extremities. Capillary refill takes more than 2 seconds. Skin perfusion and capillary refill may be altered by hypothermia or preexisting peripheral vascular disease. Delayed capillary refill should be considered in light of other assessment findings for determining shock or impending shock.

Normal urinary output is 0.5 to 1 ml/kg/hr. In shock, urinary output falls secondary to renal hypoperfusion and release of ADH. Urine specific gravity increases with reabsorption of water in the renal distal tubules. Reduction in hourly urine output with a rise in specific gravity may signify shock. Blood urea nitrogen (BUN) and creatinine increase as renal perfusion decreases.

Box 34-5 SYMPATHETIC RESPONSE EFFECTS

CARDIAC OUTPUT

$\beta1$ ↑ Heart rate — chrontropy
$\beta1$ ↑ Contractility — inotropy
$\beta1$ Attempt ↑ cardiac output
$\beta2$ Coronary artery vasodilation
$\beta1$ ↑ O_2 demand

VENTILATION

$\beta2$ Bronchodilation
↑ Respiratory rate

RENAL FUNCTION

Decreased renal blood flow
Renin response stimulated
ADH and aldosterone stimulation
↑ Na+ and water reabsorption
↑ Circulating volume
↓ Urine output
Prolonged hypotension leads to ATN

GASTROINTESTINAL/HEPATIC FUNCTION

Decreased gastrointestinal blood flow
Hepatic vasoconstriction
Hypoactive/absent bowel sounds
Slowing/cessation of peristalisis
↑ Serum amylase
↑ Blood glucose
↓ Conversion of lactate to bicarbonate

ADH, Antidiuretic hormone; *ATN,* acute tubular necrosis.

Box 34-6 ACID BASE DEVIATIONS

RESPIRATORY ACIDOSIS

Hypoventilation results in CO_2 retention, carbonic acid excess, and ↓ pH
Causes include CNS depression, pneumothorax, pulmonary edema

METABOLIC ALKALOSIS

↑ pH due to excess base or acid deficits
Causes include vomiting and diarrhea, excessive diuresis

METABOLIC ACIDOSIS

Excess fixed acids results in ↓ pH
Causes include lactic acid accumulation from anaerobic metabolism (shock, cardiac arrest), renal disease

RESPIRATORY ALKALOSIS

Hyperventilation results in ↑ CO_2 exhaled, reducing carbonic acid with ↑ pH
Causes include panic attacks, fever (especially in pediatric patient), early salicylate overdose

CNS, Central nervous system.

Vasoconstriction leads to hypoperfusion of the gastrointestinal tract. Clinical manifestations include hypoactive or absent bowel sounds, leakage of pancreatic enzymes with an elevated serum amylase, and inability of the liver to metabolize substrates such as lactic acid. In addition, peristalsis ceases increasing the risk for a paralytic ileus or necrosis of the gastrointestinal tract. Concurrently there is hypoperfusion and alteration of hepatic function that results in decreased conversion of lactate to bicarbonate and mobilization of glycogen stores resulting in increased blood glucose levels. These effects worsen metabolic acidosis found in the patient in shock. See Box 34-5 for a summary of sympathetic responses.

Initial Stabilization and Management

Stabilization is critical for a positive patient outcome. Adequate oxygenation and circulatory support to correct hypoxia and inadequate tissue perfusion are essential. An effective airway should be obtained or maintained along with support of effective breathing. Supplemental oxygen at 100% should be provided. Endotracheal intubation and mechanical ventilation should be anticipated. Management of circulation is directed toward augmentation of circulating volume and improving cardiac output through administration of crystalloids, colloids, or blood as appropriate. Peripheral veins including the antecubital veins, external jugular veins, and saphenous veins should be cannulated with the largest gauge catheter possible. Central venous access can be obtained through the internal jugular veins and the subclavian veins. Warmed intravenous fluids are preferable in order to avoid hypothermia, which can inhibit resuscitative efforts to reverse metabolic acidosis. Options to enhance cardiac output and myocardial contractility include administration of inotropic medications such as dopamine or dobutamine; however, these should be used only after hypovolemia has been corrected and preload optimized.

Acid-Base Balance

In early shock, respiratory alkalosis occurs because of tachypnea, the body's attempt to increase oxygen levels. Unfortunately, carbon dioxide is blown off as respirations increase in the effort to take in more oxygen. Concurrently, continuing anaerobic metabolism increases serum lactic acid, which culminates in metabolic acidosis. Base deficit is a sensitive indicator of shock. A value of -5mEq/L (normal value is -2 to $+2$ mEq/L) or lower represents tissue hypoperfusion and the formation of lactate. At this time respiratory rate drops and respiratory acidosis occurs. Management includes hyperventilation and administration of 100% oxygen. Administration of sodium bicarbonate is considered for metabolic acidosis documented by measurement of arterial blood gases and after hyperventilation and oxygenation. Box 34-6 outlines acid base deviations.

Hemodynamic Monitoring

Hemodynamic monitoring is now available in most emergency departments. Pulse oximetry and noninvasive blood pressure (NIBP) monitoring are as commonplace as the cardiac monitor. These monitoring avenues are an invaluable part of caring for the patient in shock; however, it is important to correlate these modalities with patient assessment.

Pulse oximetry is a noninvasive method of determining hypoxia through measurement of arterial hemoglobin saturation. Light is transmitted through tissue to a light detector attached to the patient's fingertip, toes, or ear. Variability of transmission is determined by pulsated arterial flow. The light absorption abilities of oxyhemoglobin and deoxyhemoglobin are calculated by the monitor to determine the percentage of arterial saturation.

Central venous pressure (CVP) is used to indirectly measure circulating volume, cardiac pump effectiveness, and vascular tone through measurement of pressures on the right side of the myocardium. Normal CVP measurements range from 4 to 10 cm H_2O pressure. A measurement lower than 4 cm H_2O indicates decreased circulating volume. A measurement greater than 10 cm H_2O signifies excessive pressures on the right side of the myocardium—often the result of pulmonary edema, fluid overload, or obstruction such as pericardial tamponade or tension pneumothorax.

Arterial pressure may be measured invasively using an arterial line or indirectly using NIBP. Mean arterial pressure is between 70 and 90 mm Hg. A pressure less than 70 mm Hg indicates inadequate circulating volume with inadequate perfusion of the brain, kidneys, and coronary arteries. This may result from hypovolemia, pump failure, obstruction, or loss of systemic vascular resistance. Intraarterial lines may be inserted percutaneously or through a surgical incision.

HYPOVOLEMIC SHOCK

Hypovolemic shock is the type of shock seen most frequently by the emergency nurse. It is a direct result of reduction in intravascular volume. Decreased circulating volume can be caused by loss or redistribution of whole blood, plasma, or other body fluids. Hypovolemic shock is a loss of preload. Redistribution or third-space sequestration occurs when fluid shifts from the intravascular compartment to the interstitial space. This can occur with changes in capillary permeability or capillary fluid pressures as in burn injuries or sepsis. Actual volume loss is associated with traumatic injury, posterior nasal bleeds, intraabdominal hemorrhage, significant vaginal bleeding, gastrointestinal bleeding, or ex-

cessive vomiting and diarrhea. DKA causes extreme diuresis, which may reduce circulating volume.

Early identification and treatment are essential because the potential for good patient outcome declines with profound hypotension and progression to decompensated shock. Table 34-1 summarizes clinical manifestations associated with various levels of volume depletion. Age and preexisting health problems also affect the potential for a good patient outcome.

Inspection of the patient may reveal injury or other source of hemorrhage and fluid loss. In cases of trauma, impaled objects or penetrating injury may be present. Blunt injuries or deformities often result in sequestering large amounts of blood because of occult bleeding. The presence of thermal injuries indicates the potential for substantial redistribution of fluid because of capillary injury. Clinical manifestations are related to the amount and rate of actual volume loss. Hypovolemia can occur suddenly or gradually, as in some cases of gastrointestinal bleeding.

Initial complete blood count analysis may be inaccurate, particularly in patients with sudden loss of large amounts of blood, because the serum to hematocrit and hemoglobin ratio does not change. Proportionate reductions in hematocrit and hemoglobin are usually demonstrated after fluid resuscitation.

Management of the patient in hypovolemic shock is directed toward controlling or preventing further loss of circulating volume and restoring intravascular volume. Control of external bleeding is accomplished with direct pressure to tamponade bleeding. Impaled objects are stabilized to prevent further movement and bleeding. Volume replacement is initiated with large-bore intravenous access and fluid replacement. Crystalloids are administered at a 3:1 ratio for calculated fluid replacement, whereas blood products are administered at a 1:1 replacement ratio.[3] Vasopressors are used if the patient remains hypotensive despite correction of volume deficits.

Blood is administered in cases of major trauma when there is no improvement in clinical status after 3 to 4 L of crystalloids.[3] Type-specific blood is always preferable; however, O-negative blood can be given in extremely critical sit-

Table 34-1	**PHYSIOLOGIC RESPONSES TO HEMORRHAGE (BASED ON 70 KG MALE)**					
CLASS % **BLOOD LOSS**	**PULSE**	**BLOOD** **PRESSURE**	**PULSE** **PRESSURE**	**LEVEL OF** **CONSCIOUSNESS**	**RESPIRATORY** **RATE**	**URINARY** **OUTPUT**
Class One (I) to 15% (up to 750 ml)	<100	Normal	Normal or increased	Slightly anxious	14-20	>30 ml/hr Up
Class Two (II) 15-30% (750-1500 ml)	>100	Normal	Decreased	Mildly anxious	20-30	20-30 ml/hr
Class Three (III) 30-40% (1500-2000 ml)	>120	Decreased	Decreased	Anxious, confused	30-40	5-15 ml/hr
Class Four (IV) >40% (>2000 ml)	>120	Decreased	Decreased	Anxious, confused	30-40	5-15 ml/hr

From Jacobs B, Hoyt K: *Trauma nursing core course*, ed 5, Park Ridge, Ill, 2000, Emergency Nurses Association.

uations when there is no time to wait for type-specific blood (O-positive blood may be given to females at some centers). Autotransfusion can be accomplished with intrapleural and mediastinal blood from a clean wound, usually with blood loss greater than 200 ml. Adequate renal and liver function is necessary given the potential for red blood cell hemolysis. Crystalloids and blood products should be warmed before infusion to avoid hypothermia.

Fluid replacement and blood transfusions for hypovolemic shock can save the patient's life but they can also complicate the patient's clinical course. Resuscitation can cause hypothermia, hyperkalemia, hypocalcemia, acidosis, alkalosis, clotting problems, and intravascular debris. These complications are summarized in Table 34-2. Patients who receive transfusions that replace more than 50% of their blood volume during a 3-hour period should be closely monitored for these adverse effects of resuscitation.

Table 34-2 ADVERSE EFFECTS OF FLUID AND/OR BLOOD REPLACEMENT

PROBLEM	DESCRIPTION
Hypothermia	Transfusion of banked blood without warming can make the patient hypothermic. Hypothermia shifts the oxyhemoglobin dissociation curve to the left (i.e., oxygen is not available for the cells).
Hyperkalemia	Lysis of red blood cells releases potassium from the intracellular space so the patient becomes hyperkalemic. Monitor the patient's serum potassium and observe for cardiac rhythm problems.
Hypocalcemia	Banked blood contains citrate, which binds with free calcium. Calcium chloride is given after 10 U of blood.
Acidosis	The pH of banked blood is 7.1. With large amounts of banked blood, acidosis can occur. Monitor arterial blood gases and watch for dysrhythmias.
Alkalosis	With large amounts of banked blood, alkalosis can develop because the citrate is converted by the liver into bicarbonate. Monitor arterial blood gases.
Clotting problems	Clotting factors are lost in most banked blood. Coagulation times may be prolonged and clotting problems occur with massive blood transfusions. Usually, 1 U of fresh-frozen plasma is given after 10 U of blood.
Intravascular debris	Banked blood contains debris as a result of processing. It is not known if this debris is harmful; therefore, blood is always given through a filter.

CARDIOGENIC SHOCK

Cardiogenic shock occurs when the heart fails as a pump, causing a significant reduction in ventricular effectiveness. Cardiac output decreases and tissue perfusion diminishes while left ventricular end-diastolic pressure increases. Injury to the myocardium impairs contractility, which decreases ventricular emptying. Cardiogenic shock carries a high mortality rate; most patients die within 24 hours; others may live only a few days. Cardiogenic shock is caused by myocardial infarction with damage to greater than 40% of the left ventricle, severe myocardial contusion, valvular heart disease, cardiomyopathies, ruptured papillary muscle, ruptured ventricular septum, and dysrhythmias such as third-degree heart block. Myocardial damage may occur as the result of a single infarction or subsequent to multiple events.

When pump failure occurs the myocardium cannot forcibly eject blood. Stroke volume decreases because of decreased contractility, which decreases cardiac output and blood pressure. Subsequent alteration in tissue perfusion precipitates myocardial ischemia and extends the region of injury, which further compromises cardiac contractility. Myocardial contractility is also affected by hypoxemia, metabolic acidosis, ventricular diastolic volume, and sympathetic nervous system stimulation. Poor myocardial contractility causes inadequate emptying of the left ventricle.

Incomplete emptying of the left ventricle during diastole elevates pressures in the left ventricle, left atrium, and pulmonary vessels. There is a corresponding increase in pulmonary pressures as pulmonary capillaries leak fluid into the alveolar spaces, causing pulmonary edema. Elevated pulmonary pressures increase right ventricular and atrial pressures, which contribute to right-sided heart failure.

Increased myocardial performance as a compensatory response to the shock translates to increased myocardial oxygen demand and increased myocardial ischemia, which further compromises cardiac output and eventually progresses to cardiovascular collapse.[5]

Clinical manifestations of cardiogenic shock resemble those seen in myocardial infarction. The patient complains of chest pain or pressure as a result of myocardial ischemia, myocardial infarct, or dyspnea. There are electrocardiogram changes, dysrhythmias, and an elevation in cardiac markers. Elevated pulmonary and myocardial pressures cause distended neck veins. Decreasing cardiac output and hypotension contribute to absent or weak, thready peripheral pulses. Auscultation reveals muffled heart sounds with rhythm irregularities. Tachypnea occurs to compensate for pulmonary edema. Diffuse crackles and wheezes are usually present. Skin is pale, cool, and clammy. Central cyanosis is often present.

Managing cardiogenic shock begins with administering high-flow oxygen and establishing intravenous access. Subsequent management is predominately pharmacologic. Vasodilating agents such as nitroglycerin are given to reduce pain, increase coronary perfusion, and reduce preload and afterload. These agents also decrease left ventricular filling pressures and increase cardiac output. Sodium nitroprusside may be given to decrease afterload. Morphine sulfate reduces pain and anxiety, eases respiratory efforts, and decreases afterload. Inotropic medications such as dopamine and dobutamine increase contractility and improve systolic pressure.

The intraaortic balloon pump, a diastolic assist device that improves cardiac output, coronary artery perfusion, and oxygen delivery without increasing myocardial oxygen consumption, may also be used.[5] Pulmonary arterial catheters are used to measure pulmonary artery wedge pressure (PAWP), a precise indication of left ventricular function and cardiac competence. These PAWP measurements guide fluid administration and titration of drugs in cardiogenic shock.

DISTRIBUTIVE SHOCK

Distributive shock, at one time referred to as vasogenic shock, results from an alteration in systemic vasculature that causes maldistribution of intravascular volume to the circulatory network and interstitial spaces. Distributive shock is characterized by extreme vasodilation in the presence of normal blood volume and cardiac function that results in a loss of afterload or systemic vascular resistance. Three categories of distributive shock based on etiology are neurogenic, septic, and anaphylactic shock.

Neurogenic Shock

Neurogenic shock is most often associated with acute spinal cord disruption from trauma or spinal anesthesia. Other causes of neurogenic shock are brain injury, hypoxia, depressant drug actions, and hypoglycemia associated with insulin shock. In neurogenic shock, outflow from the vasomotor center in the medulla is inhibited or depressed, causing loss of sympathetic vasomotor regulation. Uncontested parasympathetic responses cause vasodilation and loss of sympathetic tone. Inhibition of sympathetic innervation impedes release of norepinephrine and interferes with the body's ability to vasoconstrict. Consequently, venous return and cardiac output decrease. Neurogenic shock is relatively uncommon. It is a transient shock state that usually requires supportive treatment only.

The combination of hypotension and loss of sympathetic innervation contributes to two manifestations unique to neurogenic shock: bradycardia and warm, dry, flushed skin. With cord disruption, skin above the disruption is pale, cool, and moist. The patient also manifests hypotension, tachypnea, and loss of sensation, mobility, or reflexes below the level of cord disruption. Rectal and bladder sphincter control are absent. Priapism is seen in male patients. Patients become poikilothermic, assuming the temperature of the surrounding environment.

Management is primarily supportive: maintaining and supporting the airway, breathing, and circulation with simultaneous spinal immobilization. Realignment and definitive spinal stabilization with halo ring device or insertion of tongs should be performed after the patient is stabilized.

Measures to warm the patient should be instituted to maintain a normothermic core temperature. Vasopressors for hypotension and atropine for symptomatic bradycardia may be needed for supportive management.

Septic Shock

The most common cause of septic shock is untreated infection. Sepsis occurs in 1 of every 100 hospitalized patients—40% will develop septic shock.[1] The mortality rate for septic shock ranges from 40% to 90%. Survival depends on promptness of treatment. Septic shock is the most common form of distributive shock and is a combination of loss of preload, afterload, or systemic vascular resistance, and to a lesser extent cardiac contractility.

The systemic response in septic shock is caused by endotoxins of the infecting organisms, immunosuppression, or inability of the immune system to respond to the bacterial assault of an overwhelming infection. The most common causative organisms are gram-negative bacilli. Gram-positive bacteria, yeast, fungi, and viruses have also been implicated in septic shock.[4] Endotoxins released by the invading organisms prompt release of hydrolytic enzymes from weakened cell lysosomes, which causes cellular destruction of bacteria and normal cells. The immune system responds by releasing histamine, prostaglandins, and chemical mediators, precipitating profound vasodilation, increased capillary permeability, and redistribution of fluid into the interstitial spaces. The resulting inadequate tissue perfusion, third-space sequestration of fluid, and altered cellular metabolism affect multiple organs.

Clinical manifestations of septic shock occur in two phases. The initial phase is the hyperdynamic or warm phase. The patient is febrile with a high cardiac output and decreased systemic vascular resistance. Skin appears flushed and petechiae may be present. The patient is tachycardic and tachypneic. This stage is followed by the hypodynamic or cold phase, characterized by decreased cardiac output and profound vasoconstriction.[4] Skin is pale, cool, and moist with mottling progressing above the knees. Temperature is subnormal and respirations are rapid and shallow, progressing to Cheyne-Stokes respirations.

Management of the overwhelming infection follows support of airway, breathing, and circulation with high-flow oxygen and intravenous fluids. It is important to identify and remove potential sources of infection. Wounds and necrotic tissue should be debrided, and existing invasive devices such as indwelling catheters should be removed. Cultures should be obtained from potential sites before antibiotics are administered. Antipyretics should be administered for temperatures above 101° F (38° C). Inotropic medications are used to augment cardiac output and blood pressure.

Anaphylactic Shock

Anaphylaxis is an acute allergic reaction after exposure to a foreign protein to which the patient has been previously sensitized. Anaphylactic shock is a profound hypersensitivity reaction with a systemic antigen-antibody response. Clinical manifestations are usually acute and sudden; however, symptoms may occasionally be mild, evolving into respiratory distress and hypotension after several hours. Antigens commonly implicated in anaphylactic shock include medications such as antibiotics, iodine contrast dyes, foods such as shellfish or nuts, food additives such as monosodium glutamate, and insect stings. Antibodies are formed on initial exposure to a foreign protein. The antigen triggers release of vasoactive mediators that act on the vascular and pulmonary systems. The effect of these mediators is smooth muscle contraction, vasodilation, increased capillary permeability, and bronchoconstriction. Redistribution of fluid interstitially in combination with vasodilation decreases intravascular volume and causes urticaria and angioedema. Fluid leakage into the alveoli leads to pulmonary congestion.

Acute onset of angioedema of the upper airway and bronchospasm may progress rapidly to airway obstruction and respiratory arrest. Initial respiratory symptoms include respiratory difficulty, stridor, bronchospasm, and wheezing. Patients initially have warm, dry skin that becomes cool and pale. Chest tightness, dysrhythmias, and cardiac irritability may also be noted.

Management is directed toward maintaining a patent airway, effective breathing, and circulatory support. High-flow oxygen and intravenous access are followed by intravenous administration of epinephrine 0.1 to 0.5 ml of 1:1000 solution, repeated in 5 to 15 minutes for profound vasoconstriction. Antihistamines such as diphenhydramine (Benadryl), famitidine (Pepcid), and cimetadine (Tagamet) are given. Bronchodilators such as albuterol or, less commonly, aminophylline may be given for bronchoconstriction and bronchospasm. Cricothyrotomy may be required for severe airway compromise.

OBSTRUCTIVE SHOCK

Obstructive shock occurs from mechanical obstruction or compression of the great veins, pulmonary arteries, aorta, or the myocardium itself, which prevents adequate circulating volume. Inadequate cardiac output and tissue hypoperfusion occur when the obstruction prevents adequate emptying of the myocardium during systole or filling during diastole. Pulmonary embolus prevents right ventricular emptying when a large portion of the pulmonary arterial cross-sectional area is obstructed. Incomplete right ventricular emptying causes decreased cardiac output, right ventricular failure, and increased right atrial pressure. Air embolus obstructs flow from the right atrium to the pulmonary outflow tract, preventing emptying of the right ventricle during systole. Pericardial tamponade prevents filling during diastole because the atria and ventricles are unable to fill. Compression on the heart decreases stroke volume. Tension pneumothorax displaces the inferior vena cava, obstructing venous return to the right atrium, thereby reducing stroke volume. Other causes of obstructive shock include aortic

aneurysm, intracardiac clot, aortic stenosis, and a gravid uterus.

Clinical manifestations of obstructive shock vary depending on the cause of obstruction. Common manifestations include pain in the chest or back, dyspnea, tachypnea, tachycardia, profound hypotension, cyanosis, and diaphoresis. Management is directed toward removal of the obstruction and support of airway, breathing, and circulation.

COMPLICATIONS ASSOCIATED WITH SHOCK

Shock places the patient at risk for complications with long-term implications, including disability and even death. Specific complications include adult respiratory distress syndrome (ARDS), disseminated intravascular coagulation (DIC), acute renal failure, and multiorgan failure. Management of these clinical syndromes is discussed in greater detail in Chapter 32, Chapter 42, and Chapter 37, respectively.

ARDS is acute pulmonary congestion and atelectasis with hyaline membrane formation associated with aggressive blood transfusions or fluid resuscitation, sepsis, trauma, pulmonary embolus, and other conditions. Hyaline membrane formation and atelectasis decrease lung compliance, reduce pulmonary surfactant, and increase lung capillary permeability. This is followed by significant interstitial and alveolar edema with mucus formation along the alveoli and acute pulmonary congestion. Ineffective oxygenation of tissues and ventilation-perfusion abnormalities worsen as hypoxemia occurs. Management is directed toward early identification of pulmonary congestion through frequent assessment of lung sounds. Endotracheal intubation and mechanical ventilation with positive end-expiratory pressure is used to manage ventilation-perfusion abnormalities and expand alveoli.

DIC is widespread microvascular coagulation followed by depletion of clotting factors. Microthrombi form and are distributed to the microvasculature of various organs, producing infarction, tissue ischemia, and hemorrhagic necrosis when secondary fibrinolysis fails to lyse the fibrin quickly. Secondary fibrinolysis reduces clotting factors. Release of fibrin degradation products that act as anticoagulants is also impaired. These processes contribute to serious bleeding tendencies. The DIC syndrome may occur after aggressive transfusion with blood products or in association with ARDS. Patients should be observed for obvious or occult bleeding, hematuria, petechiae, and ecchymosis.

Acute tubular necrosis occurs from renal hypoperfusion, myocardial compromise, or fluid and electrolyte depletion and is characterized by oliguria, elevated BUN and creatinine levels, hyperkalemia, hyponatremia, azotemia, and acidosis. Oliguria occurs in response to extracellular volume depletion and myocardial compromise.[4] Compensatory responses stimulate sodium and water reabsorption, cause a drop in glomerular filtration rate, and eventually lead to renal tubular dysfunction. This syndrome is often associated with DIC in the shock patient.

SPECIAL POPULATIONS

It is important for the emergency nurse to recognize that pediatric, elderly, or pregnant patients respond differently to volume depletion and other causes of shock. These varied responses are due to normal growth and physiologic differences found in these patients. Table 34-3 highlights some of these differences. Emergent conditions in these populations are covered in greater detail in other chapters of this text.

SUMMARY

Shock is a progressive, pervasive process caused by inadequate tissue perfusion and oxygenation. Regardless of etiology, the cellular effects of shock are the same. Nursing assessment, early recognition, and appropriate management are essential to prevent or reverse the shock process and ensure a positive patient outcome. Box 34-7 outlines the most critical nursing diagnoses for the patient in shock.

Box 34-7	NURSING DIAGNOSES RELATED TO SHOCK
Cardiac output, Decreased	
Fluid volume, Deficient	
Gas exchange, Impaired	
Tissue perfusion, Ineffective	

References

1. Allen ML: Shock. In Phipps WJ, Sands JK, Marekl JF: *Medical surgical nursing: concepts and clinical practice,* St. Louis, 1999, Mosby.
2. Emergency Nurses Association: *Trauma nursing core course: instructors manual,* ed 5, Des Plaines, Ill, 2000, The Association.
3. Emergency Nurses Association: *Emergency nursing core curriculum,* ed 5, Philadelphia, 2000, WB Saunders.
4. Ignatavicius DD, Workman ML, Mishler MA: *Interventions for clients in shock: medical-surgical nursing across the health care continuum,* ed 3, Philadelphia, 1999, WB Saunders.
5. Jones KM, Bucher L: *Shock: critical care nursing,* Philadelphia, 1999, WB Saunders.

Table 34-3	SHOCK IN THE PEDIATRIC, ELDERLY, OR PREGNANT PATIENT
PATIENT	**DESCRIPTION**
Pediatric	Increases cardiac output by increasing heart rate; fixed stroke volume; sustains arterial pressure despite significant volume loss; loses 25% of circulating volume before signs of shock occur; hypotension and lethargy are ominous signs: early clinical manifestations are tachycardia, tachypnea, pallor, cool mottled skin, and delayed capillary refill; volume replaced with 20 ml/kg bolus of crystalloid
Elderly	Shock progression often rapid; normal physiologic changes of aging reduce compensatory mechanisms; predisposed to hypothermia; pre-existing disease states contribute co-morbities
Pregnant	Hypervolemia of pregnancy means patient can remain normotensive with up to a 1500-ml blood loss; compression of inferior vena cava by gravid uterus reduces circulating volume by 30%; place patient on left side, manually displace uterus to the left or elevate right hip with towel; risk for aspiration resulting from decreased gastric motility and decreased gastric emptying; treat suspected hypovolemia to prevent placental vasoconstriction associated with catecholamine release; potential for fetal distress exists despite maternal stability

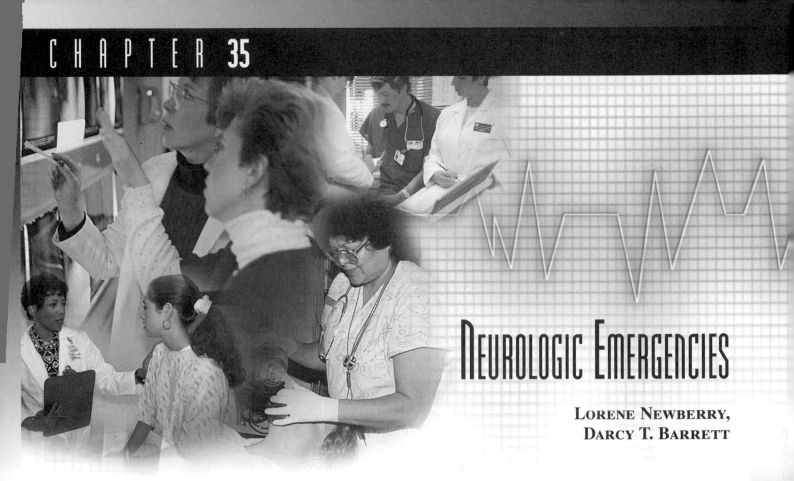

CHAPTER 35

NEUROLOGIC EMERGENCIES

LORENE NEWBERRY,
DARCY T. BARRETT

The emergency nurse encounters a variety of neurologic emergencies related to illness or injury, including stroke, head injury, spinal cord injury, headache, and meningitis. Regardless of etiology, a neurologic emergency is one that causes severe temporary or permanent disability or is an immediate threat to the patient's life. This chapter focuses on assessment and treatment of neurologic conditions caused by disease or pathologic abnormality. Patient assessment, anatomy, and physiology are also reviewed. Neurologic emergencies secondary to injury (i.e., head injury and spinal cord injury) are covered in Chapters 21 and 22, respectively.

ANATOMY AND PHYSIOLOGY

The nervous system coordinates, interprets, and controls interactions between the individual and the surrounding environment. The central nervous system (CNS) and the peripheral nervous system regulate most other body systems.

Central Nervous System

The CNS consists of the brain and spinal cord. Functional units of the CNS are neurons, cells that relay signals between the body and the brain. Figure 35-1 illustrates a generic neuron and identifies essential neuronal structures. More than 100 billion neurons relay signals that control the body's various systems.[1] Signal relay between neurons is controlled by neurotransmitters located at the synapse, or junction, between two neurons. Examples of neurotrans-

mitters include acetylcholine, dopamine, norepinephrine, epinephrine, histamine, insulin, glucagon, serotonin, and angiotensin II. Signal movement along the neuron itself is an electrical phenomenon enhanced by the presence of myelin.

Brain

The adult brain weighs approximately 3 pounds, or 2% of total body weight. Brain tissue is the most energy-consuming tissue in the body, receiving approximately 20% of the cardiac output and using approximately 20% of the body's oxygen supply. Structurally the brain consists of external gray matter and internal white matter. The brain has three distinct parts—the cerebrum, brainstem, and cerebellum (Figure 35-2). The cerebrum, divided into two hemispheres, represents almost 90% of the brain's weight. Bands of connective tissue, called the corpus callosum, relay information between the two hemispheres. Each hemisphere consists of lobes named for the adjacent portion of the skull (i.e., frontal, temporal, parietal, and occipital). The brainstem is continuous with the spinal cord and serves as an important relay and reflex center for the CNS. Nuclei for the cranial nerves are found in the brainstem. These essential nerves control respiration, the cardiovascular system, gastrointestinal functions, equilibrium, and eye movement.[1] The cerebellum controls activities below the level of consciousness (e.g., posture, equilibrium). Within the brain a series of interconnected cavities called ventricles produce cerebrospinal fluid (CSF).

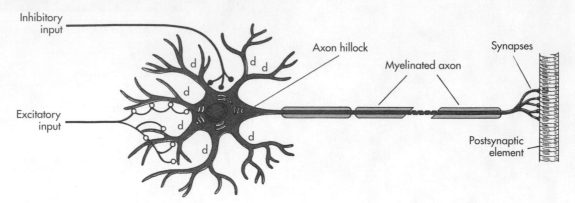

FIGURE 35-1   Schematic diagram of an idealized neuron and its major components. *d,* Dendrites. (From Berne RM, Levy MN: *Physiology,* ed 3, St. Louis, 1993, Mosby.)

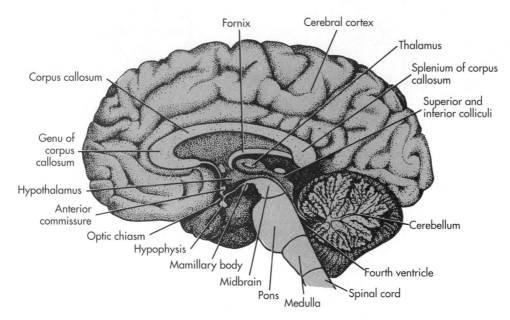

FIGURE 35-2   Midsagittal section of the brain. Note the relationships among the cerebral cortex, cerebellum, thalamus, and brainstem and the location of various commissures. (From Berne RM, Levy MN: *Physiology,* ed 3, St. Louis, 1993, Mosby.)

In addition to the cranium, three connective tissue layers, called meninges, surround and protect the brain. Figure 35-3 illustrates the dura mater, arachnoid, and pia mater and their relationship to the brain. The dura forms a tent over the brain and separates the cerebrum from the cerebellum. (This is the basis for the term supratentorial.) The subarachnoid space contains sinuses that collect venous blood from the brain and return blood to the internal jugular veins. The pia mater extends below the spinal cord to form the filum terminale.

Cranial Nerves

Twelve pairs of cranial nerves arise directly from the brainstem. Each nerve is identified with a Roman numeral and name. Cranial nerves may be sensory, motor, or both. Cranial nerve functions are not consciously controlled; there-

fore, assessment of cranial nerves provides an accurate picture of brainstem activity and neurologic function. Table 35-1 lists cranial nerves and their function.

Cerebral Blood Flow

Two pairs of arteries anastomose to form the circle of Willis, which provides collateral circulation to the brain. The internal carotid arteries supply the anterior brain and vertebral arteries supply the posterior brain. Figure 35-4 illustrates arterial blood supply to the brain. Venous blood drains from the brain through sinuses in the dura mater into the internal jugular veins.

The brain occupies 80% of the cranium. Vascular volume and CSF account for the remaining 20%. Cranial rigidity limits the brain's ability to tolerate increases in any compo-

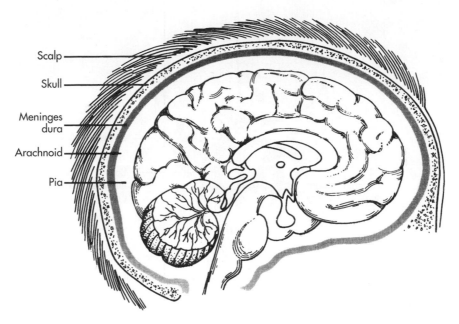

FIGURE 35-3   Cross-section of the head. (From Sheehy SB, Lenehan GP: *Manual of emergency care,* ed 5 St. Louis, 1999, Mosby.)

Table 35-1	CRANIAL NERVES AND THEIR FUNCTIONS	
NUMBER	**NAME**	**FUNCTION**
I	Olfactory	Smell
II	Optic	Vision
III	Oculomotor	Elevate upper lid, pupillary constriction, most extraocular movements
IV	Trochlear	Downward, inward movement of the eye
V	Trigeminal	Chewing, clinching the jaw, lateral jaw movement, corneal reflexes, face sensation
VI	Abducens	Lateral eye deviation
VII	Facial	Facial motor, taste, lacrimation, and salivation
VIII	Acoustic	Equilibrium, hearing
IX	Glossopharyngeal	Swallowing, gag reflex, taste on posterior tongue
X	Vagus	Swallowing, gag reflex, abdominal viscera, phonation
XI	Spinal accessory	Head and shoulder movement
XII	Hypoglossal	Tongue movement

nent. If one component increases, the other components must decrease to prevent pressure on the brain. This tenet of cerebral function is called the Monro-Kelly hypothesis. Cerebral blood flow changes with cerebral perfusion pressure (CPP) and size of the cerebrovascular bed. CPP is a product of mean arterial pressure (MAP) minus intracranial pressure (ICP) (CPP = MAP − ICP). Normal CPP is 60 mm Hg; normal ICP is 10 to 15 mm Hg.

Cerebrospinal Fluid

CSF is produced in the ventricles by the choroid plexus at a rate of 7 to 10 ml/hr. CSF protects the brain and spinal cord by forming a shock-absorbing cushion, providing nutrition via glucose transport, and removing metabolic waste products. CSF also compensates for changes in pressure and volume within the cranium. Table 35-2 summarizes normal CSF characteristics.

Spinal Cord

The spinal cord lies in the spinal canal of the vertebral bodies and is covered by meningeal layers. The adult spinal cord is approximately 16 to 18 inches long and extends from the brainstem to the intervertebral disk between L-1 and L-2. Sensory and motor neurons in the spinal cord conduct impulses to and from the brain. Unlike the brain, the spinal cord has white matter on the exterior and gray matter on the interior. Figure 35-5 illustrates the spinal cord in cross-section. Reflex arcs into the spinal cord operate without voluntary or conscious control. Table 35-3 lists these reflexes.

Peripheral Nervous System

The peripheral nervous system consists of 31 spinal nerves and the autonomic nervous system. Spinal nerves innervate skeletal muscle and a segment of skin called a dermatome. Figure 35-6 shows these dermatomes with distinct borders; however, there is significant overlap between adjacent segments. In certain areas spinal nerves form a network called a plexus; for example, the brachial plexus innervates the upper extremity.

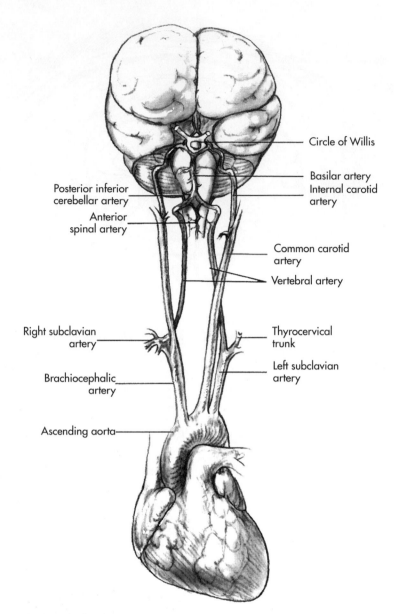

FIGURE **35-4** Origin and course of arterial supply to the brain. (From Davis JH, Drucker WR et al: *Clinical surgery,* vol 1, St. Louis, 1987, Mosby.)

Table 35-2	NORMAL CEREBROSPINAL FLUID	
QUALITY	VALUE-DESCRIPTION
Appearance	Clear, colorless, odorless
Cell count	WBC count 5/mm³
	RBC count 0/mm³
Pressure	80-180 mm H$_2$O
Glucose	60-80 mg/100 ml (2/3 serum glucose value)
Protein	15-45 mg/100 ml (lumbar)
pH	7.35-7.40
Sodium	140-142 mEq/L
Chloride	120-130 mEq/L
Volume	125-150 ml

WBC, White blood cell; *RBC,* red blood cell.

Autonomic Nervous System

The autonomic nervous system controls the body's visceral functions. There is no sensory component; functions are entirely motor. The cerebral cortex, hypothalamus, and the brainstem regulate activity. Two major divisions, the sympathetic and parasympathetic nervous systems, respond to stressors such as fear or blood loss to provide extra energy or conserve existing energy stores. The sympathetic nervous system provides the body energy, creating the fight-or-flight response. Receptors are scattered throughout the body, including the skin. Parasympathetic nervous system receptors distributed primarily in the head, chest, abdomen, and pelvis conserve the body's energy. Table 35-4 compares activities of these opposing systems.

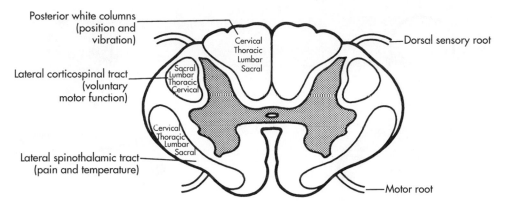

FIGURE 35-5 Cross-section of the cervical spinal cord. (From Rund DA, Barkin RM, Rosen P: *Essentials of emergency medicine,* ed 2, St. Louis, 1996, Mosby.)

Table 35-3 SPINAL REFLEXES	
REFLEX	SEGMENTAL LEVEL
Biceps	C5-6
Brachioradialis	C5-6
Triceps	C7-8
Knee	L2-4
Ankle	S1-2
Superficial abdominal (above the umbilicus)	T8-10
Superficial abdominal (below the umbilicus)	T10-12
Cremasteric	L1-2
Plantar	L4-5, S1-2

PATIENT ASSESSMENT

The most reliable indicator of neurologic function is the patient's level of consciousness (LOC). Follow initial assessment with continuous evaluation to detect changes. Question the patient's family and significant other about changes in behavior, mood, or physical ability. Evaluate for signs of increasing ICP such as headache, nausea, vomiting, or altered LOC. Assess cranial nerve function and pupil size, equality, reactivity, and accommodation. The pupil dilates when increased ICP causes pressure on Cranial nerve III; however, this is a late indicator of increasing ICP. Serial assessment is essential to identify subtle changes that may indicate impending herniation. A universal tool such as the Glasgow Coma Scale is recommended (Box 35-1). Evaluating motor strength requires comparison of the patient's dominant hand with the evaluator's dominant hand. Sensory evaluation should include differentiation of dull and sharp objects. Assessment should also include identification of existing deficits such as muscle weakness, pupil abnormality, and gait disturbances.

Stabilization of the patient with a neurologic emergency begins with the airway, breathing, and circulation (ABCs). Specific interventions depend on patient complaint and

acuity. The patient with a severe migraine headache has different priorities than does a comatose patient. A patient with severe migraine requires pain management; the comatose patient needs support of the ABCs, management of increased ICP, and monitoring for impending herniation. Herniation occurs when increased ICP forces the brain downward through the foramen magnum. Compression of the brainstem impairs respiratory and cardiovascular function, ultimately causing death. Figure 35-7 illustrates this process. Controlling increased ICP includes use of medications such as osmotic diuretics, sedatives, and analgesics. Elevating the patient's head facilitates venous drainage and decreases ICP; however, cervical spine injury must be ruled out before elevation. Decreasing stimulation such as noise and certain procedures such as suctioning can also affect ICP.

SPECIFIC NEUROLOGIC EMERGENCIES

Specific neurologic emergencies represent a threat to the patient's life, integrity of specific functions such as vision, or quality of the patient's life. Specific emergencies include headache, seizures, stroke, meningitis, Guillain-Barré syndrome, and myasthenia gravis. A brief review from the emergency nurse's perspective is presented.

Headache

Headache is one of the most common complaints seen in the emergency department (ED), with only 1% to 2% not related to trauma.[4] It is important for the emergency nurse to remember that headache is a symptom of an underlying disorder rather than a diagnosis. The headache may be minor or represent a life-threatening situation such as subarachnoid hemorrhage; therefore, careful assessment is essential. Box 35-2 highlights key assessment questions for these patients.

Headaches may be caused by an extracranial or intracranial condition. Extracranial causes include acidosis, dehydration, hypoglycemia, uremia, and hepatic disorders.

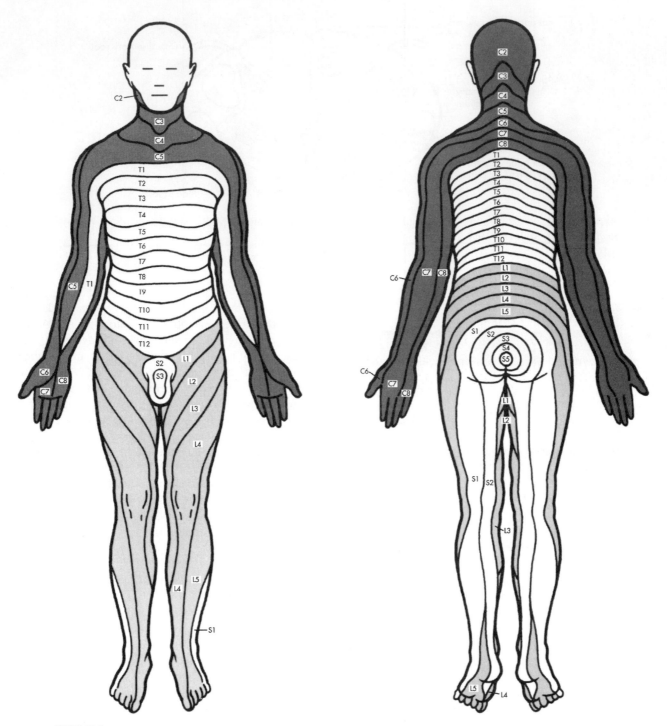

FIGURE 35-6 Sensory dermatomes. (From Rund DA, Barkin RM, Rosen P: *Essentials of emergency medicine,* ed 2, St. Louis, 1996, Mosby.)

Ophthalmic causes of headache include glaucoma, refractory errors, inflammation, or allergic reactions (see Chapter 46). Poisoning and toxicologic emergencies also cause headache (see Chapter 43). Other extracranial causes include ear infection, upper respiratory infection, sinus congestion, facial trauma, temporomandibular joint syndrome, toothache, anemia, polycythemia, electrolyte imbalance,

and systemic infection. Identification and treatment of extracranial causes should relieve the headache.

Specific headaches related to intracranial conditions include migraine headache, tension headache, and temporal arteritis. Traumatic headaches may occur as an emergency or nonemergency. Nonemergency conditions include postconcussion or contusion headaches. Emergent conditions

Table 35-4	AUTONOMIC NERVOUS SYSTEM FUNCTIONS	
SYMPATHETIC NERVOUS SYSTEM	**PARASYMPATHETIC NERVOUS SYSTEM**
Pupil dilation	Pupil constriction
Increased heart rate	Decreased heart rate
Increased conduction velocity	Decreased conduction velocity
Increased contractility	Decreased contractility
Coronary vasodilation	
Skeletal muscle vasodilation	Minimal peripheral vascular effects
Abdominal and cutaneous vasoconstriction	
Bronchodilation	Bronchoconstriction
Increased glucose release from liver	Slight glycogen synthesis
Decreased peristalsis	Increased peristalsis
Decreased gastric tone	Increased gastric tone
Increased basal metabolic rate (BMR)	No change in BMR rate
Increased coagulation	No effect on coagulation
Diaphoresis	Sweating of palms only
Piloerection	No effect on body hair

Box 35-1	GLASGOW COMA SCALE	
EYE OPENING	
Spontaneous	4
To verbal command	3
To pain	2
No response	1
BEST MOTOR RESPONSE	
Obeys commands	6
Localizes pain	5
Withdraws from pain	4
Abnormal flexion	3
Abnormal extension	2
No response	1
BEST VERBAL RESPONSE	
Oriented	5
Confused	4
Inappropriate words	3
Incomprehensible sounds	2
No response	1
TOTAL	3-15

that cause severe headache include intracranial injury (see Chapter 21). Women have reported headaches associated with the start of menses or during the premenstrual period.

Migraine Headache

Twenty-three million Americans suffer migraine headaches.[7] Diagnosis of migraine headache is based on the patient's history and presenting symptoms. Headache is never the only symptom. Before the diagnosis is made, other causes should be ruled out. Migraine symptoms include nausea, vomiting, and visual disturbances. Approximately 12% of the US population have migraine headaches, and almost 70% of those with migraines have a positive family history.[7]

Migraine headaches are classified as vascular or nonvascular. Muscular contraction or tension headache is an example of a nonvascular migraine headache. Skeletal muscle contraction in the head or neck produces steady, pulsatile pain and limited motion of the head, neck, and jaw. Pressure over contracted muscles worsens the pain. Pain also worsens with vasoconstrictive drugs such as ergotamines. Treatment includes mild analgesia with identification and treatment of the underlying cause.

Vascular headaches occur suddenly and are described as intense, sharp, and piercing or pounding and throbbing. Table 35-5 describes specific vascular migraine headaches. Vascular migraine headaches have three distinct phases. During the prodromal phase the patient may experience an aura. Fifteen percent of migraine patients experience an aura.[7] Author Lewis Carroll saw the distorted figures in *Alice in Wonderland* as part of a migraine attack. Most auras are visual; however, any sign or symptom of brain dysfunction can be a feature of an aura. During the second phase, in-flammation and cerebral vasodilation cause the characteristic headache. The third phase, or recovery phase, is characterized by extreme temporal and cranial tenderness. Migraines can be caused by changes in sleep patterns, physical exertion, sudden changes in barometric pressure, increased stress, dieting, heat, lights, cyclic estrogen levels, and certain foods, such as alcohol, caffeine, monosodium glutamate, ripened cheeses, and coffee.

Pharmacologic therapy used during a migraine attack includes analgesics, antiinflammatory agents, β-adrenergic blockers, serotonin antagonists, vasoconstrictors, and antidepressants. Diuretics, antihistamines, anticonvulsants, and short courses of steroids may also be used. Female patients with migraines should avoid oral contraceptives. Other interventions include biofeedback, relaxation training, assertiveness training, family counseling, dietary counseling, allergy testing, and education.

Temporal Arteritis

Temporal arteritis is inflammation of branches of the carotid artery that usually occurs in patients older than 50 years of age. Women are affected 4 times more often than men. Headache is the most frequent and severe symptom of temporal arteritis. Pain is severe and stabbing in one or both temporal regions, with decreased visual acuity. The patient may have difficulty sleeping and opening or closing the mouth because of pain. Weight loss, night sweats, aching joints, fever, and red nodules over the temporal region also occur. Untreated, this condition can result in blindness. Definitive diagnosis is biopsy of the temporal artery. ED management includes steroids and pain management with antiinflammatory drugs or stronger agents as necessary.[7]

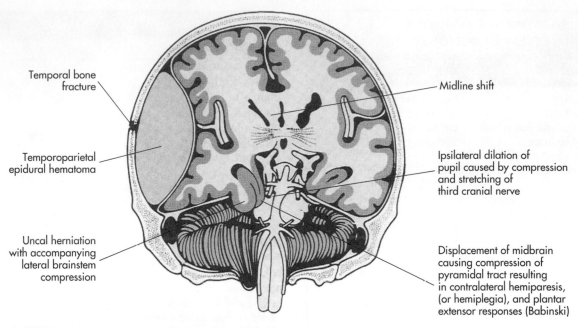

Temporal bone
fracture

Temporoparietal
epidural hematoma

Uncal herniation
with accompanying
lateral brainstem
compression

Midline shift

Ipsilateral dilation of
pupil caused by compression
and stretching of
third cranial nerve

Displacement of midbrain
causing compression of
pyramidal tract resulting
in contralateral hemiparesis,
(or hemiplegia), and plantar
extensor responses (Babinski)

FIGURE 35-7   Cross-section showing herniation of lower portion of temporal lobe (uncas) through tentorium caused by temporoparietal epidural hematoma. Herniation may occur also in the cerebellum. Note mass effect and midline shift. (From Meeker MH, Rothrock JC: *Alexander's care of the patient in surgery,* ed 10, St. Louis, 1995, Mosby.)

BOX 35-2   KEY ASSESSMENT QUESTIONS RELATED TO HEADACHE

Is this the patient's first headache?
Is this the worst headache the patient has ever had?
Is the headache generalized or localized to one area?
When did this headache start?
Has the patient been injured recently?
Have there been any personality changes?
Has the patient experienced any memory loss?
Has the patient had a recent infection?
Does the patient have any problems with vision?
Has the patient had any recent neurologic problems?
Does the patient have hypertension? For how long?
Does the patient have any emotional problems?
What medication is the patient currently taking?
What measures has the patient taken to relieve the pain?
Has the patient ever had a seizure?

Seizures

Approximately 1% to 2% of the US population have a seizure disorder.[7] Seizure is a symptom of an underlying problem rather than an independent diagnosis. Defined as an abnormal period of electrical activity in the brain, seizures are classified as partial, generalized, or unclassified. Unclassified seizures are seizures that do not fall into other categories.

Initial treatment focuses on protection of the patient's ABCs and prevention of injury during the seizure. Oxygen therapy should be initiated and intravenous access obtained. Glucose level should be checked immediately because hypoglycemia can cause seizures. Additional treatment depends on the type of seizure and the underlying cause. Intravenous midazolam (Versed), diazepam (Valium), and lorazepam (Ativan) in conjunction with intravenous phenobarbital and phenytoin (Dilantin) are used to control seizure activity. Dextrose 50% and naloxone are administered as indicated.

Partial Seizures

Partial, or focal, seizures are limited to one specific body part and may be further classified as simple or complex. The patient's mental status is not affected in a simple partial seizure, whereas there is loss of consciousness in a complex partial seizure. A partial seizure may consist of focal motor activity, somatic sensory symptoms, or disturbances in the patient's vision, hearing, smell, or taste. Focal motor activity can occur in a specific area or begin in one area and progress to surrounding areas in an organized manner (Jacksonian seizure). Somatic sensory symptoms include tingling or numbness.

Temporal lobe seizures are often preceded by an aura, such as foul smell, metallic or bitter taste, buzzing, ringing, or hissing sounds, or vague visceral feelings in the chest and abdomen. Feelings of familiarity in an unfamiliar setting (deja vu) or unfamiliarity in a familiar setting (jamais vu) have been reported. The most characteristic symptom of temporal lobe seizure is semipurposeful patterns of movement (automatism) such as lip-smacking, chewing, patting hands, or facial grimacing.

Partial seizures can occur with secondary generalized seizures. Seizure activity originates locally and progresses until the entire body is involved. There is an associated loss of consciousness.

Table 35-5	TYPES OF VASCULAR MIGRAINE HEADACHES
TYPE	**DESCRIPTION**
Classic migraine	Aura that lasts 15 to 20 minutes; clears more quickly than it develops; severe pain, usually unilateral, can be bilateral; lasts 30 minutes to several days; photophobia, sound sensitivity, nausea, vomiting, and anorexia; worsened by walking, straining, or sudden changes in body position; occurs during increased stress and pregnancy. Treatment includes ergotamines, sumatriptan (Imitrex)
Common migraine	Euphoria, hunger, depression, irritability, intense yawning, generalized edema, and photophobia present; usually does not occur in pregnancy. Treatment includes ergotamines, sumatriptan
Cluster headache	Ten times more common in men; closely grouped attacks over several weeks followed by remission of months or years; may have 12 or more headaches per day; more frequent in spring and fall; excruciating, unilateral pain, usually behind eye or in temporal region; may travel to ear, nose, and cheek; facial flushing, nasal congestion, lacrimation, rhinorrhea, and salivation may be present; may wake patient from deep sleep or occur during periods of rest after exhaustion. Treatment includes oxygen, ergotamines, sumatriptan, prednisone, and in some cases, lithium
Ophthalmoplegic migraine	Begins during infancy or early childhood; headache and paralysis of Cranial nerve III; if untreated, prominent visual field defects or blindness may occur. Treatment includes ergotamines, sumatriptan, and steroids
Hemiplegic migraine	Visual field defects, numbness of mouth or extremities, and various paresthesias; unilateral extremity weakness or paralysis; family history positive for migraine. Treatment includes rest, sedation, analgesia, and increasing carbon dioxide levels; ergotamines contraindicated
Facial migraine	Unilateral episodic facial pain; associated with cluster headache or common migraine
Migraine equivalent	All features of migraine present except headache; symptoms include vomiting, abdominal migraines, menstrual syndromes, precordial migraines, and periodic diarrhea, fever, mood changes, and sleep or trancelike states

Generalized Seizures

There are two major types of generalized seizures—absence (petit mal) and tonic-clonic (grand mal) seizures. Absence seizures usually occur in children 4 to 12 years of age. Episodes are characterized by abrupt cessation of activity with momentary loss of consciousness, duration less than 15 seconds, and may be accompanied by automatism.

Tonic-clonic seizures begin with sudden loss of consciousness followed by major tonic contractions of large muscle groups. Arms and legs extend stiffly as the person falls to the ground. A shrill cry may precede the event. During the tonic phase the person is apneic, pupils are dilated and unresponsive, and bowel and bladder incontinence occur. The individual may also bite his or her tongue. During the clonic phase strenuous, rhythmic muscle contractions occur. Hyperventilation, profuse sweating, tachycardia, and excessive salivation with frothing are usually present. A postictal phase follows as muscles relax. Deep breathing and a depressed level of consciousness are present. The person awakens confused with complaints of headache, muscle aching, and fatigue. There is generalized amnesia concerning the event and the person may sleep for hours afterward.

Status Epilepticus

Status epilepticus is a series of consecutive seizures or a single seizure that does not respond to conventional therapy. Uncontrolled seizure activity increases the patient's temperature, blood pressure, and pulse; interferes with cerebral blood flow; and increases the risk for hypoxic brain damage. Control of seizure activity is critical. Therapeutic interventions begin with the ABCs. Endotracheal intubation is used to maintain the airway and oxygenate the patient. Patient should be protected from injury with restraints and other seizure precautions. Naloxone, dextrose 50%, and thiamine may be given. Sedation (e.g., Versed and Ativan) and anticonvulsant medications (e.g., phenobarbital and phenytoin) are given until seizure activity is controlled. If these medications fail general anesthesia is considered.

Stroke

Decreased cerebral blood flow or cerebral perfusion pressure deprives the brain of oxygen and glucose. This leads to cellular ischemia and, ultimately, cerebral infarction. Strokes may be ischemic or hemorrhagic; however, 80% to 85% of all strokes are ischemic.[7] Ischemic strokes are caused by occlusion of cerebral vessels by a thrombus or embolus. Hemorrhagic strokes occur with ruptured aneurysms, leaking venous malformations, or subarachnoid hemorrhage. Factors that increase the patient's risk of stroke are hypertension, diabetes mellitus, atherosclerosis, cardiac valve disease, and smoking. Approximately 500,000 Americans suffer a stroke each year, with a 20% mortality rate the first year.[7]

Approximately half of all strokes are caused by cerebral thrombosis. Thrombotic strokes occur as atherosclerotic plaque accumulates within the vessel. Carotid stenosis is a major cause of thrombotic stroke. Symptoms occur slowly as cerebral blood flow gradually decreases. Neurologic deficits depend on the area of the brain affected. Embolic strokes occur when a free-floating substance travels to the brain and occludes a vessel. Substances tend to fragment as

Table 35-6	STROKE CLASSIFICATION
TYPE	**DESCRIPTION**
Transient ischemic attack (TIA)	Temporary disturbance of blood supply causes transient neurologic deficit; symptoms present less than 24 hours; no permanent neurologic deficit
Reversible ischemic	Neurologic deficits last a few days or weeks; minimal permanent neurologic deficits
Stroke in evolution	Progressive neurologic deterioration occurs; residual neurologic deficit present
Completed stroke	Patient appears stable with neurologic deficit permanent and unchanging

Box 35-3	FIBRINOLYTIC THERAPY FOR ISCHEMIC STROKE	
MEDICATION		**ADMINISTRATION**
Alteplase		**IV administration**
Total dose 0.9 mg/kg IV		Must be started within 3 hours of symptom onset
Maximum IV dose is 90 mg		**Intraarterial administration**
Bolus is 10% of the total dose − given IV over 1 minute		May be given up to 6 hours after symptom onset
		Given by the radiologist
Remainder of the total dose is given IV over 60 minutes		Requires cannulization of the femoral or brachial artery

Data from Hazinski MF, Cummins RO, Field JM: *Handbook of emergency cardiovascular care for health care providers,* Dallas, 2000, American Heart Association.
IV, Intravenous.

they float, so multiple areas of the brain are affected. Multifocal neurologic deficits occur. Free-floating substances include blood clots, tumor particles, fat, air, or vegetation from a diseased heart valve. Patients with atrial fibrillation are at risk for embolic stroke because of clot formation on the mitral valve.

Cerebral infarction, or stroke, may occur anywhere in the brain. Symptoms and lethality are determined by location and size of the infarction. Surrounding the area of infarction is an area of ischemia called the penumbra.[5] Recognition and treatment of stroke focus on preservation and reperfusion of this ischemic area to prevent further cellular destruction. Duration of symptoms is a crucial factor in treatment. Table 35-6 describes four types of strokes by duration of symptoms.

Treatment of stroke patients begins with the ABCs. Significant respiratory impairment occurs when the stroke affects the respiratory center. The unconscious patient or one who is unable to manage oral secretions is also at risk for respiratory compromise. Endotracheal intubation may be required to ensure a patent airway. If the patient is hypertensive (>220 mm Hg systolic, or ≥120 mm Hg diastolic), antihypertensive agents such as nitroprusside (Nipride) should be used. However, precipitous reduction of blood pressure is not recommended. Sudden rapid decrease in blood pressure can impair cerebral perfusion and reduce perfusion to the penumbra, thereby converting an area of ischemia to an area of infarction.[7]

Identification of stroke type is critical to successful treatment. Several prehospital scores (the Cincinnati Prehospital Stroke Scale and the Los Angeles Stroke Screen) have been successfully used to identify possible stroke patients before they arrive in the ED. This can greatly decrease the door to computed tomography (CT) time. CT scans must be done quickly to determine if the stroke is hemorrhagic or ischemic. This difference is essential because treatment for ischemic stroke (i.e., anticoagulant therapy) is contraindicated in hemorrhagic stroke. In a few centers, Alteplase, recombinant (tPA), is used to treat thromboembolic strokes. There is a very narrow window of opportunity for use of tPA therapy. Box 35-3 highlights administration.[2] The agent is given in-

Table 35-7	SELECTED AGENTS FOR TREATMENT OF STROKE
CATEGORY	**AGENTS***
Fibrinolytic agents	rt-PA
Antithrombotic agents	Fraxiparine
Antioxidants	PNA
NMDA receptor antagonists	Cerestat, ACPC, ACEA, GV150526
Opiate antagonists	Cervene
GABA-A agonists	Chlomethiazole
Defibrinogenating agents	Ancrod
Other neuroprotective agents	Enlimomab, Citicoline, Lubeluzole, calpain inhibitors, kinase inhibitors

Data from National Stroke Association: *The stroke/brain attack reporter's handbook,* Englewood, Colo, 1997, The Association.
rt-PA, Recombinant prurokinase.
*Includes agents currently in use and those under investigation.

travenously in many centers across the nation and is also given arterially in a small number of centers. There is some controversy as to the effectiveness of tPA therapy—reversal of symptoms may simply be due to resolution of a TIA. Hemorrhagic stroke usually requires surgical intervention to control hemorrhage and manage increased ICP.

A number of neuroprotective agents have been approved for use in cases of ischemic stroke. These agents preserve cerebral function by increasing perfusion of the penumbra.[3] Mechanism of action varies with type of agent. Table 35-7 reviews medications being studied. Some agents remove oxygen-free radicals, whereas others increase movement of calcium across the cell membrane. Agents are usually time-limited and must be given within 6 to 12 hours of symptom onset. As more research occurs in this area, additional

Table 35-8	CEREBROSPINAL FLUID RESULTS IN MENINGITIS		
RESULT	**BACTERIAL**	**VIRAL**	**FUNGAL**
Leukocytes	1000-20,000	10-1000	<500
Leukocyte differential	Mostly neutrophils	Neutrophils initially with lymphs noted >24 hours	Lymphocytes
Glucose	<40% of serum glucose	Elevated	Low
Protein	>200 mg/dl	<200 mg/dl	>200

agents with a longer window of opportunity for administration are anticipated.

Meningitis

Meningitis is inflammation of the meningeal layers surrounding the brain and spinal cord; it is a neurologic emergency and an infectious disease emergency. Infection may be viral, bacterial, or fungal. Viral meningitis is usually less acute, with gradual onset of symptoms. Bacterial meningitis has acute onset of symptoms and is fatal in 50% of patients. Common bacterial agents include *Streptococcus pneumoniae, Neisseria meningitides, Haemophilus influenzae,* group B streptococci, and *Listeria monocytogenes.* Fungal meningitis usually occurs in immune-compromised individuals; agents include *Aspergillus* and *Candida* organisms. Noninfectious causes of meningitis include drugs, toxic exposure, and neoplasms.

Symptoms of meningitis are fever, headache, photophobia, nuchal rigidity, lethargy, seizures, vomiting, and chills. The classic triad of fever, stiff neck, and altered LOC is noted in approximately two thirds of adult patients but rarely in infants.[6] The clinical presentation in patients with acquired immunodeficiency syndrome (AIDS) is not as dramatic. The patient may have isolated fevers and a chronic headache.[6] The patient may arrive at the ED with mild headache and severe confusion or comatose with shock. Patients with meningococcemia can have purpura, petechiae, splinter hemorrhages, and pustular lesions. The clinical progression is characterized by rapid deterioration in the patient with meningicoccal meningitis.

Diagnosis is confirmed with lumbar puncture (LP) and CSF cultures. Results of note for CSF are white blood cell count, glucose, protein, leukocyte differential, and protein. Results vary with the cause of the meningitis (Table 35-8). Latex agglutination may also be ordered. This test is useful for patients on previous antibiotic therapy but is not effective in ruling out bacterial infection.[6] If a brain abscess is suspected, LP is contraindicated because of the potential for herniation. A CT scan may be obtained before the LP. Treatment includes support of the patient's ABCs, immediate administration of appropriate antibiotics, antipyretics, and anticonvulsants as indicated. Serial neurologic assessment is critical to identify changes in level of consciousness. The patient with bacterial meningitis should be isolated. Prophylactic antibiotics are given for intimate contact or documented exposure such as needle stick.

Guillain-Barré Syndrome

Guillain-Barré syndrome is an acute paralytic disease caused by decreased myelin at the nerve roots and in peripheral nerves. Individuals in their 20s and 30s are affected most often. Symptoms usually follow an acute febrile episode.[5] Signs and symptoms are tingling sensation in the extremities lasting for hours to weeks, severely decreased deep tendon reflexes, and a symmetric paralysis that begins in the lower extremities and ascends. This classic pattern is seen in 90% to 95% of patients diagnosed with Guillain-Barré syndrome.[6] Paralysis eventually affects the diaphragm and intercostal muscles, causing respiratory paralysis and death. Emergency management focuses on support of the ABCs. Endotracheal intubation and ventilator support are often required. Use of succinylcholine is contraindicated because of the potential for lethal hyperkalemia. Therapy is initially plasmapheresis with immunoglobulin considered as a secondary therapy. Provide general supportive care until the disease has run its course. Patients who survive this disease usually require a long program of rehabilitation.

Myasthenia Gravis

Myasthenia gravis (MG), a defect in neuromuscular transmission, occurs more frequently in women. The disease can occur at any age, but is predominant in adults age 20 to 30 years (an estimated 5 to 10 cases per 100,000 population).[7] Ocular dysfunction is the most common initial symptom, seen in 70% of the cases.[6] Ocular symptoms include ptosis, diplopia with sustained directional gaze, and difficulty keeping the eye closed. It is important to note that MG never affects the pupil. An MG crisis has a sudden onset, causing respiratory paralysis and arrest. Patients experience increasing fatigue; delayed muscle strength recovery; weak eye, facial, and jaw muscles; weak pharyngeal muscles; diplopia; dysphagia; and inability to swallow. Therapeutic intervention is support of ABCs, with possible endotracheal intubation and ventilator management. Pharmacologic therapy is pyridostigmine bromide (Mestinon), barbiturates, opiates, quinidine, quinine, corticotropin, corticosteroids, aminoglycosides, antibiotics, and muscle relaxants. Differentiation of "myasthenic crisis" from "cholinergic crisis" may be accomplished with administration of edrophonium (Tensilon), an anticholinesterase inhibitor. If the patient's condition worsens after edrophonium, cholinergic crisis should be suspected.[7]

SUMMARY

Neurologic emergencies represent a significant challenge for the emergency nurse. Life-threatening neurologic emergencies require rapid, organized assessment with simultaneous intervention. Patients with neurologic problems that are not life-threatening may fear loss of function or cognitive ability, or pain. Patients require supportive, therapeutic care to minimize discomfort and facilitate recovery. Box 35-4 summarizes nursing diagnoses for patients with neurologic emergencies.

Management of neurologic emergencies is undergoing rapid change. Old treatments such as hyperventilation to decrease ICP are being questioned. Research in management of stroke and preservation of cerebral function in other neurologic problems—for example, head injury—is rapidly changing. Changes represent an opportunity for improved patient outcomes with decreased mortality and morbidity. Diligence by the emergency nurse is essential to maintain a current knowledge base in the face of this rapidly changing information.

Box 35-4 NURSING DIAGNOSES FOR NEUROLOGIC EMERGENCIES

Anxiety
Breathing pattern, Ineffective
Fear
Pain
Tissue perfusion, Ineffective
Verbal communication, Impaired

References

1. Guyton AC, Hall JE: *Textbook of medical physiology,* ed 10, Philadelphia, 2000, WB Saunders.
2. Hazinski, MF, Cummins RO, Field JM: *2000 Handbook of emergency cardiovascular care for health care providers,* Dallas, Tex, 2000, American Heart Association.
3. Hilton G: Experimental neuroprotective agents: nursing challenge, *Dimen Crit Care Nurs* 14(4):181, 1995.
4. Rakel RE: *Conn's current therapy,* Philadelphia, 1997, WB Saunders.
5. Rosen P, Barkin R: *Emergency medicine: concepts and clinical practice,* ed 4, St. Louis, 1998, Mosby.
6. Rosen P, Barkin RM, Hayden SR, et al: *The 5 minute emergency medicine consult,* Philadelphia, 1999, Lippincott Williams & Wilkins.
7. Tintinalli JE, Ruiz E, Krome RL: *Emergency medicine: a comprehensive study guide,* ed 4, New York, 1996, McGraw-Hill.

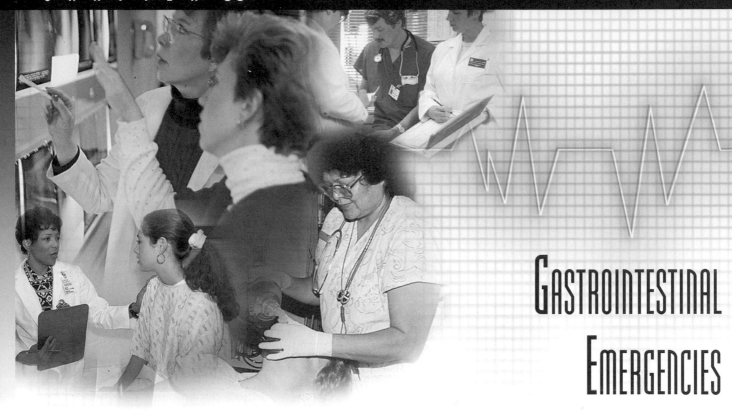

CHAPTER 36

Gastrointestinal Emergencies

Lorene Newberry

Gastrointestinal (GI) emergencies vary from minor problems to more serious, potentially life-threatening problems. Complaints of a GI nature are a common reason for visits to the emergency department (ED). Classic indications of a problem in the GI system include heartburn, nausea, vomiting, constipation, diarrhea, belching, bloating, chest pain, abdominal pain, and bleeding.[11] This chapter focuses on those conditions seen most often in the ED. A brief review of anatomy and physiology is followed by discussion of specific GI conditions (i.e., gastroenteritis, gastrointestinal bleeding, bowel obstruction, diverticulitis, gastroesophageal reflux disease [GERD], appendicitis, cholecystitis, and pancreatitis). Trauma of the GI system is discussed in Chapter 24.

ANATOMY AND PHYSIOLOGY

Normal GI function requires ingestion of nutrients and fluids and is followed by elimination of waste products formed from metabolic activities. Major organs and structures of the GI system are the esophagus, stomach, intestines, liver, pancreas, gallbladder, and peritoneum (Figure 36-1).

Esophagus

The major function of the esophagus is movement of food. The esophagus, a straight, collapsible tube, approximately 25 cm long and up to 3 cm in diameter, extends from the pharynx to the stomach. Distinct esophageal layers are the

mucous membrane, submucosa, and muscular layer. Secretions from mucous glands scattered throughout the submucosa keep the inner lining moist and lubricated. Striated muscle in the upper esophagus is gradually replaced by smooth muscle in the lower esophagus and GI tract. The upper esophageal sphincter is at the proximal end of the esophagus with the lower esophageal sphincter (also called the cardiac sphincter) at the distal junction of the esophagus and stomach. The lower esophageal sphincter prevents regurgitation from the stomach into the esophagus.

Stomach

Stomach functions include food storage, combining food with gastric juices, limited absorption, and moving food into the small intestine. The stomach is a J-shaped organ located below the diaphragm between the esophagus and small intestine. Recognized regions of the stomach are pylorus, fundus, body, and antrum (Figure 36-2). The pyloric sphincter controls food movement from stomach to duodenum. Distinct layers of the stomach wall are outer serosa, muscular layer, submucosa, and mucosa. The mucosal layer contains multiple wrinkles called rugae that straighten as the stomach fills to accommodate more volume. Completely relaxed, the stomach holds up to 1.5 L.[5] Gastric juices containing pepsin, hydrochloric acid, mucus, and intrinsic factor are secreted by glands in the submucosa. These agents begin food breakdown. Acids in the stomach maintain the pH of gastric juices at 1.0.

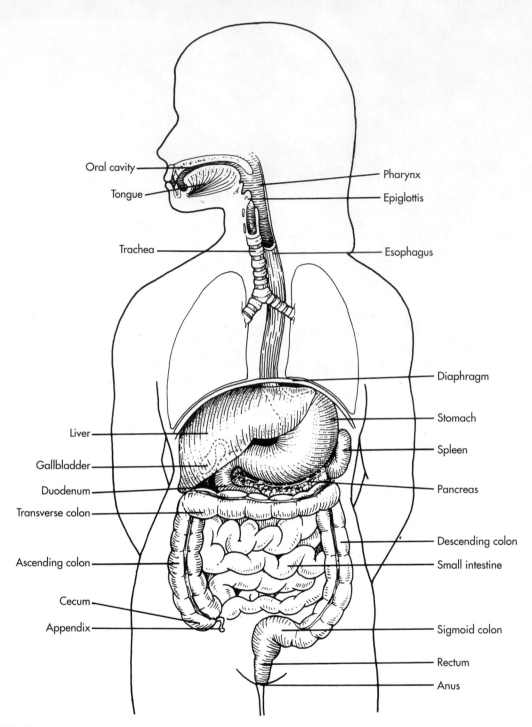

FIGURE 36-1   Anatomy of the gastrointestinal system. (From Society of Gastroenterology Nurses and Associates [SGNA]: *Gastroenterology nursing: a core curriculum,* ed. 2, St. Louis, 1998, Mosby.)

Intestines

The small intestine is a tubular organ extending from the pyloric sphincter to the proximal large intestine. Secretions from the pancreas and liver complete digestion of nutrients in chyme—the semiliquid mixture of food and gastric secre-

tions. The small intestine absorbs nutrients and other products of digestion and transports residue to the large intestine. Segments of the small intestine are the duodenum, jejunum, and ileum. The duodenum attaches to the stomach at the pyloric sphincter in the retroperitoneal space and represents the only fixed portion of the small intestine. The duodenum is approx-

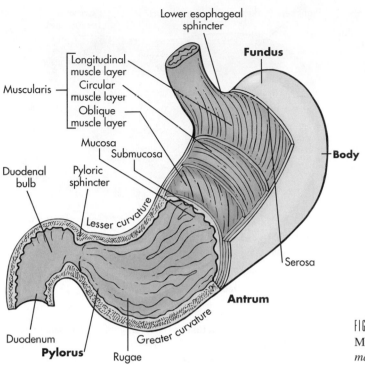

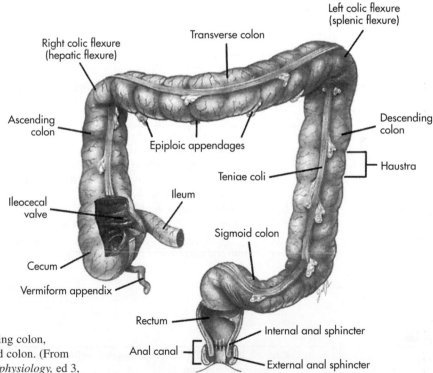

FIGURE **36-2** Parts of the stomach. (From Lewis SM, Heitkemper MM, Dirksen SR: *Medical-surgical nursing: assessment and management of clinical problems,* ed 5, St. Louis, 2000, Mosby.)

FIGURE **36-3** Large intestine showing the ascending colon, transverse colon, descending colon, and sigmoid colon. (From Seeley RR, Stephens TD, Tate P: *Anatomy and physiology,* ed 3, New York, 1995, McGraw-Hill.)

imately 25 cm long and 5 cm in diameter. The jejunum and ileum are mobile and lie free in the peritoneal cavity.

Segments of the large intestine are the cecum, colon, rectum, and anal canal. The large intestine is approximately 1.5 m long, beginning in the lower right side of the abdomen where the ileum joins the cecum. The colon is di-vided into ascending colon, transverse colon, descending colon, and sigmoid colon (Figure 36-3). Primary functions of the large intestine are absorption of water and elec-trolytes, formation of feces, and storage of feces. Approxi-mately 1500 ml of chyme pass through the ileocecal valve each day.[5]

Liver

The liver, located in the right upper quadrant of the abdomen, is divided into right and left lobes (Figure 36-4). Functional units of the liver called lobules contain sinusoids and Kupffer cells. Each lobule is supplied by a hepatic artery, sublobular vein, bile duct, and lymph channel (Figure 36-5). The liver is extremely vascular; approximately 1450 ml of blood flow through the liver each minute, accounting for 29% of resting cardiac output.[5] Sinusoids in lobules act as a reservoir for overflow of blood and fluids from the right ventricle. A thick capsule of connective tissue known as Glisson's capsule covers the liver. The liver is involved in hundreds of metabolic functions, including metabolism of nutrients, gluconeogenesis, and drug metabolism. Table 36-1 summarizes functions related to nutrition and waste removal. Production of bile is a major function of the liver; 600 to 1200 ml of bile are secreted each day. Bile is essential for digestion, absorption, and excretion of bilirubin and excess cholesterol. Bilirubin is an end product of hemoglobin destruction. Figure 36-6 illustrates processes involved in bilirubin conjugation.

Pancreas

The pancreas is a lobulated organ behind the stomach that contains endocrine and exocrine cells. The organ is di-

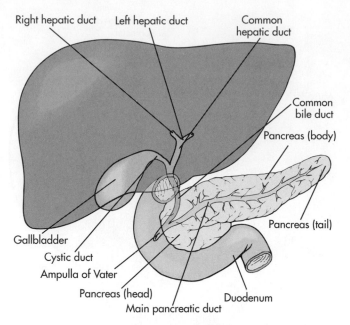

FIGURE 36-4   Gross structure of the liver, gallbladder, pancreas, and duct system. (From Lewis SM, Heitkemper MM, Dirksen SR: *Medical-surgical nursing: assessment and management of clinical problems,* ed 5, St. Louis, 2000, Mosby.)

Table 36-1 MAJOR FUNCTIONS OF THE LIVER	
FUNCTION	**DESCRIPTION**
METABOLIC FUNCTIONS	
Carbohydrate metabolism	Glycogenesis (conversion of glucose to glycogen), glycogenolysis (process of breaking down glycogen to glucose), gluconeogenesis (formation of glucose from amino acids and fatty acids)
Protein metabolism	Synthesis of nonessential amino acids, synthesis of plasma proteins (except γ-globulin), synthesis of clotting factors, urea formation from NH_3 (NH_3 formed from deamination of amino acids and by action of bacteria on proteins in colon)
Fat metabolism	Synthesis of lipoproteins, breakdown of triglycerides into fatty acids and glycerol, formation of ketone bodies, synthesis of fatty acids from amino acids and glucose, synthesis and breakdown of cholesterol
Detoxification	Inactivation of drugs and harmful substances and excretion of their breakdown products
Steroid metabolism	Conjugation and excretion of gonadal and adrenal steroids
BILE SYNTHESIS	
Bile production	Formation of bile, containing bile salts, bile pigments (mainly bilirubin), and cholesterol
Bile excretion	Bile excretion by liver about 1 L/day
STORAGE	
	Glucose in form of glycogen; vitamins, including fat-soluble (A, D, E, K) and water-soluble (B_1, B_2, cobalamin, and folic acid); fatty acids; minerals (iron and copper); amino acids in form of albumin and β-globulins
MONONUCLEAR PHAGOCYTE SYSTEM	
Kupffer cells	Breakdown of old RBCs, WBCs, bacteria, and other particles, breakdown of hemoglobin from old RBCs to bilirubin and biliverdin

From Lewis SM, Heitkemper MM, Dirksen SR: *Medical-surgical nursing: assessment and management of clinical problems,* ed 5, St. Louis, 2000, Mosby.)
RBC, Red blood cell; *WBC,* white blood cell.

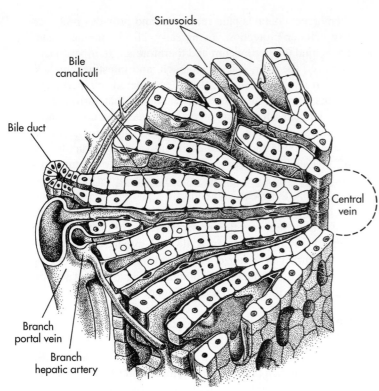

FIGURE 36-5   Microscopic structure of liver lobule. (Redrawn from Bloom W, Fawcett DW: *A textbook of histology,* ed 10, Philadelphia, 1975, WB Saunders. In Berne RM, Levy MN, editors: *Principles of physiology,* ed 3, St. Louis, 1993, Mosby.)

FIGURE 36-6   Bilirubin metabolism and conjugation. (From Lewis SM, Heitkemper MM, Dirksen SR: *Medical-surgical nursing: assessment and management of clinical problems,* ed 5, St. Louis, 2000, Mosby.)

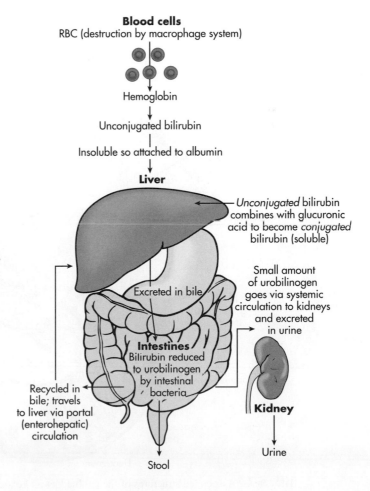

vided into the head, body, and a thin, narrow tail (Figure 36-7). Cells in the islets of Langerhans secrete insulin and regulate glucose levels. Exocrine cells called pancreatic acini secrete pancreatic juices for digestion of fats, carbohydrates, proteins, and nucleic acids. Pancreatic enzymes (i.e., lipase and amylase) enter the intestines through the pancreatic duct at the same juncture as the bile duct from the liver and gallbladder. Pancreatic and bile ducts join at a short dilated tube called the ampulla of Vater. A band of smooth muscles called the sphincter of Oddi surrounds this area and controls exit of pancreatic juices and bile.

Gallbladder

The gallbladder is a pear-shaped sac located in a depression on the inferior surface of the liver. The organ's main functions are collection, concentration, and storage of bile. Maximum volume is 30 to 60 ml; however, input from the liver can reach 450 ml over 12 hours. Concentration of bile in the gallbladder can be 5 to 20 times that of bile in the liver.[5] Bile is 80% water, 10% bile acids, 4% to 5% phospholipid, and 1% cholesterol.[17]

Peritoneum

The peritoneum is a serous membrane covering the liver, spleen, stomach, and intestines that acts as a semipermeable membrane, contains pain receptors, and provides proliferative cellular protection. Technically, all abdominal organs are behind the peritoneum and therefore are retroperitoneal; however, the liver, spleen, stomach, and intestines are suspended into the peritoneum and considered intraperitoneal organs. Omenta are folds of peritoneum that surround the stomach and adjacent organs. The greater omentum drapes the transverse colon and loops of small intestine. It is extremely mobile and spreads easily into areas of injury to seal off potential sources of infection. The lesser omentum covers parts of the stomach and proximal intestines but is not as movable as the greater omentum.

The peritoneum is permeable to fluid, electrolytes, urea, and toxins. Somatic afferent nerves sensitize the peritoneum to all types of stimuli. In acute abdominal conditions the peritoneum can localize an irritable focus by producing sharp pain and tenderness, voluntary or involuntary abdominal muscle rigidity, and rebound tenderness.

PATIENT ASSESSMENT

Assessment of a patient with a GI emergency should initially focus on airway, breathing, and circulation (ABCs) with primary survey completed before focused assessment. Determination of chief complaint, social or medical history, reason for seeking treatment, and treatment before arrival follows.

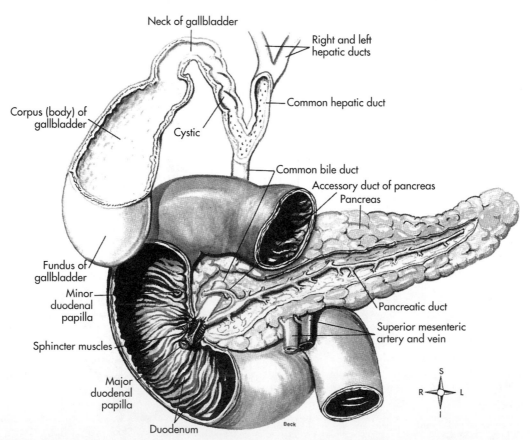

FIGURE 36-7 Associated structures of the gallbladder and exocrine pancreas. (From Huether SE, McCance KL: *Understanding pathophysiology,* St. Louis, 1996, Mosby.)

Table 36-2	PQRST ASSESSMENT OF ABDOMINAL PAIN	
COMPONENT	**DESCRIPTION**
Provocation	What makes pain better? Worse? Position? Vomiting?
Quality or character	What does pain feel like? Burning? Tight? Crushing? Tearing? Pressure? Cramping?
Radiation, location, referral	Where does pain radiate? Where is it most intense? Where does it start?
Severity	How severe is pain on a scale of 0 to 10?
Time	When did pain start? When did it end? How long did it last?

Information may be gleaned from the patient, family members, significant other, friends, emergency medical services personnel or old medical records.[6] Historical assessment should include questions related to gynecologic and genitourinary (GU) symptoms because many gynecologic or GU conditions cause abdominal pain, nausea, and vomiting. Information related to food intake and alcohol consumption should be obtained during assessment of patient history.

Evaluate the patient for abnormal skin color, abdominal wall abnormalities, pain, and alterations in bowel patterns. Abdominal pain is a common chief complaint in the ED that may be caused by an acute event or related to a chronic process. Abdominal pain may be visceral, somatic, or referred.

Visceral pain, caused by stretching of hollow viscus, is described as cramping or a sensation of gas. Pain intensifies, then decreases, and is usually centered on the umbilicus or below the midline. Diffuse pain makes localization of pain difficult. Diaphoresis, nausea, vomiting, hypotension, tachycardia, and abdominal wall spasms may be present. Conditions associated with visceral pain are appendicitis, acute pancreatitis, cholecystitis, and intestinal obstruction.

Somatic pain is produced by bacterial or chemical irritation of nerve fibers. Pain is sharp and usually localized to one area. A patient lies with legs flexed and knees pulled to the chest to prevent stimulation of the peritoneum and subsequent increase in pain. Associated findings include involuntary guarding and rebound tenderness.

Referred pain occurs at a distance from the original source of the pain and is thought to be caused by development of nerve tracts during fetal growth and development. Biliary pain can be referred to the subscapular area, whereas a peptic ulcer and pancreatic disease can cause back pain.

Assessment of abdominal pain must consider individual and cultural variations in expressions of pain. Each person reacts differently to pain—elderly patients may not exhibit the same level of pain as younger patients; men may hide pain because expression of pain is not considered masculine in many cultures. Conversely, dramatic expression of pain may be expected in some cultures. Emergency nurses must remember that pain is a symptom—not a diagnosis. Interventions should focus on identification and treatment of the source of pain.

A systematic approach is recommended for assessment of abdominal pain. The PQRST mnemonic can be used to

Table 36-3	POTENTIAL SOURCES OF ABDOMINAL PAIN BY LOCATION	
LOCATION	**POTENTIAL CAUSE**	
Right upper quadrant	Cholecystitis	Hepatomegaly
	Hepatic abscess	Pancreatic abscess
	Hepatitis	Duodenal ulcer perforation
		Right lung pneumonia
		Right renal pain
Left upper quadrant	Pancreatitis	Pericarditis
	Splenic rupture	Left lung pneumonia
	Myocardial infarction	
	Gastritis	
	Left renal pain	
Right lower quadrant	Appendicitis	Ovarian cyst
	Cholecystitis	Pelvic inflammatory disease
	Perforated ulcer	Endometriosis
	Intestinal obstruction	Right ureteral calculi
	Meckel's diverticulum	Incarcerated hernia
	Abdominal aortic aneurysm, dissection, or rupture	Gastric ulcer perforation
	Ruptured ectopic pregnancy	Colon perforation
	Twisted right ovary	Urinary tract infection
		Pelvic inflammatory disease
Left lower quadrant	Appendicitis	Endometriosis
	Intestinal obstruction	Left ureteral calculi
	Diverticulum of the sigmoid colon	Left renal pain
	Ruptured ectopic pregnancy	Urinary tract infection
	Twisted left ovary	Incarcerated hernia
	Ovarian cyst	Perforated descending colon
		Regional enteritis

Table 36-4	DESCRIPTION OF PAIN ASSOCIATED WITH CERTAIN CLINICAL CONDITIONS	
PAIN DESCRIPTION	**ASSOCIATED CLINICAL CONDITIONS**
Severe, sharp pain	Infarction or rupture
Severe pain controlled by medication	Pancreatitis, peritonitis, small bowel obstruction, renal colic, biliary colic
Dull pain	Inflammation, low-grade infection
Intermittent pain	Gastroenteritis, small-bowel obstruction

obtain appropriate historical information (Table 36-2). Identification of essential characteristics of pain, such as location, description, and provocation, provides valuable clues to etiology of pain. Potential causes based on location of pain are listed in Table 36-3; Table 36-4 reviews pain descriptions associated with certain clinical conditions.

Table 36-5	DRUG THERAPY FOR NAUSEA AND VOMITING	
CLASSIFICATION	**GENERIC NAME**	**TRADE NAME**
Antiemetic and antipsychotic	Chlorpromazine	Thorazine
	Haloperidol	Haldol
	Perphenazine	Trilafon
	Prochlorperazine	Compazine
	Promazine	Sparine
	Trifluoperazine	Stelazine
	Triflupromazine	Vesprin
Antihistamine	Buclizine	Bucladin-S
	Cyclizine	Marezine, meclizine
	Dimenhydrinate	Dramamine
	Diphenhydramine	Benadryl
	Promethazine	Phenergan
Prokinetics	Metoclopramide	Reglan
	Ondansetron	Zofran
	Granisetron	Kytril
	Cisapride	Propulsid
	Dolasetron	Anzemet
Antimuscarinic	Scopolamine transdermal	Transderm-Scop
Others	Benzquinamide	Emete-Con
	Diphenidol	Vontrol
	Thiethylperazine	Torecan
	Trimethobenzamide	Tigan

From Lewis SM, Heitkemper MM, Dirksen SR: *Medical-surgical nursing: assessment and management of clinical problems,* ed 5, St. Louis, 2000, Mosby.

Box 36-1	HISTORICAL INFORMATION RELEVANT TO DIARRHEA
CHARACTER OF STOOLS	**EXOGENOUS FACTORS—cont'd**
Amount	Institutionalization
Consistency	Sexual habits
Color	Daily activities
Odor	
Mucus	**ASSOCIATED SYMPTOMS**
Blood	Fever
Pus	Anorexia
	Nausea
TEMPORAL CHARACTERISTICS	Vomiting
Acute	Constipation
Chronic	Flatulence
Recurrent	Abdominal pain
Frequency	Tenesmus
Time of day	Weight loss
Nocturnal	Fluid intake and urine flow
Duration	
Urgency	**RELATED HISTORY**
Relationship to meals	Known gastrointestinal disease
	Acute cardiorespiratory
EXOGENOUS FACTORS	disease
Diet	Acute central nervous system
Medications	disease
Travel	Endocrine
Emotional stress	Hyperthyroidism
Exposure to others with same	Hypoparathyroidism
symptoms	Diabetes mellitus
Poisons or toxins	Adrenal insufficiency
Operations	Uremia
Irradiation	

From Rosen P et al: *Emergency medicine,* vol 2, ed 3, St. Louis, 1992, Mosby.

Another common finding with most GI emergencies is nausea and vomiting. Specific treatment varies with the underlying cause and with physician preference. Table 36-5 identifies various drugs that may be used for nausea and vomiting.

Abdominal assessment uses a sequence of inspection, auscultation, percussion, and palpation. Patient position should be noted because patients assume positions of comfort. Observe facial expression for signs of discomfort. Note skin color, temperature, and moisture. Inspect the abdominal wall for pulsations, movement, masses, symmetry, or surgical scars.

Auscultate bowel sounds in all four quadrants, determining frequency, quality, and pitch. Normal bowel sounds are irregular, high-pitched gurgling sounds occurring 5 to 35 times per minute. Decreased or absent bowel sounds suggest peritonitis or paralytic ileus, whereas hyperactive bowel sounds associated with nausea, vomiting, and diarrhea suggest gastroenteritis. Frequent, high-pitched bowel sounds occur with bowel obstruction. Vascular sounds such as venous hums or bruits are abnormal findings. Auscultation should always be done before palpation to prevent the creation of false bowel sounds by palpation.

Percussion is performed in all four quadrants. Dull sounds occur over solid organs or tumors, whereas tympanic sounds occur over air masses. Tympany is the normal sound heard when percussing the abdomen.

Palpation is the last step in abdominal assessment. Initially, palpate in an area away from areas of pain, noting ar-

eas of tenderness, guarding, or rigidity. Assess for abnormal masses and rebound tenderness.

Concurrent findings such as fever and chills are usually found with bacterial infection, appendicitis, or cholecystitis. Other signs associated with pain are nausea, vomiting, and anorexia. Intractable vomiting or feces in emesis suggest bowel obstruction. Blood in emesis occurs with gastritis or upper GI bleeding. Assess bowel patterns for abnormalities such as diarrhea or constipation, noting stool color and consistency. Diarrhea occurs with gastroenteritis; black, tarry stools suggest upper GI bleeding; and clay-colored stools are found with biliary tract obstruction. Fatty, foul-smelling, frothy stools occur with pancreatitis. Box 36-1 presents pertinent historical data related to assessment of diarrhea, Box 36-2 reviews causes of diarrhea, and Table 36-6 describes causes of infectious diarrhea.

SPECIFIC GASTROINTESTINAL EMERGENCIES

Infection, structural abnormalities, or pathologic processes may cause GI emergencies. Heredity and lifestyle also play a role. For example, excessive alcohol consumption can lead to GI bleeding, cirrhosis, or esophageal varices. Regardless

Box 36-2 CAUSES OF DIARRHEA

DECREASED FLUID ABSORPTION

Oral intake of poorly absorbable solutes (e.g., laxatives)
Maldigestion and malabsorption
  Mucosal damage: tropical sprue, Crohn's disease, radiation injury, ulcerative colitis, ischemic bowel disease
Pancreatic insufficiency
Intestinal enzyme deficiencies (e.g., lactase)
Bile salt deficiency
Decreased surface area (e.g., intestinal resection)

INCREASED FLUID SECRETION

Infectious: bacterial endotoxins (e.g., cholera; *Escherichia coli; Shigella, Salmonella,* or *Staphylococcus* species; *Clostridium difficile;* viral agents [rotavirus]; parasitic agents [*Giardia lamblia*])
Drugs: laxatives, antibiotics, suspensions or elixirs containing sorbitol (e.g., acetaminophen)
Hormonal: vasoactive intestinal polypeptide secretion from adenoma of the pancreas; gastrin secretion caused by Zollinger-Ellison syndrome; calcitonin secretion from carcinoma of the thyroid
Tumor: villous adenoma

MOTILITY DISTURBANCES

Irritable bowel syndrome
Diabetic enteropathy
Visceral scleroderma
Carcinoid syndrome
Vagotomy

From Lewis SM, Heitkemper MM, Dirksen SR: *Medical-surgical nursing: assessment and management of clinical problems,* ed 5, St. Louis, 2000, Mosby.

Table 36-6 CAUSES OF ACUTE INFECTIOUS DIARRHEA

	ONSET	DURATION	SYMPTOMS AND SIGNS
VIRAL			
Rotavirus, Norwalk	18-24 hours	24-48 hours	Explosive, watery diarrhea; nausea; vomiting; abdominal cramps
BACTERIAL			
Escherichia coli	4-24 hours	3-4 days	Four or five loose stools per day, nausea, malaise, low-grade fever
Enterohemorrhagic *E. Coli* (0157:H7)	4-24 hours	4-9 days	Bloody diarrhea, severe cramping, fever
Shigella species	24 hours	7 days	Watery stools containing blood and mucus, fever, tenesmus, urgency
Salmonellae species	6-48 hours	2-5 days	Watery diarrhea, fever, nausea, vomiting, abdominal cramps, fever
Campylobacter species	24 hours	<7 days	Profuse, watery diarrhea; malaise; nausea; abdominal cramps; low-grade fever
Clostridium perfringens	8-12 hours	24 hours	Watery diarrhea, abdominal cramps, vomiting
Clostridium difficile	4-9 days after start of antibiotics	24 hours	Associated with antibiotic treatment; symptoms range from mild, watery diarrhea to severe abdominal pain, fever, leukocytosis, leukocytes in stool
PARASITIC			
Giardia lamblia	1-3 weeks	Few days to 3 months	Sudden onset; malodorous, explosive, watery diarrhea; flatulence; epigastric pain and cramping; nausea
Cryptosporidium species	4 days	Weeks to months	Frequent soft stools with blood and mucus (in severe cases, watery stools), flatulence, distention, abdominal cramps, fever, leukocytes in stool
Entamoeba histolytica	2-10 days	1-6 months	Watery diarrhea, nausea, vomiting, abdominal cramps, weight loss in acquired immunodeficiency syndrome

From Lewis SM, Heitkemper MM, Dirksen SR: *Medical-surgical nursing: assessment and management of clinical problems,* ed 5, St. Louis, 2000, Mosby.

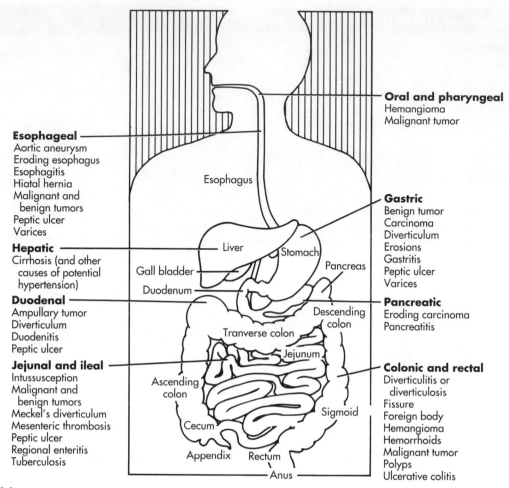

Esophageal
Aortic aneurysm
Eroding esophagus
Esophagitis
Hiatal hernia
Malignant and
benign tumors
Peptic ulcer
Varices

Hepatic
Cirrhosis (and other
causes of potential
hypertension)

Duodenal
Ampullary tumor
Diverticulum
Duodenitis
Peptic ulcer

Jejunal and ileal
Intussusception
Malignant and
benign tumors
Meckel's diverticulum
Mesenteric thrombosis
Peptic ulcer
Regional enteritis
Tuberculosis

Oral and pharyngeal
Hemangioma
Malignant tumor

Gastric
Benign tumor
Carcinoma
Diverticulum
Erosions
Gastritis
Peptic ulcer
Varices

Pancreatic
Eroding carcinoma
Pancreatitis

Colonic and rectal
Diverticulitis or
diverticulosis
Fissure
Foreign body
Hemangioma
Hemorrhoids
Malignant tumor
Polyps
Ulcerative colitis

Esophagus
Liver
Stomach
Pancreas
Gall bladder
Duodenum
Descending colon
Tranverse colon
Jejunum
Ascending colon
Sigmoid
Cecum
Appendix
Rectum
Anus

FIGURE 36-8 Sites and causes of gastrointestinal bleeding. (From SGNA: *Gastroenterology nursing: a core curriculum,* St. Louis, 1993, Mosby.)

of etiology, nontraumatic GI emergencies are a common occurrence in any ED—ranging from minor inconvenience to life-threatening problems.

Gastrointestinal Bleeding

Bleeding can originate anywhere in the GI tract and can occur at any age. The age group most often affected is individuals 50 to 80 years of age. Bleeding is functionally categorized by location—upper or lower GI bleeding. Figure 36-8 highlights various sites and causes of GI bleeding. Upper GI bleeding is more common in males, whereas lower GI bleeding is seen more often in females. Patients may have bright red blood from mouth or rectum or black, tarry stools. Bleeding stops spontaneously in 80% of hospitalized patients.[7]

Upper GI Bleeding

Upper GI bleeding refers to blood loss between the upper esophagus and duodenum at the ligament of Treitz. Bleeding is categorized as variceal or nonvariceal. The risk for death is greater with variceal bleeding because of the occurrence of hemorrhage in these patients.[13] Gastroesophageal varices are enlarged, venous channels that are dilated by portal hyper-

tension. As portal hypertension increases, varices continue to enlarge and eventually rupture, causing massive hemorrhage. The number one cause of portal hypertension in the United States is alcoholic cirrhosis, with schistosomiasis the leading cause worldwide. Figure 36-9 highlights systemic manifestations of cirrhosis. Bleeding from varices requires immediate intervention and close observation following initial control of bleeding. More than 40% of patients with variceal bleeds rebleed within 48 to 72 hours.[13]

Nonvariceal bleeding is disruption of esophageal or gastroduodenal mucosa with ulceration or erosion into an underlying vein or artery. Ulcerations or erosions occur when hyperacidity, pepsin, or aspirin inhibit mucosal prostaglandins and overwhelm protective factors of the esophagus (i.e., esophageal motility, salivary secretions, and the lower esophageal sphincter) and gastric mucosa (i.e., mucus, rapid epithelial renewal, and tissue mediators). Peptic ulcer disease, an infectious process caused by *Helicobacter pylori,* is the most common cause of upper GI bleeding in adults and children.[14] Other causes include drug-induced erosions and retching and vomiting with bulimia.

Clinical signs and symptoms are variable. Presenting symptoms may include pallor, dizziness, weakness, and

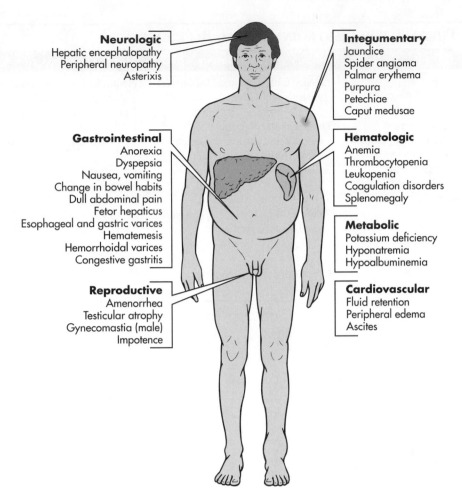

Neurologic
Hepatic encephalopathy
Peripheral neuropathy
Asterixis

Integumentary
Jaundice
Spider angioma
Palmar erythema
Purpura
Petechiae
Caput medusae

Gastrointestinal
Anorexia
Dyspepsia
Nausea, vomiting
Change in bowel habits
Dull abdominal pain
Fetor hepaticus
Esophageal and gastric varices
Hematemesis
Hemorrhoidal varices
Congestive gastritis

Hematologic
Anemia
Thrombocytopenia
Leukopenia
Coagulation disorders
Splenomegaly

Metabolic
Potassium deficiency
Hyponatremia
Hypoalbuminemia

Reproductive
Amenorrhea
Testicular atrophy
Gynecomastia (male)
Impotence

Cardiovascular
Fluid retention
Peripheral edema
Ascites

FIGURE 36-9   Systemic clinical manifestations of liver cirrhosis. (From Lewis SM, Heitkemper MM, Dirksen SR: *Medical-surgical nursing: assessment and management of clinical problems,* ed 5, St. Louis, 2000, Mosby.)

lethargy. Abdominal pain, nausea, vomiting, hematochezia, or melena can be present. Signs of hypovolemia such as tachycardia, orthostatic hypotension, and syncope may also occur. Mental confusion, jaundice, or ascites occur most often with variceal bleeding.

Management begins with maintenance of the ABCs. Administer high flow oxygen via nonrebreather mask for patients with hemodynamic compromise or decreased oxygen saturation. Fluid replacement begins with normal saline or lactated Ringer's solution followed by blood (packed red blood cells [PRBCs] or whole blood) replacement if the patient's condition does not improve. Using a cardiac monitor and continuous pulse oximetry is recommended for patients with significant blood loss or bright red bleeding. Elderly patients can experience myocardial infarction secondary to ischemia caused by hypovolemia. Monitor vital signs and level of consciousness for signs of hemodynamic compromise. A nasogastric tube is inserted for gastric lavage with saline solution to remove blood clots. Lavage also serves to clear the GI tract, which facilitates endoscopy. A urinary catheter is inserted to monitor output and fluid status.

Baseline laboratory studies include complete blood count (CBC), type and cross-match (for a minimum of 2 U), electrolytes, blood urea nitrogen (BUN), creatinine,

and serum glucose. Normal creatinine with increased BUN suggests bleeding with breakdown of blood in the gut, dehydration, or diuretic therapy. Liver function and coagulation studies are also recommended to rule out coagulopathies or liver disease. An upright chest radiograph can provide valuable information if perforation is suspected; however, this is not feasible if significant hemodynamic compromise is present. An electrocardiogram should be obtained to assess for dysrhythmias or ischemic changes related to blood loss.

Additional treatment modalities include medications, endoscopic control of bleeding, and surgical interventions. Medical therapy for nonvariceal bleeding includes administration of antacids and H_2 antagonists (Table 36-7). Gastroesophageal variceal bleeding is treated with intravenous (IV) vasopressin (20 U in 200 ml saline at 0.25 to 0.5 U/min) or Sengstaken-Blakemore, Minnesota, or Linton balloon tube to tamponade bleeding. Peptic ulcer disease is treated endoscopically with thermal coagulation or injection therapy, whereas gastroesophageal varices are treated endoscopically with injection sclerotherapy or variceal band ligation. Endoscopic procedures may be done on a limited basis in EDs across the country. Surgical intervention may be necessary for variceal or nonvariceal bleeding.[10] Complications related

Table 36-7   **DRUG THERAPY FOR GASTROINTESTINAL BLEEDING**

DRUG	SOURCE OF GI BLEEDING	MECHANISM OF ACTION
Antacids	Duodenal ulcer, gastric ulcer, acute gastritis (corrosive, erosive, and hemorrhagic)	Neutralizes acid and maintains gastric pH above 5.5, elevated pH inhibits activation of pepsinogen
Histamine H_2-receptor antagonists: Cimetidine (Tagamet), ranitidine (Zantac), famotidine (Pepcid), nizatidine (Axid)	Duodenal ulcer, gastric ulcer, esophagitis, acute gastritis (especially hemorrhagic), esophageal varices	Inhibits action of histamine at H_2 receptors of parietal cells and decreases acid secretion
Proton pump inhibitors: Omeprazole (Prilosec), lansoprazole (Prevacid), pantoprazole (Pantoloc)	Same as above	Inhibits the cellular pump that is necessary for secretion of HCl acid
Vasopressin	Acute gastritis (corrosive, erosive, and hemorrhagic)	Causes vasoconstriction and increases smooth muscle activity of the GI tract, reduces pressure in the portal circulation, and arrests bleeding
Somatostatin analogue octreotide (Sandostatin)	Upper GI bleeding, esophageal varices	Decreases splanchnic blood flow, decreases acid secretion via decrease in release of gastrin

From Lewis SM, Heitkemper MM, Dirksen SR: *Medical-surgical nursing: assessment and management of clinical problems,* ed 5, St. Louis, 2000, Mosby.
GI, Gastrointestinal; *HCl,* hydrochloric acid.

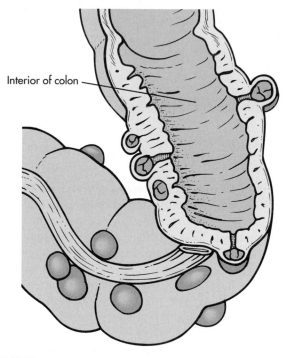

Interior of colon

FIGURE 36-10   Diverticula are outpouchings of the colon. When they become inflamed, the condition is diverticulitis. The inflammatory process can spread to the surrounding area in the intestine. (From Lewis SM, Heitkemper MM, Dirksen SR: *Medical-surgical nursing: assessment and management of clinical problems,* ed 5, St. Louis, 2000, Mosby.)

to upper GI bleeding include aspiration, pneumonia, respiratory failure, and hypovolemic shock.

Lower GI Bleeding

Lower GI bleeding is bleeding that occurs below the ligament of Treitz. Common causes are hemorrhoids, diverticulitis, angiodysplasia, colonic polyps, colon cancer, or colitis. Diverticulosis and angiodysplasia are common causes of lower GI bleeding in the elderly, whereas hemorrhoids, anal fissures, and inflammatory bowel disease occur most often in younger patients. Diverticulosis refers to pouch-like herniations on the colon (Figure 36-10). Figure 36-11 depicts internal and external hemorrhoidal veins, where hemorrhoids often erupt. Internal hemorrhoids are rarely associated with pain, whereas external hemorrhoids can cause significant discomfort. [13] Eighty-five percent of patients with lower GI bleeding experience acute bleeds that are self-limiting and do not cause significant changes in hemodynamic status. Most patients with mild lower GI bleeding who are hemodynamically stable may be evaluated on an outpatient basis. Treatment includes identifying the source of bleeding with anoscopy, flexible sigmoidoscopy, or air-contrast barium enema. Patients with severe symptomatic lower GI bleeding require hospital admission for resuscitation, diagnosis, and treatment. Colonoscopy may be performed to determine the source of bleeding after the patient is stabilized. [16]

The cardinal sign of lower GI bleeding is hematochezia. Patients may have maroon stools or occult blood in the stool. Cramplike abdominal pain may be present. Explosive diarrhea with foul odor is frequently present. Painless bleeding also occurs. Pallor, diaphoresis, and decreased capillary refill are present with significant bleeding. Orthostatic changes in pulse or blood pressure occur in many patients. Pedal edema can occur with chronic bleeding because of protein depletion.

Baseline laboratory studies include CBC, platelet count, and coagulation studies. The first priority is management of the ABCs followed by IV fluid resuscitation with normal saline or lactated Ringer's solution via large-bore catheter. Administration of PRBCs may be necessary in cases of significant blood loss. Determining the source of bleeding is a

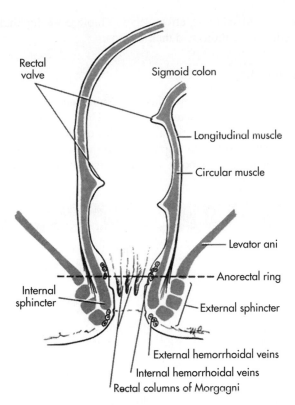

Rectal valve

Sigmoid colon

Longitudinal muscle

Circular muscle

Levator ani

Anorectal ring

Internal sphincter

External sphincter

External hemorrhoidal veins

Internal hemorrhoidal veins

Rectal columns of Morgagni

FIGURE 36-11   Anatomy of rectum and anus showing internal and external hemorrhoidal veins. (From Price SA, Wilson LM: *Pathophysiology: clinical concepts of disease processes,* ed 5, St. Louis, 1997, Mosby.)

Gastroesophageal Reflux Disease

Transient gastroesophageal reflux is a normal physiologic event that occurs at various intervals without causing disease or symptoms. Scott describes patients with hourly gastroesophageal reflux, whereas Rosen suggests that it occurs daily in 7% of patients and at least monthly in 15%. Regardless, patients who experience increased frequency of reflux experience some type of symptoms. GERD occurs in 25% to 35% of the U.S. population over their lifetime.[2] Conditions associated with GERD are decreased lower esophageal sphincter (LES) pressure, decreased esophageal motility, and increased gastric emptying time. Box 36-3 lists specific causes for each situation. It is of interest that acid secretion does not increase in patients with GERD.

Chest pain or heartburn is the most common symptom associated with this condition. Patients may experience only occasional discomfort; however, 10% report heartburn on a daily basis.[13] Relaxation of the LES during pregnancy increases the occurrence of heartburn during pregnancy. At least 25% of pregnant women experience daily heartburn. Chest pain as the only symptom of GERD is reported in 10% of patients with the disease.[14] A key aspect of pain associated with GERD is that it radiates, usually to the neck,

---

Box 36-3   FACTORS AND MEDICATIONS ASSOCIATED WITH GERD

DECREASED LES PRESSURE

Foods

Fatty foods
Chocolate
Peppermint, spearmint
Tea, coffee
Onions, garlic
Alcohol

Medications/Chemicals

Nitrates
Calcium channel blockers
Nicotine
Caffeine
Anticholinergics
Theophylline
Diazepam (Valium)
Morphine sulfate
β-adrenergic blocking drugs
Progesterone, estrogen, pregnancy

DECREASED ESOPHAGEAL MOTILITY

Presbyesophagus
Diabetes mellitus
Scleroderma
Achalasia

INCREASED GASTRIC EMPTYING TIME

Diabetic gastroparesis
Anticholinergics
Fatty foods
Gastric outlet obstruction

Modified from Lewis SM, Heitkemper MM, Dirksen SR: *Medical surgical nursing: assessment and management of clinical problems,* ed 5, St. Louis, 2000, Mosby; Rosen P, Barkin RM, Hockberger RS et al: *Emergency medicine: concepts and clinical practice,* ed 4, St. Louis, 1998, Mosby.

jaws, shoulders, arms, and abdomen. Similarities to the clinical presentation of ischemic heart disease require thoughtful consideration. It is often difficult to distinguish between these very different conditions in the ED. The emergency nurse should pay close attention to patient history and to the patient for changes in condition. Characteristics unique to GERD include worsening of symptoms with stooping, lying, or leaning forward.[14] Other symptoms associated with GERD are summarized in Box 36-4.

Management of GERD begins with elimination of other conditions that are more lethal (i.e., ischemic heart disease and esophageal perforation). Studies such as electrocardiogram, chest radiograph, and CBC are primarily used to rule out other conditions. Additional imaging studies include endoscopy and barium studies. Specific treatment in the ED includes symptomatic relief through use of antacids, H_2 blockers, and other medications. Antacids are given with viscous

---

priority. Colonoscopy, bleeding scans, or angiography may be performed with surgical intervention required in some cases.

Table 36-8	DRUG THERAPY FOR GERD
MECHANISM OF ACTION	**EXAMPLES**
INCREASE LES PRESSURE	
Cholinergic	Bethanechol (Urecholine)
Dopamine antagonist	Metoclopramide (Reglan)
Serotonin antagonist	Cisapride (Propulsid)
ACID NEUTRALIZING	
Antacids	Gelusil, Maalox, Mylanta
ANTISECRETORY	
Histamine H₂-receptor antagonists	Ranitidine (Zantac)
	Cimetidine (Tagamet)
	Famotidine (Pepcid)
	Nizatidine (Axid)
Proton pump inhibitors	Omeprazole (Prilosec)
	Lansoprazole (Prevacid)
	Pantoprazole (Pantoloc)
CYTOPROTECTIVE	
Alginic acid-antacid	Gaviscon
Antacids	Gelusil, Maalox, Mylanta
Acid-protective	Sucralfate (Carafate)

From Lewis SM, Heitkemper MM, Dirksen SR: *Medical-surgical nursing: assessment and management of clinical problems,* ed 5, St. Louis, 2000, Mosby.
LES, Lower esophageal sphincter.

lidocaine to increase effectiveness. Table 36-8 highlights specific medications and their actions.

Appendicitis

Obstruction of the appendiceal opening decreases blood supply and leads to bacterial invasion. Untreated, inflammation progresses so that the appendix becomes nonviable and gangrenous, eventually rupturing into the peritoneal space. Appendicitis affects both sexes and all ages, is most com-

Box 36-4	CLINICAL SYMPTOMS OF GERD	
TYPICAL		**ATYPICAL**
Chest pain		Noncardiac chest pain
Heartburn		Asthma
Dysphagia		Persistent cough
Odynophagia		Hiccups
Regurgitation		Hoarseness
Water brash		Frequent throat clearing
Belching		Nocturnal choking
Early satiety		Sleep apnea
Nausea		Recurrent pneumonia
Anorexia		Recurrent ENT infections
Weight loss		Loss of dental enamel
		Halitosis

GERD, Gastroesophageal reflex disease; *ENT,* ear-nose-throat.

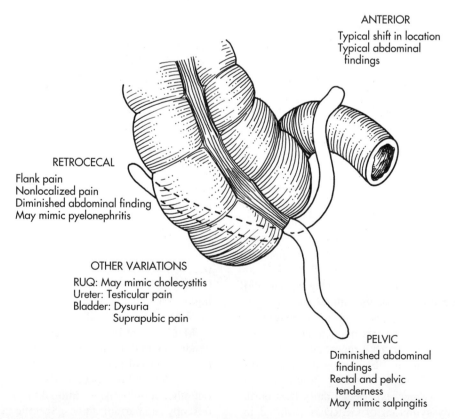

ANTERIOR
Typical shift in location
Typical abdominal findings

RETROCECAL
Flank pain
Nonlocalized pain
Diminished abdominal finding
May mimic pyelonephritis

OTHER VARIATIONS
RUQ: May mimic cholecystitis
Ureter: Testicular pain
Bladder: Dysuria
    Suprapubic pain

PELVIC
Diminished abdominal findings
Rectal and pelvic tenderness
May mimic salpingitis

FIGURE 36-12   Variable position of appendix. (From Rosen P et al: *Emergency medicine,* vol 2, ed 3, St. Louis, 1992, Mosby.)

mon in males 10 to 30 years of age, and rarely occurs in infants less than 2 years of age. Appendicitis is the most common problem requiring surgery in children. Approximately 6% of the population develops appendicitis in their lifetime. One in 2200 pregnant women develops appendicitis, making it the most common surgical procedure during pregnancy.[14,17] Surgical removal of the appendix was first documented in 1735.[14]

Patients may have abdominal pain or abdominal cramping, nausea, vomiting, tachycardia, malaise, and anorexia. Chills and fever also occur. Abdominal pain may be initially diffuse and periumbilical and may later become intense and localized to the lower right quadrant. Classic pain associated with appendicitis is located just inside the iliac crest at McBurney's point. Elderly patients are often afebrile and do not exhibit this classic pain. Pressure on the lower left abdomen intensifies pain in the right lower quadrant (Rovsing's sign).[1] Pain may not always occur in this classic location because of normal variations in the location of the appendix (Figure 36-12). The position of comfort for most patients is supine with hips and knees flexed. Women may exhibit tenderness when the cervix is moved.[14]

If the appendix ruptures, peritoneal signs increase and involuntary guarding develops. Increased fever and rebound tenderness occur when the appendix abscesses or ruptures. Diagnosis is made by assessment of clinical signs and symptoms in concert with physical examination. Diagnostic data include elevation of white blood cell (WBC) count greater than 10,000 cells/mm³ with increased neutrophils, specifically bands. WBC count is rarely greater than 20,000 cells/mm³. Ultrasound may occasionally demonstrate an enlarged appendix or collection of periappendicial fluid, with 75% to 90% sensitivity and 86% to 100% specificity.[17] Urinalysis should be performed to rule out GU problems. Computed tomography (CT) has been used effectively in certain patients, but its broad use as a diagnostic tool for appendicitis has not been established.

Definitive therapy for appendicitis is surgical intervention with laparoscopic surgery as the preferred method. Obtain IV access, administer prophylactic broad-spectrum antibiotic, and instruct the patient not to eat or drink. Narcotic pain medication is usually withheld until diagnosis is made. Complications such as perforation, peritonitis, and abscess formation can occur when treatment is delayed.

Cholecystitis

Inflammation of the gallbladder causes distention as the cystic duct becomes obstructed. Bacterial invasion, usually by *Escherichia coli,* streptococcus, or salmonella, also causes cholecystitis. Gallstones may exacerbate cholecystitis; however, 2% to 12% of patients do not have gallstones.[14] Conversely, cholecystitis occurs in 16 to 20 million Americans, with 1 million new cases each year.[17] Cholecystitis usually affects obese, fair-skinned women of increasing age and parity.

Symptoms include sudden onset abdominal pain—usually after ingestion of fried or fatty foods. Pain may radiate from the epigastrium to the right upper quadrant or may be referred to the right supraclavicular area. Patients usually describe pain as colicky. Local and rebound tenderness may also be present. Marked tenderness and inspiratory limitation on deep palpation under the right subcostal margin (Murphy's sign) may also be present.[9] Low-grade fever (38° C or 100.4° F), tachycardia, nausea, vomiting, and flatulence are common findings. If the common bile duct is obstructed, the patient may appear slightly jaundiced. Table 36-9 highlights clinical signs associated with obstructed bile flow.

Diagnostic tests include urinalysis, CBC, serum electrolytes, BUN, creatinine, serum glucose, and serum bilirubin levels; however, results are often normal.[17] An elevated amylase suggests pancreatitis rather than cholecystitis. Ultrasound is extremely useful in the emergency setting for detection of a thickened gallbladder wall, gallstones, and pericholecystic fluid.[4]

Treatment of cholecystitis includes administration of IV crystalloid solution and medications for nausea and vomiting. A nasogastric tube may be necessary for gastric decompression. Monitor vital signs and intake and output. Broad-spectrum antibiotics are indicated for potential microbial infection. Narcotic analgesics are recommended for pain control. Meperidine (Demerol) may be more beneficial than other narcotics because of its effect on the sphincter of Oddi. Definitive treatment for cholecystitis is surgery with traditional laparotomy or laparoscopic cholecystectomy.[4]

Table 36-9 CLINICAL MANIFESTATIONS CAUSED BY OBSTRUCTED BILE FLOW	
CLINICAL MANIFESTATION	**ETIOLOGY**
Obstructive jaundice	No bile flow into duodenum
Dark amber urine, which foams when shaken	Soluble bilirubin in urine
No urobilinogen in urine	No bilirubin reaching small intestine to be converted to urobilinogen
Clay-colored stools	Same as above
Pruritus	Deposition of bile salts in skin tissues
Intolerance for fatty foods (nausea, sensation of fullness, anorexia)	No bile in small intestine for fat digestion
Bleeding tendencies	Lack of or decreased absorption of vitamin K, resulting in decreased production of prothrombin
Steatorrhea	No bile salts in duodenum, preventing fat emulsion and digestion

From Lewis SM, Heitkemper MM, Dirksen SR: *Medical-surgical nursing: assessment and management of clinical problems,* ed 5, St. Louis, 2000, Mosby.

Acute Pancreatitis

Acute pancreatitis results from inflammation of the pancreas; however, the exact mechanism is not clear. Theories include bile or duodenal reflux, bacterial infection, pancreatic enzyme activation with autolysis, and ductal hypertension. Etiology can be traced to biliary disease or alcohol consumption. Seventy percent to 80% of pancreatitis cases are due to biliary disease,[3,4] probable obstruction of the common bile duct resulting in ductal hypertension, and pancreatic enzyme activation. Alcohol abuse causes toxic metabolites that injure the pancreas, leading to inflammation. Other causes include chronic hypercalcemia, surgery, abdominal trauma, infections (mumps, cytomegalovirus infection), drugs, toxins (organophosphate insecticides, scorpion venom), or endoscopic retrograde cholangiopancreatography.[3] Box 36-5 highlights various causes of pancreatitis. More than 85 drugs have been identified as causative agents for pancreatitis (Box 36-6). Regardless of mechanism, pancreatitis is characterized by acinar cell damage that leads to necrosis, edema, and inflammation. Acute pancreatitis affects 1.5 people per 100,000 population, but varies with the population.[4] Pancreatitis is the second most frequent pancreatic emergency seen in the ED, a frequency exceeded only by diabetes mellitus.[14]

A clinical hallmark in 95% of patients with pancreatitis is abdominal pain originating in the epigastric region and radiating to the back. Abdominal tenderness, rebound, and guarding are usually present. Nausea, vomiting, and abdominal distention may be present. Patients may be febrile with tachycardia, tachypnea, and hypotension. Decreased gastric motility causes hypoactive or absent bowel sounds.

Certain laboratory values can aide in diagnosis of acute pancreatitis (Table 36-10). Elevated serum amylase and li-

---

Box 36-5 ETIOLOGY OF ACUTE PANCREATITIS

Alcohol (ethanol, methanol)	*Mycoplasma* sp.
Biliary tract disease	*Legionella* sp.
Drugs	Ascariasis
(see Box 36-6)	Pancreas divisum
Hypercalcemia	Penetrating peptic ulcer
Hyperlipidemia	Postoperative
Idiopathic	Postpancreatography
Infectious agents	Pregnancy
Mumps	Scorpion bites
Coxsackie virus	Trauma
Hepatitis B virus	Tumor

From Rosen P, Barkin R, Hockberger RS et al: *Emergency medicine: concepts and clinical practice,* ed 4, St. Louis, 1998, Mosby.

Box 36-6 DRUG-INDUCED PANCREATITIS

DEFINITE

Azathioprine	Tetracycline
Cisplatin	Thiazides
Furosemide	Sulphonamides
1-Asparaginase	

PROBABLE

Acetaminophen	Mefenamic acid
Cimetidine	Opiates
Estrogens	Phenformin
Indomethacin	Valproic acid

POSSIBLE

Bumetanide	Ethacrynic acid
Carbamazepine	Isoniazid
Chlorthalidone	Isoretinoin
Clonidine	Methyldopa
Colchicine	Metronidazole
Corticosteroids	Nitrofurantoin
Clotrimaxozole	Pentamidine
Cyclosporin	Piroxicam
Cytarabine	Procainamide
Diaxozide	Rifampin
Enalapril	Salicylates
Ergotamine	Sulindac

From Rosen P, Barkin R, Hockberger RS et al: *Emergency medicine: concepts and clinical practice,* ed 4, St. Louis, 1998, Mosby.

Table 36-10 DIAGNOSTIC STUDIES FOR ACUTE PANCREATITIS

LABORATORY TEST	ABNORMAL FINDING	ETIOLOGY
PRIMARY TESTS		
Serum amylase	Increased (>200 U/L [3.34 μkat/L])	Pancreatic cell injury
Serum lipase	Elevated	Pancreatic cell injury
Urinary amylase	Elevated	Pancreatic cell injury
SECONDARY TESTS		
Blood glucose	Hyperglycemia	Impairment of carbohydrate metabolism resulting from β-cell damage and release of glucagon
Serum calcium	Hypocalcemia	Saponification of calcium by fatty acids in areas of fat necrosis
Serum triglycerides	Hyperlipidemia	Release of free fatty acids by lipase

From Lewis SM, Heitkemper MM, Dirksen SR: *Medical-surgical nursing: assessment and management of clinical problems,* ed 5, St. Louis, 2000, Mosby.

pase levels are pathognomonic for pancreatitis. Amylase levels "tend to be higher" in the patient with pancreatitis secondary to biliary disease rather than alcohol.[13] Leukocytosis, decreased hematocrit, hyperglycemia, and glucosuria may also be present. Continuing decreases in hematocrit suggest hemorrhagic pancreatitis.[17] Serum calcium is decreased, whereas serum glutamic oxaloacetic transaminase is elevated. Persistent hypocalcemia is associated with poor prognosis.[17]

Radiographic studies are useful in diagnosing acute pancreatitis. A chest radiograph may reveal pleural effusions or pulmonary infiltrates, and ileus may be detected on abdominal radiographs. Abdominal ultrasound can identify gallstones as an underlying cause. Abdominal CT scan may also contribute to the diagnosis of acute pancreatitis by identification of pancreatic edema or fluid around the pancreas.[17]

Management includes maintaining strict NPO status. Obtain IV access for fluid and electrolyte replacement with balanced salt solution to ensure renal perfusion. Antiemetics are administered for nausea, vomiting, and to minimize further fluid loss. Pain control is a high priority for the patient with pancreatitis. Meperidine is less likely than morphine to increase pressure in the sphincter of Oddi, a suspected source of pain.[3] Table 36-11 highlights drugs used for management of acute pancreatitis. Nasogastric suction helps alleviate nausea, vomiting, and abdominal distention. Ongoing monitoring of respiratory, cardiovascular, and renal functions is recommended. Prophylactic administration of antibiotics should be considered.

Severe life-threatening complications with acute pancreatitis are pleural effusion and adult respiratory distress syndrome. Rosen reports pulmonary complications in 18% to 30% of pancreatic patients.[14] Significant hypovolemia can lead to hypovolemic shock and ischemia of lungs, heart, and kidneys. Electrolyte imbalances such as hyperglycemia and hypocalcemia also occur. Septic complications include formation of pancreatic abscess.

Diverticulitis

Diverticula are small pouches that develop in the large intestines secondary to aging (see Figure 36-10). This condition, called diverticulosis, occurs in about half of all Americans age 60 to 80 years and is found in almost all Americans older than age 80 years. Weakened areas that predispose the colon to herniation of inferior tissue layers in combination with a low-fiber diet lead to this primarily painless disorder. Less than 10% of patients with diverticulosis experience pain. However, pain is the most-reported complaint when diverticula become inflamed and diverticulitis develops. Inflammation develops when fecal material is trapped in the pouches, causing trauma to the intestinal lining, which ultimately leads to inflammation. Persistent pain associated with diverticulitis is localized in the left lower quadrant. Inflamed loops of bowels called phlegmon may be palpated as a left lower quadrant mass.[15] Fever, chills, nausea, and vomiting are seen when infection is present. Other symptoms include cramping and constipation. The elderly, those on corticosteroids, and patients who are immunosuppressed usually have an unremarkable clinical examination.[15] Complications of diverticulitis include intestinal obstruction, hemorrhage, perforation, abscess, stricture, and fistula.[12]

Table 36-11 DRUGS USED IN TREATMENT OF ACUTE PANCREATITIS	
DRUG	**MECHANISMS OF ACTION**
Meperidine (Demerol)	Relief of pain
Nitroglycerin or papaverine	Relaxation of smooth muscles and relief of pain
Antispasmodics (e.g., dicyclomine [Bentyl], propantheline bromide [Pro-Banthine])	Decrease of vagal stimulation, motility, pancreatic outflow (inhibition of volume and concentration of bicarbonate and enzymatic secretion); contraindicated in paralytic ileus
Carbonic anhydrase inhibitor (acetazolamide [Diamox])	Reduction in volume and bicarbonate concentration of pancreatic secretion
Antacids	Neutralization of gastric secretions; decrease in hydrochloric acid stimulation of secretin, which stimulates production and secretion of pancreatic secretions
Histamine H_2-receptor antagonists (cimetidine [Tagamet], ranitidine [Zantac])	Decrease in hydrochloric acid by inhibiting histamine (hydrochloric acid stimulates pancreatic activity)
Calcium gluconate	Treatment of hypocalcemia to prevent or treat tetany
Corticosteroids	Use only for seriously ill patients with hypotension or shock
Aprotinin (Trasylol)	Antitryptic and antikallikreinic actions
Glucagon	Reduction in pancreatic inflammation and decrease in serum amylase, suppression of pancreatic secretions
Somatostatin	Inhibition of pancreatic secretions

Modified from Lewis SM, Heitkemper MM, Dirksen SR: *Medical-surgical nursing: assessment and management of clinical problems,* ed 5, St. Louis, 2000, Mosby.

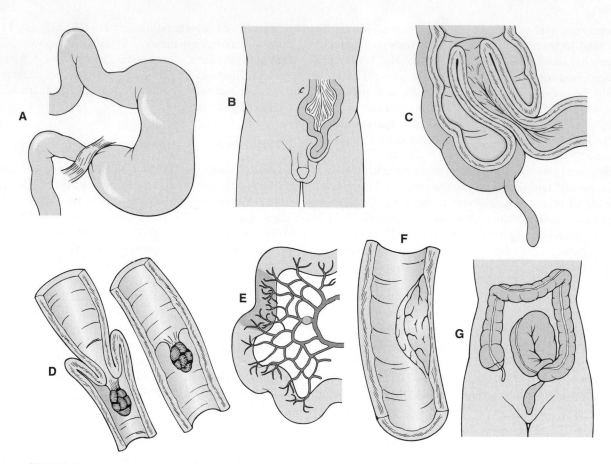

FIGURE 36-13   Bowel obstructions. **A,** Adhesions. **B,** Strangulated inguinal hernia. **C,** Ileocecal intussusception. **D,** Intussusception from polyps. **E,** Mesenteric occlusion. **F,** Neoplasm. **G,** Volvulus of the sigmoid colon. (From Lewis SM, Heitkemper MM, Dirksen SR: *Medical-surgical nursing: assessment and management of clinical problems,* ed 5, St. Louis, 2000, Mosby.)

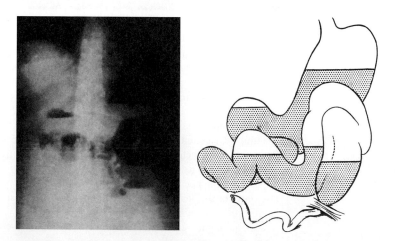

FIGURE 36-14   Mechanical bowel obstruction. Localized air-fluid levels seen on upright film of abdomen. Diagram shows dilated proximal bowel and stomach air-fluid levels and adhesive band causing obstruction.(From Liechty RD, Soper RT: *Fundamentals of surgery,* ed 6, St. Louis, 1989, Mosby.)

Diagnostic evaluation includes CBC and urinalysis. Results of the CBC show a left shift resulting from infection. The presence of WBCs and RBCs in urine is also a common finding. Supine and upright abdominal radiographs are obtained to rule out perforation or obstruction. Abdominal CT is the preferred diagnostic modality because it is more effective in identification of processes outside the colon's lumen (i.e., diverticulitis). Barium cnema, endoscopy, and ultrasonography may also be used.

Treatment of patients with diverticulitis includes rehydration with a saline solution, resting the bowel by making the patient NPO, and inserting a gastric tube if persistent vomiting is present. Anticholinergics are used to reduce colonic spasms, with opiates reserved for more aggressive pain management. Oral or parenteral antibiotics may be given depending on clinical presentation. Emergent surgery is required when there is evidence of peritonitis. [15]

Bowel Obstruction

Bowel obstruction occurs in either sex, at any age, and from a variety of causes.[3] The most common cause is adhesions from previous abdominal surgery, followed by incarcerated inguinal hernia.[17] Other causes include foreign bodies, volvulus, intussusception, strictures, tumors, congenital adhesive bands, fecal impaction, gallstones, and hematomas (Figure 36-13).

Bowel obstructions are classified as mechanical or nonmechanical. Mechanical obstruction results from a disorder outside the intestines or blockage inside the lumen of the intestines (Figure 36-14). Intussusception, telescoping of the bowel within itself by peristalsis, is an example of a mechanical obstruction (Figure 36-15). Figure 36-16 is a radiographic illustration of a small bowel obstruction. Nonmechanical obstruction results when muscle activity of the intestine decreases and movement of contents slows (i.e., paralytic ileus) (Figure 36-17).

When obstruction occurs, bowel contents accumulate above the obstruction. This leads to rapid increase in anaerobic and aerobic bacteria, which causes an increase in methane and hydrogen production.[15] Rosen indicates that "the more proximal the obstruction, the greater the discomfort" and the shorter the time between symptom onset and presentation.[14] Peristalsis increases so more secretions are released, which worsens distention, causes bowel edema, and increases capillary permeability. Plasma leaks into the peritoneal cavity with fluid trapped in the intestinal lumen, so absorption of fluid and electrolytes decreases.

Clinical signs vary with the location of the obstruction. Table 36-12 compares clinical manifestations of obstructions in the large and small intestines. Symptoms include colicky, crampy, intermittent, and wavelike abdominal pain. At times pain may be severe. Abdominal distention may also be present. Patients may have diffuse abdominal tenderness, rigidity, and constipation. Hyperactive bowel sounds (borborygmi) or absent bowel sounds may be noted. The patient may also be febrile, tachycardic, and hypotensive with nausea and vomiting. Emesis (secondary to reverse peristalsis) usually has an odor of feces from proliferation of bacteria.[14]

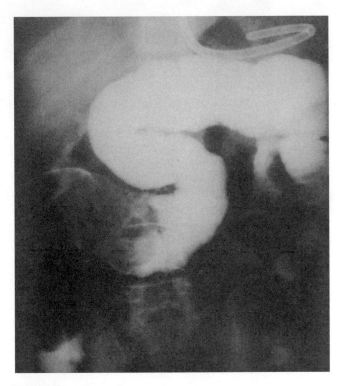

FIGURE 36-15 Intussusception with thin layer of barium around invaginating intestine. (From Rosen P et al: *Emergency medicine,* ed 4, St. Louis, 1998, Mosby.)

Table 36-12	CLINICAL MANIFESTATIONS OF SMALL AND LARGE INTESTINAL OBSTRUCTIONS	
CLINICAL MANIFESTATION	SMALL INTESTINE	LARGE INTESTINE
Onset	Rapid	Gradual
Vomiting	Frequent and copious	Rare
Pain	Colicky, cramplike, intermittent	Low-grade, crampy abdominal pain
Bowel movement	Feces for a short time	Absolute constipation
Abdominal distention	Minimally increased	Greatly increased

From Lewis SM, Heitkemper MM, Dirksen SR: *Medical-surgical nursing: assessment and management of clinical problems,* ed 5, St. Louis, 2000, Mosby.

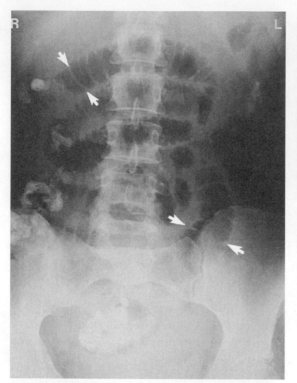

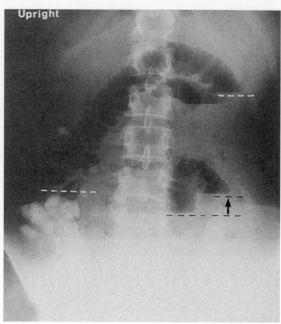

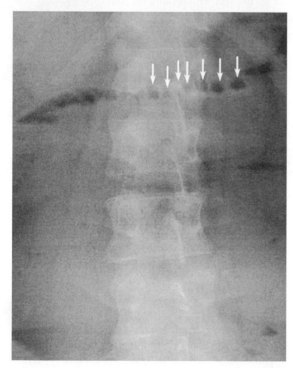

FIGURE **36-16** Radiographic illustration of a small bowel obstruction. (From Mettler FA, Guibertereau MJ, Voss CM et al: *Primary care radiology,* Philadelphia, 2000, WB Saunders.)

Laboratory studies include CBC, BUN, serum glucose, electrolytes, serum creatinine, and arterial blood gas measurements. A WBC count greater than 20,000/mm³ suggests bowel gangrene, whereas elevations greater than 40,000/mm³ occur with mesenteric vascular occlusion.[17] Abdominal radiographs show dilated, fluid-filled loops of bowel with visible air-fluid levels. Table 36-13 highlights radiographic differences with specific obstructions. Management includes IV access for fluid and electrolyte replacement using crystalloid solution to maintain hemodynamic values and renal perfusion. Intake, output, and patient response to therapy should be monitored to prevent fluid overload. Bowel sounds should be evaluated frequently to identify changes. A nasogastric tube is inserted

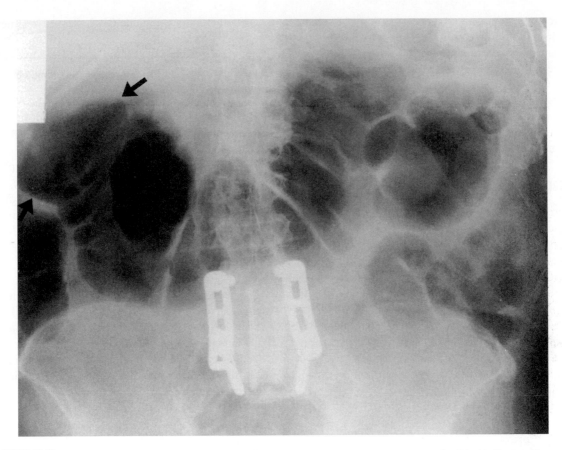

FIGURE 36-17 Ileus on abdominal radiograph. Note dilated loops of bowel. (From Dettenmeier PA: *Radiographic assessment for nurses,* St. Louis, 1995, Mosby.)

Table 36-13	RADIOGRAPHIC AND CLINICAL EVIDENCE OF SPECIFIC BOWEL OBSTRUCTIONS	
TYPE	**RADIOGRAPHIC FINDINGS**	**CLINICAL SIGNS AND SYMPTOMS**
Bowel obstructions (general)	Air-fluid levels may appear as "string of beads" and thus serve as important diagnostic clue to mechanical obstructions. More than two air-fluid levels reflect mechanical obstruction, adynamic ileus, or both. Fluid-filled loops form a proximal impediment and are indicative of bowel obstruction Routine films or contrast studies show air-fluid levels, distortion, abscess formation, narrow lumens, mucosal destruction, distension, and deformities at site of torsion	Pain, distension, vomiting, obstipation, and constipation
Strangulation obstruction	"Coffee bean" sign appears on radiograph (dilated bowel loop bent on itself, assuming shape of coffee bean) Gas- and fluid-filled loops may have unchanging locations on multiple projection films Pseudotumor (closed-loop obstruction filled with water that looks like tumor) may be present	Abdominal tenderness, hyperactive bowel sounds, leukocytosis, rebound tenderness, fever
Gallstones	Air in gallbladder tree, distension of small bowel, and visualization of stone	
Hernia		Extraabdominal or intraabdominal hernia may be present: in men, most commonly inguinal; in women, right-sided femoral hernias
Volvulus		Torsion of mesenteric axis creating digestive disturbances
Intussusception	"Coiled spring" appearance seen on contrast radiograph	

to decompress the stomach and reduce vomiting.[8] Evaluate pain for worsening of the condition. Prophylactic administration of antibiotics is recommended. Surgical intervention may be required for some patients. Life-threatening complications of bowel obstruction include peritonitis, bowel strangulation or perforation, renal insufficiency, aspiration, hypovolemia, intestinal ischemia or infarction, and death. Untreated obstruction that progresses to shock has a 70% mortality rate.[17]

Gastroenteritis

Gastroenteritis is inflammation of the stomach and intestinal lining caused by viral, protozoal, bacterial, or parasitic agents (Table 36-14). Bacterial infection accounts for 20% of acute diarrheal disease.[17] Table 36-15 highlights bacterial gastroenteritis, a common source of epidemics. Gastroenteritis may be caused by an imbalance of normal flora (*E. coli*) resulting from the ingestion of contaminated food. Patients have nausea, vomiting, diarrhea, and abdominal cramps. Hyperactive bowel sounds, fever, and headaches are also present. Anal excoriation occurs with frequent episodes of diarrhea. Diarrhea accounts for 5 to 10 million deaths annually in Asia, Africa, and Latin America.[17]

Laboratory data include CBC, electrolytes measurement, stool for ova and parasites, and stool culture. Obtain IV access for replacement of fluid and electrolytes. Administer antiemetics and analgesics as needed. Antibiotics are determined by patient history and presenting symptoms. Successful treatment is based on identifying the causative agent and resting the intestinal tract. Oral hydration with clear liquids is possible in most patients. Suggested fluids include cola, ginger ale, apple juice, tea, broth, and electrolyte replacement drinks such as Gatorade. Fluid replacement in children is critical to prevent dehydration. Rice, applesauce, bananas, and toast can be started as soon as diarrhea subsides. Feeding should begin as soon as possible in children and adults.

SUMMARY

GI emergencies can be minor or life-threatening. Most GI emergencies present with similar clinical manifestations, so triage history and physical assessment play an important role in management of these patients. Ability to differentiate conditions that require immediate attention is a requisite skill for the emergency nurse. Box 36-7 highlights selected nursing diagnoses for GI emergencies.

Table 36-14	ETIOLOGY OF GASTROENTERITIS	
TYPE	**EXAMPLE**	
Bacteria	*Salmonella, Escherichia coli, Clostridium difficile, Clostridium botulinum, Campylobacter fetus jejuni*	
Virus	Rotavirus, parvovirus, enterovirus	
Protozoa	*Giardia lamblia*, cryptosporidium	

Box 36-7	NURSING DIAGNOSES FOR GASTROINTESTINAL EMERGENCIES
Anxiety	
Fluid volume, Deficient	
Gas exchange, Impaired	
Infection, Risk for	
Knowledge, Deficient	
Pain	

Table 36-15	EPIDEMIOLOGIC ASPECTS OF INVASIVE BACTERIAL GASTROENTERITIS			
	SOURCE	**INCUBATION PERIOD**	**FEATURES**	**DURATION**
Shigella species	Person to person, fecal-oral	24-48 hours	Confined populations; poor personal hygiene and sanitation	4-7 days
Salmonella species	Poultry, eggs, water, and domestic pets	8-24 hours	Family and cafeteria-type outbreaks common	2-5 days
Campylobacter fetus	Poultry, wild birds, water	2-5 days	High relapse rate; summer months; cases sporadic	5-14 days
Yersinia enterocolitica	Food or drink and person to person	12-48 hours (?)	Appendicitis; mesenteric adenitis-like syndromes; winter months	10-14 days
Vibrio parahaemolyticus	Seafood, especially shellfish	8-24 hours	High attack rates; summer months	24-48 hours

From Rosen P et al: *Emergency medicine*, ed 4, vol 2, St. Louis, 1998, Mosby.

References

1. Cummings SP, Cummings PH: Abdominal emergencies. In Jordan KS, editor: *Emergency nursing core curriculum,* ed 5, Philadelphia, 2000, WB Saunders.

2. Grendell JH: Acute pancreatitis. In Grendell JH, McQuaid KR, Freidman SL, editors: *Current diagnosis and treatment in gastroenterology,* Stamford, Conn, 1996, Appleton & Lange.

3. Grendell JH: Miscellaneous disorders of the stomach and small intestine. In Grendell JH, McQuaid KR, Freidman SL, editors: *Current diagnosis and treatment in gastroenterology,* Stamford, Conn, 1996, Appleton & Lange.

4. Guss D: Disorders of the liver, biliary tract, and pancreas. In Rosen P, Barkin RM, Hockberger RS et al, editors: *Emergency medicine: concepts and clinical practice,* ed 4, St. Louis, 1998, Mosby.

5. Guyton AC, Hall J: *Textbook of medical physiology,* ed 10, Philadelphia, 2000, WB Saunders.

6. Heiser R: Abdominal conditions. In Kidd PS, Sturt P, editors: *Mosby's emergency nursing reference,* St. Louis, 1996, Mosby.

7. Henneman PL: Gastrointestinal bleeding. In Rosen P, Barkin RM, Hockberger RS et al, editors: *Emergency medicine: concepts and clinical practice,* ed 4, St. Louis, 1998, Mosby.

8. Hockberger RS, Henneman PL, Boniface K: Disorders of the small intestine. In Rosen P, Barkin RM, Hockberger RS et al, editors: *Emergency medicine: concepts and clinical practice,* ed 4, St. Louis, 1998, Mosby.

9. Jacobson IM: Gallstones. In Grendell JH, McQuaid KR, Freidman SL et al, editors: *Current diagnosis and treatment in gastroenterology,* Stamford, Conn, 1996, Appleton & Lange.

10. Jutabha R, Jensen DM: Acute upper gastrointestinal bleeding. In Grendell JH, McQuaid KR, Freidman SL et al, editors: *Current diagnosis and treatment in gastroenterology,* Stamford, Conn, 1996, Appleton & Lange.

11. Kearney DJ, McQuaid KR: Approach to the patient with gastrointestinal disorders. In Grendell JH, McQuaid KR, Freidman SL et al, editors: *Current diagnosis and treatment in gastroenterology,* Stamford, Conn, 1996, Appleton & Lange.

12. Lewis SM, Heitkemper MM, Dirksen SR: *Medical surgical nursing: assessment and mangement of clinical problems,* ed 5, St. Louis, 2000, Mosby.

13. Rakel RE: *Conn's current therapy 1998,* Philadelphia, 1998, WB Saunders.

14. Rosen P, Barkin RM, Hockberger RS et al: *Emergency medicine: concepts and clinical practice,* ed 4, St. Louis, 1998, Mosby.

15. Rosen P, Barkin RM, Hayden SR et al: *The 5 minute emergency medicine consult,* Philadelphia, 1999, Lippincott Williams & Wilkins.

16. Savides TJ, Jensen DM: Acute lower gastrointestinal bleeding. In Grendell JH, McQuaid KR, Freidman SL et al, editors: *Current diagnosis and treatment in gastroenterology,* Stamford, Conn, 1996, Appleton & Lange.

17. Tintinelli JE, Ruiz E, Krome RL: *Emergency medicine—a comprehensive study guide,* ed 4, New York, 1996, McGraw-Hill.

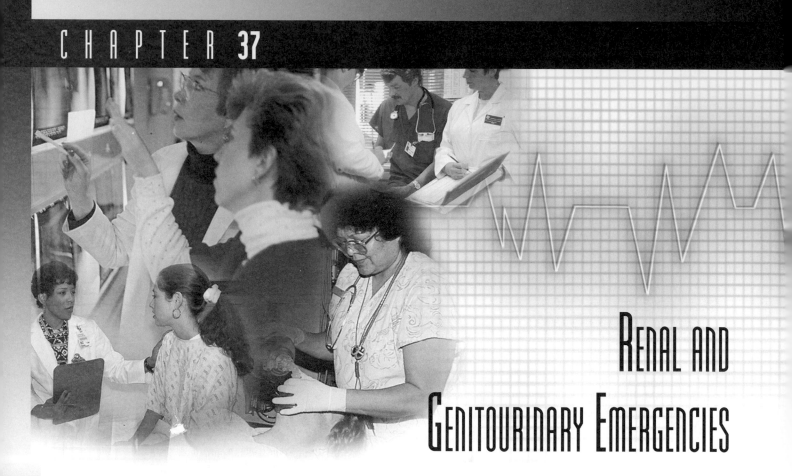

CHAPTER 37

RENAL AND GENITOURINARY EMERGENCIES

BILLIE JEAN BARRETT-WALTERS

Genitourinary (GU) problems are a common complaint in the emergency department (ED). Urinary tract infections (UTIs) are the third most common infection in ambulatory patients. Up to 3% of all females experience one or more infections a year.[2] Renal calculi affect up to 6% of the American population and account for 7 of 1000 hospitalizations.[6] Sexually transmitted diseases (STDs) are increasing in the United States, especially among low-income, urban, minority adolescents.[4] Incidence of end-stage renal disease (ESRD) is rising in all industrialized nations, although etiology of this increase is not clear. ESRD affects blacks three times more often than whites, and is most prevalent in those with diabetes or hypertension, occurring six times more often in those with hypertension. In people 65 years of age or older, incidence of renal failure increases sixfold; however, 66% of all diabetes-induced renal failure occurs before age 64. Males account for 65% of the ESRD population.[3] Acute tubular necrosis, the most common type of acute renal failure, accounts for 5% of all hospital admissions. Patients with compromised renal function often arrive at the ED with life-threatening fluid and electrolyte imbalances.

Genitourinary emergencies also occur secondary to trauma (Chapter 25). Specific GU emergencies discussed in this chapter are acute azotemia, rhabdomyolysis, UTIs, urinary calculi, testicular torsion, epididymitis, priapism, and

STDs. Refer to Chapter 44 for additional discussion of STDs in women.

ANATOMY AND PHYSIOLOGY

The genitourinary tract consists of the kidneys, ureters, urinary bladder, urethra, and external genitalia. Urine is produced by the kidneys as a way to regulate fluid volume and electrolyte balance. Ureters transport urine to the bladder for temporary storage. The urine is drained from the bladder to the outside by the urethra. Figure 37-1 shows structures of the GU system. External structures of the male GU system have reproductive functions.

The kidneys are located on the posterior abdominal wall behind the peritoneum on either side of the vertebral column. Figure 37-2 shows the kidney in cross-section. On the medial aspect of each kidney is the hilum, where the renal artery and nerve enter and renal vein and ureter exit. The hilum opens into the renal pelvis, an enlargement of the urinary channel. Renal calyces, shaped like the cup of a flower, open into the renal pelvis. Each kidney contains 20 minor calyces that open into 2 to 3 major calyces. The kidney has an outer cortex and inner layer or medulla. Cone or triangular-shaped structures called medullary pyramids located in the renal medulla open into a minor calyx. The cortex surrounds the medulla and extends between pyramids in columns to the renal

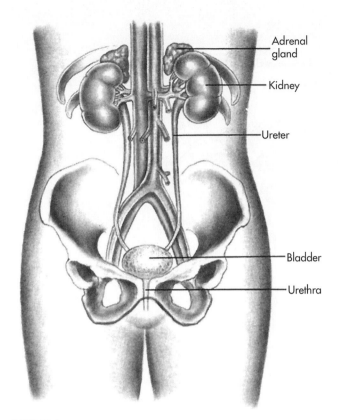

FIGURE 37-1   Components of the urinary system. (From Thompson JM, McFarland GK, Hirsch JE et al: *Mosby's clinical nursing,* ed 5, St. Louis, 2001, Mosby.)

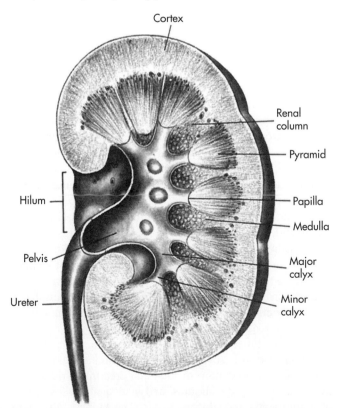

FIGURE 37-2   Cross-section of kidney. (From Thompson JM, McFarland GK, Hirsch JE et al: *Mosby's clinical nursing,* ed 5, St. Louis, 2001, Mosby.)

pelvis. Blood flow to the kidney is supplied by the renal artery, which branches off the abdominal aorta and enters the kidney through the renal sinus. Blood leaves the kidney through the renal vein, which empties into the abdominal inferior vena cava.

The nephron, the functional unit of the kidney, is composed of the renal corpuscle, proximal convoluted tubule, Henle's loop, distal convoluted tubule, and collecting ducts (Figure 37-3). Each kidney contains an estimated 1 million nephrons that are individually capable of producing urine. These nephrons cannot be reproduced once destroyed. The renal corpuscle contains the glomerulus, a web of tightly convoluted capillaries, and Bowman's capsule, which surrounds and supports these structures. Blood flows through the afferent arteriole into the glomerulus and out the efferent arteriole. Renal blood flow accounts for 21% of cardiac output, or 1200 ml/min.[1] Specialized cells called juxtaglomerular cells are located at the entrance to the glomerulus of the afferent arteriole in 15% of nephrons. Juxtaglomerular cells form a cuff and combine with the macula densa, a portion of the distal convoluted tubule that lies adjacent to the renal corpuscle between afferent and efferent arterioles. The juxtaglomerular cells and the macula densa form the juxtaglomerular apparatus, which senses changes in pressure and sodium concentration and plays a role in the renin-angiotensin-aldosterone (RAA) system. Juxtaglomerular nephrons have a greater capacity to concentrate urine because they have longer Henle's loops, which extend into the medulla.

Filtration of plasma in the renal corpuscle is the first step in urine production and helps the kidneys rid the body of wastes and retain water and essential solutes. Pressure generated as blood courses through the tight web of capillaries in the glomerulus, along with oncotic pressure within the blood, is greater than pressure created by Bowman's capsule, so plasma or filtrate and small solutes cross the semipermeable epithelial capillary lining. Injury to the glomerulus, such as ischemia or inflammation, increases permeability of the capillary membrane and allows larger molecules (red blood cells [RBCs], epithelial casts, protein, or white blood cells [WBCs]) to cross. Decreased oncotic pressure, often the result of decreased serum albumin levels, or decreased pressure within the glomerulus produced by systemic hypotension decreases glomerular filtration rate (GFR) and eventually urine output. GFR in the average adult is 125 ml/min or 180 L/day.

Tubules, Henle's loop, and collecting ducts excrete waste products (e.g., urea, nitrogen, creatinine, drug metabolites), reabsorb water and solutes (potassium, sodium, chloride, hydrogen, glucose, and amino acids) from filtrate, and secrete excess solutes the body doesn't need into filtrate. Osmosis, diffusion, and active transport occur between the nephron and surrounding capillaries. Hormonal control regulates reabsorption and secretion in the nephron.

The RAA system (Figure 37-4) and antidiuretic hormone (ADH) are feedback loop systems within the body that maintain homeostasis. Serum osmolarity increases and causes stimulation of the hypothalamus, which releases ADH. Nephron permeability increases, so additional water

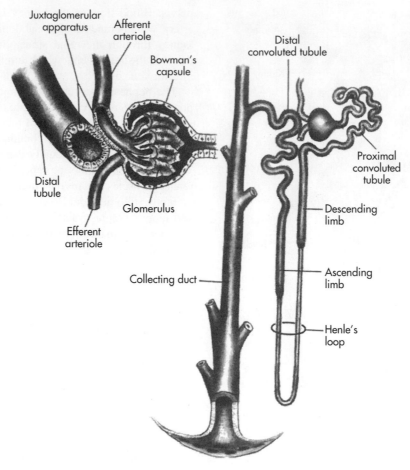

FIGURE 37-3 Components of nephron. (From Thompson JM, McFarland GK, Hirsch JE et al: *Mosby's clinical nursing,* ed 4, St. Louis, 1997, Mosby.)

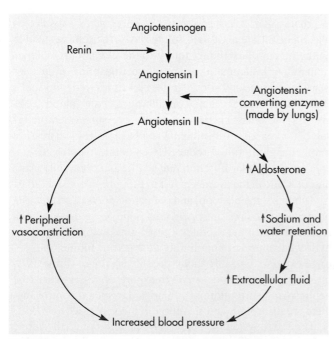

FIGURE 37-4 Renin-angiotensin-aldosterone mechanism. (From Lewis SM, Heitkemper MM, Dirksen SR: *Medical-surgical nursing: assessment and management of clinical problems,* ed 5, St. Louis, 2000, Mosby.)

is absorbed, serum osmolarity returns to normal, and ADH release stops. Pressure changes in the glomerulus are overcome by vasodilation and constriction of the afferent arteriole by a process called autoregulation. This autoregulation keeps pressure in the glomerulus within a wide range of systolic blood pressures. When range is exceeded, autoregulation fails and epithelial damage occurs with eventual scarring and sclerosis followed by decreased permeability, GFR, and urine output. Inadequate nephron perfusion stimulates the juxtaglomerular apparatus to secrete renin that converts angiotensin to angiotensin I, which stimulates aldosterone release from the adrenal cortex and reabsorption of sodium and water by the nephron. Conversion of angiotensin I to angiotensin II by an enzyme in the lung causes peripheral vasoconstriction. Perfusion increases to the nephron and the cycle is altered.

Without a functioning kidney and adequate urine production, homeostasis is severely impaired. Fluid and electrolyte imbalance, accumulation of urea and creatinine, decreased excretion of drug metabolites, and inadequate reabsorption of amino acids and glucose occur. The kidneys also help convert vitamin D into the active form (1, 25-vitamin D_3) to ensure calcium absorption from intestines and secrete erythropoietin for stimulation of RBC production in bone mar-

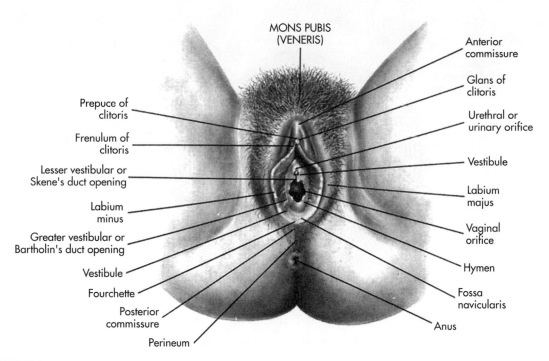

FIGURE 37-5 External female genitalia. (From Lowdermilk DL: *Maternity and women's health care,* ed 6, St. Louis, 1997, Mosby.)

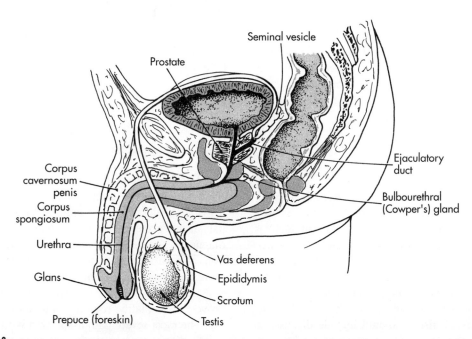

FIGURE 37-6 External and internal male genitalia. (From Price SA, Wilson LM: *Pathophysiology: clinical concepts of disease processes,* ed 5, St. Louis, 1997, Mosby.)

row. Consequently, altered renal function decreases bone mineralization and oxygen-carrying capacity of the blood.

The renal pelvis narrows to enter the ureter, where urine is moved to the bladder by peristaltic contractions. The muscular bladder stores urine until release to the urethra by the micturition reflex.

External genitalia are also part of the GU system. Female genitalia consist of the vestibule, the space into which the

urethra and vagina open, and surrounding labia minora and majora (Figure 37-5). Anatomic position and the short length of the female urethra are responsible for the high frequency of UTIs in females.

Male external genitalia include penis, scrotum, and scrotal contents (Figure 37-6). Scrotal contents include the testes, tubules that carry developing sperm cells and secrete testosterone, and the epididymis, which lies along the posterior

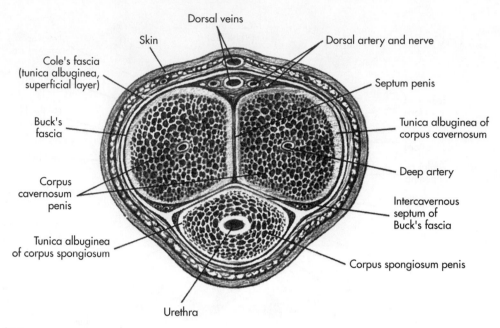

FIGURE 37-7 Cross-section of penis. (From Thompson JM, McFarland GK, Hirsch JE et al: *Mosby's clinical nursing,* ed 5, St. Louis, 2001, Mosby.)

testes and is the final maturation area for sperm. The prostate is glandular and muscle tissue that surrounds the urethra at the base of the bladder. Enlargement of the prostate can cause outlet obstruction and urinary retention. The penis consists of three columns of erectile tissue that become engorged with blood, producing erection (Figure 37-7). Two columns of corpora cavernosa form the dorsum and sides of the penis and the corpus spongiosum forms the base and glans. Clinical manifestations of GU disease frequently involve external genitalia.

PATIENT ASSESSMENT

Assessment of the GU system should determine history of hypertension, diabetes, previous infections, prostatitis, urethritis, bladder or urethral damage during childbirth, history of renal calculi, and recurrent urinary tract infections. A detailed drug list, including prescription, over-the-counter (OTC), and illegal drugs should be obtained. Identification of any history of exposure to occupational chemicals or toxins may identify contact with substances that could cause nephrotoxicicity. Sexual history should include discussion of risk factors that can cause GU symptoms (e.g., use of contraceptive jellies or creams, multiple partners, abnormal penile or vaginal discharges, unsafe sexual practices, history of STDs). GU complaints often arise from changes in urinary patterns; for example, frequency, dysuria, urgency, dribbling, or incontinence.

Hematuria, the presence of blood in the urine, may be the primary complaint or may accompany other symptoms. A detailed medication and diet history may uncover other causes for discoloration of urine. Box 37-1 highlights possible causes of red or dark red urine. Hematuria can be confirmed by urinalysis (UA); however, microscopic hematuria on a single test is common. Early-stream hematuria suggests

Box 37-1	NONHEMATURIC CAUSES OF RED OR DARK RED URINE
FOOD	**DRUGS**
Beets	Cascara
Rhubarb	Desferol
Blackberries	Adriamycin
	Phenothiazides
	Phenytoin (Dilantin)
	Rifampin

bleeding from the urethra, hematuria throughout the stream indicates upper GU tract bleeding, and bleeding at the end suggests bladder neck or urethral bleeding. Complete urinalysis and urine cytology may indicate the need for further diagnostic testing for urologic cancer, renal disease, infection, or renal calculi as the source of hematuria. Box 37-2 highlights drugs and chemicals that cause hematuria.

Pain should be assessed using the PQRST mnemonic—provocation, quality, region or radiation, severity, and timing. The most severe pain associated with the GU system is renal colic caused by calculi. Increased pressure and dilation of the kidney and urinary collecting system cause sudden, unbearable pain. The patient usually presents with restlessness, pallor, and complains of flank pain that often radiates to the abdomen and groin. If the stone lodges in the bladder, urinary frequency and urgency develop. Pain can cause tachypnea and tachycardia with elevated blood pressure. Relief of renal colic requires substantial amounts of narcotics, so drug seekers may feign renal colic pain and give a history of allergy to intravenous pyelography (IVP) dye.

Oliguria, defined as urine output less than 400 ml in 24 hours, or anuria, less than 75 ml in 24 hours, may be the presenting symptom. The cause is usually obstruction; however, blood chemistries should be evaluated for azotemia, which indicates renal failure from prolonged obstruction leading to hydronephrosis or other causes. If the patient has a urinary catheter in place, patency should be assessed. A physical ex-

amination can identify urinary retention by palpating the bladder as a firm mass above the symphysis pubis, with an urge to void on palpation. History should be obtained to identify drugs that contribute to retention, including OTC nasal decongestants containing anticholinergic ingredients. A neurologic examination should be performed to rule out spinal cord injury or disease that can interfere with the micturition reflex. The prostate is examined for enlargement as the cause of obstruction. After the patient has attempted to void, a urethral catheter may be inserted for residual volume. If the catheter cannot be inserted without force, a suprapubic bladder tap or assistance from a urologist may be necessary. With residual volume greater than 500 ml, the catheter may be left in place to allow the bladder to regain muscle tone. If residual volume is minimal, further diagnostic evaluation is aimed at identifying the cause.

SPECIFIC CONDITIONS

Acute Azotemia

Azotemia, or uremia, refers to accumulation of nitrogen waste products in the blood. Acute azotemia generally refers to the patient with acute renal failure (ARF), usually over a period of days; however, chronic renal failure patients (CRF) can experience acute episodes because of noncompliance or other medical conditions. Causes of ARF, specific pathophysiology, general treatment, and diagnostic markers are listed in Box 37-3. Table 37-1 highlights clinical manifestations of ARF; Figure 37-8 describes clinical manifestations of chronic uremia or renal failure.

Box 37-2 DRUGS AND CHEMICALS THAT CAUSE HEMATURIA

ANTIBIOTICS

Amphotericin
Ampicillin
Colistimethate
Kanamycin
Methicillin
Penicillin
Polymyxin
Sulfonamides

ANTICOAGULANTS

Heparin
Warfarin

DRUGS

Amitriptyline
Aspirin (acetylsalicylic acid)
Benztropine (Cogentin)
Cantharides
Chlorothiazide
Chlorpromazine
Colchicine

Corticosteroids
Cyclophosphamide
Indomethacin
Methenamine
Phenacetin
Phenylbutazone
Probenecid
Trifluoperazine (Stelazine)

METALS

Arsenic
Copper sulfate
Gold
Lead
Phosphorus

ORGANIC SOLVENTS

Carbon tetrachloride
Phenol
Propylene glycol
Turpentine

From Kendall AR, Karafin L: *Urology,* New York, 1973, Harper & Row.

Box 37-3 COMMON CAUSES OF ACUTE RENAL FAILURE

PRERENAL	INTRARENAL	POSTRENAL
Hypovolemia caused by:	Nephrotoxic injury from the following:	Calculi formation
Hemorrhage	Drugs (aminoglycosides [gentamicin, tobramycin,	Benign prostatic hyperplasia
Burns	amikacin], amphotericin B, cisplatin)	Prostate cancer
Dehydration	Radiographic contrast agents	Bladder cancer
Prolonged diarrhea or vomiting	Hemolytic blood transfusion reaction (hemoglobin	Trauma (to back, pelvis, or perineum)
Decreased cardiac output caused by:	blocks tubules)	Strictures
Myocardial infarction	Severe crushing injury (myoglobin released from	Spinal cord disease
Cardiac dysrhythmias	muscles blocks tubules)	
Congestive heart failure	Chemicals (ethylene glycol, mercuric chloride,	
Cardiogenic shock	carbon tetrachloride, lead, arsenic)	
Pericardial tamponade	Acute glomerulonephritis	
Surgery (e.g., open heart)	Acute pyelonephritis	
Decreased peripheral vascular	Toxemia of pregnancy	
resistance caused by:	Malignant hypertension	
Septic shock	Systemic lupus erythematosus	
Anaphylaxis	Interstitial nephritis	
Neurologic injury	Allergic (antibiotics [sulfonamides, rifampin],	
Renal vascular obstruction caused by:	nonsteroidal antiinflammatory drugs, ACE	
Thrombosis of renal arteries	inhibitors)	
Bilateral renal vein thrombosis	Infection (bacterial [e.g., acute pyelonephritis],	
Embolism	viral [e.g., CMV], fungal [e.g., candidiasis])	

From Lewis SM, Heitkemper MM, Dirksen SR: *Medical-surgical nursing: assessment and management of clinical problems,* ed 5, St. Louis, 2000, Mosby.
ACE, Angiotensin-converting enzyme; *CMV,* cytomegalovirus.

Table 37-1	CLINICAL MANIFESTATIONS OF ACUTE RENAL FAILURE	
BODY SYSTEM	**CLINICAL MANIFESTATIONS**
Urinary	↓ Urinary output
	Proteinuria
	Casts
	↓ Specific gravity
	↓ Osmolality
	↑ Urinary sodium
Cardiovascular	Volume overload
	Congestive heart failure
	Hypotension (early)
	Hypertension (after development of fluid overload)
	Pericarditis
	Pericardial effusion
	Dysrhythmias
Respiratory	Pulmonary edema
	Kussmaul's respirations
	Pleural effusions
Gastrointestinal	Nausea and vomiting
	Anorexia
	Stomatitis
	Bleeding
	Diarrhea
	Constipation
Hematologic	Anemia (development within 48 hr)
	Leukocytosis
	Defect in platelet functioning
Neurologic	Lethargy
	Convulsions
	Asterixis
	Memory impairment
Others	↑ Susceptibility to infection
	↑ BUN
	↑ Creatinine
	↑ Potassium
	↓ pH
	↓ Bicarbonate
	↓ Calcium
	↑ Phosphate

From Lewis SM, Heitkemper MM, Dirksen SR: *Medical-surgical nursing: assessment and management of clinical problems,* ed 5, St. Louis, 2000, Mosby.
BUN, Blood urea nitrogen.

Symptoms of ARF include short-term weight gain or loss, nausea and vomiting, hematemesis, melena, dysrhythmias, dyspnea, stupor, or coma. Compromise of airway, breathing, circulation, and neurologic function requires intervention. Fever may be associated with infectious or inflammatory events. Reducing measures should be instituted to prevent continued rise of nitrogenous waste products by catabolic effect of fever.

Hyperkalemia, hyponatremia, hypocalcemia, hyperphosphatemia, and volume overload are the most common fluid and electrolyte imbalances resulting from loss of the kidney's ability to excrete potassium and phosphorus, conserve sodium, and eliminate excess volume. Calcium is inversely related to phosphorus and decreases secondary to rise in phosphorus, along with inability of the kidney to convert vitamin D to the active form for calcium absorption from the gut. Electrocardiogram (ECG) may reveal tall peaked T waves, widened QRS, and prolonged PR interval secondary to hyperkalemia. Administration of intravenous (IV) calcium may be needed to antagonize the membrane and improve cardiac conductivity until removal of excess potassium by emergency dialysis can be initiated. Intravenous calcium works within minutes, but duration is short, as evidenced by return of ECG changes. Administration of IV sodium bicarbonate ($NaHCO_3$), glucose, and insulin redistributes extracellular potassium into the intracellular fluid, works within 15 to 30 minutes, and lasts approximately 4 hours. Potassium can be removed by cation exchange resin (Kayexolate), but onset of action is 60 minutes when given rectally and 120 minutes for oral administration.

Urine output may be increased or decreased. If ARF is nonoliguric, large volumes of fluid can be lost, so the patient may be dehydrated and hypotensive. Volume replacement with normal saline or volume expanders is guided by monitoring jugular vein distention and vital signs or by invasive lines such as central venous pressure and pulmonary artery catheters to avoid further ischemic injury to renal tissue. If ARF presents with oliguria, the patient may be volume overloaded and hypertensive, so minimal fluid is given until the volume can be removed by diuretics or through hemodialysis. Metabolic acidosis occurs because renal tubules can no longer regulate concentration of hydrogen ions. Intravenous $NaHCO_3$ may be used unless contraindicated by volume status.

Indications for emergency dialysis include stupor or coma (caused by rising nitrogen waste products in blood and metabolic changes), volume overload and pulmonary edema, dangerous hyperkalemia, and acidosis. Emergency hemodialysis requires vascular access (usually a temporary femoral or subclavian dual lumen catheter or internal shunt) and an artificial kidney (dialyzer) to act as a semipermeable membrane. The dialysate must be low in ions, which the body needs to excrete, and high in those to be reabsorbed. A blood pump is required to move blood through the dialyzer (Figure 37-9).

After initial stabilization, history and diagnostic testing focus on identifying the cause of ARF. Tests include serial blood chemistries, UA with sodium and potassium concentrations, chest radiograph, renal ultrasounds and Doppler studies, or computed tomography (CT) scan. Imaging procedures are usually done without contrast media because of toxic effects of the media on renal tubules.

Dialysis Access Complications

Major etiologies of CRF are vascular changes caused by diabetes, hypertension, or progressive glomerulonephritis. Renal replacement therapy may be provided by peritoneal dialysis or hemodialysis. Peritoneal dialysis involves in-

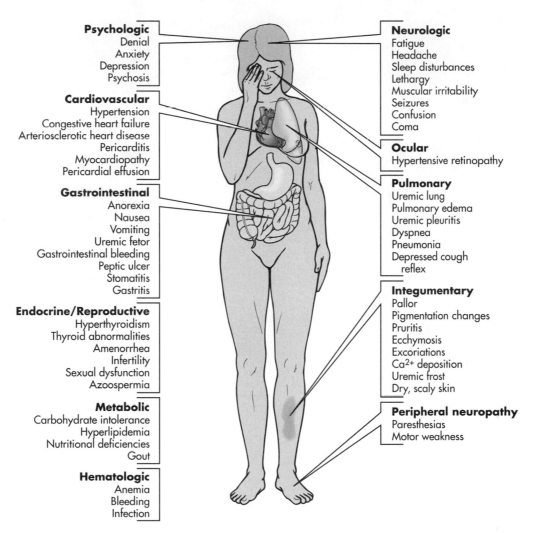

Psychologic
Denial
Anxiety
Depression
Psychosis

Cardiovascular
Hypertension
Congestive heart failure
Arteriosclerotic heart disease
Pericarditis
Myocardiopathy
Pericardial effusion

Gastrointestinal
Anorexia
Nausea
Vomiting
Uremic fetor
Gastrointestinal bleeding
Peptic ulcer
Stomatitis
Gastritis

Endocrine/Reproductive
Hyperthyroidism
Thyroid abnormalities
Amenorrhea
Infertility
Sexual dysfunction
Azoospermia

Metabolic
Carbohydrate intolerance
Hyperlipidemia
Nutritional deficiencies
Gout

Hematologic
Anemia
Bleeding
Infection

Neurologic
Fatigue
Headache
Sleep disturbances
Lethargy
Muscular irritability
Seizures
Confusion
Coma

Ocular
Hypertensive retinopathy

Pulmonary
Uremic lung
Pulmonary edema
Uremic pleuritis
Dyspnea
Pneumonia
Depressed cough
    reflex

Integumentary
Pallor
Pigmentation changes
Pruritis
Ecchymosis
Excoriations
Ca^{2+} deposition
Uremic frost
Dry, scaly skin

Peripheral neuropathy
Paresthesias
Motor weakness

FIGURE 37-8   Clinical manifestations of chronic uremia. (From Lewis SM, Heitkemper MM, Dirksen SR: *Medical-surgical nursing: assessment and management of clinical problems,* ed 5, St. Louis, 2000, Mosby.)

stilling 1 to 2 L of dialysate fluid containing varying amounts of glucose, magnesium, calcium, chloride, and lactate into the abdomen. The peritoneal membrane acts as a semipermeable pathway for exchange of solutes and water between the vascular peritoneal space and dialysate by osmosis and diffusion (Figure 37-10). Access to the peritoneal cavity is achieved through a plastic catheter held in place by a Dacron cuff (Figure 37-11). Peritonitis and exit site infections may bring the patient to the ED with complaints of abdominal pain, nausea and vomiting, fever, and cloudy dialysate fluid. Antibiotics may be given IV and added to dialysate. If this is unsuccessful the catheter should be removed and hemodialysis initiated until peritonitis clears. Unless scarring impairs permeability of the peritoneal membrane, the catheter can be surgically replaced and peritoneal dialysis reinitiated.

Clotted vascular access frequently brings patients with CRF to the ED. Arteriovenous fistulas are surgical connections of a native artery and vein in an extremity or insertion of Gortex graft material to form the connection (Figure 37-12). Available sites suitable for vascular access become ex-

hausted, so permanent subclavian dual lumen catheters are placed for hemodialysis. Clotted vascular access should be emergently declotted with use of locally instilled or infused fibrinolytics or surgery. Grafts, fistulas, and insertion sites also become infected and may progress to septicemia. Local symptoms include redness, drainage, or edema. Blood cultures and a complete blood count (CBC) should be obtained to rule out systemic infection. Access removal may be necessary, so temporary subclavian or femoral access (replaced every 2 or 3 days) can be used until blood is free of infection.

Rhabdomyolysis

Skeletal muscle destruction with subsequent release of myoglobin into the circulatory system causes rhabdomyolysis, which can lead to acute renal failure.[7] There are many different etiologies, including crush injuries, drug or toxin ingestion, infection, burns, or metabolic disturbances. Crush injuries may be caused by entrapment, such as prolonged compression of the abdomen or a limb after a motor vehicle crash.

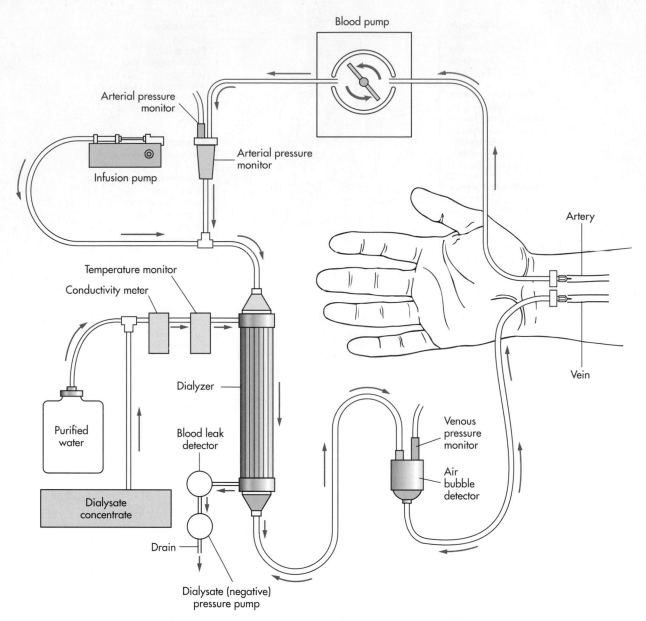

FIGURE 37-9 Components of a hemodialysis system. (From Thelan LA, Urden LD, Lough ME et al: *Critical care nursing: diagnosis and management,* ed 3, St. Louis, 1998, Mosby.)

When a crush injury occurs there is breakdown of muscle tissue with subsequent release of myoglobin into plasma circulation. Fluid shifts from the intravascular space into the interstitial space can cause the patient to become profoundly hypovolemic. Dehydration results from hypovolemia and causes hypoperfusion of the kidneys, thereby decreasing the GFR. Electrolyte imbalances are also associated with the fluid shift. Hypocalcemia, hyperkalemia, and hyperuricemia are also present. There is an increase in serum creatinine phosphokinase.[5] Urine sample collection shows concentrated urine with a reddish brown color. Proteinuria and hematuria are also noted on urinalysis; however, no RBCs are seen during microscopic examination.

Presenting signs and symptoms include complaints of muscle aches or acute muscle pain. General malaise, fever,

and muscle tenderness may occur. The urine has a characteristic reddish brown color and often a foul odor.

Treatment of rhabdomyolysis consists of volume replacement, monitoring, and maintenance of electrolyte balance. Increasing the urine output helps flush myoglobin through the kidneys. Sodium bicarbonate is added to IV fluids to increase excretion of myoglobin. If the patient progresses to acute renal failure, hemodialysis may be considered.

Urinary Tract Infections

Common symptoms of GU tract infection include pyuria, hematuria, chills and fever, leucocytosis, nausea, vomiting, and signs of bladder irritability such as frequency, dysuria, and urgency. With renal involvement, dull flank pain and

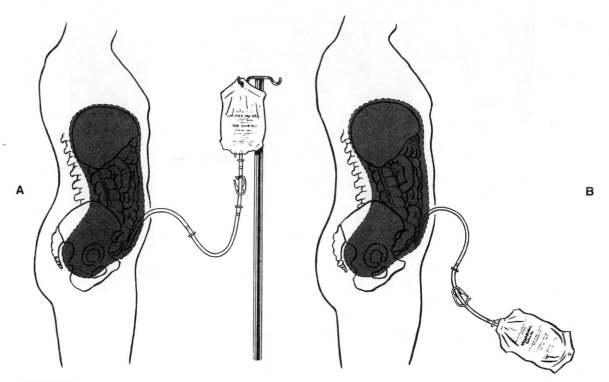

FIGURE 37-10   Peritoneal dialysis. *A,* Inflow. *B,* Outflow (drains to gravity). (From Thompson JM, McFarland GK, Hirsch JE et al: *Mosby's clinical nursing,* ed 5, St. Louis, 2001, Mosby.)

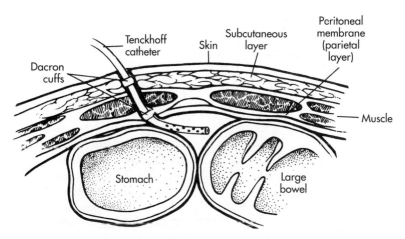

FIGURE 37-11   Peritoneal catheter. (From Thompson JM, McFarland GK, Hirsch JE et al: *Mosby's clinical nursing,* ed 5, St. Louis, 2001, Mosby.)

costovertebral angle tenderness may also be present. Figure 37-13 illustrates infectious processes of the urinary system. Diagnosis is made by history, presenting signs, UA, urine culture and sensitivity, and CBC with differential. A KUB (kidneys-ureters-bladder) radiograph may show a hazy outline of the kidney secondary to edema. Blood urea nitrogen (BUN), creatinine, and electrolyte values are obtained to rule out alteration in renal function. Persistent microscopic or gross hematuria, symptoms of obstruction, or presence of urea-splitting bacteria associated with staghorn renal calculi require work up with renal ultrasound, cystogram, or IVP. Infection with *Chlamydia trachomatis* or *Neisseria gonor-*

rhoae should be considered with urethral infection and pyuria that has negative culture. Table 37-2 compares common GU tract infections that present to the ED.

Urinary Calculi

A primary risk factor for calculi is hypercalciuria; however, there is also an association with UTI, gout, excessive ingestion of certain foods, family history, dehydration, and pregnancy (Box 37-4). Seventy-five percent of stones are composed of calcium combined with oxalate or phosphate; the remaining 25% are composed of struvite, cystine, or

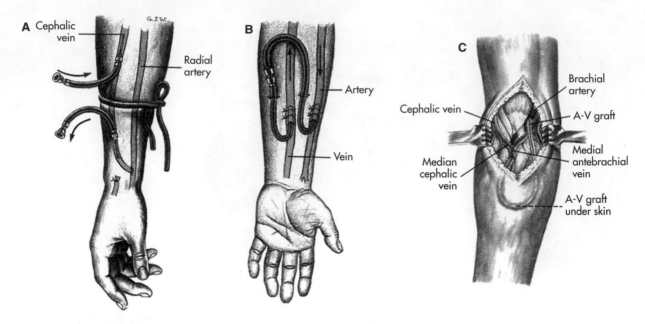

FIGURE 37-12   Circulatory access for hemodialysis. **A,** External (temporary) arteriovenous cannula (shunt). **B,** Internal (permanent) arteriovenous fistula. **C,** Internal (permanent) arteriovenous graft. (From Thompson JM, McFarland GK, Hirsch JE et al: *Mosby's clinical nursing,* ed 5, St. Louis, 2001, Mosby.)

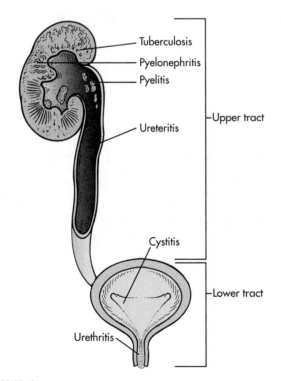

FIGURE 37-13   Sites of infectious processes in the urinary tract. (From Lewis SM, Heitkemper MM, Dirksen SR: *Medical-surgical nursing: assessment and management of clinical problems,* ed 5, St. Louis, 2000, Mosby.)

uric acid (Table 37-3). Calculi are asymptomatic until movement causes intermittent backache, urge to void, dysuria, renal colic, and hematuria. Bacteremia and proteinuria may also be present. Diagnostic studies include CBC, BUN, creatinine, electrolytes, uric acid, UA with culture and sensitivity (C and S), KUB, and IVP. Helical CT scans

are also used. Figure 37-14 shows staghorn calculus on a KUB radiograph. Ninety percent of stones exit spontaneously; however, if unpassed, they may be removed by laparoscopy, lithotripsy, or surgically. Figure 37-15 illustrates shock wave lithotripsy.

Nursing interventions include intake and output measurement, straining all urine, sending solid material for lab analysis, and increased fluids. Pain assessment and management is critical in these patients because of the severity of their pain. Narcotics such as Morphine and Dilaudid may be used; however, non–narcotics such as Toradol are equally effective in many patients. Complications include ischemia at obstructive site, altered elimination, and UTI. Criteria for admission include need for frequent pain medicine, large-diameter stones, solitary kidney, ileus, bladder stones, and infection. If the patient is discharged, information should be provided to him or her about returning to the ED in case of increasing pain, excessive vomiting, or fever and chills. Dietary restrictions should also be included (see Box 37-4).

Testicular Torsion

Testicular torsion causes vascular compromise of the testes within 6 to 12 hours and can lead to infarction with resultant atrophy and loss of spermiogenesis. Most cases occur in adolescent males, 50% during sleep, and are associated with congenital abnormality of the tunica vaginalis, the canal from which the testes descend. Clinical manifestations include upwardly retracted testes with redness and edema to the site of the torsion, abdominal pain, and nausea and vomiting. Figure 37-16 compares normal testicular structures with testicular torsion. Manual detorsion under local anesthesia or surgery must be performed within 48 hours or orchiectomy may be

Table 37-2	COMMON GENITOURINARY INFECTIONS			
TYPE	**DESCRIPTION**	**ADDITIONAL SIGNS AND SYMPTOMS**	**INTERVENTIONS**	**COMPLICATIONS AND COMMENTS**
Pyelonephritis	Involves renal parenchyma and pelvis Usually unilateral Kidneys enlarged by edema More prevalent in women and diabetics Most commonly caused by ascending *Escherichia coli* infection from lower GU tract		Antibiotics specific to C and S Antipyretics and antiemetics Adequate hydration Monitor intake and output Bed rest	Complications uncommon but may include septicemia Follow-up urine C and S to ensure effective antibiotic therapy Recurrence may require continuous antibiotic prophylactic suppression
Urethritis	More common in women; *E. coli* most common organism Associated behavioral factors include sexual intercourse, diaphragm and/or spermicide use, not voiding within 10-15 minutes after intercourse		Short-term antibiotics May need continuous antibiotic, prophylactic suppression, or postcoital antibiotic	Associated behaviors UTIs Direction of wiping after defecation Tampon use Bubble bath Douche Tight clothing Carbonated beverages, coffee, alcohol Resisting urge to void Decreasing PO fluids Synthetic underwear
Epididymitis	Bacterial infection in older men Usually preceded by STD or urethritis in young men	*P* lifting, sexual excitement, trauma *Q* Dull ache, sharp *R* Scrotum, lower abdomen *S* Increased with sex, decreased with elevation and support *T* Gradual onset Scrotum red, swollen, and warm	Antibiotics Posttreatment culture Bed rest Scrotal support Avoid heavy lifting and straining	Teach safe sex and condom use, complete antibiotic regimen
Prostatitis	Expressed prostate secretions have more WBCs than urine	May have bladder outlet obstruction Low back pain Tender, boggy, hot prostate on manual exam	Antibiotics, UA C and S and expressed prostate fluid C and S	
Nonspecific urethritis	Causative agents: *E. coli, Staphylococcus, Klebsiella, Pseudomonas*	White discharge Urethral itching Perineal, suprapubic, or testicular pain	Antibiotics as result of discharge C and S	

GU, Genitourinary; *C and S,* culture and sensitivity; *UTIs,* urinary tract infections; *PO,* oral; *STD,* sexually transmitted disease; *WBCs,* white blood cells; *UA,* urinalysis.

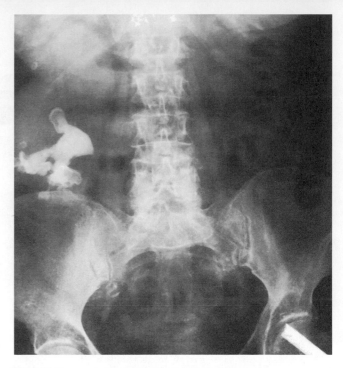

FIGURE 37-14 Radiograph of a staghorn calculus. (Courtesy Harborview Medical Center, University of Washington, Seattle.)

Table 37-3 **TYPES OF URINARY TRACT CALCULI**

URINARY STONE	INCIDENCE (%)	CHARACTERISTICS	PREDISPOSING FACTORS	THERAPEUTIC MEASURES
Calcium oxalate*	35-40	Small, often possible to get trapped in ureter; more frequent in men than in women	Idiopathic hypercalcuria, hyperoxaluria, independent of urinary pH, family history	Increase hydration. Reduce dietary oxalate. Give thiazide diuretics. Give cellulose phosphate to chelate calcium and prevent GI absorption. Give potassium citrate to maintain alkaline urine. Give cholestyramine to bind oxalate. Give calcium lactate to precipitate oxalate in GI tract.
Calcium phosphate	8-10	Mixed stones (typically), with struvite or oxalate stones	Alkaline urine, primary hyperparathyroidism	Treat underlying causes and other stones.
Struvite ($MgNH_4PO_4$)	10-15	Three to four times as common in women than men, always in association with urinary tract infections, large staghorn type (usually)	Urinary tract infections (usually *Proteus* organisms)	Administer antimicrobial agents, acetohydroxamic acid. Use surgical intervention to remove stone. Take measures to acidify urine.
Uric acid	5-8	Predominant in men, high incidence in Jewish men	Gout, acid urine, inherited condition	Reduce urinary concentration of uric acid. Alkalinize urine with potassium citrate. Administer allopurinol. Reduce dietary purines.
Cystine	1-2	Genetic autosomal recessive defect, defective absorption of cystine in GI tract and kidney, excess concentrations causing stone formation	Acid urine	Increase hydration. Give α-penicillamine and tiopronin to prevent cystine crystallization. Give potassium citrate to maintain alkaline urine.

From Lewis SM, Heitkemper MM, Dirksen SR: *Medical-surgical nursing: assessment and management of clinical problems,* ed 5, St. Louis, 2000, Mosby.

GI, Gastrointestinal.

*Calcium stones can exist as calcium oxalate, calcium phosphate, or a mixture of both. Calcium stones account for the majority of all stones.

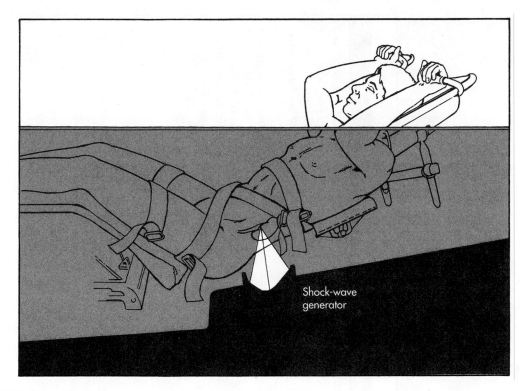

FIGURE 37-15   Patient positioned for shock-wave lithotripsy. Area of flank is exposed for efficient shock-wave conduction. (From Brundage DJ: *Renal disorders,* St. Louis, 1992, Mosby.)

necessary. Prehn's sign may be helpful in differentiating testicular torsion from epididymitis. To assess for Prehn's sign, the scrotum is gently elevated to the level of the symphysis. In testicular torsion, pain increases; however, in epididymitis, a decrease in pain is noted.

Epididymitis

Epididymitis results from inflammation of the epididymitis secondary to an STD. It is most common in sexually active males younger than age 35 years. The causative organism is most often *Chlamydia trachomatis* or *Neisseria gonorrhae.*[7] Extreme physical strain or exertion can also cause epididymitis. Signs and symptoms of epididymitis include severe scrotal pain, which can radiate into the abdomen, tenderness along the spermatic cord, edema, fever, pyuria, and possibly, urethral discharge. A positive Prehn's sign may also be observed. On laboratory assessment of the CBC, an elevated WBC count will be present, and urinalysis will reveal bacteria.

Treatment of epididymitis includes administration of antibiotics, antipyretics, and analgesics. Bed rest is indicated for approximately 3 to 4 days. A scrotal support should be worn to assist in pain relief. Sexual activity and physical strain should be avoided.

Priapism

Priapism is persistent, painful erection not associated with sexual desire. Engorgement is limited to the corpora caver-

nosa; the corpus spongiosum and glans are not involved. Obstruction of venous drainage causes build up of viscous deoxygenated blood, interstitial edema, and eventual fibrosis. Pain severity increases with duration. With urinary obstruction and bladder distention, pain can last as long as 24 hours. Etiologies include sickle cell crisis, spinal cord injury, multiple sclerosis, psychotropic drugs, or prolonged sexual activity. Priapism from use of papaverine for impotence is occurring more frequently.

Pharmacologic management of priapism includes subcutaneous terbutaline.[7] Acute detumescence is accomplished

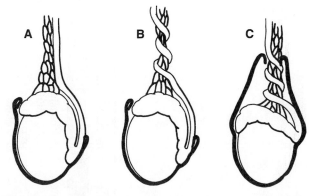

FIGURE 37-16   Testicular torsion. **A,** Normal tunica vaginalis insertion. **B,** Extravaginal torsion. **C,** Intravaginal torsion with abnormally high vaginal insertion. (From Price SA, Wilson LM: *Pathophysiology: clinical concepts of disease processes,* ed 5, St. Louis, 1997, Mosby.)

Table 37-4 COMMON SEXUALLY TRANSMITTED DISEASES

VIRUS	EPIDEMIOLOGY	CLINICAL PRESENTATION	DIAGNOSIS	TREATMENT
Herpes simplex	Most common cause of nongonococcal proctitis in sexually active homosexual men Incubation 1-12 days for first episode Recurrence in 60% of cases, usually less severe HSV1 can occur genitally but HSV2 is more common; both can occur orally	Pain, itching, dysuria, vaginal or urethral purulent discharge Classic small painful vesicles on erythematous base that may ulcer Crusting of vesicles indicates healing Lymph enlargement occurs with primary infection 33% develop meningitis	Culture lesions Serum test for virus	Acyclovir topically, orally, or IV to decrease time of viral shedding, local symptoms, and healing time 400 mg TID or 200 mg 5 times a day for 7-10 days 6-8 recurrences/year; need suppressive therapy 200 mg TID or 400 mg TID to decrease recurrence
Cytomegaly	Viral member of herpes family Primary infection followed by latency and may recur with immunosuppression Transmitted via secretions of the oropharynx, vagina, cervix, urine, breast milk, semen, and blood High prevalence in HIV-positive patients	Fever, fatigue, arthralgia, myalgia, headache, hepatitis Immunosuppressed patients may have life-threatening illness	Serum test for virus	Gancyclovir—may have increased benefit with retinitis and GI CMV
Gonorrhea	Gram-negative diplococcus bacteria Asymptomatic carriage in pharynx, urethra, rectum, and cervix common 3-5 day incubation	Urethritis in men with dysuria and mucoid drainage Endocervicitis usual form of infection in women with dysuria, frequency, abnormal discharge Anorectal infection from pruritus to proctitis Pharyngitis may occur Yellow mucopurulent drainage	Gram stain exudate on Thayer-Martin medium (prewarmed) in ED (or transported directly to lab) Resistant strains increasing in incidence	Ceftriaxone drug of choice 125-150 mg IM
Chlamydia	Intracellular parasitic infection with C. trachomatis 5-10+ days incubation period	Pelvic inflammatory disease in women Epididymitis in men Urethritis with mucopurulent drainage	Cytology of discharge	Doxycycline 100 mg BID for 7 days Erythromycin 500 mg QID for 7 days Azithromycin 1 g for one dose

Disease	Etiology/Incubation	Clinical Features	Diagnosis	Treatment
Condyloma acuminatum (venereal warts)	Incubation 3-6 months	No discharge Pink-gray soft lesions, singular or grouped Lesions are tall and may bleed		Topical 10%-25% podophyllin in tincture of benzoin OR 50% trichloroacetic acid or liquid nitrogen (treatment of choice for pregnancy)
Trichomonas vaginalis	Incubation period of 1 week	Copious, thin, frothy, greenish, gray, foul-smelling discharge Severe pruritus Edema and redness of vagina Worse following menstrual bleeding	Culture and sensitivity	Metronidazole
Gardnerella vaginalis	Incubation period 5-10 days	Fishy odor Gray, white, frothy discharge in lesser amounts than with *T. vaginalis* Mild itching	Culture and sensitivity	Metronidazole or ampicillin
Syphilis	Spirochete infection with *Treponema pallidum* Transmitted via sexual contact with moist skin lesions 3-6 weeks incubation for the primary stage (chancre) 6-8 weeks later secondary stage with disseminated bacteremia Tertiary stage if untreated with endocarditis and granuloma formation	Papule that progresses to indurated ulcer that is painless and associated with lymphadenopathy	VDRL serology Lesion culture	PCN 2.4 million units IM Doxycycline 100 mg BID for 14 days Erythromycin 500 mg PO QID for 14 days
Chancroid	Caused by *Haemophilus ducreyi* 3-14 days incubation	Acute painful ulcers that are nonindurated with nonspecific edges Inguinal tender lymphadenopathy Dysuria	Culture and gram stain of lesion	Ceftriaxone 250 mg IM for one dose Azithromycin 1 g PO for one dose Erythromycin 500 mg PO QID for 7 days Ciprofloxacine 500 mg PO BID for 3 days

HSV, Herpes simplex virus; *TID*, three times a day; *HIV*, human immunodeficiency virus; *GI*, gastrointestinal; *CMV*, cytomegalovirus; *ED*, emergency department; *BID*, two times a day; *QID*, four times a day; *PCN*, penicillin; *IM*, intramuscularly; *PO*, orally.

surgically with a large-bore needle after a regional nerve block with an adrenergic agent, such as Neosynephrine, is administered. Surgical stenting may be necessary by tissue removal to relieve obstruction or by anastomosis of veins between glans and cavernosa. CBC with increased reticulocyte count may identify sickling cells as the underlying cause, so supplemental oxygen along with transfusion may be effective. Fifty percent of cases require a urinary catheter for bladder obstruction and distention. Development of fibrosis and scarring in cavernous spaces related to the duration of priapism and decompression can cause impotence.

Sexually Transmitted Diseases

STDs spread through intimate sexual contact can present with a variety of symptoms. History should be elicited to include location, color, smell, character, and quantity of discharge. Pruritus and burning at the urethra, vagina, perineum, or pharynx can be mild to severe, and with associated lesions. Sexual activity, medical history, and date of the last menstrual period should be obtained. A pelvic examination may be performed with warm water employed as the only lubricant. A rectal examination and sigmoidoscopy may also be indicated. Diagnostic studies include C and S of lesions or drainage, VDRL, wet mount (saline and KOH), UA with C and S, and cytology smear. Along with antibiotics, discharge teaching should include abstinence until treatment is completed and lesions are healed, need for partner treatment, use of condoms, 7- to 10-day follow up, and consideration of human immunodeficiency virus testing. Complications of untreated STDs include endocarditis, arthralgias, meningitis, salpingitis, chronic pelvic inflammatory disease, severe proctitis, and sterility. Table 37-4 compares common STDs excluding acquired immunodeficiency syndrome, which is reviewed further in Chapter 40.

SUMMARY

GU emergencies require evaluation of renal function to rule out renal involvement. The GU system functions to maintain

---

> **Box 37-5 NURSING DIAGNOSES RELATED TO GENITOURINARY EMERGENCIES**
>
> Anxiety
> Electrolyte imbalance
> Fluid volume, Deficient
> Fluid volume, Excess
> Infection, Risk for
> Knowledge, Deficient
> Pain
> Tissue perfusion, Ineffective
> Urinary elimination, Impaired

homeostasis, so disruption of renal function interrupts almost all organ systems, as evidenced by the priority nursing diagnoses listed in Box 37-5. Emerging strains of resistant bacteria are challenging health care professions in treatment and prevention. Public education regarding safe sexual practice should be included in all discharge teaching for STDs. The emergency nurse has many opportunities to play an important role in the detection and prevention of GU diseases.

References

1. Carriere SR, Elsworth T: Found down: compartment syndrome, rhabdomyolysis, and renal failure, *J Emerg Nurs* 24(3):214, 1998.
2. Galejs LE: Diagnosis and treatment of the acute scrotum, *Am Fam Phys* 59(4): 817, 1999.
3. Gillenwater JY, Grayhack JT, Howards SS et al: *Adult and pediatric urology*, ed 3, St. Louis, 1996, Mosby.
4. Guyton AC, Hall J: *Textbook of medical physiology*, ed 10, Philadelphia, 2000, WB Saunders.
5. Kracun MD, Wooten CL: Crush injuries: a case of entrapment, *Crit Care Nurs Q* 21(2):81, 1998.
6. Schrier RW, Gottschalk CW: *Diseases of the kidney*, ed 6, Boston, 1997, Little, Brown.
7. Tanagho EA, McAninch JW: *Smith's general urology*, ed 14, Norwalk,1995, Appleton & Lange.

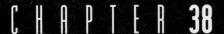
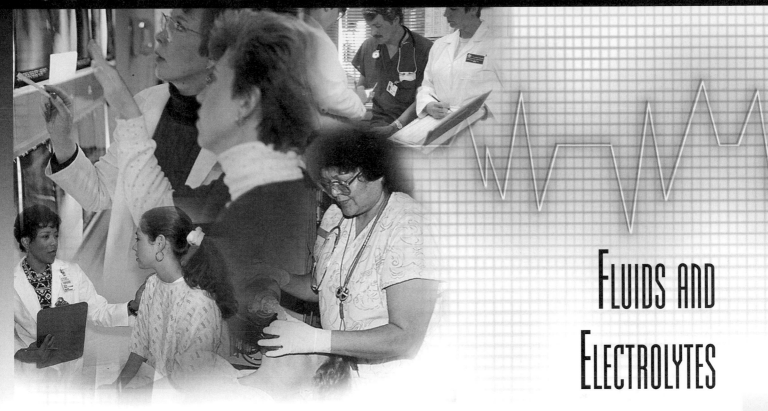

CHAPTER 38

FLUIDS AND ELECTROLYTES

KIMBERLY A. WOMACK

Water is the most abundant fluid medium in the body, composing 60% of total body weight for the average adult, 80% in an infant, and as little as 40% in an elderly adult (Figure 38-1).[5] In a healthy physiologic state this fluid medium has a constant balance of electrolytes controlled by a unique system of checks and balances. Effects of fluid and electrolyte disturbances are often a primary or secondary reason for many emergency department (ED) visits. Gastrointestinal, urologic, cardiac, respiratory, and endocrine diseases and many forms of traumatic injury cause fluid and electrolyte abnormalities.

This chapter describes the interrelation of water, water metabolism, and electrolyte composition. Fluid and electrolyte control mechanisms, signs and symptoms, etiology, and treatment of specific fluid and electrolyte abnormalities are discussed.

PATHOPHYSIOLOGY

Water and electrolytes are interdependent. Pathophysiology of one affects function and value of the other. Normal fluid and electrolyte levels are the result of structural, physiologic, and environmental factors.

Water

Water has many important metabolic functions, including transport of nutrients and other essential substances, removal of metabolic waste products, normal cellular metabolism, and maintenance of normal body temperature. Age, weight, body fat, and environmental factors such as ambient temperature determine individual fluid requirements. Fat is virtually water free; therefore, increases in body fat are associated with decreases in body water. The average adult ingests 1500 to 3000 ml of water per day through the gastrointestinal tract.[1] Water intake attributed to oxidation of hydrogen in food is approximately 150 to 250 ml/day, depending on individual metabolic rate. Water output is dependent on factors such as ambient temperature and activity level. An average resting adult in an ambient temperature of 68° F loses approximately 1400 ml of water per day in urine, 100 ml in sweat, 100 ml in feces, and 700 ml in insensible water loss. Conditions such as vomiting, diarrhea, denuding of skin (i.e., burns), increased ambient temperature, or intense physical exercise significantly increase water loss.

Total body water (TBW) is distributed between extracellular and intracellular compartments. Extracellular fluid (ECF) constitutes one third of TBW, or approximately 15 L.

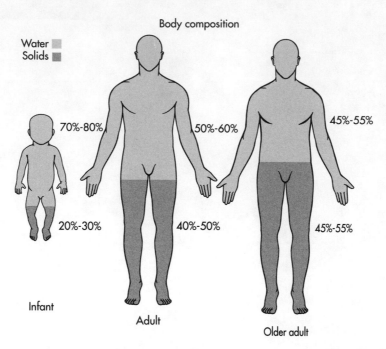

Body composition

Water ▢
Solids ▢

70%-80%   50%-60%   45%-55%

20%-30%   40%-50%   45%-55%

Infant   Adult   Older adult

FIGURE 38-1   Changes in body water content correlated with age. (From Lewis SM, Heitkemper MM, Dirksen SR: *Medical-surgical nursing: assessment and management of clinical problems,* ed 5, St. Louis, 2000, Mosby.)

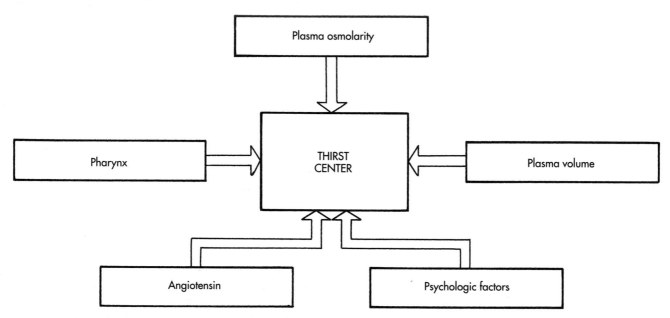

FIGURE 38-2   Stimuli affecting the thirst mechanism. (Modified from Groer MW: *Physiology and pathophysiology of the body fluids,* St. Louis, 1981, Mosby.)

Plasma, interstitial fluid, cerebrospinal fluid, intraocular fluid, fluids of the gastrointestinal tract, and fluids of potential spaces (i.e., pleural space, peritoneal space) are examples of ECF. Intracellular fluid (ICF) accounts for two thirds of TBW and represents the sum of fluid content for all the cells in the body, approximately 25 L.

Two regulatory mechanisms influential in maintaining normal water volume and tonicity or osmotic pressure are thirst and renal function. Thirst, the primary regulator for intake of water, is defined as the "conscious desire for water."

Thirst ensures adequate replacement of fluid losses and is stimulated by ECF hypertonicity and decreased ICF volume. Conversely, thirst is depressed by ECF hypotonicity and increased ICF volume. Any factor that causes intracellular dehydration stimulates a small area in the hypothalamus called the thirst center and promotes water consumption. Figure 38-2 illustrates stimuli that affect the thirst mechanism. Because the thirst mechanism is triggered by increased osmolarity, thirst is not effective in hypotonic or hyponatremic dehydration, in which water and sodium loss are equal. Factors

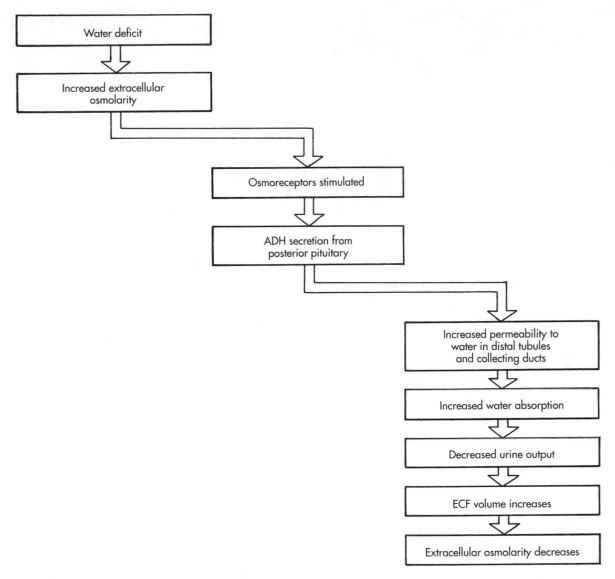

FIGURE **38-3** Osmoreceptor-antidiuretic hormone (ADH) feedback mechanism for regulating osmolarity in response to water deficit. *ECF,* Extracellular fluid.

that adversely affect the thirst mechanism include brain injury and psychosocial factors such as depression, confusion, and fear of incontinence.

Renal regulation of water balance is twofold, affecting both tonicity and body water. When glomerular filtrate is hypertonic, osmoreceptors in the hypothalamus are stimulated, and antidiuretic hormone (ADH) is released by the pituitary gland. ADH makes renal collecting tubules more permeable to water, so water is reabsorbed into the body, diluting blood and concentrating urine (Figure 38-3). If plasma or glomerular filtrate is hypotonic, ADH secretion is inhibited and collecting tubules reabsorb less water. Blood becomes concentrated and the urine is diluted as more water exits the kidneys.

The kidneys, through the renin-angiotensin-aldosterone system (Figure 38-4), regulate volume of body water. When ECF volume, specifically blood volume, is low, receptors in the kidneys secrete an enzyme called renin. Renin stimulates angiotensinogen (a normal plasma protein) to release angiotensin I, which is then converted to angiotensin II by an-

other enzyme, primarily in the lungs. Angiotensin II stimulates the adrenal cortex to secrete aldosterone, which increases sodium reabsorption from glomerular filtrate in exchange for potassium and hydrogen ions. This exchange increases plasma tonicity, which leads to ADH secretion, water retention, and increased volume. With excessive ECF volume (blood volume), aldosterone secretion is depressed so tubular reabsorption of sodium and water decreases (Figure 38-5).

Electrolytes

An electrolyte is a substance capable of carrying an electrical charge. An electrolyte with a positive charge is called a cation, whereas an electrolyte with a negative charge is an anion.[7] Electrolytes are found in varying concentrations in ECF and ICF (Figure 38-6). For the purposes of this chapter, serum electrolyte measurements are equivalent to extracellular electrolyte values (Table 38-1). Direct measurement of intracellular electrolyte concentrations in the clinical set-

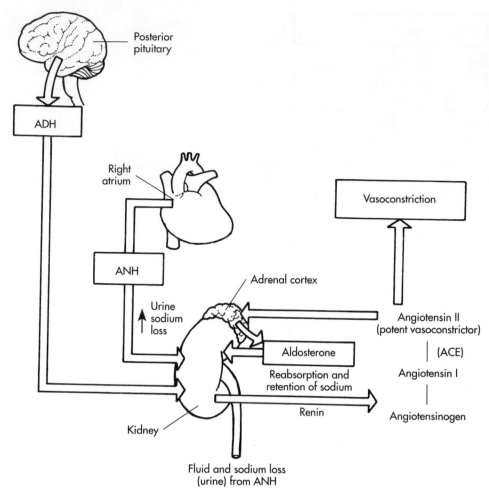

FIGURE 38-4   Renin-angiotensin-aldosterone system. *ADH,* Antidiuretic hormone; *ANH,* atrial natriuretic hormone; *ACE,* angiotensin-converting enzyme. (From Huether SE, McCance KL: *Understanding pathophysiology,* St. Louis, 1996, Mosby.)

ting is not yet feasible, so ICF electrolyte concentrations must be inferred from serum electrolyte values.

All fluids outside the cells are collectively referred to as the ECF. Electrolytes in the ECF, from greatest to least concentration, are sodium, chloride, potassium, bicarbonate, and hydrogen. ECF also contains oxygen, carbon dioxide, proteins, and a few miscellaneous anions.

ICF represents fluid found in approximately 75 trillion cells in the body, about 25 L. Electrolytes in the ICF, from greatest to least concentration, are potassium, phosphate, and sulphate combined; magnesium; and last sodium, hydrogen, and bicarbonate in equal concentrations. The ICF also contains a number of proteins.

The delicate balance of water and electrolytes between intracellular and extracellular compartments is an ongoing process of checks and balances easily disturbed by disease or injury. Regulatory processes and the role of each electrolyte are described in the following sections.

Sodium

Sodium, the principal cation in ECF, is primarily responsible for osmotic pressure. Forty percent of the body's sodium

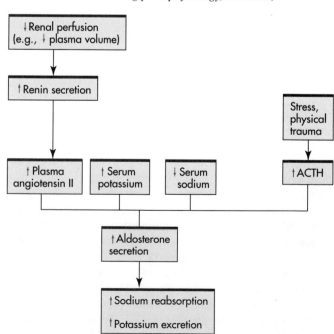

FIGURE 38-5   Influences of aldosterone secretion. (From Lewis SM, Heitkemper MM, Dirksen SR: *Medical-surgical nursing: assessment and management of clinical problems,* ed 5, St. Louis, 2000, Mosby.) *ACTH,* adrenocorticotropic hormone.

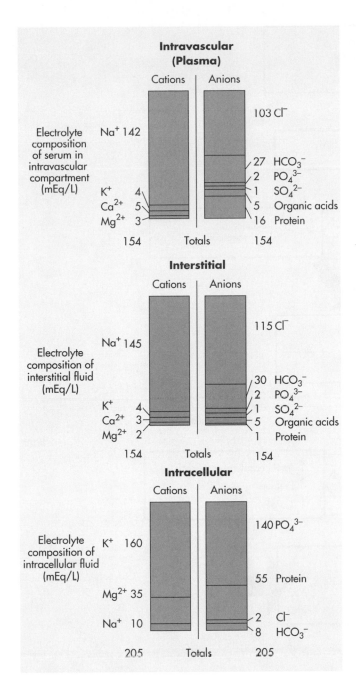

FIGURE **38-6** Electrolyte content of fluid compartments. (From Lewis SM, Heitkemper MM, Dirksen SR: *Medical-surgical nursing: assessment and management of clinical problems,* ed 5, St. Louis, 2000, Mosby.)

Table 38-1	NORMAL SERUM ELECTROLYTE VALUES
ANIONS	**NORMAL VALUE**
Bicarbonate (HCO_3^-)	20-30 mEq/L (20-30 mmol/L)
Chloride (Cl^-)	96-106 mEq/L (96-106 mmol/L)
Phosphate (PO_4^{3-})	2.8-4.5 mg/dl (0.90-1.45 mmol/L)
Protein	6-8 g/dl (60-80 g/L)
CATIONS	**NORMAL VALUE**
Potassium (K^+)	3.5-5.5 mEq/L (3.5-5.5 mmol/L)
Magnesium (Mg^+)	1.5-2.5 mEq/L (0.75-1.25 mmol/L)
Sodium (Na^+)	135-145 mEq/L (135-145 mmol/L)
Calcium (Ca^+) (total)	4.5-5.5 mEq/L (2.25-2.75 mmol/L)
Calcium (ionized)	4.5-5.5 mg/dl (1.13-1.38 mmol/L)

From Lewis SM, Heitkemper MM, Dirksen SR: *Medical-surgical nursing: assessment and management of clinical problems,* ed 5, St. Louis, 2000, Mosby.

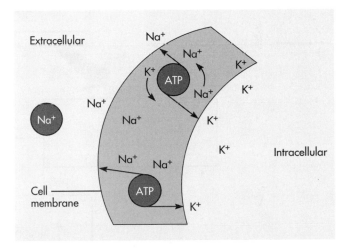

FIGURE **38-7** Sodium-potassium pump. As sodium diffuses into the cell and potassium out of the cell, an active transport system supplied with energy delivers sodium back to the extracellular compartment and potassium to the intracellular compartment. *ATP,* Adenosine triphosphate. (From Lewis SM, Heitkemper MM, Dirksen SR: *Medical-surgical nursing: assessment and management of clinical problems,* ed 5, St. Louis, 2000, Mosby.)

is in blood and ECF; the remainder is intracellular and in bone and connective tissue. Sodium is exchangeable across cell membranes to maintain sodium and water balance and normal arterial pressure. Sodium and chloride play an important role in maintaining body water; movement of glucose, insulin, and amino acids across cell membranes; and maintaining muscle strength, neural function, and urinary output. Sodium is essential for the sodium-potassium pump, which moves sodium and potassium across the cell membrane during repolarization (Figure 38-7).

Sodium levels are maintained through the renin-angiotensin-aldosterone system, sympathetic nervous system, and a less well-defined system mediated by atrial natriuretic factor. Decreased fluid volume decreases blood flow and arterial pressure, which stimulates baroreceptors in the kidneys (Figure 38-8). Baroreceptors stimulate the sympathetic nervous system, which leads to vasoconstriction of renal arterioles, decreased glomerular filtration rate, and retention of sodium and water. The opposite sequence of events occurs when fluid intake (or blood volume) rises above normal.

Atrial natriuretic hormone (ANH), released from the atria in response to increased arterial pressure, produces

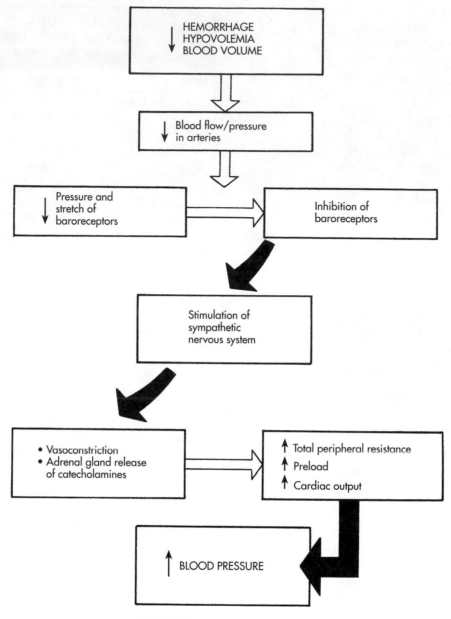

FIGURE 38-8   Baroreceptor response.

natriuresis (excretion of abnormal amounts of sodium in the urine), diuresis, vasodilation, decreased thirst, and antagonistic effects on ADH release, renin, and aldosterone.[3] The resulting increase in sodium excretion eliminates excess volume.

Chloride

Chloride, the principal anion of blood and ECF, is secreted in various body fluids along with other electrolytes. Sodium and chloride are excreted in sweat, bile, pancreatic fluids, and intestinal fluids. Gastric juice contains chloride and hydrogen. As with sodium, chloride plays a cooperative role in maintaining acid-base balance and takes part in the exchange of oxygen and carbon dioxide in red blood cells.[7]

Serum chloride levels are passively regulated by serum sodium levels. When serum sodium increases, serum chloride also increases. However, chloride levels are inversely related to bicarbonate levels because chloride is sacrificed in the kidneys to produce more bicarbonate.

Potassium

Potassium is the most abundant cation in the body, with 98% in the intracellular space and 2% in the extracellular space. Potassium is primarily responsible for cell membrane potential and is the counterpart to sodium in the sodium-potassium pump. Potassium governs cell osmolality and volume and is secreted in sweat, gastric juice, pancreatic juice, bile, and fluids of the small intestine.

Potassium level is primarily controlled through secretion of potassium by the distal and collecting tubules in the kidney. Potassium secretion increases in response to increased ECF potassium concentration, aldosterone levels, and distal tubular flow. A rise in ECF potassium stimulates the sodium-potassium pump located in the renal tubules. This pump maintains a low intracellular sodium concentration through exchange of potassium across the cell membrane. Increased extracellular potassium also triggers aldosterone secretion by the adrenal cortex. Aldosterone increases the rate at which tubular cells secrete potassium and permeability of the renal tubular lumen for potassium. This is a negative feedback system regulated by the serum potassium level. Finally, increased distal tubular flow causes rapid secretion of potassium into the urine.

Alkalosis temporarily decreases serum potassium by driving potassium into the cells in exchange for hydrogen ions.[7] Conversely, the major factor that decreases potassium secretion and increases serum potassium is acute acidosis. Acute acidosis increases hydrogen ion concentration in the ECF, so potassium moves out of the cell in exchange for excess hydrogen ions.

Calcium

Approximately 99% of the body's calcium is found in bone, with 1% in ICF and 0.1% in ECF. Bone acts as a large reservoir for calcium when ECF calcium levels fall. Calcium is transported in the blood in two forms. Half is bound to plasma proteins, usually albumin, and the rest exists as an ionized form that is free and metabolically active. A small amount of nonionized calcium forms complexes with anions such as phosphate, citrate, and sulfate. Most ionized calcium is found in the ECF. Because of the large amount of calcium bound to plasma proteins, assessment of total serum calcium without simultaneous measurement of serum proteins has limited value in determining hypo- or hypercalcemia.

Calcium has many important functions—smooth and skeletal muscle contraction, bone and brain metabolism, blood clotting, and as a primary ingredient in lung surfactant. Calcium is essential for membrane polarization and depolarization, action potential generation, neurotransmission, and muscle contraction. Calcium channels in myocardial cells allow transmembrane calcium transport.

The most important regulatory factors for calcium homeostasis are parathyroid hormone (PTH), calcitonin, and vitamin D. When ECF calcium falls below normal levels, parathyroid glands release PTH, which acts directly on bones to stimulate the release of large amounts of calcium into ECF. With an elevated calcium ion concentration, PTH secretion decreases, so excess calcium is deposited into bones.

Bones rely on proper intake and absorption of calcium to maintain calcium stores. Calcium absorption in the gastrointestinal tract and kidneys is regulated by PTH levels. In hypocalcemic states PTH activates vitamin D_3, the form of vitamin D necessary to increase intestinal calcium reabsorption. PTH also directly stimulates the kidneys to increase renal tubular calcium reabsorption, which prevents loss of calcium in the urine.

Another factor that influences calcium reabsorption is plasma concentration of phosphate. Serum calcium levels are inversely related to serum phosphate levels. Increases in plasma phosphate stimulate PTH, which increases calcium reabsorption by renal tubules and reduces calcium loss in the urine.

The thyroid gland secretes a hormone called calcitonin in response to elevated calcium levels. The effect of calcitonin on plasma calcium levels is directly opposite that of PTH. Calcitonin decreases plasma calcium levels by increasing calcium deposits in bone and decreasing formation of new osteoclasts, the cells responsible for breakdown and removal of bone. Calcitonin also has minor effects on calcium absorption in the renal tubules and gastrointestinal tract.

Phosphate/Phosphorus

Phosphorus, the major anion in the ICF, is essential for metabolism of carbohydrate, lipids, and protein. Phosphate also plays a role in hormonal activities and acid-base balance and has a close relationship to calcium in maintaining homeostasis. Clinical studies have shown that changing the phosphate level in ECF far below or far above normal levels does not cause immediate effects on the body. However, even minute increases or decreases in calcium ions in ECF cause significant physiologic effects.

Renal tubules maintain a normal phosphate level by an "overflow" mechanism. When the phosphate level in the glomerular filtrate falls below this set level, essentially all filtered phosphate is reabsorbed. When extra phosphate is present in the glomerular filtrate, excess phosphate is excreted in the urine.

PTH also plays a significant role in phosphate regulation. When PTH is present bones dump phosphate salts and calcium into the ECF. PTH then stimulates the kidneys to dump more phosphate into the urine.

Magnesium

Magnesium is the second most important intracellular cation. More than half the body's magnesium is stored in bones, with the rest in cells, particularly muscle. Only a small fraction of the body's magnesium is found in the ECF. Magnesium is involved in numerous biochemical processes in the body, so normal concentrations must be carefully maintained. Although the exact mechanism is unclear, magnesium excretion is probably regulated by altering renal tubular reabsorption. With excess magnesium, renal tubules allow excretion of extra magnesium in the urine. In magnesium depletion, renal excretion dramatically decreases.

FLUID AND ELECTROLYTE ABNORMALITIES

Imbalances in fluid and electrolytes may be due to physiologic abnormalities, injury, or stress (Figure 38-9). Fluid and electrolyte levels are closely related. For example, sodium

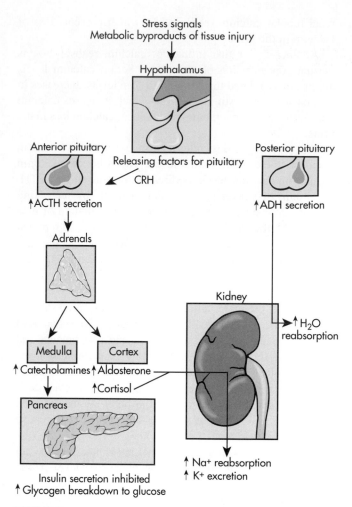

Stress signals
Metabolic byproducts of tissue injury

Hypothalamus

Anterior pituitary

Releasing factors for pituitary
CRH

Posterior pituitary

↑ACTH secretion

↑ADH secretion

Adrenals

Kidney

↑H₂O reabsorption

Medulla   Cortex

↑Catecholamines ↑Aldosterone

↑Cortisol

Pancreas

↑ Na⁺ reabsorption
↑ K⁺ excretion

Insulin secretion inhibited
↑ Glycogen breakdown to glucose

FIGURE 38-9   Effects of stress on fluid and electrolyte balance. *ACTH,* Adrenocorticotropic hormone; *ADH,* antidiuretic hormone; *CRH,* corticotropin-releasing hormone. (From Lewis SM, Heitkemper MM, Dirksen SR: *Medical-surgical nursing: assessment and management of clinical problems,* ed 5, St. Louis, 2000, Mosby.)

BOX 38-1	CAUSES OF ECF VOLUME IMBALANCES
ECF VOLUME DEFICIT	**ECF VOLUME EXCESS**
Increased loss	**Increased retention**
Vomiting	Congestive heart failure
Diarrhea	Cushing's syndrome
Fistula drainage	Chronic liver disease with
GI tract suction	portal hypertension
Excessive sweating	Long-term use of corti-
Third-space fluid shifts (e.g.,	costeroids
burns, intestinal obstruction)	Renal failure
Overuse of diuretics	
Hemorrhage	
Decreased intake	**Increased intake**
Nausea	Rare with adequate renal
Anorexia	function
Inability to drink	Excessive IV administration
Inability to obtain water	of fluids

From Lewis SM, Heitkemper MM, Dirksen SR: *Medical-surgical nursing: assessment and management of clinical problems,* ed 5, St. Louis, 2000, Mosby.
ECF, Extracellular fluid; *GI,* gastrointestinal; *IV,* intravenous.

losses are almost always associated with water losses, just as sodium retention is associated with water excess.

Fluid and electrolyte therapy has three objectives—maintain daily requirements, restore previous losses, and prevent further losses. Oral electrolyte replacement is preferred. However, most patients who present to the ED with vomiting, diarrhea, and other fluid losses can no longer treat losses orally. Treatment of electrolyte abnormalities focuses on slowly restoring previous balance and carefully correcting the underlying cause. Electrolyte levels, hydration, and cardiovascular, renal, and neurologic function should be carefully monitored.

Water Abnormalities

Water abnormalities may be due to underlying disease, iatrogenic causes, environmental factors, or psychologic abnormalities (Box 38-1). Determining the cause should occur concurrently with fluid replacement. Table 38-2 describes specific fluid imbalances.

Water Depletion

Water depletion may be due to reduced water consumption, diarrhea, vomiting, excessive sweating, excessive respiration, renal disease, ADH deficiency (i.e., diabetes insipidus) excessive diuretic use, and diabetic ketoacidosis (DKA). Water deficiency is almost always associated with loss of sodium. True water deficiency without concurrent sodium loss is rarely seen in the ED.

Signs and symptoms of water deficiency include thirst, loss of eyeball and skin turgor, dry mucous membranes, flushed skin, decreased urinary output, increased urine-specific gravity, increased temperature, tachycardia, delirium, and coma. Most patients with water deficiency are also deficient in sodium and other electrolytes, so oral or parenteral fluid replacement must be determined on an individual basis. Frequently selected fluids to replenish water and sodium loss include normal saline (0.9%) and hypotonic half-normal saline (0.45%). Serial electrolyte and plasma osmolarity levels are required to determine appropriate fluid replacement. With true water depletion and normal serum sodium, 5% dextrose in water (D₅W) may be used.[1] Table 38-3 describes various crystalloids used for fluid replacement.

Water Excess

Water excess is characterized by weight gain, muscle twitching and cramps, pulmonary and peripheral edema, hyperventilation, confusion, hallucination, coma, and convulsions. Water excess may be due to increased water ingestion,

Table 38-2	FLUID IMBALANCES		
IMBALANCE	**CLINICAL SIGNS AND SYMPTOMS**	**THERAPY**	**PRECURSORS**
Dehydration	Thirst; anxiety; weight loss; poor skin turgor; slow vein filling; elevated temperature; tachycardia; dry mucous membranes; decreased level of consciousness; and increased hematocrit, level of blood urea nitrogen, and red blood cell concentration	Volume replacement	Any condition in which water output exceeds intake; vomiting, diarrhea
Edema	Weight gain exceeding 5%, rales, dyspnea, puffy eyelids, swollen ankles, bounding pulse	Salt-poor albumin, exchange resins, diuretics	Protein deficiency, venous obstruction, heart failure, obstructed lymphatic system, toxin ingestion, liver disease, renal disease
Third space syndrome	Hypotension, tachycardia, peripheral vasoconstriction, oliguria, no weight loss, increased hematocrit with no evidence of fluid loss	Plasma, salts, water replacement, diuretics, paracentesis, thoracentesis	Ascites, cellulitis, crush injuries, vascular occlusion intestinal obstructions

excessive intravenous therapy, renal disease, excess ADH, and inadequate water transport to the kidney (e.g., shock, congestive heart failure).[8]

Treatment includes fluid restriction, with some patients limited to 1000 ml or less per day. In clinical emergencies, hypertonic saline may be used, followed by a diuretic such as furosemide to eliminate excess salt and water. If water excess is due to compulsive water consumption, psychiatric evaluation is recommended as soon as the patient's condition permits.

Electrolyte Abnormalities

Electrolyte abnormalities may be caused by an underlying disease or may be the result of starvation, therapeutic drugs, drug overdose, or other iatrogenic cause (Table 38-4). Electrolyte abnormalities are almost always associated with some degree of neuromuscular dysfunction (Table 38-5). Cardiac abnormalities are another common occurrence with many electrolyte abnormalities (Table 38-6).

Anion Gap

The balance between positive and negative electrolytes is measured by calculating the anion gap (Box 38-2). This measurement is particularly useful in determining whether metabolic acidosis is due to acid excess or bicarbonate loss. Normal anion gap is 12 ± 4.[1] Abnormalities in the anion gap may be due to a change in unmeasured anions or cations or an error in measurement of sodium, chloride, or bicarbonate.

An anion gap greater than 16 is associated with increased acids, as seen in DKA, alcoholic ketoacidosis, uremic acidosis, dehydration, salicylate intoxication, GI fistula, and renal failure. A normal anion gap is seen in diarrhea, renal tubular acidosis, Addison's disease, and metabolic acidosis caused by diuretics. Albumin administration causes a falsely elevated anion gap.[4] A decreased anion gap may be due to error in electrolyte measurement.

Sodium Abnormalities

Sodium and chloride travel together across most membranes, so sodium abnormalities are usually associated with chloride abnormalities. For the purpose of this discussion, abnormalities are described separately. Clinical manifestations of sodium abnormalities and various causes are presented in Table 38-7.

Hyponatremia. Hyponatremia is probably the most common electrolyte imbalance seen in the clinical arena. Hyponatremia is characterized by vague signs and symptoms, so diagnosis can rarely be made from clinical evaluation. Clinical manifestations are due to decreased osmolarity and cerebral edema and include anorexia, nausea, weakness, confusion, agitation, and disorientation. As serum sodium falls below 110 mEq/L, seizures, coma, or death can occur.

Mild hyponatremia does not require treatment. If the primary cause of hyponatremia is fluid imbalance, normal saline is the treatment of choice. In severe symptomatic hyponatremia, hypertonic (3%) saline solution may be cautiously administered, usually 250 ml or less, with an infusion pump.[2] The patient should be carefully monitored for fluid overload secondary to sodium replacement. Furosemide may be administered concurrently to reduce the likelihood of fluid overload. Any potassium deficits that occur as a result of treatment should be corrected.

Hypernatremia. Hypernatremia is a significant risk for infants, the elderly, and the debilitated because of their inability to independently replace fluid losses. Clinical signs and symptoms are similar to those seen with hyponatremia but are secondary to hyperosmolarity and cellular dehydration. The patient is thirsty and appears dehydrated. Early symptoms include anorexia, nausea, and vomiting. As serum sodium rises above 160 mEq/L, neurologic symptoms such as agitation, irritability, lethargy, coma, muscle twitching, and hyperreflexia may occur. Intracranial hemorrhages can result from shrunken brain tissue or engorged vasculature.

Treatment of sodium excess focuses on restoring normal fluid volume and osmolarity. Fluid replacement is the first step when hypovolemia is the cause of sodium excess. The patient initially requires administration of normal saline until the blood pressure stabilizes.[2] Treatment is followed by half-normal saline solution. Patients with

Table 38-3 COMPOSITION AND USE OF COMMONLY PRESCRIBED CRYSTALLOID SOLUTIONS

SOLUTION	TONICITY	mOsm/L (MMOL/L)	GLUCOSE (G/L)	INDICATIONS AND CONSIDERATIONS
DEXTROSE IN WATER				
5%	Isotonic	278	50	• Provides free water necessary for renal excretion of solutes • Used to replace water losses and treat hypernatremia • Provides 170 calories/L • Does not provide any electrolytes
10%	Hypertonic	556	100	• Provides free water only, no electrolytes • Provides 340 calories/L
SALINE				
0.45%	Hypotonic	154	0	• Provides free water in addition to Na^+ and Cl^- • Used to replace hypotonic fluid losses • Used as maintenance solution although it does not replace daily losses of other electrolytes • Provides no calories
0.9%	Isotonic	308	0	• Used to expand intravascular volume and replace extracellular fluid losses • Only solution that may be administered with blood products • Contains Na^+ and Cl^- in excess of plasma levels • Does not provide free water, calories, other electrolytes • May cause intravascular overload or hyperchloremic acidosis
3.0%	Hypertonic	1026	0	• Used to treat symptomatic hyponatremia • Must be administered slowly and with extreme caution because it may cause dangerous intravascular volume overload and pulmonary edema
DEXTROSE IN SALINE				
5% in 0.225%	Isotonic	355	50	• Provides Na^+, Cl^-, and free water • Used to replace hypotonic losses and treat hypernatremia • Provides 170 calories/L
5% in 0.45%	Hypertonic	432	50	• Same as 0.45% NaCl except provides 170 calories/L
5% in 0.9%	Hypertonic	586	50	• Same as 0.9% NaCl except provides 170 calories/L
MULTIPLE ELECTROLYTE SOLUTIONS RINGER'S SOLUTION	Isotonic	309	0	• Similar in composition to plasma except that it has excess Cl^-, no Mg^{++}, and no HCO_3^- • Does not provide free water or calories • Used to expand the intravascular volume and replace extracellular fluid losses
LACTATED RINGER'S (HARTMANN'S) SOLUTION	Isotonic	274	0	• Similar in composition to normal plasma except does not contain Mg^{++} • Used to treat losses from burns and lower gastrointestinal tract • May be used to treat mild metabolic acidosis but should not be used to treat lactic acidosis • Does not provide free water or calories

From Lewis SM, Heitkemper MM, Dirksen SR: *Medical-surgical nursing: assessment and management of clinical problems,* ed 5, St. Louis, 2000, Mosby.

pure water loss should receive oral hydration, intravenous D_5W, or hypotonic saline. Normovolemic patients with hypernatremia should receive D_5W and furosemide.[2] In all cases slow correction of the imbalance is essential to avoid neurologic problems such as cerebral edema and seizures.

Chloride Abnormalities

Chloride abnormalities rarely occur independently but usually occur in conjunction with sodium or potassium abnormalities.

Hypochloremia. Hypochloremia occurs in conjunction with hyponatremia and may also be seen with hyperkalemia caused by excretion of potassium chloride. Symptoms of chloride deficiency are basically the same as hyponatremia with the additional problems of profound muscle weakness, twitching, tetany, slow shallow respirations, and respiratory arrest. Treatment includes chloride and sodium replacement with careful monitoring of serum levels to determine effectiveness.

Hyperchloremia. Hyperchloremia produces all the signs and symptoms seen with hypernatremia but also causes deep, labored breathing. Causes of hyperchloremia are the same factors that cause hypernatremia, with two exceptions:

ammonium chloride ingestion and salicylate intoxication cause hyperchloremia but do not affect serum sodium. Treatment of hyperchloremia is essentially the same as for hypernatremia.

Potassium Abnormalities

Potassium is subject to multiple influences within the body. Alkalosis, aldosterone, insulin, and β2-agonists drive potas-

Table 38-4	IATROGENIC ELECTROLYTE ABNORMALITIES	
CAUSE	**EFFECT ON ELECTROLYTES**
Diuretic therapy	Hyponatremia, hypochloremia, hypokalemia, hypomagnesemia, elevated serum proteins, normal or elevated HCO_3^-
Starvation	Normal potassium or hyperkalemia, normal elevated H^-, decreased HCO_3^-, decreased protein, normal or decreased pH
Milk-alkali syndrome*	Hypokalemia, hypocalcemia, elevated HCO_3^-, hypercalcemia, elevated pH
Salicylate intoxication	Normal sodium or hypernatremia; hyperchloremia; normal potassium or hypokalemia; decreased HCO_3^-; early pH elevation, which later drops; early decrease in H^-, followed by increased H^-
Barbiturate intoxication	Hypochloremia, elevated H^-, elevated HCO_3^-, decreased pH, increased pCO_2

*Syndrome caused by ingestion of large amounts of nonabsorbable antacids such as calcium carbonate with or without milk.
pCO_2, Carbon dioxide pressure.

Table 38-6	ECG CHANGES ASSOCIATED WITH ELECTROLYTE ABNORMALITIES	
ELECTROLYTE ABNORMALITY	**ECG CHANGES**
Hypokalemia	Flattened or inverted T waves, depressed ST segment, U waves, ventricular ectopy
Hyperkalemia	Tall, peaked T waves; widened QRS complexes; prolonged PR interval; loss of P waves; sine wave or biphasic tracing; dysrhythmias including sinus bradycardia, sinus arrest, first degree heart block, nodal rhythm, idioventricular rhythm, ventricular fibrillation, and rarely asystole
Hypocalcemia	Prolonged QT interval
Hypercalcemia	Shortened QT interval
Hypomagnesemia	Torsades de pointes, ventricular tachycardia, ventricular fibrillation
Hypermagnesemia	Heart block, asystole

ECG, Electrocardiogram.

Box 38-2	ANION GAP CALCULATION
Anion gap $= Na^+ - (Cl^- + HCO_3^-)$	

Table 38-5	NEUROMUSCULAR MANIFESTATIONS OF ELECTROLYTE ABNORMALITIES								
	HYPO-KALEMIA	**HYPER-KALEMIA**	**HYPO-PHOSPHATEMIA**	**HYPO-MAGNESEMIA**	**HYPER-MAGNESEMIA**	**HYPO-CALCEMIA**	**HYPER-CALCEMIA**	**HYPO-NATREMIA**	**HYPER-NATREMIA**
Weakness	++	+	++	+	+	+	++	+	+
Paralysis	+	+	−	−	+	−	−	−	−
Myalgias	+	−	+	+	−	+	−	−	+
Fasciculations	+	+	+	+	−	+	−	+	−
Cramps	+	−	−	+	−	+	−	+	+
Restless legs	+	−	−	−	−	−	−	−	−
Tetany	−	−	−	+*	−	+	−	−	−
Myotonia	−	+†	−	−	−	−	−	−	−
Areflexia	+	+	+	−	−	−	−	−	−
Hyperreflexia	−	+	−	+	−	+	+	+	+
Choreoathetosis	−	−	−	+	−	−	−	−	−
Rhabdomyolysis	+	−	+	+‡	−	−	−	+|	+

From Knochel JP: Neuromuscular manifestations of electrolyte disorders, *Am J Med* 72:521, 1982.
*Indefinite, may be due to associated hypocalcemia.
†Myotonia may occur in familial hyperkalemic periodic paralysis.
‡Experimental animals (dog, rat) only.
|Biochemical evidence only (creatine phosphokinase increase, creatinuria).

sium into the cell, whereas acidosis and hyperosmolarity cause potassium to leave the cell.[1] Table 38-8 highlights the causes and clinical manifestations of potassium abnormalities. Potassium abnormalities are almost always associated with electrocardiogram (ECG) changes, which may or may not correlate with severity (Figure 38-10).

Hypokalemia. Hypokalemia is characterized by muscle weakness, cramps, paralysis, hyporeflexia, paralytic ileus, paresthesia, latent tetany, cardiac dysrhythmias, and hyposthenuria (inability to form urine with a high specific gravity).[8] Muscle weakness is usually more pronounced in the lower extremities and proximal muscle groups. Respiratory muscle weakness may lead to respiratory failure and arrest. Rhabdomyolysis may also occur. ECG changes such as flattened or inverted T waves and U waves do not correlate well with clinical severity (see Figure 38-10). Ventricular ectopy is the most common dysrhythmia. Hypokalemia is the result of decreased potassium intake or shifts of potassium from the ECF to the cells. Vomiting, diarrhea, intestinal obstruction, gastrointestinal suctioning, renal insufficiency, nephritis, DKA, diuretics, aldosteronism, Cushing's syndrome, and steroid therapy are all associated with hypokalemia.

Treatment is recommended when potassium is lower than 3.5 mEq/L. Potassium chloride is administered at 10 to 30 mEq/hr over 3 to 4 hours through a large-bore peripheral or central intravenous catheter.[9] An infusion pump is recommended when the entire amount of potassium in the intravenous bag exceeds 40 mEq. Potassium is extremely irritating to the veins, so concentration infused through peripheral veins should not exceed 80 mEq/250 ml with the rate less

Table 38-7	**WATER AND SODIUM IMBALANCES: CAUSES AND CLINICAL MANIFESTATIONS**	
WATER EXCESS/HYPONATREMIA ($Na^+ < 135$ MEQ/L [MMOL/L])	**WATER DEFICIT/HYPERNATREMIA** ($Na^+ > 145$ MEQ/L [MMOL/L])	
CAUSES		
Sodium loss	**Water loss**	
GI losses: Diarrhea, vomiting, fistulas, gastric suction	Increased insensible water loss or perspiration (high fever, heat-stroke)	
Renal losses: Diuretics, adrenal insufficiency, Na^+ wasting, renal disease	Diabetes insipidus	
Skin losses: Burns, wound drainage	Osmotic diuresis	
Water gain	**Sodium gain**	
SIADH	IV hypertonic NaCl	
Congestive heart failure	IV sodium bicarbonate	
Excessive hypotonic IV fluids	IV excessive isotonic NaCl	
Primary polydipsia	Primary aldosteronism	
	Saltwater near drowning	
CLINICAL MANIFESTATIONS		
Decreased ECF volume (sodium loss)	**Decreased ECF volume (water loss)**	
Irritability, apprehension, confusion	Intense thirst, dry, swollen tongue	
Postural hypotension	Restlessness, agitation, twitching	
Tachycardia	Seizures, coma	
Rapid, thready pulse	Weakness	
Decreased CVP	Postural hypotension, decreased CVP	
Decreased jugular venous filling	Weight loss	
Nausea, vomiting		
Dry mucous membranes		
Weight loss		
Tremors, seizures, coma		
Normal or increased ECF volume (water gain)	**Normal or increased ECF volume (sodium gain)**	
Headache, lassitude, apathy, weakness, confusion	Intense thirst	
Nausea, vomiting	Restlessness, agitation, twitching	
Weight gain	Seizures, coma	
Increased blood pressure, increased CVP	Flushed skin	
Muscle spasms, convulsions, coma	Weight gain	
	Peripheral and pulmonary edema	
	Increased blood pressures, increased CVP	

From Lewis SM, Heitkemper MM, Dirksen SR: *Medical-surgical nursing: assessment and management of clinical problems,* ed 5, St. Louis, 2000, Mosby.

CVP, Central venous pressure; *ECF,* extracellular fluid; *GI,* gastrointestinal; *IV,* intravenous; *SIADH,* syndrome of inappropriate antidiuretic hormone.

Table 38-8 POTASSIUM IMBALANCES: CAUSES AND CLINICAL MANIFESTATIONS

HYPOKALEMIA (K^+ <3.5 mEq/L [mmol/L])	HYPERKALEMIA (K^+ > 5.5 mEq/L [mmol/L])	HYPOKALEMIA (K^+ <3.5 mEq/L [mmol/L])	HYPERKALEMIA (K^+ > 5.5 mEq/L [mmol/L])
CAUSES		**CARDIOVASCULAR—cont'd**	
Vomiting	Renal failure	Bradycardia, first- and second-degree heart block, atrial dysrhythmias	Complete heart block
Diarrhea	Early stage of burns		Ectopic beats
Potent diuretics	Adrenal insufficiency	PVCs, especially for patients on digitalis	Ventricular fibrillation → ventricular standstill
Aldosterone-producing tumor	Massive crushing injury	Postural hypotension	
Potassium-free IV solutions	Excess IV administration of K^+	**GASTROINTESTINAL**	
Recovery phase of diabetic acidosis	Metabolic acidosis	Anorexia, nausea	Nausea
Fistulas		Paralytic ileus	Vomiting
Metabolic alkalosis		Constipation	Cramping pain
Anorexia			Diarrhea
Starvation		**NEUROMUSCULAR**	
Malnutrition		Hyporeflexia	Twitching
APPEARANCE		Muscle weakness → paralysis	Seizures
Drowsiness	No specific findings	Muscle cramps and paresthesias	Paresthesias
BEHAVIOR			Paralysis when severe
Confusion	No alteration in mentation	**URINARY FINDINGS**	
Irritability	Irritability	Urinary output ↑	Urine potassium ↑
Lethargy		Specific gravity ↓	
Depression		May have decreased output because of urinary retention	
CARDIOVASCULAR		**SERUM VALUES**	
ECG changes	ECG changes	Serum potassium ↓	Serum potassium ↑
ST depression	Peaked T waves	pH ↑	pH ↓
T wave inversion or flattening	PR interval prolongation		
	Disappearance of P wave		
U waves	Widening of QRS		

From Lewis SM, Heitkemper MM, Dirksen SR: *Medical-surgical nursing: assessment and management of clinical problems,* ed 5, St. Louis, 2000, Mosby.
ECG, Electrocardiogram; *IV,* intravenous; *PVC,* premature ventricular contractions.

than 40 mEq/hr. Additional potassium can be added to intravenous maintenance fluids at 10 to 40 mEq/L.[4] Frequent assessment of potassium levels and vital signs is necessary. Cardiac monitoring and serial evaluation of potassium levels are recommended to prevent inadvertent hyperkalemia secondary to potassium replacement. In less acute situations oral potassium may be used or potassium may be added to enteral feedings. Serum magnesium levels should be checked because both electrolytes can be depleted with persistent hypokalemia.

Hyperkalemia. Hyperkalemia is characterized by prominent cardiac changes (see Table 38-8) and neuromuscular effects such as paresthesia and muscle weakness leading to flaccid paralysis. Various ECG changes correlate well with severity in hyperkalemia. Elevated T waves occur when serum potassium reaches 7 mEq/L, whereas prolonged PR interval and widened QRS complexes are evident when the level reaches 9 to 10 mEq/L. Dysrhythmias include sinus bradycardia, sinus arrest, first-degree heart block, nodal rhythm, idioventricular rhythm, and ventricular fibrillation. Asystole may also occur. Hyperkalemia may be due to increased oral or intravenous intake, acute renal disease, potassium-sparing diuretics, adrenal insufficiency, acidosis, anoxia, and hyponatremia.[8]

Intravenous calcium chloride or calcium gluconate is the most rapid method for neutralizing neuromuscular effects of hyperkalemia. Serum potassium is rapidly reduced by administration of glucose, insulin, and sodium bicarbonate, which drives potassium into the cell in exchange for sodium. However, this intervention provides only temporary reduction in serum potassium. Urinary potassium excretion is promoted with loop or osmotic diuretics. If these efforts fail, renal dialysis may be needed for significant hyperkalemia. Ion exchange resins such as sodium polystyrene sulfonate (Kayexalate, oral or rectal) may be used in nonemergency situations. Continuous cardiac monitoring and serial potassium levels are essential for the patient with hyperkalemia.

Calcium Abnormalities

Calcium abnormalities may be due to diet, medications, injury, or disease (Table 38-9). Bones provide a large reservoir

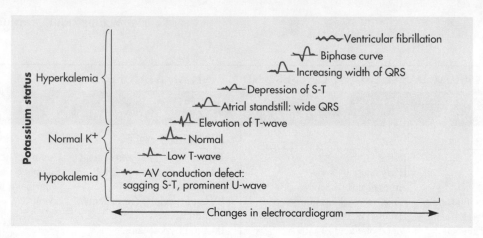

FIGURE 38-10 Electrocardiogram changes associated with alterations in potassium status. (From Lewis SM, Heitkemper MM, Dirksen SR: *Medical-surgical nursing: assessment and management of clinical problems,* ed 5, St. Louis, 2000, Mosby.)

Table 38-9	CALCIUM IMBALANCES: CAUSES AND CLINICAL MANIFESTATIONS		
HYPOCALCEMIA (<9 MG/DL [2.25 MMOL/L])	HYPERCALCEMIA (>11 MG/DL [2.75 MMOL/L])	HYPOCALCEMIA (<9 MG/DL [2.25 MMOL/L])	HYPERCALCEMIA (>11 MG/DL [2.75 MMOL/L])
CAUSES		**CARDIOVASCULAR**	
Acute pancreatitis	Excess milk-product ingestion	Electrocardiogram changes	Electrocardiogram
Primary hypoparathyroidism	Hyperparathyroidism	Prolonged QT interval	Depressed T waves
Steatorrhea	Prolonged immobilization	Dysrhythmias	Shortened QT interval
Generalized peritonitis	Multiple myeloma		Hypertension
Chronic renal failure	Thyrotoxicosis		Cardiac arrest
Vitamin D deficiency	Vitamin D excess		
Surgical removal of para-thyroids		**GASTROINTESTINAL**	
Excess administration of citrated blood		Colicky discomfort	Anorexia
Diuretic therapy		Diarrhea	Nausea
Alcoholism			Constipation
Malabsorption			Paralytic ileus
Total parenteral nutrition			
		NEUROMUSCULAR	
APPEARANCE		Hyperreflexia	Decreased muscle strength
Tonic and clonic convulsions	Lethargy	Muscle cramps	Depressed reflexes
	Weight loss	Numbness and tingling in extremities	
	Dehydration	Carpopedal spasms	
		Chvostek's sign	
BEHAVIOR		Trousseau's sign	
Personality changes	Decreased intellectual function	Seizures	
Depression	Malaise	Tetany	
Irritability	Confusion		
Easy fatigability	Psychosis	**RESPIRATORY**	
Anxiety	Coma	Laryngeal spasm	Hypoventilation
Confusion	Increased thirst	Respiratory arrest	
	Impaired memory		
	Fatigue	**URINARY FINDINGS**	
		No specific findings	Increased urinary output
MUSCULOSKELETAL		**SERUM VALUES**	
Bone pain	Bone pain	Overcorrection of acid pH (may precipitate symptomatic hypocalcemia)	
Fractures	Fractures	↓Serum albumin (patient may not have symptoms despite decreased Ca²⁺)	
Rickets	Pseudogout		

From Lewis SM, Heitkemper MM, Dirksen SR: *Medical-surgical nursing: assessment and management of clinical problems,* ed 5, St. Louis, 2000, Mosby.

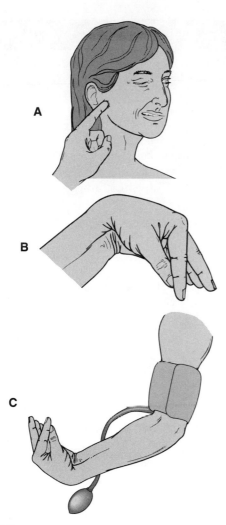

FIGURE 38-11 Tests for hypocalcemia. **A,** Chvostek's sign is a contraction of facial muscles in response to a light tap over the facial nerve in front of the ear. **B,** Trousseau's sign is a carpal spasm induced by **C,** inflating a blood pressure cuff above the systolic pressure for a few minutes. (From Lewis SM, Heitkemper MM, Dirksen SR: *Medical-surgical nursing: assessment and management of clinical problems,* ed 5, St. Louis, 2000, Mosby.)

of calcium; however, adequate dietary intake is necessary to maintain stores. Calcium abnormalities are often associated with phosphorus and magnesium abnormalities.

Hypocalcemia. Hypocalcemia makes the nervous system more excitable, which can lead to cardiac dysrhythmias, constipation, and lack of appetite. In skeletal muscle, excitability can lead to tetanic muscle contractions. Seizures are occasionally seen as a result of increased excitability of brain tissue. Clinical signs include a positive Trousseau's sign and a positive Chvostek's sign (Figure 38-11). Other manifestations include muscle twitching and cramping; facial grimacing; numbness and tingling of fingers, toes, nose, lips, and earlobes; hyperactive deep tendon reflexes; and abdominal pain. The ECG may show a prolonged QT interval, and the patient may appear anxious, irritable, and even psy-

chotic. More severe symptoms include laryngospasms, bronchospasms, seizures, and cardiac failure.

Calcium abnormalities occur with hypoparathyroidism, hypovitaminosis D, malabsorption syndrome, malnutrition, chronic nephrotic syndrome, chronic nephritis, Cushing's syndrome, and metastatic carcinoma of the bone. Overdose of calcium channel blockers can also cause hypocalcemia. Multiple blood transfusions, usually more than 10 units, are associated with hypocalcemia because citrate in banked blood binds with calcium, making it inactive.

Before treatment for hypocalcemia is begun, hypomagnesemia should be excluded because patients with low serum magnesium respond poorly to calcium replacement. Hypocalcemia is easily managed with intravenous calcium. One to two ampules of 10% calcium gluconate mixed in D_5W is administered over 10 to 20 minutes.[9] In severe deficits a continuous infusion may be necessary after the initial bolus. Calcium levels, cardiac rhythm, and blood pressure should be carefully monitored during calcium administration.

Hypercalcemia. Hypercalcemia is characterized by vague symptoms such as headache, irritability, fatigue, malaise, difficulty concentrating, anorexia, nausea, vomiting, and constipation. Neurologic effects are often the primary symptoms. Patients may be lethargic, confused, and have a depressed level of consciousness. Deep tendon reflexes may be depressed, the QT interval may be prolonged, and the patient may have polyuria, polydipsia, or an ileus. Chronic hypercalcemia is associated with renal lithiasis, peptic ulcer, and pancreatitis.

Although rarely seen in the ED, serum calcium levels that exceed 14 to 15 mg/dl are considered a medical emergency. Correction of hypercalcemia includes treating the underlying cause and increasing renal excretion of calcium with intravenous hydration and loop or osmotic diuretics. Other therapeutic options depend on the specific clinical situation and include glucocorticoid administration to decrease intestinal calcium absorption and increase urinary calcium excretion. Administration of calcitonin or phosphate inhibits bone reabsorption. In life-threatening emergencies agents such as ethylenediaminetetraacetic acid are used to chelate ionized calcium.

Phosphate Abnormalities

Phosphate abnormalities are associated with a reciprocal calcium abnormality. Phosphate elevations occur with calcium losses, whereas phosphate depletion occurs with calcium excess. The patient with a phosphate abnormality should be carefully monitored for the effects of calcium abnormality. Causes of phosphate abnormalities are listed in Box 38-3.

Hypophosphatemia. Hypophosphatemia has a variable clinical presentation ranging from no symptoms to anorexia and muscle weakness, rhabdomyolysis, respiratory failure, hemolysis, and altered mental status. Causes include hyperparathyroidism, vitamin D deficiency, intestinal malabsorption, and renal tubular acidosis.

Box 38-3   CAUSES OF PHOSPHATE IMBALANCES

HYPOPHOSPHATEMIA (PO_4^{3-} <2.8 mg/dl [0.9 mmol/L])	HYPERPHOSPHATEMIA (PO_4^{3-} >4.5 mg/dl [1.45 mmol/L])

Causes

Malabsorption syndrome	Renal failure
Nutritional recovery syndrome	Chemotherapeutic agents
Glucose administration	Enemas containing phosphorus (e.g., Fleet Enema)
Total parenteral nutrition	Excessive ingestion (e.g., milk, phosphate-containing laxatives)
Alcohol withdrawal	Large vitamin D intake
Phosphate-binding antacids	Hypoparathyroidism
Recovery from diabetic ketoacidosis	
Respiratory alkalosis	

Clinical Manifestations

Central nervous system dysfunction (confusion, coma)	Hypocalcemia
Rhabdomyolysis	Muscle problems; tetany
Renal tubular wasting of Mg^{+2}, Ca^{+2}, HCO_3^-	Deposition of calcium-phosphate precipitates in skin, soft
Cardiac problems (arrhythmias, decreased stroke volume)	tissue, cornea, viscera, blood vessels
Muscle weakness, including respiratory muscle weakness and	
difficulty weaning	
Osteomalacia	

Modified from Lewis SM, Heitkemper MM, Dirksen SR: *Medical-surgical nursing: assessment and management of clinical problems,* ed 5, St. Louis, 2000, Mosby.

Treatment of severe hypophosphatemia begins with intravenous phosphate (20 mmol over 4 to 6 hours).[9] Potential complications of phosphate administration include hypocalcemia and hypotension, so patients with less severe deficiency are treated with enteric or oral phosphate preparations.

Hyperphosphatemia. Hyperphosphatemia is associated with a reciprocal fall in serum calcium and the resultant clinical effects of hypocalcemia. Hyperphosphotemia is also associated with and can even produce acute renal failure. The most serious effect of excess phosphate relates to precipitation of calcium phosphate crystals in soft tissues such as the cornea, lung, kidney, and blood vessels. Causes include hypoparathyroidism, chronic renal disease, Addison's disease, leukemia, sarcoidosis, osteolytic metastatic bone tumor, and milk-alkali syndrome.

Treatment includes limiting phosphate intake, using oral phosphate binding agents such as aluminum hydroxide, and increasing excretion. Intravenous hydration with saline is followed by diuretics to enhance excretion.

Magnesium Abnormalities

Specific causes of magnesium abnormalities are identified in Box 38-4. Magnesium abnormalities are frequently associated with other electrolyte abnormalities. Clinically, hypomagnesemia and hypermagnesemia have the same effect on release of PTH and calcitonin as hypocalcemia and hypercalcemia. Calcium and magnesium excretion are interdependent. A sudden calcium load causes excretion of both calcium and magnesium.

Hypomagnesemia. Hypomagnesemia may result from malabsorption syndrome, ulcerative colitis, ileal bypass, cirrhosis, alcoholism, chronic renal disease, DKA, diuretic

---

Box 38-4   CAUSES OF MAGNESIUM IMBALANCES

HYPOMAGNESEMIA	HYPERMAGNESEMIA
Diarrhea	Renal failure (especially if
Vomiting	patient is given magnesium
Chronic alcoholism	products)
Impaired gastrointestinal	Excessive administration of
absorption	magnesium for treatment of
Malabsorption syndrome	eclampsia
Prolonged malnutrition	Adrenal insufficiency
Large urine output	
Gastric suction	
Diabetic ketoacidosis	
Hyperaldosteronism	

From Lewis SM, Heitkemper MM, Dirksen SR: *Medical-surgical nursing: assessment and management of clinical problems,* ed 5, St. Louis, 2000, Mosby.

---

therapy, and malnutrition. Symptoms include nausea, vomiting, sedation, decreased deep tendon reflexes, and muscle weakness. With significant hypomagnesemia, hypotension, bradycardia, coma, respiratory paralysis, and cardiac arrest may occur.[3] Severe hypomagnesemia can also exist in the absence of clinical symptoms. When symptoms do occur, they are usually confined to the neuromuscular and cardiovascular systems. Generalized weakness, muscle fasciculations, and positive Trousseau's and Chvostek's signs may be seen (Figure 38-11). Dysrhythmias such as torsades de pointes, ventricular tachycardia, and ventricular fibrillation have been associated with hypomagnesemia.

Treatment depends on severity of symptoms. Magnesium sulfate, 1 to 2 g, is administered intravenously over 1 minute followed by a continuous infusion.[9] Vital signs, deep tendon reflexes, fluid intake, urinary output, and magnesium levels should be carefully monitored.

Hypermagnesemia. Hypermagnesemia may result from reduced excretion secondary to advanced renal failure and adrenocortical insufficiency, overdose of therapeutic magnesium, or routine doses of magnesium in the patient with renal compromise. Treatment of hypermagnesemia also depends on severity of symptoms. Calcium chloride, 100 to 200 mg every 3 to 5 minutes until symptoms are reversed, is followed by a continuous infusion.[4] Saline diuresis and furosemide may also be used. In severe cases hemodialysis may be required. Serial magnesium levels, vital signs, and deep tendon reflexes should be closely monitored.

SUMMARY

Whether caring for a trauma patient, chronically ill geriatric patient, or previously healthy person with acute simple gastroenteritis, the emergency nurse should anticipate electrolyte abnormalities. Recognition of abnormalities and potential adverse effects is essential for effective treatment and prevention of complications. Box 38-5 identifies nursing diagnoses appropriate for patients with fluid and/or electrolyte abnormalities.

Box 38-5 NURSING DIAGNOSES FOR FLUID AND ELECTROLYTE ABNORMALITIES

Bowel incontinence
Breathing pattern, Ineffective
Cardiac output, Decreased
Constipation
Fluid volume, Deficient
Fluid volume, Excess
Gas exchange, Impaired
Nutrition, Imbalanced
Urinary elimination, Impaired

References

1. Ayers S, Grenvik A, Holbrook PR et al: *Textbook of critical care,* ed 4, Philadelphia, 2000, WB Saunders.
2. Collins RD: *Illustrated manual of fluid and electrolyte disorders,* ed 2, Philadelphia, 1983, JB Lippincott.
3. Guyton AC, Hall JE: *Textbook of medical physiology,* ed 10, Philadelphia, 2000, WB Saunders.
4. Harrison TR: *Harrison's principles of internal medicine,* ed 14, New York, 1998, McGraw-Hill.
5. Hazinski MF, Cummins RO, Fields JM: *2000 handbook of emergency cardiovascular care for healthcare providers,* Dallas, 2000, American Heart Association.
6. Jordan KS: *Emergency nursing core curriculum,* ed 5, Philadelphia, 2000, WB Saunders.
7. Kokko JP, Tannen RL: *Fluids and electrolytes,* ed 3, Philadelphia, 1996, WB Saunders.
8. Rosen P: *The 5 minute emergency medicine consult,* Philadelphia, 1999, Lippincott Williams & Wilkins.
9. Rosen P, Barkin R: *Emergency medicine: concepts and clinical practice,* ed 4, St. Louis, 1998, Mosby.

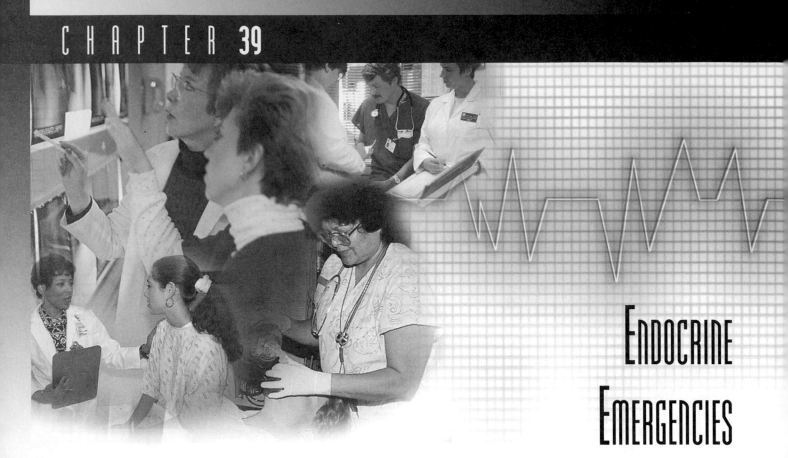

CHAPTER 39

ENDOCRINE EMERGENCIES

CHRIS M. GISNESS

The endocrine system is a regulatory system that uses hormones to control metabolic, renal, and neural functions. Endocrine disturbances lead to critical physiologic consequences if not promptly identified and treated. Most common endocrine emergencies involve diabetes and alcohol-related illnesses; however, thyroid and adrenal crises also have potentially serious outcomes. Specific endocrine emergencies described are alcoholic ketoacidosis (AKA), adrenal crisis, diabetic ketoacidosis (DKA), hyperosmolar hyperglycemic nonketotic coma (HHNC), hypoglycemia, thyroid storm, myxedema coma, and syndrome of inappropriate antidiuretic hormone (SIADH). A brief review of anatomy and physiology is provided to facilitate understanding of clinical material.

ANATOMY AND PHYSIOLOGY

The endocrine system consists of the hypothalamus, pituitary, thyroid, parathyroids, adrenals, testes, and ovaries (Figure 39-1). Each gland produces and stores one or more hormones that have specific, unique functions. Table 39-1 identifies the hormones produced by the major endocrine glands, their target tissue, and their functions. Activities of the testes and ovaries are discussed in Chapters 37 and 44.

Hormone activity is the result of feedback loops, nerve stimulation, and intrinsic rhythms. Renal and liver function; external factors such as pain, fear, and stress also affect hormone release. Circulating hormone levels above or below normal activate negative feedback loops.[7] Excessive amounts of circulating hormones inhibit hormone release, whereas low levels lead to increased hormone release. Neural stimulation triggers increased glandular activity and release of hormones such as glucagon. Intrinsic rhythms vary from hours to weeks and provide another method of hormone control.

Hypothalamus

The hypothalamus creates part of the walls and floor of the third ventricle. Various centers in the anterior and posterior hypothalamus control most endocrine functions and many emotional behaviors. Table 39-2 reviews these control centers and target areas or processes. Nerve tracts from the hypothalamus join the posterior pituitary, which lies just below (Figure 39-2). Posterior pituitary hormones are actually synthesized in the hypothalamus and then transferred along axons for storage in the posterior pituitary. The hypothalamus regulates anterior pituitary action by inhibiting or releasing certain hormones.

Pituitary

The pituitary gland, approximately 1 cm in all directions, lies within the sella turcica of the middle cranial fossa (see Figure 39-2). Two physiologically distinct areas are found in the pituitary. The anterior pituitary contains secretory cells,

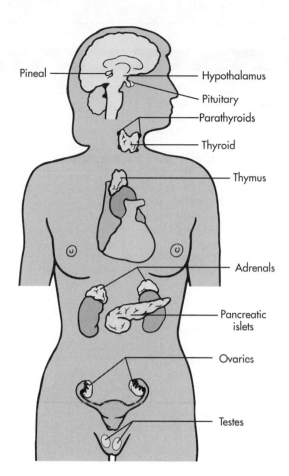

FIGURE 39-1 Location of the major endocrine glands. Parathyroid glands actually lie on the posterior surface of the thyroid. (From Lewis SM, Heitkemper MM, Dirksen SR: *Medical-surgical nursing: assessment and management of clinical problems,* ed 5, St. Louis, 2000, Mosby.)

whereas the posterior pituitary consists of neural cells that serve as a supporting structure for nerve fibers and nerve endings. Hormones secreted by the anterior pituitary include growth hormone, adrenocorticotropic hormone (ACTH), thyroid-stimulating hormone (TSH), prolactin, follicle-stimulating hormone, and luteinizing hormone. Hormones secreted by the posterior pituitary are antidiuretic hormone (ADH) and oxytocin.

Thyroid

The thyroid gland consists of two lobes connected by an isthmus (Figure 39-3). This butterfly-shaped gland in the anterior neck below the cricoid cartilage partially surrounds the trachea. Thyroid hormone release is regulated through a complex feedback system between the hypothalamus and anterior pituitary. This main metabolic regulator contains follicular cells that secrete thyroxine (T4) and triiodothyronine (T3) in response to stimulation by the pituitary. Calcitonin originating in parafollicular cells in the thyroid affects calcium metabolism.

Adrenals

The adrenal glands, located in the retroperitoneal area above the upper pole of each kidney (Figure 39-4), consist of an outer cortical layer and inner medullary layer. The adrenal cortex produces the mineralocorticoids, aldosterone, glucocorticoids, and androgens. Aldosterone is critical for maintaining internal fluid balance, whereas glucocorticoids are major players in the body's ability to resist stress. The adrenal medulla releases the catecholamines epinephrine and norepinephrine in response to sympathetic stimulation. Epinephrine is 5 to 10 times more potent than norepinephrine; however, norepinephrine has a longer duration of action. Table 39-3 summarizes the major functions of these catecholamines.

Pancreas

The pancreas is situated behind the stomach in the retroperitoneal space. The body of the pancreas extends horizontally across the abdominal wall with the head in the curve of the abdomen and the tail touching the spleen (Figure 39-5). Exocrine and endocrine cells are found in the pancreas. Acini are exocrine cells that release amylase, lipase, and other enzymes that aid in digestion. Three types of endocrine cells within the islet of Langerhans produce hormones that regulate serum glucose levels. Alpha cells secrete glucagon, beta cells produce insulin, and delta cells secrete somatostatin, which inhibits glucagon and insulin release.[4] Table 39-4 describes the physiologic actions of insulin.

PATIENT ASSESSMENT

Arrival of an unresponsive patient in the emergency department (ED) creates a flurry of activity that begins with assessment and stabilization of the airway, breathing, and circulation (ABCs) followed by assessment, treatment, and reassessment of patient condition (Figure 39-6). After a diagnosis is reached, individualization of care can begin. An important aspect of care common to all endocrine emergencies is identification of the stressor or precipitating event. Identification may come through patient history, family interviews, laboratory findings, radiographic analysis, and other diagnostic procedures.

SELECTED ENDOCRINE EMERGENCIES

Endocrine emergencies represent a significant threat to the patient's life. Conditions covered in this chapter include those situations most likely to be encountered by the emergency nurse.

Alcoholic Ketoacidosis

Alcohol is associated with 15% of the nation's health care costs. It is estimated that 50% of alcoholics go undiagnosed. Alcohol is associated with up to 200,000 deaths per year in

Table 39-1 MAJOR ENDOCRINE GLANDS AND HORMONES

HORMONES	TARGET TISSUE	FUNCTIONS
ANTERIOR PITUITARY (ADENOHYPOPHYSIS)		
Growth hormone (GH) or somatotropin	All body cells	Promotes protein anabolism (growth, tissue repair) and lipid mobilization and catabolism
Thyroid-stimulating hormone (TSH) or thyrotropin	Thyroid gland	Stimulates synthesis and release of thyroid hormones, growth and function of thyroid
Adrenocorticotropic hormone (ACTH) or corticotropin	Adrenal cortex	Fosters growth of adrenal cortex; stimulates secretion of glucocorticoids
Gonadotropic hormones Follicle-stimulating hormone (FSH) Luteinizing hormone (LH)	Reproductive organs	Stimulates sex hormone secretion, reproductive organ growth, reproductive processes
Melanocyte-stimulating hormone (MSH)	Melanocytes in skin	Increases melanin production in melanocytes to make skin darker in color
Prolactin	Ovary and mammary glands in females	Stimulates milk production in lactating women; increases response of follicles to LH and FSH; has unclear function in men
POSTERIOR PITUITARY (NEUROHYPOPHYSIS)		
Oxytocin	Uterus; mammary glands	Stimulates milk secretion, uterine motility
Antidiuretic hormone (ADH) or vasopressin	Renal tubules, vascular smooth muscle	Promotes reabsorption of water
THYROID		
Thyroxine (T_4)	All body tissues	Precursor to T_3
Triiodothyronine (T_3)	All body tissues	Regulates metabolic rate of all cells and processes of cell growth and tissue differentiation
Calcitonin (CT)	Bone tissue	Regulates calcium and phosphorus blood levels, lowering of blood Ca^{2+} levels
PARATHYROIDS		
Parathyroid hormone (PTH) or parathormone	Bone, intestine, kidneys	Regulates calcium and phosphorus blood levels (bone demineralization and increased intestinal absorption)
ADRENAL MEDULLA		
Epinephrine (adrenalin)	Sympathetic effectors	Enhances and prolongs effects of sympathetic nervous system
Norepinephrine	Sympathetic effectors	Response to stress; enhances and prolongs effects of sympathetic nervous system
ADRENAL CORTEX		
Corticosteroids (e.g., cortisol, hydrocortisone)	All body tissues	Promotes metabolism, response to stress
Androgens (e.g., testosterone and androsterone) and estrogen	Sex organs	Promotes masculinization in men, growth and sexual activity in women
Mineralocorticoids (e.g., aldosterone)	Kidney	Regulates sodium and potassium balance and thus water balance
PANCREAS		
Islets of Langerhans Insulin (from beta cells)	General	Promotes movement of glucose out of blood and into cells
Glucagon (from alpha cells)	General	Promotes movement of glucose from storage and into blood
Somatostatin	Pancreas	Inhibits insulin and glucagon secretion
GONADS		
Women: Ovaries		
Estrogen	Reproductive system, breasts	Stimulates development of secondary sex characteristics, preparation of uterus for fertilization and fetal development; stimulates bone growth
Progesterone	Reproductive system	Maintains lining of uterus necessary for successful pregnancy
Men: Testes		
Testosterone	Reproductive system	Stimulates development of secondary sex characteristics, spermatogenesis

From Lewis SM, Heitkemper MM, Dirksen SR: *Medical-surgical nursing: assessment and management of clinical problems,* ed 5, St. Louis, 2000, Mosby.

Table 39-2	CONTROL CENTERS OF THE HYPOTHALAMUS		
POSTERIOR HYPOTHALAMUS		**ANTERIOR HYPOTHALAMUS**	
CONTROL CENTER	EFFECT	CONTROL CENTER	EFFECT
Posterior hypothalamus	Increased BP; pupillary dilation; shivering	Paraventricular nucleus	Oxytocin release; water conservation
Dorsomedial nucleus	GI stimulation	Medical preoptic area	Bladder contraction; decreased heart rate; decreased BP
Perifornical nucleus	Hunger; increased BP; rage	Supraoptic nucleus	Vasopressin release
Ventromedial nucleus	Satiety; neuroendocrine control	Posterior preoptic and anterior hypothalamic area	Temperature regulation; panting, sweating, thyrotropin inhibition
Mamillary body	Feeding reflexes		
Arcuate nucleus and periventricular zone	Neuroendocrine control		
Lateral hypothalamic area	Thirst, hunger		

From Guyton AC, Hall JE: *Textbook of medical physiology,* ed 10, Philadelphia, 2000, WB Saunders.
BP, Blood pressure; *GI,* gastrointestinal.

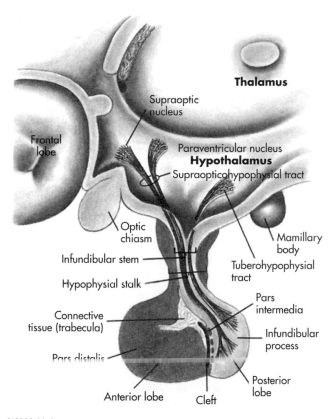

FIGURE 39-2   Anatomy of the hypothalamus and pituitary. (From Thompson JM, McFarland GK, Hirsch JE et al: *Mosby's clinical nursing,* ed 5, St. Louis, 2001, Mosby.)

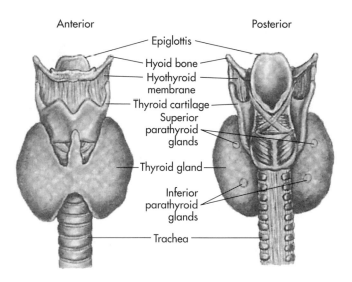

FIGURE 39-3   Thyroid gland. (From Thompson JM, McFarland GK, Hirsch JE et al: *Mosby's clinical nursing,* ed 5, St. Louis, 2001, Mosby.)

the United States.[1] Alcohol-related emergencies include acute intoxication and withdrawal; injuries related to domestic violence, motor vehicle collisions, homicides, suicides, and other accidents; gastrointestinal bleeding, pancreatitis, liver failure, and diverse acute and chronic conditions; and various psychiatric crises.

Increased amounts of adipose tissue place women at higher risk for AKA because estrogen appears to increase fatty acid production in adipose tissue. AKA typically occurs 24 to 36 hours after a patient who is ingesting large amounts of alcohol stops drinking. During this time there has been poor food intake or vomiting. More than likely the patient has had more than one episode of AKA.[15]

Major aggravating factors for development of AKA are insulin deficiency, decreased glycogen stores, and volume depletion. Liver and pancreatic damage secondary to chronic alcohol consumption decreases glycogen stores and insulin levels. Glycogen stores are further diminished by starvation or inadequate nutritional stores. Inadequate glycogen leads to utilization of fat and muscle tissue for energy. Subsequent increased fatty acid production enhances

Table 39-3	CATECHOLAMINE FUNCTIONS		
CLASS AND FUNCTION	**α-ADRENERGIC**	**β-ADRENERGIC**	**DOPAMINERGIC**
Agonist	Norepinephrine	Epinephrine	Dopamine
Antagonist	Phentolamine	Propranolol	Haloperidol
Actions			
Heart		Inotropic and chronotropic	Inotropic
Smooth muscle	Contracts	Relaxes	Mixed
Metabolic		Lipolysis	
		Glycogenolysis	
		Gluconeogenesis	
Molecular	Decreases cAMP	Increases cAMP	Increases cAMP

cAMP, Cyclic adenosine monophosphate

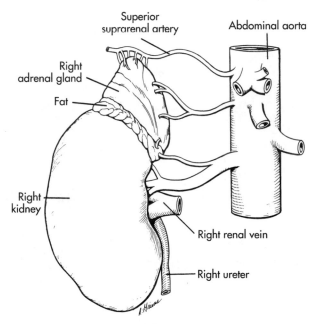

FIGURE 39-4   Adrenal gland. (From Seeley RS, Stephens TD, Tate P: *Anatomy and physiology,* ed 2, St. Louis, 1992, Mosby. Used with permission of the McGraw-Hill Companies.)

an existing acidotic state. Decreased insulin availability decreases glucose utilization, which also leads to increased fatty acid levels and acidosis. Actual alcohol metabolism decreases gluconeogenesis and compounds the altered metabolic state. Profound dehydration increases circulating levels of epinephrine, cortisol, and growth hormones, which alter glucose utilization; as a result, the ketoacidotic cycle continues.

Patients present awake with abdominal pain, nausea, and vomiting. Physical findings include tachypnea, tachycardia, mild to moderate abdominal tenderness, and some alteration in mental status, which is often assumed to be secondary to alcohol intoxication rather than ketoacidosis. The skin may be cool and dry and the patient may have a strong odor of ketones on the breath. Initial laboratory studies

show decreased pH, normal to slightly decreased potassium, hypoglycemia, elevated liver function test results, and an elevated amylase. Alcohol levels are low or undetectable. Hypomagnesemia, hypocalcemia, and hypokalemia are commonly found in chronic alcoholics.[2]

Management in the ED is symptomatic, focusing on correction of volume and glycogen depletion to restore metabolic functions. Moderate fluid replacement, usually with 5% dextrose in normal saline at 125 to 250 ml/hr, increases the serum bicarbonate level; therefore, sodium bicarbonate administration may not be necessary except in severe cases. Glucose administration triggers increased insulin production, which interrupts ketogenesis. Consequently, intravenous fluids with dextrose often produce quicker results than saline alone unless the patient is hyperglycemic. Diabetic ketoacidosis should be ruled out when hyperglycemia is present. Potassium supplements may be necessary if fluid therapy and shifting glucose molecules lead to hypokalemia. Magnesium replacement helps correct calcium and potassium disturbances and also forestalls acute alcohol withdrawal. Thiamin is given before glucose administration to prevent Wernicke's syndrome. Table 39-5 identifies drugs used in treatment of alcohol withdrawal. The patient with AKA needs close monitoring and supportive care. Frequent assessment of vital signs, intake and output, neurologic status, and electrolyte values is necessary to monitor effectiveness of therapy and to ensure an uncomplicated return to the patient's normal metabolic state.

Adrenal Crisis

Adrenal crisis is a rare occurrence with life-threatening potential that develops when acute stressors deplete adrenal glucocorticoids and mineralocorticoids. Long-term steroid therapy patients can experience adrenal crisis after abrupt discontinuation of medications. Prolonged steroid use suppresses adrenal activity so the system cannot compensate sufficiently with abrupt removal of steroids. Other stressors include trauma, infection, hemorrhage, surgery, hypothermia, metastatic disease of the adrenal glands, and patients

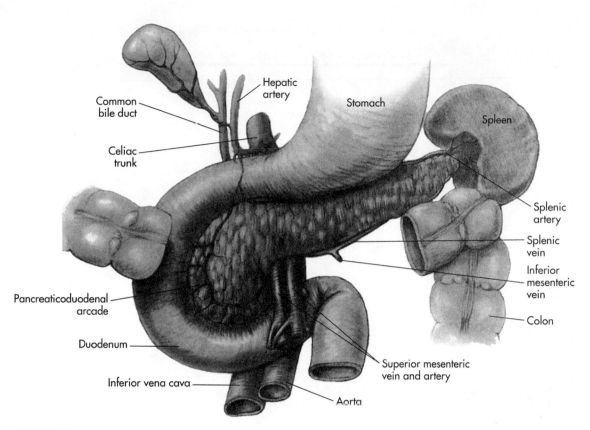

FIGURE 39-5   The pancreas and surrounding structures. (From Davis JH et al: *Surgery: a problem-solving approach,* ed 2, vol 2, St. Louis, 1995, Mosby.)

Table 39-4	ACTION OF INSULIN		
	LIVER	**ADIPOSE TISSUE**	**MUSCLE**
ANTICATABOLIC EFFECTS			
	Decreased glycogenolysis	Decreased lipolysis	Decreased protein catabolism
	Decreased gluconeogenesis		Decreased amino acid output
	Decreased ketogenesis		Decreased amino acid oxidation
ANABOLIC EFFECTS			
	Increased glycogen synthesis	Increased glycerol synthesis	Increased amino acid uptake
	Increased fatty acid synthesis	Increased fatty acid synthesis	Increased protein synthesis
			Increased glycogen synthesis

From Ellenberg M, Rifkin H, editors: *Diabetes mellitus: theory and practice,* ed 3, New York, 1983, Medical Examination Publishing. By permission of The McGraw-Hill Companies.

affected with acquired immunodeficiency syndrome (AIDS).[12] Stress increases cortisol output from the adrenal system; therefore, inability to meet these increased demands begins the sequence of events that leads to crisis.

When the adrenal system fails the resulting decrease in cortisol and aldosterone levels leads to massive sodium and water loss from the kidneys and gastrointestinal tract. Water loss results in hypotension and hypovolemia, which can progress to hypovolemic shock, coma, and death. As sodium decreases, serum potassium increases, leading to hyperkalemia and potentially fatal dysrhythmias.

Gluconeogenesis, the normal hepatic response to stress, fails without sufficient levels of cortisol; therefore, hypoglycemia can occur in concert with adrenal crisis. Decreased cortisol levels also alter activities of the adrenal medulla, which normally responds to stress through release of catecholamines to increase heart rate and serum glucose. Without a catecholamine response the severity of hypoglycemia and hypotension is magnified (Figure 39-7).

The patient in acute adrenal crisis presents with multiple symptoms, including weakness, fatigue, nausea, vomiting, abdominal pain, and palpitations. The patient may also describe

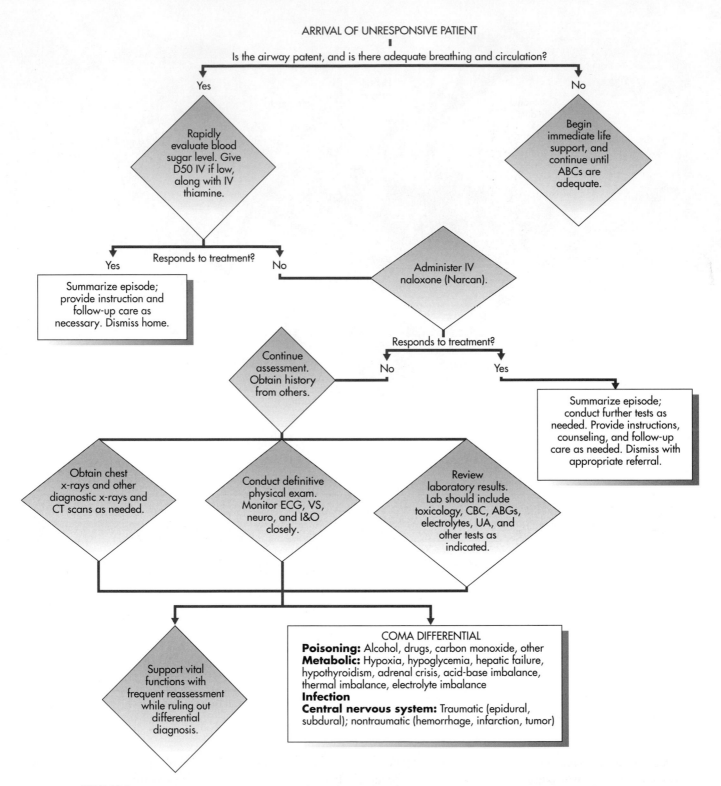

ARRIVAL OF UNRESPONSIVE PATIENT

Is the airway patent, and is there adequate breathing and circulation?

Yes

No

Rapidly evaluate blood sugar level. Give D50 IV if low, along with IV thiamine.

Begin immediate life support, and continue until ABCs are adequate.

Responds to treatment?

Yes

No

Summarize episode; provide instruction and follow-up care as necessary. Dismiss home.

Administer IV naloxone (Narcan).

Responds to treatment?

No

Yes

Continue assessment. Obtain history from others.

Summarize episode; conduct further tests as needed. Provide instructions, counseling, and follow-up care as needed. Dismiss with appropriate referral.

Obtain chest x-rays and other diagnostic x-rays and CT scans as needed.

Conduct definitive physical exam. Monitor ECG, VS, neuro, and I&O closely.

Review laboratory results. Lab should include toxicology, CBC, ABGs, electrolytes, UA, and other tests as indicated.

Support vital functions with frequent reassessment while ruling out differential diagnosis.

COMA DIFFERENTIAL
Poisoning: Alcohol, drugs, carbon monoxide, other
Metabolic: Hypoxia, hypoglycemia, hepatic failure, hypothyroidism, adrenal crisis, acid-base imbalance, thermal imbalance, electrolyte imbalance
Infection
Central nervous system: Traumatic (epidural, subdural); nontraumatic (hemorrhage, infarction, tumor)

FIGURE **39-6**   Management of the unresponsive patient. *D50,* 50% Dextrose; *IV,* intravenous; *ABCs,* airway, breathing, and circulation; *CT,* computed tomography; *ECG,* electrocardiogram; *VS,* vital signs; *neuro,* neurologic status; *I&O,* intake and output; *CBC,* complete blood count; *ABGs,* arterial blood gases; *UA,* urinalysis.

Table 39-5	MEDICATIONS FOR ALCOHOL WITHDRAWAL		
MEDICATIONS	INDICATION	DOSE AND ROUTE	CONSIDERATIONS
Atenolol (Tenormin)	Minor withdrawal	50-100 mg PO	Provides symptomatic relief; contraindicated in congestive heart failure, diabetes, bronchospasm
Chlordiazepoxide (Librium)	Minor withdrawal; anticonvulsant	25-100 mg PO	Titrate dose to achieve sedation
Clonidine (Catapres)	Minor withdrawal	0.1-0.4 mg PO	Provides symptomatic relief
Diazepam (Valium)	Delirium tremens; anticonvulsant	5-10 mg IV; may be given PO for minor symptoms	Titrate dose to achieve sedation; may need repeat doses; large doses may be necessary; watch for respiratory depression; IV rate is 5 mg/min
Lorazepam (Ativan)	Delirium tremens; minor withdrawal	1-5 mg PO, IV, or IM	Recommended for elderly patients or patients with liver disease
Phenytoin (Dilantin)	Anticonvulsant	100-300 mg PO; 500-1000 mg IV loading dose	Not usually needed for simple alcohol-related seizures; IV rate <50 mg/min; do not mix with other drugs or dextrose solutions; with IV use, monitor heart rate and rhythm, blood pressure, and central nervous system

PO, By mouth, *IV,* intravenously.

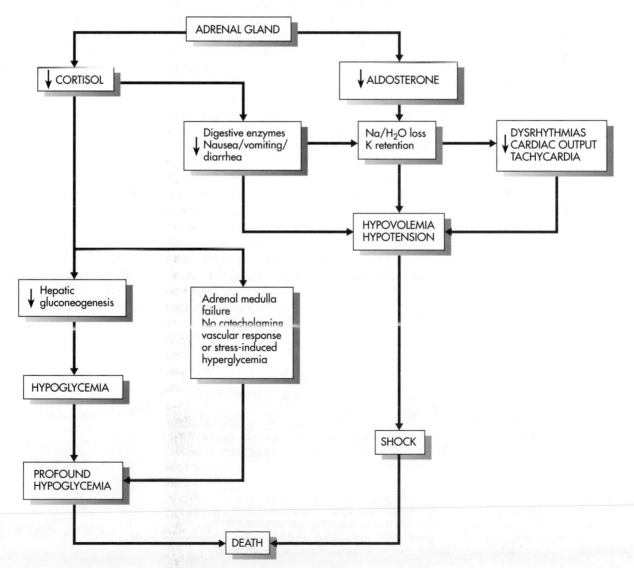

FIGURE 39-7 Pathophysiology of acute adrenal insufficiency.

salt craving. An accurate history of prior illnesses (e.g., asthma with steroid therapy), recent medication changes, recent surgery, or injury helps determine precipitating factors.

Objective findings include poor skin turgor; cool, dry mucous membranes; signs of hypovolemic shock (hypotension, tachycardia, and tachypnea); electrocardiogram changes (elevated T waves with progression to widened QRS complexes); fever related to predisposing infection; and confusion or lethargy.[9]

Hyponatremia, hyperkalemia, hypoglycemia, and hypercalcemia are usually present. Hyperkalemia, the most sensitive of these conditions, is related to aldosterone deficiency. Decreased volume also increases blood urea nitrogen (BUN). An ACTH challenge does help with diagnosis but is not useful in the emergency setting. This challenge consists of obtaining a baseline serum cortisol level, administering synthetic ACTH, and then repeating the serum cortisol level 6 to 8 hours later. If the adrenal glands are functioning appropriately, the repeat cortisol level should be at least twice the baseline level.[15]

Maintenance of ABCs, replacement of glucocorticoids, and correction of fluid and electrolyte disturbances are cornerstones of care in the patient with adrenal crisis. Oxygen should be administered to alleviate increased oxygen demands caused by tachycardia. Hydrocortisone is given as the primary glucocorticoid replacement to stimulate gluconeogenesis, inhibit inflammatory response, and allow the body to increase its response to stress. Mineralocorticoids (e.g., dexamethasone) are used as secondary replacers because of the potential for excessive sodium retention.

Rapid intravenous fluid replacement assists in correcting volume deficit. Intravenous insulin and 50% dextrose (D50) drive potassium from vascular spaces into the cell so serum potassium levels decrease. Kayexalate administration may also facilitate serum potassium reduction. Efforts to reverse hyperkalemia are made with the knowledge that total body stores of potassium are low so hyperkalemia will resolve with intravenous fluids and replacement of glucocorticoid. Close cardiac monitoring is essential. Frequent reassessment of electrolyte levels is necessary to evaluate care and prevent complications. Observation of neurologic function, intake and output, and vital signs provides information on patient response to treatment.

The patient with acute adrenal insufficiency is critically ill, so care must focus on fluid replacement, electrolyte correction, and revitalization of the adrenal system. Maintaining ABCs and providing the patient and family with necessary support and information lead to a positive outcome. The clinical picture of shock should improve within 6 to 12 hours and the patient should stabilize in 7 to 10 days.

Diabetic Ketoacidosis

DKA develops when a patient experiences relative or absolute depletion of circulating insulin. Occurring primarily in type I diabetes, DKA accounts for 10% of all diabetic-related hospital admissions. This potentially life-threatening condition occurs in patients with new-onset diabetes, so acute presentation can lead to the initial diagnosis of diabetes. Infection, illness, pregnancy, or situational stressors can lead to gluconeogenesis, which creates a relative insulin deficiency. Excess circulating glucose secondary to poor dietary management can overwhelm an already stressed system in some patients. Absolute deficiency can occur in the noncompliant patient who experiences stress and fails to follow the prescribed insulin regimen or who becomes ill and fails to take insulin. The latter example demonstrates why diabetic education is critical.

After prolonged insulin deficiency the patient can present with four acute problems: hyperglycemia, dehydration, electrolyte depletion, and metabolic acidosis. Stress causes release of regulatory hormones, which leads to onset of gluconeogenesis (Figure 39-8). Gluconeogenesis progresses to severe hyperglycemia and, ultimately, osmotic diuresis. The resulting excessive losses of water, sodium, and potassium usually lead to hypovolemia. Profound hyperglycemia overwhelms available insulin so the body is unable to metabolize glucose. Fats and muscle proteins are metabolized for energy. The ensuing lipolysis leads to buildup of fatty acids, which overcomes the body's natural buffering system, leading to ketoacidosis.

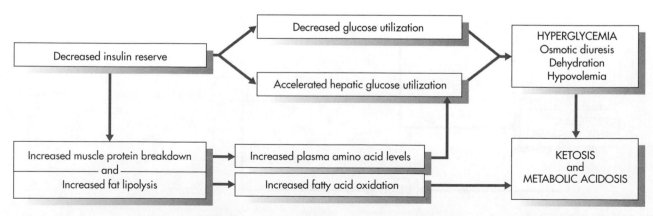

FIGURE 39-8 Pathophysiology of diabetic ketoacidosis.

DKA develops over a relatively short time, usually 2 to 3 days. The condition occurs most often in young adults, usually resulting from infection and stress. The patient describes a steady progression of symptoms including polydipsia, polyuria, fatigue, and weakness. Patients with new-onset diabetes report recent weight loss. As ketoacidosis worsens, nausea, vomiting, decreased appetite, and abdominal discomfort occur. The patient appears in moderate to severe distress with possible altered level of consciousness, confusion about recent events, or slow response to questions. Rapid, deep Kussmaul respirations are present and a fruity odor is usually noted on the breath. This acetone smell indicates worsening ketoacidosis. The skin is usually hot and dry, skin turgor is diminished, and mucous membranes are dry. The most frequently seen cardiac rhythm is sinus tachycardia, but dysrhythmias related to electrolyte disturbances also occur. Table 39-6 summarizes the clinical presentation of DKA. This is a grave situation in the pregnant woman because of deleterious effects on the fetus. Early identification and aggressive interventions are critical to minimize effects on the fetus and the mother.

Laboratory studies should be obtained early with fluid therapy started on arrival. Serum glucose higher than 300 mg/dl and normal or elevated potassium levels are usually present. Creatinine and BUN levels are also elevated as a result of dehydration. Serum osmolality is greater than 310 mOsm/kg, and serum acetone titrations are positive. Monitoring serum ketone levels is not helpful. More hydroxybutyrate is converted to acetoacetate, so measured ketones will increase despite improvement.[6] Urinalysis results include elevated ketones and glucose. Blood gas results show normal arterial oxygen pressure (PaO_2), respiratory alkalosis, and metabolic acidosis.

Treatment focuses on correction of hyperglycemia, dehydration, electrolyte imbalances, and metabolic acidosis. Close monitoring with frequent reassessment is essential to prevent complications. Oxygen therapy should be initiated for any signs of hemodynamic compromise or altered mental status.

Intravenous fluid replacement should start immediately with 1 to 2 L of normal saline over the first 1 to 2 hours of treatment. The patient may require 8 to 10 L of fluid to replace lost volume. After serum glucose reaches 250 to 300 mg/dl,

Table 39-6	CLINICAL MANIFESTATIONS OF DIABETIC KETOACIDOSIS
SYSTEM	**CLINICAL MANIFESTATIONS**
Neurologic	Lethargy, confusion, coma, hyperthermia
Pulmonary	Kussmaul's respirations, fruity acetone breath
Cardiovascular	Tachycardia, hypotension, dysrhythmias
Integumentary	Flushed skin, dry membranes, poor skin turgor
Renal	Polyuria, ketonuria, glucosuria
Gastrointestinal	Nausea, vomiting, abdominal cramps, ileus

fluids should be converted to 5% dextrose in normal saline to provide fuel until the patient is able to eat. Close observation of intake and output should be stressed. Rapid fluid infusion creates the potential for complications. Urinary catheter placement ensures accurate output assessment and helps with early identification of complications.

An insulin drip (normal saline with regular insulin) at 0.1 U/kg/hr should be initiated as soon as the serum glucose level is known.[3] The short duration of action for regular insulin allows better control of serum glucose levels. Insulin drip rates are generally low (5 to 10 U/hr) with sliding-scale parameters to cover frequent glucose monitoring. The serum glucose level is reduced gradually, usually 75 to 100 mg/dl/hr. Intravenous tubing should be flushed with 50 to 60 ml of insulin solution before administration because regular tubing absorbs part of the insulin.

Acidosis is treated with sodium bicarbonate if pH is less than 7.0 to 7.1. Bicarbonate given with higher pH causes rebound alkalosis, which can worsen hypokalemia. With higher pH levels, acidosis generally corrects with insulin therapy. By decreasing hyperglycemia, insulin helps decrease circulating amino and fatty acids, the cause of ketoacidosis.

Fluid replacement dilutes serum potassium, so potassium replacement should begin after the initial liter of intravenous fluids, even when initial values are normal. Serum potassium decreases as insulin forces potassium out of the vascular area into the cells. Cardiac dysrhythmias can develop with significant hypokalemia.

Management in the ED should be aggressive. Controlling nausea and vomiting not only improves patient comfort but prevents worsening dehydration. The patient may require analgesia to relieve abdominal pain, headaches, or other somatic complaints. Providing a quiet, calm environment can improve patient comfort. Stress reduction plays an important part in patient recovery. Thorough explanation of treatment, medications, and plan of care can alleviate stress related to hospitalization.

Infection can precipitate DKA so blood cultures and urine culture should be obtained when infection is suspected. After cultures are obtained, antibiotic therapy should begin. Radiographs may also be required to determine the primary site of infection.

Potential complications include hypoglycemia, hypokalemia, dysrhythmias, and cerebral edema. Monitor laboratory values, vital signs, intake and output, and neurologic status carefully. If the serum glucose level falls rapidly, the resulting fluid shift can lead to cerebral edema, which is associated with higher mortality rate. Cerebral edema is a greater threat for children than for adults. If the patient exhibits signs of hypoglycemia, the insulin drip should be discontinued and the physician should be notified.

Hyperosmolar Hyperglycemic Nonketotic Coma

Hyperosmolar hyperglycemic nonketotic coma (HHNC), also referred to as hyperosmolar syndrome, threatens non–insulin-dependent (type II) diabetic patients with mortality rates as high as 20% to 60%.[12] Delayed diagnosis in undiagnosed type II diabetes, alcoholics, and dialysis patients place these groups at the greatest risk. Type II diabetic patients are typically more than age 50 years with other contributing health problems, so it is necessary to search for other underlying illness. When stressed with illness, surgery, or injury the body responds with increased glucose levels. Type II diabetics produce enough insulin to avoid ketoacidosis but not enough to prevent profound hyperglycemia, dehydration, and hyperosmolality, which are the hallmarks of HHNC.[10] Figure 39-9 illustrates the pathophysiology of HHNC and Table 39-7 summarizes clinical manifestations.

Increased serum glucose levels act as osmotic diuretics, leading to severe dehydration. Patients are unable to replace lost fluids, so their condition progressively worsens. Severe dehydration also predisposes patients to thrombus formation, which can lead to disseminated intravascular coagulation. Lack of sufficient circulating insulin causes the body to metabolize fat and muscle tissues, which increases amino acid levels. The resulting hepatic gluconeogenesis compounds existing hyperglycemia.

Onset of symptoms in HHNC is much longer than with DKA, developing over days or even weeks. Subtlety of symptoms may account for delay in seeking treatment. The patient may notice vague abdominal pain, decreased appetite, polydipsia, and polyuria. As the disease progresses, headaches, blurred vision, and confusion develop. Changes in level of consciousness, seizures, or coma also occur. Tachycardia, dysrhythmias, and hypotension may also be present. Respirations may be increased but do not have the fruity smell associated with DKA. It is the decrease in mental status that usually brings the patient to the hospital.

Laboratory analysis includes complete blood count (CBC), electrolytes, urinalysis, and arterial blood gases. Blood gas analysis indicates normal PaO_2 unless respiratory infection is the stressor. Slightly decreased to normal serum pH may be present. Urinalysis shows positive glucosuria without ketonuria. Elevated white blood cell (WBC) count is present with infection. The serum glucose level is usually greater than 600 mg/dl and often greater than 1000 mg/dl.

Serum sodium and potassium may be normal or elevated depending on the level of dehydration.

Correction of hyperglycemia, dehydration, electrolyte imbalances, and a search for the underlying illness is the focus for treatment. If the patient exhibits respiratory compromise or altered level of consciousness, oxygen therapy should be initiated immediately. Rapid intravenous fluid replacement is initiated with half-normal or normal saline in adults or normal saline in children and the elderly. Dehydration in HHNC can require 12 L or more of intravenous fluid. Continual assessment and reassessment are the key to preventing complications associated with fluid therapy. Most patients are more than age 50 years, so circulatory overload is a marked risk with rapid fluid therapy. Urinary catheter placement assists with intake and output monitoring. Intravenous potassium supplements help prevent hypokalemia from hemodilution and insulin therapy. Cardiac monitoring allows observation for potential cardiac complications related to the potassium deficits.

After the serum glucose level is known, an insulin drip may be started but is not always necessary. Serum glucose should be lowered gradually because reductions greater than 100 mg/dl/hr may predispose the patient to cerebral edema from associated fluid shifts. After serum osmolality begins to normalize or the serum glucose level reaches 200 to 300 mg/dl, intravenous fluids are converted to 5% dextrose in normal or half-normal saline to provide energy until oral intake improves.

Table 39-7	CLINICAL MANIFESTATIONS OF HYPEROSMOLAR HYPERGLYCEMIC NONKETOTIC COMA	
SYSTEM	**CLINICAL MANIFESTATIONS**	
Neurologic	Confusion, lethargy, seizures, coma	
Pulmonary	Shallow or normal respirations	
Cardiovascular	Tachycardia, elevated T waves, dysrhythmias	
Renal	Polyuria, glucosuria	
Gastrointestinal	Mild abdominal discomfort, nausea, vomiting	

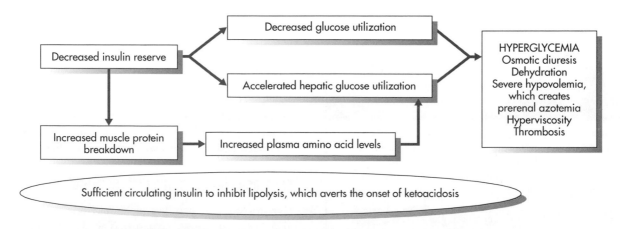

FIGURE 39-9 Pathophysiology of hyperosmolar hyperglycemic nonketotic coma.

Table 39-8	COMPARISON OF HYPERGLYCEMIC HYPEROSMOLAR NONKETOTIC COMA (HHNC) AND DIABETIC KETOACIDOSIS (DKA)	
CLINICAL PICTURE	**HHNC**	**DKA**
General	More dehydrated, not acidotic	More acidotic and less dehydrated
	Frequently comatose	Rarely comatose
	No hyperventilation	Hyperventilation
Age frequency	Usually elderly	Younger patients
Type of diabetes mellitus	Type II or non–insulin-dependent	Type I or insulin-dependent
Previous history of diabetes mellitus	In only 50%	Almost always
Prodromes	Several days' duration	Less than 1 day
Neurologic symptoms and signs	Very common	Rare
Underlying renal or cardiovascular disease	About 85%	About 15%
Laboratory findings		
Blood sugar	More than 800 mg/dl	Usually less than 800 mg/dl
Plasma ketones	Less than large in undiluted specimen	Positive in several dilutions
Serum sodium	Normal, elevated, low	Usually low
Serum potassium	Normal or elevated	Elevated, normal, or low
Serum bicarbonate	More than 16 mEq	Less than 10 mEq
Anion gap	10-12 mEq	More than 12 mEq
Blood pH	Normal	Less than 7.35
Serum osmolality	More than 350 mOsm/L	Less than 330 mOsm/L
Serum BUN	Higher than DKA ($\uparrow\uparrow\uparrow$ to $\uparrow\uparrow\uparrow\uparrow$)	Not as high as in HHNC ($\uparrow\uparrow$)
Free fatty acids	Less than 1000 mEq/L	More than 1500 mEq/L
Complications		
Thrombosis	Frequent	Very rare
Mortality	20%-50%	1%-10%
Diabetes treatment after recovery	Diet alone or oral agents (sometimes)	Always insulin

Modified from Kozak G, editor: *Clinical diabetes mellitus,* Philadelphia, 1982, WB Saunders.

Differentiation between HHNC and DKA may be initially difficult; however, this should not alter the basic course of treatment. Intravenous fluid therapy should begin immediately. Nursing actions are similar in both instances and include close observation of vital systems to prevent complications of therapy. Table 39-8 compares the clinical pictures of HHNC and DKA.

Hypoglycemia

Of three specific diabetic emergencies, hypoglycemia progresses the most quickly. Prompt nursing assessment and action are imperative to avoid fatal consequences. Type I diabetics are more susceptible because of insulin's quick onset of action. Hypoglycemia should be considered a causative agent in any unresponsive patients until established otherwise. Factors that contribute to hypoglycemia include lack of dietary intake, increased physical stress, liver disease, changes in type of insulin or oral agents, pregnancy, alcohol ingestion, and certain drugs (e.g., nonsteroidal antiinflammatory drugs, phenytoin, thyroid hormone, propranolol).

Serum glucose levels lower than 60 mg/dl indicate hypoglycemia. However, hypoglycemia can occur at a higher level, depending on the patient's "normal" glucose level. The axiom "treat the patient, not the monitor" is applied here—that is, treat the patient's symptoms, not just the serum glucose level.

Rapid decline in glucose deprives the body of normal compensatory responses; for example, glucagon and epinephrine. Normally the body senses declining serum glucose, so glucagon and epinephrine are released to increase release of glycogen stored in the liver. Glycogen functions as an alternate energy source; however, in acute hypoglycemia, glycogen stores cannot be broken down quickly enough to overcome insulin. Epinephrine release decreases utilization of existing glucose.

Mild symptoms of palpitations, tachycardia, shakiness, perspiration, and hunger are attributed to epinephrine. The known diabetic patient can usually recognize these symptoms and self-treat. β-Blocker therapy masks the sympathetic response, so these patients may not recognize onset of hypoglycemia.

Moderate symptoms include altered level of consciousness, slurred speech, headache, and decreased reaction time. As neuroglycopenia worsens, confusion with decreased ability to make decisions occurs. The patient may or may not be able to self-treat or seek treatment at this point. Without treatment moderate hypoglycemia can lead to disorientation, seizures, and eventually coma (Table 39-9). Family education is critical. Often the family must initiate treatment after recognizing changes in the patient's behavior. Patients on insulin pumps are particularly vulnerable.

Treatment of the conscious patient consists of oral intake of 10 to 15 g of carbohydrates followed by a more complex

Table 39-9	CLINICAL MANIFESTATIONS OF HYPOGLYCEMIA
SYSTEM	**CLINICAL MANIFESTATIONS**
Neurologic	Confusion, combativeness, seizures, coma
Pulmonary	Hyperventilation, shallow respirations
Cardiovascular	Palpitations, tachycardia
Integumentary	Cool, pale, clammy, diaphoretic
Gastrointestinal	Hunger, severe hypoglycemia

Box 39-1	QUICK GLUCOSE SOURCES

The following foods provide a quick glucose source (approximately 10 to 15 g of carbohydrates):

4 to 6 oz of orange juice, apple juice, or ginger ale
5 to 6 Lifesaver candies
½ to ¾ cup of nondiet soda
6 oz of milk
2 to 3 glucose tablets

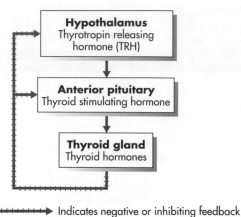

Indicates negative or inhibiting feedback

FIGURE **39-10** Thyroid regulation. (From Lewis SM, Heitkemper MM, Dirksen SR: *Medical-surgical nursing: assessment and management of clinical problems,* ed 5, St. Louis, 2000, Mosby.)

carbohydrate snack or small meal (Box 39-1). In the lethargic or unconscious patient, rapid administration of intravenous glucose (1 ampule of D50) remains the treatment of choice.[3] If intravenous access cannot be obtained, intramuscular glucagon should be administered. Glucagon, 1 mg intramuscularly, stimulates the liver to release glycogen, which is converted to glucose. If the patient has an insulin pump, the pump must be stopped immediately. If the patient has a seizure, protect the patient from injury by placing in the recovery or left lateral position to maintain the airway. In the hospital setting, priorities include ensuring patient safety and initiating oxygen therapy.

Laboratory study results obtained before glucose administration provide helpful information; however, administration of D50 should not be delayed to obtain laboratory samples. Severe neurologic deficits can result if the central nervous system is left without glucose. Once alert, the patient should be given a diet tray to provide complex carbohydrates as the D50 begins to wear off. After this meal and a glucose recheck, the patient is usually discharged if the cause of the episode is found unless the patient is on oral antihyperglycemic medications that have a longer half-life.

Thyroid Storm

Thyroid emergencies are rare but can be life-threatening. The thyroid gland regulates the body's metabolic rate, so hyperactivity or hypoactivity causes multisystem symptoms. Thyroid storm commonly occurs as a complication of Graves' disease (thyroid hyperactivity or thyrotoxicosis) and is seen primarily in women 30 to 40 years old.

The hypothalamic-pituitary-thyroid counterregulatory system is responsible for normal thyroid function. Thyroid crisis occurs when any part of the circuit malfunctions. Thyroid gland activity depends on the hypothalamus secreting

thyrotropin-releasing hormone (TRH), which is responsible for release of thyrotropin or TSH by the anterior pituitary, which causes T3 and T4 release. Circulating T4 also converts to T3 (Figure 39-10). The amount of TSH depends on the amount of TRH, which can be influenced by physical stressors such as surgery, infection, and extremely cold temperatures. Circulating levels of T3 and T4 also affect the amount of TRH released.

Hyperthyroidism can be divided into three categories. True hyperthyroidism is characterized by an overactive thyroid gland and excessive production of thyroid hormones. In Graves' disease, thyroid-stimulating immunoglobulins increase thyroid activity. Tumors and thyroid nodules also increase thyroid activity. A type of thyrotoxicosis occurs with an increased amount of circulating hormones without concurrent overactivity from the thyroid, as in thyroiditis or ingestion of thyroid hormones (intentionally or unintentionally). Certain drugs, especially iodine and iodine-containing agents such as amiodarone and lithium, induce hyperthyroidism.

Thyroid storm occurs with rapid elevation in thyroid hormone levels. Congestive heart failure is a common presentation. The patient appears toxic with temperature elevations to 105.8° F (41° C) and diaphoresis. Thyroid storm is actually a clinical diagnosis.[11] The end result is a hypermetabolic state characterized by hyperthermia, agitation, and tachydysrhythmias. Elevated hormone levels occur in response to hospitalization, surgery, infection, emotional stressors, trauma, childbirth, sudden discontinuation of antithyroid medications, and overmanipulation of the thyroid.

Gathering a concise history regarding illnesses and current medications is important. The patient may have recently discontinued a medication or experienced a recent change in therapy. The patient usually has a history of Graves' disease. Patients often report recent weight loss despite increased appetite and increased caloric intake. Complaints of abdominal pain are common.

The patient is restless with shortened attention span and may switch topics of conversation frequently. Tremors and

Table 39-10	CLINICAL MANIFESTATIONS OF THYROID STORM
SYSTEM	**CLINICAL MANIFESTATIONS**
Neurologic	Nervousness, restlessness, tremors, confusion
Pulmonary	Tachycardia, dysrhythmias, hypertension
Respiratory	Shortness of breath, dyspnea, rales, congestive heart failure
Gastrointestinal	Hyperactive bowel, abdominal pain, decreased appetite, weight loss, diarrhea, jaundice
Ocular	Exophthalmus, lid lag, staring gaze
Integumentary	Hyperthermia, flushed, diaphoresis, poor turgor

manic behaviors are also common. In late stages the patient may have altered mental status progressing to coma. Hyperthermia may be extreme with temperatures reaching 105° (40.5° C) to 106° F (41° C). Tachycardia with rates as high as 200 to 300 beats/min increases the patient's risk for cardiac failure and arrest.[11] Rales secondary to cardiac failure may be heard. The skin often progresses from warm and diaphoretic to hot and dry as dehydration worsens. Nausea, vomiting, and diarrhea are caused by increased gastric motility. Hepatic tenderness, jaundice, and thinning hair may occur. Goiter, an enlarged thyroid gland, develops as the condition progresses. Eyes become protuberant, periorbital edema develops, and the patient has a staring gaze with heavy eyelids. Table 39-10 summarizes the clinical manifestations of thyroid storm.

Thyroid hormone levels may help differentiate the causative factor but are not readily available and make it difficult to differeniate between throid strorm and thyrotoxicosis. If thyroid storm is suspected, rapid, aggressive therapy is essential to reduce hormone levels and preserve hemodynamic integrity.

Immediate goals for management of thyroid storm include inhibiting thyroid hormone synthesis, slowing thyroid hormone release, blocking peripheral thyroid hormone effects, and general supportive care.[8] Propranolol is given intravenously in doses of 1 mg/min up to 10 mg to achieve a heart rate of 90 to 110 beats per minute. Large doses of propranolol (160 to 480) may be required, especially in younger patients and those in severe crisis. Propanolol blocks conversion of T4 to T3. In cases where β-blockers are contraindicated (e.g., diabetes, asthma, pregnancy) digitalis may be used. Guanethidine and reserpine are used to deplete catecholamine stores and block further release.

Propylthiouracil and methimazole may be used to block further synthesis of the hormone. Both are given orally or through a gastric tube. Onset of action is within 1 hour but their full effect is not evident until 3 to 6 weeks. Iodine should be given 1 hour after antithyroid medications to slow release of stored thyroid hormone from the thyroid gland. If given sooner, iodine may actually be used to create new hormone. Iodine is given orally (Lugol's) or by slow intravenous infusion. Lithium carbonate has been used to prevent T4 release but has a narrow safety margin.[11]

Patients with Graves' disease and thyroid crisis metabolize and use cortisol faster than normal, so administration of glucocorticoids has been shown to increase survival rates. Glucocorticoids prevent adrenal compromise and inhibit T4 conversion to T3.[14]

Small amounts of diuretics may be required to help prevent or minimize fluid overload. Intake and output should be closely monitored to ensure fluid balance and assess response to therapy. If the causative agent is overload of thyroid medications, they can be removed through lavage or peritoneal dialysis.

Increased body temperature raises metabolic demands, which increases the percentage of free T4. Acetaminophen is preferred over salicylates, which displace thyroid hormones from binding sites and worsen the situation. Cool cloths to the axilla and groin and fans are helpful with reduction of hyperthermia. Keep the patient from shivering because this increases the metabolic rate. Chlorpromazine often is administered. Fluid replacement therapy replenishes fluids lost through hyperthermia, vomiting, and diarrhea. Administration of antiemetic and antidiarrheal agents helps the patient conserve fluids. The patient's hemodynamic status and electrolyte levels determine the fluid of choice. Providing supplemental oxygen assists with increased multisystem oxygen demands.

After the patient stabilizes, close evaluation and assessment are necessary to identify the aggravating agent or illness. Laboratory analysis includes cultures, toxicology screens, thyroid functions, electrolyte levels, and CBC. Radiographs may be ordered to rule out infectious sources; head and neck computed tomography scans may be ordered to identify existing neoplasms or structural abnormalities. Antibiotic therapy may be started when infection is suspected as a causal agent.

Myxedema Coma

Myxedema coma affects elderly women with long-standing hypothyroidism or those with undiagnosed hypothyroidism. The latter situation freqently occcurs during the winter months. Survival rates increase when patients receive prompt hormone replacement with intensive supportive care; however, mortality still approaches 50%.[13]

Untreated hypothyroidism progresses over months to years before culminating in myxedema coma. All patients who develop myxedema coma have hypothyroidism.[14] Dysfunction may be related to autoimmune thyroiditis, ablation therapy (treatment for hyperthyroidism), iodine deficiency, tumor activity, or drug therapy. Medications such as lithium, amiodarone, and certain anticonvulsants can create hypothyroid conditions. Secondary hypothyroidism stems from pituitary dysfunction. Alterations in pituitary function decrease TSH release, which lowers thyroid hormone secretion. Tertiary hypothyroidism occurs when the hypothala-

Table 39-11	CLINICAL MANIFESTATIONS OF MYXEDEMA COMA
SYSTEM	**CLINICAL MANIFESTATIONS**
Neurologic	Confusion, lethargy, coma
Pulmonary	Decreased stroke volume, decreased cardiac output, bradycardia, peripheral vasoconstriction, inverted T waves, prolonged QT interval
Respiratory	Macroglossia, obesity-related sleep apnea, pneumonia, hypoventilation, hypercarbia
Gastrointestinal	Hypoglycemia, constipation
Renal	Decreased renal blood flow, decreased sodium reabsorption, hyponatremia

mus secretes inadequate amounts of TRH or TRH fails to reach the pituitary gland.

With a hypoactive thyroid the entire system slows down. Fever, tachycardia, and diaphoresis are absent, so the crisis state may not be noticed initially. The patient may complain of pronounced fatigue, decreased activity tolerance, episodes of shortness of breath, and weight gain. Tongue swelling or macroglossia may also occur. Patients may answer questions slowly and exhibit significant confusion. Altered mental status can progress to coma. "Myxedema madness" refers to associated psychiatric symptoms such as hallucinations, paranoia, depression, combativeness, and decreased concern for personal appearance.

The tongue may be thick and can obstruct the airway in a semiconscious or unconscious patient. Weak respiratory effort with decreased respiratory drive leads to alveolar hypoventilation and can predispose the patient to infections. Alveolar hypoventilation also leads to hypercarbia, which can cause altered mental status. Obesity-related sleep apnea can further compromise the respiratory system. Table 39-11 summarizes the clinical manifestations of myxedema.

Cardiac changes include bradycardia, decreased stroke volume, and decreased cardiac output. There may be widespread ST- and T-wave changes with prolonged QT intervals. Peripheral vasoconstriction is the body's attempt to conserve heat, so skin is cool and pale, and body temperature is low.

In myxedema, coma renal blood flow and glomerular filtration rates decrease, yet sodium reabsorption also decreases. Patients cannot excrete the usual amount of fluid; however, urine osmolality does not reflect serum hypoosmolality. Generalized nonpitting edema may be observed. Occasionally, hypoglycemia develops as a result of increased insulin sensitivity and decreased oral intake. Systemic slowing affects the gastrointestinal tract, so constipation occurs. Oral medications in initial stages may not be adequately absorbed because of decreased gastric motility.

Diagnostic tests reveal decreased WBC count, decreased hemoglobin and hematocrit (caused by low erythropoietin),

and decreased thyroid levels. Creatinine kinase may be elevated with elevations of MM bands.

Care focuses on thyroid hormone replacement after the ABCs have been stabilized. The patient may require mechanical ventilation to secure the airway, correct increased carbon dioxide levels, and improve oxygenation. Hormone replacement may take the form of intravenous levothyroxine (T4). Large doses saturate empty sites and replenish peripheral circulating levels. T4 avoids the adverse cardiac effects that might occur with sudden increase in T3. Some clinicians recommend a combination of T4 and T3 therapy.[8] T3 does have a quicker onset of action, but controversy still exists related to increased mortality associated with sole T3 use.[8,14] After the patient can tolerate oral fluids, oral T4 therapy may begin. Glucocorticoid administration may help prevent adrenal crisis in patients with compromised adrenal systems.

Infection, hypothermia, and drug effects are the most common precipating factors[8] that contribute to hypothyroid crisis. Scans, radiographs, and further diagnostic tests are performed after the patient stabilizes. Severe systemic slowing exhibited in myxedema coma should not be underestimated. Nursing care focuses on ABC stabilization, medication administration to correct thyroid hormone deficiencies, close observation to avoid complications, and initiation of patient education.

Slow warming is recommended because increased oxygen demands related to warming can add stress to an overstressed system. Passive warming with blankets or heated, humidified mist is preferred. Supportive care includes analgesic administration, urinary catheter placement, and a nasogastric tube to decrease abdominal pressure and distention.

Syndrome of Inappropriate Antidiuretic Hormone

SIADH occurs when the pituitary gland releases excessive amounts of ADH because ADH's negative feedback system fails (Figure 39-11). Any disease process that alters the hypothalamic osmoreceptors or hypothalamic-pituitary-adrenal circuit can precipitate SIADH. Eighty percent of patients with SIADH have small cell cancer or pancreatic cancer. Thyroid and pituitary lesions place the patient at increased risk for SIADH.[5] Narcotics, tricyclic antidepressants, oral hypoglycemics, and certain anticonvulsants (carbamazepine) also precipitate SIADH. Other associated disorders include abscesses, pneumonia, tuberculosis, hypothyroid disorders, porphyria, and head injury. Other groups at risk are infants who are only given tap water, elderly patients on diuretics, patients with AIDS, and psychiatric patients. Box 39-2 summarizes causes of SIADH.

ADH is generated in the hypothalamus and stored in the pituitary gland. Increased distal renal tubular permeability to water resulting from ADH decreases urine volume and returns water to the systemic circulation. Serum osmolality and circulating blood volume influence ADH release. Hypothalamic osmoreceptors sense increased serum concentra-

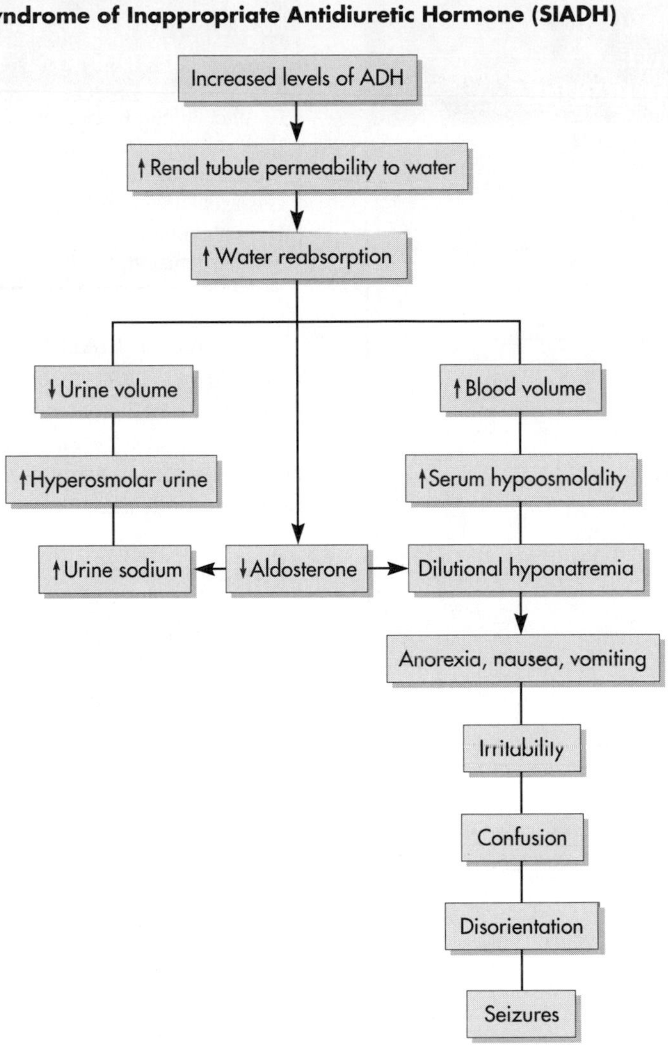

Syndrome of Inappropriate Antidiuretic Hormone (SIADH)

```
                    Increased levels of ADH
                              │
                              ▼
              ↑ Renal tubule permeability to water
                              │
                              ▼
                    ↑ Water reabsorption
                              │
          ┌───────────────────┼───────────────────┐
          │                   │                   │
          ▼                   │                   ▼
    ↓ Urine volume            │             ↑ Blood volume
          │                   │                   │
          ▼                   │                   ▼
  ↑ Hyperosmolar urine        │          ↑ Serum hypoosmolality
          │                   │                   │
          ▼                   ▼                   ▼
   ↑ Urine sodium  ◄──  ↓ Aldosterone  ──►  Dilutional hyponatremia
                                                  │
                                                  ▼
                                      Anorexia, nausea, vomiting
                                                  │
                                                  ▼
                                             Irritability
                                                  │
                                                  ▼
                                              Confusion
                                                  │
                                                  ▼
                                            Disorientation
                                                  │
                                                  ▼
                                              Seizures
```

FIGURE 39-11 Pathophysiology of syndrome of inappropriate antidiuretic hormone (SIADH). (From Lewis SM, Heitkemper MM, Dirksen SR: *Medical-surgical nursing: assessment and management of clinical problems,* ed 5, St. Louis, 2000, Mosby.)

tion and stimulate release of ADH. Serum concentration decreases when the kidneys respond with increased water reabsorption. As circulating volume expands, urinary output diminishes. The resulting hemodilution creates fluid overload with associated hyponatremia.

Baroreceptors in the left atrium sensitive to blood pressure changes respond to increased blood volume by inhibiting release of ADH, which leads to increased urinary output so blood volume returns to normal. The reverse actions occur when baroreceptors sense decreased blood pressure. Disturbances in this feedback loop may be responsible for ADH crisis.

Subjective complaints include weakness, nausea, vomiting, diarrhea, abdominal and muscle cramps, sudden weight gain without edema, and confusion. The patient may also note decreased urinary output despite regular oral intake; the greatest changes, however, may be in neurologic function. The patient appears confused and disoriented with seizures

noted as hyponatremia worsens. Severe hyponatremia leads to fluid shifts, which cause cerebral edema and brainstem herniation syndrome.[6] Deep tendon reflexes decrease.

Laboratory tests reveal marked hyponatremia (less than 120 mEq/L) and low serum osmolality. BUN and creatinine levels are low to normal. Urine specific gravity below 1.002 demonstrates serum dilution. Renal function tests are usually normal.

Management of SIADH is related to the severity of hyponatremia. Free water restriction is sufficient in mild cases.[12] Restrictions often start at 800 to 1000 ml/day; however, restrictions as severe as 500 ml/day are seen. The importance of accurate intake and output monitoring cannot be overemphasized. Fluid replacement therapy consists of hypertonic solutions such as 3% or 5% normal saline, which helps move fluid out of edematous cerebral tissue. Intravenous therapy begins at 75 to 125 ml/hr. Close monitoring is necessary for early identification of circulatory overload.

Box 39-2	CAUSES OF SYNDROME OF INAPPROPRIATE ANTIDIURETIC HORMONE

MALIGNANT NEOPLASMS

Small-cell carcinoma of lung
Carcinoma of pancreas and duodenum
Lymphosarcoma, reticulum cell sarcoma, Hodgkin's disease
Thymoma

NONMALIGNANT PULMONARY DISEASES

Tuberculosis
Lung abscess
Pneumonia
Empyema
Chronic obstructive pulmonary disease

CENTRAL NERVOUS SYSTEM DISORDERS

Skull fracture
Subdural hematoma
Subarachnoid hemorrhage
Cerebral vascular thrombosis
Cerebral atrophy
Encephalitis
Meningitis
Guillain-Barré syndrome
Systemic lupus erythematosus

DRUGS

Chlorpropamide
Vincristine
Vinblastine
Cyclophosphamide
Carbamazepine
Oxytocin
General anesthesia
Narcotics
Tricyclic antidepressants

MISCELLANEOUS CAUSES

Hypothyroidism
Positive pressure mechanical ventilation

From Moses A, Streeten D: Disorders of the neurohypophysis. In Isselbacher K et al, editors: *Harrison's principles of internal medicine,* ed 13, New York, 1994, Mosby. Used with permission of the McGraw-Hill Companies. From National Asthma Education Program: *Guidelines for the diagnosis and management of asthma: speaker's kit,* 1992, National Heart, Lung, and Blood Institute.

Small amounts of loop diuretics increase urinary output and may prevent overload. Serial electrolyte evaluations help avoid complications in therapy and assist in monitoring therapy progress. Administration of demeclocycline, 600 to 1200 mg/day, interferes with ADH action; however, this simply augments fluid restriction therapy. Ultimately, serum sodium and osmolality should improve. After the patient stabilizes, identification and treatment of the precipitating event become a primary goal.

Box 39-3	NURSING DIAGNOSES FOR ENDOCRINE EMERGENCIES

Cardiac output, Decreased
Fluid volume, Deficient
Fluid volume, Excess
Gas exchange, Impaired
Hyperthermia
Tissue perfusion, Ineffective

Uncorrected, SIADH has serious consequences. Failure of the ADH regulatory feedback loop leads to vascular water overload with severe serum hyponatremia. Fluid restriction is the primary management tool, with close observation and timely management to ensure patient safety and prevention of complications.

SUMMARY

Endocrine emergencies affect all body systems because of the diversity of hormones and their effects. Support of hemodynamic functions and identification of precipitating events are essential for survival of these patients. Box 39-3 highlights priority nursing diagnoses for the patient with an endocrine emergency.

References

1. Aaron C, Brunell T: Complication of alcohol abuse. In Harwood-Nuss A, Wolfson A, editors: *The clinical practice of emergency medicine,* ed 3, Philadelphia, 2001, Lippincott Williams & Wilkins.
2. Adams S, Bontempo L: Alcoholic ketoacidosis. In Harwood-Nuss A, Wolfson A, editors: *The clinical practice of emergency medicine,* ed 3, Philadelphia, 2001, Lippincott Williams & Wilkins.
3. Adler J, Plantz S, Stearns D et al: *NMS clinical manual emergency medicine,* Baltimore, 1999, Lippincott Williams & Wilkins.
4. Carroll R: The metabolic system. In Black J, Hawks J, Keene A, editors: *Medical surgical nursing,* ed 6, Philadelphia, 2001, WB Saunders.
5. Craig S, Marx J: Disorders of sodium, water & metabolism. In Harwood-Nuss A, Wolfson A, editors: *The clinical practice of emergency medicine,* ed 3, Philadelphia, 2001, Lippincott Williams & Wilkins.
6. English D, Howton JC: Diabetes and complications. In Schwartz G, editor: *Principles & practice of emergency medicine,* ed 4, Baltimore, 1999, Lippincott Williams & Wilkins.
7. Guyton A, Hall J: *Textbook of medical physiology,* ed 10, Philadelphia, 2000, WB Saunders.
8. Howton JC: Hyperthyroidism & thyroid storm. In Schwartz G, editor: *Principles & practice of emergency medicine,* ed 4, Baltimore, 1999, Lippincott Williams & Wilkins.
9. Larson A: In Black J, Hawks J, Keene A: *Medical surgical nursing,* ed 6, Philadelphia, 2001, WB Saunders.
10. Pope D, Zun L: Hyperosmolar hyperglycemic nonketotic coma. In Harwood-Nuss A, Wolfson A, editors: *The clinical practice of emergency medicine,* ed 3, Philadelphia, 2001, Lippincott Williams & Wilkins.

11. Ragland T, Urbanic R: Thyroid emergencies. In Harwood-Nuss A, Wolfson A, editors: *Clinical practice of emergency medicine,* ed 3, Philadelphia, 2001, Lippincott Williams & Wilkins.

12. Sabatine M: *Pocket medicine,* Philadelphia, 2000, Lippincott Williams & Wilkins.

13. Sercombe C, Ling L: Adrenal & pituitary disorders. In Harwood-Nuss A, Wolfson A, editors: *The clinical practice of emergency medicine,* ed 3, Philadelphia, 2001, Lippincott Williams & Wilkins.

14. Tietgens S, Leinaneg M: Thyroid storm, *Med Clin North Am* 79(1): 169, 1995.

15. Tintinalli J, Kelen G, Stapczynski J: *Emergency medicine: a comprehensive study guide,* ed 5, New York, 2000, McGraw-Hill.

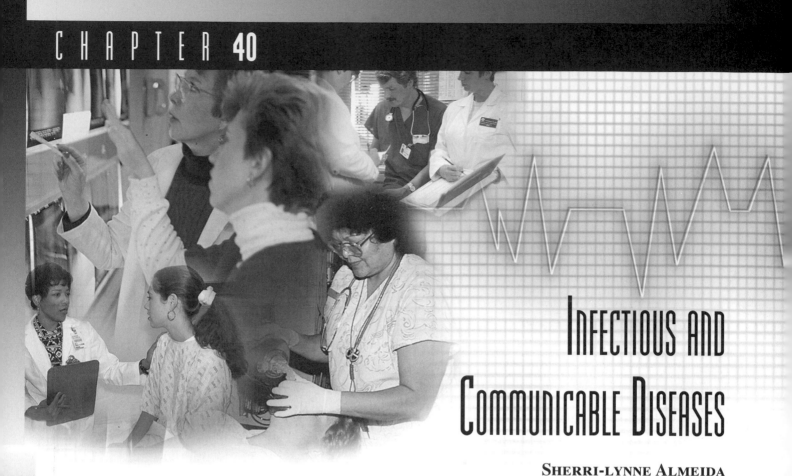

INFECTIOUS AND COMMUNICABLE DISEASES

SHERRI-LYNNE ALMEIDA

Infection is entry and development or multiplication of an infectious agent in the body. Three factors form the chain of infection: agent, host, and mode of transmission.[10] The agent or microorganism can be a bacterium, virus, fungus, or parasite. The property of an infectious agent that determines the extent to which overt disease is produced or the power of an organism to produce disease is called pathogenicity. Some agents are highly pathogenic and almost always produce disease, whereas others multiply without invasion and rarely cause disease.

A susceptible host is one who lacks effective resistance to a pathogenic agent. Characteristics that influence susceptibility include age, sex, medical history, underlying pathology, lifestyle, nutrition, immunizations, medications, and specific insult to the body, such as trauma.

Transmission is the interaction between an infectious agent and susceptible host. Major modes of transmission are direct, indirect, and airborne exposure. Direct transmission occurs when person-to-person contact occurs between an infected source and susceptible host with a receptive portal through which human or animal infection can enter. Direct contact includes touching, biting, kissing, sexual intercourse, direct inoculation with contaminated blood (needlestick injury), or direct projection of droplet spray onto conjunctiva of the eye, nose, or mouth during sneezing, coughing, spitting, or vomiting.[3] Indirect transmission occurs when susceptible hosts come in contact with a contaminated object. Any substance by which an infectious agent is transported and introduced into a susceptible host through a suitable portal of entry is vehicle-borne.

Vehicle-borne agents are contaminated, inanimate materials such as patient care equipment, soiled linen, surgical instruments, dressings, food, water, milk, and biologic products such as blood, serum, plasma, tissues, or organs. *Vector-borne* transmission occurs with injection of saliva during biting, regurgitation, or dermal exposure to feces or other material capable of penetrating nonintact skin. And finally, *airborne* transmission is defined as dissemination of microbial aerosols through a portal, usually the respiratory tract. Close contact with an infected source who is coughing or sneezing can transmit large infectious particles through the air. Factors that influence airborne transmission include ambient airflow, proximity, and spatial orientation to the person who is coughing or sneezing.

PREVENTION OF INFECTION

In the hospital environment, transmission of an infectious agent to a susceptible host occurs by direct and indirect contact.[2] Nosocomial infection, the most common form of hospital infection, is an infection acquired by a patient who had no infection at the time of arrival at the hospital. Inappropriate or lack of hand washing is the most significant reason for development of nosocomial infections. In the absence of a true emergency, personnel should always wash their hands before patient contact. Box 40-1 highlights critical times

---

Box 40-1 HAND-WASHING ESSENTIALS

Before performing invasive procedures (i.e., intravenous catheter insertion, ureteral catheterization, or tracheal suctioning)

Before caring for susceptible patients (i.e., the immunosuppressed patient, newborns, or the elderly)

Before and after touching wounds

When exposure to microbial contamination may occur (i.e., contact with mucous membranes, blood, body fluids, secretions, or excretions)

After touching contaminated inanimate objects (e.g., suction equipment, urine collection devices)

Between contact with patients

After removing protective gloves

Box 40-2 UNIVERSAL PRECAUTIONS

DO APPLY

Blood, semen, vaginal secretions, cerebrospinal fluid, synovial fluid, pleural fluid, peritoneal fluid, pericardial fluid, amniotic fluid

DO NOT APPLY

Feces, nasal secretions, sputum, sweat, tears, urine, vomitus (unless contaminated with blood)

---

when hand washing should occur. Products containing antimicrobial agents such as foams and rinses can be used when water is not available.

There will always be patients in the emergency department (ED) with infections or infectious diseases. Risk to the emergency nurse is probably no greater for these infections than risk to the community. Emergency nurses have a greater risk of exposure to bloodborne pathogens such as hepatitis B virus (HBV), hepatitis C virus (HCV), and human immunodeficiency virus (HIV) because of frequent exposure to blood and the unknown status of the patient. The emergency nurse must use universal precautions, treating all blood and most body fluids as infectious. Blood is the single most important source of HIV, HBV, HCV, and other bloodborne pathogens; however, universal precautions also apply to other body fluids. Box 40-2 identifies precautions for various body fluids. Box 40-3 summarizes guidelines to minimize exposure to bloodborne pathogens.

SPECIFIC TYPES OF INFECTIOUS DISEASES

The emergency nurse may encounter a number of infectious and communicable diseases, depending on where he or she works and how mobile the patient population is. This chapter focuses on infectious diseases that are most prevalent: hepatitis, acquired immunodeficiency syndrome (AIDS), and tuberculosis. Childhood illnesses such as measles, mumps, and chickenpox are discussed in Chapter 48 (Pediatric Emergencies).

Box 40-3 GUIDELINES TO MINIMIZE EXPOSURE TO BLOODBORNE PATHOGENS

Do not perform direct patient care or handle contaminated equipment without barrier protection when open skin lesions are present.

Use special caution if pregnant when working with patients or contaminated equipment, supplies, or materials.

Use disposable gloves when performing arterial or venous punctures, aspirating blood from existing arterial or venous catheters, handling blood or body fluid specimens, hanging or changing blood bags or transfusion tubing, emptying bedpans and urinals, and providing stoma care.

Remove damaged gloves. Wash hands and then don new gloves.

Wash hands immediately if exposed to blood or body fluids, between patient contacts, after touching contaminated objects, and after removing gloves.

Wear impervious gowns, masks, or eye covering when extensive blood or body fluid exposure is possible (e.g., trauma resuscitation, emergency delivery, gastric lavage).

Use artificial airways and resuscitation masks rather than mouth-to-mouth ventilations.

Do not recap, bend, or break needles. Do not place needles on the bed or drop on the floor. Discard needles in an appropriate sharps container.

Carry nondisposable sharp instruments in a puncture-resistant container.

Scrub reusable equipment to remove debris and blood (wear gloves).

Wipe contaminated surfaces with absorbent toweling to remove excess material and then wash with an appropriate germicide. Clothing may be washed in the regular laundry.

Remove contaminated gloves before touching a telephone or other nonclinical surfaces.

Hepatitis

Hepatitis is an acute or chronic viral infection of the liver that may be mild or life-threatening. Five types of hepatitis are currently recognized: hepatitis A, B, C, D, and E (Table 40-1). Hepatitis E is not discussed beyond this table because the condition is not common to the United States and Canada. It is limited to outbreaks in developing countries. Emergency nurses are more likely to develop hepatitis than HIV infection from an occupational injury. Universal precautions are the first line of protection against this and other infectious processes.

Hepatitis A

Hepatitis A virus (HAV) continues to be one of the most frequently reported vaccine-preventable diseases in the United States, despite licensure of hepatitis A vaccine in 1995.[4]

Acquisition of HAV infection occurs primarily by the fecal-oral route through person-to-person contact or ingestion of contaminated food or water. On rare occasions HAV infection has been transmitted by transfusion of blood or

Table 40-1	CHARACTERISTICS OF HEPATITIS VIRUSES			
	INCUBATION PERIOD	MODE OF TRANSMISSION	SOURCES OF INFECTION AND SPREAD OF DISEASE	INFECTIVITY
Hepatitis A virus (HAV)	15-50 days (average 28)	Fecal-oral (fecal contamination and oral ingestion)	Crowded conditions; poor personal hygiene; poor sanitation; contaminated food, milk, water, and shell-fish; persons with sub-clinical infections; infected food handlers; sexual contact	Most infectious during 2 weeks before onset of symptoms; infectious until 1-2 weeks after symptoms start
Hepatitis B virus (HBV)	45-180 days (average 56-96)	Percutaneous (parenteral)/ permucosal exposure to blood or blood products Sexual contact Perinatal transmission Human bile	Contaminated needles, syringes, and blood products; sexual activity with infected partners; asymptomatic carriers Tattoo/body piercing, bites	Before and after symptoms appear; infectious for 4-6 months; in carriers continues for patient's lifetime
Hepatitis C virus (HCV)	14-180 days (average 56)	Percutaneous (parenteral)/ permucosal exposure to blood or blood products High-risk sexual contact Perinatal contact	Blood and blood products, needles and syringes, sexual activity with infected partners	1-2 weeks before symptoms; continues during clinical course; indefinitely with carriers
Hepatitis D virus (HDV)	2-26 weeks HBV must precede HDV; chronic carriers of HBV are always at risk	Can cause infection only together with HBV; routes of transmission same as for HBV	Same as HBV	Blood is infectious at all stages of HDV infection
Hepatitis E virus (HEV)	15-64 days (average 26-42 days in different epidemics)	Fecal-oral Outbreaks associated with contaminated water supply in developing countries	Contaminated water; poor sanitation; found in Asia, Africa, and Mexico; not common in the United States and Canada	Not known; may be similar to HAV

From Lewis SM, Heitkemper MM, Dirksen SR: *Medical-surgical nursing: assessment and management of clinical problems,* ed 5, St. Louis, 2000, Mosby.

blood products collected from donors during the viremic phase of their infection.[9,12] Depending on conditions, HAV can be stable in the environment for months.

The illness caused by HAV infection typically has an abrupt onset of symptoms that can include fever, malaise, anorexia, nausea, abdominal discomfort, dark urine, and jaundice. The likelihood of being symptomatic with HAV infections is related to the person's age. When present, these signs and symptoms usually last less than 2 months. With an average incubation period of 28 days (range 15 to 50 days), the infectious agent reaches peak levels during the 2-week period before onset of jaundice or elevation in liver enzymes. Concentration of the virus in stool declines after jaundice appears.

The disease varies in clinical severity from a mild illness lasting 1 to 2 weeks to a severe, disabling disease lasting several months (rare). In general, severity increases with age, but complete uncomplicated recovery without recurrence is the norm. Many infections are asymptomatic. Mild cases can occur without jaundice, especially in children. Diagnosis is made by identification of immunoglobulin (Ig)M antibodies against HAV (IgM anti-HAV) in the serum of the acutely or recently ill patient. Antibodies remain detectable up to 6 months after infection. Epidemiologic evidence can provide support for diagnosis if laboratory analysis is not available.

Better hygienic and sanitary conditions and development of the hepatitis A vaccine has led to a decline in the overall incidence of hepatitis A in the United States over the past several decades. Two inactivated hepatitis A vaccines have been licensed in the United States; HAVRIX (manufactured by SmithKlineBeecham Biologicals) and VAQTA (manufactured by Merck & Co., Inc.). An inactive hepatitis A vaccine has been shown to be safe, immunogenic, and efficacious. Protection against clinical HAV may begin in some people 14 to 21 days after a single dose of vaccine; nearly all have protective antibodies by 30 days. Hepatitis A immunization is recommended for anyone who plans to travel repeatedly or reside for long periods in areas where people are at risk for infection and for children living in communities with the highest rates of infection and disease. Individuals employed in hospitals or day care centers should also be immunized.

For proven cases of hepatitis A, enteric precautions are necessary during the first 2 weeks of illness but for no more than 1 week after onset of jaundice. Passive immunization with intramuscular immune globulin (IG), 0.02 mL/kg of body weight, should be given as soon as possible after exposure to all household and sexual contacts. In a day care center, IG should be given to all classroom contacts, including staff. Immunizations are not recommended after 2 weeks of illness.

Hepatitis B

HBV is a widely distributed pathogen that produces acute and chronic infection. Chronically infected people represent the major source of infection. Individuals have an increased risk of mortality and morbidity associated with chronic liver disease and primary hepatocellular carcinoma. HBV is a worldwide problem existing even in the most remote and isolated populations of the world. Prevalence of HBV infection varies widely. The disease is highly endemic in most of the developing world but is minimally endemic in developed countries. An estimated 300 million people worldwide are chronically infected with HBV; more than 250,000 die annually from HBV-associated acute and chronic liver disease.[1] Acute and chronic consequences of HBV infection are major health problems in the United States. Each year an estimated 300,000 people, primarily young adults, are infected with HBV. The reported incidence of acute HBV increased by 37% from 1979 to 1989. One quarter of patients with HBV develop jaundice, more than 10,000 patients require hospitalization, and, on average, 250 die of fulminant disease. Approximately 4000 to 5000 people die annually from chronic liver diseases.[1]

HBV is a major infectious occupational hazard for health care workers. Risk of infection is associated with exposure to blood or potentially infectious body fluids contaminated with blood. Correcting for underreporting and subclinical infection, the Centers for Disease Control and Prevention (CDC) estimate that approximately 15,000 HBV infections are associated with health care workers each year. Fortunately, the number of cases of HBV reported in health care workers has dropped since 1985.

In the United States most people with HBV acquire the infection as adolescents or adults. Specific modes of transmission include sexual contact, especially among homosexual men and people with multiple heterosexual partners; parenteral drug use; occupational exposures; household contact with an individual who has an acute infection or is a carrier; receipt of certain blood products; and hemodialysis. The virus is passed directly from those already infected or indirectly through their body fluids. The most common modes of HBV transmission are through the skin by way of cuts, scrapes, needle sticks, or needle sharing; through the eyes, mouth, or nose by exposure to blood or other body fluids; sexual contact; and contact between an infected mother and her newborn child during birth and early infancy.

The incubation period averages 60 to 80 days, with the norm 45 to 180 days; however, the incubation period can range from 2 weeks to 6 to 9 months when hepatitis B surface antigen (HBsAg) appears. Extreme variation in the incubation period is related in part to the amount of virus in the inoculum, mode of transmission, alteration of viral pathogenicity by chemical or physical means, administration of a specific antibody, and unusual virus-host interactions.

All people who are HbsAg- and hepatitis Be antigen (HBeAg)-positive are potentially infectious. Both antigens are detectable 1 to 3 weeks after exposure and 4 to 5 weeks before onset of jaundice. Infectivity of chronically infected individuals varies from highly infectious (HbeAg-positive) to sparingly infectious (anti–Hbe-positive).

Diagnosis of HBV is based on clinical, serologic, and epidemiologic findings. Detection of HBV infection serologic markers—HbsAg—confirms hepatitis B infection. Infection may present with a variety of symptomatology: acute illness with jaundice followed by recovery, subclinical infection followed by recovery, acute illness that progresses to chronic active hepatitis, subclinical infection followed by chronic active hepatitis, and fulminant disease.[8] Viral hepatitis is the most common infectious etiology of jaundice. A short prodromal phase, varying from several days to more than a week, may precede onset of jaundice. Typical symptoms include anorexia, weakness, and fatigue. Nausea, vomiting, and diarrhea may also occur. Many patients complain of right upper quadrant abdominal pain. The preicteric phase may be characterized by fever (usually 103° F (39° C) or more), malaise, myalgia, and headache. Other symptoms are similar to serum sickness: arthritis, arthralgia, and urticaria or maculopapular rash.[8] The icteric phase begins with appearance of dark urine resulting from bilirubinuria, followed by light or gray stools and yellowish discoloration of mucous membranes, sclerae, conjunctivae, and skin. Jaundice becomes apparent when total bilirubin levels exceed 2.0 to 3.0 mg/dl. Hepatic tenderness and hepatomegaly are also present.[6] Recovery begins with disappearance of jaundice and other symptoms. HBsAg and HbeAg also disappear. The appearance of antibodies (anti-HBs and anti-HBc) indicates the infection is subsiding. Liver failure may occur in 1% to 3% of patients with acute hepatitis B. This potentially fatal disease is characterized by mental confusion, emotional instability, bleeding manifestations, and coma. Overall survival rate varies with age—7% in the elderly, 37% in patients younger than age 16 years.

The Occupational Safety and Health Administration has stated that the most effective method of infection control against hepatitis B is the hepatitis B vaccine. More than 90% of all people vaccinated develop immunity to HBV. Vaccines available in the United States contain no blood or blood products; they are made from yeast cells changed by genetic engineering. Current prevention strategy in the United States includes screening all pregnant women for the presence of HBsAg; hepatitis B IG and hepatitis B vaccine for infants of HBsAg-positive mothers; hepatitis B vaccine for susceptible household contacts; routine hepatitis B immunization for all infants; catch-up immunization for children 1 to 10 years of age in groups with high rates of chronic HBV infection; catch-up immunization for adolescents 11 to 12 years of age; and intense efforts to immunize high-risk adolescents and adults. Health care workers are reminded that universal precautions should be employed when caring for all patients when there is potential for exposure to blood or body fluids.

Hepatitis C

HCV is transmitted parenterally. This infection has been found in every part of the world. It is estimated that as many as 170 million people worldwide may be infected with HCV. HCV is the most common chronic bloodborne infection in the United States, with data indicating that approximately 1.8% of Americans have been infected.

HCV is transmitted primarily through large or repeated direct percutaneous exposures to blood. In the United States the relative importance of the two most common exposures associated with transmission of HCV—blood transfusion and injecting drug use—has changed. Blood transfusion, which accounted for a substantial proportion of HCV infections acquired greater than 10 years ago, rarely accounts for recently acquired infections. Since 1994 risk for transfusion-transmitted HCV infection has been extremely low. In contrast, injection drug use has consistently accounted for a substantial proportion of HCV infections and currently accounts for 60% of HCV transmission in the United States.[13]

As in HBV infection, contaminated needles and syringes are important vehicles of viral spread, especially among parenteral drug users and dialysis patients. Health care workers frequently contact blood, so there is increased risk for infection. However, prevalence of HCV infection among health care workers is no greater than the general population, averaging 1% to 2%, and is 10 times lower than that for HBV infection. Household or sexual contact with people who previously had hepatitis has also been documented in some studies as risk factors for acquiring HCV. The importance of person-to-person contact and sexual activity in transmission of this disease has not been well-defined. Transmission from mother to child appears to be uncommon; however, only small numbers of infants have been studied. More than 40% of HCV-infected patients have no obvious route or source of transmission.

The average time period from exposure to symptom onset is 6 to 7 weeks, whereas the average time period from exposure to seroconversion is 8 to 9 weeks. The period of communicability may range from 1 or more weeks before the onset of first symptoms and may persist indefinitely. Based on infectivity studies in chimpanzees, the titer of HCV in blood appears to be relatively low. Peaks in virus concentration appear to correlate with peaks in serum alanine transaminase (ALT) activity.

Onset is usually insidious, with severity ranging from those without apparent disease to rare fulminating, fatal cases. Symptoms include anorexia, vague abdominal discomfort, nausea, and vomiting. Symptoms progress to jaundice less frequently than with hepatitis B. The disease is usually less severe in the acute stage but chronicity is common, occurring more frequently than with hepatitis B in adults. Chronic infection may be symptomatic or asymptomatic. Chronic hepatitis C may progress to cirrhosis; there also appears to be an association between HCV infection and hepatocellular carcinoma.

Diagnosis depends on identification of anti-HCV. Anti-HCV can be detected in 80% of patients within 15 weeks after exposure, in greater than or equal to 90% within 5 months after exposure, and in greater than or equal to 97% by 6 months after exposure. Rarely, seroconversion is delayed until 9 months after exposure.[11]

General control measures against bloodborne pathogens apply. Available data regarding prevention of HCV infection with IG indicate that IG is not effective for postexposure prophylaxis of hepatitis C.[4] No assessments have been made of postexposure antiviral agents (e.g., interferon) to prevent HCV infection.

Hepatitis D

Hepatitis delta virus (HDV) is a defective virus that causes infection only in the presence of active HBV infection. HDV infections occurs as either coinfection with HBV or superinfection of an HBV carrier. Coinfection usually resolves, whereas superinfection frequently causes chronic HDV infection and chronic active hepatitis.

The prevalence of HDV varies widely, occurring epidemically and endemically in populations at high risk of acquiring HBV. Mode of transmission is thought to be similar to HBV, including exposure to blood and serous body fluids, needles, syringes, plasma derivatives, and sexual contact. Blood is potentially infectious during all phases of active HDV infection. Peak infectivity probably occurs before the onset of acute illness.

Onset is usually abrupt, with signs and symptoms resembling those of HBV infection. Symptoms may be severe and are always associated with a coexisting HBV infection. An HDV infection may be self-limiting or may progress to chronic hepatitis. Diagnosis is made by detection of total antibody to HDV (anti-HDV). ALT, alkaline phosphatase, and bilirubin are usually elevated.

General control measures against bloodborne pathogens apply. Prevention of HBV infection with hepatitis B vaccine prevents infection with HDV. However, hepatitis B immune globulin, immune globulin, and hepatitis B vaccine do not protect HBV carriers from infection by HDV.

Acquired Immunodeficiency Syndrome

AIDS was first reported in 1981; however, isolated cases occurred in the United States and other areas of the world during the 1970s.[7] HIV and AIDS have been recorded in virtually all countries among all races, ages, and social classes. Worldwide, the Joint United Nations Programme on HIV/AIDS estimates that by the end of 2000, 36.1 million people were living with HIV or AIDS. Of these, 34.7 million are adults, 16.4 million are women, and 1.4 million are children younger than age 15 years. Worldwide, it is estimated that 21.8 million people have died from AIDS since the epidemic began. As of December 31, 2000, the CDC reported the cumulative number of AIDS cases in the United States as 774,467, which resulted in 448,060 deaths. The number of people living with AIDS (322,865) is the highest ever reported. Of these, 79% were men, 61% were black or Hispanic, and 41% were infected through male-to-male sex. Male-to-male sex has been the most common mode of exposure among persons with AIDS (46%), followed by injection drug use (25%) and heterosexual contact (11%).

Epidemiologic data indicate that transmission of HIV is limited to sexual, parenteral, and maternal-infant routes. Routes of transmission are analogous to those of HBV. There is no evidence supporting other routes of HIV transmission. Substantial evidence indicates transmission does not occur through casual contact, despite reports that HIV has been isolated in small amounts from saliva and tears. From 15% to 30% of infants born to HIV-infected mothers are infected before, during, or shortly after birth. Treatment of pregnant women has resulted in a marked reduction of infant infections. Breast-feeding by HIV-infected women can transmit infection to the infant.

Direct exposure of health care workers to HIV-infected blood through percutaneous exposure is associated with seroconversion in approximately 0.3% of the cases.[5] After mucous membrane exposure, seroconversion is 0.09%, which is much lower than the risk of HBV infection (about 25%) after a similar exposure.[2]

Since 1992 scientists have estimated that half of those with HIV develop AIDS within 10 years. This time varies greatly from person to person and can depend on many factors, including a person's health status and their health-related behaviors.

The period of communicability is unknown but is presumed to begin soon after onset of HIV infection and extend throughout life. Epidemiologic evidence suggests infectivity increases with increasing immune deficiency, clinical symptoms, and presence of other sexually transmitted diseases. Recent studies suggest infectiousness may be high during the initial period after infection.[2]

AIDS is a severe, life-threatening clinical condition. This syndrome represents the late clinical stage of infection with HIV and is most often the result of progressive damage to the immune and other organ systems. Within several weeks to months after infection with HIV, many individuals develop an acute self-limited mononucleosis-like illness lasting for 1 to 2 weeks. Infected individuals may then be free of clinical signs or symptoms for months to years. Onset of clinical illness is usually insidious with nonspecific symptoms such as lymphadenopathy, anorexia, chronic diarrhea, weight loss, fever, and fatigue. More than a dozen opportunistic infections are considered AIDS infections (see Table 40-2), including several cancers, pulmonary and extrapulmonary tuberculosis (TB), recurrent pneumonia, wasting syndrome, neurologic disease (HIV dementia or sensory neuropathy), and invasive cervical cancer.

The most commonly used screening test for HIV, enzyme-linked immunoassay, is highly sensitive and specific. When this test is reactive, an additional test such as the Western blot

or indirect IFA should be obtained. Most individuals infected with HIV develop detectable antibodies within 1 to 3 months after infection. Postexposure prophylaxis is given to individuals with apparent or documented exposure (e.g., needle stick involving known HIV source).[5]

Management of the patient with AIDS in the ED is based on treatment of the specific opportunistic infection that may be present. Care should be provided in a nonjudgmental manner to support the patient, family, and significant other. For health care workers, universal precautions are the most available method to control transmission of HIV.

Tuberculosis

TB is caused by *Mycobacterium tuberculosis* and usually infects the lungs (pulmonary TB) or respiratory system. TB can spread to other organs including the kidneys, bones and joints, skin, intestines, peritoneum, eyes, lymph nodes, pericardium, and pleura. Extrapulmonary TB occurs frequently in people infected with HIV. TB should be initially considered in anyone with respiratory symptoms including fatigue, weight loss, fever, cough, chest pain, hemoptysis, and hoarseness. A person's general immune status affects the risk of TB infection. Advanced age, corticosteroid medication, chemotherapy, HIV infection, malnutrition, or chronic illness can reduce immunity and increase the risk for TB infection.

Prevalence of TB is not distributed evenly throughout the US population. Some subgroups or individuals have a higher risk for TB because they are more likely than others in the general population to be exposed and infected or because their exposure is more likely to progress to active TB. Groups with a higher prevalence of TB infection include intimate contact with individuals with active TB, foreign-born people from areas with a high prevalence of TB, medically underserved populations, homeless people, current or former correctional facility inmates, alcoholics, parenteral drug users, and the elderly.

The number of new tuberculosis cases reported in the United State declined by 7% from 1999 to 2000, continuing an 8-year downward trend since the TB epidemic peaked in 1992, according to final data released by the CDC. A total of 16,377 TB cases were reported in 2000, an all-time low. Unfortunately, the incidence of TB is on the rise worldwide. The growing global TB epidemic could affect the declines made in the United States if TB defense systems are not maintained.

Transmission of TB is a recognized risk in health care facilities. The magnitude of risk varies considerably with type of health care facility, prevalence of TB in the community, patient population served, health care worker's occupational group, area of the health care facility in which the health care worker works, and effectiveness of TB infection control interventions. Nosocomial transmission of TB has been associated with close contact with people who have infectious TB and performance of procedures such as bronchoscopy, endotracheal intubation, suctioning, open

Table 40-2 COMMON OPPORTUNISTIC DISEASES ASSOCIATED WITH AIDS*

ORGANISM/DISEASE	CLINICAL MANIFESTATIONS	DIAGNOSTIC TESTS	TREATMENT
RESPIRATORY SYSTEM			
Pneumocystis carinii pneumonia (PCP)	Nonproductive cough, hypoxemia, progressive shortness of breath, fever, night sweats, fatigue	Chest x-ray, induced sputum for culture, bronchoalveolar lavage	Trimethoprim-sulfamethoxazole (Bactrim), pentamidine, dapsone + trimethoprim, clindamycin (Cleocin) + primaquine, atovaquone (Mepron), trimetrexate (Neutrexin) + folinic acid +/− dapsone, corticosteroids
Histoplasma capsulatum	Pneumonia, fever, cough, weight loss; disseminated disease	Sputum culture, serum or urine antigen assay	Amphotericin B, itroconazole (Sporanox), fluconazole (Diflucan)
Mycobacterium tuberculosis	Productive cough, fever, night sweats, weight loss	Chest x-ray, sputum for AFB stain and culture	Isoniazid (INH), ethambutol (Myambutol), rifampin (Rifadin), pyrazinamide, streptomycin
Coccidioides immitis	Fever, weight loss, cough	Sputum culture, serology	Amphotericin B, fluconazole (Diflucan), itroconazole (Sporanox)
Kaposi's sarcoma (KS)	Dyspnea, respiratory failure	Chest x-ray, biopsy	Cancer chemotherapy, alpha-interferon, radiation
INTEGUMENTARY SYSTEM			
Herpes simplex, type 1 (HSV1) and type 2 (HSV2)	Orolabial mucocutaneous ulcerative lesions (type 1), genital and perianal mucocutaneous ulcerative lesions (type 2)	Viral culture	Acyclovir (Zovirax), famciclovir (Famvir), valacyclovir (Valtrex), foscarnet (Foscavir)
Varicella zoster virus (VZV)	Shingles, erythematous maculopapular rash along dermatomal planes, pain, pruritis	Viral culture	Acyclovir, famciclovir, valacyclovir, foscarnet
Kaposi's sarcoma (KS)	Firm, flat, raised or nodular, hyperpigmented, multicentric lesions	Biopsy of lesions	Cancer chemotherapy, alpha-interferon, radiation of lesions
Bacillary angiomatosis	Erythematous vascular papules, subcutaneous nodules	Biopsy of lesions	Erythromycin, doxycycline
EYE			
Cytomegalovirus (CMV) retinitis	Lesions on the retina, blurred vision, loss of vision	Ophthalmoscopic exam	Ganciclovir (Cytovene), foscarnet, cidofovir (Vistide)
Herpes virus, type 1 (HSV1)	Blurred vision, corneal lesions, acute retinal necrosis	Ophthalmoscopic exam	Acyclovir, famciclovir, valacyclovir, foscarnet
Varicella zoster virus (VZV)	Ocular lesions, acute retinal necrosis	Ophthalmoscopic exam	Acyclovir, famciclovir, valacyclovir, foscarnet
GASTROINTESTINAL SYSTEM			
Cryptosporidium muris	Watery diarrhea, abdominal pain, weight loss, nausea	Stool exam, small bowel or colon biopsy	Antidiarrheals, paromomycin (Humatin), azithromycin (Zithromax), atovaquone (Mepron), octreotide (Sandostatin)

From Lewis SM, Heitkemper MM, Dirksen SR: *Medical-surgical nursing: assessment and management of clinical problems,* ed 5, St. Louis, 2000, Mosby.

*Opportunistic diseases are reported in this table by systems frequently affected. However, it is important to note that in HIV infection, dissemination is common.

AFB, Acid-fast bacilli; *CNS,* central nervous system; *CSF,* cerebrospinal fluid; *CT* scan, computed tomography; *GI,* gastrointestinal; *MRI,* magnetic resonance imaging.

Table 40-2	COMMON OPPORTUNISTIC DISEASES ASSOCIATED WITH AIDS—cont'd		
ORGANISM/DISEASE	**CLINICAL MANIFESTATIONS**	**DIAGNOSTIC TESTS**	**TREATMENT**
GASTROINTESTINAL SYSTEM—cont'd			
Cytomegalovirus (CMV)	Stomatitis, esophagitis, gastritis, colitis, bloody diarrhea, pain, weight loss	Endoscopic visualization, culture, biopsy, rule out other causes	Ganciclovir (Cytovene), foscarnet, cidofovir
Herpes simplex, type 1 (HSV1)	Vesicular eruptions on tongue, buccal, pharyngeal, or perioral esophageal mucosa	Viral culture	Acyclovir, famciclovir, valacyclovir, foscarnet
Candida albicans	Whitish-yellow patches in mouth, esophagus, GI tract	Microscopic exam of scraping from lesion, culture	Fluconazole, nystatin, clotrimazole (Lotrimin), itraconazole, Amphotericin B
Mycobacterium avium complex (MAC)	Watery diarrhea, weight loss	Small bowel biopsy with AFB stain and culture	Clarithromycin (Biaxin), rifampin (Rifadin), ciprofloxacin (Cipro), Rifabutin (Mycobutin), amikacin, azithromycin
Isospora belli	Diarrhea, weight loss, nausea, abdominal pain	Stool exam, small-bowel or colon biopsy	Trimethoprim-sulfamethoxazole, pyrimethamine + folinic acid
Salmonella spp.	Gastroenteritis, fever, diarrhea	Blood and stool culture	Ciprofloxacin, ampicillin, amoxicillin, trimethoprim-sulfamethoxazole
Kaposi's sarcoma (KS)	Diarrhea, hyperpigmented lesions of mouth and GI tract	GI series, biopsy	Cancer chemotherapy, alpha-interferon, radiation
Non-Hodgkin's lymphoma	Abdominal pain, fever, night sweats, weight loss	Lymph node biopsy	Chemotherapy
NEUROLOGIC SYSTEM			
Toxoplasma gondii	Cognitive dysfunction, motor impairment, fever, altered mental status, headache, seizures, sensory abnormalities	MRI, CT scan, toxoplasma serology, brain biopsy (usually deferred)	Pyrimethamine + folinic acid + sulfadiazine, clindamycin, azithromycin, clarithromycin
JC papovavirus	Progressive multifocal leukoencephalopathy (PML) mental and motor declines	MRI, CT scan, brain biopsy	Effective antiretroviral therapy may help
Cryptococcal meningitis	Cognitive impairment, motor dysfunction, fever, seizures, headache	CT scan, serum antigen test, CSF analysis	Amphotericin B, flucytosine (Ancobon), fluconazole, itraconazole
CNS lymphomas	Cognitive dysfunction, motor impairment, aphasia, seizures, personality changes, headache	MRI, CT scan	Radiation, chemotherapy
AIDS-dementia complex (ADC)	Insidious onset of progressive dementia	CT scan	Effective antiretroviral therapy may help

abscess irrigation, and autopsy. Sputum induction and aerosol treatments that induce coughing may also increase the potential for transmission. Several TB outbreaks among people in health care facilities have been reported. Many outbreaks involve transmission of multidrug-resistant strains of TB to both patients and health care workers. Mortality associated with these outbreaks was high (range, 43% to 93%). Factors contributing to outbreaks include delayed diagnosis, recognition of drug resistance, and initiation of effective therapy.

In general, people infected with TB have an approximate 10% risk for developing active TB during their lifetime. Risk is greatest during the first 2 years after infection. TB is carried in airborne particles or droplet nuclei generated when people with pulmonary or laryngeal TB sneeze, cough, speak, or sing.[2] Infection occurs when a susceptible person inhales droplet nuclei containing TB. Droplet nuclei traverse the mouth or nasal passages, upper respiratory tract, and bronchi to reach the alveoli of the lungs.

The incubation period from infection to demonstrable primary lesion or significant tuberculin reaction is about 4 to 12 weeks. Subsequent risk of progressive pulmonary or extrapulmonary TB is greatest within the first year or two after infection. Latent infection may persist for life.

Table 40-3 DRUG THERAPY USED IN TUBERCULOSIS

DRUG	MECHANISMS OF ACTION	SIDE EFFECTS	COMMENTS
FIRST-LINE DRUGS			
Isoniazid (INH)	Interferes with DNA metabolism of tubercle bacillus	Peripheral neuritis, hepatotoxicity, hypersensitivity (skin rash, arthralgia, fever), optic neuritis, vitamin B_6 neuritis	Metabolism primarily by liver and excretion by kidneys, pyridoxine (vitamin B_6) administration during high-dose therapy as prophylactic measure, use as single prophylactic agent for active TB in individuals whose PPD converts to positive, ability to cross blood-brain barrier
Rifampin (Rifadin)	Has broad-spectrum effects, inhibits RNA polymerase of tubercle bacillus	Hepatitis, febrile reaction, GI disturbance, peripheral neuropathy, hypersensitivity	Most common use with isoniazid, low incidence of side effects, suppression of effect of birth control pills, possible orange urine
Ethambutol (Myambutol)	Inhibits RNA synthesis and is bacteriostatic for the tubercle bacillus	Skin rash, GI disturbance, malaise, peripheral neuritis, optic neuritis	Side effects uncommon and reversible with discontinuation of drug, most common use as substitute drug when toxicity occurs with isoniazid or rifampin
Streptomycin	Inhibits protein synthesis, is bactericidal	Ototoxicity (eighth cranial nerve), nephrotoxicity, hypersensitivity	Cautious use in older adults, those with renal disease, and pregnant women; must be given parenterally
Pyrazinamide	Bactericidal effect (exact mechanism is unknown)	Fever, skin rash, hyperuricemia, jaundice (rare)	High rate of effectiveness when used with streptomycin or capreomycin
SECOND-LINE DRUGS			
Ethionamide (Trecator)	Inhibits protein synthesis	GI disturbance, hepatotoxicity, hypersensitivity	Valuable retreatment of resistant organisms, contraindication in pregnancy
Capreomycin Capastat)	Inhibits protein synthesis and is bactericidal	Ototoxicity, nephrotoxicity	Cautious use in older adults
Kanamycin (Kantrex) and amikacin	Interferes with protein synthesis	Ototoxicity, nephrotoxicity	Use in selected cases for retreatment of resistant strains
Para-aminosalicylic acid (PAS)	Interferes with metabolism of tubercle bacillus	GI disurbance (frequent), hypersensitivity, hepatotoxicity	Interference with absorption of rifampin, infrequent use
Cycloserine (Seromycin)	Inhibits cell-wall synthesis	Personality changes, psychosis, rash	Contraindication in individuals with a history of psychosis, use in retreatment of resistant strains

From Lewis SM, Heitkemper MM, Dirksen SR: *Medical-surgical nursing: assessment and management of clinical problems,* ed 5, St. Louis, 2000, Mosby.
DNA, Deoxyribonucleic acid; *GI,* gastrointestinal; *PPD,* purified protein derivative; *RNA,* ribonucleic acid; *TB,* tuberculosis.

Degree of communicability depends on the number of bacilli in the droplets, virulence of the bacilli, adequacy of ventilation, exposure of bacilli to sun or ultraviolet light, and opportunities for aerosolization. Theoretically, as long as viable tubercle bacilli are discharged in the sputum, the person may be infectious. Diagnosis is confirmed by recovery of TB from a sputum sample, positive chest radiograph, and positive tuberculin skin test.

TB prevention and control programs should be established in all institutional settings in which health care is provided. Therapeutic interventions include respiratory isolation to prevent spread, administration of antituberculin drugs, and supportive care. Controlled airflow rooms are recommended for isolation of these patients. Triage guidelines should include identification of potential TB patients (Box 40-4). Table 40-3 summarizes current therapy for tuberculosis. Additional treatment includes antipyretics for fever and increased fluid intake to thin secretions.

SUMMARY

Recognition of the potential for infectious disease is paramount in the care of any ED patient. Box 40-5 highlights potential nursing diagnoses for these patients. With the prevalence of life-threatening infectious diseases, one must assume that any patient may be a potential source of infection and employ universal precautions whenever a potential for exposure exists. Careful attention to this matter reduces the spread of infection and contamination.

Box 40-4 TRIAGE ASSESSMENT FOR POSSIBLE TUBERCULOSIS

HISTORICAL AND SOCIAL INFORMATION

Homeless

Live in crowded, unsanitary conditions

Recently moved from or traveled to a high-risk country in Asia, Africa, Latin America

Previous history of tuberculosis with no treatment or poor compliance with treatment regimen

Resident of long-term care facility, nursing home, correctional institution, mental hospital, homeless shelter

Close contact with an infected person

Intravenous drug abuse or alcohol abuse

Health care worker

OBJECTIVE CLINICAL INFORMATION

Weight loss, anorexia, malaise

Cough worsening over weeks or months

Productive cough with mucopurulent or blood-streaked sputum

Night sweats, chills, low-grade fevers

Malnourished

Coinfection with human immunodeficiency virus

Preexisting medical conditions (i.e., diabetes mellitus, hematologic disorders, end-stage renal disease)

Prolonged steroid or immunosuppressive therapy

Box 40-5 NURSING DIAGNOSES FOR INFECTIOUS DISEASES

Fluid volume, Deficient

Fluid volume, Excess

Infection

Nutrition: less than body requirements, Imbalanced

References

1. Alter MJ: Epidemiology of hepatitis C, *Hepatology* 26:62S, 1997.
2. Bensenson A: *Control of communicable diseases in man,* ed 16, Washington, DC, 1995, The American Public Health Association.
3. Berg R, editor: *The APIC curriculum for infection control practice,* vol III, Dubuque, Ia, 1988, Kendall/Hunt.
4. Centers for Disease Control and Prevention: Recommendations for follow-up of healthcare workers after occupational exposure to hepatitis C virus, *MMWR* 46:606, 1997.
5. Centers for Disease Control and Prevention: Public health service guidelines for the management of health-care worker exposures to HIV and recommendations for postexposure prophylaxis, *MMWR* 47:1, 1998.
6. Centers for Disease Control and Prevention: Summary of notifiable diseases, United States, 1997, *MMWR* 46:1, 1998.
7. Centers for Disease Control and Prevention: First report of AIDS, *MMWR* 50:430445, 2001.
8. Hollinger F: Features of viral hepatitis. In Fields BN et al, editors: *Virology,* New York, 1985, Raven.
9. Lemon SM: The natural history of hepatitis A: the potential for transmission by transfusion of blood or blood products, *Vox Sang* 67(suppl 4):19, 1994.
10. Mandell G, Douglas R, Bennett J, editors: *Principles and practices of infectious diseases,* ed 3, New York, 1990, Churchill Livingstone.
11. Ridzon R, Gallagher K, Ciesielski C et al: Simultaneous transmission of human immunodeficiency virus and hepatitis C virus from a needle-stick injury, *New Engl J Med* 336:919, 1997.
12. Soucie JM, Roberston BH, Bell BP et al: Hepatitis A virus infections associated with clotting factor concentrate in the United States, *Transfusion* 38:573, 1998.
13. Villano SA, Vlahov D, Nelson KE et al. Incidence and risk factors for hepatitis C among injection drug users in Baltimore, Maryland, *J Clin Microbiol* 35:3274, 1997.

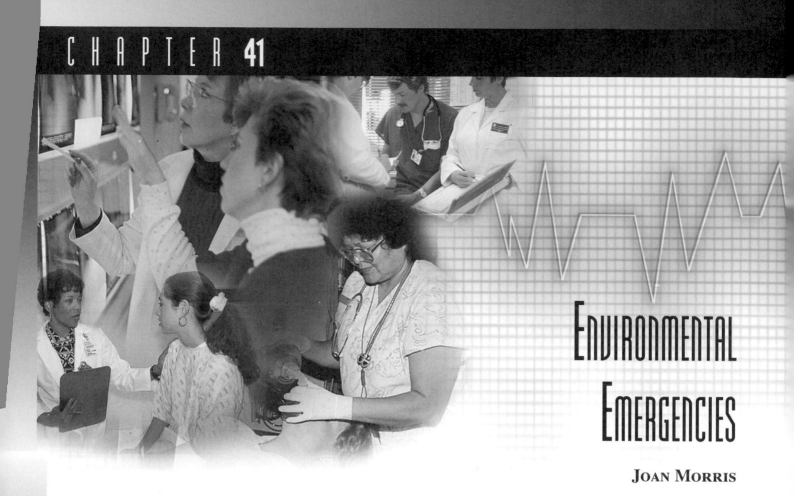

CHAPTER 41

ENVIRONMENTAL EMERGENCIES

JOAN MORRIS

Outdoor activities are extremely popular with individuals of all ages. Activities such as hiking, jogging, biking, swimming, and diving, however, place the individual at risk for illness and injury secondary to the weather, the activity, and various animals. Environmental hazards may be encountered during voluntary participation in an outdoor activity or involuntary exposure caused by confusion, mental illness, alcohol, or drugs. Specific environmental emergencies discussed in this chapter are related to heat and cold stress, water immersion, bites, and stings.

HEAT-RELATED EMERGENCIES

Many cases of heat illness are reported annually in the United States. Only head injury, spinal cord injury, and heart failure are responsible for more deaths in athletes than heat illness.[28] Regardless of physical condition, anyone can suffer ill effects from heat stress if the exposure is intense or prolonged. The effects of environmental heat stress can be mild or severe, depending on the degree of heat and length of exposure.

Ambient temperature is a product of environmental temperature and moisture in the air. For example, an environmental temperature of 90° F (32° C) creates an ambient temperature of 93° F (34° C) when the dew point is 65° F (18° C); however, ambient temperature increases to 111° F (44° C) if the dew point is 83° F (28° C). Table 41-1 presents ambient temperature for various thermometer readings and dew point in degrees Fahrenheit.

Emergencies related to heat stress include heat edema, heat cramps, heat exhaustion, and heat stroke. Heat edema is the least acute situation, usually a minor inconvenience for most individuals. Heat stroke, however, is life-threatening.

Heat Edema

Heat edema occurs in nonacclimated individuals during prolonged periods of standing or sitting. Characteristic swelling of feet and ankles resolves in a few days. Treatment includes rest, elevation of the legs, and support hose. Heat edema is self-limiting and generally does not require further treatment.

Heat Cramps

Heat cramps are severe cramps (brief and intermittent) of specific muscles, usually in the shoulders, thighs, and abdominal wall. Associated symptoms include weakness, nausea, tachycardia, pallor, profuse diaphoresis, and cool, moist skin. The person's core temperature may be normal or slightly elevated. Heat cramps develop suddenly when the victim is resting after exertion in a hot environment or one with high humidity. Salt depletion secondary to excessive perspiration in combination with excessive water consumption

Table 41-1 HEAT INDEX CHART

Dew point	TEMPERATURE (°F)															
	90	91	92	93	94	95	96	97	98	99	100	101	102	103	104	105
65	93	94	95	97	98	99	100	101	103	104	105	106	107	108	110	111
66	94	95	96	97	99	100	101	102	103	104	106	107	108	109	111	112
67	94	95	97	98	99	100	102	103	104	105	106	108	109	111	112	113
68	95	96	98	99	100	101	102	104	105	106	107	108	110	112	113	114
69	96	97	98	99	101	102	103	104	106	107	108	109	111	112	114	115
70	96	97	99	100	101	103	104	105	107	108	109	110	112	113	114	116
71	97	98	100	101	102	104	105	106	108	109	110	111	113	114	115	117
72	98	99	101	102	103	105	106	107	109	110	111	112	114	115	116	118
73	99	100	102	103	104	106	107	108	110	111	112	113	115	117	118	119
74	100	101	103	104	105	107	108	109	111	112	113	115	116	118	119	121
75	101	102	104	105	106	108	109	111	112	113	115	116	117	119	120	122
76	102	103	105	106	108	109	110	112	113	115	116	117	119	120	122	123
77	103	105	106	107	109	110	112	113	114	116	117	119	121	122	123	125
78	104	106	107	109	110	112	113	115	116	118	119	121	122	123	124	126
79	105	107	109	110	112	113	114	116	118	119	121	122	124	125	126	128
80	107	108	110	111	113	115	116	117	119	121	122	124	125	127	128	129
81	108	110	111	113	115	116	118	119	121	123	124	126	127	128	130	132
82	109	111	113	115	116	118	119	121	123	124	126	127	129	130	132	133
83	111	113	115	117	118	120	121	123	125	126	128	129	130	132	133	135

leads to muscle cramping. Increased water intake does not replace sodium losses caused by perspiration.[1] Instead, water dilutes serum sodium, causing hyponatremia, the key factor in the development of heat cramps.

Treatment includes removal from heat, rest, and electrolyte replacement with oral or parenteral fluids. Discharge instructions should stress the importance of drinking commercially prepared electrolyte supplements (e.g., Gatorade, Powerade, All Sport) when working outdoors or participating in strenuous recreational activities during hot weather. Strenuous activity should be avoided for at least 12 hours after discharge.

Heat Exhaustion

Heat exhaustion is a clinical syndrome caused by prolonged heat exposure, usually over hours or days. Excessive perspiration and inadequate fluid and electrolyte replacement lead to fluid loss, electrolyte depletion, and dehydration. Heat exhaustion occurs most often in individuals working in hot environments.[22] Hett and Brechtelsbauer assert that the elderly and very young are also at risk because they cannot increase fluid intake sufficiently to compensate for increased fluid losses from sweating.[12]

Heat exhaustion is characterized by rapid onset (within minutes) of extreme thirst, general malaise, muscle cramping, headache, nausea, vomiting, anxiety, and tachycardia—ultimately leading to syncope and collapse. Associated dehydration may cause orthostatic hypotension and mild to severe temperature elevation (98.6° to 105° F [37° to 40.6° C]). Diaphoresis may or may not be present. Untreated, heat exhaustion can progress to heat stroke.

Initial treatment begins with moving the patient to a cool, quiet environment and removing constricting clothing. When significant hyperthermia is present, moist cloths placed on the patient reduce temperature by evaporation. Fluid and electrolyte replacement should be initiated. Oral replacement with a balanced commercial salt preparation can be used if the patient is not nauseated. Intravenous 0.9% saline solution should be used if the patient is nauseated or vomiting. Salt tablets are not recommended because of potential gastric irritation and hypernatremia. Monitor the patient's temperature carefully during treatment. Hypotension may be corrected initially with a 300- to 500-ml bolus of 0.9% normal saline, with subsequent infusions correlated to clinical and laboratory findings. Patients with hypotension or a history of cardiac disease should be placed on a cardiac monitor because heat exhaustion can rapidly evolve into heat stroke. Admission should be considered for any patient who does not improve significantly with 3 to 4 hours of emergency treatment.

Heat Stroke

Heat stroke is the least common but most severe presentation of heat illness. Mortality as high as 70%[2] is directly related to the speed and effectiveness of diagnosis and treatment. With heat stroke core temperature exceeds 105° F (40.6° C). Heat stroke occurs when exposure to severe heat stress destroys the thermoregulatory system. Environmental factors and the patient's ability to dissipate heat affect the outcome of heat stroke.

Heat stroke occurs in one of two forms: classic heat stroke and exertional heat stroke. Classic heat stroke occurs during prolonged exposure to sustained high ambient temperatures and humidity. It commonly affects the elderly, chronically ill, and those who live in poorly ventilated homes without air conditioning. Children locked in cars on hot days are extremely vulnerable and at great risk for heat stroke. Poor dissipation of environmental heat is the underlying cause of classic heat stroke.

In contrast, those patients with exertional heat stroke are usually young and healthy, often athletes and military recruits. In these individuals heat production overcomes the internal heat dissipation mechanisms. Common predisposing factors associated with heat stroke are summarized in Box 41-1. Individuals with one or more risk factors are at much greater risk for hyperthermia when exacerbating environmental conditions are present.

Onset of heat stroke is usually sudden; however, the elderly and patients in predisposing environments can develop heat exhaustion several hours before heat stroke develops. Heat stroke may present with changes in neurologic function such as anxiety, confusion, hallucinations, loss of muscle coordination, combativeness, and coma. Direct thermal damage

Box 41-1	RISK FACTORS ASSOCIATED WITH HEAT STROKE

AGE

Elderly
Infants

ENVIRONMENTAL CONDITIONS

High environmental temperatures
High relative humidity
Low wind

PREEXISTING ILLNESS

Cardiovascular disease
Previous stroke/central nervous system lesions
Obesity
Diabetes
Cystic fibrosis
Skin disorders (e.g., large burn scars)

PRESCRIPTION DRUGS

Anticholinergics
Phenothiazines
Butyrophenones
Tricyclic antidepressants
Antihistamines
Antispasmodics
Diuretics
Antiparkinsonian drugs
Beta-blockers

STREET DRUGS

Lysergic acid diethylamide (LSD)
Jimsonweed
Amphetamines
Phencyclidine (PCP)
Alcohol

to the brain combined with decreased cerebral blood flow can lead to cerebral edema and hemorrhage. The brain, particularly the cerebellum, is extremely sensitive to thermal injury; therefore, the range of neurologic symptoms is broad.

Management of heat stroke is directed at reducing core temperature as rapidly as possible and treating subsequent complications. Heat stroke is often fatal despite rapid treatment. Maintenance of airway, breathing, and circulation (ABCs) is crucial for patient recovery. Establish an airway and administer supplemental oxygen by the method most appropriate for the patient's level of consciousness. Fluid volume is not depleted in most victims of hyperthermia; therefore, 1 to 2 L of isotonic saline solution during the first 4 hours is usually adequate. Lacted Ringer's solution is not recommended because the liver may not be able to metabolize lactate. Careful hemodynamic monitoring is indicated until normal vital signs are restored. After the ABCs are secured, rapid, aggressive cooling is the primary intervention.

Prehospital treatment starts with removing the patient from the external source of heat and stripping all clothing. Aggressive ice or cold-water cooling should be avoided in the field to prevent shivering and seizure activity that will only increase the core body temperature. Spray the patient with tepid water while fanning the entire body to promote cooling by evaporation. Well-padded ice packs in vascular areas such as the groin, axilla, and neck are also useful. After the patient is in the emergency department (ED), aggressive cooling measures such as ice water and gastric and peritoneal lavage can be used.

Cooling blankets may be used; however, cooling from wet skin is 25 times more effective than cooling from dry skin. Immersion in an ice water bath is contraindicated. In addition to being unpleasant for the patient and caregiver, access to the patient is limited. Ice water immersion can also cause shivering, which dramatically increases oxygen consumption and can increase body temperature. Intravenous chlorpromazine (Thorazine), 10 to 25 mg, may be used to prevent shivering during the cooling process. Massive peripheral vasoconstriction from ice water immersion can act as an insulator and prevent adequate cooling.

Cooling should be continued until rectal temperature is 102° F (39° C) or less. The core temperature should be monitored frequently during the cooling phase to prevent inadvertent hypothermia. Aspirin and acetaminophen have not proved effective in reducing hyperthermia secondary to heat stroke. Corticosteroid therapy, usually with methylprednisolone, may be used to treat cerebral edema. Intracranial pressure monitoring may be helpful for some patients. To increase renal blood flow, intravenous mannitol, 0.25 g/kg, is recommended in patients whose urinary output is less than 50 ml/hr.

High-output cardiac failure may develop with heat stroke; therefore, patients should be placed on a cardiac monitor. Central venous pressure and pulmonary capillary wedge pressure monitoring may be considered in the critical phase to evaluate fluid status. Protecting the kidneys and liver from thermal and low-flow damage is critical. Myoglobinuria and poor renal perfusion put the kidneys at risk for renal failure; therefore, urine should be carefully monitored for color, amount, pH, and myoglobin.

COLD-RELATED EMERGENCIES

According to Cochrane,[5] approximately 800 fatalities occur annually from cold exposure. Most deaths do not occur in the extreme northern areas but are reported in temperate regions, urban areas in poorly heated apartments, and among the homeless. Urban cold exposure is usually related to alcohol or a preexisting condition such as diabetes.

Injuries related to cold exposure are localized or generalized. Localized cold emergencies include chilblains, immersion foot, and frostbite, whereas hypothermia is a generalized cold emergency. Cold-related emergencies occur with prolonged exposure to cold ambient temperatures, immersion in cold water, or as a result of factors such as alcohol. Ambient temperature is a product of air temperature and wind speed: the greater the wind speed, the lower the ambient temperature (Table 41-2). Heat loss occurs 32 times more quickly with immersion in cold water.[3]

Chilblains

Chilblains, also known as pernio, are localized areas of itching and redness accompanied by recurrent edema on exposed or poorly insulated body parts such as the ears, fingers, and toes. Chilblains are usually seen in cool, damp climates with temperatures above freezing. Chilblains are probably a mild form of frostbite with gradual onset of symptoms. There is generally no pain; however, the patient may experience transient numbness and tingling. Initial pallor or redness of the nose, digits, or ears may evolve into plaques and small, superficial ulcerations over chronically exposed areas.

Prehospital treatment begins with removal to a warm area in conjunction with covering the affected area with a warm hand or placing fingers under the axilla.[22] Elevation of the affected area decreases edema, which increases circulation

and allows gradual warming at room temperature. Never rub or massage injured tissue. Avoid direct heat application. Tissue damage is rarely seen with chilblains; however, the patient should be instructed to protect the area from injury and further environmental exposure and to watch for signs of secondary infection.[14]

Immersion Foot

Immersion foot, or trench foot, refers to prolonged or constant contact between a wet foot and cold temperature, usually when the patient is wearing a watertight boot that does not allow normal evaporative "breathing." This condition is commonly seen in hunters and soldiers on outdoor maneuvers. Feet initially are cold, damp, numb, and edematous but appear warm within 24 to 48 hours. Vasodilation and hyperemia resulting from warming causes intense burning and tingling. Prolonged and repeated exposure can lead to lymphangitis, cellulitis, thrombophlebitis, and liquification gangrene.

Therapeutic interventions include drying the feet and changing frequently into dry socks. After the patient is in a controlled environment, rewarm injured areas gradually by exposing them to air or soaking them in warm water (100° to 105° F [38° to 41° C]) before drying. Some clinicians recommend daily air-drying of the feet for 8 hours.[26] Immersion foot is reversible with timely treatment. Patients are usually hospitalized for observation and prevention of complications.

Frostbite

Danzel identifies frostbite as the most prevalent injury caused by extreme cold. Ice crystals form in intracellular spaces as tissue freezes.[7] These crystals enlarge and compress cells, causing membrane rupture, interruption of enzymatic activity, and altered metabolic processes. Histamine release increases capillary permeability, red cell aggregation, and microvascular occlusion.[1] After frostbite occurs, damage is irreversible. Further exposure to extreme cold or trauma

Table 41-2	**WINDCHILL INDEX***														
WIND SPEED (MPH)	**AIR TEMPERATURE (° F)**														
	35	**30**	**25**	**20**	**15**	**10**	**5**	**0**	**−5**	**−10**	**−15**	**−20**	**−25**	**−30**	**−35**
4	35	30	25	20	15	10	5	0	−5	−10	−15	−20	−25	−30	−35
5	32	27	22	16	11	6	0	−5	−10	−15	−21	−26	−31	−36	−42
10	22	16	10	3	−3	−9	−15	−22	−27	−34	−40	−46	−52	−58	−64
15	16	9	2	−5	−11	−18	−25	−31	−38	−45	−51	−58	−65	−72	−78
20	12	4	−3	−10	−17	−24	−31	−39	−44	−51	−59	−66	−74	−81	−88
25	8	1	−7	−15	−22	−29	−36	−44	−51	−59	−66	−74	−81	−88	−96
30	6	−2	−10	−18	−25	−33	−42	−49	−56	−64	−71	−79	−86	−93	−101
35	4	−4	−12	−20	−27	−35	−43	−52	−58	−67	−74	−82	−89	−97	−105
40	3	−5	−13	−21	−29	−37	−45	−53	−60	−69	−76	−84	−92	−100	−107

*Shaded area indicates increasing danger from freezing of exposed flesh within 1 minute of exposure.

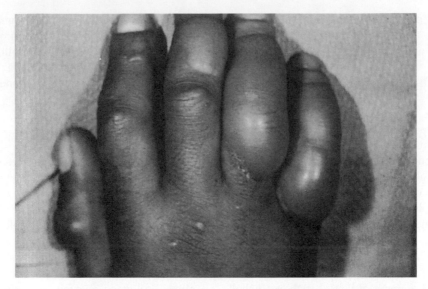

FIGURE **41-1**   Large, clear frostbite blisters on the right hand. (From Rosen P, Barkin RM, Hockberger RS et al, editors: *Emergency medicine: concepts and clinical practice,* ed 4, St. Louis, 1998, Mosby.)

Box 41-2	FACTORS AFFECTING SEVERITY OF FROSTBITE

Skin color (dark-skinned people are more prone to frostbite)
Lack of acclimatization
History of frostbite injury
Poor peripheral vascular status
Anxiety
Exhaustion

worsens the injury and increases tissue damage. The patient with frostbite may also have hypothermia. Treatment of hypothermia takes priority over management of frostbite. Frostbite can be superficial or deep, depending on severity of the cold and length of exposure. Estimation of the extent of injury may not be possible until several days after exposure.

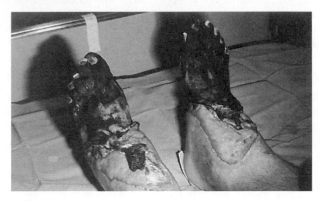

FIGURE **41-2**   Gangrenous necrosis resulting from frostbite injury. (From Auerbach P, editor: *Wilderness medicine: management of wilderness and environmental emergencies,* ed 4, St. Louis, 2001, Mosby.)

Superficial Frostbite

Superficial frostbite involves skin and subcutaneous tissue and is similar to a superficial burn. Fingertips, ears, nose, toes, and cheeks are the areas most commonly affected. Symptoms include tingling, numbness, burning sensation, and white, waxy color. Frozen skin feels cold and stiff. After the tissue thaws, the patient may feel a hot, stinging sensation. Affected areas become mottled and blisters develop within a few hours. Frostbite tissue is extremely sensitive to subsequent exposure to cold and heat and therefore susceptible to repeated frostbite injury.

Injured tissue is friable, so recovery depends on very gentle handling. Do not rub the affected area. Apply warm soaks (104° to 110° F [40° to 43° C]) and elevate the extremity. Place the patient on bed rest for several days until the full extent of the injury has been evaluated and normal circulation has returned. The patient's room should be warm; however, heavy blankets should be avoided because friction and weight on the affected area can lead to sloughing.

Deep Frostbite

Deep frostbite occurs when the temperature of a limb is lowered. Deep frostbite usually involves muscles, bones, and tendons. The degree of frostbite depends on ambient temperature, windchill factor (see Table 41-2), duration of exposure, whether the patient was wet while exposed or in direct contact with metal objects, and the type of clothing worn. Other factors that may contribute to the severity of frostbite are outlined in Box 41-2.

Deep frostbite appears white or yellow-white and is hard, cool, and insensitive to touch.[1] The patient has a burning sensation followed by a feeling of warmth then numbness. Blisters appear 1 to 7 days after injury. Edema of the entire extremity occurs and may persist for months (Figure 41-1). A gray-black mottling eventually progresses to gangrene (Figure 41-2).

Prehospital treatment includes transport with gentle handling and moderate elevation of the affected part.[22] Rewarming is deferred until the patient reaches the ED. Do not rub

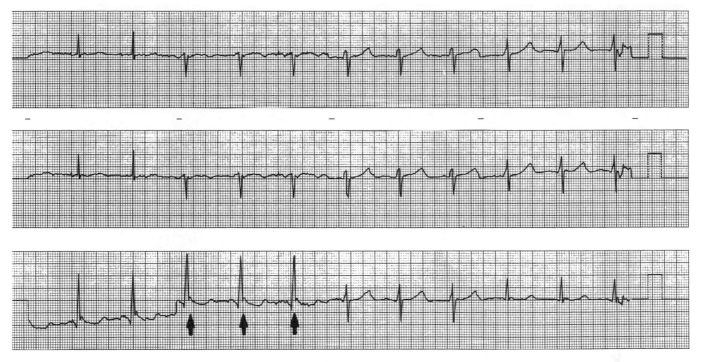

FIGURE 41-3 Hypothermic J waves with QT prolongation. (From Rosen P, Barkin RM, Hockberger RS et al: *Emergency medicine: concepts and clinical practice,* ed 3, vol 1, St. Louis, 1992, Mosby.)

the part with snow or ice. If the extremity has thawed, keep it immobile. Prevent heat loss by removing wet clothing, covering the patient with dry blankets, and removing the patient from the cold environment. If the patient is transported in a ground or air ambulance, warmed oxygen is recommended. Wool head coverings help prevent further heat loss.

Rapid rewarming under controlled conditions is the ideal treatment for maintaining tissue viability. Rewarming the patient with hypothermia and severe frostbite should occur with strict medical control. After the patient reaches the ED, obtain a baseline core temperature (rectal or esophageal), then immerse the affected area in warm (104° to 110° F [40° to 43° C]) water. Thawing frozen tissue is extremely painful, so liberal administration of parenteral narcotics is needed in severe cases. Warm intravenous fluids before administering them. Assess tetanus immunization status and consider antibiotic therapy for deep infections. If hypothermia is not present, administer warm oral liquids. Cover the patient with warm blankets, but avoid friction and pressure on the affected area. Protect the thawed part with a large, soft, bulky dressing. Elevate the affected area to minimize edema.

If severe vasoconstriction is present, escharotomy may be required. Final determination of the depth of injury may not be possible for several weeks; therefore, amputation is not considered in the ED.

Hypothermia

Hypothermia is defined as a core temperature below 95° F (35° C). Severe hypothermia is a core temperature less than 90° F (32.2° C). The American Heart Association[11] has established 86° F (30° C) as the temperature for initiation of aggressive internal rewarming procedures. Johnson maintains that death usually occurs when core temperature falls below 78° F (25.6° C).[13]

The body's metabolic responses depend on a normal temperature. As the core temperature drops there is progressive decrease in cellular activity and organ function. When the temperature drops by 18° F (10° C), the basal metabolic rate drops two to three times the normal rate. The most obvious response is seen in the central nervous system (CNS). The patient becomes apathetic, weak, and easily fatigued, with impaired reasoning, coordination, and gait. The patient's speech is slow or slurred. Renal blood flow decreases so glomerular filtration rate declines. Impaired water reabsorption leads to dehydration. Decreased respiratory rate and effort lead to carbon dioxide retention, hypoxia, and acidosis. Shivering consumes glucose stores so the patient becomes hypoglycemic. Insulin levels fall, so available glucose decreases, forcing the body to metabolize fat for energy. Drug metabolism in the liver is sluggish, so medications may last longer.

The cardiovascular system is also dramatically affected. Cold heart muscle is irritable and prone to dysrhythmias. The characteristic Osborne or J wave may be seen on an electrocardiogram (Figure 41-3). The most common dysrhythmias are atrial and ventricular fibrillation. The cold patient is in great danger of ventricular fibrillation when core temperature falls below 82° F (28° C). Ventricular fibrillation at these extremely cold temperatures does not respond to conventional treatment without prior rewarming. Defibrillation is limited to three shocks until core temperature is greater than 86° F (30° C).[11] Intravenous medications are also limited to those patients whose core temperature is

Table 41-3 REWARMING TECHNIQUES	
EXTERNAL REWARMING PROCEDURES	INTERNAL REWARMING PROCEDURES
PASSIVE	**PASSIVE**
Move the patient to a warm area	Warmed humidified oxygen
Remove patient's wet clothing	Warmed intravenous fluids
Cover the patient with blankets	
ACTIVE	**ACTIVE**
Radiant heat lamps	Peritoneal lavage with KCL-free fluid
Heating blankets	
Bair Hugger warming blanket	Gastrointestinal irrigation
Hot water bottles	Extracorporeal rewarming
Heating pads	Cardiopulmonary bypass
	Hemodialysis
	Esophageal rewarming tubes
	Continuous arteriovenous rewarming tubes (CAVR)

KCL, Potassium chloride.

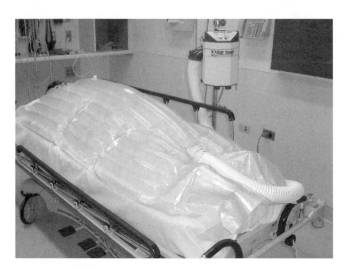

FIGURE **41-4** Bair Hugger Warming Blanket.

greater than 86° F (30° C). Careful handling of hypothermic patients, especially when their temperatures reach the vulnerable mid-80's range, is imperative because even turning may cause ventricular fibrillation. Rewarming procedures are active or passive, based on external warming or internal warming. Table 41-3 lists various procedures by category.

The goal in mild hypothermia (84° to 94° F [29° to 34° C]), in which the patient is still shivering, alert, and oriented, is to prevent further heat loss and rewarm the patient as rapidly as possible.[16] Passive external rewarming techniques such as moving the patient to a warm environment, replacing wet clothing with dry material, and wrapping with warm blankets may be effective. However, many patients require internal rewarming using warmed, humidified oxygen. Giving the patient warmed, oral fluids that contain glucose or other sugars provides more heat through calories. Passive rewarming raises

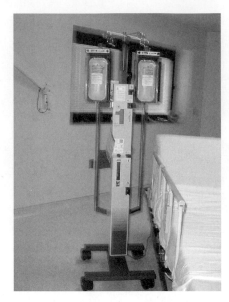

FIGURE **41-5** Sims Level I System 1025 Fluid and Blood Warmer.

the temperature 1° to 4° F (0.5° to 2.0° C) per hour. Gradual rewarming minimizes the risk of active rewarming shock.

In moderate hypothermia (78.8° to 89.4° F [26° to 31.9° C]), rewarm truncal areas at 1° F (0.5° C) per hour using heating blankets such as Bair Hugger Therapy (Figure 41-4), radiant heating lamps, and hot water bottles. Monitor closely for marked vasodilatation and subsequent hypotension. American Hospital Association guidelines recommend active internal rewarming when core temperature is less than 86° F (30° C) (see Table 41-3). Heated inhalation via endotracheal tube, mechanically warmed intravenous fluid (Figure 41-5), peritoneal lavage, gastrointestinal irrigation, bladder irrigation, extracorporeal rewarming cardiopulmonary bypass, and hemodialysis may all be used.

In severe hypothermia (lower than 78.8° F [26° C]), active internal (core) rewarming in conjunction with active external rewarming procedures is essential to prevent rewarming shock. Rewarming shock can occur when core temperature continues to drop after rewarming is initiated as cold peripheral blood returns to the central circulation. Circulation of cold blood through the heart also increases ventricular irritability and leads to fibrillation. Rewarming may also cause peripheral vasodilatation, which can precipitate hypotension and cardiovascular collapse.

Successful rewarming depends on the patient's age and general condition before the hypothermic event, length of his or her exposure, and careful handling by the ED team. To prevent hyperthermia secondary to aggressive rewarming, discontinue active rewarming when core temperature reaches 89.6° to 93° F (32° to 34° C).

DROWNING AND NEAR-DROWNING

In the United States drowning claims approximately 8,000 lives per year, with an additional 50,000 near-drownings reported annually.[21] According to the National Safety Council, drowning is the third leading cause of accidental death, with 40% of victims younger than age 5 years.[17] Toddlers and young children are at risk because of their naturally inquisitive nature and inadequate supervision. Near-drowning is defined as survival from potential drowning. Rapid identification and initiation of resuscitation measures are vital for survival. Many victims of cold water immersion have a good chance of survival without neurologic sequelae when basic cardiac life support is initiated early.

Drowning stimulates various physiologic responses; however, the actual cause of death is hypoxia secondary to asphyxiation. In any near-drowning or drowning event, the victim is immersed in water for a prolonged time. Asphyxia causes relaxation of the airway so water is swallowed and aspirated into the lungs as the victim becomes unconscious. Fluid-induced bronchospasm may also contribute to hypoxia.

Dry drowning occurs secondary to intense laryngospasm; 10 to 20 percent of the victims do not aspirate water.[24] Death is secondary to airway obstruction rather than pulmonary edema. Mortality is essentially the same for dry and wet drowning victims.

Freshwater and saltwater drowning victims present with similar clinical pictures—pulmonary edema. The difference is how the pulmonary edema develops. With freshwater drowning, water is absorbed across the alveolar-capillary membrane because of hypotonicity relative to plasma. Hypervolemia occurs as more and more water moves into the capillaries. Red cells absorb excess water, so lysis may account for hemoglobinuria found in some freshwater near-drowning victims. Dilutional electrolyte problems (i.e., decreased sodium and chloride) accompany even mild hypervolemia. Electrolyte abnormalities resolve when blood volume normalizes.

Damage to the delicate alveolar membranes is a greater concern. Surfactant activity decreases, so lung compliance is impaired. Alveoli may rupture or become engorged, which leads to pulmonary edema. Decreased gas exchange, hypoxemia, acidosis, and decreased compliance ultimately cause death. Hanke, Schwartz, and Gerace found that development of adult respiratory distress syndrome (ARDS) and multiple organ system failure contributes to the high risk of death in near-drowning victims.[10]

Saltwater aspiration causes hypovolemia secondary to hypertonicity of plasma. Plasma is pulled across the alveolar-capillary membrane into the lungs, causing pulmonary edema, impaired gas exchange, and hypoxemia. The resulting hemoconcentration increases electrolyte concentration (e.g., sodium, potassium). These electrolyte abnormalities can be reversed with restoration of adequate circulating volume.

Secondary drowning can occur up to 72 hours after the initial insult; therefore, every near-drowning victim should be taken to the hospital for observation, regardless of how he or she appears immediately after the event. Inflammatory reactions in the lung injure the alveolar-capillary membrane and alter surfactant function. Approximately 10% to 15% of

Box 41-3	**ESSENTIAL GUIDELINES FOR NEAR-DROWNING MANAGEMENT**

Determine duration of submersion.

Clear airway using cervical spine precautions, assess breathing, and provide rescue ventilations as soon as possible.

Assess circulation. If pulse is not palpated, begin chest compressions immediately. If advanced cardiac life support is available, proceed with gentle intubation.

Assess carefully for associated injuries when indicated by history and mechanism of injury.

Remove victim's wet clothing and gently wrap him or her in dry blankets.

Do not attempt to warm victim if medical facility is less than 15 minutes away.

Initiate warming techniques (e.g., warm oxygen, warm intravenous fluids, or well-padded heat packs) if medical facility is more than 15 minutes away.

Transport the victim to a medical facility even if he or she recovers at the scene.

deaths associated with drowning are due to secondary drowning.[24] Near-drowning victims should be observed for at least 24 hours.

Immersion in cold water can cause sudden death from cardiac dysrhythmias rather than drowning. Immersion syndrome occurs when cold water stimulates the vagus nerve, causing bradycardia or cardiac arrest. Alcohol is a significant factor in immersion syndrome because of altered judgment and impaired coordination. According to Cummings and Quan, 60% of all teenage drownings involve alcohol.[6]

Presenting symptoms with near-drowning vary with length of submersion, water temperature, quality of water, associated injuries, onset of cardiopulmonary resuscitation, and the patient's resuscitative response. Occasionally near-drowning victims may be asymptomatic; however, most present with mild dyspnea, a deathlike appearance with blue or gray coloring, apnea or tachypnea, hypotension, heart rate as slow as 4 to 5 beats per minute or pulselessness, cold skin, dilated pupils known as fish eyes, hypothermia, and vomiting.

Field resuscitation of the near-drowning victim is crucial for survival. Performing immediate cardiopulmonary resuscitation (CPR) on the victim after his or her removal from the water has been cited as a significant factor in survival. Regardless of advanced life support availability, increased survival results from excellent, prompt, field-initiated CPR. Initial resuscitation focuses on correcting hypoxia, acidosis, and hypotension. Box 41-3 highlights essential prehospital resuscitation. There is a high incidence of cervical spine injury in drowning victims, so cervical spine precautions are essential.

After the victim reaches the medical facility, resuscitation efforts emphasize stabilization of the ABCs and continued warming. Box 41-4 summarizes factors affecting survival. Rewarming efforts should be aggressive if the victim's

| Box 41-4 | NEAR-DROWNING SURVIVAL |

FACTORS THAT INCREASE SURVIVAL

Immediate, quality cardiopulmonary resuscitation
Colder water ($<70°$ F)
Cleaner water
Shorter immersion time
Less struggle
No associated injuries

FACTORS THAT HAVE NO EFFECT ON SURVIVAL

Sex
Race
Swimming ability
Eating a meal before the event
Type of water (saltwater or freshwater)
Use of the Heimlich maneuver during resuscitation attempts
Concurrent illnesses (i.e., cardiac or pulmonary disease)

| Box 41-5 | ESSENTIAL ED RESUSCITATION FOR NEAR-DROWNING |

Obtain history of the event, treatment, and progress during transport.
Establish airway and provide ventilation as rapidly as possible.
Continue CPR and begin active rewarming as indicated.
Perform endotracheal intubation as soon as possible and provide high-flow oxygen with positive pressure ventilation.
Handle victim gently to prevent hypothermia-induced ventricular dysrhythmias.
Monitor core temperature continuously. Anticipate further decrease in core temperature with continued rewarming.
Intubate and provide assisted ventilation with PEEP if there is evidence of pulmonary edema.
Insert a nasogastric tube to prevent gastric dilatation and possible aspiration.
Administer antibiotics for fever secondary to pneumonitis. (Prophylactic antibiotics are contraindicated for aspiration unless infection is present.)
Treat bronchospasm with a beta-agonist such as albuterol by metered dose inhaler.
Anticipate profound neurologic depression. Treat with hyperventilation, intraventricular monitoring, diuretics, and possibly barbiturates. Treat hypoxic seizures with oxygen, ventilation, diazepam, and phenytoin. Corticosteroids have no proven benefit in treatment of anoxic brain injuries and should not be routinely used.

ED, Emergency department; *CPR*, cardiopulmonary resuscitation; *PEEP*, positive end-expiratory pressure.

core temperature is below $90°$ F ($32°$ C). The heart is resistant to drug therapy and electroconversion when the core temperature is lower than $86°$ F ($30°$ C); therefore, early rewarming is essential to prevent ventricular fibrillation. Box 41-5 outlines essential steps for hospital resuscitation.

Complications associated with near-drowning are the direct result of the hypoxic event. Primary complications are pulmonary, cerebral, and cardiovascular, including pulmonary edema, pneumonitis, ARDS, anoxic encephalopathy, and cardiopulmonary arrest. Later complications include cerebral edema, disseminated intravascular coagulation, acute tubular necrosis, and renal failure.

DIVING EMERGENCIES

Over the past few decades self-contained underwater breathing apparatus (scuba) diving has enjoyed increased popularity. As equipment comfort and safety have improved, the recreational market has expanded significantly. Nearly 200,000 Americans receive scuba instruction each year. There are thousands of commercial and military divers; however, most of the 5 million scuba divers in the United States are recreational divers.[4] As the number of divers increase, dive-related accidents increase. Most accidents occur because the human body is not designed for the marine environment. Cold water, lack of available oxygen, and inability to run from hazards are intrinsic problems for which the diver must compensate. Diving accidents are increasing in all areas of the country, not just warm coastal resort areas. The most serious injuries discussed in this section are air embolism, nitrogen narcosis, and decompression sickness.

Divers are exposed to pressure changes related to water. Water is denser than air so that pressure changes are greater under water, even at relatively shallow depths (Table 41-4). Boyle's law states that gas volume is inversely related to pressure at a constant temperature. For the diver this means volume decreases and pressure increases as he or she descends. This principle is the mechanism behind all types of barotrauma, the most common medical problem that occurs with divers. Table 41-5 illustrates this principle using the lung as an example. When a diver uses a scuba tank of pressurized air, lung volume remains constant at various depths. If the diver ascends but does not exhale, water pressure decreases and gas in the lungs expands, greatly increasing pressure in the lungs (Table 41-6).

Air Embolism

Air embolism is the most serious and dangerous of all diving emergencies, second only to drowning as cause of death among divers. As gas expands, lungs expand to the point of rupture, causing pneumothoraces. High-pressure air is forced into the circulatory system, producing air embolism. Exhaling during controlled, slow ascent prevents air embolism. Divers risk injury when they ascend too rapidly or when they hold their breath during ascent.

Air embolism appears within seconds to minutes of ascent, usually less than 10 minutes from time of alveolar rupture. Symptoms are neurologic and may include vertigo, limb paresthesias, unilateral or bilateral sensory loss or paralysis, seizures, confusion, and loss of consciousness. Other signs and symptoms include chest tightness; shortness of breath; pink, frothy sputum; simple pneumothorax; and tension pneumothorax.

Table 41-4	PRESSURE-VOLUME RELATIONSHIPS ACCORDING TO BOYLE'S LAW				
	DEPTH (FEET)	GAUGE PRESSURE (ATMOSPHERES)	ABSOLUTE PRESSURE (ATMOSPHERES)	GAS VOLUME (%)	BUBBLE DIAMETER (%)*
Air	0	0	1	100	100
Seawater	33	1	2	50	79
	66	2	3	33	69
	99	3	4	25	63
	132	4	5	20	58
	165	5	6	17	54

*Bubble diameter is probably a more important variable than gas volume when considering the ability of recompression to restore circulation to a gas-embolized blood vessel.

Table 41-5	LUNG VOLUMES DURING DESCENT
DEPTH (FEET)	LUNG VOLUME UNDER PRESSURE (CC)
Sea level	1000
33	500
100	200
233	123

Table 41-6	LUNG VOLUMES DURING ASCENT WITHOUT EXHALATION
DEPTH (FEET)	LUNG VOLUME UNDER PRESSURE (CC)
233	1000
100	2000
33	4000
Sea level	8000

Table 41-7	GAS TOXICITIES IN DIVING	
GAS	SIGNS AND SYMPTOMS	THERAPEUTIC INTERVENTIONS
Oxygen (100%)	Twitching, nausea, dizziness, tunnel vision, restlessness, paresthesias, seizures, confusion, pulmonary edema, atelectasis, shock lung	Maintain ABCs, intubation, controlled ventilation to reduce FiO_2, decompression, positive end-expiratory pressure
Carbon dioxide (8%-10%)	Dizziness, lethargy, heavy labored breathing, unconsciousness	Ascent to surface, ABCs, 100% oxygen
Carbon monoxide (from contaminated tank)	Dizziness, pink or red lips and mouth, euphoria	Ascent to surface, ABCs (CPR if necessary), 100% oxygen in hyperbaric chamber at 3 atmospheres for 1 hour

ABCs, Airway, breathing, and circulation; *FiO₂,* fraction of inspired oxygen; *CPR,* cardiopulmonary resuscitation.

Death is an immediate threat to the diver with air embolism. The unconscious patient should be intubated immediately. Ensure proper ventilation with positive pressure ventilation and 100% oxygen. Perform needle thoracentesis for tension pneumothorax. Place the patient in the left lateral position to avoid cerebral embolism. If air transport is necessary, cabin altitude should not exceed 100 feet. Definitive treatment is prompt recompression and controlled decompression in a hyperbaric chamber.

Complications of air embolism depend on the end point of air bubbles. If bubbles enter the coronary arteries, the patient may have signs of myocardial infarction, whereas an embolism entering the cerebral circulation causes neurologic symptoms. Other complications include blocked vascular flow to the spinal cord with subsequent spinal cord injury, altered blood coagulation leading to disseminated intravascular coagulation, and hemoconcentration. Table 41-7 highlights gas toxicities related to diving.

Nitrogen Narcosis

Solubility of any gas in a liquid is almost directly proportional to pressure of the liquid at a constant temperature (Henry's law). The composition of room air is 79% nitrogen. Nitrogen narcosis occurs when nitrogen becomes dissolved in solution because pressures are greater than normal. Symptoms begin to appear at depths of 100 feet or more and resolve with ascent (see Table 41-6). Experienced divers usually have fewer problems than novices, although nitrogen narcosis is an inescapable problem for all divers.

Dissolved nitrogen has neurodepressant effects similar to alcohol. The "martini" rule is used to evaluate effects of dives to different depths. Every 50 feet of descent is comparable to one martini. Initially the diver may exhibit impaired judgment, a feeling of alcohol intoxication, slowed motor response, loss of proprioception, and euphoria. Below 200 feet nitrogen narcosis renders the diver unable to work;

however, individual divers have varying tolerance levels for nitrogen narcosis. Loss of consciousness occurs at approximately 300 feet.

Nitrogen narcosis has no real metabolic significance. The risk lies with impairment of the diver's judgment. Jacques Cousteau aptly described this condition as "rapture of the deep." Divers become euphoric, silly, and unaware of the dangerous situation and the need to surface. Ascent to the surface causes symptoms to disappear completely, so no further therapy is required. Nitrogen narcosis can be avoided by limiting the depth of dives.

Decompression Sickness

Decompression sickness, also called the bends, dysbarism, caisson disease, and diver's paralysis, is the most common form of diving emergency. Symptoms occur after rapid ascent. Speed of safe ascent is defined for each dive, depending on the depth-time relationship of the dive using standard U.S. Navy air decompression tables. According to Henry's law, gradual ascent allows the ambient pressure of nitrogen to reach an equilibrium that permits nitrogen to escape through respired air. Decompression sickness occurs during ascent and only when equilibrium cannot be established. Bubbles are squeezed into blood and tissues, obstructing flow and impairing tissue perfusion. Effects are seen in almost every organ of the body.

Typically, symptoms of decompression sickness begin within 30 minutes of ascent but may be delayed up to 36 hours. Some individuals (30%) exhibit symptoms before or on surfacing.[23] Factors that increase severity are described in Box 41-6. Nitrogen bubbles can develop in any tissue. The most significant mechanical effect is vascular occlusion in any tissue (e.g., supersaturation of lymphatic tissue with nitrogen causes lymphedema, cellular distention, membrane rupture). Biophysical effects are poor tissue perfusion and ischemia. Other symptoms characteristic of decompression sickness include cough, shortness of breath, and dyspnea (chokes); joint pain (bends); and neurologic symptoms such as fatigue, diplopia, headaches, dizziness, unconsciousness, paresthesias, and seizures.

Initial treatment begins with high-flow oxygen (100%) via nonrebreather mask to improve oxygenation and eliminate nitrogen. Fluid replacement is performed with intravenous normal saline or lactated Ringer's solution until urine output is 1 to 2 ml/kg/hr. Narcotic analgesics should be avoided because of their respiratory depressant effect. Steroids are often recommended to reduce progression and reoccurrence. Aspirin (325 to 650 mg) is given prophylactically for its antiplatelet activity. Treat patients for symptomatic nausea, vomiting, or headache. Definitive treatment is immediate transfer to a recompression facility. When more information is required, 24-hour assistance is available through the National Divers Alert Network at Duke University, the local health department, or the nearest naval facility.

Bends can occur at depths less than 33 feet, or 1 atmospheric pressure, if ascent is too rapid. Any joint pain within 24 to 48 hours of a dive should be treated as decompression sickness. Upper extremities are affected more often than lower extremities. A simple test for "joint bends" is inflation of a blood pressure cuff to 150 to 200 mm Hg or greater around the affected joint. Pain from the bends subsides as long as the cuff remains inflated.

Complications of decompression sickness are often related to failure to report symptoms, treat when the cause is unclear, or identify severe symptoms that result from a dive-related accident. Complications similar to air embolism may occur, such as spinal cord and cerebral lesions.

Remaining within a safe range of depth and time during repeated dives prevents decompression sickness. Gradual ascent with delays at certain depths allows nitrogen absorption and can be accomplished with decompression tables to calculate rate of nitrogen absorption. The depth and length of each dive should be limited. The diver should carry a scuba identification card for at least 48 hours after a dive.

Other Diving Problems
The Squeeze

The squeeze occurs when air is trapped in hollow chambers such as the ears, sinuses, pulmonary tree, gastrointestinal tract, teeth, and added air space such as the face mask or diving suit. Severe, sharp pain occurs when external pressure in these spaces exceeds internal pressure. The squeeze occurs if the diver descends to depths without exhalation. Symptoms include pain, edema, capillary dilation, rupture, and bleeding.

Treatment for all squeeze-related problems is gradual ascent to shallow depths to decrease pressure and maintenance of the ABCs. Symptomatic therapy with decongestants, both oral and nasal, is indicated for sinus squeeze. Pain control should be instituted with nonsteroidal antiinflammatory drugs.

Middle-ear squeeze is caused by a blocked eustachian tube or paranasal sinus with inability to equalize pressure in these spaces. Diving should be avoided when these chambers are congested from colds or allergies. When diving, gradual descents allow pressures in air-filled chambers to equalize. If the symptoms are mild, decongestants are recommended. If moderate, a short course of oral steroids is often prescribed. If the tympanic membrane is ruptured, consider antibiotics for otitis media.

Box 41-6 FACTORS THAT INCREASE SEVERITY IN DECOMPRESSION SICKNESS

Extremes in water temperature
Increasing age
Obesity
Fatigue
Poor physical condition
Alcohol consumption
Peripheral vascular disease
Heavy work during diving

A more serious but less common type of aural squeeze is inner-ear barotrauma. Structures of the inner ear may rupture with sudden pressure changes between the middle and inner ear. Permanent nerve damage and deafness can occur. Consultation with an otolaryngologist is recommended for the dive patient with tinnitus, vertigo, or deafness.

Barotrauma of Ascent
Barotrauma of ascent is the reverse of the squeeze. Although air-filled chambers may equalize during descent, air trapped in these spaces expands as atmospheric pressure decreases during ascent. If air cannot escape, barotrauma occurs. This condition is uncomfortable; however, no treatment is required because the condition subsides with time as the pressure gradually equalizes.

Hyperpnea Exhaustion Syndrome
Diver fatigue is usually responsible for hyperpnea exhaustion syndrome. Symptoms include tachypnea, anxiety, feeling of impending doom, difficulty floating, and exhaustion. Treatment consists of returning to the surface and rest.

CARBON MONOXIDE POISONING

Carbon monoxide (CO) gas is odorless and colorless. Most severe cases of CO intoxication are associated with inhalation of smoke from house fires; however, engine exhaust, improperly vented stoves, and faulty stoves or heating sys-

tems are also significant causes of accidental poisoning. Poisoning occurs primarily during the winter, usually because of faulty heating systems. CO poisoning is the most frequent source of poisoning in the United States, with CO poisoning from engine exhaust a common means of suicide. Accidental and intentional CO poisoning accounts for 3500 to 4000 deaths annually. Easley found a mortality rate of 30%.[8] Many victims die before transport to the hospital.

The most significant effect of CO exposure is hypoxia. Toxicity is the result of hemoglobin's affinity for CO, altered oxygen-hemoglobin dissociation curve, and impaired cytochrome oxidase systems. Hemoglobin's affinity for CO is 200 times greater than for oxygen. Hemoglobin preferentially binds with CO, so oxygen-carrying capacity is diminished even when oxygen is available. Carboxyhemoglobin (HbCO), formed when hemoglobin binds with CO, can be measured to determine severity of CO poisoning. HbCO is measured in parts per million, with concentration indicated by percentage (Table 41-8). CO also binds with myoglobin at a rate 40 times greater than oxygen. Consequently, hypoxia occurs at the tissue level and in the oxygen transport system. Pulse oximetry indicates adequate saturation despite the presence of hypoxia.

Generally, oxygen diffuses from the blood into the tissues. The oxygen-hemoglobin dissociation curve describes this process. Any event that shifts the curve to the left or right affects cellular oxygenation. Hypoxia that results from a shift in the HbCO dissociation curve is more significant

Table 41-8 SIGNS AND SYMPTOMS OF CARBON MONOXIDE EXPOSURE		
EXPOSURE LEVEL	**SIGNS AND SYMPTOMS**	**TREATMENT**
MILD		
10%-25% HbCO when no cardiac or neurologic involvement	Throbbing headache, nausea, impaired function for complex tasks	Maintain airway; administer IV fluids; use cardiac monitor; ensure oxygen administration by tight-fitting mask for 4 hours or until HbCO <5%
MODERATE		
20%-30% HbCO; less if cardiac or neurologic involvement is present	Severe headache, irritability, weakness, visual problems, palpitations, loss of dexterity, nausea and vomiting, ECG abnormalities, confusion, and lethargy	Hyperbaric oxygen administration at 3 atmospheres for 46 minutes; repeat in 6 hours if full CNS recovery does not occur; maintain airway; administer IV fluids; use cardiac monitor
SEVERE		
40%-50% HbCO	Tachycardia, tachypnea, collapse, syncope	As above
LIFE-THREATENING		
50%-60% HbCO	Coma, Cheyne-Stokes respirations, intermittent convulsions, cherry red mucous membranes	As above
LETHAL		
Greater than 60% HbCO	Cardiac and respiratory depression, likely cardiac arrest	CPR and as above

HbCO, Carboxyhemoglobin; *IV*, intravenous; *ECG*, electrocardiogram; *CNS*, central nervous system; *CPR*, cardiopulmonary resuscitation.

than hypoxia that results from a simple reduction in functional hemoglobin. HbCO shifts the oxygen curve so that partial pressure needed to unload oxygen from blood to the tissue is lower than in normal tissue.

CO also interferes with cytochrome oxidase systems. Decreased function of these systems impairs cellular respiration by displacing oxygen, particularly in high-rate metabolic organs (i.e., the brain and heart). Oxygen displacement is responsible for dysrhythmias and many CNS symptoms seen in CO poisoning.

Symptoms may be initially vague but worsen with increased exposure. Variability of symptoms in individuals with identical exposure exists; the longer the time between exposure and presentation, the greater the variability. Children may have increased susceptibility to CO toxicity. A child's higher metabolic rate may cause syncope and lethargy at HbCO levels of 25%. Specific signs and general management of CO poisoning are discussed in Table 41-8. The cornerstone for all treatment is high-flow oxygen to displace CO from hemoglobin. The half-life of CO is 5 to 6 hours on room air. Half-life is reduced to 1 hour with 100% oxygen and less than 20 minutes with hyperbaric oxygen therapy.

CO promotes dysrhythmias and myocardial ischemia. Alterations in the alveolar-capillary membrane may lead to pulmonary edema and hemorrhage. Neurologic deficits include seizures, cerebral edema, and coma. Renal failure occurs secondary to myoglobinuria. Patients with HbCO levels greater than 25% or signs of cardiac ischemia and neurologic deficits should be admitted for observation. If patients are discharged, instructions should include discussion of neurologic sequelae such as headache, loss of memory and concentration, irritability, personality changes, and excessive fatigue. Hyperbaric oxygen therapy may be required if symptoms return.

BITES AND STINGS

Specific environmental emergencies related to bites and stings include bites from snakes, animals, spiders, and ticks and stings from scorpions and hymenopterans (i.e., bees, wasps, hornets, and fire ants). Table 41-9 summarizes bites and stings. Lethality is the result of poisonous venom and stings or secondary to anaphylaxis. Respiratory distress and anaphylactic shock are discussed in Chapters 32 and 34.

Snakebites

There are 3000 species of snakes. Of these, 375 species from five different families are venomous: Crotalidae, Elapidae, Viperidae, Colubridae, and Hydrophidae. Two families of poisonous snakes indigenous to the United States are Crotalidae or pit vipers (rattlesnakes, copperheads, and cottonmouths) and Elapidae (coral snakes). Cobras and mambas belong to the Elapidae family but are not indigenous to the United States. Figure 41-6 summarizes the differences between poisonous and nonpoisonous snakes. More than

45,000 snakebites occur annually in the United States. Envenomation occurs in only 8000 cases. The most common poisonous snake in the United States is a pit viper (95%), usually the rattlesnake. Fortunately, fewer than 15 deaths occur per year.[20] Venom is a complex substance containing enzymes, glycoproteins, peptides, and other substances capable of causing tissue destruction—cardiotoxic, neurotoxic, hemotoxic, or any combination of these. Pit viper venom is primarily hemotoxic, whereas coral snake venom is primarily neurotoxic. Venom is manufactured in salivary glands and stored in the ducts of the fangs located in the anterior mouth. Envenomation occurs when venom is injected into the victim's subcutaneous tissue through the fangs.

Signs and symptoms of snakebites depend on the type and size of the snake, size and age of the patient, location and depth of the bite, number of bites, and amount of venom injected. The patient may also have a specific sensitivity to the venom that makes the reaction worse. The snake's teeth contain numerous microorganisms, so a bite can cause secondary infection. Major signs and symptoms are divided into local and systemic reactions. Local reactions have one or two fang marks, teeth marks, edema around the bite site 1 to 36 hours after the bite, pain at the site, petechiae, ecchymosis, loss of function of the limb, and necrosis 16 to 36 hours after the bite. Systemic reactions include nausea, vomiting, diaphoresis, syncope, and a metallic or rubber taste. The patient may develop paralysis, excessive salivation, difficulty speaking, visual disturbances, muscle twitching, paresthesia, epistaxis, blood in the stool, vomitus or sputum, and ptosis. Neurologic symptoms include constricted pupils and seizures. Life-threatening systemic reactions include severe hemorrhage, renal failure, and hypovolemic shock.

Initial assessment includes a history of the snakebite; for example, the size of the snake, location and depth of the injury, number of bites, and amount of venom injected (if known). Document the time of injury and all interventions employed before ED arrival. Prehospital interventions include stabilization of ABCs and keeping the patient calm and supine to minimize exertion. Immobilize the limb at or below the level of the heart to reduce blood flow. Do not apply ice or a tourniquet. Place a band 4 inches proximal to the bite to impede lymphatic flow while preserving arterial and venous flow. Remove potentially constrictive jewelry or tight-fitting clothing. Do not cut or attempt to suck venom from the wound.

Incision for venom suction is rarely indicated. If incision and suction are performed within the first 5 to 15 minutes, 10% of the venom may be removed; effectiveness drops dramatically 30 minutes after the bite. Ice has not proved beneficial and may impair absorption of antivenin and increase necrosis secondary to decreased circulation. Drinking coffee or alcohol and smoking cause vasodilation and increase absorption of the venom.

Hospital interventions begin with the ABCs. Initiate aggressive intravenous infusion of normal saline or lactated Ringer's solution to maintain renal blood flow and fluid vol-

Table 41-9 BITES AND STINGS

TYPE OF ARTHROPOD	SIGNS AND SYMPTOMS	MANAGEMENT
STINGING		
Honeybee *(Apis mellificus)* Bumblebee *(Bombus)*	Painful injection wound; stinger often visibly protruding. Edema and itching may be apparent.	Remove stinger by scraping with dull object. Do not grasp and pull; this contracts venom sac, releasing more toxin. Cleanse site and apply antiseptic. Apply ice and elevate part. Oral antihistamines and steroids may be indicated.
Yellow jacket *(Vespula maculifrons)* Wasp *(Chlorion ichneumonica)*	Painful injection wound. Does not leave stinger behind; stings repeatedly. Wheal formation, edema, and itching may be present.	See bee sting (above). Watch for anaphylaxis.
Hornet *(Vespula maculata)* Velvet ant *(Mutilla sacken)* Fire ant *(Solenopsis geminata)*	Painful injection wound with wheal that expands to large vesicle; as purulence develops, reddening of area occurs; scarring and crusting follow reabsorption of pustule.	See bee sting (above). Watch for anaphylaxis.
Scorpions *(Centruroides sculpturatus, Centruroides vittatus, and Centruroides gertschi)*	Lethal: No visible local effect. Sharp pain, hyperesthesia followed by hypoesthesia itching, and speech disturbances are common. Jaw muscle spasms, nausea, vomiting, incontinence, and seizures follow. Death may occur from cardiovascular or respiratory failure.	Apply tourniquet as near to sting site as possible, and pack area in ice well beyond the tourniquet. After 5 minutes, loosen tourniquet and reapply.
	Nonlethal: Sharp burning pain at sting site with edema and discoloration; anaphylaxis is rare.	Caution: Morphine and opiates are contraindicated; they enhance toxic effects.
BITING AND PIERCING		
Tick *(Dermacentor variabilis)*	Victim unaware of presence; local irritation and possible infection when body removed but head remains in tissue; some species (which transmit Rocky Mountain Spotted Fever) cause flaccid paralysis from neurotoxin. Initial symptoms are paresthesias and pain in lower extremity. Respiratory failure results from bulbar paralysis.	Remove offending ticks. Apply gasoline, ether, or hot (not burning) match to the tick body. Wait 10 minutes for disengagement. Do not manually remove; squeezing the body may inject more virus into victim. Paralysis will dramatically subside after removal.
Centipedes Eastern house centipede *(Scutigera cleoptratu)* Western house centipede *(Scolopendra heros)*	Wound site red, edematous, and painful; sometimes tissue necrosis occurs.	Cleanse wound. Employ analgesics and antibiotics if indicated.
Spiders Black widow *(Latrodectus mactans)* (hourglass spider, female)	Pricking sensation followed by dull, numbing pain. Edema and tiny red fang marks may become visible. Chest and abdominal pain may be evident adjacent to site of the bite. Pain and rigidity of muscles subside after 48 hours. Blood pressure, temperature, and white blood count may be elevated. Hematuria rarely develops. Spinal fluid may have increased pressure.	Use ice locally to slow absorption of toxins. Employ muscle relaxants and 10% calcium gluconate IV to reduce spasms. Use antivenin (Latrodectus mactans). Do skin test before administration of the horse serum. Symptoms subside 1-3 hours after antivenin administration.
Brown recluse *(Loxosceles reclusa)* (fiddleback)	Local reaction begins 2-8 hours after bite with pain, edema, bleb formation, and ischemia. On third or fourth day after bite, central area turns dark and is firm to touch. In second week central area becomes depressed and demarcated with open ulceration formation. Healing may take place in about 3 weeks. Fever, chills, malaise, weakness, nausea, vomiting, joint pain, and petechiae may also be noted. Blood dyscrasias such as hemolytic anemia and thrombocytopenia rarely occur.	Immediate excision of wound with toxins may be useful. Steroids, antihistamines, and antibiotics are to be employed as indicated. Skin grafting may be necessary if healing does not take place.

IV, Intravenous; *ECG,* electrocardiogram.

*Antivenins for most aquatic bites and stings (e.g., stonefish, jellyfish, sea snake) are available from Commonwealth Serum Laboratories, Melbourne, Australia.

Continued

Table 41-9 BITES AND STINGS—cont'd

TYPE OF ARTHROPOD	SIGNS AND SYMPTOMS	MANAGEMENT
True bugs		
Kissing bug (Conenose triatoma)	Mild or no pain at wound site. Redness, edema, itching, or nodular hemorrhagic lesions, depending on sensitivity.	Cleanse wound with soap and water. Oral antihistamines may be indicated. Anaphylaxis has been reported.
Assassin bug (Arilus christatus) (wheel bug)	Intense pain at wound site. Usually lasts 2-5 hours. Localized edema, itching, and redness can occur.	Cleanse wound with antiseptic solution. Anaphylaxis is rare.

VESICATING OR URTICATING

Blister beetles	Clear amber fluid (cantharidin) released from the insects' knee joints, prothorax, and genitalia. Mild burning sensation may become apparent as a result of fluid released at site.	Cleanse area with soap and water as soon as possible.
Lepidoptera (larva) Lo caterpillar (Automeris lo) Puss caterpillar (Megalopyge opercularis) Saddle back caterpillar (Sibine stimulea) Range caterpillar (Hemileuca oliviae)	Distinct row of released spines may be seen at site of intense pain. Nausea, vomiting, headache, and fever may be present.	Remove spines with adhesive tape, if possible. Apply ice to the wound; analgesics may be indicated. Unremoved spines could cause infection.
Aquatic organisms* Stingray	Wound contains venom sacs from furrowed spine of stingray tail. Fainting, nausea, vomiting, and diarrhea occur with occasional progression to muscle paralysis, respiratory distress, seizures, and even death.	Immediately irrigate wound with normal saline to remove venom sacs. Follow initial irrigation with immersion in hot water for 30 minutes (110°-114° F [43.3°-45.5° C]) to inactivate venom. Antibiotics recommended; antihistamines and steroids may also be indicated. For severe cases, have ventilatory support and resuscitation equipment at hand. Surgical closure of wounds may be necessary in some instances.
Catfish	Wound from dorsal spine causes pain and infection.	Use deep irrigations of hydrogen peroxide. Employ antibiotics as indicated.
Portuguese man-of-war (Physalia physalis)	Tentacles become embedded in skin. Welts, burned areas, or streaks may be present. Pain may be intense enough to produce shock and collapse. Headache, cramps, and paralysis also noted.	Tourniquet may be tried. Remove tentacles with alcohol and sodium bicarbonate scrub (prevents further stinging and neutralizes acid). Leave alcohol on for 6-8 min. Follow with sodium bicarbonate, allowing it to dry. Employ antihistamines and steroids locally and systemically. General anesthesia may be necessary to control pain.
Stings (cone shell snails, sea anemones, corals, and jellyfish)	Acid wound produced.	Cleanse wound with alkali (ammonia, sodium bicarbonate).
Bites (sea snake and octopus)	Wounds contain neurotoxin. Muscle stiffness, paralysis, myoglobinuria, and death from respiratory arrest can occur.	Apply tourniquet. Control shock. Use indicated resuscitation measures.
Scorpion fish	Intense pain, edema, shock, and ECG changes.	See stingray injuries (above) for wound cleansing and heat application. Give antivenin.
Sea urchins	Painful injection site with erythema, edema, numbness, and paralysis. Respiratory distress and death may occur.	Use heat as described under stingray. Do not attempt to remove spines initially. Attempt to locate with x-ray films. Granulomatous lesions often develop from embedded spines.

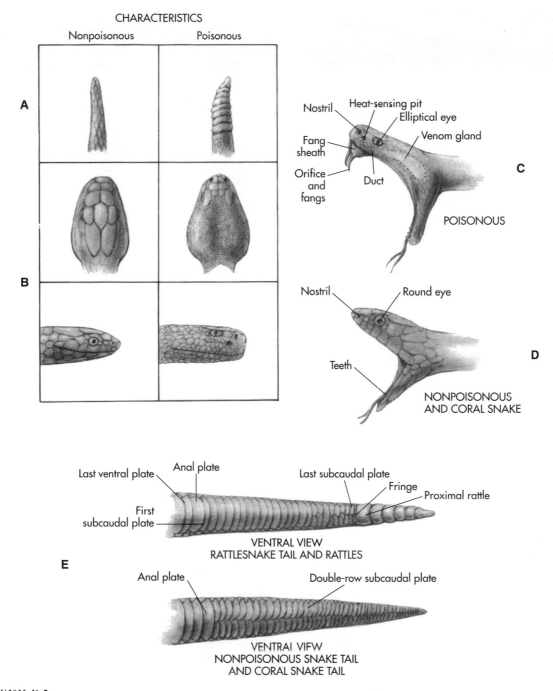

FIGURE 41-6 Comparison of venomous and nonvenomous snakes. **A,** Tail. **B,** Head shape. **C,** Absence or presence of heat-sensing facial pit between the eye and the nostril. **D,** Absence or presence of well-developed venom glands, duct, and fangs. **E,** Belly scales leading up to the tail. (From Davis JH et al: *Surgery: a problem solving approach,* ed 2, vol 1, St. Louis, 1995, Mosby.)

ume. Obtain a complete blood count; coagulation studies; electrolyte, blood urea nitrogen, creatinine, creatinine phosphokinase levels; blood type; and cross-match. Clean the wound and clearly mark and time edges of envenomation. Administer analgesics for pain, preferably acetaminophen because hemorrhage can occur with aspirin or nonsteroidal antiinflammatory drugs. Avoid narcotics because of the risk of respiratory depression. Administer tetanus prophylaxis if the patient's immunization history is incomplete or out-

dated. Plain films of the extremity may reveal retained teeth or fangs in the wound.

Suspect compartment syndrome if the extremity becomes increasingly tense because of edema and third-space fluid accumulation. Compartment pressures should be measured in this situation and an orthopedist consulted for possible fasciotomy to relieve pressure. Fasciotomy is usually indicated if compartment pressures remain persistently higher than 30 mm Hg despite appropriate use of antivenin.

Table 41-10	ANTIVENIN DOSAGE REGIMEN	
SIGNS AND SYMPTOMS	DEGREE OF ENVENOMATION	DOSE
Fang marks; no local swelling or paresthesia	None	No skin test or antivenin required
Fang marks; local swelling of hands or feet; pain; no systemic responses	Minimal	3-5 vials*
Fang marks; progressive swelling beyond site of bite; mild systemic symptoms	Moderate	5-10 vials*
Multiple fang marks; progressive swelling, pain, and ecchymosis; marked systemic symptoms, hypotension, fasciculations, or clotting deficits	Severe	10-20 vials*

*Dilute antivenin in half-normal saline at a 1:4 ratio. Infuse within 2 hours. Repeat dose every 2 hours until symptoms subside. Children generally require 50% more antivenin.

Antivenin therapy is reserved for life-threatening snakebites because there is a high incidence of sensitivity reaction and anaphylaxis. If antivenin is administered the patient should be closely monitored. Resuscitation equipment and emergency medication should be readily available. Antivenin is prepared in horse serum; therefore, the patient should be questioned carefully about allergies to horse serum. Perform a skin test for antivenin if the patient will receive the medication, has had no previous antivenin treatments, and is not allergic to horse serum. Inject 0.02 ml of a 1:1000 dilution intradermally. Observe for 15 to 30 minutes and then check for wheals. After a negative skin test, administer antivenin by slow intravenous drip. (Table 41-10 provides dosage regimen.) Insufficient dosage is the most common cause of treatment failure. Administer antivenin until symptoms subside.

The physician may elect to give the antivenin despite a positive skin reaction. Monitor closely for systemic reactions such as urticaria, wheezing, or other symptoms of progressing anaphylaxis. Meticulous patient observation and slow administration of the medication are essential. Explain the risks of treatment to the patient. A consent may be required in some areas. Administration of antivenin is not a common ED procedure in most areas of the country; therefore, consultation with a professional poison control center is advised.

Lizard Bites

The iguana is a member of the family Iguanidae. The bite is generally nontoxic, causing pain without systemic reactions.

Two venomous varieties, however, are the Gila monster (Heloderma) and the Mexican bearded lizard. Gila toxin is released in saliva. Symptoms may begin with pain and swelling, progressing to systemic symptoms of nausea, vomiting, weakness, hypotension, syncope, shock, and anaphylaxis. No antivenin is currently available for Gila toxin. Treatment includes wound care, tetanus prophylaxis, and analgesics. Meperidine enhances the effect of Gila toxin and should be avoided. Provide supportive care for systemic response.

Animal Bites

An estimated 1 to 3 million animal bites occur annually in the United States. The number of animal bites peak during the spring, with the incidence greater in urban areas than rural areas. Dogs and cats are the most frequent offenders, with wild rodents and pet rodents ranked second. Treatment of animal bites includes cleaning the wound, tetanus prophylaxis, copious irrigation with saline solution, and analgesics as necessary.

Dog Bites

Dog bites account for 80% to 90% of all bites occurring to humans in the United States.[18] Most victims own the dogs that bite them, with children the population at greatest risk. The most common sites of injury are the extremities. Dog bite wounds may be simple punctures or major deforming lacerations, tears, avulsions, or soft-tissue crush injuries. Tissue necrosis may occur with a crush injury. The type of injury usually depends on the size of the dog and the body area where the wound is inflicted.

Therapeutic intervention focuses on reducing the possibility of infection and neutralizing rabies virus. Potentially disfiguring wounds of the face, particularly eyelids, lips, and ears, should be cleansed gently before evaluation for repair by a reconstructive surgeon. Irrigate the wound with copious amounts of normal saline using a pressure irrigation set or 20-gauge intravenous catheter. In general 100 to 200 ml of irrigation solution (normal saline or 1% povidone solution) per inch of wound is required. Heavily contaminated wounds may require more. Anticipate debridement of nonviable tissue. Puncture wounds are left open, whereas lacerations are loosely sutured. The extremity should be splinted and immobilized. Prophylactic antibiotic therapy is used with high-risk injuries such as hand and foot bites, puncture wounds, and wounds greater than 6 to 12 hours old. Report the incident to the local animal control or public health authorities. The dog should be quarantined for 10 days if immunization history is unknown or rabies is suspected.

Aftercare instructions for wound care should be given to the patient and family with careful explanation of signs and symptoms of infection. If a bite is not treated, infection, cellulitis, osteomyelitis, and residual neurovascular damage may occur. Puncture wounds have a higher rate of infection because of the depth of the wound. An estimated 5% of all dog bites become infected. Other complications include rabies. Fortunately, rabies is not a routine outcome of dog bites because of effective canine immunization programs.

Cat Bites and Scratches

Cat bites account for 5% to 15% of all bites inflicted on humans in the United States each year.[25] Cats are notorious for scratches because of their sharp claws. Cat scratches cause the same complications as bites and are treated in the same manner. Cat bites cause deep puncture wounds that can involve the victim's tendons and joint capsules. There is little incidence of crush injury because cats' teeth are sharp, narrow, and long and the jaw lacks power. Incidence of wound infections from cat bites is greater than in dog bites. Cats are hunters and often come in contact with bacteria-infested rodents, which contaminate their mouths with *Pasteurella multocida*. Consequently, rapid onset of infection can occur after the bite. Nearly all infections are from mixed organisms. Cats also use their paws to groom themselves and may have considerable bacteria on their claws. Treatment for cat bites is the same as for dog bites. Osteomyelitis, septic arthritis, and tenosynovitis have been reported. Cat-scratch disease may cause lymphadenitis of the extremity days to weeks after the scratch. Because risk of infection is so great, thorough wound care instructions with clear instructions for follow-up are essential.

Human Bites

Human bites have the highest rate of infection and tissue damage of all bite injuries. The human mouth has great crushing ability and also harbors more than 40 potential pathogens. The most common sites for bites are the fingers, hands, ears, and tip of the nose. A human bite may cause a laceration, puncture, crush injury, soft-tissue tearing, or even amputation. Boxer's fractures are often associated with an open wound over the knuckles that occurred when the fist impacted another person's teeth. Treatment is similar to other bites, with the exception that the patient always receives prophylactic antibiotics. If infection is already present, the patient is usually admitted for parenteral antibiotic therapy. Human bites have an increased risk of osteomyelitis, cellulitis, and septic arthritis. Human bites are reported to the local police in some states.

Spider (Arachnid) Bites

All spiders inject venom when they bite. Most venom causes itching, stinging, swelling, or a combination of symptoms in a local area. Despite the vast number of arthropod bites and stings occurring on a daily basis, systemic reactions occur in only 4% of the population, with anaphylaxis in only 0.4%. In the United States approximately four deaths per year are reported as a result of spider bites.[19] Tarantula bites usually cause only local reactions (i.e., slight pain and stinging). Black widow spider venom and brown recluse spider venom may cause systemic reactions and anaphylaxis.

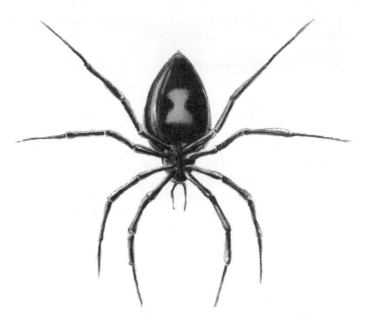

FIGURE 41-7 Female black widow spider (*Latrodectus mactans*) with typical hourglass marking on the abdomen. (From Davis JH et al: *Surgery: a problem solving approach,* ed 2, vol 1, St. Louis, 1995, Mosby.)

Black Widow Spider Bites

Black widow spiders are usually found in damp, cool places, such as under rocks or in woodpiles. They are recognizable by their shiny black body and the bright red hourglass marking on their abdomen (Figure 41-7). The black widow spider's venom is neurotoxic. A local reaction begins within minutes, including pain out of proportion to the size of the bite. Two tiny red fang marks appear at the point of venom entry surrounded by a small papule. Multiple bites rule out spider envenomation, for spiders rarely bite more than once. Systemic reactions develop within 1 hour and include nausea, vomiting, hypertension, hyperactive deep tendon reflexes, and elevated temperature. Patients may also have respiratory difficulty, headache, syncope, weakness, and chest and abdominal pain or spasms. Seizures and shock may also develop. Symptoms from envenomation peak 2 to 3 hours after onset but can last several days.

Reactions may be minor and require only local wound care; however, severe systemic responses also occur. Interventions begin with stabilization of the ABCs. Apply ice to the bite area to slow action of the neurotoxin. Steroid ointment can be applied for comfort. Administer muscle relaxants such as methocarbamol (Robaxin) or diazepam (Valium) and give calcium gluconate (10 ml of 10% solution) for muscle spasms, rigidity, and pain. Narcotic analgesics may be required for severe pain. Tetanus immunization should be updated with all black widow spider bites. Consider antivenin therapy for severe reactions or high-risk individuals (e.g., young children, adults with hypertension or cardiac disease). Contact a poison control center for further consultation. With aggressive, supportive therapy, symptoms usually subside within 48 hours; however, hypertension and muscle spasms may recur for 12 to 24 hours.

Brown Recluse Spider Bites

Brown recluse spiders, also known as fiddleback or violin-back spiders, have a light brown color with a dark brown fiddle-shaped mark that extends from the six white eyes down the back (Figure 41-8). These spiders are found in the southeastern, south central, and southwestern United States; however, they can appear anywhere in the country if the spider crawls into luggage or a car. They prefer hot, dry, dark areas such as basements, garages, closets, and boxes. They are most active at night, from spring to fall.

The venom of the brown recluse spider is cytotoxic and hemolytic. Characteristic symptoms occur within minutes to several hours. A mild stinging occurs at the time of the bite and progresses to severe pain a few hours later. Local edema, a bluish ring around the bite (bull's eye), and a bleb develop. Erythema, local ischemia, and tissue necrosis appear on the third or fourth day. Eschar forms on the fourteenth day; however, the patient may have an open sore for days or even weeks. The wound should heal within 21 days. Systemic reactions rarely occur. Symptoms, if present, begin 24 to 48 hours after envenomation and include fever, chills, nausea, vomiting, weakness, general malaise, arthralgia, joint pain, and petechiae. In light of recent world events, cutaneous anthrax should also be considered in patients with these symptoms.

Management is supportive and includes ice, elevation, and rest of the affected area. Consider antihistamines for itching. Systemic or local steroids may be used. Local debridement with skin grafting may be indicated after the wound is stabilized. Antibiotics may decrease the local inflammatory response and the resulting skin necrosis. Discharge instructions should include wound care training and cooling of lesion for the first 72 hours. Patient should soak the wound daily and have daily wound checks until the lesion resolves.

Dapsone, a polymorphonuclear leukocyte inhibitor, has been highly effective in the management of crater lesions in adults. The recommended oral dosage is 50 mg 2 times per day for 10 days. This drug should be used cautiously because of potential blood dyscrasias. Intolerance in patients with glucose-6-phosphate dehydrogenase (G6PD) deficiency has been reported; therefore, G6PD screening and complete blood count monitoring must accompany administration.

Scorpion Stings

Scorpions are found primarily in the warm southwestern states and exotic pet shops across the country. Stings occur most often in the early evening and night hours. Scorpions appear to sting in self-defense; they are not by nature aggressive creatures. There are several kinds of scorpions, but only one is considered lethal—Centruroides sculpturatus,

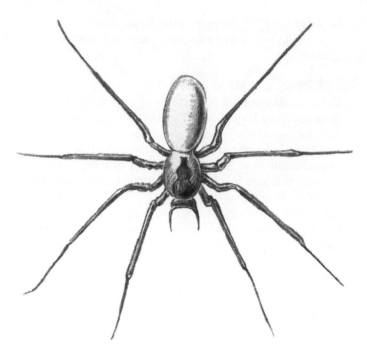

FIGURE 41-8   Brown recluse spider (*Loxosceles reclusa*) with typical dark violin-shaped marking on the cephalothorax. (From Davis JH et al: *Surgery: a problem solving approach,* ed 2, vol 1, St. Louis, 1995, Mosby.)

also known as "bark scorpions" because they dwell in tree bark.

The tail of the scorpion contains a telson where venom is produced and stored. A stinger injects a neurotoxic venom, which produces immediate local pain at the sting site, edema, discoloration, hyperesthesia, numbness, and agitation. Anxiety, restlessness, itching, speech disturbances, tachycardia, hypertension, and tachypnea occur with extensive envenomation. Systemic reactions include wheezing, respiratory stridor, profuse salivation, visual disturbances, ataxic gait, incontinence, muscle spasms of the jaw muscles, nausea and vomiting, dysphagia, seizures, and anaphylaxis. Pain and numbness resolve without treatment in a few hours; however, systemic responses may last several days. Patients with severe envenomation may exhibit complicated neuromuscular and autonomic symptoms.

Treatment includes supporting the ABCs. Apply ice or cool compresses to relieve pain. Only mild analgesics are recommended because narcotic analgesics have been reported to increase the toxic effect of the venom. Immobilize the extremity to slow venom absorption. Antihistamines are indicated for some patients. Scorpion antivenin is available from the Antivenin Production Laboratories of Arizona State University; however, the antivenin is not approved by the Food and Drug Administration. The antivenin is effective only for severe stings from the Centruroides exilcicauda found in the United States. Specific antivenin for local species is available in other countries.

Hymenopteran Stings (Bee, Wasp, Hornet, and Fire Ant)

Hymenopterans are an insect family found in temperate regions and includes the honeybee, wasp, hornet, and fire ant. Stings are more common in the summer months. Hymenopteran venom varies among species and may be cytotoxic, hemolytic, allergenic, or vasoactive. Hymenopteran stings cause 40 to 150 deaths annually in the United States.[15]

Hymenopteran stings cause a variety of reactions ranging from mild local reactions to anaphylactic shock depending on the type and amount of venom and the patient's sensitivity to the venom. Reactions can occur at the time of the sting and up to 48 hours later. Stings are usually cumulative. The greater the number of stings, the more severe the reaction. With the exception of the honeybee, most hymenopterans sting repeatedly. Fire ants have a painful sting that causes a wheal that expands to a large vesicle. The area then reddens and a pustule forms. When the pustule is reabsorbed, crusting and scar formation occur.

Symptoms vary from mild stinging or burning sensations, swelling, and itching to severe local reactions such as edema of the entire extremity. The patient may also have severe systemic reactions, including urticaria, pruritus, edema, bronchospasm, laryngeal edema, and hypotension.

Treatment begins with removal of the stinger as quickly as possible to prevent absorption of the venom. The stinger actively injects venom into the wound for 1 minute after the sting. Do not grasp or squeeze the stinger with tweezers because this squeezes out more venom. Scrape the stinger away using a dull object such as the side of a credit card or needle. Apply ice packs to the site. Further treatment is determined by severity of the reaction. If the reaction is mild, minimal medications are required—usually oral antihistamines block effects of some venom and the effects of endogenously released histamine. If the reaction is severe, medications such as epinephrine, Benedryl, Pepcid, and Becadron may be required. Most stings resolve with no residual complaints.

Tick Bites

Most tick bites are harmless; however, tick bites can cause Rocky Mountain spotted fever, Lyme borreliosis, and tick paralysis. Regardless of the species and subsequent illness, principal management consists of tick removal followed by supportive therapy.

Rocky Mountain Spotted Fever

Rocky Mountain spotted fever is caused by *Rickettsia rickettsii*. Occurring across the country, the disease is most prevalent in the south Atlantic and south central states. Most cases have been reported when ticks are most active, from April to September. Incubation period is 2 to 14 days. Major symptoms include fever, chills, malaise, myalgias, and headache. During the first 10 days the patient develops a pink, macular, or petechial rash over the palms, wrists, hands, soles, feet, and ankles. However, the rash may involve any part of the body. Treatment includes antibiotic therapy. Recovery occurs within 20 days. Goddard found the mortality, if untreated, is between 8% and 25%.[9]

Lyme Disease

Lyme disease, the most widespread tickborne disease, is transmitted via the Ixodes tick and caused by the spirochete *Borrelia burgdorferi*. Incubation is 3 to 32 days. In 1992 more than 90% of reported cases occurred in the northeastern and midwestern states.[15] Most cases occur in the spring and summer.

Within days of the tick bite, symptoms develop in three distinct stages. During the first stage, erythema migrans, the patient experiences an expanding circular area of redness or rash at least 5 cm in diameter and flulike symptoms. This stage may last 2 months. First-line treatment recommendation is doxycycline for 14 to 21 days. However, the rash generally disappears without treatment. The second stage occurs days to weeks after the tick bite. Patients may exhibit neurologic, cardiac, and musculoskeletal complications such as meningitis, hepatitis, cranial neuropathies, atrioventricular blocks, cardiomyopathies, and arthralgia. Ceftriaxone is the most widely used agent in treating acute neurologic complications and third-degree heart block and Lyme arthritis. Patients with first- and second-degree heart block are treated with doxyclycline. The third and final stage may last months or years. In this stage the patient primarily manifests musculoskeletal and neurologic symptoms such as chronic arthritis and peripheral radiculoneuropathy. Lyme disease appears to respond to various medications; however, the most effective regimen remains controversial. In addition, only 1% of untreated patients develop Lyme disease after a tick bite. Thus, the Infectious Disease Society of America does not recommend or support the use of routine or selective treatment.[27] The committee recommends that the patient be evaluated and treated for any symptoms with the recommendations discussed previously.

Tick Paralysis

Tick paralysis is a neurotoxic disease transmitted by a bite from a female Dermacentor andersoni (wood tick) or Dermacentor variabilis (dog tick). Incubation is 5 to 7 days. Most cases occur in the southeastern and northwestern United States. Tick paralysis is primarily an ascending motor paralysis occurring over 1 to 2 days. Symptoms include ataxia, lower extremity weakness progressing to upper extremities, paresthesia, decreased to absent reflexes, and eventually respiratory failure.

Treatment begins with tick removal. Gently grasp the tick with forceps at the point of entry and pull upward in a steady motion. Other methods include covering the tick with alcohol, mineral oil, or petroleum jelly or killing the tick with ether or a hot match. After the tick is removed, symptoms should gradually improve. Supportive care is necessary until symptoms resolve, usually within 48 to 72 hours.

SUMMARY

Environmental emergencies cover a broad spectrum of diseases arising from a variety of environmental factors. These emergencies can occur in any geographic area and at any time of the year. Morbidity and mortality are directly related to the magnitude and duration of the exposure, regardless of the source. Box 41-7 highlights nursing diagnoses for these patients. Prevention is the key to management of environmental emergencies. Those at greatest risk require information on protection against environmental dangers, use of good judgment, survival skills, and awareness of early signs and symptoms for specific emergencies.

Box 41-7   NURSING DIAGNOSES FOR ENVIRONMENTAL EMERGENCIES

Airway clearance, Ineffective
Fluid volume, Deficient
Gas exchange, Impaired
Knowledge, Deficient
Skin integrity, Impaired
Thermoregulation, Ineffective
Tissue perfusion, Ineffective

References

1. Auerbach PA: *Wilderness and environmental emergencies,* ed 4, St. Louis, 2001, Mosby.
2. Blum LN, Bresolin LB, Williams MA: Heat-related illness during extreme weather emergencies, *JAMA* 279(19):1514, 1998.
3. Bristow GK: Disturbances due to cold. In Rakel RE, editor: *Conn's current therapy 2000,* ed 52, Philadelphia, 2000, WB Saunders.
4. Carvalho MD, Shockley TW: Diving emergencies. In Rosen P, Barkin RM, Hockberger RS et al, editors: *Emergency medicine: concepts and clinical practice,* ed 4, St. Louis, 1998, Mosby.
5. Cochrane DA: Hypothermia: a cold influence on trauma, *Int J Trauma* 7(1):8, 2001.
6. Cummings P, Quan L: Trends in unintentional drowning: the role of alcohol and medical care, *JAMA* 281(23):2198, 1999.
7. Danzel D: Frostbite. In Rosen P, Barkin RS, Hockberger RS et al, editors: *Emergency medicine: concepts and clinical practice,* ed 4, St. Louis, 1998, Mosby.
8. Easley RB: Open air carbon monoxide poisoning in a child swimming behind a boat, *South Med J* 93(4):430, 2000.
9. Goddard J: *Physician's guide to arthropods of medical importance,* ed 3, Boca Raton, Fla, 1999, CRC Press.
10. Hanke BK, Schwartz GR, Gerace JE: Near drowning. In Schwartz GR, editor: *Principles and practice of emergency medicine,* ed 4, Baltimore, 1999, Williams & Wilkins.
11. Hazinski MF, Cummins RO, Field JM, editors: *2000 handbook of emergency cardiovascular care for healthcare providers,* Dallas, Tex, 2000, American Heart Association.
12. Hett HA, Brechtelsbauer DA: Heat related illness, *Postgrad Med* 103:107, 1998.
13. Johnson L: Hypothermia. In Schwartz GR, editor: *Principles and practice of emergency medicine,* ed 4, Baltimore, 1999, Williams & Wilkins.
14. Kazenbach TL, Dexter WW: Cold injury: protecting your patient from the dangers of hypothermia and frostbite, *Postgrad Med* 105:72, 1999.
15. Kemp ED: Bites & stings of the arthropod kind, *Postgrad Med* 103:88, 1998.
16. Lazer HL: The treatment of hypothermia, *New Engl J Med* 337:1545, 1997.
17. National Safety Council: *Injury facts,* Itasca, Ill, 1999, The Council.
18. Newton E: Mammalian bites. In Schwartz GR, editor: *Principles and practice of emergency medicine,* ed 4, Baltimore, 1999, Williams & Wilkins.
19. Otten EJ: Venomous animal injuries. In Rosen P, Barkin RM, Hockberger RS et al, editors: *Emergency medicine: concepts and clinical practice,* ed 4, St. Louis, 1998, Mosby.
20. Roberts JR: Diagnosis and treatment of snakebites. In Schwartz GR, editor: *Principles and practice of emergency medicine,* ed 4, Baltimore, 1999, Williams & Wilkins.
21. Sachdeva RC: Near-drowning, *Crit Care Clin* 15(2):281, 1999.
22. Sanders MJ: Environmental conditions. In Sanders MJ, editor: *Mosby's paramedic textbook,* ed 2, St. Louis, 2000, Mosby.
23. Schwartz GR, Sipsey J, Hanke BK: Diving and altitude emergencies. In Schwartz GR, editor: *Principles and practice of emergency medicine,* ed 4, Baltimore, 1999, Williams & Wilkins.
24. Weinstein MD, Krieger BP: Near-drowning: epidemiology, pathophysiology, and initial treatment, *J Emerg Med* 14(4):461, 1996.
25. Whal RP, Eggleston J, Edlich RF: Puncture wounds and animal bites. In Tintinalli JS, Ruiz E, Kromes RL, editors: *Emergency medicine: a comprehensive study guide,* New York, 1996, McGraw-Hill.
26. Wilson RF: Temperature-related (non-burn) injuries. In Wilson RF, Walt AJ, editors: *Management of trauma: pitfalls and practice,* ed 2, Baltimore, 1996, Williams & Wilkins.
27. Wormser GP, Nadelman RB, Dattwyler RJ: Practice guidelines for the treatment of lyme disease, *Clin Infect Dis* 31:S1, 2000.
28. Yarbrough B, Bradham A: Heat illness. In Rosen P, Barkin RM, Hockberger RS et al, editors: *Emergency medicine: concepts and clinical practice,* ed 4, St. Louis, 1998, Mosby.

Suggested Reading

Hanania NA, Zimmerman JL: Accidental hypothermia, *Crit Care Clin* 15:235, 1999.
Murphy LV, Banwell PE, Roberts AH et al: Frostbite: pathogenesis and treatment, *J Trauma* 48(1):171, 2000.
Sheehy SB: Environmental emergencies. In Sheehy SB, editor: *Manual of emergency care,* ed 5, St. Louis, 1999, Mosby.

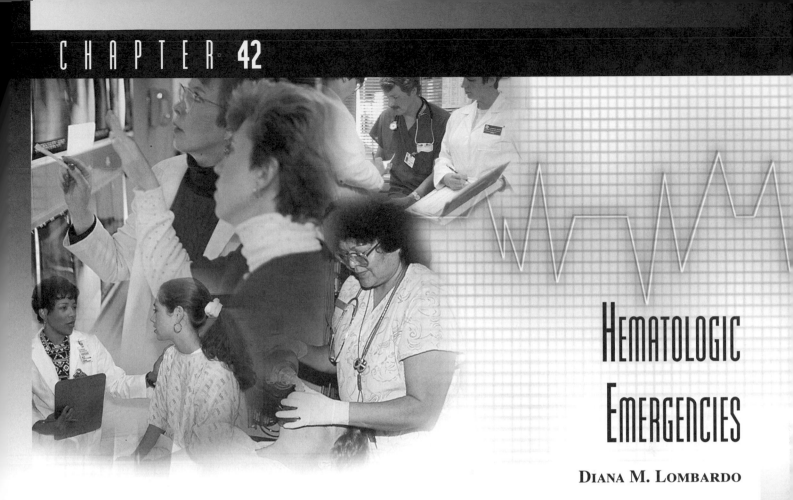

CHAPTER 42

HEMATOLOGIC EMERGENCIES

DIANA M. LOMBARDO

Hematologic emergencies represent acute onset of a new condition or sudden exacerbation of an existing disease. Knowledge of the disease process and astute assessment skills enhance ability of the emergency nurse to care for individuals with a hematologic emergency. This chapter provides an overview of blood physiology, discusses general assessment of individuals with hematologic emergencies, and describes specific hematologic emergencies, including anemia, hemophilia, sickle cell disease, disseminated intravascular coagulation (DIC), leukemia, and thrombocytopenia.

ANATOMY AND PHYSIOLOGY

Blood is a suspension of erythrocytes, leukocytes, platelets, and other particulate material in an aqueous colloid solution. This suspension provides a medium for exchange between fixed cells in the body and the external environment. Nutrients such as oxygen are carried to each cell, whereas cellular wastes such as nitrogen are removed. Other essential functions include regulation of pH, temperature, and cellular water; prevention of fluid loss through coagulation; and protection against toxins and foreign microbes. Table 42-1 summarizes basic characteristics of blood.

Plasma

Plasma is a clear, yellow fluid containing blood cells, electrolytes, gases, amino acids, glucose, fats, and nonprotein nitrogens such as urea, creatine, and uric acid.[11] These and other substances may be dissolved in the plasma or may bind with various plasma proteins for transport. Albumin, the primary plasma protein, maintains blood volume by providing colloid osmotic pressure, regulates pH and electrolyte balance, and transports substances including many drugs. Other major plasma proteins include globulins and fibrinogen.

Erythrocytes

Adults have approximately 5 million erythrocytes or red blood cells (RBCs) per microliter of blood. The number of RBCs is slightly higher in men. Natives living at altitudes greater than 14,000 feet may have as many as 7 million/μl. The primary role of RBCs is transport of oxygen and carbon dioxide. Erythrocytes have no nucleus and cannot reproduce. Their life span is only 120 days, so new cells must be constantly produced.[5] The normal rate of hematopoiesis, or RBC production, is 2 million RBCs per second. Production

633

Table 42-1	CHARACTERISTICS OF BLOOD
CHARACTERISTIC	**DESCRIPTION/VALUE**
COLOR	
Arterial	Bright red
Venous	Dark red
pH	
Arterial	7.35-7.45
Venous	7.31-7.41
SPECIFIC GRAVITY	
Plasma	1.026
Red blood cells	1.093
VISCOSITY	
	3.5-4.5 times thicker than water
VOLUME	
	5.5 L in the average adult

Table 42-2	TYPES OF HEMOGLOBIN (HB)
TYPE	**SIGNIFICANCE/OCCURRENCE**
Hb A	92%Adult hemoglobin
Hb A$_{1c}$	5% Adult hemoglobin
Hb A$_2$	2% Adult hemoglobin
Hb F	Fetal hemoglobin, thalassemia after 6 months
Hb C	Hemolytic anemia
Hb S	Sickle cell anemia
Hb M	Methemoglobinemia

Table 42-3	RED CELL INDICES IN ADULTS	
COMPONENT	**DESCRIPTION**	**NORMAL VALUE**
MCV	Ratio of hematocrit (packed cell volume) to RBC count	80-95 m^3
MCH	Hemoglobin/RBC ratio; gives weight of hemoglobin in average red cell	27-31 pg
MCHC	Ratio of hemoglobin weight to hematocrit; defines volume of hemoglobin in average red cell	32-36 g/dl

MCV, Mean corpuscular value; *RBC,* red blood cell; *MCH,* mean corpuscular hemoglobin; *MCHC,* mean corpuscular hemoglobin concentration.

occurs in the bone marrow but is regulated by the kidneys. When oxygen levels drop, the kidneys release erythropoietin, which stimulates RBC production by the bone marrow. Reticulocytes are erythrocyte precursors that mature within 24 to 48 hours of release into the circulation. Increased reticulocytes indicate increased bone marrow activity.

Erythrocytes are soft pliable cells that change shape easily, thereby increasing the cell's oxygen-carrying capability by increasing surface area. The outer stroma of the cell contains antigens A, B, and Rh factor, whereas the inner stroma contains hemoglobin, the primary vehicle for oxygen transport. Hemoglobin molecules are so small they would leak across the blood vessel's endothelial membrane if left floating free in plasma. There are 300 different types of genetically determined hemoglobin (Hb). With the exception of Hb F, Hb A, and Hb S, hemoglobins are identified by sequential letters of the alphabet. Abnormal hemoglobin molecules are produced in response to molecular abnormalities within blood. Tests such as hemoglobin electrophoresis are used to differentiate normal and abnormal hemoglobin. The most common hemoglobins are described in Table 42-2.

Red cell indices provide information about the size and weight of average red cells and are used to differentiate acute and chronic anemias (Table 42-3). Mean corpuscular volume, mean corpuscular hemoglobin, and mean corpuscular hemoglobin concentration values provide information on how well red cells function.

Erythrocyte sedimentation rate (ESR) measures the time required for erythrocytes in a whole blood specimen to settle to the bottom of a vertical tube. ESR is a product of red cell volume, surface area, density, aggregation, and surface charge.[2] Increased ESR occurs with widespread inflammation, red cell aggregation, pregnancy, and some malignancies, whereas polycythemia, sickle cell disease, and decreased plasma proteins are associated with decreased ESR.

Leukocytes

The body's primary defense against infection is leukocytes, or white blood cells (WBCs). Six types of leukocytes normally occur in the blood: neutrophils, eosinophils, basophils, monocytes, lymphocytes, and, occasionally, plasma cells (Table 42-4). The WBC count quantifies the total number of leukocytes in the circulation, whereas the differential count quantifies the percentage of each type. This count is based on 100 WBCs; therefore, a differential count should always total 100%. The ratio of RBCs to WBCs is 700:1.

Neutrophils

Neutrophils are the primary defense against bacterial infection. Bone marrow contains a reserve approximately 10 times greater than daily neutrophil production. About one half of all mature neutrophils adhere to vessel walls and are not measured by the traditional WBC count. The bone marrow reserve and the number of neutrophils on vessel walls account for sudden increases in the WBC count in response to stress or infection. After being released into the circulation, neutrophils live 4 to 8 hours. Immature neutrophils are called bands (also called stabs); mature neutrophils are called polymorphonuclear neutrophil leukocytes (PMNs or segs). An increased number of bands indicates acute infection.

Eosinophils

Eosinophils accumulate at the site of allergic reactions. Increases also occur during asthma attacks, drug reactions, and parasitic infections. Eosinophils decrease in response to

Table 42-4 LEUKOCYTES: FUNCTIONS AND CHARACTERISTICS

Name	Percent of total WBCs	Function	Circulatory life span
Neutrophils	62.0	Attack and destroy bacteria and viruses through phagocytosis	4-8 hr
Eosinophils	2.3	Attach to surface of parasites, then release substances that kill the organism; detoxify inflammatory substances that occur in allergic reactions	4-8 hr
Basophils	0.4	Prevent coagulation and speed fat removal from blood after a fatty meal	4-8 hr
Monocytes	5.3	Consume bacteria, viruses, necrotic tissue, and other foreign material	10-20 hr
Lymphocytes	30.0	Provide immunity against acquired infections; basis for antibody formation	2-3 hr
Plasma cells	—	Produce γ-globulin antibodies in response to specific antigens	Varies with need for antibodies

WBCs, White blood cells.

Table 42-5 TYPES OF T-CELL LYMPHOCYTES

Name	Function
Helper T cells	Regulate immune functions by forming lymphokines or protein mediators such as interleukin and interferon; inactivated or destroyed by AIDS virus
Cytotoxic T cells	Also called killer T cells; capable of direct attack on microorganisms and on the body's own cells; role in destroying cancer cells and heart transplant cells
Suppressor T cells	Protect from attack by the person's own immune system; suppress helper and cytotoxic T-cell functions

AIDS, Acquired immunodeficiency syndrome.

stressors such as trauma, shock, or burns. Cell half-life is approximately 4.5 to 5 hours after release into the circulation.

Basophils

Basophils contain histamine, heparin, bradykinin, serotonin, and lysosomal enzymes. During allergic reactions, basophils rupture and release these substances into surrounding tissue. This accounts for many of the typical manifestations of an allergic reaction. The number of basophils also increases in chronic inflammation and during times of stress.

Monocytes

Monocytes remain in the circulation less than 20 hours before moving into surrounding tissue to become macrophages. A macrophage acts as a "garbage collector," consuming bacteria and other debris in areas such as the spleen, lungs, and lymph nodes. Macrophages can live for months or even years. Monocytes are the body's second line of defense and are usually associated with chronic infection.

Lymphocytes

Lymphocytes play a major role in immunity against acquired infections. Their life span may be weeks, months, or years, depending on the body's needs. Two types of lymphocytes provide essential protection against bacteria and viruses: B-cell lymphocytes become antibodies and are re-

sponsible for humoral immunity; T-cell lymphocytes are responsible for cell-mediated immunity. At least three major types of T-cell lymphocytes have been identified: helper T cells, cytotoxic T cells, and suppressor T cells (Table 42-5).[5] Lymphocyte increases are associated with viral infection.

Plasma Cells

Plasma cells produce γ-globulin antibodies in response to a specific antigen. Production continues until plasma cells die from exhaustion days or even weeks later.

Platelets

Platelets, or thrombocytes, provide hemostasis at the site of injury. These granular, disk-shaped fragments form when a parent cell breaks into thousands of cell fragments. The parent cell has no nucleus, so it cannot divide. Platelet life span is 9 to 12 days. Approximately one third of the body's platelets are stored in the spleen as a reserve. Clotting factors V, VIII, and IX are found on the platelet's surface. Platelets provide hemostasis by clumping at the site of injury to form a platelet plug and seal bleeding capillaries. Substances such as ethanol and salicylates interfere with platelet aggregation by impairing their ability to clump. Decreased platelet aggregation leads to increased bleeding.

Hemostasis

Hemostasis refers to processes that prevent blood loss after vascular damage (i.e., vascular spasm, platelet aggregation, coagulation, and fibrinolysis). When injury occurs the initial response is reflex vasoconstriction. Arterioles contract, decreasing blood flow by decreasing vessel size and pressing endothelial surfaces together. Next, serotonin and histamine release cause immediate vasoconstriction and decrease blood flow to the injured area.[9] Vasoconstriction is followed by platelet aggregation at the injury site. This temporary measure prevents bleeding by sealing capillaries.

Platelet aggregation is followed by clot formation, which requires activation of the coagulation cascade (Figure 42-1). The coagulation cascade is a complex network of 12 different clotting factors (Table 42-6). A defect of any clotting

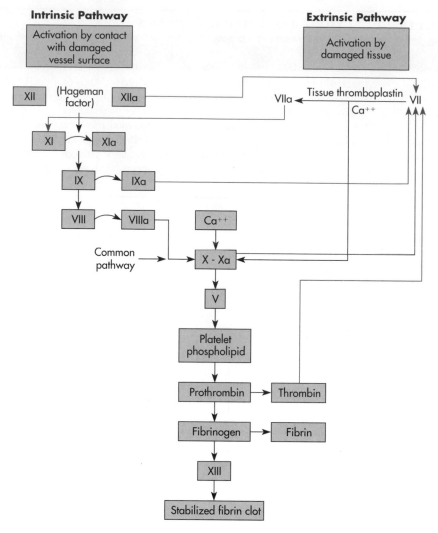

FIGURE **42-1** The coagulation cascade. (From Huether SE, McCance KL: *Understanding pathophysiology,* ed 2, St. Louis, 2000, Mosby.)

Table 42-6	COAGULATION FACTORS	
FACTOR	**SYNONYMS**	**DESCRIPTION/FUNCTION**
I	Fibrinogen	Fibrin precursor
II	Prothrombin	Activates prothrombin
III	Tissue thromboplastin	Thrombin precursor
IV	Calcium	Essential for prothrombin activation and fibrin formation
V	Labile factor, proaccelerin	Accelerates conversion of prothrombin to thrombin
VII	Prothrombin conversion accelerator	Accelerates conversion of prothrombin to thrombin
VIII	Antihemophilic factor A (AHF)	Associated with factors IX, XI, and XII; essential for thromboplastin formation
IX	Christmas factor, antihemophilic factor B	Associated with factors VIII, XI, and XII; essential for thromboplastin formation
X	Thrombokinase factor, Stuart-Prower factor	Triggers prothrombin conversion; requires vitamin K
XI	Plasma thromboplastin antecedent, antihemophilic factor C	Formation of thromboplastin in association with factors VIII, IX, and XII
XII	Contact factor, Hageman factor	Activates factor XI in thromboplastin formation
XIII	Fibrin stabilizing factor	Strengthens fibrin clot

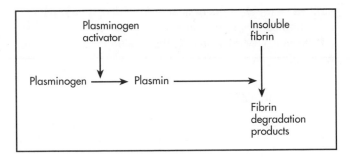

FIGURE 42-2 Fibrinolysis system.

factor or an injury that overwhelms the entire system can cause failure of the coagulation cascade and lead to life- or limb-threatening hemorrhage. The cascade may be activated by intrinsic factors, such as damage to a vessel wall, or extrinsic factors, such as damage to surrounding tissue. Regardless of the method of activation, the end result of the coagulation cascade is formation of a clot—a protein mesh made of fibrin strands.

The final step in hemostasis is clot resolution via the fibrinolytic system. Clot resolution maintains blood in a fluid state by removing clots that are no longer needed (Figure 42-2). Without this system, circulation to affected areas may be permanently lost because of obstructed blood vessels.

PATIENT ASSESSMENT

The type and severity of hematologic emergency depend on the individual's situation. Assessment is often complicated by vague complaints (e.g., fatigue, headache, fever, syncope, dyspnea on exertion). Therefore it is important to observe the patient for clues to hematologic problems, such as pale, jaundiced, or cyanotic skin. Ecchymosis, purpura, petechia, and ulcerations may also be present. Evaluate skin for temperature, diaphoresis, warmth, coolness, texture, and turgor. Observe for joint deformity, edema, redness, limitation of movement, and difficulty or inability to ambulate. Obtain vital signs, including orthostatic blood pressure and pulse.

Note new onset of fever, weakness, cough, rash, dyspnea, and increased or unusual bruising. Does the patient complain of spontaneous bleeding, such as epistaxis or menorrhagia? Are bleeding gums, hematemesis, melena, dark urine, or hemoptysis present? These symptoms suggest a hematologic problem and indicate the need for more detailed evaluation.

Identify existing hematologic diseases and family history of hematologic diseases. Obtain medication history, including use of prescription and over-the-counter medications. It is also important to query the patient about herbals that may affect clotting. For example, evening primrose, garlic, and skull cap increase clotting time, whereas ginseng, cinnamon, and parsley decrease clotting time. Document allergies, exposure to toxic substances, and dietary history.

SPECIFIC HEMATOLOGIC EMERGENCIES

Anemia

Anemia is a reduction in the total number of RBCs or a deficiency in the cells' ability to transport oxygen. Anemia may be acute or chronic. Severity depends on the patient's ability to compensate for RBC loss and provide essential oxygen to the cells. Oxygenation depends on blood flow and on hemoglobin's oxygen-carrying capacity and affinity for oxygen. A defect in any of these factors affects cellular oxygen.

Acute Anemia

Acute anemia is usually the result of blood loss. Causes include trauma, gastrointestinal hemorrhage, vaginal bleeding, and uterine rupture. Response to blood loss depends on the patient's age, physical condition, and rapidity of blood loss. Signs and symptoms include cool, clammy skin, tachycardia, decreased blood pressure, narrowing pulse pressure, tachypnea, postural hypotension, and decreased urinary output. Thirst and complaints of "feeling cold" are early clues to acute blood loss. A decreased level of consciousness may also occur.

Treatment begins with stabilization of the patient's airway, breathing, and circulation. Large-bore intravenous catheters and fluid resuscitation with normal saline or lactated Ringer's solution are used for volume replacement. Initial laboratory studies include complete blood count (CBC), type and cross-match, prothrombin time (PT), partial thromboplastin time (PTT), international normalized ratio (INR), and serum electrolytes. Supplemental oxygen is indicated because these patients have lost a source of oxygen. Blood replacement therapy may be necessary in severe anemia.

Other causes of anemia include sickle cell disease, massive burns, DIC, toxins, infections, ABO incompatibility, transfusion reactions, carbon monoxide poisoning, and medications. Most chemotherapy agents affect RBC production in some manner. Sickle cell disease and DIC are discussed later in this chapter.

Chronic Anemia

Chronic anemia is not considered life-threatening, has an insidious onset, and is often diagnosed before an emergency department (ED) visit. Patients complain of fatigue, headache, irritability, dizziness, and shortness of breath. Diagnosis is made by clinical assessment, history, and laboratory analysis, including a CBC with leukocyte differential, RBC indices, peripheral smear, and reticulocyte count. Patients are usually treated as outpatients unless they have acute shortness of breath, chest pain, severe dizziness, or altered level of consciousness.

Diminished RBC production occurs in iron deficiency anemia, thalassemia, lead poisoning, vitamin B_{12} deficiency, chronic liver disease, and hypothyroidism.[4] Decreased bone marrow production causes aplastic anemia. Other causes include increased destruction of RBCs resulting from enzyme defects (e.g., glucose-6-phosphate dehydrogenase deficiency), cell membrane abnormalities, or abnormalities of the hemoglobin molecule (e.g., sickle cell disease).

Hemophilia

Hemophilia refers to a number of clotting disorders, including hemophilia A, hemophilia B, and von Willebrand's disease.[6] Hemophilia is an inherited, sex-linked disorder that occurs almost always in males. Females carry the disease and pass it on to their children. Severity ranges from mild to severe. The primary defect in hemophilia is absence or dysfunction of a specific clotting factor.

Hemophilia A, or classic hemophilia, is due to a factor VIII disorder. In the majority of patients with hemophilia A, factor VIII is not missing. It may even be present in excess quantities; however, available factor VIII does not function adequately. Disease severity is directly related to the functional activity of factor VIII.

Hemophilia B, or Christmas disease, occurs less often than hemophilia A. It is caused by the absence or functional deficiency of factor IX.

Von Willebrand's disease is usually less acute than hemophilia A or B and occurs in both sexes. The specific coagulation defect in this type of hemophilia is defective platelet adherence and decreased levels of factor VIII.

Hemophilia A and hemophilia B have similar clinical presentations. Patients with von Willebrand's disease exhibit less severe symptoms, with a lower incidence of bleeding into joints and deeper tissues. When a patient has hemophilia, even minor trauma can cause major bruises, visceral bleeding, and subdural hematomas. With the exception of lacerations or major trauma, one of the worst features of hemophilia is hemarthrosis—bleeding into a joint. Hemarthrosis usually begins in adolescence and involves primarily the knees, ankles, and elbows. Patients almost always come to the ED because of severe pain associated with hemarthrosis rather than actual bleeding. Improperly managed hemarthrosis can lead to arthritis and ultimately joint destruction. Platelet-mediated hemostasis does not depend on factor VIII or factor IX; therefore, the affected extremity should be elevated whenever possible. Identification of the specific type of hemophilia is crucial because hemophilia A and hemophilia B present the same clinical picture but require treatment with different clotting factors. A bleeding history should be obtained from all patients with abnormal bleeding. A screening coagulation panel should also be considered.

Fresh frozen plasma (FFP) has been used to treat hemophilia A and von Willebrand's disease. Unfortunately, FFP contains relatively small amounts of factor VIII per unit of volume, so large quantities are required for successful treatment. Cryoprecipitate is rich in factor VIII per unit of volume; however, it has been associated with transmission of hepatitis and human immunodeficiency virus (HIV). Fortunately, recent product modifications have reduced this transmission risk and are also less expensive. Antibody-

purified factor IX is the treatment for hemophilia B patients with limited prior exposure to cryoprecipitate who are HIV-negative. Mild to moderate bleeding may be treated with FFP.

Sickle Cell Disease

Sickle cell disease is a genetically determined, inherited disorder that occurs in approximately 1 in 500 black Americans. Although sickle cell disease is primarily found in those of equatorial African descent, it also occurs in people of Mediterranean, Indian, and Middle Eastern lineage.[13] Several states including Georgia test every newborn for sickle cell disease. RBCs contain Hb S, an abnormal hemoglobin that precipitates into long crystals when exposed to low oxygen concentrations. The resulting sickle shape of the cell gives the disorder its name. Sickle cell anemia occurs in people whose parents have the Hb S gene. If only one parent has the Hb S gene, the offspring can have sickle cell trait and may pass the gene to his or her offspring. Hemoglobin electrophoresis shows a predominance of Hb S, variable amounts of Hb F, and no Hb A. In a person with sickle cell trait, Hb S and Hb A are both present.

As cells become hypoxic and sickling occurs, the cells clump in various parts of the body. The resulting ischemia causes a painful sickle cell crisis, occurring most often in long bones, large joints, and the spine. It may be precipitated by exposure to cold, infection, or acidosis. Prolonged ischemia leads to local tissue necrosis. Priapism may occur in males if sickling prevents exit of blood from the penis after normal erection. Treatment includes analgesia, oxygen, hydration with intravenous solutions, treatment of existing infections, local heat, and folic acid supplements.

Individuals with sickle cell disease rarely survive adolescence because of various physiologic sequelae and complications of their disease. Ongoing research into the disease may change this dismal outlook through use of stem cell transplants and other emerging treatment options. These patients develop hepatomegaly, hepatic infarctions, and jaundice. There is a high risk for pneumonia, meningitis, salmonellosis, osteomyelitis, pulmonary emboli, cor pulmonale, and chronic skin ulcers. Complications include recurrent sickle cell crisis, hemolytic anemia, transient aplastic crisis, cholelithiasis, cholecystitis, delayed sexual maturation, renal disease, bone disease, cardiac failure, and autosplenectomy. There is also a high incidence of spontaneous abortion, prenatal mortality, and maternal mortality.

Sickle cell crisis or vasoocclusive crisis is the most common painful complication of sickle cell disease and the main reason for seeking medical care in the ED. Acute episodes cause severe pain; however, providers are often reluctant to give patients adequate doses of narcotics.[1,15] Pain crisis is the hallmark of sickle cell disease; acute chest syndrome (ACS) is the second most common cause of hospitalization and the leading cause of mortality and morbidity in this disease entity.[14] The hallmark of ACS is that the illness is self-limited; it presents symptoms of chest pain, dyspnea, cough, fever, and causes pulmonary infiltrates that show up as a total white-out on chest x-ray.

Pain management in sickle cell disease should be individualized and treatment should be driven by patient assessment. The ED nurse handling pain management also needs to remember that drug therapy should be adjusted for drug tolerance. Combination therapy to enhance efficacy includes antiinflammatory agents or antihistamines used with opioids.[1] According to Wethers morphine is preferred over Demerol because it can be given subcutaneously when intravenous access is not readily available.[1] In addition, Demerol is not indicated for long-term pain management and may cause seizures after a few days of administration.[14]

Hydroxyurea (HU) is an effective therapy for adults with sickle cell disease. A recent study by Kinney demonstrated that HU was safe and effective in children when treatment was directed by a pediatric hematologist.[7] Phase III trials are warranted to determine if HU can prevent chronic organ damage in children.[7] HU in children induces similar laboratory changes as seen in adults.[7] Hydroxyurea, a cytotoxic drug with carcinogenic potential, retards deoxynucleic acid replication and consequently, cell division. Research has established that hydroxyurea stimulates Hb F production; however, its mechanism of action is not fully understood.[3] Hydroxyurea toxicities that can occur are hematologic, renal, and hepatic; therefore, monitoring lab values for patients with previous or current hydroxyurea therapy is indicated for those who present to the ED.

Disseminated Intravascular Coagulation

Disseminated intravascular coagulation (DIC) involves simultaneous clotting and bleeding. Associated conditions include infection, neoplasm, obstetric complications, thrombosis, trauma, hypoxia, and liver disease. In DIC, activation of the coagulation cascade leads to accelerated clotting, which triggers thrombosis as excessive fibrin is released in the circulation, especially in the small vessels. As coagulation continues at this accelerated rate the fibrinolysis system also functions at an accelerated rate. Consequently, platelets, clotting factors, and fibrinogen are consumed faster than the body can replace them. As the system becomes overwhelmed, simultaneous hemorrhage and clotting occur.

Patients with DIC may have acute bleeding or gradual blood loss, including epistaxis, hemoptysis, bleeding gums, menorrhagia, ecchymosis, purpura, and hematuria. Other signs associated with DIC are cough, dyspnea, confusion, fever, tachypnea, and cyanosis. Diagnostic laboratory studies include PT, PTT, fibrinogen levels, platelet levels, and fibrin split products.

Treatment focuses initially on the precipitating condition. After that problem is controlled the next step is restoration of depleted coagulation factors. Platelets, FFP, and cryoprecipitate are recommended. Heparin therapy is contraindicated in some types of DIC but is used when there is evidence of organ damage or loss of life or limb is imminent. Because DIC is characterized by prolonged PTT, fibrinogen levels are used to monitor effectiveness of heparin therapy. Hirudin therapy is considered experimental. Fluid replacement is used to maintain circulation, restore blood pressure, and ensure urinary output. The clinical picture of DIC can be further complicated by development of renal failure, shock, cardiac tamponade, hemothorax, and gangrene.

The cornerstone of treatment in DIC is recognizing and treating the underlying cause. Use of blood and blood products should be guided by the clinical picture. Patients with bleeding as a major symptom should receive FFP to replace clotting factors and platelet concentrates to correct thrombocytopenia.[4] Use of heparin during bleeding is still controversial.[4,10] Heparin is contraindicated in patients with central nervous system injury, fulminant liver failure, and most obstetrical events.[10]

Leukemia

Leukemia is a malignant disorder of blood and blood-forming organs characterized by excessive, abnormal growth of leukocyte precursors in the bone marrow. An uncontrolled increase in immature leukocytes decreases production and function of normal leukocytes.

Leukemia is classified as lymphogenous or myelogenous. Lymphogenous leukemias are caused by cancerous production of lymphoid cells, whereas myelogenous leukemias begin as the cancerous growth of myelogenous cells in the bone marrow. Both types may be acute or chronic. Acute leukemia has an abrupt, rapid onset and is characterized by a massive number of immature leukocytes. Life expectancy for these patients may be as short as 6 months; however, life expectancy for all types of leukemia has increased. Chronic leukemia has a slower disease progression with longer life expectancy.

Regardless of type, leukemic cells invade the spleen, lymph nodes, liver, and other vascular regions. Clinical manifestations include fatigue, fever, and weight loss. The patient may also complain of bone pain. Elevated uric acid levels, lymph node enlargement, hepatomegaly, and splenomegaly are usually present. Neurologic findings include headache, vomiting, papilledema, and blurred vision.

Treatment includes chemotherapy, immunotherapy, and bone marrow transplants. Blood transfusions, antibiotics, antifungal agents, and antiviral agents are also used. These patients are at significant risk for infection from their disease and their treatment; therefore, it is critical that the patient is protected against exposure to potential infectious agents.

Thrombocytopenia

Normal platelet count is 150,000 to 450,000/ml. Thrombocytopenia is an abnormal decrease in the number of platelets.[6] The platelet count is affected by menses, nutrition, and severe deficiencies in iron, folic acid, or vitamin B_{12}. Infectious disorders (sepsis), tumors, medications (acetylsalicylic acid), and bleeding can also affect platelet count.[9]

Thrombocytopenia may be secondary to congenital or acquired disorders such as decreased bone marrow production, increased splenic sequestration, or accelerated destruction of platelets.[6] Idiopathic thrombocytopenic purpura (ITP), the most common form of thrombocytopenia, is an acquired disease caused by increased platelet destruction. Immune complexes containing viral antigens bind to iron receptors on platelets, or antibodies produced against viral antigens react with platelets.[6]

Acute ITP usually occurs in children several weeks after a viral infection such as rubella, rubeola, or chickenpox. It can also follow immunizations for these same viruses. Acute ITP occurs equally in males and females, is self-limiting, and resolves spontaneously within 6 months. Peak incidence is between 2 and 4 years of age.

Bruising and petechiae are considered universal presenting symptoms for ITP. Patients may also present with purpura, epistaxis, bleeding gums, gastrointestinal bleeding, and hematuria. A small percentage of patients may have severe manifestations, such as massive purpura, profuse epistaxis, and retinal hemorrhage. Differential diagnosis is based on clinical findings of isolated thrombocytopenia without evidence of another hematologic disorder. Bone marrow aspiration is used to rule out acute leukemia.

Observation may be all that is needed for acute ITP. Glucocorticoids are given if conservative measures prove ineffective. Intravenous immune globulins are used to rapidly increase platelet count. Splenectomy is only recommended for children with severe bleeding symptoms related to their thrombocytopenia. In rare cases, plasmapheresis may be required.

Neutropenia

Neutropenia can be the result of toxic or therapeutic effects of a specific drug, infection, hematologic neoplasm, metastatic disease, chronic idiopathic neutropenia, or cyclic neutropenia.[10] Neutropenic patients are especially prone to gram-negative bacteria.[12] The agents with the greatest success in achieving gram-negative prophylaxis are fluoroquinolones.[12] Febrile neutropenia is considered a medical emergency and demands hospitalization, culturing of body fluids, and intravenous antibiotics.[10] Patients should be placed in protective isolation to avoid contact with others who may complicate the neutropenic condition and compromise the patient. Prophylactic antibiotic therapy is still controversial.[10]

SUMMARY

Hematologic emergencies cover an array of clinical conditions and represent a broad spectrum of patient acuity. Pri-

Box 42-1	NURSING DIAGNOSES FOR HEMATOLOGIC EMERGENCIES

Anxiety
Fluid volume, Deficient
Infection, Risk for
Injury, Risk for
Knowledge, Deficient
Pain
Tissue perfusion, Ineffective

oritization of patient care is essential to ensure optimal patient outcome. Box 42-1 identifies the most critical nursing diagnoses for the patient with a hematologic emergency.

References

1. Benjamin LJ, Swinson GI, Nagel RL: Sickle cell anemia day hospital: an approach for the management of uncomplicated painful crisis, *Blood* 95(4):1130, 2000.
2. Beutler E et al: *Williams hematology,* ed 5, New York, 2000, McGraw-Hill.
3. Day SW, Wynn LW: Sickle cell pain & hydroxyurea, *Am J Nurs* 100(11):34, 2000.
4. Fauci AS, Braunwald E, Isselbacher KJ et al: *Harrison's principles of internal medicine,* ed 14, New York, 1998, McGraw-Hill.
5. Guyton AC, Hall JE: *Textbook of medical physiology,* ed 10, Philadelphia, 2000, WB Saunders.
6. Hoffbrand AV, Pettit JE: *Essential hematology,* ed 3, London, 2000, Blackwell Scientific Publications.
7. Kinney TR, Helms RW, O'Branski EE et al: Safety of hydroxyurea in children with sickle cell anemia: results of the HUG-KIDS study, a phase I/II trial, *Blood* 94(5):1550, 1999.
8. Lewis SM, Heitkemper MM, Dirksen SR: *Medical-surgical nursing: assessment and management of clinical problems,* ed 5, St. Louis, 2000, Mosby.
9. McCance KL, Heuther SE: *Pathophysiology: the biologic basis for disease in adults and children,* ed 3, St. Louis, 1994, Mosby.
10. Rakel RE: *Saunders' manual of medical practice,* ed 2, Philadelphia, 2000, W.B. Saunders.
11. Rippe JM et al: *Intensive care medicine,* ed 3, vol 1, Boston, 1996, Little, Brown.
12. Shoemaker WC, Ayes SM, Grenvik A et al: *Textbook of critical care,* ed 3, Philadelphia, 1995, W.B. Saunders.
13. Stuart MJ, Setty B: Sickle cell acute chest syndrome: pathogenesis and rational treatment, *Blood* 94(5):1555, 1999.
14. Wethers DL: Sickle cell disease in childhood, *Am Fam Phys* 62(6):1309, 2000.
15. Yale SH, Nagib N, Guthrie T: Approach to the vaso-occlusive crisis in adults with sickle cell disease, *Am Fam Phys* 61(5):1349, 2000.

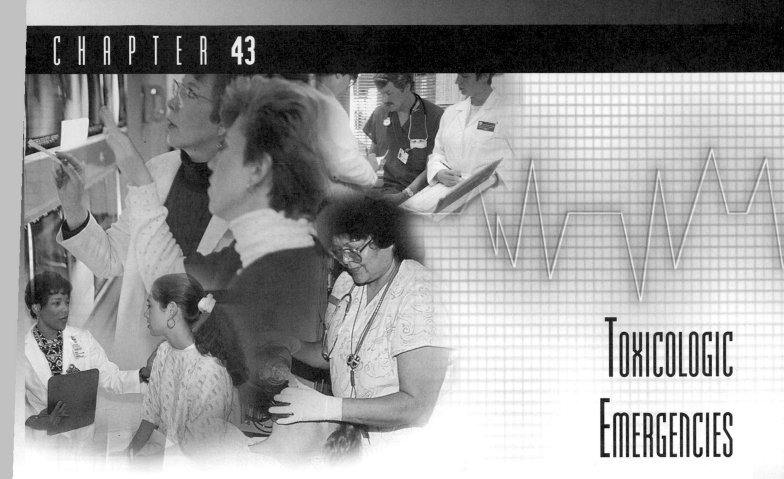

CHAPTER 43

Toxicologic Emergencies

LAURA M. CRIDDLE

Poisonings are responsible for more than 1 million emergency department (ED) visits annually in the United States.[27] Children account for approximately two thirds of all human toxic exposures reported to the American Association of Poison Control Centers.[7] Toxic agents are manufactured or naturally occurring chemicals that have deleterious effects on humans. Toxins can enter the body through ingestion, inhalation, injection, mucosal absorption, ocular exposure, or dermal contact. The quantity of toxin required to produce symptoms varies widely among substances. Exposure may be accidental or intentional and related to recreation or occupation.

Management of the poisoned patient involves continuous respiratory and hemodynamic support, careful evaluation of toxicosis potential, interventions to reduce toxin absorption and promote excretion, and substance-specific therapy, including use of antidotes. An overview of assessment and management of the patient with a toxicologic emergency is followed by discussion of specific, common poisonings. See Chapter 17 for discussion of decontamination systems.

PATIENT MANAGEMENT

Determining the precise agent or agents involved in a toxicologic emergency can be a daunting task because of the vast number of potentially injurious substances. Poison control centers are an excellent resource for information on various drugs, potential toxicity, and patient management. Poison control centers, located across the nation, provide both professionals and the public with 24-hour telephone advice.[44]

Symptoms of toxic exposures range from subtle to dramatic and vary widely with the causative agent, dose, and extent of exposure. Toxins are capable of affecting any tissue in the body, with effects seen in every body system (Table 43-1). Assess the patient carefully by obtaining a detailed history from the patient, family, or prehospital care providers. Table 43-2 describes essential assessment information related to toxic exposure.

General Interventions

Stabilization of the airway, breathing, and circulation is the first priority when caring for an individual with a poisoning emergency. Protect the airway, ensure adequate oxygenation and ventilation, and support the cardiovascular system while attempting to identify specific toxins involved. Interventions can be as simple as positioning the patient, providing supplemental oxygen, or washing the skin. More significant exposures may require endotracheal intubation, mechanical ventilation, and vasoactive medications.

Significant substance-to-substance variations in toxicologic management exist; however, the need to ensure patient safety and provide emotional support is common to all poisonings (Table 43-3). Beyond issues of safety and psychologic

Table 43-1	POTENTIAL SYSTEMIC EFFECTS OF TOXIC SUBSTANCES	
SYSTEM	**POTENTIAL EFFECTS**
Neurologic	Altered level of consciousness, abnormal pupillary response, euphoria, depression, confusion, coma, hallucinations, agitation, violence, seizures
Pulmonary	Hyperventilation, hypoventilation, acid-base disturbances
Cardiovascular	Tachycardia, bradycardia, dysrhythmias, conduction abnormalities, decreased cardiac output, altered contractility, blood pressure instability
Gastrointestinal	Nausea, vomiting, diarrhea, abnormal liver function, coagulopathies
Renal/genitourinary	Renal failure, electrolyte disturbances

Table 43-3	SAFETY AND SUPPORT IN TOXIC EMERGENCIES	
ACTION	**DISCUSSION**
Maintain patient safety	Individuals with an altered level of consciousness are predisposed to injury. Patients with intentional overdose or chronic substance abuse are at increased risk for self-destructive behavior.
Protect others	Confusion, agitation, aggressiveness, and violent behavior place others at risk for injury.
Support the patient	Provide basic emotional care, psychiatric evaluation, family intervention, referral to substance abuse programs, or information on self-help groups.

Table 43-2	ESSENTIAL ASSESSMENT INFORMATION FOR TOXIC EXPOSURE	
ITEM	**DESCRIPTION**
Substance	If possible, visually confirm substance(s) involved. Ask what medications the patient takes at home.
Time of exposure	Time since exposure influences both symptoms and treatment.
Acute or chronic	Acute exposures have different presenting symptoms and are managed differently than chronic exposures.
Amount of toxin	Determine the maximum quantity possible. Count pills in the bottle; confirm when the prescription was filled.
Signs and symptoms	Assess for symptoms in all systems. Toxins can affect every tissue in the body.
Prior treatment	Clarify any interventions provided by lay and prehospital personnel. Some home remedies can be detrimental.
Intentional or accidental	Poisoning is a popular form of suicide and suicidal gesture. Have there been previous suicide attempts? Does the patient have a history of depression or preexisting mental health problems? Was the poisoning recreational? Is this a possible homicide attempt?

Box 43-1 PRIORITIES IN THE MEDICAL MANAGEMENT OF TOXIC EXPOSURES

STABILIZE THE PATIENT

Airway
Breathing
Circulation

LIMIT ABSORPTION

Induced emesis
Gastric lavage
Activated charcoal
Dermal decontamination
Ocular decontamination

ENHANCE ELIMINATION

Repeat-dose activated charcoal
Cathartic administration
Whole-bowel irrigation
Forced diuresis
Hemodialysis and hemoperfusion

SUBSTANCE-SPECIFIC INTERVENTIONS

Antidote administration
pH manipulation

assistance, medical management focuses on limiting toxin absorption, enhancing drug elimination, and providing toxin-specific interventions (Box 43-1).

Limit Absorption

Options to reduce toxin absorption include emesis, gastric lavage, activated charcoal, dermal cleansing, and eye irrigation. Specific interventions are determined by patient condition and the precise toxin involved.

Gastrointestinal Decontamination. Although considered standard therapy for many years, there is little evidence to support gut-emptying procedures for treatment of oral poisonings. Studies indicate that, in the average overdosed patient, rapid administration of activated charcoal is at least as effective as the traditional regimen of gut emptying followed by charcoal.[32]

INDUCED EMESIS. Emesis is most commonly induced with syrup of ipecac, which causes both gastric irritation and stimulates the vomiting center in the brainstem.[38] Once a mainstay of poison management, this treatment has become increasingly less popular. Ipecac is rarely used in the ED because it is ineffective if time since ingestion is greater than 30 to 60 minutes. The average adult dose is 15 to 45 ml followed by 250 to 500 ml of water. Emesis should occur within 20 to 30 minutes.[38] Ipecac is not recommended for infants younger than age 6 months.

There is a low overall rate of drug return with induced vomiting. Further, ipecac is not effective for drugs that are rapidly absorbed. This agent has an unpredictable onset of action and intensity of effect. Violent, protracted vomiting (in response to ipecac) predisposes the patient to fluid loss, acid-base abnormalities, electrolyte disturbances, and Mallory-Weiss tears, and delays administration of activated charcoal and oral antidotes. Avoid ipecac in patients who have the potential for a rapidly deteriorating level of consciousness or seizures, which would place vomiting patients at risk for aspiration. Use of syrup of ipecac for hydrocarbon or caustic ingestion increases the incidence of oral, upper airway, and pulmonary injury. Apomorphine and other emetics are unsafe and should not be used.[32]

GASTRIC LAVAGE. Gastric lavage should not be routinely employed in management of poisoned patients. There is no evidence that its use improves clinical outcome, and it may cause significant morbidity. Generally, gastric lavage is only considered when a patient has ingested a potentially life-threatening amount of poison and the procedure can be undertaken within 60 minutes of consumption. Even when used within this time frame, clinical benefit has not been confirmed in controlled studies.[42] After consumption of agents that slow gastric emptying (e.g., anticholinergics, opiates), lavage may possibly be useful several hours postingestion.

Before initiating lavage, place the patient in a left lateral position or elevate the head of the bed 30 to 45 degrees to decrease risk of aspiration. If the gag reflex is diminished, protect the airway with endotracheal intubation before lavage.[40] Monitor for bradycardia secondary to vagal stimulation during tube placement. For patients with pill ingestion, insert a large-diameter (36F-40F) orogastric tube with a bite-block to prevent tube occlusion. Smaller tubes may be inserted in patients who ingested a liquid substance.[15]

With mechanical suction or a catheter tip syringe, withdraw as much of the gastric contents as possible. Some authorities recommend administering a dose of activated charcoal (1 mg/kg) down the tube before beginning lavage. To perform lavage, repeatedly instill and remove 200 to 250 ml aliquots of tepid tap water or normal saline until the return is clear. Do not exceed a total of 2 L. For pediatric patients administer 10 to 15 ml/kg in 50 ml boluses through a 24F to 28F tube.[38,41]

Lavage is not contraindicated in people with caustic ingestions and can be used to remove corrosive materials from the stomach to prepare patients for endoscopy.[32] When large amounts of lavage solution are required, serious fluid, electrolyte, and acid-base imbalances can occur. Other adverse effects include epistaxis, esophageal perforation, aspiration, and hypothermia. Lavage does not remove all pill frag-

BOX 43-2	SUBSTANCES POORLY ABSORBED BY CHARCOAL
Acids	Lead
Alkali	Lithium
Cyanide	Mercury
Ethanol	Methanol
Ethylene glycol	Mineral acids
Fluoride	Organic solvents
Iron	Potassium

ments. In fact, only a small percentage of ingested material is retrieved through gastric lavage. Even the widest tube may not accommodate pill clumps, whole tablets, or extremely large fragments.

ACTIVATED CHARCOAL. Activated charcoal (AC) appears to be the single most important therapeutic intervention for management of most toxic ingestions. Charcoal is "activated" by exposure to high temperatures that dramatically increase its surface area. This permits AC particles to bind many times their weight in toxins. The newer "super" activated charcoal has an even greater drug affinity.[7] Binding prevents absorption into the portal circulation, allowing toxins to be eliminated in feces. Studies suggest that, used alone, activated charcoal administration is as effective or even more effective than AC after emesis or gastric lavage procedures.[32]

AC readily absorbs most poisons except heavy metals, toxic alcohols, and inorganic salts (Box 43-2). Gastric emptying is associated with significant risks, low rate of return, and lower effectiveness as time passes, whereas AC continues to absorb toxins in the intestines and the stomach. Contraindications to charcoal administration include diminished bowel sounds, an ileus, or ingestion of a substance poorly absorbed by charcoal. Adverse effects of AC include nausea, vomiting, gastrointestinal obstruction, and pulmonary aspiration.

AC is given orally or through a gastric tube in doses of 50 to 100 g (1 g/kg for children).[17] If the quantity of an ingested substance is known, give at least 10 times the ingested dose of toxin (by weight) to prevent desorption of the substance in the lower intestine. Administration of one or two follow-up doses at 1 to 2 hour intervals is common.

Dermal decontamination. Skin decontamination is indicated for dermal exposure to any toxin. Remove contaminated clothing and jewelry as soon as possible and flush areas of contact for 10 to 15 minutes with copious amounts of water or saline. Brush dry substances from the body before washing. Neutralizing agents should not be applied because the resulting chemical reaction produces heat and can increase tissue damage. Depending on substance and amount, both clothing and irrigant fluids may be considered hazardous waste. Individuals with dermal toxic exposures also represent a risk to others. Health care personnel should wear protective clothing (gloves, gowns, and goggles) to avoid secondary contamination.

Ocular Decontamination. Ocular decontamination involves vigorous eye irrigation with copious amounts of water or normal saline. Prolonged flushing may be necessary after exposure to caustic substances, particularly alkalines. An ophthalmologist should be consulted if ocular complaints persist after irrigation. Refer to Chapter 46 for discussion of eye irrigation and ocular burns.

Enhance Elimination

After initial efforts to limit absorption, enhancing elimination of absorbed toxins is the next priority in managing the poisoned patient. Techniques to enhance toxin elimination include repeat-dose AC, cathartic administration, whole-bowel irrigation, forced diuresis, hemodialysis, charcoal hemoperfusion, and continuous hemofiltration.

Repeat-dose Activated Charcoal. In rare cases, 8 to 10 additional doses of AC (0.5-1 g/kg every 2-4 hours) may be needed. Repeat-dose AC is used in cases of theophylline, phenobarbital, paraquat, salicylate, dapsone, digoxin, phenylbutazone, and carbamazepine toxicity.[17,38] Even when parenterally administered, these agents may be effectively removed with AC in a process that is distinctly different from AC's usual gastrointestinal decontamination effect. Not only does charcoal bind toxins in the intestines and prevent absorption, but AC can also facilitate elimination by decreasing serum concentrations of certain already absorbed poisons through a process of "gastrointestinal dialysis." This occurs as a result of the concentration gradient between charcoal in the gut and the toxin in the blood. Because of the intestine's tremendous blood supply, AC can draw select poisons from the circulation and bind them for elimination in feces, a process enhanced with repeated doses of charcoal.

Cathartic Administration. Cathartics, such as sorbitol and magnesium citrate, can be mixed with AC to aid with elimination of ingested toxins by stimulating intestinal motility. Although few data exist to support their efficacy, cathartics are commonly used in management of the orally poisoned patient. Without concomitant use of a cathartic, charcoal may cause constipation, leaving both charcoal and toxins in the gut. Many practitioners believe this creates the potential for toxin unbinding and systemic absorption. Cathartic use is contraindicated after corrosive ingestion and when vomiting, diarrhea, or ileus are present. Half the original cathartic dose may be repeated if there has been no charcoal stool within 6 to 8 hours. Multiple doses of cathartic agents should be avoided because the subsequent diarrhea has been associated with fatal electrolyte imbalances, particularly in children. Occasionally, cathartics are used without AC to remove largely nontoxic materials or substances with poor affinity for charcoal, such as iron tablets or hydrocarbons. All cathartics should be used with caution in pediatric patients.[7] Sorbitol is not recommended for infants because of potential fluid and electrolyte abnormalities.

Whole-bowel Irrigation. Whole-bowel irrigation (WBI) can dramatically decrease gastrointestinal transit time by ef-

fectively emptying the entire large and small intestine. WBI is accomplished with an isotonic polyethylene glycol and electrolyte solution (GoLYTELY, COLYTE) administered by mouth or gastric tube in volumes of approximately 2 L/hr (500 ml/hr or 35 ml/kg/hr in children), or until rectal effluent is clear. This process efficiently flushes out heavy metals, enteric-coated medications, or slowly dissolving tablets.[38] Swallowed foreign bodies such as cocaine-filled balloons or condoms have also been retrieved with this technique.[17] Be prepared for large-volume stools within 1 to 2 hours. WBI is not without problems. Despite use of electrolyte-balanced formulas, WBI can cause fluid and electrolyte disturbances, particularly in pediatric patients, and is contraindicated in the presence of ileus or intestinal obstruction.

Forced Diuresis. Diuresis is occasionally useful for removal of substances such as amphetamines, isoniazid, lithium, phencyclidine, phenobarbital, and salicylates. Large intravenous volumes of saline (3-6 ml/kg/hr) can increase elimination of toxins that are primarily excreted by the kidneys. Adding mannitol or furosemide to the therapeutic regimen further enhances renal excretion; however, forced diuresis carries a significant risk of fluid overload and electrolyte problems.

Hemodialysis, Hemoperfusion, and Hemofiltration. Hemodialysis, hemoperfusion, and hemofiltration not only remove toxins and their metabolites from the circulation, but also rapidly and effectively correct acid-base and electrolyte disturbances. Substances such as alcohols, lithium, salicylates, and phenobarbital can be removed with dialysis (Box 43-3). Hemodialysis is generally reserved for poisonings associated with severe acidosis because of requirements for vascular access, equipment, and skilled personnel. Hemoperfusion is similar to hemodialysis but binds toxins as blood moves across a charcoal or resin filter rather than the traditional hemodialysis filter and dialysate. Hemoperfusion achieves greater clearance rates than does hemodialysis and is particularly effective for severe cases of poisoning with paraquat, theophylline, phenytoin, and some sedative-hypnotic agents.[20] Continuous arteriovenous and venovenous hemofiltration have been suggested as alternatives to conventional hemodialysis when the need for rapid drug removal is less urgent. The role of these modalities in management of the acutely poisoned patient remains uncertain.

Box 43-3 POISONS THAT RESPOND TO HEMODIALYSIS

Acetaminophen	Lithium
Antibiotics (various)	Methanol
Bromide	Paraquat
Ethanol	Phenobarbital
Ethylene glycol	Salicylates
Isopropanol	Theophylline

Substance-Specific Interventions

In addition to minimizing absorption and enhancing excretion, key interventions in managing toxic emergencies include intubation, mechanical ventilation, cardiovascular stabilization, antidote administration, and pH manipulation.

Antidote Administration

Usefulness of antidote administration is limited to a few select poisonings because there are only a small number of true antidotes. Many recommended agents are only minimally or moderately effective and often carry their own toxic potential.[8] The antidotes oxygen, vitamin K, and naloxone are inexpensive, safe, and effective, whereas agents such as physostigmine, deferoxamine, and Fab fragments are costly, relatively ineffective, and even dangerous. Table 43-4 summarizes antidotes currently used in most EDs.

pH Manipulation

The pH can be altered by respiratory or metabolic manipulation. Some toxins produce acidosis or alkalosis that can benefit from correction. Others are simply better excreted at a higher- or lower-than-normal body pH. Intubation and mechanical ventilation, along with sodium bicarbonate administration, is used to manipulate pH. Urinary elimination of

Table 43-4	RECOGNIZED ANTIDOTES
ANTIDOTE	**INDICATION**
Amyl nitrite	Cyanide
Atropine	Organophosphates
BAL/dimercaprol	Heavy metals
Calcium chloride/ calcium gluconate	Calcium channel blockers
Deferoxamine	Iron
Ethylenediaminetetraacetic acid	Heavy metals
Ethanol	Ethylene glycol, methanol
Fab fragments	Digitalis
Flumazenil	Benzodiazepines
Fomepizole	Ethylene glycol, methanol
Glucagon	Beta-blockers, calcium channel blockers
Insulin and glucose	Calcium channel blockers
Methylene blue	Nitrites
N-acetylcysteine	Acetaminophen
Naloxone	Opiates
Octreotide	Sulfonylureas
Oxygen	Carbon monoxide
Penicillamine	Heavy metals
Physostigmine	Anticholinergics
Pralidoxime (2-PAM)	Organophosphates
Pyridoxine	Isoniazid
Sodium bicarbonate	Tricyclic antidepressants
Sodium nitrite	Cyanide
Sodium thiosulfate	Cyanide
Vitamin K	Warfarin

mildly acidic toxins, such as phenobarbital, sulfonylureas, formaldehyde, and salicylates, can be facilitated by addition of sodium bicarbonate to intravenous fluids. Amphetamines, quinidine, and phencyclidine elimination is enhanced in a moderately acidic environment. However, because these toxins also predispose patients to rhabdomyolysis, acidification (which aggravates myoglobinuric renal failure) is generally avoided. Alkalinization of urine to a pH of 7 is helpful in treatment of rhabdomyolysis secondary to drug toxicity.

SPECIFIC TOXIC EMERGENCIES

Patients may present with toxicity from a single agent or from ingestion of multiple drugs. Caregivers should never assume the overdose patient took only one pill or one type of pill. Specific toxic emergencies are reviewed in the following section.

Salicylates

Salicylates have potent analgesic, antiinflammatory, and antipyretic properties, making them frequent components of both prescription and nonprescription drugs. Aspirin (acetylsalicylic acid) is the most readily available salicylate. Oil of wintergreen (methyl salicylate) is a liquid, highly toxic form of salicylate used in products such as Ben-Gay. Bismuth subsalicylate is an ingredient in Pepto-Bismol. The incidence of acute salicylate ingestion has dropped in the United States over the last two decades because of increased use of acetaminophen and ibuprofen. However, acute and chronic overdoses continue to occur.

Acute salicylate ingestions, with serum salicylate concentrations greater than 150 mg/kg, are associated with the development of toxic clinical symptoms. Severe intoxication is likely after acute ingestion of 300 to 500 mg/kg.[21] Salicylates affect the brainstem, stimulating hyperventilation and respiratory alkalosis. They also decrease adenosine triphosphate (ATP) production, which leads to metabolic acidosis. Direct gastrointestinal irritation causes nausea, protracted vomiting, and hematemesis. Effects on the clotting cascade increase prothrombin time (PT) and can lead to bleeding disorders. Other effects include ototoxicity (i.e., tinnitus).

Clinical findings vary significantly with patient age, amount of salicylate consumed, and whether ingestion was chronic or acute. Acidosis, electrolyte abnormalities, and impaired ATP synthesis lead to dysrhythmias and cardiac failure. Neural disturbances range from lethargy and confusion to seizures and cerebral edema. Signs of acute toxicity are vomiting, hyperventilation, upper gastrointestinal bleeding, diaphoresis, ketonuria, coagulopathies, hyperthermia, abdominal pain, and dysrhythmias. Chronic toxicity may occur with ingestion of more than 100 mg/kg/day for 2 or more days. Symptoms include lethargy, confusion, dehydration, hallucinations, pulmonary edema, elevated liver enzymes, and prolonged PT. Patients may also exhibit hyperthermia, renal failure, tinnitus, and hypoglycemia.

Diagnostic studies include serial measurement of salicylate levels, arterial blood gases, electrolytes (particularly potassium), glucose, blood urea nitrogen (BUN), creatinine, PT, and urine pH. Traditionally, the Done nomogram has been used to predict salicylate toxicity; however, its usefulness is restricted to the patient with a recent, one-time, acute ingestion of non–enteric-coated salicylates. Because of these limitations, most toxicologists no longer recommend use of this nomogram. Obtain serial serum levels until values drop to asymptomatic levels (<40 mg/dl). In chronic ingestions salicylates move from blood to tissues, so serum levels do not accurately reflect total body drug content.

If implemented within 30 minutes, gastric emptying may limit salicylate absorption in acute ingestion. Administer AC either after or in lieu of lavage. Enhanced elimination can be achieved with multiple doses of AC at 3- to 5-hour intervals until levels are clearly falling. Fluid administration enhances salicylate excretion but should be used cautiously in patients prone to pulmonary edema. Alkalinization also promotes urinary elimination. This can be accomplished by adding 100 mEq of sodium bicarbonate to each liter of D5¼ NS, infusing at 200 ml/hr. Systemic acidemia should be avoided because a low pH increases brain salicylate concentrations and worsens toxicity.[21] Hemodialysis is very effective for poisonings that do not respond to simpler measures. Patients are frequently dehydrated and require intravenous fluid replacement. Monitor serum potassium levels closely and administer potassium as needed. Use a short-acting benzodiazepine for emergency treatment of salicylate-induced seizures.

Acetaminophen

As with salicylates, acetaminophen (APAP) is a common ingredient in many over-the-counter analgesics, antipyretics, and cold remedies. APAP overdoses are usually accidental in the pediatric patient and intentional in adults. Although initial symptoms are mild, severe acetaminophen poisoning causes life-threatening hepatotoxicity.

APAP is rapidly absorbed from the gut and broken down by the liver, forming a toxic metabolite. In therapeutic doses endogenous hepatic enzymes rapidly detoxify this intermediary product. However, toxic doses deplete these essential enzymes, damaging both the liver and kidneys as metabolites accumulate. Serum APAP levels 140 mg/kg or greater are considered toxic. Individuals at risk for APAP toxicity at lower doses include those with malnutrition, preexisting hepatic dysfunction, and taking anticonvulsant medications or isoniazid.[17]

Signs and symptoms of APAP toxicity develop slowly and can be overlooked until significant damage has occurred. Symptoms are divided into four phases according to elapsed time from ingestion (Table 43-5). Initial APAP levels should be drawn 4 hours after ingestion. Plotting the 4-hour APAP value on the Rumack-Matthew nomogram (Figure 43-1) determines whether the patient is potentially hepatotoxic. This nomogram is only useful for acute, single-dose poisonings not combined with other agents (such as opioids or anticholinergics) that delay absorption. Obtain liver function studies, PT, complete blood count, BUN, and creatinine levels on patients who present with clinical symptoms and those whose level falls within the "probable hepatic toxicity" range on the nomogram. If a patient's 4-hour level remains below the line, no further treatment is required. Serial APAP levels are unnecessary.[31]

Gastric emptying can be avoided if charcoal is given promptly. Do not administer AC if more than 3 or 4 hours

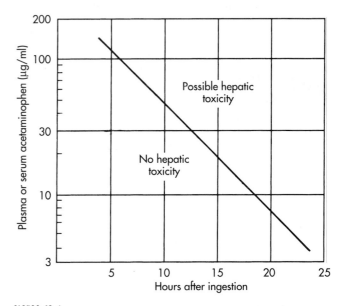

FIGURE 43-1   Rumack-Matthew nomogram. (From American Academy of Pediatrics: *Pediatrics* 55:871, 1975.)

Table 43-5	ACETAMINOPHEN TOXICITY	
STAGE	TIME FRAME	SYMPTOMS
I	0-24 hours	May be asymptomatic or experience lethargy, diaphoresis, mild gastric upset including nausea, vomiting, anorexia
II	24-48 hours	May have no complaints or develop liver failure, abnormal liver function tests, prolonged PTT, increasing bilirubin levels, right upper quadrant pain, hepatomegaly, oliguria
III	72-96 hours	Massive hepatic dysfunction, liver enzymes >100 times normal, hypoglycemia, jaundice, patient appears acutely ill, can progress to hepatic failure, encephalopathy, and death
IV	4 days-2 weeks	If patient survives Stage III, enters recovery phase characterized by slow resolution of hepatic dysfunction

PTT, Partial thromboplastin time.

Table 43-6	CLINICAL EFFECTS OF CNS STIMULANTS
DEGREE OF INTOXICATION	**EFFECTS**
Mild	Insomnia, talkativeness, restlessness, garrulousness, agitation, aggression, tremor, hyperactivity
Moderate	Mydriasis, headache, nystagmus, hypertension, tachycardia, chest pain, dysrhythmias, hallucinations
Severe	Paranoia, shock, hyperthermia, rhabdomyolysis, acute tubular necrosis, acidosis, hyperkalemia, seizures, coma, myocardial infarction
Late	Chronic abusers may be exhausted after bingeing due to intense exertion and dopamine depletion; may sleep for hours; can be difficult to awaken but, when aroused, the patient is oriented

CNS, Central nervous system.

have lapsed since time of ingestion unless delayed absorption is suspected. Multiple doses of charcoal do not decrease serum APAP concentration but may be used to treat cotoxicities. N-acetylcysteine (NAC, Mucomyst), the antidote for APAP poisoning, can be alternated with charcoal every 2 hours. Because effective therapy depends on early initiation of oral NAC, it is important to treat vomiting with antiemetics such as prochlorperazine and metoclopramide. All patients with a serum APAP level that falls in the "possible hepatic toxicity" range should receive NAC. Patients in whom significant poisoning is suspected should begin NAC therapy on arrival without waiting for results of the serum APAP level.[5]

NAC works by replenishing the liver's supply of essential enzymes, allowing removal of APAP metabolites. The earlier the therapy is begun, the better the prognosis; however, NAC may still be effective when initiated up to 24 hours after ingestion. Although AC absorbs NAC, this effect does not appear to be clinically significant. The standard initial dose is 140 mg/kg, followed by half the calculated amount every 4 hours for 17 additional doses. Continue to treat if the patient remains symptomatic. Several alternate dosing regimens are under investigation.[31] Because of the foul taste and odor, NAC is usually given through a gastric tube or diluted in fruit juice or soft drinks. If the patient vomits within 1 hour of ingestion, the dose should be repeated. An intravenous form of NAC is available in Canada and Europe.[6] Liver dialysis has shown promise in treatment of severe poisoning, and transplantation has been attempted in APAP overdose patients when other therapies fail.[5]

Central Nervous System Stimulants

Central nervous system (CNS) stimulants are a loosely related group of legal and illegal drugs that act by simulating or mimicking the sympathetic branch of the autonomic nervous system. Illicit CNS stimulants include cocaine, methamphetamines, phencyclidine (PCP), and agents with street names such as ectasy, ice, and crank.[26] Some CNS stimulants are available by prescription for the treatment of narcolepsy, obesity, and attention deficit disorder in children. Other CNS stimulants such as caffeine, phenylpropanolamine, and pseudoephedrine are common ingredients in over-the-counter diet pills, cold remedies, and alertness aids. Legitimate CNS stimulants are less potent and produce fewer euphoric or psychotic effects than their illegal counterparts; however, sufficient doses produce similar physiologic responses. CNS stimulants can be ingested, injected, inhaled, snorted, and absorbed rectally or vaginally.

Although CNS stimulants are not all the same, their actions, side effects, and hazards are similar. Street drugs, such as cocaine and amphetamines, are often diluted or "cut" with other CNS stimulants (e.g., caffeine, phenylpropanolamine, or PCP), making precise identification of specific agents difficult. CNS stimulants are rapidly absorbed from the gut, with onset of action minutes after injection or inhalation. These stimulants have relatively short half-lives and produce varying degrees of sympathetic nervous system innervation of α-, β_1-, and β_2-adrenergic receptors.

Patients present with a wide range of responses and symptoms related to the drug and quantity consumed (Table 43-6). The patient may experience a sense of omnipotence, excitement, hyperalertness, hyperactivity, hypersexuality, anxiety, agitation, aggression, hallucinations, mania, or paranoia. Tachycardia, hypertension, cardiac dysrhythmias, hemorrhagic stroke, coronary artery spasms, and myocardial infarction also occur. Neurologic effects include pupil dilation, tremor, restlessness, delirium, seizures, and coma. Stimulation of the gastrointestinal tract produces nausea, vomiting, and diarrhea. Other effects include hyperthermia, rhabdomyolysis, piloerection (goose bumps), and coagulopathies.[22]

The toxic dose is highly variable and depends on the agent or agents involved, route of entry, individual tolerance, and drug amount. Toxicologic screening of urine or blood provides a rapid qualitative test for common CNS stimulants; quantitative measures do not correlate well with clinical status. Basic care is symptomatic and addresses the airway, breathing, and circulatory needs of the patient on a case-by-case basis. Because of an increased metabolic rate, diaphoresis, and drug-induced diuresis, this population is frequently dehydrated. Adequate fluid volume is essential to minimize complications such as tachycardia, hyperthermia, and myoglobinuric renal failure.[17]

Orally ingested tablets or capsules may be removed by gastric lavage only if ingestion was very recent and the risk of seizure is low. Administer a single dose of AC as soon as possible. Gastric decontamination has no benefit when drugs are inhaled, snorted, or injected. "Body-packers" who have ingested cocaine-filled balloons or condoms should receive AC to absorb cocaine from the gastrointestinal tract in case the containers rupture.

No specific measures are used to promote CNS stimulant elimination. Urinary acidification enhances excretion of some CNS agents but places patients at risk for rhabdomyolysis. WBI has been used successfully to remove swallowed body-packed or body-stuffed drugs. Endoscopic or surgical removal may be necessary if packets rupture.

Treatment of CNS stimulant toxicosis is largely symptomatic. Symptoms can progress rapidly, mandating diligent observation. Continuous cardiac and blood pressure monitoring detect tachycardia, dysrhythmias, and hypertension. A 12-lead electrocardiogram (ECG) is indicated for patients with chest pain or shock. Because of the potential for rapid development of severe hyperthermia, check body temperature frequently until symptoms subside.

The patient with a significant CNS stimulant overdose can be paranoid, incredibly strong, and anesthetized to pain. Prevent injury to the patient and others by sedating psychotic patients with benzodiazepines, droperidol, or haloperidol. Exclusive use of physical restraints can cause extreme agitation and intense muscle activity, contributing to hyperthermia and rhabdomyolysis. After the patient is under control, provide a minimal-stimulation environment.

CNS stimulants affect the sympathetic nervous system, so a β-blocker (e.g., propranolol, esmolol) may be used for treatment of significant overdoses, sometimes given in combination with a vasodilator. Intense muscle activity and increased metabolic rate can rapidly produce core temperatures greater than 104° F (40° C). Cool patients aggressively.

Intravenous benzodiazepines are the agents of choice for treatment of actual or impending seizures. Adequate seizure control is essential because strenuous muscle use contributes significantly to hyperthermia. Phenytoin, phenobarbital, and even a neuromuscular blocking agent may be required.

Opiates and Opioids

Originally derived from the opium poppy, opiates are among the oldest known analgesic agents. They have been both used and abused for thousands of years. Today, opium is refined into many different drugs. Numerous synthetic opioids are also available. In the United States, single-agent and multidrug formula opiates can be legally obtained only by prescription. Narcotic toxicosis is often associated with intravenous abuse. Overdoses result from both pharmacologically prepared and "street drug" versions. Illicitly obtained opiates may be cut with caffeine, amphetamines, mannitol, phencyclidine, strychnine, lactose, or powdered sugar. Cointoxicants may be responsible for many of the patient's symptoms.

Although there are significant differences among opiate agents, all act on the CNS, producing variable degrees of sedation, euphoria, analgesia, and amnesia. Their psychic effects make opiates popular drugs of abuse. CNS depression, sufficient to induce coma, can occur with large drug doses or with relatively small amounts in novice users. Tolerance and

Table 43-7	EFFECTS OF NARCOTIC ABUSE AND TOXICITY
ETIOLOGY	POTENTIAL EFFECTS
Narcotic	Pinpoint pupils, respiratory depression, mental changes, hypotension, visual hallucinations, analgesia, amnesia, sleep, coma
Lifestyle	Skin abscesses, cellulitis, endocarditis, septicemia, track marks, malnutrition, dental disease, hepatitis, human immunodeficiency virus infection, tuberculosis, pulmonary edema, fecal impaction, septic arthritis, frequent trauma
Withdrawal	Rhinorrhea, tearing, yawning, dilated pupils, abdominal pain, diarrhea, diaphoresis, nasal congestion, vomiting, headache, piloerection, chills, fever, joint pain, agitation, confusion, hyperactivity

dependence are common phenomena; addiction may follow chronic abuse.

Opiates also act on the respiratory center in the brainstem, producing depression and apnea. These agents slow the gastrointestinal system, making constipation a common side effect. Opiates, such as paregoric and diphenoxylate hydrochloride with atropine (Lomotil), are prescribed specifically for this action. Signs and symptoms of opiate toxicity and abuse can be related to specific effects of the agent, substance abuse lifestyle, or acute drug withdrawal (Table 43-7).[19]

A qualitative toxicologic screen documents recent opiate use but levels do not correlate with clinical presentation because of the number of substances available and the wide range of individual tolerance. Oral ingestions of opiates should be treated as soon as possible with AC, which effectively binds and reduces absorption into the circulation. Gastric emptying is not necessary if AC can be given promptly. Cathartic agents, in conjunction with charcoal, are particularly useful for enhancing drug elimination in opiate toxicity because of drug-induced intestinal hypomotility.[2]

A naloxone (Narcan) challenge serves as both a diagnostic tool and therapeutic intervention. A dose of 2 mg—given intravenously, intramuscularly, subcutaneously, intratracheally, or injected under the tongue—antagonizes opiate receptor sites in the CNS, reversing opioid effects, and rapidly awakening patients with narcotic-induced CNS depression. Occasionally doses up to 10 mg are required. Titrate naloxone to a level where the patient is breathing easily and can be awakened. Full and sudden awakening is rarely desirable. Each opiate's duration of action is very drug specific; sufentanil effects disappear within minutes, whereas methadone effects may last more than 24 hours. Naloxone has a 2- to 3-hour duration of action, which may be considerably less than that of the particular narcotic involved. Repeat doses, or continuous intravenous naloxone infusions, are frequently indicated and should be titrated to clinical response. A newer narcotic antagonist, nalmefene hydrochloride (Revex), has a much longer duration of effect than naloxone (24-72 hours versus 20-90 minutes), allowing many patients to be treated with a single dose and safely discharged sooner than with naloxone therapy.[2]

Benzodiazepines

Benzodiazepines are commonly prescribed anxiolytic and sedative-hypnotic agents. This class contains a large number of substances that vary widely in their indications, potency, and duration of effect (Table 43-8). Fortunately, the level of toxicity associated with these drugs is generally mild. In overdose situations benzodiazepines ingested with other CNS depressants (e.g., ethanol, opiates, barbiturates) produce a more severe poisoning.

Benzodiazepines potentiate effects of the inhibitory neurotransmitter γ-aminobutyric acid, producing CNS depression. The toxic effects of benzodiazepines are an extension of their therapeutic effects and a milligram-per-kilogram toxic dose has not been established.

Qualitative serum benzodiazepine levels confirm the presence of these agents. Quantitative levels are not particularly useful because of significant individual variability. Therefore interventions are dictated by the patient's clinical status rather than by serum drug levels.

Benzodiazepines cause drowsiness, lethargy, ataxia, hypothermia, and mild coma with midposition or small pupils that do not respond to naloxone. Profound coma suggests involvement of other CNS depressants. Significant circulatory compromise after isolated benzodiazepine ingestion is rare, so other causes should be considered. Hypotension has been associated with rapid intravenous administration of diazepam (particularly in children) related to its propylene glycol diluent. This condition usually responds to supine positioning and intravascular volume replacement. With pure benzodiazepine ingestion, respiratory depression is not a common finding but it has occasionally been associated with high-dose, intravenous bolus injection of a potent, short-acting agent.

Gastric emptying is of no additional value if AC can be given promptly. Administer a cathartic agent, along with the charcoal, to counteract gastrointestinal hypomotility and enhance fecal drug elimination. Hemodialysis and charcoal hemoperfusion have little benefit in benzodiazepine overdose. Flumazenil (Romazicon) is an effective antagonist agent that competes directly with benzodiazepines at their receptor sites. Administering flumazenil produces a rapid change in level of consciousness in patients with benzodiazepine toxicosis, making it an effective diagnostic tool and a therapeutic agent. However, flumazenil administration can induce seizures in those with benzodiazepine addiction and in those with concomitant tricyclic antidepressant overdose. Because benzodiazepine toxicosis is associated with a low morbidity and mortality, the decision to administer flumazenil must be considered carefully.

Table 43-8	BENZODIAZEPINES
GENERIC NAME	BRAND NAME
Alprazolam	Xanax
Chlordiazepoxide	Librium
Clonazepam	Klonopin
Chlorazepate dipotassium	Tranxene
Diazepam	Valium
Estazolam	ProSom
Flunitrazepam	Rohypnol
Flurazepam	Dalmane
Halazepam	Paxipam
Lorazepam	Ativan
Midazolam	Versed
Oxazepam	Serax
Prazepam	Centrax
Quazepam	Doral
Temazepam	Restoril
Triazolam	Halcion

Tricyclic Antidepressants

There are a variety of tricyclic antidepressant (TCA) drugs available, including amitriptyline (Elavil), imipramine (Tofranil), and desipramine (Norpramin). Widely prescribed for depression, TCA overdoses are usually associated with suicidal intent.[16] Table 43-9 lists common TCAs.

Each TCA has varying degrees of anticholinergic, adrenergic, and α-blocking properties. They are well absorbed from the gastrointestinal tract and are difficult to remove from the body once absorbed. Toxicity is not closely associated with a milligram-per-kilogram ingested dose; therefore, serum levels do not correlate well with clinical effects. A qualitative urine study is sufficient to confirm ingestion.

Because TCAs produce neurotoxicity, cardiotoxicity, and anticholinergic effects, signs and symptoms of TCA poisoning fall into three general categories. Neurotoxicity is characterized by both CNS depression and irritability. Common findings are lethargy, delirium, hallucinations, coma, myoclonic jerking, and seizure activity. Cardiac manifestations include hypotension and numerous ECG changes such as ST- and T-wave abnormalities, prolonged QT intervals, conduction blocks, tachycardia, bradycardia, ventricular dysrhythmias, and pulseless electrical activity. In fact, TCA poisoning should be suspected in any patient with lethargy, coma, or seizures accompanied by QRS prolongation.[11]

Anticholinergic effects include mydriasis, flushed skin, dry mucous membranes, anxiety or psychosis, tachycardia, elevated body temperature, and urinary retention. A mnemonic commonly used to recall the signs of anticholinergic toxicity is "Blind as a bat. Red as a beet. Dry as a bone. Mad as a hatter, and hotter than Hades."

Respiratory arrest can occur without warning, and death from TCA toxicity usually happens within a few hours of admission. AC should be administered as soon as possible.

Table 43-9	CYCLIC ANTIDEPRESSANTS	
GENERIC NAME	**BRAND NAME**	**TOXICITY**
Amitriptyline	Elavil, Endep	A, C, S
Amoxapine	Asendin	S
Clomipramine	Anafranil	A, C, S
Desipramine	Norpramin	A, C, S
Doxepin	Sinequan, Adapin	A, C, S
Imipramine	Tofranil	A, C, S
Maprotiline	Ludiomil	C, S
Nortriptyline	Aventyl, Pamelor	A, C, S
Protriptyline	Vivactil	A, C, S
Trimipramine	Surmontil	A, C, S

A, Anticholinergic; *C,* cardiovascular; *S,* seizures.

Do not attempt to induce vomiting because CNS depression can develop rapidly. For large overdoses protect the patient's airway with endotracheal intubation, then perform lavage. AC effectively binds TCAs, dramatically reducing their half-life. Gastric emptying is not necessary if AC can be given promptly. Because of TCAs' anticholinergic effects, intestinal transit time is significantly lengthened, making cathartic use a common adjunctive therapy for increasing drug elimination and preventing gastrointestinal obstruction. TCAs are highly tissue-bound, so forced diuresis, hemodialysis, and charcoal hemoperfusion are not effective. There are some data to suggest that TCA overdose patients benefit from the "gastrointestinal dialysis" effect of repeat-dose charcoal.

Continuous cardiac monitoring is imperative for all significant TCA ingestions. Dysrhythmias include sinus tachycardia secondary to anticholinergic effects and widening of the QRS complex, which can progress to ventricular irritability and conduction disturbances.[1] Treat ventricular dysrhythmias with amiodarone or lidocaine. Do not administer procainamide (Pronestyl) or other type 1A antidysrhythmic agents. Serious conduction blocks may respond to an external pacemaker.

Systemic alkalinization of serum with sodium bicarbonate is cardioprotective and can quickly reverse life-threatening conduction disturbances and ventricular dysrhythmias. Sodium bicarbonate is administered initially as a 1 mEq/kg bolus. Further doses are titrated to maintain a systemic pH of 7.5. This can be accomplished by the addition of sodium bicarbonate to intravenous fluids, guided by arterial blood gas values. Potassium chloride 10 to 20 mEq may be added to IV fluids to prevent hypokalemia secondary to sodium bicarbonate administration. Hypotension is initially managed with crystalloid boluses; however, catecholamine vasopressors (dopamine, norepinephrine, or phenylephrine) are necessary for refractory hypotension. Treat seizures acutely with a short-acting benzodiazepine such as diazepam or lorazepam. After seizure activity is controlled, a loading dose of phenytoin can be initiated, with subsequent maintenance doses as needed.[1]

Toxic Alcohols

In addition to ethanol, three other alcohols can cause severe poisoning. Toxic alcohols exist in many common household products not generally considered dangerous. Methanol, also known as "wood alcohol," is found in windshield wiper fluid, canned fuel (Sterno), and solvents such as paint removers. Isopropanol is a major component of rubbing alcohol, disinfectants, cleansers, and nail polish removers. Ethylene glycol is an odorless substance contained in antifreeze, detergents, paints, polishes, and coolants. Its sweet taste and fluorescent color are particularly appealing to children and pets. Toxic alcohol ingestions can be accidental, recreational, suicidal, or may occur in desperate alcoholics unable to obtain ethanol.[29] In addition to oral ingestion, toxic alcohols may be inhaled or topically absorbed.

These alcohols are relatively nonpoisonous before hepatic conversion by the enzyme alcohol dehydrogenase to their toxic metabolites. The toxins—glycolaldehyde (ethylene glycol), formaldehyde, formic acid (methanol), and acetone (isopropanol)—produce widespread damage and metabolic dysfunction.[45]

Clinical findings of alcohol intoxication include CNS and respiratory depression. Methanol toxicity causes nausea, vomiting, abdominal pain, blindness, and coma. The patient with isopropanol ingestion presents with an acetone breath odor, vomiting, and possibly significant hypotension. Ethylene glycol causes seizures, ataxia, coma, nystagmus, cardiac conduction disturbances, and dysrhythmias. Profound acidosis, renal failure, and pulmonary edema may also occur.[13]

Perform appropriate laboratory studies to detect the following predicted abnormalities. In methanol intoxication, pronounced metabolic acidosis results from accumulation of formic acid. Isopropanol poisoning causes elevated serum acetone levels with ketones present in blood and urine. Hyperglycemia may also occur. With significant ethylene glycol toxicity, both anion gap metabolic acidosis and a large osmolal gap are evident. Expect hypocalcemia along with elevated BUN and creatinine levels.[45]

Gastric lavage may be used in severe cases to remove any alcohol remaining in the stomach. Because of the rapid absorption of alcohols, effectiveness of gastric lavage and activated charcoal is limited. The lungs are responsible for eliminating a significant amount of toxic alcohols; therefore, intubation and mechanical ventilation can be used to maximize respiratory excretion in severe poisoning. Hemodialysis both effectively removes toxic metabolites and reverses acidosis.[29]

Ethanol, and each of the toxic alcohols, relies on the enzyme alcohol dehydrogenase for metabolism; however, the liver preferentially metabolizes ethyl alcohol. Therefore administration of intravenous ethanol (100 mg/kg/hr) saturates available alcohol dehydrogenase molecules and slows methanol and ethylene glycol degradation, preventing accumulation of toxic metabolites. Ethanol infusions must be continued during dialysis with the rate increased to maintain serum ethanol level of 100 mg/dl. A relatively new antidote, fomepizole (Antizol), can be substituted for ethanol in the treatment of ethylene glycol and methanol poisoning.[3] Neither fomepizole nor ethanol are indicated for isopropanol toxicity.

Other treatable causes of altered level of consciousness such as hypoglycemia and opiate ingestion cannot be overlooked. $D_{50}W$ is given to reverse hypoglycemia; however, thiamin should be given concurrently because it allows the brain to metabolize the glucose. Narcan is used to reverse opiate toxicity.

Organophosphates and Carbamates

Organophosphates and carbamates are major active ingredients in hundreds of insecticides found in most American homes, including ant sprays, flea sprays, and insect sprays, powders, and liquids. Toxicity varies significantly among chemical formulations.[35] Organophosphates can be ingested, inhaled, or absorbed topically. Mass poisoning occasionally occurs from ingestion of unwashed produce or airborne contamination during crop spraying. Sarin gas, and other chemical warfare substances classed as "nerve agents," fall in the organophosphate category.[18]

The neurotransmitter acetylcholine is released into synaptic junctions in response to parasympathetic and sympathetic impulses. Normally, cholinesterase enzymes rapidly break down acetylcholine, halting its action until another stimulus is received. Organophosphates aggressively bind to cholinesterase molecules, inhibiting their effect, and allowing acetylcholine to remain unopposed in the neural synapse. Organophosphate-cholinesterase bonds do not spontaneously reverse. After 24 to 48 hours of continuous binding, cholinesterase molecules are destroyed. Complete regeneration of cholinesterase can take weeks or even months.[18] Carbamates produce a similar effect; however, their acetylcholinesterase binding is transient and usually self-limited.

Two tests of cholinesterase, serum and red blood cell, should be performed but results may not be available for several days. These studies indicate the percent of cholinesterase that remains functional.[74] Dermal exposures necessitate removal of all clothing and jewelry, followed by copious soap and water skin cleansing. Contaminated irrigant should be considered hazardous waste. Suction or lavage ingested agents from the stomach; once absorbed, organophosphates are difficult to eliminate. AC effectively reduces organophosphate absorption and must be given promptly. Because of toxin-induced diarrhea, patients seldom require concomitant cathartic administration.

Clinical findings depend on the specific organophosphate, amount of poison involved, and patient size. Symptoms range from mild to severe and are usually evident within 12 hours of contact. A few lipophilic organophosphates may not produce significant distress for 24 to 36 hours. Generalized effects include fatigue, lethargy, fasciculations, blurred vision, dizziness, diaphoresis, headache, delirium, seizures, and coma. The patient is weak and presents with tremors, fasciculations, and inability to stand. Gastrointestinal effects include nausea, vomiting, anorexia, drooling, abdominal cramping, and diarrhea. Cough, bronchorrhea, and wheezing are also evident. Classically, bradycardia is prominent, but tachycardia, atrioventricular blocks, dysrhythmias, and ST-wave abnormalities are not uncommon. Other effects include a garlic odor, diaphoresis, pinpoint pupils, hypertension, urinary incontinence, and respiratory muscle paralysis that can lead to sudden respiratory arrest.[35]

Interventions are largely supportive. Effective antidote therapy counteracts organophosphate effects, although recovery requires synthesis of new cholinesterase. Because organophosphates produce a cholinergic syndrome, anticholinergics are the treatment of choice. Immediate therapy includes administration of intravenous atropine titrated to clinical effect. Cases of severe poisoning may necessitate up to 5 mg of atropine every 15 to 30 minutes. Continue boluses until signs of atropinization (dilated pupils, decreased secretions, tachycardia, and dry, flushed skin) appear. The presence of tachycardia is not a contraindication to atropine administration in the organophosphate-poisoned patient. After full atropinization is achieved, initiate intravenous pralidoxime (2-PAM; Protopam) therapy. Pralidoxime has an anticholinergic effect, and doses are titrated to severity. An initial bolus is followed by additional boluses every 1 to 2 hours or by a continuous infusion.[35]

The organophosphate-intoxicated individual is at significant risk for contaminating others. Perform resuscitation and decontamination in a well-ventilated, isolated area. All people coming into contact with the poisoned individual require full protective gear, including gloves and goggles. Special decontamination gloves should be used if available; if not, wear two pairs of gloves. The patient's clothing is considered contaminated. Vomitus, gastric lavage material, and stool must be handled with caution, followed by careful disposal, to avoid secondary contamination.

Hallucinogens

Lysergic acid diethylamide (LSD), mescaline, nutmeg, morning glory seeds, and tetrahydrocannabinol (the active ingredient in marijuana and hashish) are among the most popular drugs in the hallucinogen category. Although some toxins are naturally occurring and have probably been used for thousands of years (e.g., psilocybin mushrooms, peyote), LSD and other synthetic agents are of recent invention.[4] Although not typically classed as hallucinogens, many medications and toxins can induce hallucinations when administered in sufficient quantities or to susceptible individuals. At high doses most CNS stimulants are hallucinatory agents. PCP, for example, is classed as an anesthetic agent but has potent hallucinogenic and sympathomimetic properties. Table 43-10 compares PCP with other drug groups.

Besides their psychedelic effects, hallucinogens have other chemical properties that are responsible for a variety of sympathomimetic or anticholinergic responses. The majority of recreational hallucinogen abusers have no reason to visit an ED. Patients who present are generally those with concomitant trauma and toxicity produced by coingestants or psychosis.

Hallucinogenic chemicals stimulate the brain, producing visual and auditory-sensory-perceptual alterations with associated behavioral changes, cognitive disturbances, and even acute psychotic reactions. The environment, mood, and circumstances a patient is in at the time of ingestion greatly influence hallucinations, which vary from pleasant to terrifying.

Patients are generally self-absorbed, exhibiting inward-drawn behavior. Other symptoms include soliloquy, auditory, and visual events experienced only by the drugged individual, paranoia, mood fluctuations, and attempts to perform superhuman feats. Physical findings, such as tachy-

cardia, hypertension, and hyperthermia, are generally a product of the sympathomimetic or anticholinergic properties associated with many hallucinogens.

A urine or serum drug screen confirms the presence of certain common hallucinogenic substances. Quantitative measurement has little clinical value. Some hallucinogens are smoked (e.g., marijuana) or ingested in such tiny quantities (e.g., LSD) that attempts at gastric emptying are unproductive. People who recently swallowed large quantities of hallucinogens (e.g., mushrooms) may benefit from gastric emptying before AC. Orally ingested PCP is sometimes treated with multiple doses of AC.

Many hallucinogen abusers are in a happy little world of their own. As long as the individual is safe, the effects of hallucinogens are not dangerous, considered self-limiting, and require little intervention for uncomplicated toxicity. Agitation and violence, frequently associated with sympathomimetic hallucinogens, can be controlled with benzodiazepines, droperidol, or haloperidol. Other supportive therapies are drug- and patient-specific.[4]

GHB

Originally an anesthetic agent, gamma hydroxybutyrate (GHB) is now legally available only for the treatment of narcolepsy. Illicit GHB, and its precursor gamma butyrolactone, are easy to manufacture, inexpensive, and widely available. Shortly after ingestion, GHB induces euphoria and sleepiness. Unconsciousness and deep coma may follow within 30 to 40 minutes.[9] When GHB is ingested alone, coma duration is 2 to 4 hours, but concominant ethanol use potentiates GHB's effect and has led to cases of fatal respiratory depression.[40]

GHB's easy accessibility, rapid onset, short duration, and purported euphoric and "fat burning" effects have made it a popular drug of abuse in dance clubs and at rave parties.[25] It has also become known as a "date rape" drug because it can produce amnesia and rapid loss of consciousness, allowing sexual assault. This anesthesia may contribute to the number of patients with recurrent GHB-related ED visits. Symptoms of intoxication include confusion, disorientation, vomiting, nystagmus, ataxia, bradycardia, coma, and apnea.[10] Frequent GHB use may produce tolerance and dependence. Laboratory tests for GHB are not readily available but levels can be obtained at a few national reference laboratories from blood or urine samples obtained within 6 to 12 hours of ingestion.[40]

Flumazenil and naloxone have no therapeutic effect on GHB but may assist with diagnosis. Treatment for GHB poisoning is largely symptomatic. Support ventilations as needed and do not attempt to induce vomiting. Both lavage and AC administration are of very limited value because of the generally small amount and rapid absorption of the drug. Consider charcoal use for recent, large ingestions or when significant coingestants are suspected. GHB elimination is not enhanced by diuresis, dialysis, or hemoperfusion.

Table 43-10	**PCP COMPARISON WITH OTHER DRUG GROUPS**	
CLASSES OF DRUGS	**SIMILARITIES**	**DIFFERENCES**
CNS depressants	Coma	Tachycardia
	Ataxia	Increased deep tendon reflexes
Sympathomimetics	Nystagmus	Hypertension
	Tachycardia	Coma
	Hypertension	Ataxia
		Muscle rigidity
		Increased secretions
		Nystagmus
Anticholinergics	Hypertension	Increased secretions
	Tachycardia	Pupils usually normal
	Hyperthermia	Nystagmus
	Bizarre behavior	Blank stare
	Seizures	Muscle rigidity
	Coma	
Cholinergics	Increased secretions	Tachycardia
	Miosis	Hypertension
	Seizures	Increased deep tendon reflex
		Muscle rigidity
Psychedelics	Bizarre behavior	Ataxia
	Tachycardia	Muscle rigidity
		Increased secretions
		Coma
		Nystagmus
		Acute brain syndrome
Opiates	Coma	No response to naloxone
	Miosis	Increased deep tendon reflex
	Hyperventilation	Muscle rigidity
	Apnea	Hypertension

From Rosen P, Barkin RM, Hockberger RS et al: *Emergency medicine: concepts and clinical practice,* ed 4, St. Louis, 1998, Mosby.
PCP, Phencyclidine; *CNS,* central nervous system.

Heavy Metals

Heavy metals involved in poisoning include lead, mercury, zinc, arsenic, and cadmium. Because heavy metals are a by-product of the industrial age, all inhabitants of developed countries have measurable heavy metal serum levels. Intoxication by these agents is often chronic and subtle, making diagnosis difficult.[36] For example, lead exposure may be related to daily use of glazed ceramic dinnerware or occasional ingestion of paint chips by a small child. Industrial exposure to button batteries, dental cement, marine paints, solder, and countless other products and manufacturing processes puts individuals at risk for heavy metal poisoning. Water pollution has caused mercury toxicity from seafood ingestion.

Absorption of these metals can occur through inhalation and ingestion. Chronic toxicities have a different presentation than acute poisonings. Exposure to an inorganic metal versus an organic metal salt also causes different effects. Heavy metal toxicosis is frequently associated with other poisons such as hydrocarbons (leaded gasoline), organophosphates (arsenic-containing pesticides), and carbon monoxide (mercury released in fuel burning). Without careful assessment and diagnostic evaluation, such polytoxicities can easily be missed.

Heavy metals have no known beneficial physiologic activity in humans and are not metabolized, so they accumulate in the tissues. The metals bind with reactive protein groups and enzymes, disrupting enzymatic function. Excretion from the body is slow, making the effects long term. Although symptoms vary with type of metal and extent of exposure, gastrointestinal disturbances—ranging from nausea, vomiting, and diarrhea to gastrointestinal hemorrhage—are frequently found. Central and peripheral nervous system effects include tremor, peripheral neuropathies, neuropsychiatric disturbances, and seizures. Acute inhalation produces chemical pneumonitis, pulmonary edema, and lung cancer. Table 43-11 summarizes toxin-specific findings.

Serum levels generally provide the best evaluation of heavy metal exposure, although urine and hair samples are sometimes tested. A plain film of the abdomen may show recently ingested metals in the gastrointestinal tract. The need for therapeutic intervention is determined by extent of exposure and patient symptomatology. With certain chronic exposures, terminating contact with the offending agent or en-

vironment is all that is required. For very recent ingestions, standard gastric emptying techniques can be employed; however, this is of no benefit for chronic ingestion or inhalation. AC does not absorb metals.

Because heavy metals accumulate in tissues and are not metabolized, chelation therapy is the best means of eliminating these substances from the body. Chelating agents—administered orally, intramuscularly, or intravenously—bind to metals, facilitating excretion. Three chelating drugs are commonly used: dimercaprol, penicillamine, and ethylenediaminetetraacetic acid. The particular agent selected and route of administration varies with the toxin involved. Dosage is dependent on patient size and symptom severity. Because of the highly individual circumstances surrounding each exposure, consultation with poison control center personnel should be undertaken before administering any chelating drug. Other supportive measures are largely determined on a patient-by-patient basis as symptoms dictate. Fluid volume deficits, anemia, cardiopulmonary dysfunction, and renal failure require intervention as appropriate.

Iron

Iron overdose is one of the most common and severe poisonings of childhood.[30] Unlike heavy metals, iron plays an important physiologic role. Its therapeutic usefulness has made iron widely available in many over-the-counter formulations containing varying amounts of elemental iron. Iron toxicity begins with a direct corrosive effect on gastrointestinal mucosa, leading to perforation, hemorrhage, and necrosis. After it is absorbed, iron initiates cellular toxicity by interfering with aerobic metabolism, causing lactic acidosis, and producing free-radical injury.[34]

Doses less than 20 mg/kg of elemental iron are generally asymptomatic. Ingestions between 20 and 30 mg/kg may produce self-limited vomiting, abdominal pain, and diarrhea. Doses higher than 40 mg/kg are considered serious, and doses greater than 60 mg/kg have been fatal.[43]

Classically, the iron-poisoned patient passes through four clinical stages. Initially, iron's effects produce gastrointestinal corrosion (Stage I). Symptoms range from nausea to massive hemorrhage. Patients who survive this phase may experience a latent period of apparent improvement over the next 12 hours (Stage II). Stage III is signaled by abrupt onset of coma, shock, seizures, metabolic acidosis, coagu-

Table 43-11	HEAVY METAL POISONING	
METAL	**POISONING TYPE**	**FINDINGS**
Lead	Acute	Lethargy, ataxia, constipation, colic, seizures, coma
	Chronic	Subtle behavioral changes, motor neuropathy, intellectual impairment
Mercury	Acute	Renal failure, gastrointestinal symptoms, irritation of the mucous membranes
	Chronic	Tremor, neuropsychiatric symptoms, irritability, memory loss
Arsenic	Acute	Garlic breath odor, tremor, seizures, severe gastrointestinal symptoms, hemolysis
	Chronic	Peripheral neuropathies, anemia, malaise, anorexia

lopathies, and hepatic failure. Survivors eventually enter stage IV, the recovery phase.

Diagnosis of iron ingestion is based on a history of exposure. Suggestive laboratory tests include elevated white blood cell count (>15,000), hyperglycemia (>150 mg/dl), and total serum iron level greater than 450 mcg/dl. Iron tablets may also be visible on abdominal radiographs.

If the acutely iron-toxic patient presents in hemorrhagic shock, early management focuses on basic stabilization. Gastric lavage may be considered if exposure was recent, tablets were chewed, or a liquid iron preparation was ingested. However, intact tablets are large and are unlikely to pass through a lavage tube. AC does not absorb iron and is not recommended unless other drugs were ingested. WBI is very effective and can be considered first-line treatment. Massive ingestions may result in bezoar formation requiring endoscopic or surgical removal.

Deferoxamine, the specific antidote for iron poisoning, is indicated in cases of serious intoxication. This chelating agent is generally given intravenously by constant infusion at a rate of 10 to 15 mg/kg/hr. The chelated deferoxamine-iron complex is excreted in urine, producing a characteristic orange or pink-red color. Therapy may be stopped when urine color or serum iron levels return to normal.

Digitalis Glycosides

Digitalis glycosides are available in pharmaceutic preparations such as digoxin and digitoxin and can also be found in homes and yards in oleander, lily of the valley, rhododendron, and foxglove plants. At therapeutic and toxic doses, digitalis glycosides block the sodium-potassium-adenosine triphosphatase pump. With high serum concentrations, both vagal and sympathetic tone increase.

Clinical symptoms can be vague and difficult to diagnose, particularly with chronic overdoses in elderly patients. Findings include drowsiness, lethargy, and coma. Cardiac conduction disturbances (first-, second-, and third-degree heart block), ventricular dysrhythmias (premature ventricular contractions, ventricular tachycardia, and ventricular fibrillation), asystole, and profound hypotension also occur. (See Chapter 33 for discussion on management of various dysrhythmias.) Visual changes include appearance of yellow or green halos around objects. The patient may experience anorexia, nausea, and vomiting, especially in cases of chronic poisoning. Elevated potassium levels are a prominent feature of cardiac glycoside poisoning, and hyperkalemia (>5.5 mEq/L) must be treated aggressively.[14]

Quantitative serum levels of digoxin or digitoxin can be useful for assessing an individual's degree of toxicity. Complete tissue distribution of cardiac glycosides requires at least 12 hours. Although serum levels are routinely drawn when toxicity is first suspected, samples collected before that time may not reflect a state of blood-tissue equilibrium. Because toxicosis can occur at various serum concentrations, symptomatology must guide therapy. AC absorbs dig-

italis glycosides from the gastrointestinal tract, decreasing systemic absorption. Multiple doses of AC have been suggested for the treatment of digoxin and digitoxin overdose, although limited clinical experience with this treatment has been reported.

High serum digitalis concentrations are an indication for antidote treatment. Digoxin immune Fab (Digibind), an ovine-derived antibody, attaches to digitalis glycosides and renders them inactive. Indications for Digibind are the presence of two or more of the following: life-threatening dysrhythmias, serum potassium levels higher than 5 mEq/L, or serum digoxin concentration greater than 10 ng/ml. The Digibind manufacturer also suggests administration if a single digitalis dose of more than 4 mg has been ingested by a child or more than 10 mg by an adult. An appropriate Digibind dosage is calculated based on a pharmacokinetic determination of total digoxin/digitoxin body load. One drawback to Digibind therapy is its high cost.[14]

Inhalants

A huge number of substances can enter the body through the inhalation route, including organophosphates (sarin gas), heavy metals (lead and mercury as byproducts of combustion), and toxic alcohols. Because of the rapid onset of effects, inhalation is a popular route for drugs of abuse. CNS stimulants (cocaine, PCP) and hallucinogens (marijuana, hashish) are all available in inhalant form. Each of these substances has been addressed in the corresponding section of this chapter.

Other inhalants of abuse do not fall clearly into one of the preceding categories. Among these are various glues, paints, aerosol propellants, cleaning agents, gases, and even food products, most of which are readily available in every home (Table 43-12). One study identified gasoline, freon, butane lighter fluid, glue, and nitrous oxide as the five most commonly abused toxins in the inhalant class.[37] Sniffed or "huffed" from plastic bags, the active components of these agents produce brief, rapid-onset intoxication.[28] These factors make inhalants particularly appealing to children and adolescents.

Systemic effects of moderate exposure include headache, nausea, vomiting, confusion, and drunkenness. Severe intoxication results in coma, ventricular dysrhythmias, myocardial infarction,[33] hepatic injury, and respiratory arrest. There is no specific antidote or treatment. Inhaled toxins are rapidly absorbed and may potentiate cardiac dysrhythmias by increasing sensitivity of myocardium to effects of catecholamines, placing abusers at risk for Sudden Sniffing Death Syndrome.[37] Care is supportive, but epinephrine or other sympathomimetic amines that might precipitate ventricular dysrhythmias should be avoided.[12,33] Tachydysrhythmias caused by increased myocardial sensitivity may be treated with a β-blocker.

In sufficient quantities, inhalants can also displace oxygen from the environment, producing hypoxemia. Freon gas causes frostbite when it comes in contact with tissue, so

Table 43-12 COMMONLY ABUSED INHALANTS

CATEGORY	HARMFUL CHEMICALS	HOUSEHOLD AND OTHER PRODUCTS
Aerosols	Butane, propane, fluorocarbon, hydrocarbon, toluene	Spray paint, hairspray, air freshener, deodorant, fabric protector, asthma inhalers, refrigeration systems
Solvents	Acetone, toluene, methylene chloride, methanol, butane, isopropane bromochlorodifluoromethane	Nail polish remover, paint remover, paint thinner, correction fluid, lighter fluid, fire extinguishers, model glue, felt tip markers, gasoline, carburetor cleaner
Cleaning agents	Tetrachloroethylene, trichloroethane trichloroethylene	Dry cleaning solution, spot removers, degreasers
Food products	Nitrous oxide	Dessert topping (whipped cream) spray, vegetable cooking spray, whippets
Gases	Nitrous oxide, butane, propane, helium halothane, enflurane, ethyl chloride, halon, freon	Anesthetic agents, analgesic spray, refrigeration systems

Table 43-13 HYDROCARBON INGESTIONS

GROUP	TYPE	COMMON FORMS	TOXICITY*
I	Hydrocarbons of high viscosity (>100 SSU)	Lubricating oil, petroleum jelly, grease, diesel oil, tar, paraffin	Low (do not empty stomach)
II	Hydrocarbons of low viscosity (<60 SSU)	Mineral seal oil, gasoline, turpentine, lighter fluid, kerosene, Stoddard solvent, petroleum, ether	Moderate (empty stomach if more than 1 ml/kg)
III	Halogenated hydrocarbons	Vinyl chloride, carbon tetrachloride, trichloroethylene, 1,1,1 trichloroethane, halothane	High (empty stomach)
IV	Aromatic hydrocarbons	Benzene, toluene, xylene	High (empty stomach)

From Rosen P et al: *Emergency medicine: concepts and clinical practice,* ed 2, vol 2, St. Louis, 1988, Mosby.
SSU, Saybolt seconds universal.
*Toxicity relative to risk of aspiration.

caregivers should examine the mouth for signs of frostbite (i.e., blackened tissue or white waxy spots).[23]

Hydrocarbons

Hydrocarbons are found in petroleum, natural gas, coal, and bitumen. Exposure may be caused by inhalation, dermal contact, or ingestion. Accidental exposures are common in children younger than 5 years of age with access to kerosene, gasoline, or lighter fluid. Adults are usually poisoned as a result of occupational contact.

The effects of hydrocarbon toxicity can be divided into pulmonary aspiration and systemic absorption. The potential for pulmonary aspiration is inversely related to the substances' viscosity—the more viscous the hydrocarbon, the less toxic the substance (Table 43-13). Aspiration of tiny amounts of low-viscosity hydrocarbons causes coughing and wheezing and can progress to a life-threatening chemical pneumonitis within hours. Systemic absorption occurs from ingestion, inhalation of hydrocarbon vapors, or dermal contact. Systemic manifestations of hydrocarbon toxicity vary widely by substance and time since exposure. Neurologic symptoms include confusion, headache, lethargy, ataxia, and coma. Hydrocarbons affect the heart's conduction system, causing complete heart block, asystole, and ventricular fibrillation. Nausea, vomiting, and gastrointestinal bleeding have also been reported. Hepatic failure, renal failure, or hemolysis can occur days or even weeks after exposure. Dermal contact causes local irritation and chemical burns.

Exposure to high-viscosity substances, with a low systemic toxicity potential, requires no treatment. Chemicals with a low potential for systemic problems, but with high risk of aspiration pneumonitis, only require observation for pulmonary embarrassment with appropriate respiratory support, should complications occur. Gastric suctioning and AC administration are indicated for recent ingestion of substances with low viscosity and high potential for systemic toxicity. A cuffed endotracheal tube must be inserted before gastric lavage to protect the patient from aspiration.[40,42] Continuous cardiac and oxygen saturation monitoring are recommended. Remove clothing and wash contaminated skin with copious amounts of soap and water. Intravenous access should be established for emergency medications; however, fluids should be administered judiciously because of the potential for pulmonary edema development. Position the patient carefully to minimize risk of aspiration. Obtain a chest radiograph to rule out early pulmonary alterations. Do not administer steroids or prophylactic antibiotics. All symptomatic patients should be observed for 24 hours for pulmonary and cardiac problems. Patients who remain asymptomatic can be discharged after 4 to 6 hours.

Toxic Plants

Many plants found in the home and surrounding environment contain toxic substances. In fact, there are more than 100 species of toxic mushrooms alone. Some plants contain hallucinogenic, narcotic, or anticholinergic toxins making them popular substances of abuse; others have neuro- or cardiotoxic effects. Many are simply gastrointestinal irritants. Plants frequently associated with accidental or intentional poisoning[39] include jimsonweed, lily of the valley, oleander, nightshade, morning glory, dieffenbachia, and poinsettia. Table 43-14 highlights some common poisonous plants.

SUMMARY

Toxicologic emergencies are a routine cause of ED visits. This chapter highlights some of the more frequently seen poisonings. The initial focus of care in any intoxicated patient is always stabilization of cardiopulmonary or hemodynamic problems. Box 43-4 summarizes potential nursing diagnoses for these patients. Treatment priorities include limiting poison absorption, enhancing substance elimination, and providing toxin- and patient-specific supportive interventions. The reader is referred to a detailed toxicology text or the experts at a poison control center for further information on any of the toxicities discussed in this chapter.

Box 43-4 NURSING DIAGNOSES FOR TOXICOLOGIC EMERGENCIES

Airway clearance, Ineffective
Breathing pattern, Ineffective
Cardiac output, Decreased
Coping, Ineffective
Family processes, Interrupted
Fluid volume, Deficient
Fluid volume, Excess
Gas exchange, Impaired
Injury, Risk for
Thermoregulation, Ineffective
Tissue perfusion, Ineffective
Violence, Risk for

Table 43-14 POISONOUS PLANTS IN THE HOUSE AND GARDEN

PLANT	TOXIC COMPONENTS	TOXIC EFFECTS
Aloe	Entire plant	Marked catharsis 6 to 12 hours after ingestion; alkaline urine may turn red; large doses cause nephritis
Bird-of-paradise	Pods and seeds	Vomiting, diarrhea, dizziness, vertigo, drowsiness
Castor bean	Leaves, pods, beans	Gastrointestinal distress, convulsions
Cherry	Pits	Dyspnea, vocal paralysis, convulsions, death
Dieffenbachia (dumbcane), philodendron, elephant ear	Entire plant	Mastication causes sudden pain followed by swelling of tongue and throat with dysphagia, blisters, and vocal cord paralysis; swallowing causes laryngeal edema
English ivy	Entire plant and berries	Skin irritation, nausea, vomiting, severe diarrhea, increased thirst and salivation, abdominal pain, dyspnea; can progress to coma
Holly	Berries and leaves	Vomiting, diarrhea, stupor, narcosis
Hunter's robe	Sap	Irritation of skin, lips, tongue; diarrhea can develop
Jack-in-the-pulpit	Leaves	Gastrointestinal irritation; swelling of tongue, lips, and palate
Jerusalem cherry	Entire plant	Stomach pain, low-grade fever, paralysis, dilated pupils, vomiting, diarrhea, depressed respiratory and circulatory function, loss of sensation, death
Lily of the valley, oleander	Entire plant	Gastrointestinal distress, conduction defects, sinus bradycardia, escape beats, hyperkalemia; digitalis-like toxicity depends on amount consumed
Mistletoe	Berries	Gastrointestinal irritation, diarrhea, bradycardia
Pencil tree	Spurges, milk sap	Severe irritation of mouth, throat, and stomach
Poinsettia	Milky sap, stem, leaves	Irritation of mouth, throat, and stomach, skin; flower bud is a significant ocular threat
Rhododendron	Leaves and sap	Oropharyngeal burning followed hours later by salivation, diarrhea, vomiting, and paresthesias; weakness, decreased vision, bradycardia, coma, seizures
Rhubarb	Leaf blades	Stomach pains, nausea, vomiting, weakness, dyspnea, oropharyngeal burning, internal bleeding, death
Star of Bethlehem	Entire plant—fresh and dried	Nausea, gastrointestinal irritation
Yew	Entire plant	Diarrhea, vomiting, tremors, pupil dilation, facial pallor, circumoral cyanosis, rash, dyspnea, muscular weakness, seizures, coma, dysrhythmia, death

References

1. Adams M, Lammon C, Stover L: Responding to tricyclic antidepressant overdose, *Dimens Crit Care Nurs* 17(2):67, 1998.

2. Albertson T: Opiates and opioids. In Olson K, editor: *Poisoning & drug overdose,* ed 3, Stamford, Conn, 1999, Appleton & Lange.

3. Barceloux D, Krenzelok E, Olson K et al: American Academy of Clinical Toxicology practice guidelines on the treatment of ethylene glycol poisoning. Ad Hoc Committee, *J Toxicol Clin Toxicol* 37(5):537, 1999.

4. Blaho K, Merigian K, Winbery S et al: Clinical pharmacology of lysergic acid diethylamide: case reports and review of the treatment of intoxication, *Am J Ther* 4(4-6):211, 1997.

5. Broughan T, Soloway R: Acetaminophen hepatotoxicity, *Dig Dis Sci* 45(8):1553, 2000.

6. Buckley N, Whyte I, O'Connell D et al: Oral or intravenous N-acetylcysteine: which is the treatment of choice for acetaminophen (paracetamol) poisoning? *J Toxicol Clin Toxicol* 37(6):759, 1999.

7. Burns M: Activated charcoal as the sole intervention for treatment after childhood poisoning, *Curr Opinions Pediatr* 12(2):166, 2000.

8. Burns M, Linden C, Graudins A et al: A comparison of physostigmine and benzodiazepines for the treatment of anticholinergic poisoning, *Ann Emerg Med* 35(4):374, 2000.

9. Chin R, Sporer K, Cullison B et al: Clinical course of gamma-hydroxybutyrate overdose, *Ann Emerg Med* 31(6):716, 1998.

10. Couper F, Logan B: Determination of gamma-hydroxybutyrate (GHB) in biological specimens by gas chromatography—mass spectrometry, *J Analytical Toxicol* 24(1):1, 2000.

11. Diaz J, Lopez M: Voluntary ingestion of organophosphate insecticide by a young farmer, *J Emerg Nurs* 25(4):266, 1999.

12. Edwards K, Wenstone R: Successful resuscitation from recurrent ventricular fibrillation secondary to butane inhalation, *Br J Anesth* 84(6):803, 2000.

13. Egbert P, Abraham K: Ethylene glycol intoxication: pathophysiology, diagnosis, and emergency management, *ANNA J* 26(3):295, 1999.

14. Gittelman M, Stephan M, Perry H: Acute pediatric digoxin ingestion, *Pediatr Emerg Care* 15(5):359, 1999.

15. Grierson R, Green R, Sitar D et al: Gastric lavage for liquid poisons, *Ann Emerg Med* 35(5):435, 2000.

16. Henry J: Epidemiology and relative toxicity of antidepressant drugs in overdose, *Drug Safety* 16(6):374, 1997.

17. Jones A, Volans G: Management of self poisoning, *Br J Med* 319(7222):1414, 1999.

18. Karalliedde L: Organophosphorus poisoning and anesthesia, *Anesthesia* 54(11):1073, 1999.

19. Karch S, Stephens B: Toxicology and pathology of deaths related to methadone: retrospective review, *West J Med* 172(1):11, 2000.

20. Kawasaki C, Nishi R, Uekihara S et al: Charcoal hemoperfusion in the treatment of phenytoin overdose, *Am J Kidney Dis* 35(2):323, 2000.

21. Kim S: Salicylates. In Olson K, editor: *Poisoning & drug overdose,* ed 3, Stamford, Conn, 1999, Appleton & Lange.

22. Kolecki P: Inadvertent methamphetamine poisoning in pediatric patients, *Pediatr Emerg Care* 14(6):385, 1999.

23. Kuspis D, Krenzelok E: Oral frostbite injury from intentional abuse of a fluorinated hydrocarbon, *J Toxicol Clin Toxicol* 37(7):873, 1999.

24. Lessenger J, Reese B: Rational use of cholinesterase activity testing in pesticide poisoning, *J Am Board Fam Pract* 12(4):307, 1999.

25. Li J, Stokes S, Woeckener A: A tale of novel intoxication: a review of the effects of gamma-hydroxybutyric acid with recommendations for management, *Ann Emerg Med* 31(6):729, 1998.

26. MacConnachie A: Ecstasy poisoning, *Intensive Crit Care Nurs* 13(6):365, 1997.

27. McCaig L, Burt C: Poisoning-related visits to emergency departments in the United States 1993-1996, *J Toxicol Clin Toxicol* 37(7):817, 1999.

28. McGarvey E, Clavet G, Mason W et al: Adolescent inhalant abuse: environments of use, *Am J Drug Alcohol Abuse* 25(4):731, 1999.

29. Meyer R, Beard M, Ardagh M et al: Methanol poisoning, *N Z Med J* 113(1102):11-13, 2000.

30. Morris C: Pediatric iron poisonings in the United States, *South Med J* 93(4):352, 2000.

31. Olson K: Acetaminophen. In Olson K, editor: *Poisoning & drug overdose,* ed 3, Stamford, Conn, 1999, Appleton & Lange.

32. Olson K: Emergency evaluation and treatment. In Olson K, editor: *Poisoning & drug overdose,* ed 3, Stamford, Conn, 1999, Appleton & Lange.

33. O'Neill J, McCarthy C: Myocardial infarction in a 14-year old-boy after butane inhalation, *Ir Med J* 92(4):344, 1999.

34. Pestaner J, Ishak K, Mullick F et al: Ferrous sulfate toxicity: a review of autopsy findings, *Biol Trace Element Res* 69(3):191, 1999.

35. Peter J, Cherian A: Organic insecticides, *Anesth Intensive Care* 28(1):11, 2000.

36. Piamphongsant T: Chronic environmental arsenic poisoning, *Int J Dermatol* 38(6):401, 1999.

37. Rohrig R: Sudden death due to butane inhalation, *Am J Forensic Med Pathol* 18(3):299, 1997.

38. Shannon M: Primary care: ingestion of toxic substances by children, *New Engl J Med* 342(3):186, 2000.

39. Southgate H, Egerton M, Dauncey E: Lessons to be learned: a case study approach. Unseasonal severe poisoning of two adults by deadly nightshade, *J Royal Soc Health* 120(2):127, 2000.

40. Timby N, Eriksson A, Bostrom K: Gamma-hydroxybutyrate-associated deaths, *Am J Med* 108(6):518, 2000.

41. Tucker J: Indications for, techniques of, complications of, and efficacy of gastric lavage in the treatment of the poisoned child, *Curr Opinions Pediatr* 12(2):163, 2000.

42. Vale J: Position statement: gastric lavage. American Academy of Clinical Toxicology; European Association of Poison Centres and Clinical Toxicologists, *J Toxicol Clin Toxicol* 35(7):711, 1997.

43. Woo O: Iron. In Olson K, editor: *Poisoning & drug overdose,* ed 3, Stamford, Conn, 1999, Appleton & Lange.

44. Youniss J, Litovitz T, Villanueva P: Characterization of U.S. poison centers: a 1998 survey conducted by the American Association of Poison Control Centers, *Vet Human Toxicol* 42(1):43, 2000.

45. Zimmerman H, Burkhart K, Donovan J: Ethylene glycol and methanol poisoning: diagnosis and treatment, *J Emerg Nurs* 25(2):116, 1999.

Suggested Reading

Bryson P: *Comprehensive review in toxicology for emergency clinicians,* ed 3, Washington, DC, 1996, Taylor & Francis.

Dart R, editor: *The 5 minute toxicology consult,* Philadelphia, 2000, Lippincott Williams & Wilkins.

Goldfrank L, Flomenbaum N, Lewin N et al, editors: *Goldfrank's toxicologic emergencies,* ed 6, Stamford, Conn, 1998, Appleton & Lange.

Haddad L, Shannon M, Winchester J, editors: *Clinical management of poisoning and drug overdose,* ed 3, Philadelphia, 1998, WB Saunders.

Olson K, editor: *Poisoning & drug overdose,* ed 3, Stamford, Conn, 1999, Appleton & Lange.

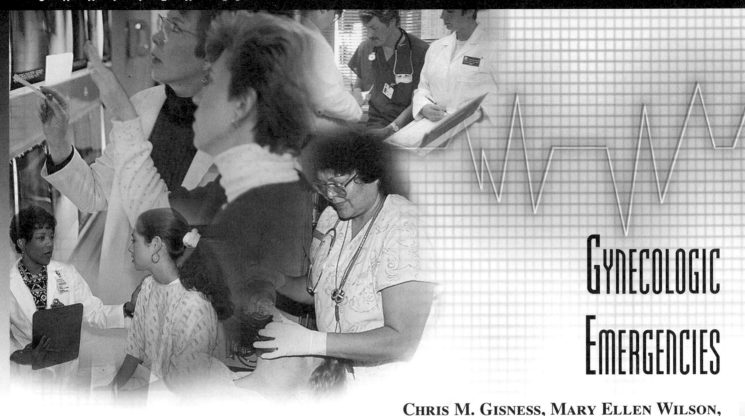

CHAPTER 44

GYNECOLOGIC EMERGENCIES

CHRIS M. GISNESS, MARY ELLEN WILSON,
LORENE NEWBERRY

Patients with gynecologic disorders are seen frequently in emergency departments (EDs) across the country. Knowledge of the normal reproductive system and its functions is necessary to assess and manage the female patient with various gynecologic complaints. Patients may not seek care or, despite seeking care, may not be forthcoming about all symptoms because of embarrassment or lack of knowledge of their own anatomy. Cultural sensitivity and the need for privacy are fundamental to any discussion of problems related to the reproductive organs. This chapter focuses on gynecologic emergencies in the nonpregnant female. Obstetric trauma, obstetric emergencies, and sexual assault are discussed in Chapters 31, 47, and 54, respectively.

ANATOMY AND PHYSIOLOGY

Gynecologic emergencies affect the nonpregnant female's ovaries, fallopian tubes, uterus, cervix, vagina, and external genitalia (Figure 44-1). External genitalia include the mons pubis, labia majora and minora, clitoris, vestibular glands, hymen, urethral opening, and perineum (Figure 44-2). The vestibule is located between the labia minora and contains the hymen, vaginal orifice, urethral orifice, ducts of the Bartholin's glands, and Skene's ducts.[14] Bartholin's glands secrete a mucus-like fluid during excitation. Skene's ducts are not present in all patients but, when found, drain urethral glands into the vestibule.[4] The perineum is a triangular-shaped area between the posterior portion of the vestibule and anus that supports portions of the urogenital and gastrointestinal tracts.

The ovaries, fallopian tubes, and uterus are located inside the peritoneal cavity (Figure 44-3). The ovaries are bilateral oval structures located between the uterus and lateral pelvic wall. During childbearing years, each ovary is 2.5 to 5.0 cm long, 1.5 to 3.0 cm wide, and 0.6 to 1.5 cm thick. Size diminishes significantly after menopause. The number of ova present in the ovaries also decreases with age—from approximately 2 million at birth to 300,000 to 400,000 by puberty.[14] During ovulation each ovary releases a single ovum that is transported down the fallopian tubes to the uterus. The fallopian tubes (approximately 10 cm long) transport the ovum to the uterus through muscle contractions. These bilateral tubes are not contiguous with the ovaries; consequently, the ovum can migrate into the peritoneal cavity. This is the basic mechanism that leads to endometriosis and to ectopic pregnancy in the peritoneal space.

The uterus is a thick-walled organ shaped like an inverted pear. It is suspended in the anterior pelvis above the bladder and in front of the rectum. Length in women who have never been pregnant is 6 to 8 cm. After pregnancy, the uterus lengthens to 9 to 10 cm.[9,14] A layer of peritoneum covers the superior portion of the uterus and forms the serous layer of the uterine wall. The middle layer of the uterine wall consists of smooth muscle with an inner mucous lining called

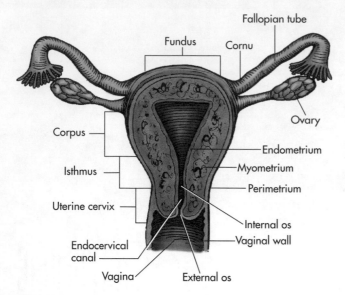

FIGURE 44-1 Female internal genitalia. (From Monahan FD, Neighbors M: *Medical-surgical nursing: foundations for clinical practice,* ed 2, Philadelphia, 1998, WB Saunders.)

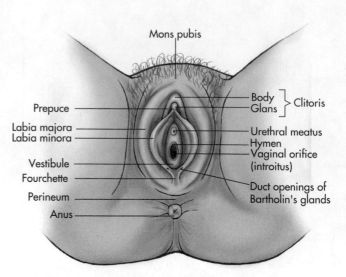

FIGURE 44-2 Female external genitalia. (From Monahan FD, Neighbors M: *Medical-surgical nursing: foundations for clinical practice,* ed 2, Philadelphia, 1998, WB Saunders.)

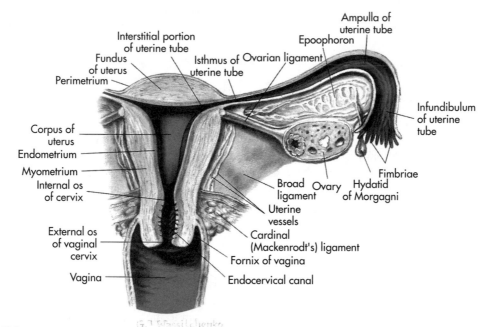

FIGURE 44-3 Female reproductive system. (From Lowdermilk DL, Perry SE, Bobak IM: *Maternity and women's health care,* ed 6, St. Louis, 1997, Mosby.)

the endometrium. The lower portion of the uterus or cervix provides entrance into the uterus. It is located in the vagina between the bladder on the anterior aspect and rectum posteriorly (Figure 44-4).

The female sexual cycle consists of ovulation and menstruation, with each cycle determined by the level of female hormones. Changes in hormone levels prepare the endometrium for implantation of a fertilized ovum. If the ovum is not fertilized, the endometrium sheds the inner lining as menstrual flow. Length of each cycle ranges from 20 to 45 days with an average of 28 days for most women. Menstrual flow lasts typically 3 to 7 days.

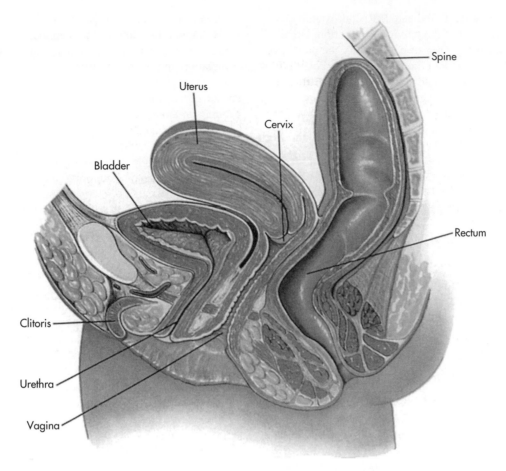

FIGURE 44-4   Sagittal section of the female pelvis. (From Sanders MJ: *Mosby's paramedic textbook*, ed 2, St. Louis, 2000, Mosby.)

ASSESSMENT

Patients with gynecologic emergencies can develop hypovolemia secondary to acute blood loss. Therefore it is imperative to assess carefully for clues to fluid volume deficits (e.g., tachycardia, diaphoresis, narrowed pulse pressure, orthostatic changes in blood pressure and pulse). After the patient's airway, breathing, and circulation have been stabilized, focused assessment of the patient's specific complaint is completed. Assessment includes detailed pain assessment (i.e., onset, quality, character, duration, radiation, precipitating events, and actions that diminish or alleviate the pain). Other pertinent historic information includes menstrual and obstetric history and any history of sexually transmitted diseases. Box 44-1 summarizes essential interview questions for these patients.

Public discussion of sexual activity and sexual history does not come easily for many women. Physical discomfort and emotional overtones related to sexuality or reproductive concerns may cause anxiety or make the patient appear withdrawn. Respecting the patient's privacy and personal dignity can help alleviate some of the patient's anxiety. Provide the patient with visual and auditory privacy during assessment. Allow the patient to undress in private before any examination.

Box 44-1 INTERVIEW QUESTIONS FOR GYNECOLOGIC EMERGENCIES

When was your last menstrual period? Was it normal?

How long does your period normally last?

Are you sexually active?

What type of birth control do you use? Do you consistently use it?

Is there a possibility you are pregnant?

Do you normally have a vaginal discharge? What is different about your discharge today?

How much are you bleeding? How many pads or tampons have you used in the last hour?

Do you have any swelling, itching, redness, or pain?

How many pregnancies have you had? How many children do you have?

Are you having other symptoms or problems?

Any female of reproductive age that presents to the ED with pelvic or lower abdominal pain should be considered pregnant until proven otherwise. The patient's abdomen should be examined for masses, palpable areas of tenderness, and signs of peritonitis. A complete pelvic examination with assessment of external genitalia, vagina, and bimanual examination of the uterus is indicated. Rectal examination may also be done as part of the pelvic examination. Urinalysis helps determine pregnancy or can identify the presence of a urinary tract infection. Wet mount slides with potassium oxide (KOH [preservative]) and normal saline are helpful for determining the cause of vaginitis. Ultrasound and computed tomography (CT) are valuable for defining a mass or abscess. Culdocentesis can confirm the presence of intraperitoneal bleeding but it has been replaced by the less-invasive modality of ultrasound. Laparoscopy is used for diagnosis as well as definitive care.[20]

SPECIFIC GYNECOLOGIC EMERGENCIES

Emergencies of the reproductive organs in the nonpregnant female fall loosely into four categories—bleeding, pain, infection, and structural abnormalities. Pain may be secondary to infection, menstruation, or structural abnormalities with infection secondary to sexually transmitted diseases or related to changes in normal vaginal pH and flora. Bleeding can be attributed to menstruation, can occur at an abnormal time in the female cycle, or can occur after menopause.

Vaginal Bleeding

In addition to pain, abnormal vaginal bleeding is one of the most common gynecologic complaints treated in the ED. Dysfunctional uterine bleeding (DUB) occurs in the pregnant and nonpregnant female. (See Chapter 47 for discussion of vaginal bleeding related to pregnancy.) The first occurrence of DUB is usually in the late teens to mid-20s, but can occur throughout the patient's 30s and 40s. Low-calorie diets, rapid weight change, obesity, and perimenopause have all been linked to DUB.[21] Medical causes of DUB include coagulopathies, hypothyroidism, cirrhosis, hypertension, and anticoagulation therapy.[18]

Hemodynamic instability secondary to DUB is rare; however, DUB can herald the presence of a life-threatening condition.[21] Historic information should differentiate normal vaginal bleeding from DUB. Determine when the bleeding began, amount of bleeding the patient is experiencing, and presence of other symptoms such as pain. Normal vaginal bleeding is 25 to 60 ml per day for 4 to 5 days with most tampons or pads holding 20 to 30 ml when fully saturated. Abnormal vaginal bleeding is considered excessive when bleeding is greater than one pad or tampon per hour for several consecutive hours.[2]

Menorrhagia is excessive bleeding associated with passage of clots. This type of bleeding is irregular flow that occurs other than at the expected time for menses. The condition is considered DUB when bleeding occurs less than 21 days from the last episode of menstrual bleeding. Irregular bleeding secondary to hormonal imbalances is not typically associated with pain; however, dysfunctional bleeding resulting from endometriosis is almost always associated with some level of discomfort.

Prepubertal and menopausal females also experience DUB. Vaginal bleeding in the prepubertal female is associated with vulvovaginitis secondary to increased estrogen stimulation and decreased progesterone levels. Conversely, bleeding in postmenopausal women suggests uterine, ovarian, or cervical tumors. Medication history is also critical; patients on anticoagulant therapy may present with vaginal bleeding or hematuria even with therapeutic anticoagulant levels.

Breakthrough bleeding with contraceptive therapy is the most common cause of abnormal uterine bleeding and usually is the result of poor compliance with the medication schedule or an inadequate daily dose. Adjusting the estrogen dose and adhering to the medication schedule can easily and quickly eliminate this type of DUB.[2,15] Depo-Provera can also cause abnormal bleeding.

Assessment includes a detailed menstrual history followed by a thorough abdominal and bimanual pelvic exam. A rectovaginal examination is also recommended. A detailed menstrual history includes date of the last period, duration of menses, and type of flow, including the presence of clots. Medication history may identify those agents that affect endometrial stimulation or ovulation. Laboratory studies that may be helpful include a complete blood count (CBC), pregnancy test, clotting studies, thyroid-stimulating hormone levels, and a type and cross-match.

Massive blood loss, regardless of etiology, requires immediate resuscitation and stabilization. For other patients the focus is on finding the source and stopping the bleeding. A 14-day regimen of oral Provera 10 mg is used if the patient is less than 35 years of age. Perimenopausal women are treated with cyclic oral contraceptives to regulate bleeding. Patients older than age 35 with DUB are referred to a gynecologist for further work-up. The stable patient who is anemic is discharged on iron supplements.

Pelvic Pain

Pelvic pain is a clinical symptom that encompasses many organ systems—it is an extremely common complaint in the ED. Detailed history and physical examination can often isolate the cause of the pain. When etiology is not immediately apparent, consider ectopic pregnancy, appendicitis, or other surgical emergency for all female patients with pelvic pain. In the adolescent patient, sexual abuse should be considered as a possible cause of pelvic pain.[20] Box 44-2 lists causes for pelvic pain that originate in the reproductive system.

Dysmenorrhea

Pain with menstruation affects a large percentage of female patients that present to the ED. Ninety percent of women experience discomfort at some point during their reproductive years, but it is most common in late teens to mid-20s.[1] Ten to eighteen percent of young females experience pain so severe that daily activities are restricted. Dysmenorrhea is categorized as primary or secondary. Risk factors include

CAUSES OF ACUTE PELVIC PAIN OF GENITAL ORIGIN

PERITONEAL IRRITATION

Ruptured ectopic pregnancy*
Ovarian cyst rupture*
Ruptured tuboovarian abscess*
Uterine perforation*

TORSION

Ovarian cyst or tumor*
Pedunculated fibroid*

INTRATUMOR HEMORRHAGE OR INFARCTION

Ovarian cyst*
Solid ovarian tumor*
Uterine leiomyoma*

INFECTION

Endometritis
PID
Trichomonas cervicitis or vaginitis
Tuboovarian abscess*

PREGNANCY-RELATED

First trimester

Ectopic pregnancy*
Abortion*
Corpus luteum hematoma*

Late pregnancy

Placental problems*
Preeclampsia*
Premature labor*

MISCELLANEOUS

Endometriosis
Foreign objects*
Pelvic adhesions
Pelvic neoplasm
Primary dysmenorrhea

From Rosen P, Barkin M, Hockberger RS et al: *Emergency medicine: concepts and clinical practice,* ed 4, St. Louis, 1998, Mosby.
PID, Pelvic inflammatory disease.
*Potentially requires surgical management.

early menarche, smoking, alcohol ingestion, long menstrual periods, and weight greater than the 90th percentile. There is some evidence linking childhood sexual abuse with the occurrence of dysmenorrhea.[10]

Primary dysmenorrhea has no structural pathology. Increased progesterone during the luteal phase of the menstrual cycle is thought to be the cause.[24] Pain begins hours before or after onset of menstruation and can last 1 to 2 days. It is described as diffuse, dull, and aching in the mid to lower abdomen, radiating to the lower back, and anterior thighs. Headache, fatigue, abdominal distension, nausea, and diarrhea frequently accompany the pain. Some patients experience mild to severe breast tenderness. Increased

prostaglandin levels have been identified in women with severe dysmenorrhea.

Secondary dysmenorrhea usually has an underlying organic cause such as endometriosis, tumors, or fibroids. Infertility is usually associated with secondary dysmenorrhea.

Management of dysmenorrhea includes nonsteroidal antiinflammatory drugs (NSAIDs) just before or at the onset of menstrual flow; narcotics should be avoided. These agents are not given during pregnancy. A heating pad to the abdominal area may also be helpful. Oral contraceptives are used to inhibit ovulation, which decreases concentration of prostaglandins and uterine contractions and consequently decreases the amount of menstrual pain and bleeding.[15] A gynecologist should evaluate patients with excessive bleeding.

Mittelschmerz

Pain with ovulation or Mittelschmerz occurs midcycle. It is always cyclic and is predictable. Patients experience unilateral adnexal pain resulting from leakage of blood from the graafin follicle.[9] Spasms of the fallopian tubes have also been implicated. The pain is described as sudden and sharp. The patient has signs of localized peritoneal irritation without concurrent hyperpyrexia, hypotension, and signs of infection. Abdominal examination is characterized by localized abdominal tenderness without adnexal mass. Laboratory studies may include CBC (to assess for systemic disease and blood loss), urinalysis, pelvic ultrasound, and abdominal or pelvic CT scan. A positive pregnancy test is not consistent with Mittelschmerz. Treatment for Mittelschmerz includes pain management with NSAIDs. Pain should resolve in 24 to 48 hours. A gynecologist should perform any follow-up care.

Vaginal Discharge

Normal vaginal discharge is composed of vaginal cells, lactic acid, and secretions from the cervical and Bartholin's glands.[9] Physiologic vaginal discharge is usually clear and typically odorless. Vaginitis, cervicitis, or sexually transmitted diseases (STDs) may cause abnormal vaginal discharge. Changes in vaginal pH caused by pregnancy, antibiotics, oral contraceptives, vaginal creams or jellies, and douches also cause an abnormal vaginal discharge. Women usually seek care for a discharge that is abnormal for them, usually abnormal in color, consistency, or odor. Color abnormalities range from white to yellow to green. A white discharge suggests *Candida albicans,* yellow discharge suggests *Neisseria gonorrhoeae,* and gray or greenish-gray discharge is associated with *Trichomonas vaginalis* or *Gardnerella vaginalis.* The discharge may be thin and watery or thick with a cottage cheese consistency. A vaginal discharge secondary to *C. albicans, T. vaginalis,* or *G. vaginalis* is widely distributed in the perineum, unlike mucopurulent cervicitis that is characterized by a viscous discharge from the cervical os.[11]

Candidiasis

The patient with a vaginal yeast infection, or candidiasis, develops a thick, white vaginal discharge that has no odor in

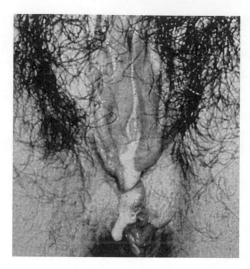

FIGURE **44-5** *Candida albicans.* (From Zitelli BJ, Davis HW: *Atlas of pediatric physical diagnosis,* ed 2, London, 1992, Gower Medical Publishing.)

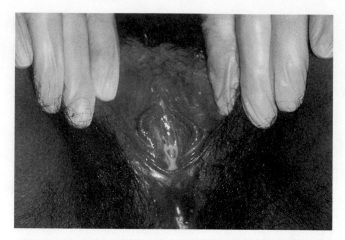

FIGURE **44-6** Trichomoniasis vaginal discharge. The discharge is profuse and watery and appears purulent. (From Monahan FD, Neighbors M: *Medical-surgical nursing: foundations for clinical practice,* ed 2, Philadelphia, 1998, WB Saunders.)

most patients. The discharge has the consistency of cottage cheese and adheres to vaginal mucosa (Figure 44-5). Other symptoms include mild to severe pruritis, dysuria, and erythema and edema of the labia. The infection is associated with oral contraceptives, antibiotic therapy, steroids, and restrictive clothing. There is a 10% to 20% increase in these infections with pregnancy.[11] Diabetes mellitus or immunosuppression should be considered in patients with refractory or recurrent candidal vaginitis.[4] An unidentified human immunodeficiency virus (HIV) infection should be considered in women with recurrent yeast infections. Treatment includes Butoconazole 2% cream 5 g intravaginally for 3 days or Fluconazole 150 mg by mouth as a single dose. Clotrimazole 1% 5 g cream intravaginally for 7 to 14 days is also used.

Trichomonas

Trichomonas is a protozoal infection affecting 3 million people annually.[13] This organism prefers an alkaline environment, so changes in normal vaginal pH make the woman more susceptible to infection. Other risk factors include an increased number of sexual partners and increased frequency of sexual activity. Men may be asymptomatic or have only minor symptoms, whereas women can develop a copious vaginal discharge (Figure 44-6). Twenty percent of nonspecific urethritis in men is caused by trichomonas. Females have a characteristic discharge that is gray or greenish-gray in color. It is foamy, frothy, and malodorous, typically described as a fishy smell. Labia may become erythematous and the patient can experience pruritis, dysuria, and dyspareunia.

Trichomonas is considered an STD; therefore, concurrent testing for gonorrhea and chlamydia is recommended.[11] Half the patients with trichomonas have a concurrent gonoccocal infection. The infection is confirmed when motile trichomonads are found on the wet prep. Both patient and sexual partner(s) must be treated. Nongravid patients and their

partners are given a single injection of metronidazole (Flagyl) 2 g or 500 mg by mouth twice a day for 7 days. If the infection does not resolve, the patient takes metronidazole 500 mg by mouth twice a day for 7 days. Avoid concomitant alcohol use while taking metronidazole and up to 1 week after treatment is completed. The combination of alcohol and metronidazole can precipitate an antabuse reaction. Metronidazole is not given to pregnant patients. The patient receives clotrimazole 100 ml tablet vaginally every night for 2 weeks. Sitz baths and occasional douches may help alleviate discomfort.

Pelvic Inflammatory Disease

Infection of the upper genital tract (cervix, endometrium, and fallopian tubes) is called pelvic inflammatory disease (PID). Risk factors for PID include early sexual activity, multiple partners, mechanical instrumentation, and use of an intrauterine device (IUD). PID occurs more often in women younger than 30 years of age. Upward migration of a genital infection or contamination during gynecologic procedures or delivery leads to infection of the fallopian tubes and surrounding structures. The infection may be an acute episode or can occur as a chronic health problem. The more widespread the infection in the genital tract and peritoneal area, the more severe the discomfort becomes. The Centers for Disease Control and Prevention has delineated criteria for confirming the presence of PID (Box 44-3). Etiology is usually the result of sexual activity but has also been linked to instrumentation and use of IUDs. The most common pathogens are *N. gonorrhea* and chlamydia. Others include gram-negative rods and streptococci.

Moderate to severe lower abdominal pain that increases with walking, urination, defecation, and sexual intercourse characterizes clinical presentation of PID. Pain causes the patient to walk stooped over or with a characteristic shuffling gait. An abnormal vaginal discharge is thick, cream-

Box 44-3	CDC CRITERIA FOR IDENTIFICATION OF PID

PAIN

Lower abdominal tenderness
Bilateral adnexal tenderness
  Cervical motion tenderness

ASSOCIATED FINDINGS

Fever higher than 100.4° F (38° C)
Gram-negative diplococci on Gram stain
WBC count >10,000 cells/mm^3
Increased sedimentation rate
Increased C-reactive protein
Cervical discharge

CDC, Centers for Disease Control and Prevention; *PID*, pelvic inflammatory disease; *WBC*, white blood cell.

Box 44-4	OUTPATIENT ANTIBIOTIC THERAPY FOR PID

One of the following regimens is recommended.
  Ceftriaxone 250 mg IM × 1 injection
  Cefoxitin 2 g IM x 1 injection *plus* probenecid 1 gm PO for
    1 dose
  Ofloxacin 400 mg PO BID for 14 days *plus* Clindamycin
    450 mg PO QID for 14 days
  Flagyl 500 mg BID for 14 days
  Spectinomycin 2 g IM × 1 injection *plus* doxycycline 100
    mg BID for 14 days.

PID, Pelvic inflammatory disease; *IM*, intramuscular; *PO*, by mouth; *BID*, twice daily; *QID*, four times a day.

Box 44-5	CRITERIA FOR HOSPITAL ADMISSION AND INTRAVENOUS ANTIBIOTICS FOR PID

Adolescents and children
Pregnancy
HIV infection
Pelvic abscess present or suspected
Temperature higher than 104° F (38° C)
Inability to eat or drink
Presence of peritonitis
Has not responded to outpatient therapy
Underlying disease has lowered the patient's resistance to infection
Diagnosis not clear (i.e., cannot exclude surgical emergencies such as ectopic pregnancy and appendicitis)
Close follow-up is not available

From Centers for Disease Control and Prevention: 1998 guidelines for treatment of sexually transmitted disease, *MMWR* 47(RR-1):1, 1998.
PID, Pelvic inflammatory disease; *HIV*, human immunodeficiency virus.

colored, and foul smelling. Vaginal bleeding is occasionally present. Dysuria and vomiting also occur. The patient is febrile with the temperature usually higher than 101° F (38.4° C). Conversely, patients with an infection secondary to *Chlamydia trachomatis* are usually afebrile and have less severe symptoms, with pain described as diffuse rather than severe.

Initial onset of PID is not considered an emergency; however, the disease can be catastrophic in reproductive terms. Untreated, the infection can scar fallopian tubes or lead to development of tuboovarian abscess. Scarring of the fallopian tubes causes infertility for many and can lead to the occurrence of ectopic pregnancy in others. Many other patients suffer from recurrent disease and chronic pain. The occurrence of Fitz-Hugh-Curtis syndrome or gonoccocal perihepatitis is a capsular inflammation of the liver associated with PID.

Laboratory analysis includes CBC, urinalysis, pregnancy test, cervical cultures, and Gram stain of any cervical discharge. Depending on severity of the infection, an elevated white count may be present. Presence of a concurrent urinary tract infection is indicated by white cells in the urine. Gram-negative diplococci on the Gram stain indicates the presence of *N. gonorrhea*, whereas *C. trachomatis* is identified through cultures. Bimanual pelvic exam demonstrates lower abdominal tenderness, bilateral adnexal tenderness, and cervical motion tenderness. Diagnostic studies such as pelvic ultrasound and abdominal or pelvic CT are generally reserved for those patients who do not respond to antibiotic therapy or those with suspected tuboovarian abscess.

Treatment for PID includes aggressive antibiotic therapy, positioning, and pain control. Elevate the patient's head 30 to 45 degrees to facilitate pooling of secretions into the lower pelvic area, localize irritants, and decrease pain. Outpatient antibiotic therapy is summarized in Box 44-4. More severe cases of PID require inpatient treatment with intravenous antibiotics (Box 44-5).

Tuboovarian Abscess

Tuboovarian abscess (TOA) occurs with PID when purulent bacteria are trapped in the fallopian tubes. The condition becomes an emergency when the abscess ruptures, spilling anaerobes into the peritoneal space. Rupture leads to peritonitis with mortality as high as 50%. Complete hysterectomy and bilateral salpingectomy may be required to save the patient's life when rupture occurs.[24]

The patient with TOA experiences lower abdominal and pelvic pain or continued PID despite antibiotic therapy. A palpable adnexal mass is also present. Diagnostic studies include CBC, urinalysis, and ultrasound. A pelvic and transvaginal ultrasound is used to confirm the presence of an unruptured TOA. Treatment before rupture includes admission and intravenous antibiotics. Surgical drainage is required when the patient does not improve after 48 hours of treatment. The patient with a ruptured TOA presents with obvious peritonitis characterized by hyperpyrexia and severe

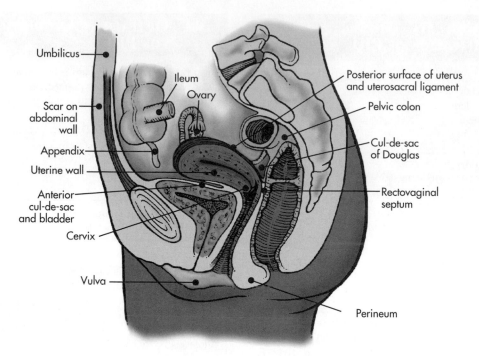

FIGURE 44-7 Common locations for endometriosis. (From Monahan FD, Neighbors M: *Medical-surgical nursing: foundations for clinical practice*, ed 2, Philadelphia, 1998, WB Saunders.)

abdominal pain. An adnexal mass is not palpable after the TOA ruptures.

Endometrial Emergencies

Emergencies related to the endometrium include endometriosis, which is a structural abnormality, and endometritis, which involves inflammation of the endometrium. Patients may present with a previously identified problem or symptoms such as pain or bleeding.

Endometriosis

Migration of endometrial tissue outside the uterus or endometriosis is typically found on the ovaries, posterior cul de sac, and uterosacral ligaments. Studies found intestinal implants in only 5% of the cases.[18] There have been rare reports of implants above the diaphragm. One or both fallopian tubes may be involved. Figure 44-7 highlights the most common locations for endometriosis. Despite its abnormal location endometrial tissue functions normally so it sloughs and bleeds just as does the uterine lining. The patient may experience mid-cycle pain with retrograde flow of endometrial tissue up the fallopian tubes or at the same time as menses. Pain may be diffuse, acute, or described as midline abdominal cramping that radiates to the anterior thighs. Associated symptoms include headache, nausea, vomiting, and diarrhea.

Diagnostic studies in the ED include CBC, pregnancy test, and urinalysis with culture and sensitivity. Blood type and cross-match is indicated when there is evidence of hypovolemia. Laparoscopy is used for definitive diagnosis of the condition but is not indicated for the ED patient unless the patient is acutely ill.[20] Primary management of endometriosis in the ED is control of pain and preservation of fertility. Oral contraceptives are used to decrease pain, minimize bleeding, and regulate the menstrual cycle. Short-term narcotic therapy may be indicated; however, NSAIDs are preferred for most patients. Danzol therapy suppresses luteinizing hormone and follicle-stimulating hormone causing amenorrhea. Stopping the menses eliminates sloughing and bleeding that causes the painful symptoms of endometriosis.

Endometritis

Inflammation of endometrial tissue or endometritis usually occurs during the postpartum period but has been reported after therapeutic or spontaneous abortion. Symptoms include fever, chills, abdominal tenderness, and decreased bowel sounds. Foul-smelling lochia is also present. The first symptoms are usually evident within 24 hours of delivery or abortion. A CBC and blood culture are obtained to assess for systemic disease. Endometritis is treated with antibiotic therapy, fever control, and pain management.

Ovarian Emergencies

Emergencies of the ovaries involve ovarian cysts or ovarian torsion. Presentation may be due to pain or severe hypovolemia with rupture. As with endometrial problems the patient may present with known diagnosis of ovarian cyst or may present with a new or an unidentified problem.

Ovarian Cyst

An ovarian cyst is a sac on the ovary that contains fluid, semifluid, or solid material. Size, consistency, and development vary. The most common cause of ovarian cyst is overgrowth of endometrial tissue. Follicular cysts are failed ovulations that occur during the first 2 weeks of the cycle. Hemorrhage of a mature corpus luteum cyst causes a blood-filled cyst in the ovarian wall. This type of cyst can cause catastrophic hemorrhage when it ruptures.

For most patients ovarian cysts are asymptomatic. Problems develop when rupture, hemorrhage, or torsion occurs. Follicular cysts tend to rupture with strenuous exercise or sexual intercourse during the first 2 weeks of the cycle.[21] Conversely, rupture of a corpus luteum cyst occurs during the last few weeks of the cycle before menses. Cysts may cause pressure or abdominal pain. A dull ache on the affected side is associated with a cyst that increases in size over time. Prolonged menstruation is present in some patients. It is important to remember that the ovaries of menopausal and premenarche patients are usually not palpable so sudden enlargement suggests ovarian hemorrhage.

Rupture of a cyst can also cause Mittelschmerz midcycle pain. Contents of small cysts are usually spontaneously reabsorbed after rupture. Management focuses on pain management with NSAIDs and reassurance. Short-term narcotic therapy may be required for some patients. Doppler ultrasonography is used to rule out ruptured ectopic pregnancy, appendicitis, and intraperitoneal bleeding in stable patients because these conditions exhibit similar symptamotology. A pregnancy test, CBC, and urinalysis are obtained.

Surgical intervention is not required unless there is evidence of hypovolemia. Circulatory compromise is more likely to occur with rupture of a blood-filled cyst. The patient presents with hypovolemia and clinical signs that range from mild tachycardia, dizziness, and syncope to severe hypotension and shock depending on blood loss. Adnexal tenderness and signs of peritonitis are usually present in patients with significant blood loss. Management for these unstable patients is surgical intervention. After the airway and breathing are stabilized, the priorities are insertion of large-bore intravenous catheters, rapid infusion of crystalloid solutions, obtaining blood for type and cross-match, and getting the patient to the operating room as quickly as possible.

Ovarian Torsion

Twisting of the ovary or fallopian tube is called ovarian torsion. The condition usually occurs with a large cyst or tumor and is more likely to occur during pregnancy from an enlarged corpus luteum cyst. Ovarian torsion is characterized by sudden, sharp intermittent pain on one side. Pain lasts a few hours to several days. Associated symptoms include

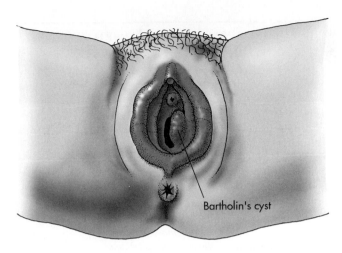

FIGURE 44-8 Bartholin's cyst. (From Ignatavicius DD, Workman, ML, Mishler MA: *Medical-surgical nursing across the healthcare continuum,* ed 3, Philadelphia, 1999, WB Saunders.)

fever, dysuria, nausea, and vomiting. Some patients report previous episodes of pain that subsides if spontaneous detorsion occurs.[23] Abdominal assessment demonstrates unilateral lower quadrant pain with a palpable adnexal mass.

Diagnostic studies include a CBC and urinalysis. Pelvic ultrasound with Doppler flow is used to identify the torsion. Patients with suspected ovarian torsion require hospital admission and close observation. Surgical intervention is required when the torsion does not spontaneously resolve. Untreated, torsion can lead to infertility, infections, and even necrosis.

Bartholin's Gland Abscess

The Bartholin's glands are located within the vestibule at the 8 and 4 o'clock positions. These glands secrete a clear viscous fluid that lubricates the vaginal vestibule.[4] Under normal circumstances the glands cannot be palpated or visualized. A small, painless lump develops when the duct is blocked. Warm sitz baths are all that is required for treatment when there is no infection; however, occlusion with mucous plugs or vaginal secretions can lead to abscess formation. Infection is primarily the result of vaginal or fecal organisms (*E. coli, G. vaginalis,* and other anaerobic bacteria); however, sexually transmitted diseases such as *N. gonorrhoeae* and *C. trachomatis* have also been cultured. Abscess of Bartholin's glands usually occurs in women 20 to 29 years of age.

The patient with an abscess of the Bartholin's gland develops a painful, erythematous swelling of the labium (Figure 44-8). Progressive swelling, fluctuant mass, and increasing pain characterize this condition. The patient has difficulty sitting or standing and usually reports dyspareunia. Spontaneous rupture does occur and is associated with purulent drainage. Treatment for a Bartholin's gland abscess

Table 44-1	COMPLICATIONS CAUSED BY SEXUALLY TRANSMITTED ORGANISMS	
COMPLICATION	**CAUSATIVE ORGANISMS**	
Salpingitis, infertility, and ectopic pregnancy	*Neisseria gonorrhoeae* *Chlamydia trachomatis* *Mycoplasma hominis*	
Reproductive loss (abortion/ miscarriage)	*Neisseria gonorrhoeae* *Chlamydia trachomatis* Herpes simplex virus *Mycoplasma hominis* *Ureaplasma urealyticum* *Treponema pallidum*	
Puerperal infection	*Neisseria gonorrhoeae* *Chlamydia trachomatis*	
Perinatal infection	Hepatitis B virus Human immunodeficiency virus Human papillomavirus *Neisseria gonorrhoeae* *Chlamydia trachomatis* Herpes simplex virus *Treponema pallidum* Cytomegalovirus Group B streptococcus	
Cancer of genital area	*Chlamydia trachomatis* Herpes simplex virus Human papillomavirus	
Male urethritis	*Mycoplasma hominis* Herpes simplex virus *Neisseria gonorrhoeae* *Chlamydia trachomatis* *Ureaplasma urealyticum*	
Vulvovaginitis	Herpes simplex virus *Trichomonas vaginalis* Bacteria causing vaginosis *Candida albicans*	
Cervicitis	*Neisseria gonorrhoeae* *Chlamydia trachomatis* Herpes simplex virus	
Proctitis	*Neisseria gonorrhoeae* *Chlamydia trachomatis* Herpes simplex virus *Campylobacter jejuni* *Shigella* species *Entamoeba histolytica*	
Hepatitis	*Treponema pallidum* Hepatitis A virus	
Dermatitis	*Sarcoptes scabiei* *Phthirus pubis*	
Genital ulceration or warts	*Chlamydia trachomatis* Herpes simplex virus Human papillomavirus *Treponema pallidum* *Haemophilus ducreyi* *Calymmatobacterium granulomatis*	

From Ignatavicius DD, Workman ML, Mishler MA: *Medical-surgical nursing across the healthcare continuum,* ed 3, Philadelphia, 1999, WB Saunders.

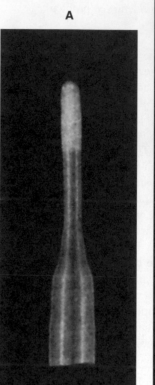 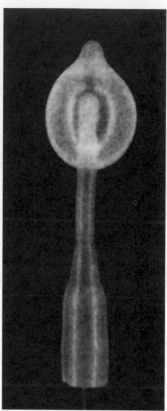

FIGURE 44-9 Word catheter. **A,** Uninflated. **B,** Inflated. (From Davis JH et al: *Clinical Surgery,* St. Louis, 1987, Mosby.)

is incision and drainage with placement of a drain or wick.[16,22] A special gland or Word catheter (Figure 44-9) is preferred because it has a small balloon that can be inflated to hold the drain in position. If this is not available, a small Penrose drain can be used. Patients are discharged with the catheter or drain in place for approximately 24 hours. The patient should avoid sexual intercourse until the catheter or drain is removed. Other discharge instructions include perineal warm soaks, sitz baths, and pain control. Pain is controlled with NSAIDs or short-term narcotic therapy. The patient is placed on oral antibiotics and reevaluated in 24 to 72 hours.

Sexually Transmitted Diseases

STDs include PID (discussed earlier in this chapter), genital herpes, genital warts, chancroid, gonorrhea, syphilis, chlamydia, HIV infection, and hepatitis. (See Chapter 40 for discussion of HIV and hepatitis). Regardless of the condition, an STD can lead to long-term sequelae. Table 44-1 summarizes complications related to various STDs. When caring for any patient with an STD, discuss high-risk behaviors such as unprotected intercourse, multiple partners, and anal intercourse. Stress the importance of barrier protection for any type of sexual intercourse (oral, vaginal, and

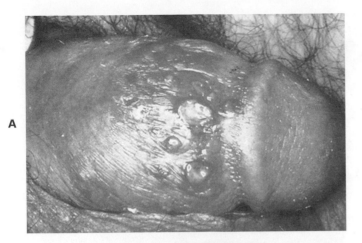

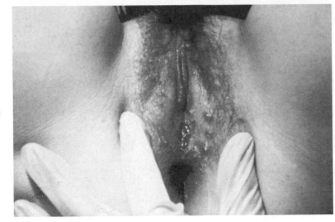

A

B

FIGURE **44-10** Genital herpes in a male (**A**) and in a female (**B**). (From Lewis SM, Collier IC, Heitkemper MM: *Medical-surgical nursing: assessment and management of clinical problems*, ed 4, St. Louis, 1996, Mosby.)

anal). Most states mandate reporting STDs to local health departments. Refer to your specific facility and state to determine who makes the report (ED, laboratory, other) and where the report goes (health department or other agency). Reference to and illustration of some STDs in males have been included in the following discussion for illustration purposes only.

Genital Herpes

An estimated 25 million people in the United States have genital herpes. This chronic, incurable STD is caused by herpes simplex virus type 2 (HSV-2) whereas herpes simplex virus type 1 (HSV-1) causes cold sores. Clinically, lesions caused by the two viruses are identical. In general, HSV-1 is associated with lesions above the waist whereas HSV-2 is associated with lesions below the waist. However, cold sores (HSV-1) can cause genital herpes (HSV-2) if the patient has oral sex.

Painful herpetic lesions develop on the genitalia, buttocks, or thighs 2 to 12 days after exposure (Figure 44-10). The most common sites in women are the cervix and vulva with the glans and prepuce the most common sites in men.

Flu-like symptoms such as fever, chills, headache, nausea, vomiting, and malaise occur during this initial period. The patient often has a stinging or burning sensation before blisters erupt. Inguinal lymphadenopathy may also be present. Urinary retention can occur secondary to pain when urine comes in contact with the ulcerated area. Symptoms normally subside 2 to 3 weeks after onset. Fifty percent of patients with genital herpes have a recurrence three to four times annually.[21]

Treatment of genital herpes is palliative and includes acyclovir, famciclovir, or valacyclovir and warm baths, topical anesthetics, and mild analgesics.[5] Recurrent attacks often occur during times of stress; therefore, rest, a balanced diet, and stress reduction are part of the treatment regimen. Table 44-2 summarizes medication regimen for primary and recurrent infections, whereas Box 44-6 highlights techniques for symptomatic relief during active infections. Barrier protection should be used during intercourse; sexual activity should be avoided altogether during infectious outbreaks and the 24-hour prodromal period. Ideally, there should be no sexual activity until all lesions are dry. Genital herpes increases the risk of cervical cancer, so female patients should have regular gynecologic examinations and annual pap smears.

Genital Warts

Approximately 5.5 million new cases of human papilloma virus (HPV) are reported annually in the United States.[7] More than 30 different types of HPV cause ano-genital warts.[13] Warts are flesh-colored papular lesions that can be flat, sessile, or pedunculated—lesions often have a cauliflower configuration.[12] Primary locations are the vulva, perineum, penis, and perianal regions (Figure 44-11). Lesions in the mouth, pharynx, and larynx have also been reported. Vaginal or cervical warts occur in one third of women with genital warts, so internal examination with a speculum should be done. Squamous cell cervical cancer is now firmly linked to HPV.[17] Warts also flourish during pregnancy.[6] Other factors that favor development of warts include HIV, smoking, poor nutrition, and fatigue.

The patient may also have a vaginal discharge and dyspareunia.[8] One third of these patients have an underlying gonococcal or chlamydia infection, so screening tests or cultures should be obtained. There is no definitive cure for HPV, treatment is not always successful, and recurrences are common. Treatment consists of painting the affected area with podophyllin in benzoin 10% to 25% or trichloroacetic acid 85% weekly.[6] Multiple applications are required and may not totally eradicate the problem. Podophyllin should never be used during pregnancy because it has significant abortion-causing properties.[6] Treatment is more successful when warts are small and present for less than 12 months.[13] Interferon has been used on a limited basis; but it is expensive and has numerous side effects.[5] Carbon dioxide lasers and electrocautery may be used for some patients. Surgical excision is used for extensive warts.

Table 44-2	MEDICATION THERAPY FOR GENITAL HERPES
DRUG	**DOSE**
Acyclovir (Zovirax)	**Intravenous** 5 mg/kg over 1 hour every 8 hours for 5-7 days Initial or recurrent infections for immune suppressed patients Severe initial clinical episode in other patients **Oral** 200 mg PO every 4 hours while awake for total of 5 capsules daily for 10 days for initial primary infection, taken intermittently for recurrent infection Chronic suppressive therapy is 400 mg TID up to 6 months but may require up to 5 capsules per day to suppress disease **Topical ointment** Cover all lesions every 3 hours or 6 times daily for 7 days
Famciclovir (Famvir)	**Oral** 250-500 mg BID for 5 days 125 mg PO BID for 5 days for suppressive therapy
Valacyclovir (Valtrex)	**Oral** 1000 mg PO BID for 5 days 500 mg PO BID for 5 days for suppressive therapy

PO, By mouth; *TID,* three times a day; *BID,* twice daily.

Box 44-6	SYMPTOMATIC RELIEF FOR GENITAL HERPES INFECTIONS

Keep lesions clean and dry.

Avoid using lubricants and creams (may prolong healing time and contribute to secondary infection).

Wear loose clothing and cotton underwear to decrease pressure and irritation.

Use drying agents such as Campho-Phenique for pain and itching.

Use soaks, sitz baths, and cool compresses for local pain relief.

Take aspirin and acetaminophen for pain control.

Modified from Monahan FD, Neighbors M: *Medical-surgical nursing: foundations for clinical practice,* ed 2, Philadelphia, 1998, WB Saunders.

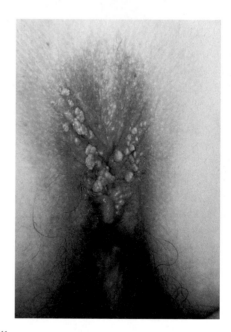

FIGURE 44-11   Genital warts (condylomata acuminata). (From Black JM, Hawks JH, Keene AM: *Medical-surgical nursing: clinical management for positive outcomes,* ed 6, Philadelphia, 2001, WB Saunders.)

Chancroid

Chancroid is a highly contagious infection that is a cofactor in HIV transmission and is associated with a high rate of HIV infection.[13] The infection is caused by *Haemophilus ducreyi*, a gram-negative bacillus that has an incubation period of 2 to 12 days. The patient develops papules or pustules that lead to deep genital ulcers (Figure 44-12). Lymphadenopathy with tenderness in the inguinal area occurs in half the cases. The patient is treated with a single dose of 1 g oral azithromycin or a single intramuscular injection of ceftriaxone 250 mg. Oral erythromycin 500 mg by mouth four times a day for 7 days, ciprofloxacin 500 mg by mouth twice a day for 7 days, or amoxicillin/clavulanic acid 500mg/125mg by mouth three times a day for 7 days may also be used.

Gonorrhea

Humans are the only known host for *N. gonorrhoaea.*[21] Gonorrhea (GC) is one of the most frequently reported communicable diseases in the United States. The condition is more likely to be transmitted from a contaminated male to a female partner. Ironically, approximately 30% of males exposed to an infected female do not develop an infection.[21] Penile and vaginal infections are most common; however, pharyngeal and anal infections also occur. Ocular infections

Table 44-3 TREATMENT OF GONORRHEA			
UNCOMPLICATED INFECTIONS (URETHRITIS, CERVICITIS, PROCTITIS)		DISSEMINATED INFECTIONS (BACTEREMIA AND ARTHRITIS)	
DRUG OF CHOICE	CONCURRENT TREATMENT FOR CHLAMYDIA	DRUG OF CHOICE	ALTERNATIVES
Cefixime 400 mg PO in a single dose	Azithromycin 1 g PO (nonallergic adults and adolescents)	Ceftriaxone 1 g IM q day	Spectinomycin 2 gm IM q 12 hr
Ceftriaxone 125 mg IM in a single dose	Doxycycline 100 mg PO BID × 7 days (nonallergic adults and children > 7 yr and > 44 kg)	Ceftizoxime 1 g IV q 8 hr	
Ciprofloxacin 500 mg PO in a single dose	Erythromycin base 500 mg PO QID × 7 days (children < 8 yr and > 44 kg)	Cefotaxime 1 g IV q 8 hr	
Ofloxacin 400 mg PO in a single dose	Erythromycin base 50 mg/kg/day in four doses × 10-14 days (children < 45 kg)		

From Rosen P, Barker RM, Hockberger RS et al: *Emergency medicine: concepts and clinical practice,* ed 4, St. Louis, 1998, Mosby.

PO, By mouth; *IM,* intramuscular; *q,* every; *IV,* intravenous; *QID,* four times a day.

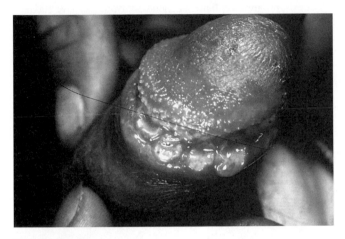

FIGURE 44-12   Chancroid lesions. (From Black JM, Hawks JH, Keene AM: *Medical-surgical nursing: clinical management for positive outcomes,* ed 6, Philadelphia, 2001, WB Saunders.)

result when the organism is transmitted from contaminated fingers to the eyes or during birth. Symptoms develop 2 to 7 days after exposure.[18] Patients with ocular GC should be seen by an ophthalmologist and hospitalized for parenteral antibiotic therapy. Many patients have a concurrent *C. trachomatis* infection.

Three patterns of disease have been identified in women with gonorrhea: asymptomatic carrier, PID, and cervicitis. Between 30% and 40% of women with the infection are asymptomatic carriers. Women with cervicitis develop a yellow or white mucopurulent discharge. The cervix becomes swollen, congested, and very fragile.[18] Abnormal vaginal bleeding, vaginal itching, and dysuria also occur. PID secondary to gonoccocal infection is characterized by abdominal pain, fever, cervical motion tenderness, bilateral adnexal tenderness, nausea, and vomiting. Refer to the discussion on PID earlier in this chapter. Vaginitis is the most common gonoccocal infection seen in children.[18]

Men are almost always symptomatic. Urethritis with a yellow-white thick discharge occurs only days after expo-sure. The patient has concurrent symptoms of a urinary tract infection. Prostatitis, epididymitis and proctitis also occur.

Fever, chills, and a rash characterize disseminated gonoccocal infections. Hemorrhagic pustules that resemble meningococcus arise. Meningitis, endocarditis, migratory tenosynovitis, arthralgia, and arthritis are associated with this type of infection. Hepatitis also occurs but the incidence is low.

Diagnostic work-up includes a Gram stain of urethral exudates in males and cervical discharge in females. Cervical, pharyngeal, and rectal cultures are obtained when appropriate. Blood cultures are obtained when disseminated GC is suspected. A CBC and urinalysis is indicated for PID. Antibiotic-resistant strains have been reported; however, there are numerous agents that are effective for gonoccocal infections. Uncomplicated infections are treated with one of several drug options. Table 44-3 identifies current treatment recommendations for gonorrhea and concurrent chlamydia infection.

Syphilis

This sexually transmitted disease occurs when *Treponema pallidum* spirochetes enter the body through mucous membranes and breaks in the skin.[21] The disease occurs in three distinct phases—primary, secondary, and tertiary or latent. Table 44-4 summarizes clinical symptoms for each phase. Figure 44-13 highlights one clinical feature of primary syphilis, whereas Figure 44-14 illustrates the classic rash found in secondary syphilis.

Early identification and antibiotic therapy is the key to stopping disease progression and preventing the catastrophic sequelae that occur in the central nervous system and cardiovascular system. The disease can also be transmitted *in utero* during the latent stage.[16] Diagnostic lab studies include rapid plasma reagent (RPR) and Venereal Disease Research Laboratory (VDRL) tests. The incubation period is usually 3 weeks with tests positive 2 to 4 weeks after the chancre develops.[6] Cultures and other studies of cerebrospinal fluid are

Table 44-4	CLINICAL SYMPTOMS OF SYPHILIS BY PHASE	
PHASE	**ONSET**	**CLINICAL FEATURES**
Primary	Occur 10-90 days after exposure	Small papule at site of the exposure
		Papule becomes a painless chancre
		Rubbery, nontender inguinal adenopathy
		Rectal chancre may be painful or painless
		Rectal irritation or discharge may be present
Secondary	6-20 weeks after exposure	Dull symmetric rash involving palms and soles of feet
		Fever and chills
		Lethargy
		Lymphadenopathy
		Flat rectal warts
		Patchy alopecia
		Lose lateral third of the eyebrows
		Nonspecific findings such as sore throat, headache, malaise
Tertiary (latent)	Years after initial infection	Neurosyphilis
		Maybe asymptomatic
		Meningitis, general paresis, progressive dementia, neuropathy, progressive ataxia, tremulous extremities
		Urinary incontinence
		Thoracic aneurysm, aortic insufficiency occur

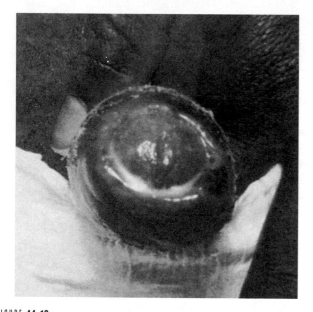

FIGURE **44-13**   Primary syphilis in the male. (From Greenberger NJ, Hinthorn DR: *History taking and physical examination: essentials and clinical correlates,* St. Louis, 1993, Mosby.)

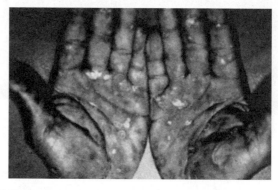

FIGURE **44-14**   Secondary syphilis. (From Goldstein BG, Goldstein AO: *Practical dermatology,* ed 2, St. Louis, 1997, Mosby.)

done when neurosyphilis is suspected. Table 44-5 highlights medical management of syphilis.

Chlamydia

Chlamydia is three to five times more common than gonorrhea, making it the most common STD in the United States.[25] This infection is the primary cause of infertility in females and the major cause of nongonoccocal urethritis in heterosexual males.[21] Chlamydia causes PID and cervicitis, has been cultured in Bartholin's gland abscesses, and has also been linked to preterm labor and postpartum en-

dometritis. The incubation period is 5 to 10 days or more. Concurrent gonococcal infections are found in 20% to 25% of patients with chlamydial infections.[6]

Females are usually asymptomatic.[3,17,19] Males develop a yellow-white thin discharge, burning with urination, urethral itching, and symptoms of epididymitis.[17] Small, shallow painless vesicles or ulcers called lymphogranuloma venereum develop in the genital area. A rectal discharge, papule, or stricture can occur. Prostatitis, epididymitis, proctitis, and Reiter's syndrome are caused by chlamydia. Reiter's syndrome is characterized by reactive arthritis, urethritis, and conjunctivitis. Pharyngitis, pneumonia, and conjunctivitis secondary to chlamydia have also been reported. Conjunctivitis 5 to 13 days after birth can lead to corneal damage and blindness if untreated.[21]

Chlamydia infection is diagnosed with cultures, deoxynucleic acid recognition test, enzyme-linked immunoassay, or direct fluorescent antibody test.[1-3,19] A urinalysis should be obtained when dysuria is present with an

Table 44-5 TREATMENT OF SYPHILIS		
PRIMARY, SECONDARY, OR EARLY LATENT	**LATE LATENT, UNKNOWN DURATION, TERTIARY (EXCLUDING NEUROSYPHILIS)**	**NEUROSYPHILIS**
ADULTS		
Benzathine penicillin G, 2-4 million units in a single dose; or (in penicillin-allergic, nonpregnant patients) doxycycline 100 mg BID PO × 14 days; or tetracycline 500 mg QID PO × 14 days	Benzathine penicillin G, 2-4 million units IM weekly × 3 weeks; or (in pencillin-allergic, nonpregnant patients) doxycycline 100 mg PO × 30 days; or tetracycline 500 mg QID PO × 30 days	Aqueous crystalline penicillin G 2.4 million units q 4 hr × 10-14 days; or procaine penicillin 2.4 million units IM q day × 10-14 days and probenecid 500 mg PO QID × 10-14 days
CHILDREN		
Benzathine penicillin G, 50,000 U/kg IM in a single dose up to 2.4 million units	Benzathine penicillin G, 50,000 U/kg IM weekly up to 2.4 million units per dose × 3 weeks	Aqueous crystalline penicillin G 50,000 U/kg IV q 6 hr × 10-14 days

From Rosen P, Barkin RM, Hockberger RS et al: *Emergency medicine concepts and clinical practice,* ed 4, St. Louis, 1998, Mosby.
PO, By mouth; *BID,* twice a day; *QID,* four times a day; *IM,* intramuscular.

RPR or VDRL to rule out concurrent syphilis infection. In addition to information on treatment of gonoccocal urethritis, cervicitis, and proctitis, Table 44-3 provides antibiotic options for these same problems when the pathogen is chlamydia. Conjunctivitis secondary to chlamydia is treated with doxycycline or tetracycline for 7 days. Lymphogranuloma venereum requires much longer antibiotic treatment—21 days of doxycycline, tetracycline, or erthromycin.[21]

SUMMARY

The patient with a gynecologic emergency may have a problem that is directly related to his or her sexual practices or lifestyle. The caregiver must focus on the patient's problem in a caring, nonjudgmental manner. Inability to do so can interfere with identification of potentially life-threatening gynecologic conditions. Recognition of potentially life-threatening conditions takes priority over other interventions. However, the caregiver must not lose sight of the long-range effect many gynecologic emergencies can have on the patient's fertility and sexuality. Box 44-7 lists the most common nursing diagnoses for these patients.

Box 44-7 NURSING DIAGNOSES FOR GYNECOLOGIC EMERGENCIES
Anxiety
Body image, Disturbed
Cardiac output, Decreased
Fear
Fluid volume, Risk for deficient
Infection, Risk for
Knowledge, Deficient
Pain
Self-esteem, Situational low

References

1. Adler J, Plantz S, Stearns D et al: *Emergency medicine,* Baltimore, Md, 1999, Lippincott Williams & Wilkins.
2. Anderson E, Mackey H: Non-pregnant vaginal bleeding. In Harwood-Nuss A, Wolfson A, editors: *The clinical practice of emergency medicine,* ed 3, Philadelphia, 2001, Lippincott Williams & Wilkins.
3. Beirstein G, Snyder M, Conly M et al: Adolescent chlamydia testing practices and diagnosed infections in a large managed care organization, *Sex Transm Dis* 28(8):477, 2001.
4. Carroll R: The reproductive system. In Black J, Hawks J, Keene A, editors: *Medical-surgical nursing,* Philadelphia, 2001, WB Saunders.
5. Centers for Disease Control and Prevention: Guidelines for treatment of sexually transmitted diseases, *MMWR* 47 (RR-1):1998.
6. Emergency Nurses Association: *Emergency nursing core curriculum,* ed 5, Philadelphia, 2000, WB Saunders.
7. Glickman J: *Health science report.* (2001). Retrieved July 13, 2001 from the World Wide Web: http://www.alotek.com.
8. Handsfield H: Clinical presentation and natural course of anogenital warts, *Am J Med* 102(5A):16, 1997.
9. Ignatavicius D, Workman M, Mishler M: *Medical-surgical nursing: a nursing process approach,* ed 2, Philadelphia, 1995, WB Saunders.
10. Jamieson D, Steege F: The association of sexual abuse with pelvic pain complaints in a primary care population, *Am J Obstet Gynecol* 177(6):1408, 1997.
11. Knoop K, Stack L, Storrow A: *Atlas of emergency medicine,* New York, 1997, McGraw-Hill.
12. Markovchick V, Pons P: *Emergency medicine secrets,* ed 2, Philadelphia, 1999, Hanley & Balfus.
13. Martin Y: Recognizing & treating the silent STD, *Advances for nurses,* Carolina/Georgia, September 3, 2001.
14. Monahan R, Neighbors M: *Medical-surgical nursing,* ed 2, Philadelphia, 1998, WB Saunders.
15. Newton E, Hochbaum S: Vaginal bleeding unrelated to pregnancy. In Rosen P, Barkin RM, Hockberger RS et al, editors: *Emergency medicine:concepts and clinical practice,* ed 4, St. Louis, 1998, Mosby.

16. Pearlman M, Tintinalli J: *Emergency care of the woman,* New York, 1998, McGraw-Hill.

17. Pirog E: Is cervical adenocarcinoma caused by HPV infection? *Contemp OB/GYN* 46(7):69, 2001.

18. Pointer J, Mulligan-Smith D: Genital Infections. In Rosen P, Barkin RM, Hockberger RS et al, editors: *Emergency medicine:concepts and clinical practice,* ed 4, St. Louis, 1998, Mosby.

19. Poulin C, Alary M, Bernier F et al: Prevalence of *Chlamydia trachomatis* and *Neisseria gonorrhoeae* among at-risk women, young sex workers, and street youth attending community organizations in Quebec city, Canada, *Sex Transm Dis* 28(8):437, 2001.

20. Ringo P: GYN causes of abdominal pain. In Harwood-Nuss A, Wolfson A, editors: *The clinical practice of emergency medicine,* ed 3, Philadelphia, 2001, Lippincott Williams & Wilkins.

21. Rosen P, Barkin R, Hayden S et al: *The 5 minute emergency medicine consult,* Philadelphia, 1999, Lippincott Williams & Wilkins.

22. Shapiro A: Vaginal bleeding. In Swartz G, editors: *Principles and practice of emergency medicine,* ed 4, Baltimore, 1999, Lipincott Williams & Wilkins.

23. Thach A, Young G: Pelvic pain. In Rosen P, Barkin RM, Hockberger RS et al, editors: *Emergency medicine—concepts and clinical practice,* ed 4, St. Louis, 1998, Mosby.

24. Wheeler S: GYN emergencies. In Swartz G, eds: *Principles and practice of emergency medicine,* ed 4, Baltimore, 1999, Lippincott Williams & Wilkins.

25. Wiest D, Spear S, Bartfield J: Empiric treatment of gonorrhea and chlamydia in the ED, *Am J Emerg Med* 19(4)274, 2001.

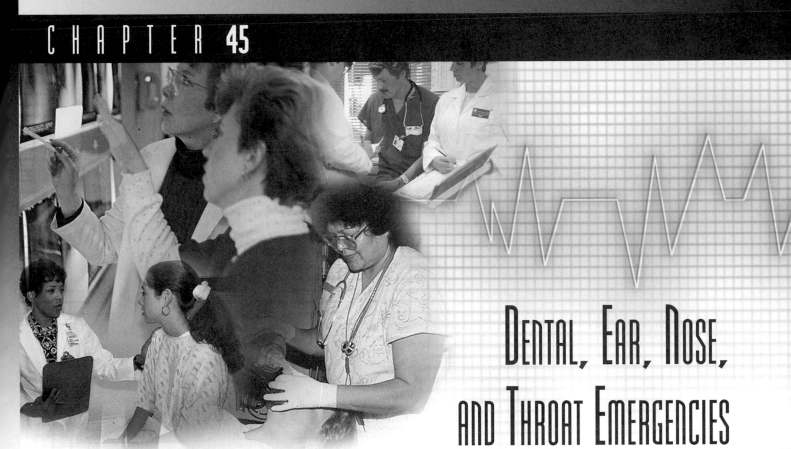

CHAPTER 45

DENTAL, EAR, NOSE, AND THROAT EMERGENCIES

CATHERINE OLSON

Most emergencies of the face, mouth, ears, nose, and throat involve discomfort and pain. However, certain conditions can become life-threatening if associated edema compromises the airway. Infectious processes in the mouth and face can spread to the brain, with potentially fatal systemic effects. Other concerns include loss of function and possible cosmetic deformities. This chapter describes conditions of the face, mouth, ears, nose, and throat that are frequently seen in the emergency department (ED). A brief review of anatomy is provided.

ANATOMY

Structures of the mouth, nose, ears, throat, and face are intimately connected. Injury to one area can affect the others, just as infection from one site can spread to adjacent areas.

Mouth

Dentition consists of two main structures: the teeth and periodontium. Teeth comprise pulp, dentin, enamel, and root (Figure 45-1). The pulp, located at the center of the tooth, provides neurovascular supply and produces dentin. Dentin is a microtubular structure that overlays the pulp, provides hydration, and cushions teeth during mastication. Enamel, which covers the crown, is the visible part of the tooth and the hardest substance in the body. The root anchors the tooth into alveolar tissue and bone. The periodontium is made up

of gingiva and the attachment apparatus. Gingiva, or gums, is a mucous membrane with supporting fibrous tissue encircling the teeth and covering teeth not yet erupted. The attachment apparatus consists of the cementum, periodontal ligament, and alveolar bone.[2] Table 45-1 describes the function of each. In children, onset of primary and permanent teeth is important in determining management of injuries.[22] Normal primary dentition begins erupting at 6 months, with 20 teeth by age 3 years. Permanent dentition begins at 5 to 6 years with eruption of the first molar and is usually completed by age 16 to 18 for a total of 32 teeth.[7]

Ears

The ear is divided into three sections: external, middle, and inner ear (Figure 45-2). The external ear consists of the auricle (pinna), ear canal, and tympanic membrane (TM). The auricle is a cartilaginous appendage attached to each side of the head that collects and directs sound to sensory organs within the ear. The S-shaped ear canal is approximately 2.5 to 3.0 cm long in adults, terminating at the TM. Glands lining the canal secrete cerumen, a yellow, waxy material that lubricates and protects the ear.[10]

The TM, or eardrum, is a thin, translucent, pearly gray oval disk separating the external ear from the middle ear. It protects the middle ear and conducts sound vibrations to the ossicles.[4] On inspection with an otoscopic light, a cone of light at the anteroinferior aspect of the TM should normally

Table 45-1 DENTAL ATTACHMENT APPARATUS	
COMPONENT	**FUNCTION**
Cementum	Functions as connective tissue covering and supporting the root of the tooth
Periodontal ligament	Fibrous structure surrounds and anchors the root into alveolar bone
Alveolar bone	Anchors tooth to oral cavity and gives shape to dentition

Data from Amsterdam JT: Dental disorders. In Rosen P, Barkin RM, Hockberger RS et al, editors: *Emergency medicine: concepts and clinical practice,* ed 4, St. Louis, 1998, Mosby.

be visible. Another landmark is the long process of the malleus (manubrium) pointing posterior and inferior and terminating in the center of the TM (Figure 45-3).

The middle ear, an air-filled cavity inside the temporal bone, consists of the ossicles, windows, and eustachian tube. Three tiny ear bones, or ossicles, are the malleus (hammer), incus (anvil), and stapes (stirrup), so named because of their appearance. Round and oval windows open into the inner ear, where sound vibrations enter. The eustachian tubes connect the middle ear with the nasopharynx, allowing passage of air to equalize pressure on either side of the TM.[13] They also provide drainage for middle ear and inner ear secretions

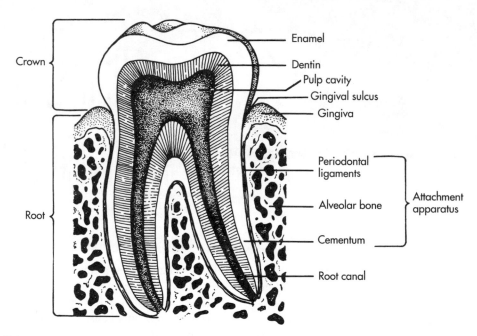

FIGURE **45-1**   Dental anatomic unit and attachment apparatus. (From Rosen P, Barkin RM, Hockberger RS et al: *Emergency medicine: concepts and clinical practice,* ed 4, St. Louis, 1998, Mosby.)

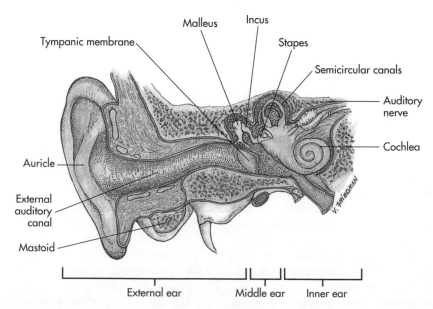

FIGURE **45-2**   Ear structures. (From Potter PA, Perry AG: *Fundamentals of nursing,* ed 5, St. Louis, 2001, Mosby.)

into the nasopharynx.[23] The inner ear contains the bony labyrinth, which holds the sensory organs for equilibrium and hearing.[10]

Nose

Externally, the nose is a triangular, mostly cartilaginous structure that warms, filters, and moistens inhaled air, provides a sense of smell, and is the primary passageway for inhaled air to the lungs (Figure 45-4). The upper third of the

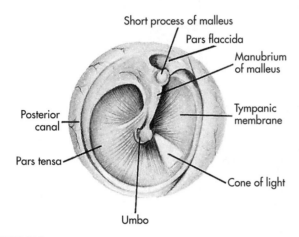

FIGURE **45-3**   Normal tympanic membrane. (From Bowers AC, Thompson JM: *Clinical manual of health assessment,* ed 4, St. Louis, 1992, Mosby.)

nose where the frontal and maxillary bones form the bridge is bony. Two nares at the base of the triangle allow air to enter and pass into the nasopharynx. The internal nose is formed by the palatine (hard palate) bones inferiorly and superiorly by the cribriform plate of the ethmoid bone. Branches of the olfactory nerve pass through the cribriform plate. The nasal cavity is separated by the septum, which forms two anterior vestibules. The septum is usually deviated slightly to one side. Lateral walls are formed by three parallel bony projections—the superior, middle, and inferior turbinates—that help increase surface area to warm inhaled air (Figure 45-5).[26]

Blood supply to the nose originates from the internal and external carotid arteries. The internal maxillary artery branch of the external carotid artery supplies the posterior nasal septum and lateral wall of the nose. As a branch of the internal carotid artery, the anterior ethmoidal artery supplies blood to the anterior septum at Kiesselbach's plexus in Little's area.[26] This area is also supplied by the septal branches on the sphenopalatine and superior labial arteries (Figure 45-6).

Throat

The throat, or pharynx, comprises the nasopharynx, oropharynx, and laryngopharynx (Figure 45-7). The nasopharynx is positioned behind the nasal cavities and extends to the plane of the soft palate. The pharyngeal tonsils, or adenoids, and eustachian tube openings are located in this

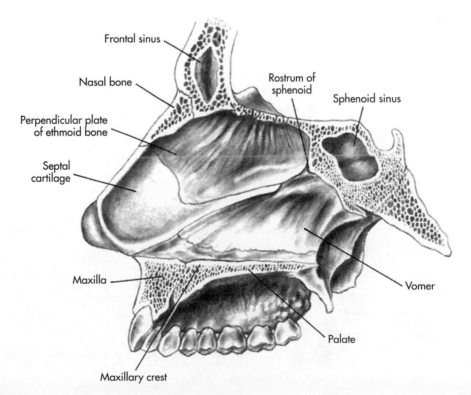

FIGURE **45-4**   Nasal structures. (From Thompson JM, McFarland GK, Hirsch JE et al: *Mosby's clinical nursing,* ed 5, 2001, Mosby.)

area.[8] The oropharynx, a common passageway for both air and food, extends downward from the inferior soft palate to the level of the hyoid bone. The palatine tonsils, lymphoid tissue that filters microorganisms to protect the respiratory and gastrointestinal tracts, are found here. The laryngopharynx extends from the hyoid bone to the opening of the larynx anteriorly and esophagus, posteriorly.[27] The pharynx allows passage of air into the larynx. Pharyngeal constrictor muscles propel food or liquid into the esophagus. These muscles are also responsible for the cough and gag reflex, which are controlled by the cranial nerves. The larynx, or voicebox, is a tubular, mostly cartilaginous structure that connects the trachea and pharynx; its main purpose is to allow air into the trachea. The epiglottis, a large, leaf-shaped piece of cartilage, lies on top of the larynx. This structure prevents aspiration by forming a lid over the glottis (the space between the vocal cords) so that liquids and food are routed into the esophagus and away from the trachea.[27] The larynx is also responsible for voice production via the vocal cords.

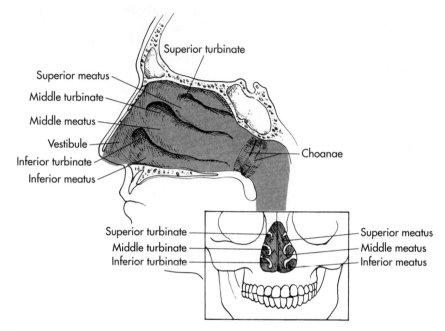

FIGURE 45-5 Nasal turbinates. (From Barkauskas et al: *Health and physical assessment,* ed 2, St. Louis, 1998, Mosby.)

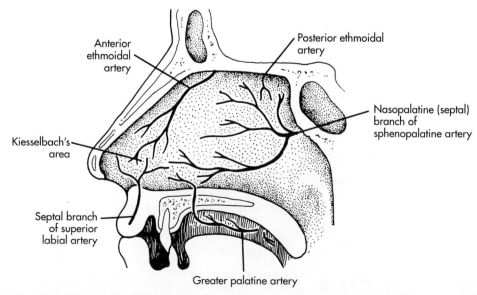

FIGURE 45-6 Arterial supply to nasal septum. (From Rosen P, Barkin RM, Hockberger RS et al: *Emergency medicine: concepts and clinical practice,* ed 4, St. Louis, 1998, Mosby.)

Face

The bony structures of the face are symmetric and consist of a single vomer and mandible and the following pairs of bones: maxillae, palatine, zygomatic, lacrimal, nasal, and inferior nasal conchae. The facial skull forms the shape of the face and provides attachment for muscles that move the jaw and control facial expressions.[27] Cranial nerves V (trigeminal) and VII (facial) are responsible for facial innervation and movement, respectively. The paranasal sinuses are sterile, air-filled pockets situated behind and around the nose, which lighten the weight of the skull, provide resonance for speech, and move secretions into the nasopharynx via ciliated mucous membranes.[10] Four pairs of sinuses are named for their craniofacial location (Figure 45-8). In children younger than 6 years, the sinuses are not fully developed.[26] The ethmoidal and frontal sinuses are fairly well developed between 6 and 7 years and mature along with the maxillary and sphenoidal sinuses during adolescence.[10]

The temporomandibular joint (TMJ) is the point where the mandible connects to the temporal bone of the skull; it can be palpated bilaterally just anterior to the tragus of the ear. The TMJ is a synovial joint that allows hinge action to open and close the jaws, gliding action for protrusion and retraction, and gliding for side to side movement of the lower jaw.[10]

DENTAL EMERGENCIES

Dental emergencies affect the teeth and gums. Specific emergencies involve infection, eruption of new teeth, or trauma. The most common emergencies seen in the ED are related to pain.

Odontalgia

Dental caries are the most frequent cause of dental pain or odontalgia (Figure 45-9).[2] Too much sugar in the diet is largely responsible for decay. Box 45-1 identifies other po-

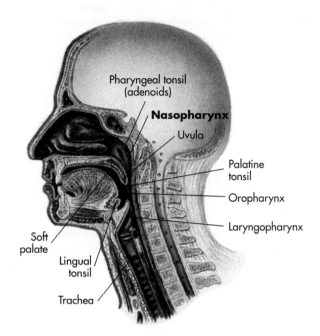

FIGURE 45-7 The pharynx. (From Wilson SF, Thompson JM: *Respiratory disorders,* St. Louis, 1990, Mosby.)

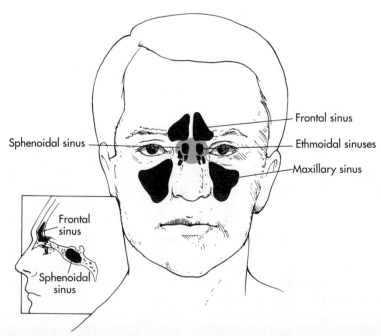

FIGURE 45-8 Paranasal sinuses. (From Barkauskas et al: *Health and physical assessment,* ed 2, St. Louis, 1998, Mosby.)

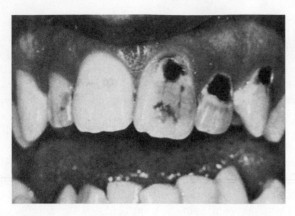

FIGURE 45-9   Dental caries. (From Grundy JR, Jones JG: *A color atlas of clinical operative dentistry crowns and bridges,* ed 2, London, 1992, Wolfe Medical Publishing.)

Box 45-1   COMMON CAUSES OF DENTAL PAIN

Dry socket (postextraction pain)
Fractured teeth
Hematoma from anesthetic injection
Maxillary sinusitis
Pericoronitis secondary to erupting wisdom teeth
Periodontal (gum) disease
Postroot canal surgery
Prosthetic device pressure
Unerupted teeth—especially in children

---

tential causes of dental pain. Dental caries are also caused by poor oral hygiene, which allows bacterial plaque to develop, which in turn form acids that break down and decalcify tooth enamel. Sodium fluoride, found in toothpaste, oral rinses, and public drinking water, helps stabilize the integrity of tooth enamel to prevent this breakdown. Affected teeth are usually tender to percussion and sensitive to heat, cold, or air.[19] If left untreated, decay progresses and invades dentin and pulp, eventually producing a hyperemic response. The pulp becomes inflamed, leading to pulpitis and finally pulpal necrosis. Occasionally, pus leaks from the apex of the affected tooth as a periapical abscess forms.[1] Toothaches accompanied by facial or neck swelling should be assessed and promptly treated to prevent spread of infection. Clinical management includes antibiotics, topical anesthetics, nerve blocks, and analgesics including parenteral narcotics as palliative treatment until the patient receives definitive care from the dentist.[2]

Tooth Eruption

Between 6 months and 3 years of age, children's primary teeth erupt, causing a variety of symptoms including pain, irritability, disrupted sleep, nasal discharge, and crying. Increased salivary gland production causes diarrhea as well as significant drooling.[1] Decreased fluid intake related to dental pain may cause dehydration and low-grade fever of 37.9° C (100.6° F). Care must be taken not to attribute sig-

nificant fevers to this relatively benign process.[1] Tonsillar or throat infections, thrush, other oral lesions, and respiratory emergencies such as epiglottitis (especially with excessive drooling) should be considered. In the second decade of life, third molars, or wisdom teeth, begin erupting, causing pain in adolescents and adults. Gingival inflammation secondary to wisdom tooth eruption may cause pericoronitis.

Topical anesthetics such as benzocaine are used sparingly to prevent sterile abscess formation. Acetaminophen is useful for analgesia in young children. To maintain hydration, popsicles are usually well received and also provide pain relief. When there is minimal oral intake, a bolus of intravenous fluids may be necessary. In adults frequent saline irrigation may be used to remove debris from the affected tooth. Nonnarcotic analgesia is effective for pain relief in adult patients. Any consistent swelling or drainage from the eruption site requires referral to a dentist or oral surgeon.

Pericoronitis

If erupting molars become impacted or crowded, food and debris lodge under the pericoronal flap, causing gingival inflammation or pericoronitis. Pericoronitis is extremely painful, especially with opening and closing of the mouth. Earache on the affected side, sore throat, and fever may also occur.[2] Surrounding tissues appear red and inflamed with submandibular lymphadenopathy and trismus noted in some patients.

Warm saline or peroxide irrigation and mouth rinses are helpful in early stages of pericoronitis. When pus is present, incision and drainage may be necessary. Antibiotic therapy, usually penicillin or erythromycin, is indicated. Follow-up with an oral-maxillofacial surgeon within 24 to 48 hours for removal of the affected third molar is highly recommended.[2]

Fractured Tooth

The most frequently seen dental emergency in the ED is a chipped or broken tooth, usually anterior maxillary teeth. Trauma to dentition occurs as a result of sports activity, motor vehicle collisions, propulsive objects, falls, convulsive seizures, and physical assaults or abuse. With children, it should be noted that 50% of physical trauma in child abuse occurs in the head and neck region.[18] The emergency nurse should assess for concurrent head injury or maxillofacial trauma. Aspiration of a tooth or fragment or an embedded tooth should also be considered. Management of fractures of the anterior teeth is determined by the relationship of the fracture to the pulp as well as patient age.[2] The Ellis classification system is used to describe location of tooth fractures. Class I fractures are the most common, involving only enamel. Injured areas appear chalky white. Cosmetic restoration is possible with dental referral within 24 to 48 hours. Class II fractures pass through the enamel and expose dentin. The fracture area appears ivory-yellow. Fractures are urgent for children because there is little dentin to protect pulp. Bacteria pass easily into pulp, causing an infection or

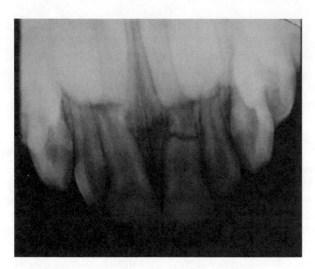

FIGURE 45-10 This radiograph reveals a root fracture in the apical third of an upper primary incisor. This was suspected clinically because of tenderness and increased mobility. (From Zitelli B, Davis H: *Atlas of pediatric physical diagnosis,* ed 3, St. Louis, 1997, Mosby.)

abscess if exposed for longer than 6 hours.[22] Adults may be treated up to 24 hours later because the pulp is protected by a thicker layer of dentin, which reduces potential for infection. Place warm, moist cotton covered by dry gauze over the exposed area as needed for discomfort secondary to thermal sensitivity. Class III fractures are a dental emergency (Figure 45-10). Injury to the enamel, dentin, and pulp cause a pink or bloody tinge to the fractured area. Exposure of pulp also exposes the nerve, causing significant discomfort. Again, dry gauze can be used to minimize discomfort from thermal sensitivity. Some practitioners apply a layer of zinc oxide or calcium hydroxide to exposed dentin, which is then covered with dental foil.[18] The patient should be referred to a dentist with follow-up within 24 hours. Oral analgesics or a nerve block are usually effective for pain control. Tetanus immunizations should be administered as appropriate. Reassure the patient that cosmetic restoration is possible with enamel-bonding plastic materials.[2]

With facial trauma, assess the airway, breathing, and circulation (ABCs) before assessing the dental problem. History should include mechanism of injury, concomitant injuries, and tissue loss. Consider abuse in children, the elderly, or disabled adults when the history does not correlate to the injury. Assess for tooth pain, thermal sensitivity, stability of the tooth in the socket, and malocclusion. Complications of tooth fractures include infection (pulpitis), malocclusion, embedded tooth fragments, aspiration of tooth fragments, color change, or loss of affected teeth.

Tooth Avulsion

Tooth avulsion is a dental emergency. When a tooth has been torn from the socket, tissue hypoxia develops, followed by eventual necrosis of the pulp.[17] Reimplantation within 30 minutes greatly increases chances for reimplantation and healing. The periodontal ligament cells die if the tooth is out of the socket for more than 60 minutes. Determine the mechanism and time of injury immediately on arrival. Handle the avulsed tooth by the crown to avoid damage to attached periodontal ligament fragments. These fragments aid in healing of the reimplanted tooth.[22] Ideally, the tooth should be rinsed and placed back in the socket as soon as possible. Immediate reimplantation is not always possible because of lack of patient cooperation, life-threatening injuries, or other factors at the scene of injury. In these cases the tooth should be transported in Hank's solution (pH-preserving fluid), milk, saline, or under the tongue of an alert patient. Use discretion with children, who may swallow or aspirate the tooth. Primary teeth (6 months to 6 years) are not reimplanted because fusion with the bone interferes with permanent tooth eruption and can cause cosmetic deformities.[2] If the tooth cannot be found, examine the oral cavity and face to ensure the tooth is not embedded in soft tissue. A chest x-ray is recommended to rule out tooth aspiration.

Symptoms include pain and bleeding at the site of the avulsion. Assess for concomitant head, neck, or maxillofacial injuries. Moist saline gauze may be applied to exposed oral tissues for comfort and to control bleeding. Administer analgesics and tetanus prophylaxis as indicated. Instruct the patient not to bite into anything with the affected tooth and to avoid hot or cold substances.[1] Referral to a dentist or oral surgeon for definitive care is recommended.

Dental Abscess

Primary dental abscesses are periapical and periodontal. Periapical abscesses occur as an extension of pulpal necrosis from a decayed tooth or traumatic injury. A pocket of plaque and food debris between the tooth and the gingiva cause localized swelling at the apex of the tooth, which leads to periodontal abscess formation.[19] Normally abscesses are confined; however, certain infectious processes can spread to facial planes of the head and neck.[2] The upper half of the face is affected with extension of infection from the maxillary teeth. Cellulitis in the lower half of the face and neck extends from the infection of the mandibular teeth.[2] With localized abscesses the patient may have severe pain unrelieved by analgesics, fever, malaise, foul breath odor, and slight facial swelling near the affected tooth. An extensive abscess causes facial and neck edema, trismus, dysphagia, difficulty handling secretions, and potential airway obstruction.

Oral or parenteral narcotics, antipyretics, and antibiotics such as penicillin or erythromycin are recommended.[9] If abscess fluctuance is present, incision and drainage with culture and sensitivity of the exudate are required. The patient should be instructed to take medications as directed, use warm saline rinses, and follow up with an oral surgeon, dentist, or ear, nose, and throat specialist within 24 to 48 hours for definitive care. Admission for further diagnostic studies and intravenous antibiotics may be necessary if the patient has abnormal vital signs or is unable to take oral medications.[19]

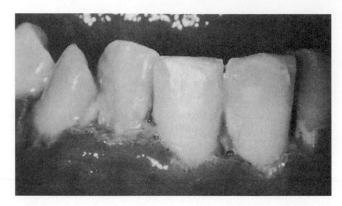

FIGURE 45-11   Acute necrotizing ulcerative gingivitis involving lower anterior teeth. (From Rosen P, Barkin RM, Hockberger RS et al: *Emergency medicine: concepts and clinical practice,* ed 4, St. Louis, 1998, Mosby.)

Gingivitis

Gingivitis, or inflammation of the gums, is usually caused by poor dental hygiene, allowing for the accumulation of food debris and plaque in crevices between the gums and teeth. This periodontal disease, along with periodontitis (loss of supporting bony structure of the teeth) affects approximately two thirds of young adults and 80% of middle-age and older adults. A large percentage of children are also affected.[29] It is the most common cause of tooth loss today.[3] Gingivitis may also occur with vitamin C deficiency or in pregnancy and puberty because of changing hormone levels.[10] If inflammation continues, alveolar bone is lost, leading to periodontitis and eventual loss of teeth. Visual evidence of gingivitis includes red, swollen gum margins and possible bleeding. Pain unrelieved by over-the-counter analgesics, difficulty chewing, and low-grade fever also occur. Topical anesthetics, analgesics, and oral antibiotic therapy are indicated. Patient teaching regarding good oral hygiene, including brushing and flossing three to four times a day with peroxide and warm water rinses every hour, is extremely important to prevent extension of gingivitis. Figure 45-11 shows a complication of chronic gingivitis.

Ludwig's Angina

Ludwig's angina is the spread of an existing, untreated dental infection or cellulitis into three mandibular spaces: submandibular, sublingual, and submental. Infection spreads downward from the jaw to the mediastinum and is characterized by bilateral, boardlike, brawny induration of involved tissues and elevation of the tongue. The inherent danger with Ludwig's angina is respiratory distress and airway obstruction.[19]

The patient develops significant swelling of the anterior and lateral neck. Swelling of the submandibular tissue displaces the tongue superiorly. Other symptoms include pain and tenderness, trismus, muffled voice, dysphagia, drooling, and fever or chills. Dyspnea and decreased oxygen pressure occur secondary to edematous tissues. The patient may be anxious or restless. Offer reassurance, check the patient frequently, and explain all procedures to ease fears.

Priorities in the ED include maintaining ABCs, pain relief, and intravenous antibiotics. Elevate the head of the bed to prevent aspiration of secretions. Administer supplemental oxygen in concert with continuous pulse oximetry monitoring. Respiratory and mental status should be continuously monitored. Provide prescribed analgesics appropriate for the patient's degree of pain. Insert an intravenous catheter for IV fluids to prevent dehydration, administer antibiotic therapy (usually high-dose penicillin), and as an access for emergency medications. Diagnostic procedures such as arterial blood gases, complete blood count (CBC) with differential, erythrocyte sedimentation rate, culture and sensitivity of exudate, and soft tissue x-rays or computed tomography (CT) scan of the neck may be ordered.[19] Definitive care by an oral-maxillofacial surgeon includes determining site of the initial infection, surgical drainage of pus with removal of necrotic tissue, and continued antibiotic therapy.[2]

EAR EMERGENCIES

Ear emergencies commonly seen in the ED involve infection, pain, foreign body in the ear canal, or injury of the TM. Most ear emergencies require instillation of some type of otic drops (Figure 45-12).

Otitis

Otitis, or inflammation of the ear, may occur in any section of the ear. Symptoms vary with location; however, almost all cases of acute otitis cause significant discomfort.[24]

Otitis externa is inflammation of the external ear canal and auricle. Also known as swimmer's ear, this condition is seen most often during the summer. Table 45-2 summarizes factors that predispose the patient to otitis externa. The infectious agent is usually bacteria such as *Pseudomonas* species, *Proteus vulgaris,* streptococci, and *Staphylococcus aureus.* Symptoms include pain, swelling, redness, and purulent drainage of the auricle and ear canal (Figure 45-13). Pain is usually worsened by chewing or movement of the tragus or pinna. Regional cellulitis, partial hearing loss, and lymphadenopathy may also be present. Basic treatment measures cure 90% of patients without complications.[30] Treatment includes keeping the ear dry; applying heat with a heating pad, heating lamp, or warm, moist compresses; and providing analgesics and antibiotics. Topical or otic antibiotics are used unless the patient has a persistent fever or regional cellulitis, in which case admission and high-dose antibiotic therapy is needed.[30] Otitis externa usually resolves in 7 days but frequently recurs. Parents should be instructed to use earplugs to protect the ear canal from water for 2 to 4 weeks.[23]

Otitis media (OM), or infection of the middle ear, occurs most often in children between 6 months and 3 years of age, and is usually preceded by a viral upper respiratory infection

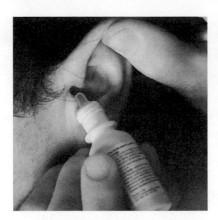
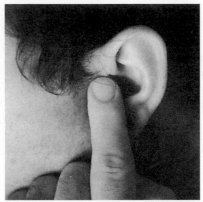

FIGURE **45-12**   Ear drop instillation. Turn the head to the side so that the affected ear faces upward. The orifice is exposed, and the drops of medicine are directed toward the internal wall of the canal. The pinna is pulled up and back in a person older than 3 years of age and down and back in a younger child. The tragus is then pushed against the ear canal to ensure that the drops stay in the canal. (From Potter PA, Perry AG: *Fundamentals of nursing,* ed 5, St. Louis, 2001, Mosby.)

Table 45-2	PREDISPOSING FACTORS FOR OTITIS EXTERNA
PREDISPOSING FACTOR	**DESCRIPTION**
Swimming in contaminated water	Cerumen creates a culture medium for microorganisms found in the contaminated water.
Cleaning the ear canal with a foreign object	Objects such as hairpins can irritate the ear canal and introduce microorganisms.
Exposure to chemical irritants	Chemicals such as hair dye can cause an allergic irritation and inflammation.
Regular use of earphones, earplugs, or earmuffs	These devices trap moisture in the ear and create a culture medium for bacteria and other organisms.
Perforated TM	Chronic drainage from a ruptured TM can lead to infection.

TM, Tympanic membrane.

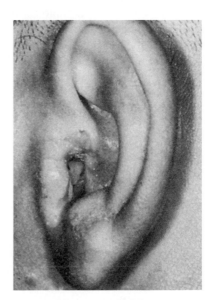

FIGURE **45-13**   Acute external otitis. Note swelling of the ear canal and lymphadenopathy in front of the tragus. (From Deweese DD et al: *Otolaryngology: head and neck surgery,* ed 8, St. Louis, 1994, Mosby.)

(URI).[28] *Streptococcus pneumoniae* and *Haemophilus influenzae* are the most common causative organisms. Acute OM is characterized by rapid onset of ear pain, headache, tinnitus, hearing loss, and nausea or vomiting. Infants and young children may present with irritability, crying, rubbing or pulling the ears, restless sleep, and lethargy. Other symptoms such as fever, rhinitis, cough, otorrhea secondary to rupture of the TM, and conjunctivitis occur at any age.[28] Visualization of the TM, necessary for diagnosis, usually reveals a distorted light reflex and whitish-yellow opacity. Bulging may also occur as the infection progresses.[15] Redness of the TM is an inconsistent finding because it may be caused by crying or fever.[28] Sinusitis and purulent rhinitis frequently accompany otitis in children and infants.[31] Uncomplicated acute OM is treated with antibiotics, antipyretics, and analgesics such as acetaminophen or ibuprofen.

Topical anesthetic otic solutions (e.g., Auralgan) for pain relief should be warmed before instilling. If not treated promptly, acute OM can cause serious complications such as ruptured TM, meningitis, acute mastoiditis, intracranial abscess, neck abscess, facial nerve damage, or permanent hearing loss.[28] Patients should complete the full course of antibiotic therapy and be reevaluated if there is no improvement in 48 to 72 hours.[30] Encourage parents to ensure children finish prescribed medications and to keep follow-up appointment. Children should be reevaluated in 14 to 21 days to confirm the infection has been eradicated or to determine if middle ear effusion (serous OM) persists. Chronic or persistent pediatric OM may require prophylactic antibiotics or referral to an otolaryngologist for myringotomy tube placement if intractable pain is present.

Labyrinthitis, or inflammation of the inner ear, is rare. Causes include acute febrile illness and chronic otitis media. The inner ear is the body's center of balance. The patient usually develops severe vertigo with nausea and vomiting, but without tinnitus and hearing loss. Vertigo usually lasts 3 to 5 days but may persist for weeks. Treatment includes bed rest, meclizine (Antivert) to control vertigo, and fluids for dehydration secondary to vomiting. Antibiotics are indicated for purulent labyrinthitis.

Ruptured Tympanic Membrane

A ruptured TM is most often the painful result of a bacterial infection—acute or chronic OM. Trauma such as skull fracture, foreign body insertion (e.g., cotton swabs, hair pins), explosions, or blows to the ear also rupture the TM. Children, especially those with chronic ear infections, are most often victims of this disorder. Symptoms include pain, bloody or purulent discharge, hearing loss, vertigo, and fever. Or the patient may be pain free because pain and pressure are relieved with rupture. In trauma-related TM rupture, ear drainage should be checked for the presence of cerebrospinal fluid, which is indicative of basilar skull fracture.[6] Otoscopic examination reveals the TM as slit-shaped or irregular. X-rays of the skull, temporal bone, and cervical spine may be indicated with trauma. Hearing loss may be present in the affected ear, so speak slowly and clearly toward the unaffected ear while facing the patient. Large perforations require myringoplasty. If the middle ear is also involved, a tympanoplasty is performed.[4] More than 90% of perforations heal spontaneously.[29]

Management includes antibiotics, analgesics, and antipyretics. Carefully clean the ear canal of blood or debris with gentle suction, and obtain a culture and sensitivity of drainage. Irrigation is contraindicated with TM rupture. Instillation of antibiotic ear drops is generally not necessary.[29] The patient should be instructed to keep water out of the ears because this provides an environment conducive to bacterial or fungal growth. A piece of cotton lightly coated with petroleum jelly and placed in the affected ear helps repel water. The patient should follow up with an otolaryngologist for definitive care.

Foreign Body

Cerumen is the most common obstructive material seen in children's ears, often caused by cotton swabs pushing wax and cotton fibers deeper into the ear canal.[5] Therefore remind parents to put "nothing smaller than an elbow into the ear."[25] Cerumen is a yellow-brown, waxy material that obstructs view of the TM and must be removed. Adults, especially older patients, are also prone to impacted cerumen. In nursing home patients the estimated incidence of cerumen impaction is almost 40%. Use of hearing aids is a contribut-

---

| Box 45-2 | IRRIGATION OF THE EAR |

EQUIPMENT

Warm tap water or 1:1 solution of hydrogen peroxide/warm water
30 cc or 60 cc syringe
Large-bore angiocath with needle removed or butterfly needle tubing cut about 3 cm from the hub
Basin to collect fluid
Towels and absorbent pad

PROCEDURE

With patient in sitting position, protect clothing with towels or pads. Tilt head with affected ear up and provide a basin to hold under the ear to be irrigated.

Place warmed 98.6° F (37° C) solution in a sterile basin and put on gloves.

Straighten ear canal by method appropriate for age.

Using 30-60 cc of solution at a time, direct stream superiorly against ear canal wall to exert back pressure on FB/cerumen, thus driving it outward, never directly against TM because rupture may occur. May require several attempts with frequent otoscopic exams to determine effectiveness of irrigation.

Discontinue procedure immediately if patient complains of dizziness, nausea, or pain.

After irrigation, dry the external canal with a cotton ball. Have patient lie with the affected side down to drain excess fluid.

Alternatively, a Water-pik device designed for dental use may be used for irrigation; however, this practice is not recommended because of excessive uncontrolled fluid pressure on the TM.

(Commercial otic devices are also available.)

From Freeman FB: Impacted cerumen: how to safely remove earwax in an office visit, *Geriatrics* 50(6):52, 1995.
FB, Foreign body; *TM*, tympanic membrane.

---

ing factor because of increased cerumen production and obstruction of natural outflow from the ear.[7]

The patient who presents with a foreign body in the ear is most often a child 9 months to 4 years of age.[25] Beads, small stones, beans, corn, and dry cereal are common culprits. Parents, often unaware of the foreign body, bring the child to the ED with an earache or purulent, foul-smelling ear discharge. Older children and adults may complain of decreased hearing and fullness in the affected ear. Insects, including roaches, can fly or crawl into the ear and become trapped, moving and buzzing in the ear, causing great distress and anxiety for the patient. Children with insects in the ear may be extremely frightened.

Before attempting removal of impacted cerumen or a foreign body, evaluate for a history of ruptured TM or current infection. Explain the procedure to the patient in terms that are appropriate for his or her age. Cooperation is elicited from a child whose trust is not violated. Conscious sedation or restraints may be required in difficult situa-

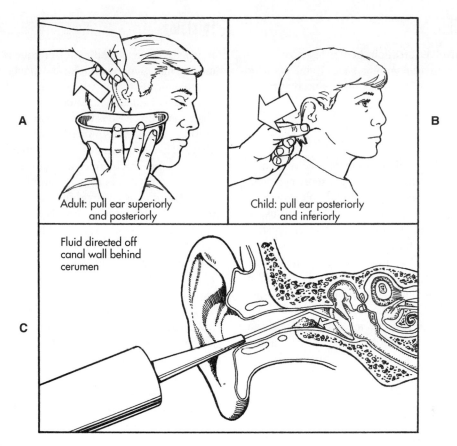

FIGURE **45-14**   Ear irrigation. **A,** The external auditory canal in the adult can best be exposed by pulling the earlobe upward and backward. **B,** The same exposure can be achieved in the child by gently pulling the auricle of the ear downward and backward. **C,** An enlarged diagram showing the direction of irrigating fluid against the side of the canal. NOTE: This is more effective in dislodging cerumen than if the flow of solution were directed straight into the canal.

tions.[15] Methods for foreign body removal include suctioning, irrigation, or use of special tools under direction visualization. A good light source such as an operating otoscope or head lamp is imperative for these procedures. To best expose the ear canal, pull the auricle up and back for adults, down and back for children. Vegetables or other soft materials that may absorb water should not be irrigated. Subsequent swelling caused by water absorption makes removal more difficult. Live insects can be killed by placing a few drops of mineral oil in the ear, or by filling the ear canal with 2% lidocaine. The dead insect can then be removed with direct instrumentation.[14] If removal is difficult, referral to an ear, nose, and throat (ENT) specialist within 24 hours is recommended.

Irrigation, often the safest[11] and most effective method for removal of impacted cerumen, is contraindicated with a history of TM rupture, infection, a soft or vegetable-like foreign body, or in children younger than age 5. Any solutions for the ear should be warmed to 98.6° F (37° C) before instillation to prevent inner ear stimulation, which may cause dizziness, nausea, and vomiting.[7] Suggested guidelines for ear irrigation are described in Box 45-2 and illustrated in Figure 45-14.

Other methods of foreign body removal include use of an ear curette, right-angle hook, Frazier suction catheter, soft flexible catheter with funnel-shaped tip, and alligator forceps (Figure 45-15).[6] Surfactant ear drops (i.e., Cerumenex, glycerin and peroxide) may soften cerumen for easier removal. If an impacted foreign body cannot be removed, refer the patient to an ENT specialist within 24 hours. Emergent referral is necessary with severe pain or presence of a caustic foreign body substance.[15] Antibiotics may be prescribed to prevent or treat an existing infection. Complications include hearing loss, TM rupture, and acute OM or otitis externa from injury during attempted foreign body removal or from retained foreign body material.

NASAL EMERGENCIES

Nasal emergencies involve infection, hemorrhage, or a foreign body. Most problems are minor such as infection or nasal fracture. However, life-threatening hemorrhage can also occur.

Rhinitis

Rhinitis is inflammation of nasal mucosa that usually accompanies the common cold. Acute rhinitis, the most prevalent disease among all age groups, is spread by droplet contact.[9] Upper respiratory viruses such as rhinovirus, adenovirus, or influenza virus are the most common causative organisms. Symptoms include copious, mucopurulent nasal secretions, red and swollen nasal mucosa, mild fever, and decreased sense of smell. Allergic rhinitis (hay fever) may be perennial or seasonal—caused by pollens, grasses, trees, or flowers. Perennial allergic rhinitis is a chronic condition caused by environmental factors such as dust, animal dander, mold, and foods.[17] Perennial rhinitis is characterized by nasal mucosa that appears pale to bluish and swollen, tearing, periorbital edema, and thin, watery nasal discharge.

The single most effective treatment for all forms of rhinitis is warm saline irrigation; however, not all patients are willing to continue this treatment on their own.[21] Systemic or topical antihistamines are used to shrink swollen nasal tissues. Box 45-3 describes effective use of nasal spray. Analgesics and antipyretics are administered as necessary. The patient should be instructed to drink plenty of clear fluids, humidify the home environment, avoid allergens, and rest. Complications associated with rhinitis include serous otitis media, nasal polyps, sinusitis, and exacerbation of asthma. Excessive use of topical medications and nose blowing may cause epistaxis.[21]

Epistaxis

Epistaxis, or nosebleed, is seen frequently in the ED. Causes include infection, trauma, local irritants, foreign bodies, anticoagulant drug therapy, hypertension, congenital or disease-induced coagulation disorders, and tumors. However, the most common cause is nose picking. Bleeding may occur anteriorly or posteriorly. Anterior bleeding is usually acute and almost always originates at Kiesselbach's plexus in Little's area, a highly vascularized area of the nose (see Figure 45-6). Posterior epistaxis is usually chronic and common in the elderly. Bleeding is more profuse, involving posterior branches of the sphenopalatine artery. Hypertension as the cause of epistaxis may be undetected if blood loss lowers blood pressure to normal.[21] In mild cases bleeding may stop spontaneously within minutes or by simply pinching the nares. Bleeding may be profuse and continuous with a potential for hypovolemia, requiring aggressive management.

The patient usually presents clutching bloody tissues or towels to the nose and can be extremely anxious. A calm, reassuring systematic approach by the emergency nurse helps ease anxiety and allows efficient management. Obtain a quick history, including duration, frequency, and amount of bleeding, recent trauma or surgery, nausea or vomiting, recreational drug use, and pertinent medical history. All staff caring for this patient should observe universal precautions

---

Box 45-3 **USING NASAL SPRAYS EFFECTIVELY**

Spray each nostril, and then lie supine for 2 minutes. Repeat the procedure.
The first dose shrinks nasal mucosa, which allows the second dose to reach the upper turbinates and sinus ostia.[4]
Using nasal sprays just prior to bedtime may enhance relief.[20]

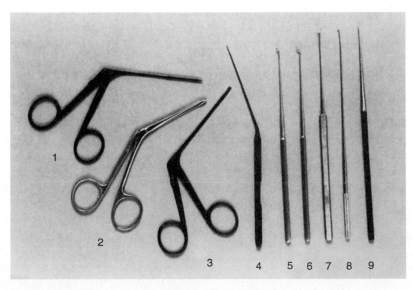

FIGURE **45-15** Useful ear foreign body tools. *1,* Alligator forceps; *2,* Hartman ear forceps; *3,* cupped forceps; *4,* Schuknecht pick; *5,* small Buck curette; *6,* large Buck curette; *7,* Sharpleigh curette; *8,* Day hook; *9,* Turner needle. (From Cummings CW et al: *Otolaryngology: head and neck surgery,* ed 3, vol 4, St. Louis, 1998, Mosby.)

including gloves, goggles, mask, and gown, because potential for blood splashing is high.

Maintain the patient in an upright seated position with the head tilted downward and nostrils pinched. Assess ABCs and initiate appropriate interventions such as suction, intravenous access, cardiac monitor, and oxygen saturation monitor. Obtain CBC, prothrombin time, partial thromboplastin time, and type and cross-match as ordered. The bleeding site is determined after clearing the nose of clots by having the patient blow the nose or with suction using an 8F or 10F Frazier catheter. A nasal speculum is required to visualize the posterior nasal cavity. Treatment of anterior epistaxis begins with identification of the bleeding site followed by application of topical vasoconstrictors (i.e., 2% to 5% cocaine hydrochloride, Neo-Synephrine), direct pressure for 5 to 10 minutes, chemical (silver nitrate) or electrical cautery, and packing if necessary.[20] Nasal packing may be done with standard petro-

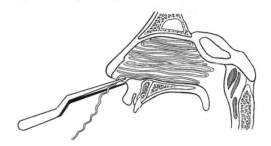

FIGURE 45-16 Anterior nasal packing.

latum-iodoform gauze (Figure 45-16) or newer commercial products such as the Merocel nasal sponge or Gelfoam, which eventually dissolve and do not require removal. Coat packing material with antibiotic ointment before insertion to help prevent sinusitis and toxic shock.[21] Anterior nasal packing is left in place 24 to 72 hours. The patient should follow up with an otolaryngologist or return to the ED immediately for persistent bleeding or dislodged nasal packing.[19]

With posterior epistaxis, bleeding is much more difficult to control. Direct pressure is ineffective, and packing often difficult. A posterior nasal pack should be inserted in anyone with posterior nasal hemorrhage (Figure 45-17).[20] Devices such as a Merocel nasal sponge, Nasostat epistaxis balloon (Figure 45-18), or 12F to 16F urinary catheter with the distal tip cut off can be used for posterior packing. These devices should be removed in 2 to 3 days. Posterior nasal packing predisposes the patient to respiratory obstruction, so admission is necessary for airway monitoring, sedation, antibiotic therapy, and humidified oxygen. Surgical ligation of vessels may be required for control of severe posterior epistaxis.[21] Antihypertensive agents may be needed for patients whose blood pressure remains elevated.

Complications of anterior and posterior epistaxis include hypoxia, dislodged nasal packing, airway occlusion, hypovolemia, severe discomfort, sinusitis, toxic shock, cardiac dysrhythmias, and respiratory or cardiac arrest. With severe blood loss, blood transfusion may be necessary. Figure 45-19

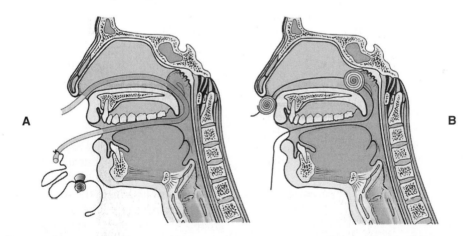

FIGURE 45-17 Method for placing posterior nasal pack. **A,** Catheter is passed through the bleeding side of the nose and pulled out through the mouth with a hemostat. Strings are tied to the catheter and the pack is pulled up behind the soft palate and into the nasopharynx. **B,** Nasal pack in position in the posterior nasopharynx. Dental roll of the nose helps to maintain correct position. (From Lewis SM, Heitkemper MM, Dirksen SR: *Medical-surgical nursing: assessment and management of clinical problems,* ed 5, St. Louis, 2000, Mosby.)

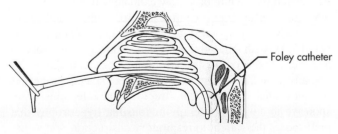

Foley catheter

FIGURE 45-18 Nasal packing for severe epistaxis.

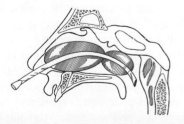

FIGURE 45-19 Anterior and posterior nasal balloon tamponade for control of both anterior and posterior epistaxis.

illustrates anterior and posterior nasal packing. Posterior epistaxis is often associated with significant atherosclerosis and can precipitate myocardial or cerebral infarction.[21]

Foreign Body

A foreign body in the nose usually occurs in children and is often discovered when a purulent nasal discharge is noticed.[5,19] Usually self-inserted, foreign bodies in the nose may also occur with trauma. Nasal cavities are easily expanded, so unusual, large, or multiple retained foreign bodies are possible. The patient may present with pain and fullness from a recently placed foreign body or with purulent, foul-smelling nasal discharge, recurrent epistaxis, sinus pain, fever, and edematous nasal mucosa.[9] Care should be taken to prevent damage to the highly vascular nasal septum and mucosa during removal of a nasal foreign body. Children may require conscious sedation or a papoose board for restraint. Ask the cooperative patient to occlude the unobstructed nostril, close the mouth, and make a forceful nasal exhalation at least 15 times.[16] If unsuccessful, apply a topical anesthetic agent and place the patient in Trendelenburg position. The object is then removed with alligator or ring forceps.[19] A Harman forceps, wire loop, or suction foreign body catheter may prove helpful. Extreme care must be taken not to dislodge or drive the foreign body deeper into the nasopharynx because aspiration may occur.[12] Complications such as epistaxis, septal hematoma, septal perforation, or inability to remove the foreign body should be referred to an otolaryngologist. (Refer to Chapter 28 for discussion of septal hematoma and nasal trauma.)

THROAT EMERGENCIES

Throat emergencies represent a threat to the patient's airway. The emergency nurse should evaluate the patient's ABCs carefully and monitor for significant changes in breathing and mentation. (Refer to Chapter 48 for assessment and management of epiglottitis.)

Pharyngitis

Pharyngitis, inflammation of the pharynx, often accompanies the common cold. Symptoms include bright red throat, swollen tonsils, white or yellow exudate on tonsils and pharynx, swollen uvula, and enlarged, tender cervical and tonsillar nodes.[8] The patient may complain of sore throat, fever, dysphagia, and halitosis (foul breath odor). Treatment for pharyngitis depends on underlying pathology.[4] A throat culture and sensitivity should be obtained to distinguish bacterial or viral cause. Many EDs use a rapid strep test to screen for streptococcal infections. Most sore throats in adults are viral and do not warrant antibiotics.[7] For bacterial pharyngitis (i.e, streptococcal pharyngitis) treatment consists of antibiotics, antipyretics, and analgesics. Encourage the patient to gargle frequently with warm saline. Stress the importance of bed rest, increased fluid intake, and completing the full

course of antibiotics. Tonsillectomy, or removal of tonsils, may be necessary in severe cases. Complications include retropharyngeal abscess, glomerular nephritis, and subacute bacterial endocarditis resulting from invasion of group A β-hemolytic streptococci.[17]

Laryngitis

Acute laryngitis, inflammation of the vocal cords, may accompany URI or can exist alone. Causes of acute laryngitis include overuse, allergies, irritants, and viral or bacterial infections.[9] Tension in the vocal cords determines the amount of vibration produced when air flows upward through the glottis. Anything that alters this tension affects the ability to speak.[17] The patient presents with partial or complete voice loss, with or without URI symptoms. Dyspnea or stridor should be evaluated and treated immediately as potential airway obstruction. Throat culture and CBC are the usual diagnostic procedures. Treatment includes voice rest, steam inhalations to thin secretions and improve moisture, increased fluid intake, and topical anesthetic throat lozenges.[7] Patient teaching should emphasize preventive therapy; avoiding airway irritants such as cigarette smoke and loud or excessive use of the voice. Gastroesophageal reflux resulting from excess acid production may also be responsible. This can be treated with diet, antacid, and H_2 inhibitors.[17] In the presence of infection administer antibiotics and instruct the patient to complete the entire course. Aspirin is contraindicated for analgesia because of its anticoagulant properties, which increase the risk of vocal cord hemorrhage and subsequent scarring and changes in voice quality.[15] Complications of laryngitis are aspiration pneumonia, decreased cough reflex, and airway compromise or obstruction.

Tonsillitis

Tonsillitis refers to inflammation of the palatine tonsils. Tonsils are lymphatic tissue that filters bacteria and other microorganisms to protect the respiratory and gastrointestinal tract.[7] Approximately 30% of tonsillitis cases are caused by group A β-hemolytic streptococci or staphylococci.[17] Viruses are also a leading cause of this contagious, airborne infection. Symptoms are similar to pharyngitis and may include a feeling of fullness in the throat, malaise, otalgia (ear pain), and swollen lymph nodes in the neck.[17] The patient may have difficulty speaking or swallowing. The tonsils may be covered by a white or yellow exudate and the patient can have foul breath. Rapid strep test, throat culture and sensitivity, CBC, monospot test, and chest radiograph may be ordered.[7] As with pharyngitis, warm saline gargles, topical anesthetic lozenges, analgesics, antipyretics, and antibiotics (usually penicillin or erythromycin) are indicated. Surgery is recommended for recurrent streptococcal infections unresponsive to antibiotic therapy or tonsillar hypertrophy that predisposes the patient to respiratory obstruction or dysphagia. Retropharyngeal and peritonsillar abscess, glomerular nephritis, and subacute bacterial endocarditis are potential complications of tonsillitis.[17]

Peritonsillar Abscess

Untreated acute or chronic suppurative tonsillitis may evolve into a peritonsillar abscess, or quinsy, caused by a perforated tonsillar capsule and extension of the infection along deeper muscle planes.[18] The abscess is usually unilateral with dysphagia, drooling, muffled voice, painful swallowing, trismus, and anxiety present.[9] Fever, malaise, and dehydration are usually seen. In mild cases, needle aspiration relieves trismus and painful swallowing; therefore, the patient is discharged on oral antibiotics with ENT follow-up.[11] In more severe cases with airway compromise, surgical incision and drainage or needle aspiration is followed by intravenous antibiotic therapy. Stability of the ABCs is a priority. Provide oxygen, monitor arterial oxygen saturations and respirations, and keep the head of the bed elevated 80 to 90 degrees. Tonsillectomy may be required to prevent recurrence of the abscess.[17] Dangerous sequelae associated with peritonsillar abscess include aspiration, airway obstruction, parapharyngeal abscess, dehydration, glomerulonephritis, and subacute bacterial endocarditis. Fortunately complications can be avoided with aggressive antibiotic treatment (penicillin based or erythromycin). Ice packs to the neck help decrease pain and edema. Encourage oral hygiene; however, gargling should be avoided because this may cause inadvertent rupture of the abscess.[17]

FACIAL EMERGENCIES

Facial emergencies affect structures of the face such as the nerves, bones, and sinuses. These emergencies may be secondary to infection or other disease processes.

Sinusitis

Acute sinusitis, inflammation of mucous membranes in any of the paranasal sinuses, generally occurs as a result of blockage and back-up of secretions. The cause is usually attributed to URI or allergic rhinitis. Other causes include foreign bodies, trauma, dental disorders, inhalation of irritants (e.g., cigarette smoke, cocaine use), deviated nasal septum, polyps, and tumors. Secretions are retained in the sinus cavity as a result of altered ciliary activity and obstruction of the sinus ostia.[17] Negative pressure and air-fluid levels result from fluid accumulation and reabsorption of air in the sinus. Fluid accumulation forms a medium for bacteria to grow and multiply, resulting in bacterial sinusitis. *H. influenzae* and *S. pneumoniae* are common causative organisms.[32]

In chronic sinusitis the mucous membrane becomes permanently thickened from prolonged or repeated inflammation or infection.[7] The patient with sinusitis complains of dull, achy pain over the affected sinus. In adults, frontal sinusitis with periorbital and forehead pain that worsens when bending over is common. Ethmoidal sinusitis, common in children, causes pain at the bridge of the nose and behind the eyes. Fever, decreased appetite, and nausea may also be present.[14] Ethmoidal sinusitis is especially serious in children because of the tendency for the infection to extend toward the retroorbital area and central nervous system.[20] The patient has tenderness to palpation over the involved sinus; swollen, erythematous mucosa with purulent nasal discharge; and diminished transillumination. Radiographic studies are not always conclusive or reliable in diagnosis of sinusitis. Findings that are most reliable include sinus opacity, air-fluid level, or 6 mm of mucosal thickening. Absence of radiographic evidence does not exclude the diagnosis of sinusitis.[20] Other diagnostic methods include CT scan, sinus endoscopy, and sinus cultures of the ostia via needle aspiration.

Over-the-counter nasal decongestant sprays (e.g., Afrin or Neo-Synephrine) may provide immediate relief; however, topical decongestants should not be used for more than 3 days because of a dangerous rebound effect.[4] Isotonic saline nose drops may also help. Encourage increased fluid intake and use of a humidifier in the home. Warm, moist compresses to the sinus areas promote drainage and comfort. Administer antibiotics and analgesics as prescribed. Instruct the patient to avoid environmental irritants and avoid bending over because this increases sinus pressure and pain. If the condition worsens despite antibiotic therapy for 3 to 5 days, the patient should return to the ED immediately or see an ENT specialist. Complications of undertreated acute sinusitis are chronic sinusitis, orbital or periorbital cellulitis or abscess, cavernous sinus thrombosis, sepsis, brain abscess, meningitis, and osteomyelitis of the frontal bone.

Temporomandibular Joint Dislocation

TMJ dislocation refers to anterior and superior bilateral displacement of the jaw. Unilateral dislocation rarely occurs. Jaw muscles attempt to close the mandible, but the resulting spasm prevents condyles from returning to normal position in the mandibular fossae.[2] TMJ dislocation usually occurs when opening the mouth too wide, as in yawning or laughing. Trauma or dystonic reaction to drugs may also be responsible. The patient usually presents with the chin protruding, the mouth open, drooling, and pain related to muscle spasms. The patient cannot close the mouth, talk, or swallow and may be extremely anxious.[4] Diagnostics include pre- and postreduction radiographs. Muscle relaxants may be administered to reduce muscle spasm and relax the patient.

To reduce the dislocation, seat the patient facing the emergency physician. The physician places the thumbs intraorally onto the lower molar ridge and applies a downward and backward pressure to return the condyle to the normal position.[2] The physician should pad the thumbs with a thick layer of gauze because the strong masseter muscles of the jaw contract with great force with reduction of the TMJ. Postreduction pain is rare and is minimal when present. Nonsteroidal antiinflammatory drugs and muscle relaxants may be helpful.[2] Instruct the patient to avoid stress on the TMJ by consuming a soft diet for 3 to 4 days.[14] Because patients with one episode of TMJ dislocation are predisposed to further dislocations, referral to an otolaryngologist is recommended.[4]

SUMMARY

Emergencies of the mouth, face, nose, and ears are a routine part of emergency nursing. Most are not life-threatening. However, the ability to discern problems that represent a potential threat to the patient's life is a requisite skill for the emergency nurse. Box 45-4 highlights nursing diagnoses for these patients.

Box 45-4	NURSING DIAGNOSES FOR DENTAL, EAR, NOSE, THROAT, AND FACIAL EMERGENCIES

Airway clearance, Ineffective
Anxiety
Breathing pattern, Ineffective
Gas exchange, Impaired
Hypovolemia
Infection, Risk for
Pain

References

1. Amsterdam JT: General dental emergencies. In Tintinalli JE, Ruiz E, Krome RL, editors: *Emergency medicine: a comprehensive study guide*, ed 4, New York, 1996, McGraw-Hill.
2. Amsterdam JT: Dental disorders. In Rosen P, Barkin RM, Hockberger RS et al, editors: *Emergency medicine: concepts and clinical practice*, ed 4, St. Louis, 1998, Mosby.
3. Beaudreau RW: Oral and dental emergencies. In Tintinalli JE, Kelen GD, Stapczynski JS, editors: *Emergency medicine: a comprehensive study guide*, ed 5, New York, 2000, McGraw-Hill.
4. Black JM, Matassarin-Jacobs E: *Medical-surgical nursing: a psychophysiologic approach*, ed 6, Philadelphia, 2000, WB Saunders.
5. Cox RJ: *Foreign bodies of the nose* (2000). In *Emerg Med/Ear, Nose & throat*. Retrieved March 15, 2001 from the World Wide Web: http://www.emedicine.com/emerg/topic186.htm.
6. Criddle LM: Maxillofacial trauma and ear, nose, and throat emergencies. In Kitt S et al, editors: *Emergency nursing: a physiologic and clinical perspective*, ed 2, Philadelphia, 1995, WB Saunders.
7. Freeman FB: Impacted cerumen: how to safely remove earwax in an office visit, *Geriatrics* 50(6):52, 1995.
8. Hackeling T, Triana R Jr: Disorders of the neck and upper airway. In Tintinalli JE, Kelen GD, Stapczynski JS, editors: *Emergency medicine: a comprehensive study guide*, ed 5, New York, 2000, McGraw-Hill.
9. Ignatavicius DD, Workman ML, Mishler MA: *Medical-surgical nursing: health across the continuum*, ed 3, Philadelphia, 1999, WB Saunders.
10. Jarvis C: *Physical examination and health assessment*, ed 3, Philadelphia, 1999, WB Saunders.
11. Kazzi AA. Peritonsillar abscess. In *Emerg Med/Ear, Nose, & throat*. Retrieved March 15, 2001 from the World Wide Web: http://www.emedicine.com/emerg/topic417.htm.
12. Kennedy E. Sinusitis. In *Emerg Med/Ear, nose, & throat*. Retrieved March 15, 2001 from the World Wide Web: http://www.emedicine.com/emerg/topic536.htm.
13. Leonard CH: *Gray's pocket anatomy*, New York, 1984, Crown.
14. Mantooth R. Ear foreign bodies. In *Emerg Med/Ear, nose, & throat*. Retrieved March 15, 2001 from the World Wide Web: http://www.emedicine.com/emerg/topic185.htm.
15. Peacock WF: Otolaryngologic emergencies. In Tintinalli JE, Ruiz E, Krome RL, editors: *Emergency medicine: a comprehensive study guide*, ed 4, New York, 1996, McGraw-Hill.
16. Peacock WF: Face and jaw emergencies. In Tintinalli JE, Kelen GD, Stapczynski JS, editors: *Emergency medicine: a comprehensive study guide*, ed 5, New York, 2000, McGraw-Hill.
17. Peng L. Avulsed dentate. In *Emerg Med/Ear, nose, & throat*. Retrieved March 15, 2001, from the World Wide Web: http://www.emedicine.com/emerg/topic125.htm.
18. Peng L. Fractures of the dentate. In *Emerg Med/Ear, nose, & throat*. Retrieved March 15, 2001 from the World Wide Web: http://www.emedicine.com/emerg/topic127.htm.
19. Peng L. Infections of the dentate. In *Emerg Med/Ear, nose, & throat*. Retrieved March 15, 2001 from the World Wide Web: http://www.emedicine.com/emerg/topic128.htm.
20. Pfaff JA, Moore GP: Ear, nose, and throat emergencies. In Rosen P, Barkin RM, Hockberger RS et al, editors: *Emergency medicine: concepts and clinical practice*, ed 4, St. Louis, 1998, Mosby.
21. Pons PT: Nasal foreign bodies. In Rosen P, Barkin RM, Hockberger RS et al, editors: *Emergency medicine: concepts and clinical practice*, ed 4, St. Louis, 1998, Mosby.
22. Rahman WM, O'Connor TJ: Facial trauma. In Barkin RM, editor: *Pediatric emergency medicine: concepts and clinical practice*, ed 2, St. Louis, 1997, Mosby.
23. Rogers JS: Eye, ear, nose, and throat disorders. In Soud TE, Rogers JS, editors: *Manual of pediatric emergency nursing*, St. Louis, 1998, Mosby.
24. Rothenhaus T. Epistaxis. In *Emerg Med/Ear, nose, and throat*. Retrieved March 15, 2001 from the World Wide Web: http://www.emedicine.com/emerg/topic806.htm.
25. SantaMaria JP, Abrunzo TJ: Ear, nose, and throat. In Barkin RM, editor: *Pediatric emergency medicine: concepts and clinical practice*, ed 2, St. Louis, 1997, Mosby.
26. Smith JA: Nasal emergencies and sinusitis. In Tintinalli JE, Ruiz E, Krome RL, editors: *Emergency medicine: a comprehensive study guide*, ed 4, New York, 1996, McGraw-Hill.
27. Tortora G: *Principles of anatomy and physiology*, ed 4, New York, 1984, Harper & Row.
28. Uphold CR, Graham MV: *Clinical guidelines in family practice*, ed 3, Gainesville, 1998, Barmarrae Books.
29. Urdaneta E, Lucchesi M: Common disorders of the external, middle, and inner ear. In Tintinalli JE, Kelen GD, Stapczynski JS, editors: *Emergency medicine: a comprehensive study guide*, ed 5, New York, 2000, McGraw-Hill.
30. Walsh M. Otitis externa. In *Emerg Med/Ear, nose, and throat*. Retrieved March 15, 2001 from the World Wide Web: http://www.emedicine.com/emerg/topic350.htm.
31. Walsh M. Otitis media. In *Emerg Med/Ear, nose, and throat*. Retrieved March 15, 2001 from the World Wide Web: http://www.emedicine.com/emerg/topic351.htm.
32. Waters TA, Peacock WF IV: Nasal emergencies and sinusitis. In Tintinalli JE, Kelen GD, Stapczynski JS, editors: *Emergency medicine: a comprehensive study guide*, ed 5, New York, 2000, Mosby.

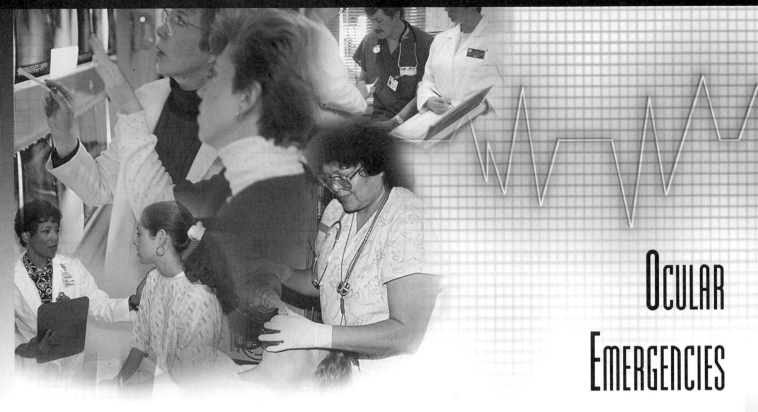

CHAPTER 46

Ocular Emergencies

Darcy Egging

Emergency nurses care for patients with eye problems on a regular basis; however, true ocular emergencies are not an everyday occurrence. The ability to identify conditions that represent a threat to the patient's vision is essential to protecting the patient's vision. This chapter provides a brief description of anatomy, ocular assessment, and common ocular emergencies encountered in the emergency department (ED).

It has been estimated that one in every thousand people will have a significant eye injury each year.[14] In the United States alone it is estimated that 2.4 million eye injures occur each year.[21] Work-related injuries constitute between 22% and 50% of all ocular trauma.[21]

True ocular emergencies, such as angle-closure glaucoma and retinal artery occlusion, usually occur in the older patient and are not typically seen in the ED. Typical ocular emergencies treated in the ED include corneal or conjunctival foreign body, conjunctivitis, and corneal abrasion. These conditions do not cause significant morbidity; however, the patient does experience discomfort and disruption of routine.

ANATOMY AND PHYSIOLOGY

The eyes are the windows of the world. Vision is often considered the most important of the five senses. Basic understanding of ocular structures facilitates assessment and treatment of ocular problems. Figure 46-1 illustrates these ocular structures. The eyes are protected by the surrounding bony structures, eyelids, and sclera. Lacrimal glands secrete tears, which continuously bathe the eye to decrease friction and remove minor irritants (Figure 46-2). Meibomian glands secrete oil, which lines eyelid margins and prevents tears from running out of the conjunctival sacs.

Light enters the eye through the cornea, passes through the lens, and is reflected off the retina. The amount of light entering the posterior chamber is controlled by the iris as it expands and contracts to open and close the pupil. Six oculomotor muscles (Figure 46-3) control movement of the eye itself.

PATIENT ASSESSMENT

Assessment of the patient with an ocular problem begins with triage and continues into the treatment area. A potential threat to vision should be triaged as emergent, whereas a patient with a red eye and no potential loss of vision could be triaged as nonurgent if no other problems exist.

After a brief assessment to ensure that the airway, breathing, and circulation (ABCs) are stable, the patient is evaluated to identify potential threats to vision. Ocular emergencies that represent a threat to the patient's vision and require immediate attention include globe penetration, retinal artery occlusion, chemical burns, and acute angle-closure glaucoma.

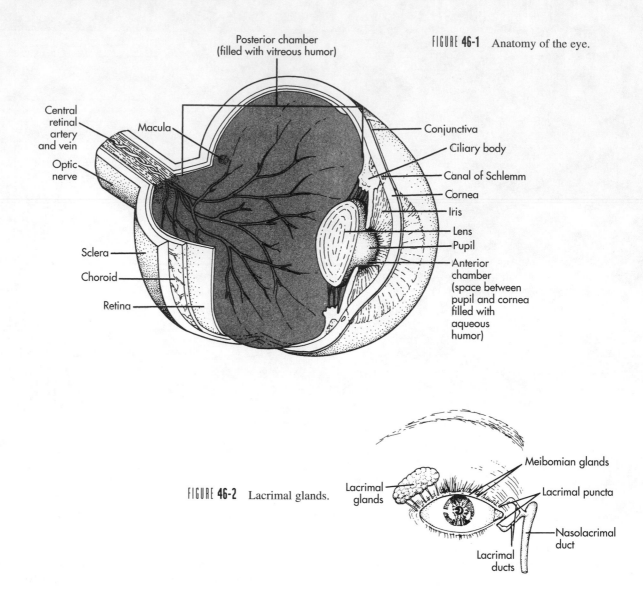

Posterior chamber
(filled with vitreous humor)

FIGURE **46-1** Anatomy of the eye.

Central retinal artery and vein

Macula

Optic nerve

Sclera

Choroid

Retina

Conjunctiva

Ciliary body

Canal of Schlemm

Cornea

Iris

Lens

Pupil

Anterior chamber
(space between pupil and cornea filled with aqueous humor)

FIGURE **46-2** Lacrimal glands.

Meibomian glands

Lacrimal glands

Lacrimal puncta

Nasolacrimal duct

Lacrimal ducts

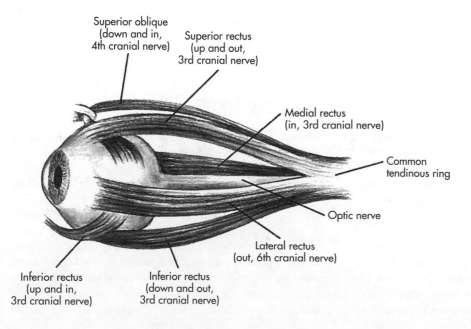

Superior oblique
(down and in, 4th cranial nerve)

Superior rectus
(up and out, 3rd cranial nerve)

Medial rectus
(in, 3rd cranial nerve)

Common tendinous ring

Optic nerve

Lateral rectus
(out, 6th cranial nerve)

FIGURE **46-3** Extrinsic muscles of the eye. (From Rudy EB: *Advanced neurological and neurosurgical nursing*, St. Louis, 1984, Mosby.)

Inferior rectus
(up and in, 3rd cranial nerve)

Inferior rectus
(down and out, 3rd cranial nerve)

Focused assessment includes determination of precipitating events, duration of symptoms, and identification of anything that worsens or improves symptoms. When the patient verbalizes discomfort, description of the discomfort helps clarify the patient's problem. Does the patient describe itching, burning, or the sensation of something in the eye? Determine the degree of pain and where the pain occurs. Clarify reported visual changes to determine if the loss is partial or complete, in one or both eyes. Biocular changes suggest a neurologic condition rather than an ocular condition, whereas the presence of floaters suggests retinal tear.

When the patient has a history of trauma, determine when the injury occurred and the mechanism of injury. Determine tetanus status. If the injury occurred because of a motor vehicle crash, did the air bag deploy? The alkaline powder in air bags can cause significant eye irritation. Question the patient regarding use of protective eyewear, glasses, or contact lenses. Evaluate medical history including ocular history, use of corrective lenses, ocular medications, past ocular surgery, and disease such as diabetes.

The primary elements of the ocular examination are visual acuity, external features, pupils, anterior segment, and extraocular motility. The physician may perform a slit lamp examination, intraocular pressure (IOP) measurement, and direct ophthalmoscopy.

Visual Acuity

Visual acuity is a vital sign for patients with an ocular emergency. This simple test is done on all patients presenting with any type of eye or vision complaint.[11] Physical examination begins with visual acuity unless the patient has been exposed to a chemical. In these situations irrigation takes priority over determination of visual acuity.

Measure visual acuity with the patient wearing corrective lenses and when the patient is not wearing corrective lenses.[2] When corrective lenses are not available, the pinhole test can be used for measurement of visual acuity. This is accomplished by punching a hole in a note card with an 18-gauge needle. Looking through a pinhole usually corrects any refractory error to at least 20/30.[11] Test the affected eye first, then the unaffected eye, and finally both eyes. The Snellen chart is the standard method for determination of visual acuity. For the examination, have the patient stand 20 feet from the chart and cover the eye without applying pressure to the orbit. Figure 46-4 shows two types of Snellen charts. Box 46-1 identifies alternate techniques for visual acuity when a Snellen chart is not available. Table 46-1 describes documentation of visual acuity for the Snellen chart and alternate techniques for visual acuity. For people who are illiterate or do not speak English, there is an E chart where the patient indicates the direction of the letter E. The Allencard of objects is used for children. Be sure to name the objects before the test so that they are identified correctly. The patient with a corneal abrasion or foreign body may have difficulty with photophobia, pain, and tearing.

Placing a drop of topical anesthetic in the affected eye may assist in accomplishing an accurate visual acuity in this patient.

External Features

External examination for ocular injury begins by observing the patient. Observe for bruising, laceration, lesions, and other differences between the eyes. Assess eyelids, lashes, and how the eyes rest in the socket. Examine the conjunctiva and sclera for abnormal color.

Pupil Examination

Pupil examination includes assessment of shape, size, and reaction. Testing should be performed in a dimly lit examination room. Pupils are normally round, black, and equal in size. Variations may indicate a potentially serious problem or may reflect a normal physiologic variation. Up to 25% of the population have unequal pupils (anisocoria) as a normal finding. An oval pupil may be caused from a tumor or retinal detachment. A pupil that is the shape of a teardrop suggests a ruptured globe, with the teardrop pointing to the rupture site.[17]

Pupil size is measured in millimeters. Assess and document the size change that occurs in each pupil in response to direct and consensual light stimulation. Normally, both pupils constrict equally when a strong light is directed at one eye (direct response in eye on which the light is shined and consensual response of the other eye).[2,17]

Anterior Segment

The anterior segment is composed of the conjunctiva, cornea, anterior chamber, iris, lens, and ciliary body. The conjunctiva or the white of the eye should be inspected for change in color, swelling (chemosis), discharge, foreign bodies, and laceration. The cornea should be clear. The cornea is stained with fluorescein to inspect for the presence of any abrasions. The anterior chamber is inspected for hyphema (blood in the anterior chamber) or hypopyon (pus in the anterior chamber). To inspect the anterior chamber, hold a light tangential or at a 90-degree angle to the eye. A slit lamp is used to perform an adequate assessment of the anterior chamber.[10]

Ocular Motility

Evaluate the patient's ability to move the eyes through six cardinal positions of gaze by asking the patient to follow your finger as you move it through these positions. Ocular movement is controlled by the cranial nerves that regulate the oculomotor muscles. Figure 46-5 shows these positions of gaze and identifies the specific oculomotor muscles and cranial nerves involved. Impaired ocular motility may occur with an entrapped muscle secondary to a blowout fracture, muscular injury, orbital cellulitis, or underlying central nervous system problem.[10] Evaluation of ocular motility in children

Box 46-1   METHODS FOR DETERMINING VISUAL ACUITY

Have patient read Rosenbaum Pocket Vision Screener held 14 inches from the nose.

Have patient read newsprint, and record the distance at which the paper must be held for the patient to read it.

Hold up a specific number of fingers, and record the distance at which the patient can see your fingers; then ask the patient how many fingers you are holding up.

Record the distance at which the patient perceives hand motion, that is, when the patient cannot see fingers moving.

Record the distance at which the patient perceives light (when the patient cannot see hand motion).

Document inability to perceive light.

requires patience and creativity. Hold toys, keys, or lights in different areas so that the child glances in that direction. Children become easily bored with the same object, so a general rule of thumb is to use a different toy for each position.

Other Examinations

Other techniques used to evaluate ocular function include fluorescein staining, measurement of IOP, and funduscopic examination. Fluorescein is used to determine if the corneal epithelium is intact. Figure 46-6 and Box 46-2 illustrate this procedure. Before staining, the patient should remove his or

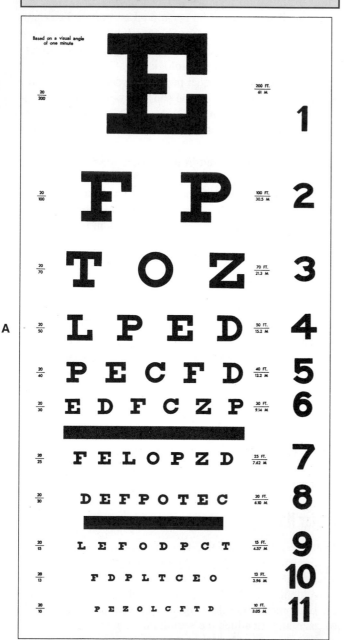

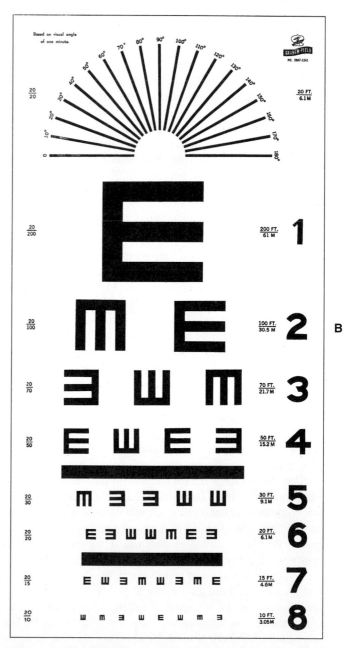

FIGURE 46-4 **A,** Snellen and **B,** E chart for assessment of visual acuity. (From Seidel HM, Ball JW, Dains JE, Benedict GW: *Mosby's guide to physical examination,* ed 4, St. Louis, 1999, Mosby.)

Table 46-1	EXAMPLES OF VISUAL ACUITY EXAMINATION
20/20	Standing at 20 feet, patient can read what the normal eye can read at 20 feet.
20/20 2	Standing at 20 feet, patient can read what the normal eye can read at 20 feet; however, missed two letters.
20/200	At 20 feet, patient can read what the normal eye can read at 200 feet. Patient is considered legally blind if reading is obtained while wearing glasses or contact lenses.
10/200	When the patient cannot read letters on the Snellen chart, have patient stand half the distance to the chart. Record findings at the distance the patient is standing from the chart over the smallest line he or she can read.
CF/3 ft	Patient can count fingers at a maximum distance of 3 feet.
HM/4	Patient can see hand motion at a maximum distance of 4 feet.
LP/position	Patient can perceive light and determine the direction from which it is coming.
LP/no position	Patient can perceive light but is unable to tell the direction from which it is coming.
NLP	Patient is unable to perceive light.

her contact lenses. Figure 46-7 illustrates removal of hard contacts; Figure 46-8 illustrates soft contact removal. Following fluorescein application, flush the eye with normal saline and instruct the patient not to insert contact lenses for at least 1 hour.

IOP is measured with a Schiøtz tonometer or a tonopen (Figure 46-9). This procedure is contraindicated in patients with possible ruptured globe. Normal IOP is 10 to 21 mm Hg.[10] The tonopen is a hand-held instrument that is gaining popularity because of its ease of use and decreased incidence of contamination.[15] The tip is covered with a sterile cover that is discarded after each patient. The Schiøtz is another instrument that can be used to measure IOP. Regardless of technique, the cornea must be anesthetized before measurement. A low reading indicates increased IOP, whereas a high reading indicates decreased IOP. Any obstruction such as glaucoma to aqueous outflow can result in an elevated IOP.[17] Box 46-3 describes the procedure for the Schiøtz tonometer.

Direct ophthalmoscopy, or funduscopic evaluation, is used to evaluate the posterior chamber of the eye using the light beam directed through the pupil. Mydriatic drops may

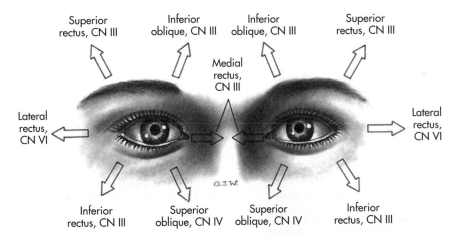

FIGURE 46-5 Innervation and movement of extraocular muscles. *CN*, Cranial nerve. (From Thompson JM, McFarland GK, Hirsch JE et al: *Mosby's clinical nursing*, ed 5, St. Louis, 2001, Mosby.)

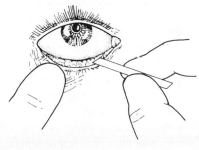

FIGURE 46-6 Fluorescein staining. Touch moistened fluorescein strip to inner canthus of lower lid.

Box 46-2 **FLUORESCEIN STAINING**

Explain the procedure to the patient.
Moisten end of sterile fluorescein strip with normal saline solution.
Pull down on lower lid.
Ask the patient to blink so tears distribute solution over the cornea.
Examine cornea with cobalt blue light. Disruptions appear as a bright yellow spot.

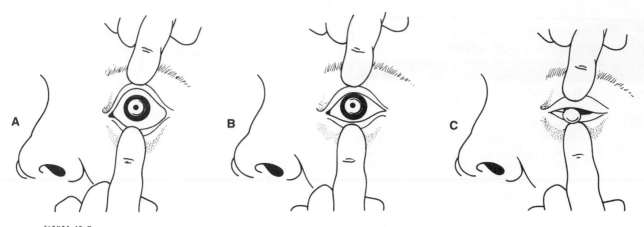

FIGURE 46-7 *Technique for removing hard corneal contact lens from eye.* **A,** Spread eyelids apart. **B,** Push lids toward center of eye under contact lens. **C,** Remove lens.

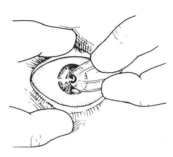

FIGURE 46-8 Soft contact lens removal. Lift lens off cornea.

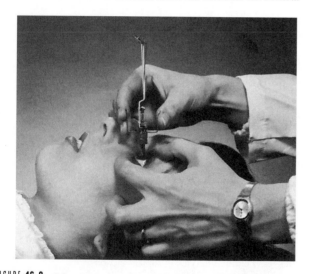

FIGURE 46-9 Measurement of ocular tension with Schiøtz tonometer. (From Newell FW: *Ophthalmology: principles and concepts,* ed 8, St. Louis, 1996, Mosby.)

Box 46-3	**INTRAOCULAR PRESSURE MEASUREMENT WITH A SCHIØTZ TONOMETER**

Explain the procedure to the patient before the test.
Assess visual acuity before the examination.
Place two drops of anesthetic in each eye.
Place the patient in a supine position.
Calibrate the tonometer before use.
Place sterile tonometer point directly on the eye and obtain reading.

Table 46-2	**COLOR CODES FOR OPHTHALMIC MEDICATIONS**	
CAP COLOR	**DRUG ACTION**	**EXAMPLES**
Red	Pupil dilation (mydriasis)	Epinephrine, atropine, neostigmine
Green	Pupil constriction (miosis)	Pilocarpine
Clear or white	Topical anesthesia	Proparacaine (Alcaine, Opthaine)
Blue	Irrigation, lubrication	Liquid tears
Yellow	Decrease aqueous humor production	Timolol

Modified from Barish RA, Naradzay JF: Ophthalmologic therapeutics, *Emerg Med Clin North Am* 13(3):652, 1995.

be administered to dilate the pupil and make visualization of the disc, retinal artery, and macula easier. Ophthalmoscopes provide different shapes and colored light beams to detect various conditions.

PATIENT MANAGEMENT

General management of ocular emergencies includes removal of contact lens, instillation of ocular medication, irrigation, and eye patching. These techniques apply to most ocular emergencies.

Eye drops and ophthalmic ointments are used to decrease pain, provide antibiotic therapy, change pupil size, reduce allergic reactions in the eye, and cleanse the eye. Topical ophthalmic medications are prepared under sterile conditions and distributed in single-dose containers. Container caps are color coded by the medication's effect on the pupil. Table 46-2 highlights this coding system. Various ophthalmic medications are described in Table 46-3.[1]

Instilling eye drops or ointments requires attention to detail to prevent contamination and minimize systemic effects of the medication. Before instilling eye drops or ointments, explain the procedure to the patient, and place the patient in the supine position. Instruct the patient not to roll his or her eyes because this can worsen injury, particularly when anesthetic drops have

Table 46-3   OPHTHALMOLOGIC MEDICATIONS

GENERIC NAME	COMMON BRAND NAMES	ACTION USE
GLAUCOMA MEDICATION		
Beta-blockers		
Betaxolol	Betoptic	Lowers IOP, decreases the production
Carteolol	Ocupress	of aqueous by the cilliary body
Levobunolol	Betagan	
Timolol	Timoptic	
Carbonic anhydrase inhibitors		
Acetazolamide	Diamox	Inhibits aqueous production
Brinzolamide	Azopt	
Dorzolamide	Trusopt	
Glaucoma agents–other		
Apraclonidine	Lopidine	
Brimonidine	Alphagan	
Dorzolamide + timolol	Cosopt	
Dipivefrin	Propine	
Echothiophate iodine	Phospholine Iodide	
Latanoprost	Xalatan	
Polocarpine	Pilocar, Pilopine HS, Isopto, Carpine	
MYDRIATICS AND CYCLOPLEGICS		
Atropine		Mydriasis—dilitation
Homatropine		Cyloplegia—loss of accommodation
Phenylephrine	Neo-synephrine	
NONSTEROIDAL ANTIINFLAMMATORIES		
Diclofenac	Voltaren	
Ketorolac	Acular	Allergic conjunctivitis
OCULAR DECONGESTANT/ANTIALLERGY		
Cromolyn sodium	Crolom	
Levocabastine	Livostin	Seasonal allergies
Naphazoline	Naphcon	Allergic ocular disorders
Naphcon-A		Ocular decongestant
Olopatadine	Patanol	Allergic conjunctivitis
ANTIBACTERIALS		
Ciprofloxacin	Ciloxan	Corneal ulcers/keratitis
Erythromycin	Ilotycin	
Gentamicin	Garamycin	
Ofloxacin	Ocuflox	Corneal ulcers/keratitis
(Polymyxin B + Bacitracin)	Polysporin	
(Polymyxin B + trimethoprin)	Polytrim	
Sulfacetamide	Sulamyd, Bleph-10	
Tobramycin	Tobrex	Mild to moderate infections
ANTIVIRAL AGENTS		
Formivirsen	Vitravene	
Trifluridine	Viroptic	Keratoconjunctivitis
CORTICOSTEROIDS		
Dexamethasone	Decadron	
Prednisolone	Pred-Forte	
(Neomycin + polymyxin + hydrocortisone)	Cortisporin	
(Dexamethasone + neomycin + polymyxin)	Maxitrol	
(Tobramycin + dexamthasone)	TobraDex	

Box 46-4 **INSTILLING EYE DROPS**

Pull the lower eyelid downward, and have the patient gaze upward.

Instill 1-2 drops of the intended solution into the cul-de-sac (the center of the inner lower lid).

Direct the patient to blink to distribute the solution.

Apply pressure to the medial canthus for several minutes to close the nasolacrimal duct and minimize systemic effects.

Instruct the patient *not* to squeeze eyelids together because this causes medication to leak out.

If more than one type of drop is ordered, wait several minutes between applications to allow maximal exposure.

Box 46-5 **INSTILLING OPHTHALMIC OINTMENT**

Pull the lower eyelid downward while the patient gazes upward.

Apply ointment in a thin line from the inner aspect of the lower lid to the outer canthus.

Have the patient slowly close and rotate the eye to expose all surfaces to the medication.

Press the medial canthus gently for several minutes to decrease rapid drainage.

Instruct the patient *not* to squeeze eyelids together because this repels the ointment.

Box 46-6 **EYE IRRIGATION**

Cleanse the entire area around the eye and eyelid.

Prepare irrigation setup and solution.

Place patient supine, or adjust the examining chair to a reclining position.

Turn the head to the affected side and pull the eyelid down.

Run solution directly over the eye and lower lid from the inner to the outer canthus.

Direct the patient to occasionally blink and look from side to side to distribute solution.

Irrigate for a minimum of 30 minutes with chemical exposure.

Evert and swab beneath the eyelid to remove residual particles.

Box 46-7 **EYE PATCHING**

Administer antibiotic ointment or solution as directed.

Ask the patient to close both eyes.

Place a folded eye patch over the affected lid followed by an unfolded eye patch.

Tape the eye patch obliquely with paper tape. Avoid nasolabial folds.

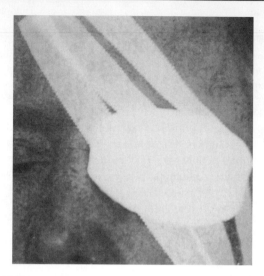

FIGURE **46-10**   Eye patch. (From Grossman JA: *Atlas of minor injuries,* St. Louis, 1993, Gower Medical Publishing.)

---

been used. Box 46-4 describes instillation of eyedrops; Box 46-5 discusses instillation of ocular ointments. Monitor patients carefully following instillation of eyedrops; systemic effects secondary to eye drops may occur.

Irrigation is used to remove chemicals, small foreign bodies, and other substances. Isotonic saline is the fluid of choice for ocular irrigation; however lactated Ringer's solution is also used. Dextrose solutions should not be used because they are sticky and irritate the eye. Irrigation is contraindicated in the patient with a possible ruptured globe. Box 46-6 describes the procedure for eye irrigation. A Morgan lens can also be used for irrigation.

The eye is patched to minimize ocular stimulation by reducing movement and limiting light exposure. Patching both eyes simulates total blindness; patching one eye alters depth perception. Box 46-7 describes the procedure for patching the eyes. Figure 46-10 shows an appropriately applied eye patch. Eye patches should not be used when there is an increased risk of a *Pseudomonas* organism infection; for example, in the contact lens wearer. When the patient is discharged with an eye patch, discharge instructions must include discussion of altered vision and the hazards of driving or using machinery.

SPECIFIC OCULAR EMERGENCIES

Injury or disease may cause ocular emergencies. Comprehensive discussion of every disease process is beyond the scope of this text; however, situations encountered most often by the emergency nurse are discussed.

Trauma

General principles pertaining to ocular examination are essentially the same for the patient with an eye injury; however, the patient's ABCs should be evaluated and stabilized before interventions for the ocular problem. Ocular injury often occurs in conjunction with head and facial trauma; therefore, the patient should be carefully evaluated for an associated eye injury. Check for contact lenses in the unconscious patient and remove them as soon as possible. Do not instill eye drops before evaluation of ocular injury. Severe

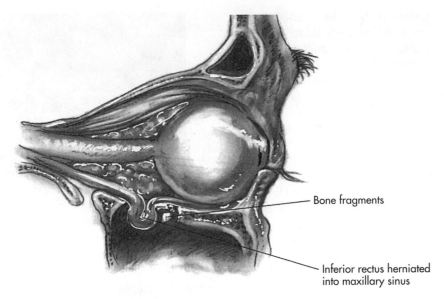

Bone fragments

Inferior rectus herniated
into maxillary sinus

FIGURE **46-11**   Mechanism of entrapment of inferior rectus muscle through an orbital floor defect. (From Davis JH et al: *Surgery: a problem-solving approach,* ed 2, vol 2, St. Louis, 1995, Mosby.)

pain associated with ocular trauma can be minimized without medication by patching both eyes. When the patient cannot blink, protect the cornea from drying with ophthalmic ointment or artificial tears. The eyes may be taped shut when ointment is used.

Obtain pertinent details of history including mechanism of injury, time of injury, energy source, material involved when there is ocular penetration, and use of protective eyewear. If the foreign material is organic, there is increased risk of infection, whereas metallic material causes vitreous and ocular reactions.

Blunt Trauma

Blunt trauma to the eye may be caused by a motor vehicle collision, assault with various weapons, or a fall. The most commonly seen ocular injury is periorbital contusion or a black eye. This injury is usually benign, but the patient should be assessed for more serious injury, such as basilar skull fracture. Symptoms usually include ecchymosis of the lids, which can make it very difficult to visualize the globe. If the globe appears intact, rule out blowout fracture and hyphema. If no obvious associated problems are identified, therapeutic interventions such as ice, head elevation, and reassurance are initiated. Resolution of noncomplicated periorbital ecchymosis usually occurs within 2 to 3 weeks.[10]

Orbital Fractures.   Orbital fractures involve the orbital floor and the orbital rim. Fractures of the orbital floor are serious and usually result from direct blunt trauma to the eye. A blowout fracture occurs when direct trauma increases IOP to the point where the orbital floor fractures (Figure 46-11). Orbital contents may herniate into the maxillary or ethmoid sinuses and trap the inferior rectus muscle in the defect. A blowout fracture is diagnosed by history and observation of periorbital ecchymosis, subconjunctival hemorrhage, periorbital edema, enophthalmos (sunken eye), an upward gaze,

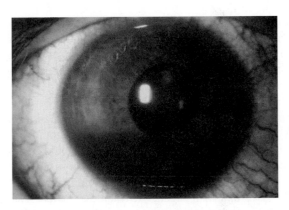

FIGURE **46-12**   Traumatic hyphema. (From Abrams D: *Ophthalmology in medicine: an illustrated clinical guide,* St. Louis, 1990, Mosby.)

and a complaint of diplopia. The latter three conditions occur when the inferior rectus and oblique muscles are trapped in the fracture. Facial radiographs, including the Caldwell view (showing orbital rim and walls) and Waters view (orbital floor and roof), are used to assist with diagnosis of a blowout fracture. Computed tomography (CT) scan is more helpful in identification of entrapment than plain radiographs.[12]

Orbital fractures are not considered an ocular emergency unless visual impairment or globe injury is present. Surgical intervention is usually delayed until swelling resolves in 10 to 14 days. Patients without eye injury or entrapment may be referred to an ophthalmologist and treated conservatively. Patients who have fractures involving the sinuses should receive a prescription of antibiotics. Discharge instructions should include ice and cautions against Valsalva maneuvers and nose blowing.[12]

Hyphema.   Hyphema refers to bleeding into the anterior chamber of the eye, usually secondary to blunt trauma (Figure 46-12). It occurs when blood vessels of the iris break and leak into the clear aqueous fluid of the anterior chamber.[18] Hyphema size varies from microscopic to total involvement of the anterior chamber. The term *eight-ball hyphema* describes a total hyphema that has begun to clot.[13] A large clot can obstruct aqueous outflow and lead to secondary glaucoma. Any patient with a hyphema requires evaluation by an ophthalmologist.

Symptoms of hyphema include pain, photophobia, and blurred vision. Blood in the anterior chamber may be easily seen in patients with lighter-colored eyes but may be extremely difficult to see in dark-eyed patients. Suspect concurrent head injury if the patient has an altered level of consciousness. Patients with bleeding disorders, anticoagulant therapy, kidney disease, liver disease, or sickle cell disease have an increased risk of complications; therefore, these patient should be monitored carefully for increased bleeding. The most common complication of hyphema is rebleeding in 10% to 25% of patients, usually within 2 to 5 days, but can occur up to 14 days after the initial injury.[13] Other complications include corneal blood staining, secondary glaucoma, loss of vision, and loss of the eye.

Management of hyphema is variable and controversial, particularly relative to activity. The controversy regards whether the patient should be allowed quiet activity or placed on strict bed rest. Regardless of the decision, when the patient is in bed, the head of the bed should be elevated 30 to 45 degrees. There is also disagreement regarding hospitalization and eye patching. Conservative therapy should be considered for those patients at risk for complications, children, and the elderly. Hospitalization should be considered when noncompliance with treatment is an issue. Pharmacologic management includes β-blockers to control elevated IOP, mydriatic agents to increase patient comfort, steroids to decrease inflammation in the anterior chamber, and an antifibrinolytic agent to delay clot dissolution and decrease the rate of rebleed.[4] Analgesics may also be used; however, aspirin and nonsteroidal antiinflammatory medications should be avoided. Antiemetics may be used to decrease the risk of vomiting if the patient is nauseated. All patients with a hyphema are referred to an ophthalmologist for follow-up.

Subconjunctival Hemorrhage. Subconjunctival hemorrhage is a harmless ocular condition that can frighten patients by its appearance. It is usually caused by trivial trauma such as a cough, sneeze, or the Valsalva maneuver. This condition is caused when a small blood vessel of the eye ruptures and bleeds (Figure 46-13). The symptoms are a painless, bright red flat patch on the sclera. Most patients usually find a subconjunctival hemorrhage by accident when looking in the mirror. Although a subconjunctival hemorrhage is benign there is a need to differentiate it from a bloody chemosis, which can be indicative of scleral rupture, conjunctivitis, iritis, or coagulopathy.[13] No treatment is required; blood will usually reabsorb in 2 to 3 weeks.

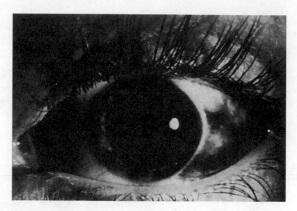

FIGURE 46-13 Subconjunctival hemorrhage. (From Stein HA, Slatt BJ, Stein RM: *The ophthalmic assistant,* ed 7, St. Louis, 2000, Mosby.)

Penetrating Trauma

Penetrating injury to the eye may occur during work or play and is often associated with lack of protective eyewear. Injury may affect surface structures such as the cornea or involve damage to the globe.

Periorbital Wounds. Periorbital wounds involve injury to the eyelids and surrounding periorbital tissue. Tissues lie in close proximity to the globe, so wounds should be examined carefully for globe penetration. Depending on mechanism of trauma, careful examination for foreign bodies should be part of the examination. Therapeutic interventions for lacerations include wound care and early closure with careful approximation of wound edges before edema develops. For major lacerations or injuries with missing tissue, a plastic surgeon is recommended. An ophthalmologist may be consulted to rule out ocular damage. The eyelid has an excellent blood supply, so trauma to the eyelid has a low incidence of infection; antibiotic treatment is rarely required.

Globe Rupture. Globe rupture is a major ocular emergency that results from blunt or penetrating trauma. Rupture occurs at a point of weakness in the ocular structures, usually insertion of the extraocular muscles or the corneoscleral junction (limbus). Penetrating injuries to the globe are caused by perforation with a sharp object such as a knife, stick, or other projectile object. Blunt forces cause globe rupture secondary to an abrupt rise in IOP.

Signs and symptoms of globe rupture include an unusually deep or shallow anterior chamber, altered light perception, hyphema, and occasionally vitreous hemorrhage. In addition, the patient may experience eye pain with nausea.[8] The pupil assumes a teardrop shape with the tip pointing to the perforation.[17] When globe rupture is suspected, further eye manipulation should be avoided. If an impaled object is present, do not remove it. Secure the object and patch the opposite eye to decrease eye movement and prevent further damage. Detailed examination is not performed until the ophthalmologist arrives. General anesthesia may be necessary to perform an adequate examination. Eye drops should not be used when globe rupture is suspected. Aggressive pain management is crucial to prevent or decrease expulsion of intraocular contents. If the patient is nauseated, antiemetics should be given. Tetanus immunization should be updated. While waiting for the ophthalmologist a fox shield or other protective device should be placed over the affected eye. Keep the patient NPO and prepare for surgery.

Superficial Trauma

Corneal Abrasion. Corneal abrasions are an extremely common injury seen in the ED. The cornea is damaged when a foreign body such as a contact lens scratches, abrades, or denudes the epithelium. Damage to the cornea exposes superficial corneal nerves, causing tearing, eyelid spasms, and pain. The patient will usually complain of a foreign body sensation, photophobia, and acute onset of pain.[13]

Instillation of a drop of topical anesthesia will assist in determing visual acuity. It will also alleviate the sensation of a foreign body and decrease pain. The upper eyelid should be everted to ensure that no foreign body is found. Diagnosis is made with fluorescein staining and examination with a cobalt light and a slit lamp examination. If the abrasion is large, cycloplegics may be prescribed to decrease ciliary spasms. Topical antibiotics are usually prescribed to prevent secondary infection. Additional medications that may be given are topical nonsteroidal agents and analgesics. Patching is no longer recommended unless there is a large defect or for comfort.[20] Patching should never be done if the patient wears contact lenses.[8,10,13] The injury should be reevaluated in 24 hours.

Corneal Lacerations. Corneal lacerations may be small or large. Small lacerations are treated as corneal abrasions. Larger corneal lacerations may require surgery to preserve the integrity of intraocular contents. An ophthalmology consult is indicated for these patients.

Foreign Body

The most common foreign body is a small particle of dust. The patient usually presents with photophobia, excessive tearing, or pain, especially when opening or closing the eye. Foreign bodies and corneal abrasions feel similar to the patient. With a foreign body, the first step is to locate the object. Local anesthesia may be required to examine the eye adequately. Good lighting and a magnification source are essential to locate and safely remove a foreign body from the eye.

With a foreign body in the conjunctiva and cornea, determine identity of the foreign body (what the patient believes is in the eye). A history of high-speed projectiles should increase the index of suspicion for an intraocular foreign body. Organic foreign bodies have a higher incidence of infection, whereas metallic objects leave a rust ring unless the object is removed within 12 hours. Inert foreign bodies do not cause infection but have a greater risk of penetration.

Therapeutic intervention includes everting the upper eyelid with a cotton-tipped swab, irrigating with normal saline solution, and gently removing the foreign body with a moistened cotton-tipped swab. Never use a dry cotton-tipped swab on the cornea because it may create a large corneal defect. If the foreign body adheres to the cornea, a topical anesthetic is applied, then a 25 to 27-gauge needle is used at a tangential angle to remove the object. Larger embedded objects are referred to the ophthalmologist for removal or follow-up.[6,17] After the foreign body is removed, the cornea should be carefully examined for other objects, rust ring, or corneal abrasion. Ocular burr drills are also used to remove rust rings and may be used to free foreign bodies stuck to the cornea. Treat subsequent corneal abrasions. If the patient has a rust ring, an ophthamologic referral should be arranged so that the patient is seen within the next 24 hours.

Intraocular Foreign Body. Intraocular foreign bodies are usually small and easily overlooked. Metal fragments and other small projectiles enter the eye at high speed and come to rest within the posterior chamber. The entry site may be small and difficult to locate. A high index of suspicion is required to prompt a vigorous evaluation for this type of injury.[5] Many patients experience only slight discomfort. Visual acuity may be significantly decreased or may be normal. The pupil may assume the shape of a cat's eye.

An intraocular foreign body is an ocular emergency. Early therapeutic intervention is essential to preserve vision. The amount of damage to the eye depends on size, shape, and composition of the foreign body. All foreign bodies in the eye are considered contaminated, so the patient is treated with antibiotics and tetanus prophylaxis as appropriate. A CT scan is the best way to locate an intraocular foreign body. Surgery is indicated for most patients to prevent further damage to the eye secondary to hemorrhage, infection, or detached retina.

Ocular Burns

Ocular burns are an immediate threat to the patient's vision. Burns to the eye may result from a chemical, heat source such as a curling iron, or radiation. Regardless of etiology, these injuries cause significant discomfort.

Chemical Trauma. Chemical burns occur at home and work. A chemical burn is the most urgent of all ocular emergencies. An alkaline, acid, or thermal source may cause burns. These substances, particularly alkalines, have a devastating effect on the eye. Acid burns cause immediate damage to the cornea by denaturing the tissue, so the cornea appears white and opaque. No further damage occurs after the initial impact because the acid is neutralized on impact. Alkalines such as concrete, lye, and drain cleaners also cause the cornea to opacify; however, alkalines continue to damage the cornea until the substance is removed.[2]

Chemical burns are the only ocular emergency in which visual acuity is temporarily postponed. Copious irrigation with normal saline should be initiated as soon as possible, preferably before the patient arrives in the ED. With alkaline burns, irrigation should continue until ocular pH reaches approximately 7. Irrigation for a minimum of 30 minutes with

2 L of fluid is the norm. With severe cases, irrigation for 2 to 4 hours may be necessary. After pH reaches the desired level, the eyelid should be everted, then the cul-de-sac swabbed and irrigated to remove any remaining particles. Patients should receive topical antibiotics, cycloplegic agents, and steroids. Parenteral or oral narcotic analgesia is also recommended. Administer tetanus as appropriate. Obtain ophthalmologic consult for all burns.[8]

Thermal Burns. Thermal burns affect the eyelids but rarely involve the globe because of reflex lid closure. Thermal burns are treated similar to other burns that occur on the body. If the lids are damaged so they do not close adequately, special attention must be given to ensure that the globe is not injured. Burns to the eyelids may cause lid contracture, which is disfiguring and affects vision. Therapeutic interventions include analgesia, sedation, eye irrigation, antibiotics, cycloplegics, and bilateral eye patches.

Radiation Burns. Radiation burns may be ultraviolet or infrared. Severity of burn depends on wavelength and degree of exposure. Ultraviolet burns occur in welders, snow skiers, ice climbers, people who read on the beach, and those who use sun lamps. Ultraviolet radiation is absorbed by the cornea and produces keratitis, conjunctivitis, or both. Pain, tearing, photophobia, and a foreign body sensation usually begin 6 to 10 hours after exposure. Ultraviolet burns are considered the most painful of all ocular burns. Visual acuity is usually decreased. Therapeutic interventions include topical antibiotics, cycloplegics, systemic analgesics, topical antibiotic ointment, and patching for 24 hours.[10] The cornea usually heals within 24 hours without residual scarring. Slit lamp examination with fluorescein staining reveals superficial punctate keratitis that looks like small microdots on the corneal surface.

Infrared radiation burns are more severe than ultraviolet radiation burns. Fortunately, infrared radiation injuries are rare since the development of protective eyewear. Infrared radiation burns cause permanent loss of vision secondary to absorption of infrared rays by the iris and increased lens temperature, which leads to cataract formation. Table 46-4 describes common infrared burns.

Medical Problems Involving the Eye

Many ocular problems that present to the ED are not related to trauma. Problems may be a minor annoyance or represent a significant threat to the patient's vision. The most common medical conditions seen in the ED are described in the following section.

Infections

Lids

HORDEOLUM. Hordeolum, or an external stye, is an infection of an eyelash oil gland of Zeis or Moll.[3] The patient develops a small external abscess, pain, redness, and swelling (Figure 46-14). Therapeutic intervention includes application of warm compresses four times per day until the abscess comes to a point. A hordeolum may rupture sponta-

Table 46-4	**INFRARED BURNS**
NAME	**DESCRIPTION**
Glassblower's cataracts	Caused by prolonged exposure to intense heat during production of glass.
Focal retinitis	Also called eclipse blindness; occurs during exposure to an eclipse or an atomic bomb.
X-ray burns	Injury proportional to penetration of rays. Soft rays produce superficial keratoconjunctivitis and dermatitis, whereas hard rays, such as gamma rays, produce retinal damage and cataracts.

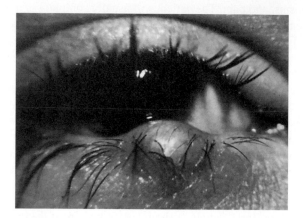

FIGURE 46-14 Acute hordeolum of the lower eyelid. (From Newell FW: *Ophthalmology: principles and concepts,* ed 8, St. Louis, 1996, Mosby.)

neously or require incision to drain the abscess. If the abscess points to the conjunctiva, the physician makes a vertical incision; if the abscess points toward the skin, a horizontal incision is made. Ophthalmic antibiotic ointment should be applied every 4 hours. The patient should be instructed not to squeeze the abscess because this can spread infection and worsen the condition.

CHALAZION. A chalazion is an internal hordeolum caused by chronic granulomatous inflammation of the meibomian gland (Figure 46-15). The patient usually presents with several weeks of painless, localized swelling. A chalazion is differentiated from a hordeolum by the absence of acute inflammation. Treatment in the early stages includes topical antibiotic ointment and incision and drainage when the chalazion affects vision.

BLEPHARITIS. Blepharitis is an ulcerative inflammation of the lid margin, usually with *S. aureus*. Symptoms include burning, stinging, and itching of the lids. The eye appears rimmed with red, and scales may appear on the lashes. Treatment consists of removing the crusts and cleaning lid margins twice daily with soap and applying an antibiotic ophthalmic ointment.

Corneal

KERATITIS. Keratitis is a generic term for inflammation of the cornea. The cornea becomes light-sensitive, red, and painful, with profuse tearing. A corneal ulcer, bacteria, or

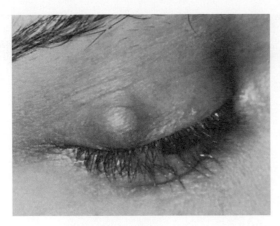

FIGURE 46-15 Chronic chalazion of meibomian gland of the upper eyelid. (From Newell FW: *Ophthalmology: principles and concepts,* ed 8, St. Louis, 1996, Mosby.)

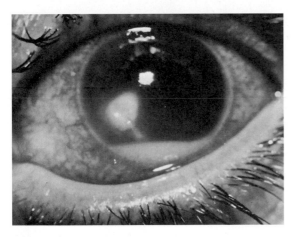

FIGURE 46-16 An acute hypopyon ulcerative keratitis caused by a *Streptococcus* organism infection in a 69-year-old patient with facial nerve paralysis that prevented adequate closure of the eyelid. Leukocytes in the anterior chamber form a hypopyon. (From Newell FW: *Ophthalmology: principles and concepts,* ed 8, St. Louis, 1996, Mosby.)

fungus may cause keratitis. The patient presents with a "white spot" on the cornea, an epithelial defect, or a corneal ulcer (Figure 46-16). Risk factors for bacterial keratitis include traumatic corneal injury and corneal injury secondary to contact lens use. The typical presentation is conjunctivitis, pain, photophobia, mucopurulent discharge, and decreased vision. Pus in the anterior chamber (hypopyon) may also be present. Culture and sensitivity should be obtained to determine the specific cause of the infection. Therapeutic interventions include warm compresses, broad-spectrum antibiotics, and possibly fungal drops. A topical cycloplegic agent may be used to control pain. The eye should not be patched because of the risk for *Pseudomonas* organism infection. Referral to an ophthalmologist within 24 hours is required to prevent further complications.[10]

VIRAL KERATOCONJUNCTIVITIS. Viral keratoconjunctivitis is an acute conjunctivitis and keratitis usually caused by

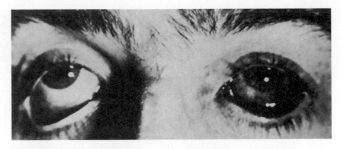

FIGURE 46-17 Acute conjunctivitis. (From Stein HA, Slatt BJ, Stein RM: *The ophthalmic assistant,* ed 6, St. Louis, 1994, Mosby.)

adenovirus. The patient complains of redness to the eye, tearing, and pain. Photophobia usually begins several days later. Eyelids and conjunctiva become swollen. In adults this condition is confined to the eye; however, children may have fever, pharyngitis, and diarrhea. Therapeutic intervention is usually symptomatic. Topical antibiotics may be started while awaiting culture results. This type of infection spreads easily; therefore, it is critical to stress scrupulous hand washing to the patient. All instruments used on the patient should be sterilized.

HERPES SIMPLEX. Herpes simplex infection can affect the eyelids, conjunctiva, and the cornea. Skin involvement is vesicular lesions while the conjunctiva becomes inflamed. Corneal findings show a dendrite of herpes keritis seen with fluorescein staining. Outbreaks on the lids and conjunctiva can be treated with Zovirax or Famvir and topical antiviral drops (Viroptic five times per day without corneal involvement and nine times per day with corneal involvement). Ophthalmology referral in 2 to 3 days is recommended.[10]

HERPES ZOSTER OPHTHALMICUS. Herpes zoster ophthalmicus represents shingles in the ophthalmic division of the trigeminal nerve. Patients will often have prodromal signs of fever and scalp tenderness on half the forehead. If the tip of the nose is involved, ocular involvement is more likely (Hutchinson's sign). The patient can develop iritis, which is treated with topical steroids when there is no corneal involvement. The patient may be given oral Zovirax or Famvir to lessen the course. At times hospitalization may be necessary for intravenous acyclovir, especially if any intracranial symptoms are present.[8,10]

CONJUNCTIVITIS. Conjunctivitis, or pink eye, is a frequent problem seen in the ED. Conjunctivitis is caused by many etiologies: bacterial, viral, or allergic.

Bacterial conjunctivitis usually presents with a purulent discharge that is yellow-green in color. Patients will usually complain that eyes are matted shut in the morning. This infection can involve one or both eyes. It is important to ask the patient if they have been exposed to someone with pink eye. Infections can be caused by *Pneumococcus, Streptococcus pneumoniae, S. aureus, Haemophilus,* and *Meningococcus* organisms.[16] Signs and symptoms of bacterial infection include purulent discharge, reddened eye, and swollen eyelid, associated with tenderness (Figure 46-17). Treatment

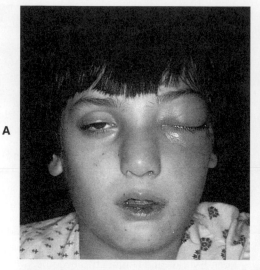

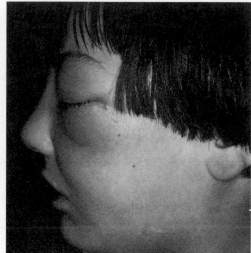

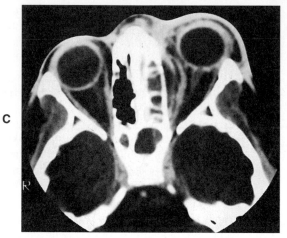

FIGURE **46-18** Orbital cellulitis. **A** and **B.** This child had a fever, severe toxicity, and marked lethargy. He experienced intense orbital and retroorbital pain, and showed a limited range of ocular motion. **C,** This CT scan shows preseptal swelling, proptosis, and lateral displacement of the globe and orbital contents by a subperiosteal abscess. (From Zitelli B, Davis H: *Atlas of pediatric physical diagnosis,* ed 3, St. Louis, 1997, Mosby.)

usually consists of a topical ocular antibiotic for 5 to 7 days. For contact wearers, a fluoroquinolone or aminoglysocide is prescribed to cover a *Pseudomonal* organism infection. Warm soaks are used to keep the lids and lashes free of debris.

Acute bacterial conjunctivitis is contagious. Detailed aftercare instructions should include how to prevent the disease from spreading. Teaching should include discussion of cross-contamination through eye makeup, pillows, washcloths, and towels. Children should be kept out of school until the discharge subsides.[16] Appropriate hand-washing techniques should also be reviewed.

Conjunctivitis secondary to *Neisseria gonorrhoeae* causes copious purulent discharge with extremely red and swollen conjunctiva. This is usually seen in sexually active adolescents and newborns. Diagnosis is made on the presence of purulent discharge from the eyes and genital discharge. A positive Thayer-Martin culture confirms the diagnosis. Therapeutic intervention is ceftriaxone 125 mg intramuscularly or intravenously.[8] Immediate referral to an ophthalmologist is essential. Other potential contacts, including sexual contact, should be treated.

Viral conjunctivitis is usually caused by the adenovirus. Viral infections are highly contagious and may accompany an upper respiratory infection. Onset is usually abrupt and unilateral and at times resembles a cold. Eye drainage is usually clear and the conjunctiva is reddened. Treatment consists of Naphcon-A.[10] A topical antibiotic may be prescribed if the diagnosis is uncertain. Detailed aftercare instructions should include how to prevent the disease from spreading.

UVEITIS/IRITIS. Uveitis/iritis is an inflammation of the uveal tract including the iris, ciliary body, and choroid. Uveal inflammation usually affects the anterior portion of the uveal tract and is categorized as iritis. Severe inflammation may decrease the patient's vision. Other symptoms include photophobia, unilateral gradual eye pain, red eye, and excessive tearing. Anterior uveitis and iritis need an ophthalmic referral. Initial treatment includes cycloplegics and topical steroids. This decreases photophobia and inflammation.

ORBITAL CELLULITIS. Orbital cellulitis (Figure 46-18), an orbital infection deep into the orbital septum, can be a life-threatening infection. Usual causes are *Streptococcus pneumoniae, S. aureus,* and *Haemophilus influenza.* There is usually an associated sinus infection. Symptoms include pain, fever, and impaired extraocular movement motility. Decreased visual acuity is a late finding. A CT

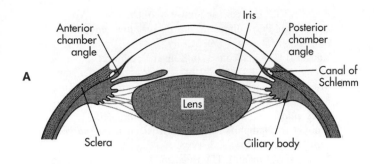

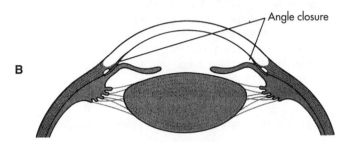

FIGURE **46-19**   Comparison of **A,** normal angle of eye with, **B,** closed angle in angle-closure glaucoma.

scan of the orbits and sinuses, blood cultures, and admission to the hospital is required. The patient is given intravenous antibiotics. Immediate ophthalmologic referral is required.[8,10,17]

Orbital cellulitis may progress to a life-threatening condition called cavernous sinus thrombosis. This is an infection that has spread from an infected sinus to the orbital area. Signs and symptoms include chills, headache, lethargy, nausea, pain, and decreased vision. The patient may also have fever, vomiting, and other signs of systemic involvement.

Retinal Emergencies

CENTRAL RETINAL ARTERY OCCLUSION.   Central retinal artery occlusion produces sudden, painless blindness and is usually limited to one eye. This is a true ocular emergency. Retinal circulation must be reestablished within 60 to 90 minutes to prevent permanent loss of vision. Occasionally, before total occlusion occurs, the patient may experience transient episodes of blindness called amaurosis fugax. This can be equated to a transient ischemia attack. The patients usually describe the episode as a shade coming down over the eye.[11] Causes include embolus (carotid and cardiac), thrombosis, giant cell arteritis, or simple angiospasm (rare) associated with a migraine or atrial fibrillation. To prevent permanent damage, treatments include ocular massage, IOP-lowering drugs, and vasodilation techniques (breathing into a paper bag).[10]

RETINAL DETACHMENT.   Retinal detachment occurs when the retina tears and allows vitreous humor to seep between the retina and the choroid. When the retina is torn, loss of blood and oxygen supply renders the retina unable to perceive light. Normal function of the retina is to perceive light and send an impulse to the optic nerve. With retinal detachment, the patient complains of "flashing lights," "floaters," and "veil" or curtain effect in the visual field. The prognosis is excellent if treated early. Therapeutic interventions include hospitalization, bed rest, and bilateral eye patches. Ophthalmologic consultation for immediate referral is necessary for a laser repair or a scleral buckling procedure.[11]

Glaucoma.   Glaucoma is the second most common cause of blindness in the United States.[11,19] Glaucoma is classified as primary or secondary and open angle or closed angle. Secondary glaucoma is associated with some type of underlying ocular or systemic condition, whereas with primary glaucoma there is no underlying or known cause. Closed-angle glaucoma is caused when the anterior chamber angle is narrowed; open-angle glaucoma has a normal anterior chamber angle. Primary open-angle glaucoma is the most common form of glaucoma. The most concerning type of glaucoma is primary angle-closure glaucoma. Acute glaucoma occurs when the aqueous humor cannot escape from the anterior chamber, so volume increases and IOP rises (Figure 46-19). Normally, aqueous humor leaves the anterior chamber and enters the vascular system via the Schlemm's canal at the junction of the iris and cornea. With glaucoma, increased anterior chamber pressure decreases circulation to the retina and increases pressure on the optic nerve. If left untreated these high pressures eventually cause blindness.

ACUTE ANGLE-CLOSURE GLAUCOMA.   The prevalence of acute angle-closure glaucoma increases with age and is more common in women. There is a higher incidence of acute angle-closure glaucoma in Asians and Eskimos. Acute angle-closure glaucoma occurs with blockage of the anterior chamber angle near the root of the iris. The patient presents with severe eye pain, a fixed and slightly dilated pupil, hard globe, foggy-appearing cornea, severe headache, complaining of halos around lights, diminished peripheral vision, and nausea and vomiting.[7] IOP greater than 60 to 70 mm Hg damages the corneal endothelium, lens, iris, optical nerve, and retina. Diagnosis may be difficult because symptoms can mimic cardiovascular or gastrointestinal processes. Therapeutic intervention focuses on decreasing IOP as quickly as possible by decreasing production and increasing removal of aqueous humor. Pilocarpine 2% should be administered every 15 minutes until pupillary constriction occurs. Timolol 0.5% will decrease IOP within 30 to 60 minutes.[9] Antiemetics and narcotics may be useful. Ophthalmologic consultation for definitive treatment is required.

SUMMARY

Most ocular emergencies do not represent a threat to the patient's life; however, these conditions represent a great threat to the patient's well-being. Once lost, vision cannot be replaced. The emergency nurse should assess the patients who present with various ocular problems and identify those patients with actual or potential threats to vision. Early recognition of true ocular emergencies is essential for preserva-

Box 46-8	**NURSING DIAGNOSES FOR OCULAR EMERGENCIES**

Anxiety
Infection, Risk for
Injury, Risk for
Knowledge, Deficient
Pain
Sensory perception, Disturbed

tion of sight. Box 46-8 summarizes nursing diagnoses for patients with an ocular problem.

References

1. Barish RA, Naradzay JF: Ophthalmologic therapeutics, *Emerg Med Clin North Am* 13(3):649, 1995.
2. Beaver HA, Lee AG: Trauma emergencies in ophthalmology, *Hosp Med* 34(8):41, 1998.
3. Birinyi F, Mauger TF: Ophthalmic conditions. In Knoop KJ, Stack LB, Storrow AB, editors: *Atlas of emergency medicine,* New York, 1997, McGraw-Hill.
4. Cakanac CJ: *Adding insight to injury.* Retrieved March 2000 from the World Wide Web: http://www.revoptom.com/OSC/re0300osc.htm.
5. Cakanac CJ: *How to deal with fractures and penetrations.* Retrieved April 2000 from the World Wide Web: http://www.revoptom.com/OSC/re0400osc.htm.
6. Easterbrook M, Johnston RH, Howcroft MJ: Assessment of ocular foreign bodies, *Physician Sportsmed* 25(2), 1997.
7. Effron D, Forcier BC, Wyszynski RE: Funduscopic findings. In Knoop KJ, Stack LB, Storrow AB, editors: *Atlas of emergency medicine,* New York, 1997, McGraw-Hill.
8. Englanoff JS: Eye pain and redness. In Davis MA, Votey SR, Greenough PG, editors: *Signs & symptoms in emergency medicine,* St. Louis, 1999, Mosby.
9. Kanski JJ: The glaucomas. In Kanski JJ, editor: *Clinical ophthalmology,* ed 3, Oxford, 1997, Butterworth Heinemann.
10. Mitchell JD: Ocular emergencies. In Tintinalli JE, Ruiz E, Krome RL, editors: *Emergency medicine: a comprehensive study guide,* ed 5, New York, 2000, McGraw-Hill.
11. Morgan A, Hemphill R: Acute visual change, *Emerg Med Clin North Am* 16(4):825, 1998.
12. Munter DW, McGuirk TD: Head and facial trauma. In Knoop KJ, Stack LB, Storrow AB, editors: *Atlas of emergency medicine,* New York, 1997, McGraw-Hill.
13. Peak DE, Chisholm CD, Knoop KJ: Ophthalmic trauma. In Knoop KJ, Stack LB, Storrow AB, editors: *Atlas of emergency medicine,* New York, 1997, McGraw-Hill.
14. Pizzarello LD: Ocular trauma: time for action, *Ophthalmic Epidemiol* 5:115, 1998.
15. Quigley M: Tonometry. In Proehl JA, editor: *Emergency nursing procedures,* ed 2, Philadelphia, 1999, WB Saunders.
16. Ruppert SD: Differential diagnosis of pediatric conjunctivitis, *Nurse Pract* 21(7):12, 1996.
17. Shingleton BJ, Mead MD: *New England Eye Center handbook of eye emergencies,* Thorofare, NJ, 1998, Slack.
18. St. Luke's Eye.com: *Hyphema* (2000). Retrieved from the World Wide Web: http://www.stlukeseye.com/hyphema.htm.
19. Whitaker R Jr, Whitaker VB, Dill C: Glaucoma: what the nurse practitioner should know, *Nurse Pract Forum* 9(1):7, 1998.
20. Wingate S: Treating corneal abrasions, *Nurse Pract* 24(6):53, 1999.
21. Wong TY, Tielsch JM: Epidemiology of ocular trauma. In *Dauane's clinical ophthalmology,* vol 5, Philadelphia, 1998, JB Lippincott.

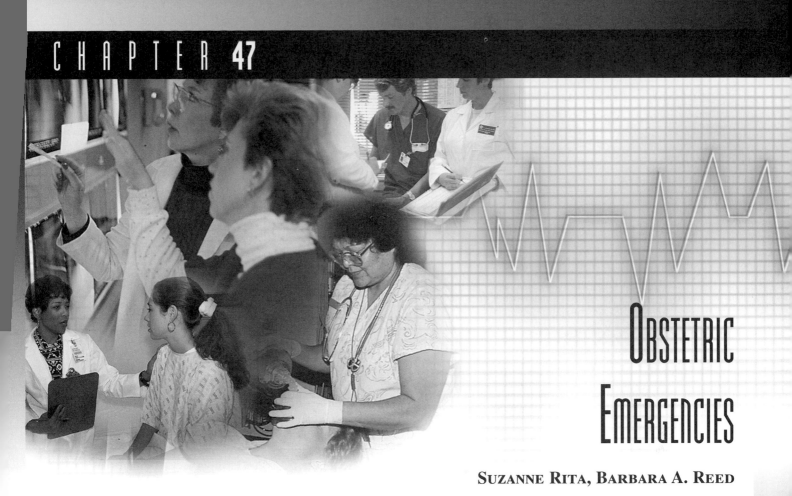

CHAPTER 47

OBSTETRIC EMERGENCIES

SUZANNE RITA, BARBARA A. REED

Pregnant women can present to the emergency department (ED) with a variety of complaints related to pregnancy. These may occur before, during, or after delivery. Management of obstetric emergencies requires acute assessment skills to identify life-threatening conditions and quickly intervene to prevent adverse outcomes for mother and baby. This chapter describes changes in pathophysiology related to pregnancy, assessment of the pregnant patient, and management of emergencies commonly associated with pregnancy. Refer to Chapter 31 for discussion of obstetric trauma.

ANATOMY AND PHYSIOLOGY

The female reproductive system consists of the fallopian tubes, ovaries, uterus, vagina, and external genitalia (Figure 47-1). The cervical os, or opening to the uterus, is located within the vagina. The vagina serves as the exit route for menstrual blood flow, entry point for sperm, and the birth canal. Physiologic activity of the reproductive system is cyclic. Each month the uterus prepares for implantation of a fertilized egg through proliferation of the uterine endometrium. Eggs are stored in the ovaries and released in a cyclic pattern. If the egg is not fertilized, the uterine lining sloughs and is shed as menstrual blood flow. If the egg is fertilized, it begins to reproduce and replicate. The embryo is

formed, transported through the fallopian tube, and embedded in the uterine wall to continue its growth.

As the pregnancy progresses, it is characterized by increasing size of the embryo and various sexual organs. Uterine size goes from about 50 g to about 1100 g.[3] Concurrently, breasts double in size, and the vagina enlarges. Total weight gain during pregnancy is about 25 pounds. Other body systems affected by pregnancy include the cardiovascular, respiratory, gastrointestinal, and genitourinary systems. Changes in these systems are summarized in Table 47-1.

PATIENT ASSESSMENT

Many EDs care for pregnant patients throughout the pregnancy, whereas others provide care only for complaints not related to pregnancy (e.g., colds, flu, sprains, strains, fractures, and lacerations). Each pregnant patient should be carefully assessed (Box 47-1).

Regardless of gestation the first priority for assessment of women with an obstetric emergency is airway, breathing, and circulation (ABCs). The age of fetal viability is considered 24 weeks' gestation. Management of obstetric emergencies after onset of fetal viability involves two patients, mother and fetus. See Chapter 48 for discussion of neonatal resuscitation. After assessment of the patient's ABCs, the next priority is determination of gestation and evaluation of

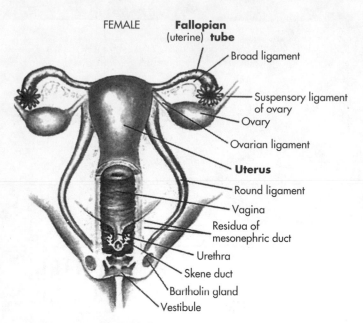

FEMALE **Fallopian** (uterine) **tube**

- Broad ligament
- Suspensory ligament of ovary
- Ovary
- Ovarian ligament
- **Uterus**
- Round ligament
- Vagina
- Residua of mesonephric duct
- Urethra
- Skene duct
- Bartholin gland
- Vestibule

FIGURE 47-1 Female reproductive system. (From Huether SE, McCance KL: *Understanding pathophysiology,* St. Louis, 1996, Mosby.)

Table 47-1 **PHYSIOLOGIC CHANGES RELATED TO PREGNANCY**

BODY SYSTEM	CHANGES
Cardiovascular	Cardiac output increases 30%-40% by week 27
	Placental blood flow is 625-650 ml/min
	Blood volume increases by 30%
Respiratory	Heart rate increases throughout pregnancy
	Respiratory rate increases
	Oxygen consumption increases by 20%
	Minute volume increases by 50%
	Arterial pCO_2 decreases secondary to hyperventilation
Urinary	Rate of urine formation increases slightly
	Sodium, chloride, and water reabsorption increases as much as 50%
	Glomerular filtration rate increases about 50%
Gastrointestinal	Smooth muscle relaxes, which increases gastric emptying time
	Intestines are relocated to the upper abdomen
Other	Anemia develops because of increased iron requirements by mother and fetus

pCO_2, Pressure of carbon dioxide.

impending delivery. Specific emergencies are divided into those associated with the first, second, and third trimester and the postpartum period.

Box 47-1 **ASSESSMENT GUIDELINES FOR THE PREGNANT PATIENT**

Last normal menstrual period
Birth control method
Gravida, parity, and abortion history
Bleeding, discharge, or tissue present
Nausea or vomiting
Urinary symptoms
Abdominal pain—location, duration, description
Estimated date of confinement
Prenatal care
Problems with present or previous pregnancies
Medications and allergies
Maternal medical and surgical history
Blood type and Rh factor if known

FIRST TRIMESTER EMERGENCIES

First trimester emergencies involve only one patient—the mother. Mortality is related to blood loss. Other issues relate to loss of pregnancy and potential loss of fertility.

Ectopic Pregnancy

Ectopic pregnancy occurs when the fertilized ovum implants anywhere other than the endometrium, such as the fallopian tube, ovary, or abdominal cavity. Ninety-five percent of all ectopic pregnancies occur in one of the fallopian tubes, with the most common site for implantation the ampulla followed by the isthmus (Figure 47-2). The ovum begins to grow but may rupture, usually after the twelfth week of pregnancy. Ectopic pregnancy is one of the major causes of maternal death, usually from hemorrhage.

On assessment the patient gives a history of being pregnant (at least 12 weeks). However, 15% of patients with ectopic pregnancy are symptomatic before the first missed period. Complaints include pelvic pain or vaginal bleeding. Pain, if present, may be mild to severe. If the ectopic pregnancy is leaking or has ruptured, the diaphragm becomes irritated from blood in the peritoneum, causing referred pain to the shoulder (Kehr's sign).

Pelvic pain and vaginal bleeding or spotting in a woman of childbearing years should be treated as an ectopic pregnancy until this life-threatening condition is ruled out. Predisposing factors for ectopic pregnancy include previous ectopic pregnancy, adhesions from previous pregnancies and surgeries, and previous pelvic infections. Presence of an intrauterine device has been noted in some patients with ectopic pregnancy.

A pregnancy test should be obtained on all women presenting with pelvic pain and vaginal bleeding or spotting. A pelvic examination is done to evaluate the cervical os and identify the amount and source of bleeding. Bimanual pelvic examination defines uterine size and allows palpation of masses outside the uterus.

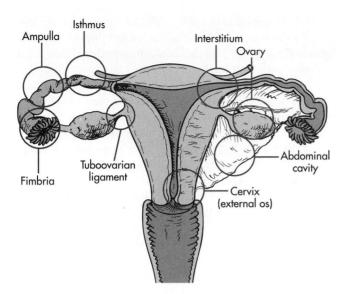

FIGURE **47-2**   Sites of implantation of ectopic pregnancies. Order of frequency of occurrence is ampulla, isthmus, interstitium, fimbria, tuboovarian ligament, ovary, abdominal cavity, and cervix (external os). (From Lewis SM, Heitkemper MM, Dirksen SR: *Medical-surgical nursing,* ed 5, St. Louis, 2000, Mosby.)

Table 47-2	TYPES OF ABORTION
TYPE	**SIGNS AND SYMPTOMS**
Threatened	Vaginal bleeding
	Mild abdominal cramping
	Closed or slightly open os
Inevitable	Heavy vaginal bleeding
	Severe abdominal cramping
	Open os
Incomplete	Heavy vaginal bleeding
	Abdominal cramping
	Some products of conception retained
Complete	Slight vaginal bleeding
	No abdominal cramping
	All products of conception passed
Missed	Usually no maternal symptoms
	Discrepancy in fetal size when compared to dates
Septic	Severe abdominal pain
	High temperature
	Malodorous vaginal discharge

If an ectopic pregnancy is suspected, intravenous access should be established with a large-bore catheter in anticipation of potential life-threatening hemorrhage. Quantitative serum β-human chorionic gonadotropin (β-hCG) level, complete blood count (CBC), and type and screen should be obtained. An abdominal ultrasound is done to identify an ectopic pregnancy.

Treatment for ectopic pregnancy includes nonoperative and operative interventions. For selected cases ectopic pregnancy can be medically managed as an alternative to surgery. Methotrexate, a folic acid antagonist that prevents further duplication of fetal cells, is administered intramuscularly, then the patient is followed as an outpatient with serial β-hCG tests. Occasionally β-hCG levels do not fall, so additional methotrexate injections may be necessary. Operative interventions are indicated when the ectopic pregnancy has ruptured, the patient is in shock, or nonoperative interventions are not appropriate.

In addition to assessment and intervention for physiologic needs, the emergency nurse must recognize the need for emotional support for the patient and the family. The patient may fear for her life and her future childbearing ability, feel concern the pregnancy is not normal, or experience personal guilt related to the pregnancy.

Abortion

Termination of pregnancy at any time before the fetus has achieved viability (24 weeks' gestation) is defined as abortion. Abortion is the number one cause of vaginal bleeding in women of childbearing years, with an estimated 10% to 15% of all pregnancies resulting in spontaneous abortion.[2] This is one of the differential diagnoses for any woman of childbearing years with vaginal bleeding. Table 47-2 summarizes the types of abortion. Causes of abortion include infection, injury, and an incompetent cervix.

The patient presents to the ED complaining of vaginal bleeding with abdominal pain frequently noted. A missed period may or may not be reported. Gynecologic history should be elicited from the patient, including amount of bleeding. Ask the patient how many pads or tampons she has used in the past hour; a general rule of thumb is a saturated pad or tampon equals 20 to 30 ml of blood loss.

Obtain a urine pregnancy test or serum β-hCG level. Palpate the patient's abdomen for pain or tenderness, which may indicate ectopic pregnancy. A pelvic examination determines the source of bleeding, visualizes any products of conception, and determines dilatation of the cervical os. Observe for vaginal discharge. A bimanual examination is performed to determine size of the uterus and other reproductive organs. Palpation of the adnexa is performed to determine tenderness. Consider pelvic ultrasound to exclude ectopic pregnancy.

Therapeutic interventions depend on the type of abortion. Fifty percent of threatened abortions result in complete or incomplete abortion within a few hours. A patient with threatened abortion should be observed closely for changes in hemodynamic status. Document the amount of blood loss. If the patient exhibits signs of shock, replace blood loss with fluids or blood. Provide emotional support to the patient, significant other, and family.

If the abortion is inevitable or incomplete, obtain blood for complete blood count, Rh type, and type and screen. Start at least one intravenous (IV) line with a large-bore catheter and administer fluids (normal saline or lactated Ringer's solution). Prepare for suction curettage.

If the patient will be discharged, aftercare instructions should include information on bed rest and instructions to return to the ED or call the primary caregiver for increased vaginal bleeding, increasing abdominal pain, passage of tissue, fever, or chills. The patient should also be told to avoid douching and intercourse while on bed rest because these can increase vaginal bleeding, worsen cramping, or cause infection if the cervical os begins to open. The patient should be instructed to follow up with the appropriate referral caregiver. RhoGam should be given within 72 hours if the mother is Rh negative.

ANTEPARTUM EMERGENCIES

Emergencies that occur during the last months of pregnancy threaten the mother and the fetus. Neurologic sequelae such as seizures and anoxic brain damage are also possible.

Pregnancy-Induced Hypertension

The term *pregnancy-induced hypertension* (PIH) refers to toxemia of pregnancy and includes preeclampsia and eclampsia. This condition usually occurs in the last few months of pregnancy (after 20 weeks' gestation) and can appear up to 72 hours after delivery. Actual etiology is unknown. The syndrome occurs most often in women who have a family history of preeclampsia, primigravida, or who are younger than 20 years and older than 40 years of age.

There is also increased risk if there is a history of chronic vascular disease, renal disease, diabetes, multiple fetuses, or hydatidiform mole. PIH can cause maternal morbidity and mortality with high fetal mortality.

PIH is characterized by hypertension, proteinuria, and edema. Systolic blood pressure is greater than 140 mm Hg or there is an increase of 30 mm Hg over the nonpregnant level. An increase of 15 mm Hg of the diastolic over baseline or diastolic blood pressure of 90 or more is classified as hypertension (HTN).[4] HTN leads to vasospasm and hemolysis and effects several organ systems.

Blood pressure elevation, the paramount symptom of preeclampsia, is compared to prenatal or early pregnancy. Proteinuria is a late sign and is an indicator of severity of the disease. Edema is the least reliable sign because of the frequency of occurrence during pregnancy. However, sudden onset of facial edema with weight gain is a significant indicator of preeclampsia (Table 47-3). Pulmonary edema may also be present. Subjective signs of preeclampsia may include visual changes, headaches, epigastric pain, and decreased urination. Preeclampsia left untreated may progress to eclampsia. In eclampsia the patient presents with seizures or coma. This situation is an immediate threat to the mother and fetus.

Treatment includes oxygen, IV access, and fetal monitoring. The woman is placed in the left lateral recumbent posi-

Table 47-3	CHARACTERISTICS OF MILD VERSUS SEVERE PREECLAMPSIA	
CHARACTERISTICS	**MILD PREECLAMPSIA**	**SEVERE PREECLAMPSIA**
Blood pressure	Greater than 140/90 mm Hg but less than 160/110 mm Hg 30 mm Hg systolic rise; or 15 mm Hg diastolic rise over baseline readings of early pregnancy (Readings are obtained after rest in a sitting position two times at least 6 hr apart)	Blood pressure greater than 160/110 mm Hg
Proteinuria (albuminuria)	300 mg/L/24 hr or two separate random daytime specimens 6 hr apart (true clean catch) of 1+, 2+	5 g or more per 24 hr, 3+, 4+ in true clean-catch or catheterized specimen
Edema	Weight gain of more than 3 lbs (1.4 kg) per week or 6 lbs (2.72 kg) per month—any sudden weight gain is suspicious Minimal or marked edema 1+, 2+ of lower extremities	Weight gain advances at accelerated rate Edema more pronounced, especially of hands, face 3+, 4+ (as condition worsens, edema of lungs, brain, and other organs)
Urine output	Not below 500 ml/24 hr	Oliguria less than 500 ml/24 hr
Neurologic signs and symptoms	Absent or only occasional headaches, blurred vision, or spots before eyes Normal peripheral reflexes	More persistent headaches, blurred vision, and spots before eyes—retinal arteriole spasms on ophthalmic examination Hyperactive knee jerk and other tendon reflexes +3, +4 with clonus Irritability, tinnitus
Other organ involvement		Liver involvement causing epigastric or right upper quadrant abdominal pain, nausea, vomiting (often said to precede convulsion/coma or onset of eclampsia) Pulmonary edema manifested by respiratory distress, rales, cyanosis

From Novak JC, Broom BL: *Ingalls and Salerno's maternal and child health nursing,* ed 9, St. Louis, 1999, Mosby.
*These criteria are not uniformly accepted by experts in the field.

tion so the gravis uterus does not cause aortocaval compression. Pharmocologic therapy to control hypertension is usually initiated when diastolic blood pressure is higher than 90 to 100 mm Hg. Magnesium sulfate is the drug of choice to prevent seizures (Box 47-2). Continuous monitoring including blood pressure, pulse, and respirations every 15 to 30 minutes is essential to identify changes in the patient's condition due to PIH and magnesium toxicity. Signs of magnesium toxicity include absent deep tendon reflexes, respirations less than 12 per minute, urine output less than 30 ml/hr

---

Box 47-2 MAGNESIUM SULFATE IN PREGNANCY-INDUCED HYPERTENSION

LOADING DOSE

4-6 g 10% magnesium sulfate in 250 ml D$_5$W solution, given IV over 15-30 minutes

MAINTENANCE DOSE

2-3 g 10% magnesium sulfate per hour

THERAPEUTIC SERUM MAGNESIUM LEVEL

4.8-8.4 mg/dl

MONITORING PARAMETERS

Cardiac monitor
Fetal monitor

URINARY OUTPUT

30 ml/hr

DEEP-TENDON REFLEXES

Loss means toxicity

CAUTIONS

Respiratory rate must be greater than 12 breaths/min
Antidote for decreased respirations is calcium gluconate 1 g (10 ml in 10% solution) given slowly IV

From Poole JH: Aggressive management of HELLP syndrome and eclampsia, *AACN Clin Issues*, 8(4), 1997.
D$_5$W, 5% Dextrose in water; *IV*, intravenous.

Box 47-3 DIFFERENTIAL DIAGNOSES OF HELLP SYNDROME

Autoimmune thrombocytopenia purpura
Chronic renal failure
Pyelonephritis
Cholecystitis
Gastroenteritis
Hepatitis
Pancreatitis
Thrombotic thrombocytopenia purpura
Hemolytic-uremic syndrome
Acute fatty liver of pregnancy

From Pearlman M, Tintinalli J: *Emergency care of the woman*, New York, 1998, McGraw-Hill.
HELLP, Hemolysis, elevated liver enzymes, and low platelets.

---

or 120 ml per 4 hr, and signs of fetal distress. If magnesium toxicity occurs, the patient is given calcium gluconate 1 g IV. Ativan can be used to control seizures. Fetal monitoring is essential. Any drop in fetal heart rate or deceleration of heart rate during contractions indicates the need for immediate emergency cesarean section.

HELLP Syndrome

The HELLP syndrome is a potentially life-threatening form of preeclampsia that occurs when the patient develops multiple organ damage. Hemolysis, Elevated Liver enzymes, and Low Platelets (HELLP) affects up to 12% of women with preeclampsia-eclampsia syndrome.[4] Unlike preeclampsia, which usually effects primigravidas, HELLP syndrome is more common among the multigravida population. The HELLP syndrome, characterized by complaints of epigastric or right upper quadrant pain, can imitate a variety of nonobstetric medical problems. Serious medical and surgical pathology must be ruled out (Box 47-3).

THIRD TRIMESTER EMERGENCIES

Fetal viability and the mother's survival are the primary focus for emergencies during the third trimester. Hemorrhage can be obvious or occult, so the emergency nurse must be alert to changes in the mother and fetus.

Placenta Previa

Previa means "in front of," so placenta previa occurs when the placenta presents before the fetus. Placenta previa is caused by implantation and development of the placenta in the lower uterine segment rather than normal implantation in the upper uterine wall. Implanting in the lower segment of the uterus puts the placenta in the zone of effacement and dilation, which causes the placenta to partially or completely cover the internal cervical os. Three types of placenta previa are defined by how much the os is covered (Figure 47-3):

Total—the placenta completely covers the os.
Partial—the placenta partially covers the os.
Marginal or low implantation—the placenta is adjacent to but does not extend beyond the margin of the os.

Although total placenta previa is rare, marginal or partial placenta previa occurs in 1 in 200 pregnancies. Seventy-five percent of placenta previa cases occur in multiparous women. Multiparity with advancing age and a rapid succession of pregnancies are believed to be predisposing factors for placenta previa.

Hemorrhage, the first and most commonly seen sign of placenta previa, is not accompanied by contractions, so there is no associated pain. Because the cervix begins to dilate and efface in the eighth month, maternal vessels tear when the patient is asleep. Bleeding may cease spontaneously or continue, depending on the size of torn vessels. After two or three hemorrhages, labor usually begins. Associated membrane rupture can lead to infection. Premature labor and an

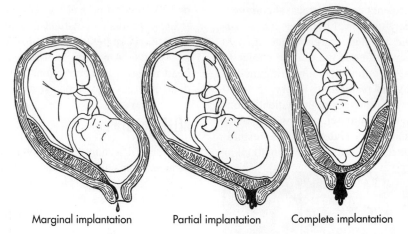

Marginal implantation   Partial implantation   Complete implantation

FIGURE **47-3** Placenta previa. (Modified from AJN/Mosby nursing boards review for NCLEX-RN, ed 10, St. Louis, 1997, Mosby.)

abnormal presenting part can further complicate delivery. In total placenta previa, bleeding occurs earlier and is more profuse. Suspect placenta previa when painless uterine bleeding occurs in the last half of the pregnancy.

Diagnostic studies include ultrasonography to determine the specific position of the placenta. A CBC, type and cross-match for several units of blood, and clotting studies should be immediately obtained. Establish a large-bore IV line, administer a crystalloid solution such as lactated Ringer's solution, and transfer the patient to labor and delivery for monitoring and, if indicated, immediate cesarean section. Pelvic examination is contraindicated because of potential perforation of the placenta and catastrophic hemorrhage.

Assessment of vital signs should always include assessment of fetal heart rate. If fetal heart tones are not heard, this finding should be reported immediately. Normal fetal heart rate is 120 to 160 beats/min. Stay with the patient and encourage her to talk. Provide necessary assistance for her husband or significant other with admitting procedures and contacting other family members.

Abruptio Placentae

Another major complication of pregnancy in the last trimester is premature separation of the placenta from the uterus, or abruptio placentae. The primary cause is unknown but there is some indication that abruptio placentae is related to PIH. Another suspected cause is increased venous pressure when the vena cava is compressed by the gravid uterus when the mother is in the supine position. Advanced maternal age (35 years and older), multiparity, a short cord, and trauma also play a large part in development of abuptio placentae. Partial separation causes occult or frank hemorrhage. Frank hemorrhage is always an emergency because of blood loss and associated hypotension and hypoxia; however, the more dangerous of the two is occult hemorrhage.

Abruptio placentae should be considered in any woman in the third trimester who presents to the ED with vaginal bleeding and abdominal pain or contractions. This is an emergency requiring immediate intervention.

Maternal assessment and assessment of vital signs and fetal heart rate are essential. At least one IV line should be started with a large-bore catheter and lactated Ringer's solution. A CBC and type and cross-match should be sent to the laboratory immediately. Fetal monitoring is essential. The patient should be sent to labor and delivery for monitoring and, if indicated, immediate cesarean section.

DELIVERY

With decreasing access to a dwindling number of obstetricians, the probability of deliveries occurring in prehospital care settings and the ED is high. If a patient in labor arrives in the ED and time permits, rapid obstetric examination should be performed and brief obstetric history obtained. An in-depth, rapid maternal assessment should be completed. And, remember that when the mother says, "The baby is coming," she is always right.

The first stage of labor is the time from onset of regular contractions until complete cervical dilation. This is generally the longest of the three stages of labor. The second stage of labor is the time from full cervical dilation until delivery of the baby. The mother may have the urge to push in this stage. The average time for stage two is 20 minutes to 1 hour. The third stage of labor is from delivery of the baby until delivery of the placenta. This stage usually lasts from 5 to 15 minutes. In cases where the placenta fails to detach from the uterine wall, it may be necessary to manually remove the placenta.

When a woman in labor arrives at the ED, if time permits, a brief physical examination should be performed. First check fetal heart tones. Normal fetal heart tones are 120 to 160 beats/min. Prolonged bradycardia or tachycardia may indicate fetal distress. When this occurs, place the mother on her left side and give supplemental oxygen at high flow. Arrange for immediate obstetric consultation for possible emergency delivery by cesarean section.

After it has been determined that the fetus is well, examine the mother's abdomen and measure uterine height. A full-term fetus elevates the uterus to xiphoid level. Palpate contractions as they occur. Help the mother to relax between contractions. The emergency nurse involved in delivery should remember that the mother does most of the work. Your basic role is to provide psychologic support, "coach" the mother, and ensure the infant, once delivered, is breathing adequately, has a good pulse, and is kept warm.

If crowning is not present, perform a manual vaginal examination to determine dilation, effacement, and station of the fetus. Use sterile technique. If fluid is present, check for amniotic fluid by determining acidity of the fluid. Amniotic fluid is neutral, whereas normal vaginal secretions are acidic. If the test is equivocal because of the presence of blood, assume the membranes have ruptured and that amniotic fluid is present.

A rapid decision should be made as to whether delivery is imminent and the baby will be delivered in the ED or if time permits transport of the mother to labor and delivery. If there is any indication that the mother will deliver imminently (i.e., crowning), keep her in the ED for delivery.

In an emergency situation place the mother on a stretcher. Equipment for an imminent delivery should be readily available. Sterile disposable delivery kits usually have most equipment necessary for the delivery. Do not place equipment between the mother's legs but on a surface beside the stretcher. Minimum essential equipment includes cord clamps, scissors, towel, and bulb syringe.

After donning appropriate attire, cover one hand with a sterile towel or a 4×4 inch dressing. Apply gentle pressure to the infant's head as it crowns to prevent explosive delivery and possible tearing of the perineum. When the head is delivered, quickly suction the infant's mouth and then the nose to prevent aspiration. At this point, check for the umbilical cord around the infant's neck. If the cord is loose, carefully slip it over the infant's head. If it is tight, clamp it in two places and cut the cord. After the head is delivered and has rotated, hold it gently in both hands. Apply gentle downward pressure to assist with delivery of the anterior shoulder and gentle upward traction to assist with delivery of the posterior shoulder. Carefully support the infant's head. After the shoulders are delivered, delivery of the rest of the infant's body usually occurs quite rapidly (Figure 47-4).

Keep the infant in a head-dependent position at the level of the introitus to prevent aspiration. Once again, suction the mouth and then the nose. If spontaneous breathing or crying does not occur, gently rub the infant's back with a towel to stimulate breathing.

Clamp the umbilical cord in two places at least 6 inches from the umbilicus. The cord can be cut as soon as it is convenient, usually when it has stopped pulsating.

Place the infant in a warmed environment. Assess airway, breathing, and circulation. If necessary, open the infant's airway with a slight chin lift, being careful not to overextend the neck. If breathing is absent or the heart rate is less than 60 beats/min, despite 30 seconds of assisted ventilation, begin resuscitation measures. A useful pneumonic, TABS, is

---

BOX 47-4   TABS PROCEDURE FOR NEWBORN RESUSCITATION

T (TEMPERATURE)

Dry and cover the neonate as soon as possible to prevent heat loss. Place in a heated environment as soon as possible.

A (AIRWAY)

Suction the mouth first, then the nose.
If breathing is absent, give positive pressure ventilation and 100% oxygen.

B (BEATS [HEART RATE])

Initiate compressions if the HR is absent or if the HR remains less than 60 beats/min despite 30 seconds of assisted ventilations. Continue ventilating the neonate.
Consider pharmacologic support with drugs such as epinephrine, atropine, naloxone, dextrose, and sodium bicarbonate.

S (SUGAR)

A blood glucose level <40 mg/dl is a critical level in a neonate. When glucose is given, administer a 25% solution at 0.5 g/kg (or 2 ml/kg of a 25% solution).

HR, Heart rate.

---

described in Box 47-4. For additional information on neonatal resuscitation, see Chapter 48.

Determine the infant's Apgar score at delivery and repeat 5 minutes after delivery (Table 47-4). The Apgar score is a system used to predict health outcomes by scoring and totaling five key factors. Each factor is scored from 0 to 2. Zero is a poor response or absence of the factor being measured, 1 indicates some response, and 2 indicates a normal finding. A total score of 10 is possible with 7 to 10 considered very good. A score of 4 to 6 indicates a moderately depressed infant, whereas a score of 0 to 3 indicates a severely depressed infant.

After ensuring health of the infant and its continued warmth, place the infant on the mother's abdomen and encourage the mother to breastfeed the infant if appropriate. Sucking stimulates the uterus to contract, reassures the mother the infant is fine, and helps to keep the infant warm. Put an identification band on the infant's wrist and ankle.

After delivery of the infant, stage three labor begins. At this point, unclamp the cord and obtain laboratory specimens from the cord for determinations of hematocrit, hemoglobin level, blood type, Rh factor, and bilirubin level. Reclamp the cord and palpate the uterus through the abdominal wall. Prepare for delivery of the placenta; this usually occurs 5 to 10 minutes after the infant is born. A sudden gush of blood occurs when the placenta separates from the uterine wall; the uterus rises into the abdomen and the umbilical cord protruding from the vagina lengthens. Do not pull on the umbilical cord; this could cause uterine inversion.

When the placenta has separated, apply slight traction to the umbilical cord and place your hand on the dome of the

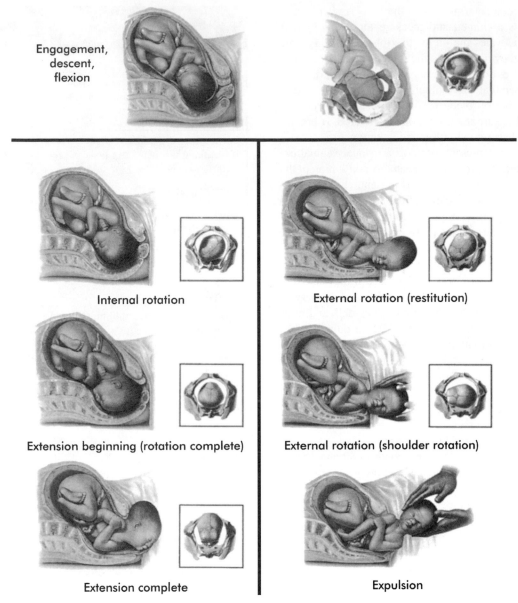

Engagement, descent, flexion

Internal rotation

External rotation (restitution)

Extension beginning (rotation complete)

External rotation (shoulder rotation)

Extension complete

Expulsion

FIGURE 47-4 Mechanism of normal labor. (Courtesy Ross Products Division, Abbott Laboratories, Inc., Columbus, Ohio.)

Table 47-4	APGAR SCORE		
		SCORE	
FACTOR	0	I	2
A Appearance (color)	Blue	Blue limbs, pink body	Pink
P Pulse (heart rate)	Absent	<100 beats/ min	>100 beats/ min
G Grimace (muscle tone)	Limp	Some flexion	Good flexion
A Activity (reflexes irritable)	Absent	Some motion	Good motion
R Respiratory effort	Absent	Weak cry	Strong cry

uterus, pressing downward slightly toward the suprapubic area. As the placenta enters the vaginal area, continue applying gentle traction to the umbilical cord and carefully remove the placenta.

Complicated Deliveries

Meconium Aspiration Syndrome

Meconium aspiration syndrome occurs when meconium enters fetal lungs during delivery. Relaxation of the anal sphincter in utero caused by fetal hypoxia leads to meconium staining of amniotic fluid. Staining is seen most often in postterm deliveries. Meconium staining of amniotic fluid is an emergency for the fetus, but delivery must be adapted to address potential fetal respiratory distress. The hypophar-

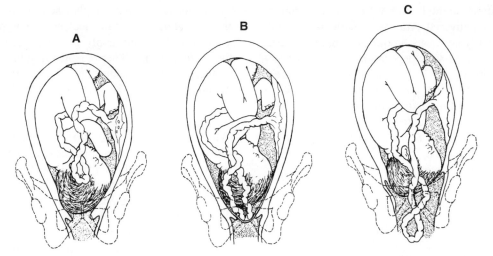

FIGURE 47-5 Prolapse of the umbilical cord. Note pressure of presenting part on umbilical cord, which endangers fetal circulation. **A,** Occult (hidden) prolapse of cord. **B,** Complete prolapse of cord. Note membranes are intact. **C,** Cord presenting in front of fetal head may be seen in vagina. (Modified from Lowdermilk DL, Perry SE, Bobak IM: *Maternity and women's health care,* ed 7, St. Louis, 2000, Mosby.)

ynx is suctioned with delivery of the head. If the infant has absent or depressed respirations, heart rate less than 100 beats/min or poor muscle tone, direct endotracheal suctioning is recommended. If the infant is vigorous, suctioning is not required.[1]

Prolapsed Cord

A prolapsed umbilical cord constitutes an obstetric emergency. The umbilical cord precedes the fetus through the birth canal, becomes entrapped when the fetus passes through the birth canal, and obstructs fetal circulation (Figure 47-5).

There are three variations of this condition. The first is a situation in which uterine membranes are intact; the cord is compressed by fetal parts but is not visible externally. This variation should be suspected when there are signs of fetal distress, most prominently bradycardia. This variation is actually called "cord presentation" rather than true prolapse.

In the second variation, the cord may not be visible but can be felt in the vagina or cervix. In the third and most extreme variation, the umbilical cord actually protrudes from the vagina.

Cord compression can be determined in two ways. On examination, the cord is felt as the presenting part. Most often, cord compression is determined when the fetus suddenly develops distress with the fetal monitor showing decreasing fetal heart rate or deceleration.

Therapeutic intervention is aimed at relieving pressure on the cord and minimizing fetal anoxia. Place the mother on the left side to relieve pressure from the huge gravid uterus on the abdominal aorta. Administer oxygen via nonrebreather mask at 100%. An exposed cord dries out so cover it with saline-moistened sterile gauze. If the cervix is completely dilated, forceps may be used to rapidly deliver the baby. If the cervix is not fully dilated, emergency cesarean section is performed.

Shoulder Dystocia

Risk factors associated with shoulder dystocia include large infants, prolonged second stage of labor, and use of high forceps during delivery. Whatever the cause, the infant's shoulder has difficulty passing through the pelvis. Shoulder dystocia is an emergency that presents in fewer than 2% of deliveries.[5] As the head is delivered, the shoulders cannot pass through the pelvis. Compression of the shoulders can lead to cord compression and subsequent fetal distress. Rapid delivery is critical! Position the mother with legs hyperflexed over the abdomen (McRobert's manuever)[6] and apply suprapubic pressure (Figure 47-6) to deliver these infants. Complications of shoulder dystocia include fractured clavicle and Erb's palsy. Although most complications are transient, some can leave permanent damage.

Breech Delivery

With breech delivery, the head—the largest fetal body part—is delivered last. A woman whose fetus is a breech presentation is often scheduled for cesarean section. Unfortunately, in the emergency setting when a woman arrives in labor with delivery imminent, even when the fetus is in a breech position, there may not be time to arrange for cesarean section. Delivery must be completed in the ED, especially if the fetus has been delivered to the level of the umbilicus.

Categories of breech presentation are frank breech, full or complete breech, and footling breech (Figure 47-7). Frank breech is the most common variation, occurring when fetal legs are extended across the abdomen toward the shoulders. Full (or complete) breech is reversal of the usual cephalic presentation. The head, knees, and hips are flexed, but the buttocks are presenting. Footling breech is when one or both feet present.

With any breech presentation, call for obstetric support if possible. It is usually best to allow the fetus to deliver spontaneously to the level of the umbilicus. If the fetus is in a front breech presentation the legs may require extraction after the buttocks are delivered. After the umbilicus is visualized, gently extract a generous amount of umbilical cord. Rotate the fetus to align shoulders in an anterior-posterior position. Place gentle traction on the fetus until the axilla are seen. Pull upward gently on the feet to allow delivery of the posterior shoulder. Carefully extract the posterior arm, then gently pull downward on the feet to deliver the anterior shoulder. Rotate the buttocks to the mother's front. Using a Mauriceau maneuver, rest the fetus on your arm, then place your index and middle finger in the fetus's mouth, gently

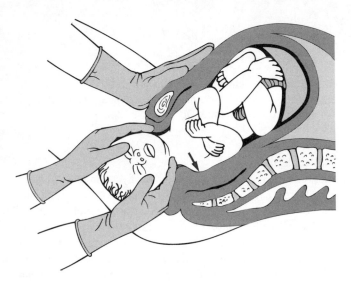

FIGURE **47-6**   Application of suprapubic pressure (From Wong DL, Perry S: *Maternal-child nursing care,* St. Louis, 1998, Mosby).

flexing the head. Do not apply traction with this hand. Grasp the fetus at the base of the neck and tip of the shoulders with your other hand and apply gentle traction. If assistance is available, have the other person apply firm, steady pressure to the top of the fundus toward the suprapubic area. The neonate should then be suctioned and the cord clamped.

Multiple Fetuses

With delivery of twins or other multiple births, there are additional concerns. Often multiple birth neonates are premature or have a host of other problems. The initial and most important objective is to ensure safe delivery of all fetuses. The best advice is to take one fetus at a time, as they come. The first may present vertex or breech. Follow the previous information for various presentations. The second fetus usually has membranes intact. If the second fetus is in the head-first position, you may rupture the membranes and allow the mother to deliver the fetus by pushing when she has a contraction. If the second fetus is breech, the feet should be delivered, then the membranes should be ruptured. Both neonates should be suctioned as they are delivered. Both cords should be clamped and both neonates should receive identification bands.

Amniotic Fluid Embolism

Amniotic fluid embolism is a catastrophic event with high maternal mortality because amniotic fluid leaks into the mother's venous circulation during labor or delivery. This embolus of squamous epithelial cells, lanugo, and vasoactive chemicals travels to the pulmonary circulation causing sudden, severe obstruction. Respiratory arrest is almost always immediately followed quickly by cardiac arrest.

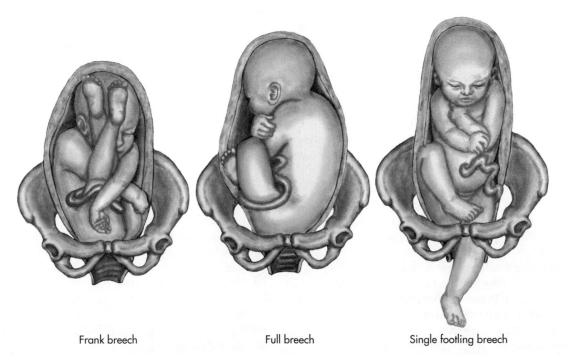

Frank breech   Full breech   Single footling breech

FIGURE **47-7**   Three variations of breech presentations. Frank breech is most common. Footling breeches may be double or single. (From Gorrie TM, McKinney ES, Murray SS: *Foundations of maternal-newborn nursing,* Philadelphia, 1998, WB Saunders.)

Amniotic fluid emboli are seen most commonly with placenta previa, abruptio placentae, precipitate labor in the multiparous woman and with intrauterine fetal death. The mother may initially demonstrate profound hypotension, tachycardia, tachypnea, cyanosis, and hypoxia followed by cardiopulmonary arrest. Coagulopathies also occur.

Therapeutic intervention must be rapid and aggressive. Administer oxygen at high flow via a nonrebreather mask. Rapid endotracheal intubation and mechanical ventilation with positive end-expiratory pressure is required for many patients. Crystalloid solutions and blood products should be administered. Fresh frozen plasma may be used in anticipation of coagulopathies.

POSTPARTUM EMERGENCIES

Disseminated Intravascular Coagulation

Disseminated intravascular coagulation is characterized by acceleration and hyperactivity of clotting mechanisms in pregnancy. This condition of simultaneous bleeding and clotting is seen most often in severe cases of abruptio placentae in the form of hypofibrinogenemia but can also occur after excessive blood loss, amniotic fluid embolus, or fetal death *in utero*. In this hypercoagulatory state, clotting factors are consumed before the liver has time to replace them. See Chapter 42 for additional discussion of DIC.

Postpartum Hemorrhage

Excessive bleeding in the postpartum period is an emergency. Bleeding can occur immediately after delivery or be delayed 7 to 14 days. The main causes of postpartum bleeding are subinvolution of the uterus, retained products of conception (pieces of the placenta or membranes), and vaginal or cervical tears incurred during delivery. Postpartum hemorrhage is usually described as blood loss in excess of 1000 ml within 24 hours of delivery.

Subinvolution usually occurs 7 to 14 days after delivery when thrombi detach from placental sites and the sites begin to bleed. If the involutional process does not return the gravid uterus to its nonpregnant state, bleeding can become excessive. Retention of membranes or placental fragments can also cause sudden hemorrhage because they interfere with the involutional process. The emergency nurse should also be aware of a condition known as placenta accreta. When the placenta fails to separate from the uterine wall after delivery because it has grown into the uterine muscle itself, postpartum bleeding results and immediate surgery is indicated. Cervical tears and vaginal lacerations can also cause postpartum hemorrhage.

When assessing the patient with postpartum bleeding, survey the patient's general condition. Note the presence or absence of pain, skin color, posture, gait, motor activity, and facial expression. The following information should be elicited when obtaining history of the problem.

- Quantity, character, and duration of bleeding. How does it compare with the patient's normal menstrual period? How many pads has she used in the past hour? How does it compare with the number she normally requires during a period?
- Menstrual history. When was the date of her last period?
- Does she have pain? What is the nature of the pain—dull, achy, cramping, constant, or radiating? Where is the pain? How long has she had it? Was onset gradual or sudden?
- Is there any history of trauma?
- When did she deliver? Has she ever had any infections of the reproductive system? Has she had previous episodes of bleeding?

Continued assessment should include vital signs, fundal palpation for firmness, and evaluation of vaginal bleeding. Check the pad the patient is wearing to objectively evaluate the amount of bleeding. Note presence or absence of clots or odor. Examine and save any clots or tissue that the patient may have brought with her for laboratory examination. Note condition of the fundus. If the fundus is boggy and relaxed, gently massage until firm.

Evaluate the patient's condition, and institute appropriate measures for stabilization. If bleeding is profuse, two IV lines with large-bore needles for warmed crystalloids and blood should be established. If respirations are labored, administer oxygen. Obtain a CBC with sedimentation rate and clot tube for type and cross-match.

While collecting data and stabilizing the patient, prepare for a vaginal examination. Explain each procedure and reassure the patient by allowing her to express her feelings.

Postpartum bleeding generally responds to administration of intravenous oxytocin (Pitocin), bed rest, and fundal massage. If bleeding continues, prepare the patient for operative evaluation of bleeding. Treatment of retained products of conception includes removal of the offending piece by dilation and curettage and a thorough exploration of the uterus after the patient is under general anesthesia. Suturing of vaginal lacerations can be performed in the ED. However, with the possibility of damage at the cervix, suturing is best performed after general anesthesia. A complete pelvic examination can also be performed after anesthesia.

Postpartum Infection

Vaginal lacerations, cervical tears, episiotomy sites, placental implant sites, and retained tissue can become host sites for infection. Patients develop fever, abdominal or pelvic pain, and occasionally have foul-smelling lochia. Therapeutic intervention includes culture of drainage and treatment with antibiotics as indicated.

OTHER EMERGENCIES

Hydatidiform Mole

Hydatidiform mole, or molar pregnancy, occurs when trophoblast villi grow very rapidly, then die. If an embryo is formed, it dies very early. As trophoblast cells degenerate, they fill with a jelly-like fluid. The cells become vesicles that look like grapes filled with fluid. Bleeding occurs early in the second trimester as these vesicles enlarge and rupture (Figure 47-8). There is a definite association between hydatidiform mole and choriocarcinoma (a rapidly growing carcinoma), so early diagnosis is critical.

Hydatidiform mole occurs in 1 in 100 pregnancies. It is noticed most often in women of poor socioeconomic status with lack of protein in their diet, mothers younger than 18 years or older than 35 years, and women of Asian background.

Because the trophoblast secretes hCG and grows very rapidly, the uterus grows larger than expected for the due date. At about 16 weeks' gestation, the woman develops vaginal bleeding. Bleeding may be mixed with clear fluid as the vesicles begin to rupture. The patient will have a positive pregnancy test with enlarging uterus; however, fetal heart tones cannot be auscultated. A viable fetus is not evident on pelvic ultrasound.

Intervention for hydatidiform mole is removal of the mole. The patient should be prepared for suction dilatation and curettage. The patient and family need much emotional support. They now know this is an abnormal pregnancy (without a fetus) and must also worry about the possibility of a tumor.

SUMMARY

The emergency nurse uses the nursing process and pertinent nursing diagnoses to assess and prioritize care for women with obstetric complaints (Box 47-5). Through this process, the emergency nurse can identify life-threatening problems and intervene quickly. The ability to do this while providing emotional support for the mother and family is the hallmark of emergency care for the obstetric patient in the ED.

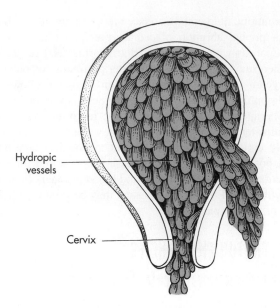

FIGURE 47-8 Hydatidaform mole with some vesicles being passed. (From Novak JC, Broom BL: *Ingalls & Salerno's maternal and child health nursing,* ed 9, St. Louis, 1999, Mosby).

Box 47-5	NURSING DIAGNOSES ASSOCIATED WITH OBSTETRIC EMERGENCIES

Anxiety
Fear
Fetal risk
Fluid volume, Deficient
Knowledge, Deficient
Tissue perfusion, Ineffective

References

1. American Heart Association: Guidelines 2000 for cardiopulmonary resuscitation and emergency cardiovascular care, *Circulation,* 102(suppl I):I-1, 2000.
2. Gorrie TM, McKinney ES, Murray SS: *Foundations of maternal-newborn nursing,* ed 2, Philadelphia, 1998, WB Saunders.
3. Guyton AC, Hall GE: *Textbook of medical physiology,* Philadelphia, 1996, WB Saunders.
4. Jarvis C: *Physical examination and health assessment,* ed 3, Philadelphia, 2000, WB Saunders.
5. Novak JC, Broom BL: *Ingalls & Salerno's maternal and child health nursing,* ed 9, St. Louis, 1999, Mosby.
6. Wright M, Grant HP: How competent are you and your staff with shoulder dystocia? *AWHONN Lifelines,* 3(1):35, 1999.

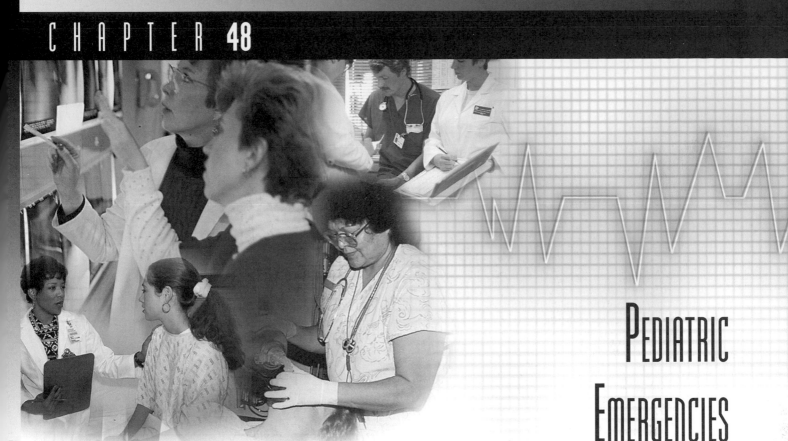

PEDIATRIC EMERGENCIES

COURTNEY COSBY

Sick children present unique challenges to health care professionals. Assessment and treatment of sick children are unique because children's perceptions may be radically different from those of adults. In a busy emergency department (ED), nurses may not always take the time to realize that children brought in for care are likely to be scared at the sight of strangers and the unknown "hurts" that lie ahead. Furthermore, depending on age, children may or may not be able to say what is bothering them. Patience and understanding are key to overcoming or averting these problems (Figure 48-1).

Communicating with a child and the family is a three-way process involving the nurse, child, and parent. For the most part, information about the child is acquired by direct observation or is communicated to the nurse by parents. Usually, it can be assumed that close contact with the child makes information imparted by the parent reliable. Assessment requires input from the child (verbal and nonverbal), information from parents, and the nurse's own observations of the child and interpretation of the relationship between child and parent. Box 48-1 outlines guidelines for communicating with children. In most cases, parents should stay with the child during all phases of the visit (Figure 48-2). Approach the child slowly while asking questions of the parent or caregiver. Fear and uncertainty surrounding the child's condition, coupled with a loss of control of the situation, add to the stress. Positive, caring interactions with the child and parent help alleviate stress and facilitate assessment of the child.

Most emergency nurses, regardless of practice area, will encounter a sick child at some stage in their career. The ability to intervene in critical situations requires a strong foundation of knowledge and assessment skills. This chapter provides an overview of pediatric assessment and common emergencies. Pediatric trauma and child abuse are discussed in Chapters 29 and 49, respectively.

TRIAGE

Pediatric patients account for approximately 25% to 35% of annual ED visits nationally. Children require careful triage for rapid identification of serious illness or injury. The triage nurse must have excellent assessment, communication, and organization skills. The emergency nurse who becomes skilled at triage develops a "sixth sense" for identifying the "really sick" infant or child. Lethargy, poor skin color, dull eyes, shallow respirations, and flaccidity are considered red flags.

A sick child in the ED usually makes nurses who are unfamiliar with children uneasy, just as an adult with chest pain causes alarm in a pediatric nurse. Triage of a child does not require familiarity with every childhood disease, medication, and neurologic reflex or a bevy of specialized equipment. Pediatric triage does require understanding of concepts related to pediatric emergencies, including the following.

- Anatomic, physiologic, and developmental differences between children and adults

719

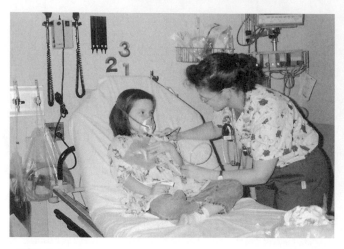

FIGURE **48-1** The child may be scared and unsure of the nurse, the equipment, and all the noises in the ED.

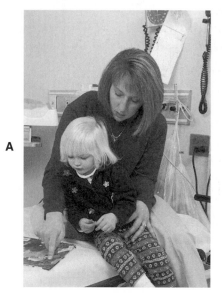

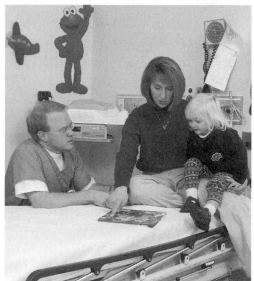

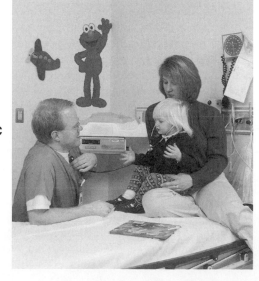

FIGURE **48-2** Take time to gain the child's and parent's trust. **A,** Mother and child look at a book. **B,** Mother and child look at the book with the nurse. **C,** Mother and child with nurse interacting with the child.

- Recognition of conditions leading to pediatric arrest (hypoxia and shock) and appropriate interventions
- Dealing with parents
- "Rules" of pediatric triage

Children are difficult to evaluate when compared with adults for several reasons. Children often have nonspecific symptoms, such as fever. Communication can be difficult because of limited vocabulary and verbal skills, so nurses must depend on the parent for history. A child's response to illness or injury depends on current developmental stage. Toddlers cling to parents, whereas adolescents are independent. Children compensate for longer periods in the face of illness; therefore, they may not be outwardly symptomatic despite the presence of a life-threatening condition. Normal vital signs do not always indicate stability in the pediatric patient.

Special Pediatric Considerations

The most important differences between children and adults are found in the respiratory and circulatory systems (i.e., airway, breathing, and circulation [ABCs]). Respiratory disorders are a common cause of illness in infants and children and are the third most common cause of death in the 1- to 12-year-old age-group after cancer and congenital malformations. Respiratory distress is the preceding event in most pediatric cardiac arrests. Pediatric differences in ABCs and nursing implications are listed in Table 48-1.

Rules of Pediatric Triage

The following unofficial rules of pediatric triage may assist triage nurses in evaluating children.

1. Parents know their children better than you do—listen to them. Parent history can give clues to the cause of illness or injury and help triage nurses determine urgency (Figure 48-2).
2. Remember the ABCs—children are different. Do not focus on the obvious; a subtle, more serious problem can be overlooked.
3. Some children can talk, walk, and still be in shock; do not depend on the child's appearance. Consider history and vital signs but do not allow normal vital signs to give you a sense of security.
4. Never tell parents their child cannot be evaluated in the ED, no matter what the chief complaint. With the development of preferred provider and health maintenance organizations, authorization for payment may be refused. Make sure parents realize authorization for payment is being denied, not authorization for care. Triage assessment and medical screening examination must still be performed to evaluate whether immediate care is needed—before referral elsewhere.

Table 48-1 PEDIATRIC DIFFERENCES IN AIRWAY, BREATHING, AND CIRCULATION	
FACTOR	**NURSING CONSIDERATIONS**
AIRWAY	
Large tongue	Airway easily obstructed by tongue; proper positioning is often all that is necessary to open the airway.
Smaller diameter for all airways (in a 1-year-old child, tracheal diameter is less than child's little finger).	Small amount of mucus or swelling easily obstructs the airway; child normally has increased airway resistance.
Cartilage of larynx is softer than in adults; cricoid cartilage is narrowest portion of larynx.	Airway of infant can be compressed if neck is flexed or hyperextended; provides a natural seal for endotracheal tube; cuffed tubes are not necessary in children less than 8-10 years of age.
BREATHING	
Sternum and ribs are cartilaginous; chest wall is soft; intercostal muscles are poorly developed; infants are obligate nose breathers for first 4 weeks of life; increased metabolic rate (about twice that of an adult); increased respiratory demand for oxygen consumption and carbon dioxide elimination.	Infant's chest wall may move inward instead of outward during inspiration (retractions) when lung compliance is decreased; greater intrathoracic pressure generated during inspiration; anything causing nasal obstruction can produce respiratory distress; respiratory distress increases oxygen demand, as does any condition that increases metabolic rate, i.e., fever.
CIRCULATION	
Child's circulating blood volume is larger per unit of body weight, but absolute volume is relatively small; 70%-80% of newborn's body weight is water (compared to 50%-60% of adult body weight); about one half of this volume is extracellular.	Blood loss considered minor in an adult may lead to shock in a child; decreased fluid intake or increased fluid loss quickly leads to dehydration.
Increased heart rate, decreased stroke volume; cardiac output is higher per unit of body weight.	Tachycardia is the child's most efficient method of increasing cardiac output if heart rate is greater than 180-200 beats/min.

Table 48-2	COMPONENTS OF BASIC PEDIATRIC ASSESSMENT	
C	**C**hief complaint	Reason for the child's ED visit and duration of complaint (e.g., fever lasting 2 days).
I	**I**mmunizations	Evaluation of the child's current immunization status: • The completion of all scheduled immunizations for the child's age must be evaluated. The most current immunization recommendations are published by the American Academy of Pediatrics. • If the child has not received immunization because of religion or cultural beliefs, document this information.
	Isolation	Evaluation of the child's exposure to communicable diseases (chickenpox, shingles, mumps, measles, whooping cough, tuberculosis): • A child with active disease or who is potentially infectious, based on a history of exposure and the disease incubation period, must be placed in respiratory isolation on arrival in the ED. • Immunosuppressed or compromised children can develop active disease even when previously immune. These children must also be protected from inadvertent exposure to viral and bacterial illness while in the ED and placed in *protective* or *reverse isolation.* • Other exposures that may be evaluated include exposure to meningitis (with or without evidence of purpura), pneumonia, and scabies.
A	**A**llergies	Evaluation of the child's previous allergic or hypersensitivity reactions: • Document reactions to medications, foods, products (e.g., latex), and environmental allergens. The type of reaction must also be documented.
M	**M**edications	Evaluation of the child's current medication regimen including prescription and over-the-counter medications: • Dose administered. • Time of last dose. • Duration of medication use.

P	**P**ast medical history	A review of the child's health status, including prior illnesses, injuries, hospitalizations, surgeries, and chronic physical and psychiatric illnesses. Use of alcohol, tobacco, drugs or other substances of abuse must be evaluated, as appropriate:
		• The medical history of the infant must include the prenatal and birth history:
		    Complications during pregnancy or delivery.
		    Number of days infant remained in hospital postbirth.
		    Infant's birth weight.
		• The medical history of the menarcheal female includes the date and description of last menstrual period.

ED, Emergency department.

Pediatric Triage Examination

Depending on the facility, triage examination may be brief, limited to determining chief complaint and looking at the child. Or, it may be more comprehensive and include obtaining vital signs and providing treatment such as antipyretics, splinting, or ice packs. Whatever triage protocols or critical pathways exist, the most important aspect is prompt assessment with observation and history.

History is an important part of the pediatric triage assessment. With small infants, history may be vague, nonspecific, and limited by the parent's ability to communicate. Medical history is important in determining if the child has a prior condition that may affect assessment (e.g., congenital heart disease, chronic respiratory condition). Ask the parents, "What does your child normally look like?" or "Does your child look normal to you?" The CIAMPEDS mnemonic describes components of basic pediatric assessment (Table 48-2).

Observation variables such as playfulness, eye contact, and attention to the environment are also important. The triage nurse can usually observe the child while obtaining the history or performing the assessment. Observation may have to be performed as a separate part of the examination to allow the child to feel comfortable.

Pediatric Primary Assessment

Primary assessment consists of evaluation of the ABCs and neurologic status. ABCs may be the only part of the assessment performed in triage if the child has an emergent condition. The primary survey includes assessment of level of consciousness; respiratory effort, rate, and quality; skin color and temperature; and pulse rate and quality.

Secondary Assessment

Secondary assessment consists of vital signs and head-to-toe survey. During triage, secondary assessment is usually limited to evaluating the area of chief complaint. The rest of the examination is performed later in a treatment room. Secondary assessment is summarized in Table 48-3. When performing secondary assessment on a child, do not focus on the obvious injury. Don't be fooled by a known patient with a chronic condition. Communicate your findings to other

Table 48-2	COMPONENTS OF BASIC PEDIATRIC ASSESSMENT—cont'd	

	Past medical history—cont'd	• The medical history for sexually active patients may include:
		    Type of birth control used.
		    Barrier protection.
		    Prior treatment for sexually transmitted disease.
		    Gravida (pregnancies) and para (births, miscarriages, abortions, living children).

	Parent's/caregiver's impression of the child's condition	Identification of the child's primary caregiver. Consider cultural differences that may affect the caregiver's impressions. Evaluation of the caregiver's concerns and observations of the child's condition.

E	Events Surrounding the Illness or Injury	Evaluation of the onset of the illness or circumstances and mechanism of injury:
		• Illness:
		    Length of illness, including date and day of onset and sequence of symptoms.
		    Exposure of others with similar symptoms.
		    Treatment provided prior to ED visit.
		    Examination by primary care provider.
		• Injury:
		    Time and date injury occurred.
		    M: Mechanism of injury, including the use of protective devices such as seat belts and helmets.
		    I: Injuries suspected.
		    V: Vital signs in prehospital environment.
		    T: Treatment by prehospital providers.
		    Description of circumstances leading to injury.
		    Witnessed or unwitnessed.

D	Diet	Assessment of the child's recent oral intake and changes in eating patterns related to the illness or injury: • Changes in eating patterns or fluid intake. • Time of last meal and last fluid intake. • Regular diet: Breast milk, type of formula, solid foods, diet for age, developmental level, and cultural differences. • Special diet or diet restrictions (e.g., American Dietetic Association diet).
	Diapers	Assessment of the child's urine and stool output: • Frequency of urination over last 24 hours (number of wet diapers); changes in frequency. • Time of last void. • Changes in odor or color of urine. • Last bowel movement; color and consistency of stool. • Change in frequency of bowel movements.
S	Symptoms associated with the illness or injury	Identification of symptoms and progression of symptoms since the onset of the illness or injury event.

personnel and document your assessment. It is also important to listen to parents; they often offer information to the triage nurse and then assume they don't have to mention it again. Consider child abuse in suspect circumstances. Know your responsibility in reporting possible abuse.

Vital Signs

All triage systems should include vital signs in the initial assessment, including temperature, pulse rate, respiration rate, blood pressure, and weight (Figure 48-3). Many EDs do not routinely obtain blood pressure in children younger than 10 to 12 years unless there is some indication of hemodynamic compromise. Weight, considered the "fifth vital sign," is necessary because all medications and fluids are based on the child's weight.

Pulse and respirations can be measured while the nurse is evaluating airway and breathing. Temperatures are easily obtained, especially with availability of thermometers that measure temperature of the tympanic membrane. Tympanic measurement in infants younger than 2 years may not be accurate because of anatomic considerations. The tympanic thermometer can be used to screen for fever in the older child in whom the degree of fever is not a factor in determining seriousness of the illness (e.g., the child with a laceration). When an accurate temperature is required to make a treatment decision, a rectal temperature is the most reliable.[3] Blood pressure measurements are often deferred because a cuff the right size is not available or because the child resists the procedure. The cuff must cover two thirds of the upper arm. A cuff that is too small gives a false high reading, whereas an oversized cuff gives a false low reading.

Weight can be obtained at triage or a recent value obtained from the parent. Weight is important for calculating medication doses, assessing dehydration, and comparing the

Table 48-3   PEDIATRIC SECONDARY ASSESSMENT

BODY AREA	CONDITION TO BE ASSESSED
Head	Presence of injuries, pain, or tenderness; anterior fontanelle—depressed, flat, bulging (most infants have an open anterior fontanelle until 18 months)
Eyes	Pupil size and reaction; tears; movement of eyes; drainage or periorbital swelling; presence of injuries; visual acuity (if appropriate)
Ears	Drainage; presence of pain, bruising behind ears
Nose	Nasal flaring, odor, mucus crusting
Throat	Do not attempt to examine if child is in severe respiratory distress; swelling or exudate of pharynx; swelling of cervical lymph nodes
Mouth	Color of oral mucosa; presence of lesions; moistness of lips and mucous membranes; odor of breath
Chest	Respiratory status as indicated during primary assessment; presence of rashes or bruising
Abdomen	Distention; bowel sounds; tenderness
Genitalia and rectum	Diaper rash; vaginal discharge or irritation; odor; rectal bleeding or tears; discharge from penis; trauma
Skin, extremities, and bilateral comparison	Presence of swelling, deformity; pain; movement; sensation; color; pulse rates; presence of rashes, bruising
Vital signs	Temperature, pulse rate, respiration rate, blood pressure, weight, oxygen saturation

Table 48-4   AVERAGE VITAL SIGNS BY AGE

	PULSE RATE (BEATS/MIN)	RESPIRATION RATE (BREATHS/MIN)	BLOOD PRESSURE (SYSTOLIC, MM HG)
Newborn	100 to 160	40 to 60	50 to 70
1 year	90 to 120	30 to 40	80 to 100
3 years	80 to 110	25 to 30	80 to 110
5 years	80 to 110	20 to 25	80 to 110
10 years	60 to 100	15 to 20	90 to 120
15 years	70 to 100	15 to 20	80 to 120

child's growth and development with normal growth and development for that age-group. Birth weight should be documented for infants younger than 8 weeks of age.

Vital signs vary with age (Table 48-4); therefore, alterations from normal must be viewed in light of the child's history and other symptoms. Some causes of alterations in vital signs are listed in Table 48-5. Infants localize infections poorly; therefore, any child younger than 3 months of age should be evaluated for possible bacterial infection. Infants cannot regulate body temperature effectively for several months after birth so every attempt should be made to keep the infant warm.

RESPIRATORY EMERGENCIES

Recognition of respiratory distress and failure in the pediatric patient is crucial because respiratory arrest is almost always the precursor to cardiac arrest in children.[2] The dyspneic child is apprehensive, restless, has expiratory stridor, is wheezing, and usually exhibits intercostal and sternal retractions. Airway obstruction in children results from a myriad of causes including congenital anomalies, peritonsillar abscess, laryngeal obstruction, elevated diaphragm, cardiac failure, cystic fibrosis, drug intoxication, pneumothorax, and foreign bodies such as coins or toy parts.

Sudden onset of respiratory distress suggests foreign body obstruction or spasms. Gradual onset of respiratory distress with coughing and perhaps hemoptysis indicates pulmonary or cardiac insufficiency. Allergies and exposure to disease processes are also considerations. When the child breathes through the mouth, has heavy nasal secretions, or both, consider adenoid infection or a foreign body. Pharyngeal infections can also produce dysphagia.

Viruses cause 80% to 90% of childhood respiratory infections with respiratory syncytial virus (RSV), rhinovirus, parainfluenza, influenza, and adenovirus the most common ones in the pediatric population. An individual virus can cause several different patterns of illness (e.g., RSV can cause bronchiolitis, croup, pneumonia or the common cold [coryza]).

When a child first arrives in the ED with any respiratory problem, rapid assessment should be completed using a sys-

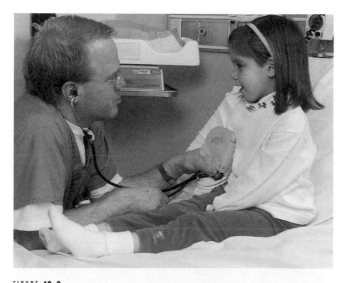

FIGURE 48-3 Vital signs include blood pressure using appropriate cuff size for child's arm.

Table 48-5   SOME CAUSES OF ABNORMAL VITAL SIGNS IN CHILDREN

VITAL SIGN AND VARIATION	CAUSES AND NURSING CONSIDERATIONS
TEMPERATURE	
Hyperthermia (fever)	Viral infections (upper respiratory, gastrointestinal); bacterial infections (pneumonia, otitis media, urinary tract infections, bacteremia, meningitis, epiglottitis); collagen vascular diseases (rheumatic fever, Schönlein-Henoch purpura) drug intoxications (salicylates, atropine, amphetamines); malignancies; hyperthermia can lead to febrile seizures
Hypothermia	Sepsis; shock; exposure; infants have an unstable temperature-regulating mechanism and can become hypothermic as a result of exposure; hypothermia can lead to metabolic acidosis, decreased respiration rates, bradycardia, and cardiopulmonary arrest
PULSE RATE	
Bradycardia	Most common cause in hypoxia (bradycardia equals hypoxia until proven otherwise); other causes include hypotension, acidosis, drug ingestions (narcotics, sedatives); bradycardia in children is always an emergency condition, possibly signaling impending arrest; supplemental oxygen should always be provided immediately, as well as any other interventions to support ABCs
Tachycardia	Earliest sign of shock is supraventricular tachycardia, the most common dysrhythmia in children[2]; other common causes include anxiety, fever, ingestions (anticholinergics, tricyclic antidepressants)
RESPIRATION RATE	
Tachypnea	"Quiet" tachypnea (occurs with no other signs of respiratory distress): diabetes, ketoacidosis, poisonings, or dehydration Other causes of tachypnea: respiratory distress, fever, and congestive heart failure in the child who has congenital heart disease
Bradypnea	Respiratory failure; shock; acidosis; hypothermia; ingestions (narcotics)
BLOOD PRESSURE	
Hypertension	Increased intracranial pressure; renal disease; cardiovascular disease (children with coarctation of the aorta have increased blood pressure in upper extremities, as compared with blood pressure in lower extremities); endocrinologic disorders; drugs (pressor agents, corticosteroids, amphetamines)
Hypotension	Shock (late sign); drug ingestions (tricyclic antidepressants, narcotics, clonidine)

ABC, Airway, breathing, circulation.

tematic approach with the least intrusive methods first. Observation is the simplest assessment tool, providing the nurse with vital information on respiratory effort and level of consciousness. Inspect the child's bare chest for structural abnormalities, symmetry of movement, and use of accessory muscles. Any movement of the head in association with respiratory effort indicates severe distress.

Assessment

Observe the child's position. A child in respiratory distress finds a position of comfort with the body leaning slightly forward and the head in the "sniffing" position, as if smelling a flower. This position allows maximum airway opening.

Respiratory Rate and Pattern

The young child's respiratory muscles are not well developed, so the diaphragm plays a critical role in breathing. Chest auscultation and observation of rise and fall of the abdomen are the best methods for assessing respiratory rate in patients younger than 2 years. Respiratory rates are often ir-

regular in small children, so the rate should be carefully assessed for 1 full minute.

Normal respiratory rates vary by age. A neonate has a normal respiratory rate from 40 to 60 breaths/min, which slows as the child ages. With respiratory distress, the child's respiratory rate initially increases. A resting respiratory rate faster than 60 breaths/min is a sign of respiratory distress in a child, regardless of age. As respiratory failure progresses and the child becomes more acidotic, mental status changes and respiratory rate slows. Bradypnea is therefore a serious sign in a pediatric patient. An adult respiratory rate (12 to 16 breaths/min) is an unusually slow rate for any preadolescent child.

Work of Breathing

Children in respiratory distress have increased work of breathing and use accessory muscles (intercostal, spinal extensor, and neck muscles) for breathing. As work of breathing increases, intercostal, substernal, and supraclavicular retractions are observed.

Inspiration is an active process in which muscles expand the chest. Exhalation is passive, relying on elasticity of the

Table 48-6	ABNORMAL BREATH SOUNDS AND THEIR SIGNIFICANCE IN CHILDREN*
BREATH SOUNDS	**SIGNIFICANCE**
Stridor, inspiratory crowing sound	Caused by upper airway obstruction; high-pitched in croup and foreign body aspiration, low-pitched and muffled in epiglottitis
Wheezing, usually inspiratory but may be expiratory	Caused by lower airway obstruction; bilateral wheezing suggests asthma or bronchiolitis; unilateral wheezing suggests foreign body aspiration
Decreased or unequal breath sounds	Airway obstruction, pneumothorax, pleural effusion, pneumonia
Grunting	Caused by early closure of the glottis during exhalation with active chest wall contraction; increases expiratory airway pressure, preventing airway collapse; creates positive end expiratory pressure (PEEP); seen in diseases with diminished lung compliance such as pulmonary edema; also occurs as a result of pain

From American Academy of Pediatrics and American College of Emergency Physicians: *Advanced pediatric life support,* Elk Grove Village, Ill, and Dallas, 1989, The Academy and College.
*Breath sounds should be assessed over the lateral chest wall and over the anterior chest. Breath sounds heard only over the anterior chest may be misleading, because the child's thin chest wall allows transmission of central airway breath sounds.

lungs and chest wall. Under normal circumstances these two processes are balanced with expiration roughly the same length as inspiration (inspiration/expiration ratio 1:1). When air passages are narrowed by inflammation or obstruction, time required for inhalation may remain the same with an increase in effort; however, exhalation takes substantially longer than inspiration (inspiration/expiration ratio 1:2 or 1:3).

Alertness, willingness to play, and consolability are important observations in assessing mental status with children. Irritability is often a sign of hypoxia; however, a restless child who becomes progressively quieter should be carefully assessed to make certain improved oxygenation rather than respiratory failure or exhaustion is causing restlessness to abate.

Quality of Breathing

Quality of breathing includes depth and sound of breathing. A child's chest should expand symmetrically; therefore, asymmetry or inadequate expansion indicates serious problems such as pneumothorax or hemothorax, foreign body obstruction, or flail chest. To auscultate a child's chest, place the stethoscope at the anterior axillary line level with the second intercostal space on either side. This helps identify the location of any abnormal breath sounds. The small size of a child's chest and thinness of the chest wall allow sounds from one side to resonate throughout the thorax (and even into the abdomen). Therefore listening to the anterior and posterior aspects of the chest may not be as useful for pediatric assessment as it is for an adult.

Breath Sounds

Various pulmonary abnormalities produce adventitious sounds that are not normally heard over the chest. Crackles result from passage of air through moisture or fluid. Wheezes are produced as air passes through airways narrowed by exudate, inflammation, spasm, or tumor. Other abnormal breath sounds include rales and rhonchi. Table 48-6 lists abnormal breath sounds and their possible significance.[1]

Monitoring

The child with a respiratory problem should be monitored carefully for changes in level of consciousness, work of breathing, and level of fatigue. Respiratory rate monitors should be used when available.

Arterial blood gas (ABG) analysis gives the clearest picture of the patient's respiratory status. For pediatric patients, ABG values must be carefully considered because additional stress brought on by the procedure is likely to cause further deterioration in patient condition.

Pulse oximetry is a useful, noninvasive means of continuously measuring oxygen saturation and correlates well with ABG measurement of this variable (Figure 48-4). Oxygen saturation of 90% to 93% is the lowest acceptable range in children. Pulse oximetry's major limitation is that carbon dioxide and acid-base balance are not evaluated. Pulse oximetry relies on analysis of hemoglobin color and may not be useful when extremity perfusion is diminished from trauma, cold ambient temperature, or vasopressors or when the number of erythrocytes is decreased, as in anemia.

Airway Obstruction by Foreign Body

Small children spend a good deal of time exploring their world. Small objects hold a special fascination for children and are likely to end up in their mouths. Foreign body aspiration can occur at any age but is most commonly seen in children younger than 3 years of age. A child brought to the ED with sudden onset of respiratory distress should be evaluated for foreign body aspiration if no other cause is apparent. Initially, a foreign body obstruction produces choking, gagging, wheezing, or coughing. After the object is lodged in the larynx, the child cannot speak or breathe. After the initial period there may be an interval of hours, days, or even weeks without symptoms. Secondary symptoms relate to the anatomic area in which the object is lodged and are usually caused by a persistent respiratory infection.

Foreign body obstruction that completely occludes the airway is an acute emergency. Initial treatment is immediate

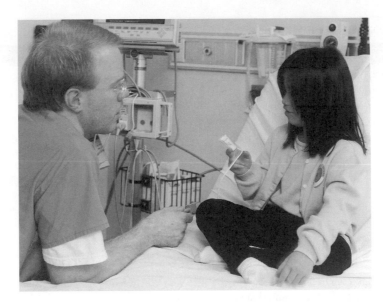

FIGURE 48-4 Use of pulse oximeter can help determine degree of respiratory distress. Explain what you are doing to the child.

removal of the object using age-appropriate maneuvers, such as finger sweeps and chest or abdominal thrusts. If these maneuvers fail, forceps may be used to remove the foreign body. Immediate cricothyrotomy or tracheostomy must be performed to open the airway if the airway remains obstructed. Cardiopulmonary resuscitation must be initiated if the child is not breathing and has no heartbeat.

If ventilation appears adequate, allow the child to assume whatever position is most comfortable. Unless the object is observed high in the upper airway, its exact location must be determined by radiograph. Bronchoscopy may be necessary for removal. A swallowed object is allowed to pass normally through the gastrointestinal tract, unless it is long and sharp. These objects present significant danger of intestinal perforation. Nickel-cadmium batteries must be removed because of the potential for toxic leakage.

Asthma

Asthma is a chronic inflammatory lung disease affecting 5% to 10% of all American children.[2] Wheezing, the most obvious sign of asthma, may range from mild to severe and is accompanied by tachycardia, chest retractions, and anxiety. Expiration may be prolonged because of narrowed airways. Obtaining a thorough history may be useful in trying to determine the cause and severity of the attack. Repeated asthma attacks are a dangerous sign because of increasing fatigue and potential complications. Recent hospitalization is likely to be an indication of a seriously ill child.

When assessing a child with asthma, evaluate respiratory rate, quality, and effort to determine the degree of respiratory distress. The child may require supplemental oxygen if saturation on room air is less than 95% and tachypnea and tachycardia are present.

Treatment of a child in the ED with moderate to severe distress involves inhaled β_2-agonist agents with oxygen (Table 48-7). Nebulized albuterol treatments are usually given every 20 minutes for three doses. Terbutaline nebulized with normal saline solution is frequently used when the child does not respond to albuterol treatments. Subcutaneous epinephrine is reserved for severe attacks. Use of intravenous aminophylline has declined because of the belief that the drug is not as effective in patients treated with β_2-agonists. Concerns over increased mortality related to β_2-agonists have increased the use of glucocorticoids. Another factor contributing to steroid management is understanding the inflammatory process of asthma.[5]

Good hydration for children with asthma is important. They are prone to fluid loss during hyperventilation. Intravenous fluids may be necessary in some patients.

Bronchiolitis

Bronchiolitis, a viral infection commonly found in infants younger than 18 months, can be a life-threatening illness. An inflammatory process causes edema in the bronchial mucosa with resultant expiratory obstruction and air trapping. Bronchiolitis has a broad spectrum of severity. Determination of when dyspnea began helps predict the course of the illness because the critical period of bronchiolitis usually occurs during the first 24 to 72 hours after onset of dyspnea. History typically includes symptoms of a cold, cough, and coryza for a few days before onset of dyspnea. Bronchiolitis is often difficult to differentiate from bronchial asthma; therefore, careful evaluation should be made in the ED including oxygen saturation, ABGs, complete blood count (CBC), and cultures from the nasopharynx. Chest radiograph may demonstrate air

Table 48-7	MEDICATIONS USED FOR ASTHMA		
MEDICATION	**DOSAGE**	**METHOD**	**COMMENTS**
Albuterol 5% solution	0.01-0.03 ml/kg in 2 ml NS (0.5-0.15 mg/kg); maximum 0.5 ml (2.5 mg)	Nebulizer	Peak onset 30-60 min; duration 4-6 hr
	2 puffs every 5 min for total of 12 puffs, then 4 puffs every 1 hr if improved	MDI (90 g/puff)	
Epinephrine 1:1000 solution	0.01 ml/kg; maximum 0.35 ml	Subcutaneous	May cause tremors, restlessness, tachycardia
Hydrocortisone	4 ms/kg	IV	
Ipratropium bromide (Atrovent)	5-10 puffs with spacer every 4-6 hr	Nebulizer	Peak onset 1-2 hr; duration 3-4 hr
Prednisone	1-2 ms/kg/day in single or divided doses for outpatients; 1-2 mg/kg every 6 hr for inpatients	PO	Onset of action: 3 hr; peak effectiveness: 6-12 hr
Methylprednisolone	1-2 mg/kg/dose every 6 hr	IV	
Epinephrine 1:1000 (1 mg/ml)	0.01 mg/kg up to 0.3 mg every 20 min × 3	Subcutaneous	May cause tremor, restlessness, tachycardia
Terbutaline (1 mg/1ml)	0.01 mg/kg up to 0.3 mg every 2-6 hr prn	Subcutaneous	Peak onset 30 min; duration 3-4 hr
	0.02 10 μg/kg over 10 min (loading dose), followed by 0.4 μg/kg/min increase prn by 0.2 μg/kg/min (expect to use 3-6 μg/kg/min)		
Aminophylline	Loading dose: 6 mg/kg (if patient not currently taking theophylline) continuous infusion: 0.5-1.2 mg/kg/hr depending on age	IV	Toxicity: nausea, vomiting, tachycardia, seizures

NS, Normal saline; *MDI,* metered-dose inhaler; *IV,* intravenous; *PO,* by mouth.

trapping. Hospitalization is necessary for infants younger than 2 months of age and those with an apneic episode.

RSV, the most common causative organism of bronchiolitis, is a highly contagious respiratory pathogen transmitted by direct contact with infected respiratory secretions or contaminated objects. The virus enters the body by contact of the hands with the nose, eye, or other mucous membranes. Aerosol spread occurs but is less common.

Aerosolized bronchodilators provide symptomatic relief of wheezing in these infants. Albuterol is the drug of choice. During administration, the infant is monitored for tolerance of the drug, including observing work of breathing, respiratory rate, and heart rate. Discharge instructions may include the administration of albuterol via nebulizer, oral syrup, or an inhaler for up to 5 to 7 days.

Carbon Monoxide Poisoning

Carbon monoxide (CO) is a colorless, odorless gas resulting from incomplete burning of organic substances, such as gasoline, coal products, tobacco, and building materials. Injury and death occur when CO interferes with or inhibits cellular respiration. When CO enters the bloodstream, it readily combines with hemoglobin to form carboxyhemoglobin, but it is released less easily. Tissue hypoxia can reach dangerous levels before oxygen is available to meet tissue needs.

Accidental poisoning is often the result of fumes from heaters or smoke from structural fires. Signs and symptoms of CO poisoning are the result of tissue hypoxia. Severity

varies with the level of carboxyhemoglobin. Mild manifestations produce irritability, headache, visual disturbances, and nausea, whereas more severe cases cause confusion, hallucinations, ataxia, and coma. Bright cherry-red lips and skin, described as classic signs of poisoning, occur less often then pallor and cyanosis.

Primary treatment is administration of 100% oxygen with a nonrebreather mask or bag-valve mask. Efforts should be made to reduce the child's metabolic demand for oxygen by keeping the child quiet and calm. Severe cases may require intubation or hyperbaric oxygen therapy. Children with suspected or known inhalation of CO are admitted for close observation and oxygen therapy. Because CO has a half-life of approximately 2 hours, oxygen therapy is needed for a prolonged period.

Croup

Croup, or laryngotracheobronchitis, is viral inflammation of the subglottic area, including the trachea and bronchi. Croup occurs most frequently in infants and children 6 months to 3 years of age but may occur in older children. It is slightly more prevalent in boys. Croup is seen most frequently in cooler months.

The inflammatory process of viral croup produces edema of the trachea and surrounding structures. Edematous airways secrete tenacious mucus, which leads to problematic removal of secretions. The child's effort to inspire air through edematous structures produces the characteristic stridor of croup.

Table 48-8	COMPARISON OF EPIGLOTTITIS AND CROUP	
	EPIGLOTTITIS (SUPRAGLOTTITIS)	**LARYNGOTRACHEITIS (CROUP)**
Age	1 to 6 years	6 months to 3 years
Onset	Rapid	Preceded by several days of upper respiratory infection, cough, or both
Usual cause	Bacteria, i.e., *Haemophilus influenzae*	Parainfluenza or other virus
Fever	>39.4° C (103° F)	Varies; often low grade
Clinical assessment	Appears ill; dyspnea, drooling, dysphagia	Upper respiratory infection, barking cough, stridor
Complications	Asphyxia caused by inflammation and obstruction in *supraglottic* area	Asphyxia caused by inflammation and obstruction in *subglottic* area
Field treatment	Oxygen; rapid transport to health care facility	Oxygen; rapid transport to health care facility
ED treatment	Calm environment; oxygen; defer IV line; prepare resuscitation equipment; possible need for ventilatory support with bag-valve-mask device, intubation, or surgical airway	Varies with severity; oxygen, mist treatment, epinephrine, racemic epinephrine; hospitalization if severe, if racemic epinephrine is given, or if caretakers are unable to treat patient at home

ED, Emergency department; *IV,* intravenous.

History usually includes an upper respiratory infection for a few days followed by nocturnal onset of the characteristic barking cough. The child may have a hoarse voice or cry. Nursing assessment should be performed carefully to keep the child calm. The stress of crying increases the work of breathing, so both stridor and retractions markedly increase. Assessment should focus on cardiorespiratory status, hydration, anxiety, or fatigue level and parental anxiety.

Nursing interventions in croup focus on relieving anxiety and reducing work of breathing. Cool, humidified oxygen should be provided in a manner comfortable for the child. Many times this is done with the child sitting on the parent's lap, where humidified oxygen is delivered close to the nose and mouth. Most anxious children become more anxious if forced to wear a face mask. Racemic epinephrine is used in severe cases to reduce mucosal edema and laryngospasm. Steroids are used with severe cases, usually methylprednisolone sodium succinate or dexamethasone. Cross-table, soft-tissue radiograph of the neck may be used to rule out epiglottitis.

Croup responds well to mist treatments—children may improve sufficiently to be able to go home. The decision for hospital admission rests on the degree of respiratory distress, ability to maintain adequate hydration, ability to rest, and degree of parental apprehension. When a child with croup is discharged, parents should be provided instructions for home care of croup including use of a cool mist vaporizer, keeping windows open at night, fever control, and offering frequent cool fluids. Parents often require considerable reassurance. Table 48-8 shows some of the differences between croup and epiglottitis (supraglottitis) and identifies emergent treatment for both.

Epiglottitis

Epiglottitis, or supraglottic laryngitis, is the most emergent acute airway obstruction of childhood. This disease produces rapid onset of inflammatory edema of the epiglottis. Epiglottitis occurs throughout the year, is seen in boys and girls with equal frequency, and usually affects children ages 2 to 5 years. Because most pediatric cases are caused by *Haemophilus influenzae* type B, the incidence of epiglottitis has significantly declined since the *H. influenzae* type B conjugate vaccine became available. A child with epiglottitis typically presents in an anxious state, with respiratory distress, drooling because of difficulty swallowing, and sitting forward with the neck extended. The child may have audible respiratory sounds and generally appears flushed and toxic with a high temperature. The epiglottis becomes swollen and cherry red, and it can cause total airway obstruction if manipulated during examination. Figure 48-5 illustrates this clinical picture. Many children with acute epiglottitis require intubation, cricothyroidotomy, or tracheostomy. Therefore necessary equipment should be on hand and ready before an examination is done.

When epiglottitis is suspected, keep the child calm and quiet. The primary focus is to maintain a patent airway. If the child is quiet in the parent's lap, let the child stay there during a brief assessment. A lateral soft-tissue radiograph of the neck is taken if the patient is stable, to identify the swollen epiglottis (Figure 48-6). The thumb sign refers to the shape of the epiglottis on the lateral soft tissue x-ray of the neck. This radiographic sign may be more apparent in older children with epiglottitis.

Most patients with severe respiratory distress from epiglottitis go directly to the operating room for intubation or tracheostomy. Oxygenation is provided as passively as possible to prevent agitation and increased edema of the epiglottis. Hospital admission is always necessary for known or suspected epiglottitis. Intravenous fluids are necessary until oral fluids can be swallowed. The preferred route for antibiotics is intravenous.

Peritonsillar and Retropharyngeal Abscess

Other diseases with signs and symptoms similar to epiglottitis include peritonsillar abscess and retropharyngeal abscess.

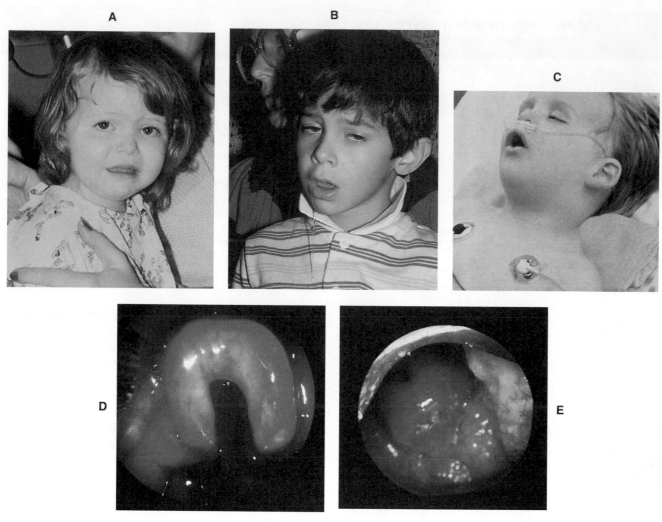

FIGURE 48-5 Epiglottitis. **A** to **C,** These three patients with acute epiglottitis demonstrate the varying degrees of distress that may be seen, depending on age and time of presentation. **A,** This 3-year-old seen a few hours after onset of symptoms was anxious and still but had no positional preference or drooling. **B,** This 5-year-old, who had been symptomatic for several hours, holds his neck extended with head held forward, is mouth breathing and drooling, and shows signs of tiring. **C,** This 2-year-old was in severe distress and was too exhausted to hold his head up. **D** and **E,** In the operating room the epiglottis can be visualized and appears intensely red and swollen. It may retain its omega shape or resemble a cherry. (From Zitelli B, Davis H: *Atlas of pediatric physical diagnosis,* ed 3, St. Louis, 1997, Mosby.)

Peritonsillar abscess on rare occasions can compromise the child's airway. Retropharyngeal abscess has a less abrupt onset than supraglottitis but also poses substantial risk to airway patency. A child with peritonsillar or retropharyngeal abscess requires the caregiver to give attention to and support of respiratory and circulatory function. Retropharyngeal abscesses require drainage in the operating room, whereas a peritonsillar abscess may sometimes be drained in the ED if there is danger of airway compromise. Both conditions are treated with intravenous antibiotics.

Pertussis

Pertussis, or whooping cough, is an acute respiratory infection caused by *Bordetella pertussis.* Whooping cough usu-

ally occurs in children younger than 4 years of age who have not been immunized. Highly contagious, whooping cough is particularly threatening to young infants, in whom there are higher morbidity and mortality rates. Incidence is highest in the spring and summer.

Pertussis is usually indistinguishable from a common cold until the paroxysmal stage. During this stage, the child has a fever, hypoxia, and cough. Petechiae above the nipple line, otitis media, atelectasis, pneumothorax, and vomiting may also be present. Hernias may appear suddenly as a result of exertion during coughing.

Excitement and crying tend to worsen the coughing paroxysms, so care should be taken to keep the child as calm as possible. Airway clearance is important in management of pertussis and may require gentle suctioning. Humidified

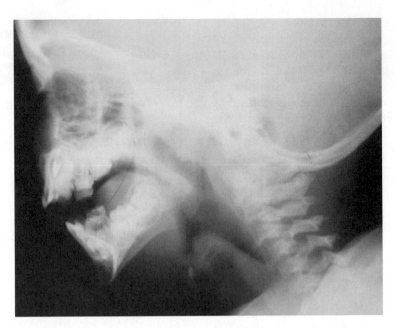

FIGURE 48-6   Mild epiglottitis or supraglottitis. The lateral neck radiograph demonstrates mild epiglottic swelling and thickening of the aryepiglottic folds. (From Zitelli B, Davis H: *Atlas of pediatric physical diagnosis,* ed 3, St. Louis, 1997, Mosby.)

oxygen should be used and the child should be isolated from other patients. Caregivers should use universal precautions, wear masks, and handle secretions carefully. Antibiotic therapy should be initiated as soon as possible. Hospitalization is recommended for those infants who exhibit respiratory distress in association with coughing paroxysms. Infants may also require intravenous fluids for dehydration secondary to inability to feed caused by coughing.[5]

Pneumonia

Pneumonia, inflammation of the pulmonary parenchyma, is common throughout childhood but occurs more frequently in infancy and early childhood. Clinically, pneumonia may occur as a primary disease or complication of other illnesses. A majority of pneumonias in children are caused by viruses, although bacterial pneumonia, usually caused by group B streptococci and gram-negative bacilli, is more likely to occur in the first weeks of life. Whether viral or bacterial, pathogens reach the lung and cause an inflammatory response that leads to accumulation of fluid in the lungs, tachypnea, cough, and fever. Bacterial pneumonia tends to have abrupt onset with high fever, 38.5° to 41° C (101.3° to 105.8° F). In viral pneumonia, fever is usually lower than 39° C (102.2° F). With bacterial pneumonia there is an increase in the number of granulocytes and bands on the white cell differential count.

Treatment varies with the child's age, suspected causative agent, severity of symptoms, and immune status of the child. Infants younger than 2 months usually require hospitalization for intravenous antibiotic treatment. Children with minimum distress who are tolerating oral fluids well can usually be treated at home with oral antibiotic therapy. Aerosolized bronchodilators may be helpful at any age.

Pneumothorax

A pneumothorax is collection of air in the pleural space caused by rupture of an alveolar bleb on the surface of the pleura that results in partial collapse of one or both lungs. A pneumothorax may occur spontaneously or secondary to obstruction, trauma, cancer, or tuberculosis. A history of a previous pneumothorax increases the likelihood of recurrence.

Symptoms depend on how much air escapes into the pleural space. Small amounts may be asymptomatic. A large amount of air prevents full expansion of the affected lung, causing tachypnea, dyspnea, grunting, hypoxia, and cyanosis. Contrary to most respiratory problems that cause retraction of chest wall musculature, a pneumothorax may cause bulging of these muscles, especially intercostal muscles over the affected area. Bilateral breath sounds are usually heard in infants and small children.

Hospital admission is almost always recommended. Oxygen administration and bed rest are used in mild cases. Children with more than 40% pneumothorax usually require a chest tube with closed drainage to evacuate air from the pleural space and reexpand the lung. The child must be continually assessed for development of tension pneumothorax, which is a life-threatening problem.

CARDIOVASCULAR EMERGENCIES

Causes of cardiovascular emergencies in the pediatric age-group differ from those in adults, but the three basic categories of cardiovascular compromise are the same: inadequate heart function, inadequate volume for circulation, and problems of fluid distribution. Table 48-9 summarizes common causes of cardiovascular emergencies in children.

Most pediatric cardiac arrests are related to respiratory arrest rather than primary cardiac arrest. Support the child's respiratory efforts and intervene early to prevent potential cardiac problems.

Cardiovascular Assessment

Blood volume in a child is 80 ml/kg, with total blood volume much less than in an adult. Loss of 1 cup of blood in a 10-kg child is equivalent to blood loss of 1 quart in an adult. With infants and children, immaturity of the sympathetic innervation of the ventricles keeps stroke volume at a relatively fixed rate. A child responds to the need for increased cardiac output with tachycardia. Tachycardia may initially increase cardiac output during periods of distress; however, prolonged tachycardia more than 200 beats/min for infants and 170 beats/min for children causes decompensation and decreases cardiac output. Close attention to heart rate, skin signs, and mental status is the key to early recognition of compensated shock. Capillary refill time is also recommended as a sensitive indicator of perfusion in the pediatric patient. Use of this parameter has not been studied extensively; however, normal capillary refill time is about 2 seconds. More than 3 seconds may indicate poor perfusion in a normothermic child.

Cardiovascular assessment should identify shock or conditions leading to shock that require the emergency nurse to intervene. A history of illness or injury is important in interpreting signs and symptoms. Observing the child plays a major role. Important elements to assess include the following:

- Skin color. Pallor may indicate decreased perfusion caused by diminished cardiac output.
- Capillary refill. A delay of 3 seconds or more is abnormal.
- Level of consciousness. Decreased perfusion to the brain may cause lethargy and confusion.
- Skin turgor. Check mucous membranes for moisture.
- Anterior fontanelle. A bulging fontanelle may indicate increased intracranial pressure, whereas a sunken fontanelle suggests dehydration.
- Peripheral pulse rates. Decreased perfusion to extremities results in weak peripheral pulse(s).
- Vital signs. Temperature, pulse rate, respiration rate, and blood pressure. Average vital signs for the pediatric patient are listed in Table 48-4.

Vital signs should be documented as part of the baseline assessment. Children in early shock may have a normal blood pressure because of their ability to compensate. Declining blood pressure is a serious sign warranting immediate intervention. A child can lose a significant amount of blood before blood pressure decreases. Table 48-4 lists average blood

Table 48-9	CAUSES OF CARDIOVASCULAR COLLAPSE IN CHILDREN
PROBLEM	**ETIOLOGY**
Inadequate heart function	Cardiac dysrhythmia
	Congestive heart failure
	Congenital heart disease
Inadequate volume	Dehydration
	Burns
	Trauma
Maldistribution of fluid	Septic shock
	Anaphylaxis
	Drug ingestion
	Sickle cell disease

pressures by age. Another method of estimating normal blood pressure is to use the following formula:

$$\text{Systolic pressure} = 80 + (\text{age in years} \times 2)$$

Inadequate Heart Function

Rhythm Disturbances

Children have young, strong hearts, so rhythm disturbances are seldom primary events. Dysrhythmias usually result from hypoxia or metabolic disturbances. Pediatric patients with rhythm disturbances from congenital cardiac problems are seen with increasing frequency in the ED, probably because of increased survival rates. The most common congenital problems causing rhythm disturbances are transposition of the great vessels and congenital mitral stenosis. Acquired cardiac diseases such as cardiomyopathies, rheumatic heart disease, and viral myocarditis may also cause rhythm disturbances.

Abnormal rhythms in this age-group are divided into three categories: fast, slow, and absent (Table 48-10). Absent rhythms are disorganized or nonperfusing rhythms. Sinus tachycardia and supraventricular tachycardia are two major rhythm disturbances found in children. Sinus tachycardia in children is a rate of 140 to 220 beats/min, whereas supraventricular tachycardia is usually higher than 220 beats/min. Bradycardia is an ominous sign in a pediatric patient. Sinus bradycardia is frequently caused by hypoxia and should be treated aggressively with ventilation and oxygenation. An infant with a rate less than 60 beats/min requires immediate cardiac compressions.[3] Junctional and idioventricular rhythms are usually terminal rhythms. Absent, disorganized, and nonperfusing rhythms require cardiopulmonary resuscitation and advanced life support procedures.

Congestive Heart Failure

Congenital heart disease accounts for the majority of children seen in the ED with congestive heart failure (CHF). Preload, afterload, and myocardial contractility are major factors in determining the amount of blood pumped through

Table 48-10 RHYTHM DISTURBANCES IN CHILDREN

RHYTHM	CAUSE	CHARACTERISTICS	TREATMENT
FAST RHYTHMS			
Sinus tachycardia	Fever, anxiety, pain, hypovolemia	Rapid sinus rhythm; rate 140-220 beats/min	Treat underlying cause.
Supraventricular tachycardia	Reentry mechanism	Paroxysmal sinus rhythm; P waves often undetectable; rate $\leq$ 230 beats/min	*Stable:* Vagal maneuvers. Consider adenosine if no response. *Unstable:* Adenosine 0.1 mg/kg rapid IV bolus (maximum single dose: 12 mg). If no response, cardioversion 0.5 J/kg. Consider alternative medications if no response (e.g., Amiodarone, Procainamide, Lidocaine [wide complex only]).
Ventricular tachycardia	Structural disease, hypoxia, acidosis, electrolyte imbalance, toxic ingestion	Rate $\leq$ 120 beats/min; wide QRS; no P waves	*Pulse:* Amiodarone 5 mg/kg IV over 20-60 min or Procainamide 15 mg/kg IV over 30-60 min or Lidocaine 1 mg/kg IV bolus. If no response, synchronized cardioversion 0.5-1.0 J/kg. *Pulseless:* Defibrillation in rapid succession—2 J/kg, 4 J/kg, 4 J/kg. Amiodarone 5 mg/kg bolus (IV/IO) or Lidocaine 1 mg/kg bolus (IV/IO/ET) or Magnesium 25-50 mg/kg (IV/IO) if torsades des pointes or hypoglycemia
SLOW RHYTHMS			
Sinus bradycardia	Hypoxemia, hypotension, shock	Sinus rhythm; slow rate (<80 beats/min in infants, <60 beats/min in children)	Ventilation, oxygenation, cardiopulmonary resuscitation. Epinephrine (1:10,000), 0.01 mg/kg IV/IO or 0.1 mg/kg ET tube. Repeat every 3-5 minutes. Atropine, 0.02 mg/kg; minimum dose 0.1 mg and a maximum single dose of 0.5 mg for children and 1.0 mg for adolescents.
Junctional rhythm, heart blocks	Hypoxemia, hypotension, acidosis	Rare in children; slow rate; P waves may or may not be present	Ventilation, oxygenation, CPR. Atropine, 0.02 mg/kg; minimum dose 0.1 mg and a maximum single dose of 0.5 mg for children and 1.0 mg for adolescents. Epinephrine (1:10,000), 0.1 ml/kg
ABSENT/DISORGANIZED/NONPERFUSING RHYTHMS			
Asystole	Hypoxia, hypovolemia, acidosis	Flat line on ECG; absent pulse; absent respirations	CPR, ALS procedures
Ventricular fibrillation	Rare in infants and children; hypoxia, acidosis	No identifiable P, QRS, or T waves; wavy line on ECG	CPR, ALS procedures (defibrillate 2 J/kg, then 4 J/kg)
Pulseless electrical activity (PEA)	Hypoxia, acidosis, tension pneumothorax, hypovolemia	Pulselessness, with organized electrical activity on ECG	CPR; treat underlying cause

CPR, Cardiopulmonary resuscitation; *ECG,* electrocardiogram; *ALS,* advanced life support; *ET,* endotracheal tube; *IV,* intravenous; *IO,* intraosseous.

the circulatory system. When the heart is not able to pump effectively because of chronic disease, rhythm disturbance, pressure on the heart, or excessive fluid volume, the fluid backs up in the system, causing signs of overload such as pulmonary edema, jugular vein distention, and enlarged liver.

Signs of CHF include tachycardia, tachypnea, cough, wheezes, cyanosis, pallor, poor appetite, and failure to thrive. Many times infants with CHF have a very rapid respiratory rate (60 to 100 breaths per minute) but do not appear in distress. Lack of distress is evidence of the infant's ability to compensate. Observe for presence and degree of other indicators of respiratory effort such as nasal flaring, intercostal retractions, head bobbing, and expiratory grunting.

Primary treatment of CHF is aimed at improving myocardial contractility and decreasing cardiac workload by using pharmacologic agents. These agents include inotropic drugs (Digoxin) that improve myocardial contractility, diuretics (Furosemide) to reduce preload, and afterload-reducing agents (sodium nitroprusside, Captopril) to reduce ventricular afterload. If dyspnea is present, the child may benefit from cool, humidified oxygen. Hospitalization is required to determine the cause of CHF and develop a treatment plan with the family.

Inadequate Volume

The major medical cause of hypovolemia in children is dehydration. A child who has been sick for even a short time with vomiting and diarrhea is at risk, as is a child who has been ill for several days with fever and decreased fluid intake. When output exceeds intake over time, dehydration becomes clinically significant and electrolyte imbalances occur. Electrolyte disturbances cause more nausea and vomiting, starting a downward spiral that can be reversed only with medical intervention. A dehydrated child looks sick, with sunken eyes, pale skin, and lethargy. When 5% or more of the child's body mass (weight) is lost, skin and mucous membranes appear dry. It is often helpful to ask the parent about intake and output; that is, the number of bottles the child has taken and the number of stools or wet diapers per day for small children. Unless fluid volume is replaced and balance between intake and output restored, the condition will progress to hypovolemic shock.

Heart rate, skin signs, and capillary refill provide the most useful information about the child's cardiovascular status. If the patient shows signs of shock, ensure adequate ventilation and oxygenation, then give 20 ml/kg of normal saline solution and repeat until improvement is seen.[1] If vascular access cannot be obtained, intraosseous access should be obtained in children 6 years of age and younger. Intraosseous vascular access is a quick, safe, and dependable route for administering fluids, medications, and blood products.

Diagnostic tests, usually CBC, electrolytes, glucose, blood urea nitrogen (BUN), and urinalysis, are used to assess hydration status, guide treatment, and determine the cause of dehydration. Patients requiring admission are those who are more than 5% to 10% dehydrated as evidenced by weight loss, dry mucous membranes, tachycardia, oliguria, urine specific gravity greater than 1.030, and elevated BUN or those who are unable to retain oral fluids. Patients with only slightly dehydration whose laboratory results are within normal limits are discharged with home care instructions unless there are other reasons for admission.

Septic Shock

Sepsis, or septicemia, is a profound, life-threatening bacterial infection in the bloodstream. Septic shock occurs in patients with septicemia when inadequate tissue perfusion occurs in the wake of massive vasodilation. The ABCs should be rapidly assessed and supported. The nurse must keep in mind that hypotension is a late sign of shock in infants and young children. When present, it indicates severe shock. The skin is often cool, especially the extremities, but can also be warm and pink because of early vasodilation. Capillary refill time may be delayed longer than two seconds. Skin should be inspected for petechia, purpura, jaundice, pallor, cyanosis, or mottling.

Management in the ED focuses on preservation of vital functions. Adequate ventilation and oxygenation are the first priority. Administer oxygen and assist with breathing if ventilation is inadequate. Institute nursing interventions to decrease oxygen demand (e.g., thermoregulation, alleviation of pain, reassurance). Allow the parent to remain with the child as much as possible. Diagnostic studies include blood culture, CBC with white cell differential, chest radiograph, and urinalysis.

Isotonic crystalloids such as normal saline are usually given for volume replacement. An indwelling urinary catheter is inserted to monitor urinary output. After the diagnosis of sepsis or septic shock is made, intravenous antibiotic therapy should be instituted immediately. Care should be taken that all cultures (blood, urine, others) are collected before antibiotic administration. The antibiotics administered vary with the child's age and the presumed source of infection. After culture results are available, antibiotic therapy can be more specific. Severe metabolic acidosis should be corrected with sodium bicarbonate (0.5-1.0 mg/kg). Sympathomimetic and inotropic drugs such as epinephrine (0.05-0.15 mg/kg/min) and dopamine (2-5 mg/kg/min) may be used to increase heart rate and cardiac output in patients with poor myocardial function and systemic perfusion despite adequate oxygenation and fluid resuscitation. Serum glucose should be carefully monitored. In younger infants and children, limited glycogen stores in the liver place the child at risk for hypoglycemia. The child is admitted, usually to the intensive care unit for continued intravenous antibiotics and monitoring.

Anaphylaxis

Anaphylaxis is an acute clinical syndrome resulting from the interaction of an allergen with a patient who is hypersensitive. Severe reactions are immediate, often life-threatening, and frequently involve multiple systems. Skin flushing and urticaria are common early signs, followed by angioedema, most notable in the eyelids, lips, and tongue. Bronchiolar constriction may follow significant narrowing of the airway.

Recovery from anaphylactic reactions depends on rapid recognition and institution of treatment. The goal of treatment is to provide ventilation, restore adequate circulation, and prevent further exposure by identifying and removing the cause. A mild reaction with no evidence of respiratory distress is managed with subcutaneous epinephrine, H_2 blockers, and antihistamines. Moderate or severe distress represents a potentially life-threatening emergency. Establishing an airway is the first concern. Epinephrine is given subcutaneously or intravenously as an antihistamine to support the cardiovascular system and increase blood pressure. Fluids are given to restore blood volume. Children with severe anaphylaxis should be hospitalized and monitored for at least 24 hours.

Sickle Cell Disease

Sickle cell disease is a hereditary blood disorder. Sickled hemoglobin molecules cause irregularly shaped red blood cells. Sickle cells clump together, occluding small blood vessels and causing tissue ischemia.

There are three major categories of sickle cell crisis. Vasoocclusive crisis occurs when small vessels in bone, soft tissue, and organs (i.e., liver, spleen, brain, lungs, penis) are occluded, causing ischemia, pain, and swelling. The first presentation of vasoocclusive crisis, usually after 2 or 3 months of age, is precipitated by infection, exposure, dehydration, or other stress. Initial signs of vasoocclusive crisis in the very young child may be warmth and swelling of one or both hands or feet. Older patients have pain in affected organs, visual disturbances, respiratory distress, and priapism.

Another problem resulting from sickle cell disease is aplastic crisis, caused by red blood cell destruction coupled with impaired red blood cell production in bone marrow. Aplastic crisis worsens anemia and leads to high-output CHF.

Sequestration crisis is the most fulminant manifestation of sickle cell disease, is less common than other crises, and can be rapidly fatal. Incidence is greater in young children, several months to 6 years of age. Blood suddenly pools in the spleen and other visceral organs, causing severe anemia and hypovolemic shock.

Because of the need for close monitoring, most patients with sickle cell disease are cared for by specialists. However, a first crisis or severe crisis may lead to treatment in the ED. Medical management is usually directed at supportive, symptomatic treatment. The main objectives are oxygenation, hydration with oral or intravenous solutions, electrolyte replacement, rest, analgesics, and blood replacement as needed and antibiotics as required. The administration of narcotics should be anticipated for pain control because sickle cell disease is a chronic painful disease. Morphine

sulfate 0.1 to 0.2 mg/kg intramuscularly or intravenously (maximum initial dose 10 mg) is the drug of choice for managing the pain associated with sickle cell disease. Refer to Chapter 42 for additional discussion.

NEUROLOGIC EMERGENCIES

Head trauma is the most common cause of neurologic emergency in children; however, seizures, shunt malfunction, and, rarely, brain tumors and congenital vascular malformations can also affect mental status in the pediatric age-group. Infectious processes such as meningitis and sepsis are another cause for neurologic changes in children. Refer to Chapter 29 for discussion of pediatric trauma.

Neurologic Assessment

When a child has altered mental status, it is important to remember the first priority is airway and ventilation. Neurologic assessment of pediatric patients presents special challenges, especially for the preverbal child. When parents say their child is "not acting normal," this should be taken seriously. Early signs and symptoms of increased intracranial pressure include altered mental status, restlessness, irritability, headache, and vomiting. Constricted or dilated pupils and decorticate or decerebrate posturing are late signs of increased intracranial pressure.

Numerous methods of assessing neurologic function in children have been proposed, including pediatric adaptations of the Glasgow coma scale (see Figure 29-3). The simplest and probably the most useful in the emergency setting is the mnemonic AVPU:

A	*Alert*
V	responds to *Verbal* stimuli
P	responds to *Painful* stimuli
U	*Unresponsive*

Serial assessment with this mnemonic, together with a description of the patient's behavior, is the clearest means for documenting changes. An accurate history from parents is also helpful. When a child has altered mental status, ask about trauma, previous medical problems, ingestions, headache, and signs and symptoms of infection. Box 48-2 presents a minineurologic examination for the pediatric patient. Evaluating history and level of consciousness can be enough to classify the child's condition as an emergency. An altered level of consciousness in any child is an emergent condition.

A commonly used mnemonic, AEIOU TIPS, is useful for identification of causes for altered level of consciousness (Table 48-11). Intussusception as a cause of altered consciousness in the infant has been added to this mnemonic because lethargy has been found to be a common symptom of this condition. Treatment of children who arrive in the ED with an altered level of consciousness includes assessment of ABCs along with assessment for injury or illnesses. The child must be evaluated for symptoms of increased intracranial pressure to prevent central nervous system injury. Lab-

Box 48-2 MINI NEUROLOGIC EXAMINATION

HISTORY

1. Time and mechanism of injury
2. Neurologic status immediately after injury; elapsed time between time of injury and arrival in hospital
3. Any neurologic change that may have occurred

LEVEL OF CONSCIOUSNESS

1. Aware: may be disoriented or confused but still awake
2. Lethargic: can be aroused to follow commands
3. Stuporous: cannot be aroused to follow commands; purposeful withdrawal in response to deep, painful stimuli
4. Semicomatose: only reflex responses to pain (i.e., decorticate or decerebrate)
5. Comatose: no response to pain

PUPILS

1. Size: equal or unequal
2. Reaction to light

RESPONSE TO PAIN

1. Purposeful
2. Semipurposeful
3. Decorticate
4. Decerebrate
5. No response

MOVEMENT OF EXTREMITIES

1. Spontaneous
2. Response to pain
3. Equal strength and movement

PLANTAR RESPONSES

1. Upgoing
2. Downgoing
3. Equivocal

FACIAL MOVEMENTS

Central or peripheral weakness may be present.

FUNDI

Describe hemorrhages. Rare to see papilledema sooner than 12-24 hours after injury.

CEREBROSPINAL FLUID OTORRHEA OR RHINORRHEA

Usually blood with or without cerebrospinal fluid in acute phase

VITAL SIGNS

Obtain baseline; monitor closely.

Table 48-11 AEIOU TIPS MNEMONIC FOR EVALUATING ALTERED LEVEL OF CONSCIOUSNESS

CAUSE	COMMENTS
Alcohol	More common in adolescents than younger pediatric patients
Encephalopathy	Hypertension, hepatic, Reye's syndrome
Endocrinology	Thyroid, adrenal
Electrolytes	Alterations in sodium, potassium, calcium, or magnesium levels
Insulin	Hypoglycemia or hyperglycemia
Intussusception	Decreased level of consciousness may be the first manifestation of intussusception before abdominal symptoms appear
Overdose	Opiates and other toxins, ingested, inhaled, or transferred to the fetus before birth
Uremia	Hemolytic uremic syndrome, chronic renal impairment
Trauma	One of the major causes; usually, head injuries and chest injuries leading to hypoxia
Infection	More common in children than in adults; meningitis, encephalitis, Reye's syndrome, and sepsis
Psychiatric	Rare in children; should be considered only after other factors are ruled out
Seizure	Postictal states, syncope

From American Academy of Pediatrics and American College of Emergency Physicians: *Advanced pediatric life support,* Elk Grove Village, Ill, and Dallas, 1989, The Academy and College.

oratory studies may be ordered to detect toxins or electrolyte abnormalities.

Seizures

Seizures are involuntary movements or alteration in sensation, behavior, or consciousness caused by abnormal electrical activity in the brain. In young children seizures associated with fever are one of the most common neurologic disorders of childhood, affecting 3% to 5% of children. Most febrile seizures occur after 6 months of age and usually before 3 years, with increased frequency in children younger than 18 months.

The cause of febrile seizures is still uncertain. In most children, height and rapidity of temperature elevation seem to be important factors. Temperature can exceed 38.8° C (101.8° F). Seizures usually occur during temperature rise rather than after prolonged elevation. Febrile seizures may accompany upper respiratory infection, gastrointestinal infection, or otitis. Between 25% and 30% of children with simple febrile seizures have a recurrence with subsequent infections.[5]

Treatment for febrile seizures consists of ensuring the child's safety during the seizure, controlling the seizure, and reducing the temperature. Parents also need reassurance of the benign nature of febrile seizures.

Other seizure disorders have numerous and varied causes. Seizure disorders are idiopathic if the cause is unknown and organic or symptomatic if the cause is identifiable.

Table 48-12	SEIZURE MEDICATIONS		
MEDICATION	DOSAGE	METHOD	SIDE EFFECTS
Lorazepam*	0.03-0.05 mg/kg; status epilepticus, 0.1 mg/kg; has longer half-life and faster onset than diazepam	IV	Respiratory depression
Diazepam*	0.2-0.5 mg/kg	IV, intramuscular, endotracheal, rectal	Respiratory depression
Paraldehyde*	0.1-0.25 mg/kg	Usually rectal (when given rectally must be mixed with equal amounts of mineral oil); may be given IV, IM, NG	Respiratory depression
Phenytoin*	18-20 mg/kg	Slow IV push, 50 mg/min; mix only with normal saline solution; monitor heart rate and rhythm	Hypotension, respiratory depression, cardiac rhythm disturbance (prolonged QT interval)
Phenobarbital*	12-20 mg/kg; maximum dose 300 mg	Slow IV push, 50 mg/min; only in normal saline solution	Hypotension, drowsiness, respiratory depression

IV, Intravenous; *IM,* intramuscular; *NG,* nasogastric.

*Lorazepam, diazepam, and paraldehyde are used in emergency situations to treat status epilepticus. Phenytoin and phenobarbital have more long-term use in preventing recurrence.

Epilepsy is the diagnosis when seizures are recurrent with no apparent cause for the seizures. Seizure patients may exhibit a wide range of behaviors, from lip smacking and staring to violent muscular contractions or sudden loss of consciousness. Urinary and bowel incontinence also occur. Status epilepticus occurs when seizure activity is prolonged or the patient has sequential seizures without regaining consciousness between each seizure. Airway management, prevention of injury, and cessation of seizure activity with drug therapy are indicated for management of seizures (Table 48-12).

Whether the patient is admitted to the hospital or discharged home depends on the patient's history, laboratory findings, and physical findings. Children with first-time febrile seizures are usually admitted for further observation and diagnostic testing. Children with previously undiagnosed seizures are also admitted for further evaluation and anticonvulsant therapy. Those with previously diagnosed seizure disorders whose condition has stabilized are often discharged home with referral to their neurologist.

Status Epilepticus

Prolonged continuous seizure activity, or status epilepticus, may be a manifestation of anoxia, infection, trauma, ingestion, or metabolic disorder. In about half the children with status epilepticus, the cause is not identified. Sustained seizure activity produces cerebral anoxia and possible ischemic brain damage, so airway maintenance, oxygenation, and rapid termination of convulsive activity are priorities. Ensure the child's safety. Insert an oral airway to keep the airway open only when the child has not clamped down. Do not attempt insertion of the airway, tongue blade, or biteblock if the child's teeth are clenched. If the child is in severe respiratory distress or stops breathing, bag-valve-mask ventilation should be used until intubation is possible. A large-bore intravenous catheter should be inserted for administration of fluids and medication. Intravenous anticonvulsant medications are given until seizure activity ceases. Laboratory tests include CBC; electrolyte, glucose, calcium, magnesium, and BUN levels; urinalysis; and toxicology screening.

GASTROINTESTINAL AND GENITOURINARY EMERGENCIES

Dehydration

Dehydration, a common disturbance in children, occurs when total fluid output exceeds total intake, regardless of underlying cause. Dehydration can result from lack of oral intake but is more often the result of abnormal fluid losses, such as vomiting or diarrhea.

Innumerable children are brought to the ED with nausea, vomiting, diarrhea, and poor feeding. Most often the problem is viral gastroenteritis or viral syndrome, so the patient can be discharged with minimal treatment. If the child has abdominal pain, an acute abdominal condition must be ruled out, so the child should not be allowed to drink any fluid until evaluation is complete. Diagnostic tests including a CBC, electrolyte, glucose, BUN levels, and urinalysis are usually obtained. Patients whose laboratory analyses are within normal limits, those who are only mildly dehydrated, and those who are able to take fluids by mouth can be discharged. Instruct parents to give the child small amounts of clear liquids at frequent intervals (a teaspoonful at a time), progressing to the BRAT (bananas, rice, applesauce, and tea and toast) diet. Apple juice should not be used because it is hyperosmolar and may worsen diarrhea. Also instruct parents to return to their physician or the ED if the patient does not improve within 24 hours, abdominal pain increases, or the child is acting strangely in any way. Severe dehydration is treated with 20 ml/kg of intravenous crystalloid solutions.

Abdominal Pain

Other illnesses causing gastrointestinal upset or abdominal pain are infection with bacterial agents and parasites; surgical emergencies such as appendicitis, strangulated hernia, intussusception, testicular torsion, bowel obstruction; urinary tract infection; and toxic ingestion. For the most part, ED treatment of the stable patient with abdominal pain focuses on assessing the patient, including history and vital signs; deciding whether the patient can be discharged or requires hospitalization; and determining if the problem needs medical or surgical management. In general, the possibility of a surgical abdomen should be considered for any patient with abdominal pain associated with palpation or movement. Basic diagnostic tests include CBC, urinalysis, and chest and abdominal radiographs. Adolescent female patients should be asked about pregnancy before radiographs are obtained. Assume that a female of childbearing age is pregnant until proven otherwise and obtain a serum pregnancy test.

Appendicitis

Appendicitis is inflammation of the vermiform appendix or blind sac of the cecum. It is the most common condition requiring surgical intervention during childhood. Primarily an acute condition, appendicitis can progress to perforation and peritonitis without appropriate treatment. Signs and symptoms of appendicitis vary greatly but may include epigastric or lower right quadrant pain with rebound tenderness, nausea, and vomiting. The most important diagnostic test is a white blood cell count and differential. With appendicitis, total white blood cell count is usually 15,000 to 20,000 cells/ml with bands present. Fever is usually present, varying from 99.5° F to 101.3° F (37.5° to 38.5° C). If the temperature is greater than 102.2° F (39° C), viral illness or perforation is likely.

Definitive treatment for appendicitis before perforation is surgical removal of the appendix, or appendectomy. However, fluid and electrolyte imbalance should be corrected before the child goes to surgery. The child should be NPO until surgery. Prophylactic antibiotics may be started before surgery for patients with evidence of perforation. Recovery from this surgery is rapid; the child may be discharged within 24 hours when the procedure is done laparscopically or within days when the traditional technique is used.

Incarcerated Hernia

A hernia is a protrusion of a portion of an organ through an abdominal opening. Classic presentation is an asymptomatic bulge that becomes more prominent with crying, defecation, coughing, or laughing.[5] Danger from herniation arises when the organ protruding through the opening is constricted to the extent that circulation is impaired. Hernias can often be manually reduced in the ED. Giving pain medication, placing the patient in Trendelenburg's position, and applying ice to the area may assist in this process. Surgical intervention is eventually required for most patients.

Intussusception

Intussusception occurs when a proximal portion of the intestine telescopes into a more distal portion of intestine. This occurs in infancy, most often between ages 3 months and 1 year. Telescoping prevents passage of intestinal contents beyond the defect. Fecal material is unable to move beyond the obstruction. Stools contain primarily blood and mucus, resulting in the currant jelly stools characteristic of intussusception.

In most cases, initial treatment is nonsurgical hydrostatic reduction by barium enema concurrent with diagnostic testing. If this does not reduce the obstruction, surgical intervention is necessary.

Testicular Torsion

A prepubertal male with sudden onset of severe scrotal pain radiating to the abdomen may have testicular torsion. Twisting of spermatic vessels causes ischemia, swelling, and a high-lying testis. The duration of pain is usually less than 24 hours. Testicular salvage is approximately 20% with more than 12 hours of pain. Patients may complain of nausea and vomiting. Scrotal edema is present, and blood pressure may be elevated because of pain and anxiety. Fever is rarely present. If the torsion has been present less than 3 or 4 hours, manual reduction by the ED physician or urologist may be possible. If surgery is indicated, keep the patient NPO and administer analgesics as ordered. Patients with suspected testicular torsion should receive a higher priority from triage because of increased recovery with early resolution of the problem.

Other Genitourinary Problems

Other pediatric genitourinary problems seen in the ED include urinary tract infection, phimosis, dysmenorrhea, and pregnancy-related problems. Treatment for these illnesses is essentially the same as for adults.

INFECTIOUS DISEASE EMERGENCIES

Children with upper respiratory infections such as colds, sore throats, sinusitis, and otitis are often brought to the ED. For the most part they are rapidly discharged and followed by their private physicians. Some of the more serious infectious diseases are described in this section.

AIDS

Infants and children with acquired immunodeficiency syndrome (AIDS) or those infected with the human immunodeficiency virus (HIV) present to the ED with numerous physical problems requiring supportive nursing care, both physiologic and psychologic. HIV has created a whole new population of chronically ill and disabled children. The virus has been found in blood and almost all body fluids, including semen, saliva, vaginal secretions, urine, breast milk, and tears. Evidence to date indicates the virus is transmitted primarily through direct contact with blood or blood products. There is no evidence that casual contact between affected and unaffected individuals can spread the virus.

In the pediatric population, three age-groups are primarily affected. These are children exposed *in utero* to an infected mother, children who received blood products infected with the virus, and adolescents infected through high-risk behaviors. The majority of children with AIDS are younger than 2 years of age and constitute a small percentage of the total AIDS population.

Children, as do adults, have a wide range of signs and symptoms related to this infection. Most children with AIDS have recurrent bacterial and fungal infections, chronic diarrhea, chronic anemia, renal disease, cardiomyopathy, neurologic deterioration, or general failure to thrive. Infection with HIV is a multisystem problem; therefore, ED presentation can vary greatly. Diagnosis of AIDS in children is suspected on the basis of clinical presentation and the presence of risk factors associated with AIDS. Clinical presentation may be failure to thrive, chronic pneumonia, respiratory distress resulting from pneumonia, liver or spleen enlargement, oral lesions, or recurrent bacterial infections. No cure for pediatric HIV or AIDS exists. Treatment is primarily supportive, aimed at prevention of infections and complications, early recognition of complications, and support of optimal general health. Current drug therapy includes zidovudine and didanosine, which are antiretroviral agents that inhibit HIV replication. Although noncurative, these drugs minimize symptoms and may prolong life if given early in the course of HIV infection.

In the ED the child and family need support dealing with this terminal disease. Family reaction to the disease may include shock, anger, fear, or guilt. Family members should be encouraged to express their feelings. Emergency nurses should listen and provide support. The emergency nurse can play a part in family education concerning the disease. Teaching in the ED should focus on the presenting problem and discussion of resources available for follow-up care.

Bacteremia

The effects of bacterial invasion of the bloodstream may range from relatively mild symptoms of infection (bacteremia) to overwhelming, life-threatening infection (sepsis or septicemia). Bacteremia and septicemia represent the two extremes on a continuum of severity rather than disparate entities.

Bacteremia may occur in association with meningitis, cellulitis, or kidney infection. It may also occur without localized findings (occult bacteremia). Bacteremia is most common in children younger than 2 years of age and may be difficult to detect in the child less than 2 months of age. Any child younger than 2 years of age should be suspected of bacteremia when there is fever and documented infection (white blood cell count greater than 15,000 cells/ml) without an observable focus of infection. Bacteremia rarely occurs in infancy and may be especially difficult to detect at this age because infants do not always respond to infection with fever. Bacteremia should be suspected when a child has fever with malaise, poor feeding, irritability, and is not playful or easily consoled. Diagnostic workup includes CBC, blood cultures, chest radiograph, urinalysis, and complete septic workup including lumbar puncture if indicated.

In the ED the child with fever more than 101.1° F (38.4° C) may be given acetaminophen (10 to 15 mg/kg) to lower temperature. Frequently, oral antibiotics are prescribed. If the patient is discharged, careful attention should be given to the parent's ability to give medication on schedule, as well as clear directions concerning danger signs of sepsis. The child should be reevaluated within 24 to 48 hours. Bacteremia can progress to sepsis if the patient is not adequately treated.

Sepsis

Sepsis is an overwhelming, life-threatening infection of the bloodstream. Overall mortality rates of 15% to 50% have been reported, depending on infectious agent. The younger the child, the higher the risk. The child with sepsis appears very ill. A child younger than age 3 months may be afebrile. Older children often have a high fever with tachycardia, abnormal skin signs, altered mental status, and sometimes petechiae or purpura. Sepsis requires immediate assessment and intervention for shock and determination of cause of infection by laboratory analysis. CBC; electrolyte, glucose, BUN, and creatinine levels; blood cultures; prothrombin time and partial thromboplastin time; aspartate transaminase and alanine transaminase; urinalysis; and chest radiograph are recommended. Intravenous antibiotics are indicated. The patient with sepsis requires a high level of care, namely, an intensive care unit.

Meningitis

Meningitis, acute inflammation of the meninges, is a common cause of death and disability in children. Annual incidence of meningitis is 1 case per 2000 children with a peak in children 2 months to 5 years.[5] Causative organism is often bacterial, but viral meningitis also occurs. With bacterial meningitis, organisms enter the bloodstream through focal infection or by routes such as open wounds, skull fractures, and surgical procedures and spreads the infection through the subarachnoid space, causing swelling and pain. Recognition and treatment are essential to prevent death and residual damage.

Increased intracranial pressure is a major concern in meningitis. As inflammation increases, expansion within the rigid skull causes direct pressure on the brain. Narrow passageways to the ventricles are occluded and cerebrospinal fluid outflow is obstructed, producing altered sensorium.

Many children present with headache, nausea, vomiting, or poor feeding. Most children have an elevated temperature; however, infants may have normal temperature or even hypothermia. A classic sign of meningitis is nuchal rigidity, which is rarely seen in infancy. Common signs and symptoms of increased intracranial pressure may be evident, including irritability, restlessness, altered mental status, and seizures. Bulging fontanelles are a late sign. A severely ill child may be in respiratory distress, exhibit cyanosis, and have a rash or petechiae.

In the late stages, meningitis requires aggressive intervention including airway management, hyperventilation to prevent increased intracranial pressure, intravenous medication (mannitol, steroids, diuretics, antibiotics), and admission to the intensive care unit. Strict isolation is required. Seizures are treated with anticonvulsant medication until seizure activity stops. Definitive diagnosis requires a lumbar puncture and laboratory analysis of cerebrospinal fluid for protein, white cells, and Gram's stain. Other laboratory tests include serum electrolyte and glucose determinations obtained before the lumbar puncture because stress of the procedure may raise the glucose level.

Meningococcemia

Meningococcemia, caused by invasion of the bloodstream with *Neisseria meningitidis,* can occur with or without meningitis. The child with meningococcemia has fever, headache, and rash (usually maculopapular rash), petechiae, and purpura. Figure 48-7 illustrates the cutaneous effects of meningococcemia. Shock and disseminated intravascular coagulation occur very quickly. Meningococcemia can be rapidly fatal. Rapid assessment and intervention are critical. Diagnostic tests include CBC, electrolytes, glucose, and urinalysis. Lumbar puncture, blood cultures, and clotting studies are also necessary.

Encephalitis

Acute encephalitis, or inflammation of brain parenchyma, may be caused by direct viral invasion or may follow an infection such as measles. Symptoms and treatment of encephalopathy vary by cause. Associated symptoms include but are not limited to headache, fever, altered sensorium, and nuchal rigidity. Supportive measures with fluid restriction and monitoring electrolytes may be all that are required for acute encephalitis. However, herpes encephalitis is a life-threatening disease requiring aggressive intervention.

Reye's Syndrome

Reye's syndrome, encephalopathy associated with fatty infiltration in the liver, is rarely seen today. This illness develops a few days after what appears to be a mild viral illness. The cause is unknown, but genetic predisposition, use of aspirin during the viral illness, and an intrinsic toxin affecting mitochondrial metabolism have all been proposed. Symp-toms of Reye's syndrome are recurrent vomiting and altered mental status, progressing rapidly to coma. Reye's syndrome requires rapid diagnosis and aggressive, complex interventions to prevent death or devastating sequelae. Standard diagnostic tests and aspartate transaminase and alanine transaminase determinations are required, but presumptive diagnosis is initially made by elevated blood ammonia level, usually with a normal bilirubin level.

Skin Rashes

Children are brought to the ED with various rashes. Most rashes, such as neonatal acne, diaper dermatitis, and viral exanthema, are not life-threatening. Other diseases have long-term consequences and should be taken seriously. Some infectious diseases that present with a skin rash are shown in Table 48-13.

Kawasaki Disease

Kawasaki disease is acute systemic vasculitis occurring mainly in children under the age of 5 years. The acute disease is self-limiting; however, without treatment, one in five children can develop cardiac sequelae. Kawasaki disease is the leading cause of acquired heart disease in children in the United States. The etiology remains a mystery. Children present with fever and irritability. Parents should be asked about any rash or erythema. The child may be dehydrated and may have nausea and vomiting.

Treatment is geared toward prevention of complications. High-dose γ-globulin (2 g/kg) has been useful in reducing the risk of coronary artery disease. High doses of aspirin, 30 to 100 mg/kg per 24 hours, are often given simultaneously. Beyond these two treatments, treatment is largely supportive. Intravenous fluids should be given to correct dehydration.

Tuberculosis

Tuberculosis (TB) is a disease controlled in most developed countries that still remains a health hazard and leading cause of death in many parts of the world. It is caused by *Mycobacterium tuberculosis,* with the source of infection in most situations a member of the household. A steady increase in new cases has occurred during the past several years attributed, in part, due to the influx of foreign-born people and recognition of the disease in the native-born population.

Clinical manifestations of TB are extremely variable. Fever, malaise, anorexia, weight loss, or cough may be present. Coinfection with HIV is also common. Most children with pulmonary TB have noninfectious disease; therefore, they seldom require isolation. Hospitalization is seldom necessary; most children can be managed at home. Antimicrobial agents cure most cases of TB, with the limiting factor being patient compliance with drug administration. Drug therapy usually lasts 6 to 9 months. Historically, TB has been regarded with fear of infection, so it is important to

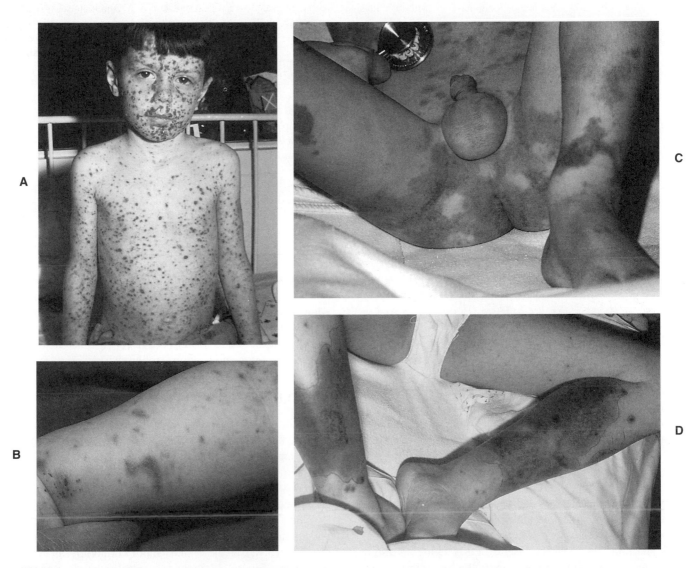

FIGURE 48-7   Meningococcemia. **A,** This child manifests the generalized purpuric and petechial rash characteristic of acute meningococcemia. **B,** Petechiae are more apparent in this closeup of an infant. Gram's stain of petechial scrapings may reveal organisms. **C** and **D,** Purpura may progress to form areas of frank cutaneous necrosis, especially in patients with DIC. (From Zitelli B, Davis H: *Atlas of pediatric physical diagnosis,* ed 3, St. Louis, 1997, Mosby.)

Table 48-13   INFECTIONS WITH SKIN RASHES

CHARACTERISTIC	MEASLES (RUBEOLA)	CHICKENPOX (VARICELLA)	SCARLET FEVER	ROSEOLA (EXANTHEMA SUBITUM)	PETECHIAL RASH (FROM MENINGITIS)
Incubation	10-11 days	10-20 days	2-4 days	10-15 days	None
Signs and symptoms	3-5 days fever, cough, coryza, toxic appearance, conjunctivitis; Koplik's spots (mucosal lesions) appear 2 days	Fever and cough, simultaneously with rash; headache; malaise	Fever for 1-2 days, sore throat, strawberry tongue, vomiting, chills, malaise	Rapid rise of high fever lasting 3-4 days in otherwise well child	May be sudden onset or preceded by fever and malaise; if sudden onset and accompanied by fever, may indicate sepsis
Exanthem (rash)	Reddish brown; begins on face, spreads downward; confluent high on body, discrete lesions in lower portions; lasts 7-10 days	Vesicles appearing in crops; trunk, scalp, face, extremities; lesions in all stages of development	Punctate, sandpaper texture; blanches on pressure; appears first in flexor areas; rash lasts 7 days	Appears discrete, rose-colored; appears after fever; begins on chest and spreads to face	Reddish purple vascular, *non-blanching* rash
Complications	Pneumonia, encephalitis, otitis media	Pneumonia, encephalitis, Reye's syndrome	Rheumatic heart disease	None	Sepsis, septic shock, long-term sequelae from increased intracranial pressure

clarify any misconceptions parents may have regarding this disease.

Lyme Disease

Lyme disease is a systemic, tickborne illness. A skin lesion, known as erythema chronicum migrans, is present in a majority of cases. Lyme disease caused by the spirochete *Borrelia burgdorferi* is carried by a tick that lives primarily on white-tailed deer and white-footed field mice. The multisystem nature and slow evolution of the illness make diagnosis difficult. In a child with suspected Lyme disease, a history of tick bite or being in a wooded area is important. The small size of the tick may prevent the patient from realizing its presence. General malaise, aching, sore throat, or fever may cause the patient to seek treatment.

Antibiotic therapy varies, depending on clinical presentation and progression of the disease. Early Lyme disease is treated with oral doxycycline, amoxicillin, or erythromycin. More serious symptoms such as Lyme carditis, neurologic manifestations, or Lyme arthritis require intravenous therapy with ceftriaxone or penicillin G. Prevention of the disease involves awareness and taking precautions before and after being in areas where the ticks are. Parents should check the child's entire body after being in a wooded area.

OTHER DISEASES WITH SKIN LESIONS
Cellulitis

An injury that breaks the skin barrier, such as insect bite, abrasion, laceration, or surgical procedure, may allow entry of organisms that cause cellulitis (e.g., *Staphyloccoccus aureus,* group A streptococci). Inflammatory response causes edema and swelling, usually without fever. Most patients are treated on an outpatient basis. Children younger than 3 years old with facial cellulitis are more likely to have bacteremia and require intravenous antimicrobial therapy.

Hair Tourniquets

Hair tourniquet syndrome is a relatively common finding in infants. The infant usually presents with excessive crying or the parent or caretaker notices redness of the extremity. It is an emergency because failure to promptly remove the hair acting as a tourniquet can lead to serious infection or even amputation.

This syndrome usually affects the toes, fingers, or external genitalia with the third toe and third finger the most commonly involved areas. Hair is more commonly associated with toes (Figure 48-8) and external genitalia, whereas threads are more often found around fingers. There is an association with older, frequently washed clothes and wearing of mittens.

Treatment includes removal with fine scissors and forceps. If unable to remove, some physicians have used depilatory agents to dissolve the hair and material. In rare incidents, surgery may be required if the thread is very deep. Usually there is no sequelae after removal.

Impetigo

Impetigo is a skin infection caused by group A streptococci. It is typically found in children younger than 6 years of age.

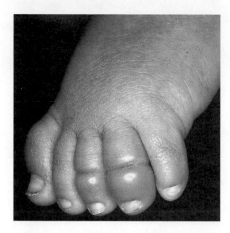

FIGURE 48-8 Hair tourniquet. The mild erythema and edema of the third and fourth toes are the result of constriction by hairs that accidentally became wrapped around them. (From Zitelli B, Davis H: *Atlas of pediatric physical diagnosis,* ed 3, St. Louis, 1997, Mosby.)

The patient has skin lesions that ooze serous fluid and crust when dry. Most cases of impetigo can be treated on an outpatient basis with oral or intramuscular antibiotics.

Scabies

Scabies is caused by the itch mite *Sarcoptes scabiei.* The major symptom of scabies is severe itching. Infestation results in eruption of wheals, papules, vesicles, and often visible threadlike burrows. Scabies is transmitted by direct contact. Application of lindane or crotamiton is the treatment for children older than 1 year. Oral antihistamines may be required to control itching. All bedding and clothing should be removed and washed.

SUMMARY

Most children seen in the ED are not critically ill or severely injured. Those who are can cause great anxiety for the emergency nurse. Developing expertise in pediatric triage, assessment, and care requires the emergency nurse to develop

---

Box 48-3 NURSING DIAGNOSES FOR THE PEDIATRIC PATIENT
Breathing pattern, Ineffective
Communication, Impaired verbal
Fluid volume, Risk for deficient
Nutrition, Imbalanced
Thermoregulation, Ineffective

a system that is comfortable, systematic, thorough, and adaptable. Box 48-3 gives just a few nursing diagnoses pertinent for the pediatric patient.

This chapter provides a brief review of medical emergencies seen in the pediatric population. In caring for pediatric illnesses, it is important to remember that the child's medical care is only one aspect of treatment. Recognition of the fundamental importance of the parent-child relationship is essential for both parent and child. This can be difficult in an emergency; however, this does not negate its importance. Showing concern and offering support for the family, including the family in the child's care whenever possible, and giving thorough, clear discharge instructions lay the groundwork for ongoing care of the child after the emergency is over.

References

1. American Academy of Pediatrics and American College of Emergency Physicians: *Advanced pediatric life support,* ed 3, Elk Grove, Ill, and Dallas, 2001, The Academy and College.
2. Barkin RM: *Pediatric emergency medicine: concepts and clinical practice,* ed 2, St. Louis, 1997, Mosby.
3. Emergency Nurses Association: *ENPC provider manual,* ed 2, Des Plaines, Ill, 1998, The Association.
4. Hazinski MF, Cummins RO, Field JM: *2000 Handbook of emergency cardiovascular care for healthcare providers,* Dallas, TX, 2000, American Heart Association.
5. Strange GR, Ahrens WR, Schafer-Meyer RW et al: *Pediatric emergency medicine: a comprehensive study guide,* New York, 1999, McGraw-Hill.
6. Wong DL: *Whaley and Wong's pediatric nursing,* ed 5, St. Louis, 1997, Mosby.

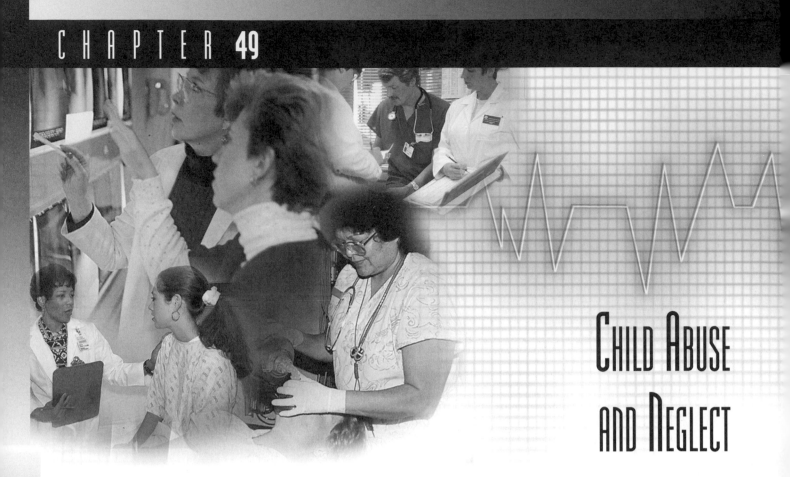

CHAPTER 49

CHILD ABUSE AND NEGLECT

KATHLEEN FOUNTAIN GRAHAM, BARBARA PIERCE

Fatalities caused by child abuse and neglect increased an estimated 11% from 1994 to 1999. Approximately 1400 children died as a result of abuse in 1999 alone. These tragic figures represent the death of four children in the United States each day. Children under the age of 5 account for four of the five deaths, with those less than 2 years accounting for two of the five deaths.[12] Actual deaths may be even higher—several researchers suggest that deaths related to maltreatment are under-reported by as much as 60%.[5,10,12]

In Chicago a 35-year-old mother kicks and throws her 16-month-old baby out a window because he would not stop crying; an Alabama couple shackles their twin daughters above the knees and locks them in a room to live in their own excrement; a Detroit drug addict sells her son to settle a $1000 crack cocaine debt; a trusted priest is sentenced to more than 30 years for sexually abusing children during his reign as youth leader; in California a teenage girl is abducted from her home and later found raped, beaten, and dead; a 4-year-old is beaten to death by her father while a neighbor reports she had to walk to another part of the house and turn up the television volume to drown out the child's screams; a 3-year-old raped by a trusted family friend is left infected with *Neisseria gonorrhoeae* and human immunodeficiency virus (HIV); and in South Carolina, the drowning of two young boys at the hand of their mother horrifies the nation. Our country is in a state of national emergency.

Child abuse and neglect is a burden to society in many ways. Abused children are more likely to develop alcoholism, abuse drugs, and suffer from depression. Tragically, abused children often grow up to be abusive adults. There is also a significant financial burden. Annual direct costs related to child abuse exceed $24 billion, whereas annual indirect costs approach $70 billion.[13] Direct costs include hospitalization, the child welfare system, and the judicial system; indirect costs encompass special education, juvenile delinquency, and adult criminality.

Child abuse and neglect are more prevalent today than ever before. In 1999 more than 3.2 million incidents of suspected child abuse and neglect were reported to child protection services, with nearly half the victims younger than age 1 year.[11,13] Reports of violence against children have almost tripled since 1976. The National Clearinghouse on Child Abuse and Neglect estimates that 9 of 10 children are maltreated by parents or family friends in some manner. The most common pattern of abuse is neglect, usually perpetrated by the female parent, whereas physical and sexual abuse is most often inflicted by a male acting alone.[13]

NEGLECT

The lack of visible bruises or broken bones belies the fact that ongoing child neglect is a silent, serious attack on children that can leave lasting mental and physical problems (Table 49-1). Neglect, defined as intentional or unintentional omission of needed care and support, may appear to the emergency nurse as a child who is unkempt, left unattended,

Table 49-1	TYPES OF CHILD NEGLECT
TYPE	**DESCRIPTION**
Medical	Caregiver fails to provide medical treatment, immunizations, recommended surgery, or other interventions necessary in a serious health problem. Often occurs when parent's religious beliefs conflict with the medical community. Issue is often resolved in court.
Physical	Failure to protect from harm or danger; failure to provide basic physical needs such as food, clothing, and shelter. Most widely recognized and reported type of neglect.
Emotional	Difficult to recognize and diagnose because of lack of physical evidence. Occurs in the home, unobserved by professionals; child is often too young to speak out. Extreme forms of emotional abuse can lead to physical illness, failure to thrive, and death. Definition of emotional abuse includes inability to meet the child's emotional needs; however, there is no universal agreement on what those needs are. Emotional abuse is often typified by child behaviors such as depression, habit disorders (sucking, biting, rocking, enuresis), conduct and learning disorders such as antisocial behaviors (e.g., cruelty).
Educational	Caregivers fail to comply with state requirements for schooling and school attendance. Can also be parental resistance to essential specialized education programs.
Mental health	Similar to medical neglect in that parent refuses to comply with recommended corrective or therapeutic measures in cases in which the child has serious emotional or behavioral problems.

Modified from Myers JB, Hendrix CT, Berliner L et al: *The American Professional Society on the Abuse of Children handbook on child maltreatment,* ed 2, Westlake Village, Calif, 1997, The Society.

Box 49-1	POTENTIAL INDICATORS OF CHILD NEGLECT
BEHAVIORAL	**PHYSICAL**
Begs or steals food	Height and weight significantly below normal for age level
Falls asleep in school, lethargic	Inappropriate clothing for weather
Poor school attendance, frequent tardiness	Poor hygiene, including lice, body odor, scaly skin
Chronic hunger	Child abandoned and left with inadequate supervision
Dull, apathetic appearance	Untreated illness or injury
Runs away from home	Lack of safe, warm, and sanitary shelter
Reports no caregiver in the home	Lack of necessary medical and dental care
Assumes adult responsibilities	

From *For kids sake: a child abuse prevention and reporting kit,* rev ed, Oklahoma City, 1992, Oklahoma State Department of Health.

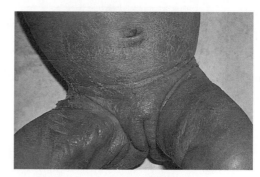

FIGURE 49-1   Neglect. An infant with severe failure to thrive has a badly neglected case of irritant diaper dermatitis. (From Zitelli BJ, Davis HW: *Atlas of pediatric physical diagnosis,* ed 3, St. Louis, 1997, Mosby.)

Failure to Thrive

Failure to thrive is defined as the condition in children younger than age 5 years whose growth persistently and significantly deviates from norms for age and sex based on national growth charts. Measurements for height, weight, and head circumference are plotted against normal childhood growth patterns. Failure to thrive children generally fall below average in all three areas. The cause of failure to thrive may be medical (e.g., *Giardia* organism infection, celiac disease, lead poisoning, malabsorption) or psychosocial.

Psychosocial causes are often linked to and reported as child neglect. Maladaptive parenting practices, chronic family illnesses, parental depression, and substance abuse among caregivers are recognized causes. Failure to thrive does not necessarily imply abuse or neglect but does require aggressive treatment and follow-up by appropriate health care professionals. Untreated, failure to thrive can lead to developmental and behavioral difficulties secondary to nutritional deprivation of the nervous system and other sys-

not dressed appropriately for the weather, malnourished, or diagnosed with "failure to thrive." Identification of neglect must recognize parental attempts to provide essentials despite limited resources. Failure to provide adequate physical protection, nutrition, or health care is generally considered neglect, but neglect can also include lack of human contact and love. Currently, 53.5% of all abuse cases involve neglect, with 44% of the deaths in 1999 attributed to neglect.[9,13] Recognizing neglect is often difficult in the emergency department (ED) because of limited, one-time contact with most patients. However, the emergency nurse should be alert for behaviors that suggest neglect (Box 49-1). Be aware that neglect can be physical, emotional, or educational. Figure 49-1 shows a case of neglect.

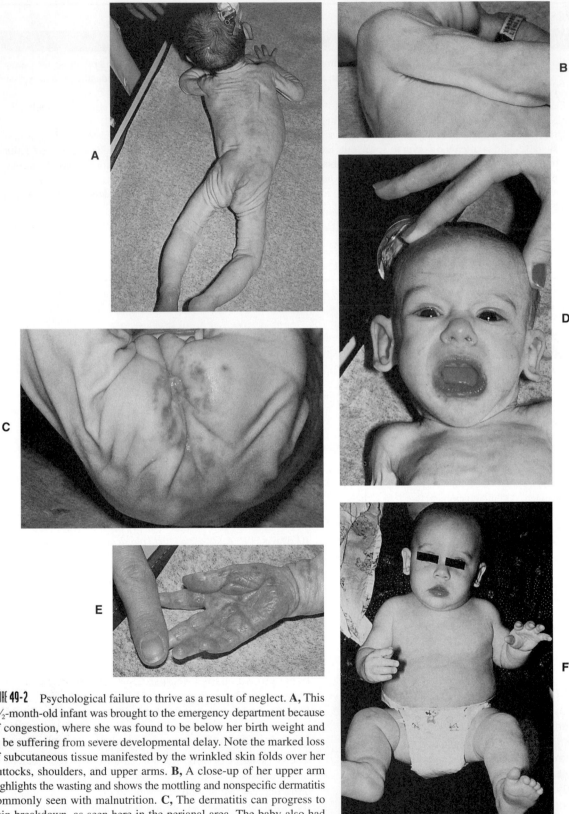

FIGURE **49-2**   Psychological failure to thrive as a result of neglect. **A,** This 4½-month-old infant was brought to the emergency department because of congestion, where she was found to be below her birth weight and to be suffering from severe developmental delay. Note the marked loss of subcutaneous tissue manifested by the wrinkled skin folds over her buttocks, shoulders, and upper arms. **B,** A close-up of her upper arm highlights the wasting and shows the mottling and nonspecific dermatitis commonly seen with malnutrition. **C,** The dermatitis can progress to skin breakdown, as seen here in the perianal area. The baby also had manifestations of multiple vitamin deficiencies, including (**D**) stomatitis; glossitis; and perioral, perinasal, and periorbital dermatitis (riboflavin, niacin, and vitamin B₆ deficiencies respectively); as well as (**E**) sharply demarcated palmar erythema with thinning of the skin (niacin deficiency). **F,** Three and a half months after removal from the home, she was well nourished and had caught up developmentally.

tems. A multidisciplinary approach in treating failure to thrive has the best opportunity for success. Family assessment, nutritional counseling, medical intervention, and family support are needed to correct failure to thrive. Table 49-2 describes medical evaluation for suspected neglect and failure to thrive. Figure 49-2 illustrates a case of failure to thrive and the benefits of intervention.

PHYSICAL ABUSE

Physical abuse is nonaccidental injury to a child younger than age 18 years by a parent or caregiver. Child abuse is typically a pattern of behavior repeated over time but it can also be a single attack. The condition is characterized by injury, torture, maiming, or use of unreasonable force. Abuse may result from harsh discipline or severe punishment. Box 49-2 identifies behavioral and physical indicators found in physical abuse. Children rarely tell anyone about physical abuse because of feelings of shame or confusion. The emergency nurse should be cognizant of reasons for failure to communicate potential abuse situations (Box 49-3).[1]

Specific Abuse Patterns

Children can experience a multitude of insults and injuries at the hands of primary caregivers or other adults. Two patterns seen with increasing frequency are shaken baby syndrome and Munchausen syndrome by proxy.

Shaken baby syndrome (SBS) occurs when infants are shaken vigorously. According to the American Academy of Pediatrics, SBS is a violent form of abuse that occurs in infants younger than 2 years but can involve children as old as 5 years.[4,11] Acceleration-deceleration of the head creates a triad of injuries: subdural hemorrhage (Figure 49-3), retinal hemorrhage (Figure 49-4), and altered level of consciousness. There are often no external signs of trauma. Babies shaken into unconsciousness are often put to bed in hopes the injuries will resolve; therefore, the window for therapeutic intervention is lost. The spectrum of symptoms may vary from vomiting and irritability in mild shakings to unconsciousness, convulsions, and even death in severe shakings. To rule out SBS, health care providers should look for any external signs of injuries such as bruises. A fundoscopic examination of the pupils should be performed to look for retinal hemorrhages. Pupil dilation may be required in some patients. A computed tomography scan should be obtained to identify brain hemorrhages. Magnetic resonance imaging, when available, is extremely helpful for detection of subdural hematoma. A skeletal survey should be obtained to rule out fractures, especially in the area of the ribs.

Table 49-2	MEDICAL EVALUATION OF SUSPECTED NEGLECT AND FAILURE TO THRIVE	
COMPONENT	**DESCRIPTION**
History	Lack of parental concern about physical illness, delayed development, or failure to thrive
	Bizarre dietary or feeding history
	Isolated or depressed parent
	Financial or social crisis
	Alcohol or drug abuse in parent
	Any evidence of organic failure to thrive
	Possible physical abuse
Physical examination	Lack of subcutaneous tissue
	Developmental delay
	Evidence of organic disease
	Signs of physical abuse
Laboratory tests	Complete blood cell count
	Renal assessment, including measurement of electrolytes and urinalysis
	Does baby gain weight when adequate intake of a regular diet is established?

Courtesy Helen Britton, MD, Primary Children's Medical Center, Salt Lake City, Utah.

Box 49-2 PHYSICAL ABUSE FINDINGS

BEHAVIORAL FINDINGS

Requests or feels deserving of punishment
Afraid to go home, or requests to stay in school or daycare
Overly shy, tends to avoid physical contact with adults, especially parents
Displays behavioral extremes (withdrawal or aggressiveness)
Cries excessively or sits and stares
Reports injury by parent or caretaker
Gives unbelievable explanations for injuries
Clings to health care worker rather than parent

PHYSICAL FINDINGS

Unexplained bruises or welts found most frequent, usually on face, torso, buttocks, back, or thighs; can reflect shape of object used (e.g., electric cord, hand, belt buckle); may be in various stages of healing
Unexplained burns often on palms, soles of feet, buttocks, or back; can reflect pattern of cigarette burn, electrical appliance, or rope burn
Unexplained fractures or dislocation involving skull, ribs, and bones around joints; may include multiple fractures or spiral fractures
Other unexplained injuries such as lacerations, abrasions, human bite, or pinch marks; loss of hair or bald patches; retinal hemorrhages; abdominal injuries

Modified from *For kids sake: a child abuse prevention and reporting kit*, rev ed, Oklahoma City, 1992, Oklahoma State Department of Health.

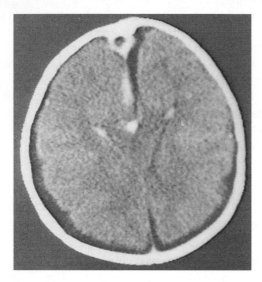

FIGURE **49-3**   Subdural hematoma secondary to shaken baby syndrome. (From Zitelli BJ, Davis HW: *Atlas of pediatric physical diagnosis,* ed 3, St. Louis, 1997, Mosby. Courtesy the division of Neuroradiology, University Health Center of Pittsburgh.)

Munchausen syndrome by proxy (MSP) is a complex condition in which a caretaker knowingly keeps a child ill for secondary gain or attention through the child's illness. The child is subjected to illnesses perpetuated by caregivers who may give ipecac or other drugs, introduce pathogens, or otherwise contribute to a child's illness. Caretakers also falsify medical histories and symptoms. Often undetected by caregivers, MSP can lead to death in extreme cases.

One difficulty in identifying abuse is the number of conditions that mimic physical abuse. Physiologic or pathologic causes for physical findings should always be considered.[2]

- Sudden infant death syndrome can appear as child abuse because of pooling of blood, mottling, and other discoloration associated with death. The definitive cause of death should be determined by autopsy.
- Clotting disorders, such as Wiskott-Aldrich syndrome, hemophilia, and thrombocytopenia purpura, cause bruises in varying stages of healing.

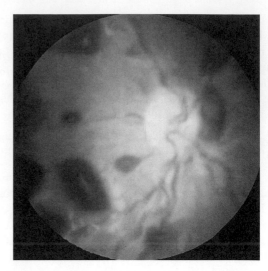

FIGURE **49-4**   Retinal hemorrhages secondary to shaken baby syndrome. (From Zitelli BJ, Davis HW: *Atlas of pediatric physical diagnosis,* ed 3, St. Louis, 1997, Mosby. Courtesy Dr. Stephen Ludwig, Children's Hospital of Philadelphia.)

- Mongolian spots are birthmarks found predominantly in Spanish Americans, southeast Asians, southern Europeans, Native American Indians, or anyone with dark pigmentation. Mongolian spots do not change coloration or size over time and have a grayer appearance than bruises.
- Multiple petechiae and purpura of the face can occur when vigorous crying, retching, or coughing increases vena cava pressure. Unlike intentional choking, there are no marks around the neck.
- Bullous impetigo may appear as an infected wound or burn. This condition may reflect neglect if caregivers are apathetic about care of lesions.
- Cultural or ethnic practices such as coining or cupping are used to treat pain, fever, or poor appetite. Coining—rubbing a coin over bony prominences—causes a striated "pseudoburn." Cupping (warming a cup, spoon, or shot glass in oil and then placing it on the neck, back, or ribs) can result in a petechial or purpuric rash over the affected area.
- Osteogenesis imperfecta is an inherited disease that can result in multiple fractures with minimal trauma and causes a tendency to bleed easily.

Interviewing Caregivers

When abuse is suspected, the caregiver should be carefully interviewed to obtain as much information as possible. Make every effort to establish rapport, conveying genuine concern and understanding. A nonjudgmental, noncritical attitude is essential. Judgmental attitudes hinder communication and limit information. Tactfully determine issues of concern to the caretaker. The person may feel desperate and inadequate. Use reflective statements, such as "You sound really frustrated right now." Do not agree or condone, merely listen and reflect, using critical listening skills.

Parents often feel intense neediness and helplessness about their inability to meet their own needs, so a child who is needy, demanding, or misbehaves proves extremely stressful. Parents may also feel intensely negative about themselves and dwell on their own worthlessness, helplessness, and incompetence. Support the caregiver but do not convey pity. Emphasize anything positive; for example, the parent sought help. Reinforce the decision to seek help; normal behavior is to withdraw without seeking help. Help parents draw on personal strengths. Helplessness and worthlessness are self-destructive, so effort should be made to draw parents away from negative feelings. Parents may be agitated, embarrassed, or tearful, so work to make them feel valued as individuals.

Parents are often distressed because of isolation and lack of a social network. Discuss places for support such as church, family, and friends. Talk about stressors the person is experiencing, including economic worries, unemployment, poverty, illness, divorce, and single-parenting concerns.

Allegations of Abuse

Allegations of child abuse sometimes arise during separation, divorce, and child custody proceedings. Perceptions exist that false allegations can be made during divorce or custody proceedings in an attempt to place one parent in a "favored" position for child custody. False accusations are sometimes made; however, all allegations of abuse or neglect during divorce proceedings deserve serious consideration because of the increased risk for abuse during this time.

Sexual allegations in divorce[11] syndrome occurs when allegations of sexual abuse arise during predivorce or postdivorce periods. A higher index of suspicion for abuse and neglect is required with divorcing families because families are experiencing increased stress and are dysfunctional as a result of the divorce process. Separation of parents increases the opportunity for sexual and physical victimization but can also provide an opportunity for a child to disclose that abuse has taken place if the abuser is out of the home. Risk for extra-familial abuse is higher because of changes in caregivers or presence of a nonbiologic caregiver in the home.

Reporting Abuse

When suspicion of nonaccidental trauma or sexual abuse is raised, appropriate agencies must be notified immediately. Each state defines child abuse and neglect differently; however, the ultimate goal, regardless of geographic location, is prevention of further injury through prompt intervention. If child endangerment is a concern, the child should be taken into protective custody. State statutes regarding protective custody vary, so become familiar with local requirements. Such statutes now exist in all 50 states. These statutes designate specific individuals (i.e., law enforcement, physicians, health care professionals, and educators) who must report suspected child abuse and neglect. State reporting laws grant immunity for good-faith reporting. In most states

liability exists only if the reporter knows the allegations are false or the individual acted with malicious purpose.

Reasonable judgment should be exercised when disclosing to caregivers that police agencies or child protective services have been contacted. Avoid inflammatory statements when relaying information to caregivers. When it is near arrival time for outside agencies, simply state the legal responsibility to report suspicions.

Treatment

Care of injury is the primary medical concern. After immediate physical needs are resolved, further assessment is then initiated. Query the child and caregivers, avoiding judgments of possible perpetrators or reasons the injury occurred. Health care providers must remember that investigation of child abuse allegations are the responsibility of police or the appropriate division of family services. Emergency nurses who suspect child abuse or neglect must report specific concerns and the reasons for those concerns.

Reassure the child and caregiver that you are there to help. Establish trust, allay fears, and lay groundwork for expression of concerns. Give the child some degree of control by providing choices. "Which color gown do you want—blue or green?" "May I listen to your heart, or do you want to listen to it first?" Be clear and explain what you are doing. Be honest; if something will hurt, say so.

Obtain a detailed history, paying close attention to the sequence of events. Is the history consistent with the child's age and nature of injury? Interview the child and parent(s) separately if the child is old enough to talk. Is the parent at high risk for abuse—isolated, abused as a child, low self-esteem? Is the child at high risk for abuse—difficult child, difficult developmental age, premature infant? Is the family experiencing a crisis—financial, social? Are other children at home at risk for abuse? Is alcohol or drug abuse present?

Physical Examination

Identify and document all injuries, old and new, comparing historical information to clinical evidence. Measure, draw, and describe location, color, induration, and scarring. Assess for limited range of motion, which may indicate old fractures. Look for pattern injuries such as cigarette burns (Figure 49-5), strap marks (Figure 49-6), electric cord marks (Figure 49-7), or spiral femur fractures in a nonambulatory child. Examine for imprint marks (Figure 49-8), bruising on the buttocks (Figure 49-9), and inflicted scald burns (Figure 49-10). Downturned mark at the corners of the mouth occur when the child has been gagged.[8] Measure height, weight, and head circumference and compare the measurements to standard growth charts. Assess developmental level of function. An ocular and funduscopic examination is required to identify retinal hemorrhages. Skeletal surveys are obtained on children younger than age 2 years to rule out existing or healed fractures. Prothrombin time, partial thromboplastin time, factor XIII, fibrinogen level, platelet count, and bleeding time results are recommended to rule out existing blood dyscrasia.

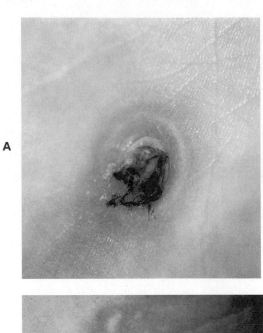

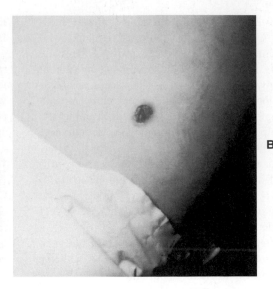

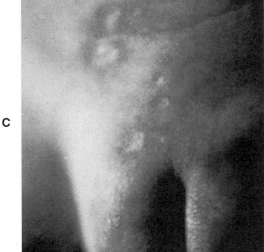

FIGURE 49-5   Cigarette burns. **A,** This sharply circumscribed burn was inflicted through the child's sock. The burn is perfectly circular with a blistered rim and a full-thickness punched-out center to which charred fabric adheres. The configuration did not fit the history that he had accidentally stepped on a cigarette. **B,** This older burn has begun to granulate. **C,** Full-thickness, punched-out scars are characteristic of healed cigarette burns. ((From Zitelli BJ, Davis HW: *Atlas of pediatric physical diagnosis,* ed 3, St. Louis, 1997, Mosby. **A,** Courtesy Dr. David Evanko, Butler, PA; **C,** Courtesy Dr. Marc Rowe, Children's Hospital of Pittsburgh.)

SEXUAL ABUSE

Child sexual abuse, involvement of children in sexual activities that violate social taboos, is usually done for gratification or profit of a significantly older person. Children do not understand these acts and are not able to give informed consent. Types of sexual abuse include, but are not limited to, fondling, digital manipulation, exhibitionism, pornography, and actual or attempted oral, vaginal, or anal intercourse. According to child protective services, more than 103,000 reports in 1998 were indicated for sexual abuse.[13] Nine percent of the confirmed cases of abuse in 1999 were sexual abuse.[11] Unfortunately, the definition of child sexual abuse varies from state to state and there is no national reporting system, so determination of actual incidence and prevalence rates is difficult.

The primary portal of entry into the health care system for children with sexual abuse is the ED. One study showed 46% of children with suspected sexual abuse were first evaluated in the ED. Without appropriate intervention there is a 50% chance of further abuse and a 10% chance for death. Physicians historically hesitate to become involved because they lack confidence in the medical examination, fear testifying in court, and are uncomfortable handling social problems that accompany a diagnosis of sexual abuse. However, legal and social systems depend heavily on medical examination to provide evidence that can withstand intense scrutiny when used to protect children from further abuse and prosecute the offender. Consequently, emergency care professionals must recognize sexual abuse and be skilled in examinations with medical and forensic strength. Screening and treatment protocols specifically addressing child sexual abuse are recommended for all EDs.

Clinical Presentation

Most children are brought to the ED by their mothers for evaluation of complaints directly related to the anogenital region such as discharge, bleeding, pain, swelling, dysuria, or difficulty stooling and nonspecific symptoms such as

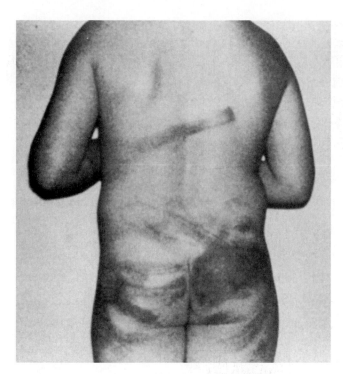

FIGURE **49-6**   Injuries from strap marks. (From Rosen PR, Barkin RM, Hockberger RS et al: *Emergency medicine: concepts and clinical practice*, ed 4, St. Louis, 1998, Mosby. Courtesy J. Brummitt, MD, Alberta Children's Hospital.)

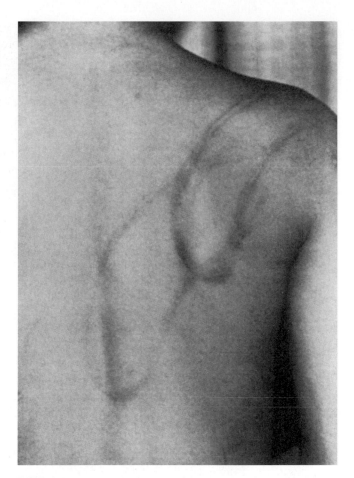

FIGURE **49-7**   Bruising caused by beating with a looped cord. (From Rosen PR, Barkin RM, Hockberger RS et al: *Emergency medicine: concepts and clinical practice*, ed 4, St. Louis, 1998, Mosby. Courtesy J. Brummitt, MD, Alberta Children's Hospital.)

headache, abdominal pain, or fatigue. Patients may present with sexually transmitted diseases such as genital herpes (Figure 49-11) and genital warts (Figure 49-12). Behavioral symptoms such as excessive masturbation, depression, inappropriate sexual expression (verbal or physical), suicidal gestures, delinquency, fearfulness, anxiety, decline in school performance, sleep disturbances, or drug and alcohol abuse may also be identified. The majority of pedophiles molest boys; however, most reported victims are girls. Male victims abused by males may be reluctant to report sexual abuse because of fear of being labeled a homosexual. Most children are sexually molested by individuals they know—a family member or close family friend. In most cases abuse has been ongoing for many years.

Urgency for medical evaluation depends on timing of the last abuse episode and presenting symptoms. Immediate examination is required if abuse occurred within 72 hours or there is bleeding, pain, or discharge. Evidence may still be present, so specimens for a rape kit are collected for law enforcement officials. Genital examination may be deferred when there is no history of acute trauma and the child is asymptomatic and considered safe. A general physical examination should be performed before patient discharge to ensure that no acute problems exist.

Emergency personnel should ascertain safety of the child and of the home environment and treat current conditions (e.g., pelvic inflammatory disease, sexually transmitted diseases [STDs]). Prophylaxis against pregnancy should be given for the pubescent female. Other responsibilities include emotional support, reporting suspected abuse to child protection authorities (including law enforcement), and involving the hospital-based child protection team or medical social worker.[10]

The most important component of sexual abuse evaluation is obtaining the patient history.[4] Physical findings or behavioral indicators rarely stand alone; they are most valuable in supporting the history given by the child.[10] The type and extent of interview are contingent on many factors. If a multidisciplinary forensic interviewing team is available, emergency health care providers should collect just enough information to complete the medical examination and make recommendations. When a team is not available, a social worker may be helpful in coordinating care. History taking requires a quiet, child-friendly environment. A health care professional should begin by interviewing the adult who accompanied the child—without the child present. A careful, comprehensive medical history should document previous traumas to the anogenital area and attempt to gain an understanding of the adult's perception and emotional response to what has occurred.

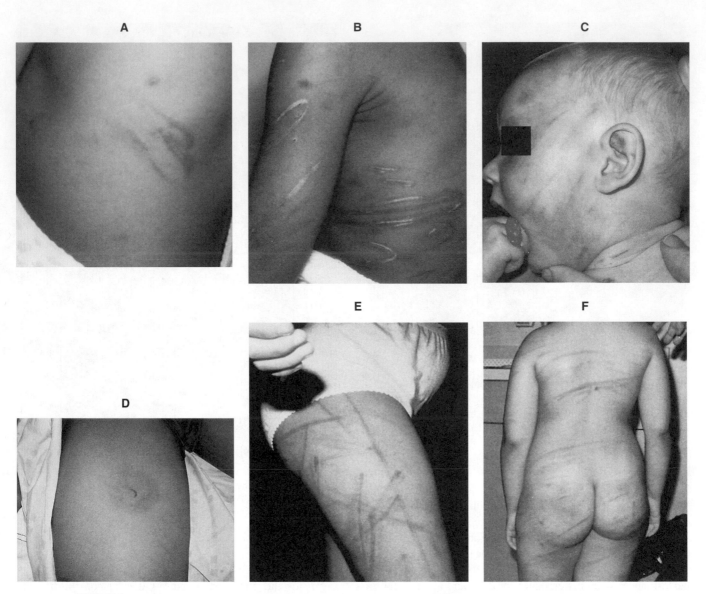

FIGURE 49-8   Imprint marks reflecting the weapons used to inflict them. **A,** Fresh looped-cord marks. **B,** Hypopigmented and hyperpigmented scars that were the result of beatings with a looped electrical cord. **C,** The characteristic pattern of parallel lines that results from blows with a belt. **D,** This contusion in the configuration of a closed horseshoe with a central linear abrasion was inflicted with a belt buckle. **E,** The red linear contusions on this child's thigh were the result of repeated blows with a switch. **F,** These acute linear contusions over the back and buttocks were inflicted with a belt and a switch. (From Zitelli BJ, Davis HW: *Atlas of pediatric physical diagnosis,* ed 3, St. Louis, 1997, Mosby.)

Although children may not exhibit external trauma, a mental health emergency may develop because victim and family are in a state of crisis.[10] Ideally the child and caregivers should be interviewed separately. Obtaining a child's statement requires an interviewer who is sensitive, nonjudgmental, nonthreatening, and trained in forensic interviewing of children. Interviewers must respond to the child's developmental and cognitive level and ask questions accordingly, using the child's terminology for body parts. Allow time for the child to ask questions. General questions should include inquiries about the caregiver, where the child lives, sleeping arrangements, school habits, friends, names for body parts, and primary care provider. Focus on specific questions by addressing hurtful touches, pain, bleeding, or other "ouches."[10] Health care professionals should not be overzealous; however, interviewers should attempt to determine what abuse occurred, who was involved, when the last abuse occurred, and where it occurred. If the child becomes uncomfortable at any time, stop the interview. Children should not be further traumatized in an attempt to collect history. Always close the interview with praise for the child and reassurance that he or she has done nothing wrong and is not at fault for someone else's actions.

G

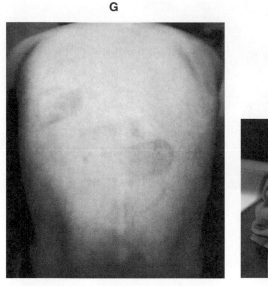

H

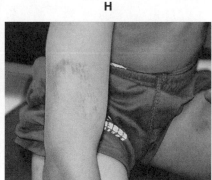

I

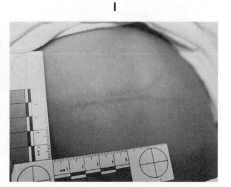

J

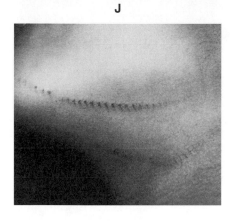

FIGURE 49-8 cont'd   Imprint marks reflecting the weapons used to inflict them. **G,** This boy was hit with a slipper with such force that the imprint of the heel is evident. **H,** The heel prints of a running shoe left on this boy's arm and thigh were distinct enough to enable identification of his abuser. **I,** This girl was hit forcefully with a spatula. **J,** This boy was struck with a chain, leaving a clear imprint of the links. (From Zitelli BJ, Davis HW: *Atlas of pediatric physical diagnosis,* ed 3, St. Louis, 1997, Mosby.)

Physical Examination

Health care providers must be confident in their ability to correctly identify anatomy and detect acute injuries, non-specific findings, scars, and healed tissue of genital trauma.[8] Physical findings in the genital area are communicated using the face of a clock. The clitoris is always at 12 o'clock with the posterior fourchette at 6 o'clock. The area of the anus closest to the posterior fourchette is always at 12 o'clock. Tanner staging determines a child's outward sexual development and helps communicate level of sexual maturity (Box 49-4). The effect of estrogen on female genitalia is described by Huffman stages (Table 49-3).[8]

Preparing the child for medical evaluation is extremely important (Table 49-4). Give the child lots of decisions to make, such as what color of gown to wear, who he or she wants in the examination room, and if he or she wants to sit on the right or left side of the table. Always tell the truth and promise only what you can control. While the child is fully clothed, explain the purpose of the examination. Most experts in the field use a colposcope, which allows magnification of the genital area up to 25 times, serves as an excellent light source, and is capable of photographing physical evi-

dence. A colposcope can be frightening to a small child and should be fully explained before use. Demonstrate the colposcope, saline, and culture swabs. Use this time to assess the developmental, behavioral, and emotional status of the child. Allow the child as much control as possible. Let the child take pictures or hold swabs.

When the child appears comfortable, begin with a general head-to-toe examination to de-emphasize the anogenital examination and look for other medical conditions. In males the penis, testes, and scrotum are examined in the standing position. Look for urethral discharge, bleeding, swelling, bruising, or bite marks. Females are placed in the supine frog-leg position (Figure 49-13) on a pelvic table, flat examination table, or mother's lap. With legs open, identify external genitalia and assess Tanner stage of development. Assess for ecchymoses, bleeding, lacerations, or abrasion. Use gloved hands to grasp the labia majora with thumb and forefinger, and apply gentle traction in a lateral, downward, and outward motion (toward the examiner). Gentle traction can best be explained as "opening double doors so we can look where you go pee-pee and make sure everything is okay." A normal hymen can exist in many shapes and forms: crescentic, annular, septated, redundant, cribriform, or

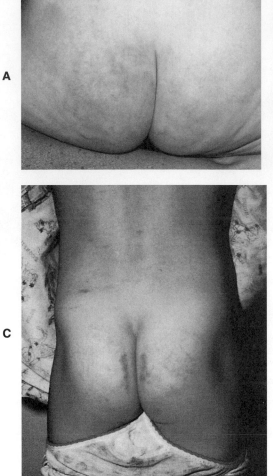

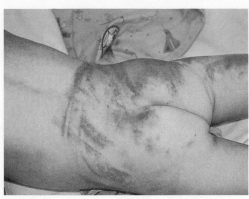

FIGURE **49-9** Buttock bruises. **A,** At first glance, this toddler appeared to have a diaper rash; on closer inspection, the lesions were found to be petechiae produced by a severe spanking. **B,** The severe contusions of the buttocks and lower back seen in this child were inflicted by hand, hairbrush, and belt. **C,** A linear pattern of petechial hemorrhages is seen on either side of the gluteal cleft in this boy who was subjected to repeated rapid-fire blows across the gluteal crease. (From Zitelli BJ, Davis HW: *Atlas of pediatric physical diagnosis,* ed 3, St. Louis, 1997, Mosby.)

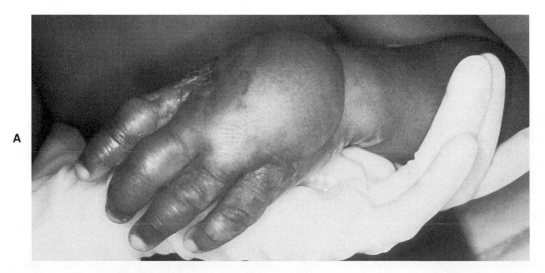

FIGURE **49-10** Inflicted scalds. **A,** This child suffered severe second-degree dip burns on both hands and wrists. (From Zitelli BJ, Davis HW: *Atlas of pediatric physical diagnosis,* ed 3, St. Louis, 1997, Mosby.)

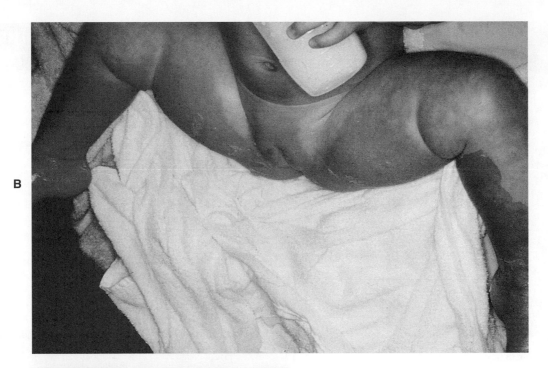

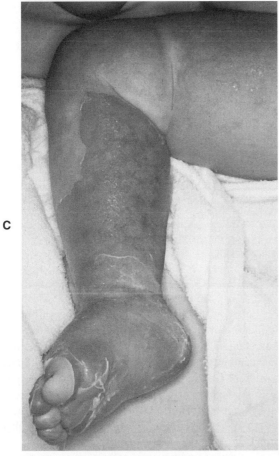

FIGURE 49-10 cont'd   Inflicted scalds. **B,** Patient seen 2 days after receiving dip burns to the lower extremities and perineum. **C,** Close-up of severe second-degree burns of the foot and lower leg. (From Zitelli BJ, Davis HW: *Atlas of pediatric physical diagnosis,* ed 3, St. Louis, 1997, Mosby.)

rarely imperforate. If the hymen does not visualize well, saline solution may be squirted on the hymen, and then a moist Dacron swab is used to tease the hymenal edge up for better view. If the edge is still difficult to visualize, place the child in the knee-chest position. The knee-chest position is often the position in which abuse occurs and may be very uncomfortable for the child. The knee-chest position uses gravity to help redundant hymenal tissue fall downward for inspection. Assess for loss of tissue, lesions, transections, tears, notches, or bumps (Table 49-5). Look for discharge or signs of foreign body. Table 49-6 depicts conditions that can be mistaken for sexual abuse. Speculum examination is not

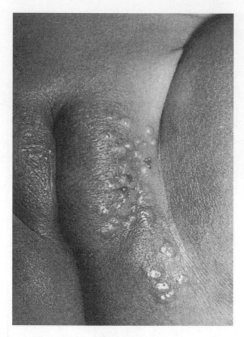

FIGURE **49-11**   Herpes genitalis in a prepubertal girl. (From Barkin RM: *Pediatric emergency medicine: concepts and clinical practice,* ed 2, St. Louis, 1997, Mosby. Courtesy N. Esterly, MD)

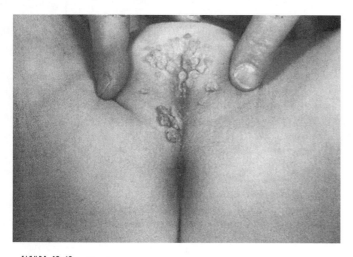

FIGURE **49-12**   Condyloma acuminata in a prepubertal girl. (From Barkin RM: *Pediatric emergency medicine: concepts and clinical practice,* ed 2, St. Louis, 1997, Mosby. Courtesy N. Esterly, MD)

Box 49-4   SECONDARY SEX CHARACTERISTICS (TANNER STAGES)

BREAST DEVELOPMENT

Stage I	Preadolescent; elevation of papilla only
Stage II	Breast and papilla elevated as small mound; areolar diameter increased
Stage III	Breast and areola enlarged; no contour separation
Stage IV	Areola and papilla form secondary mound
Stage V	Mature; nipple projects; areolar part of general breast contour

NOTE: Stages IV and V may not be distinct in some patients.

GENITAL DEVELOPMENT (MALE)

Stage I	Penis, testes, and scrotum preadolescent
Stage II	Enlargement of scrotum and testes, texture alteration; scrotal sac reddens; penis usually does not enlarge
Stage III	Further growth of testes and scrotum; penis enlarges and becomes longer
Stage IV	Continued growth of testes and scrotum; scrotum becomes darker; penis becomes longer; glans and breadth increase in size
Stage V	Genitalia adult in size and shape

PUBIC HAIR (MALE AND FEMALE)

Stage I	None; preadolescent
Stage II	Sparse growth of long, slightly pigmented downy hair, straight or only slightly curled, chiefly at base of penis or along labia
Stage III	Considerably darker, coarser and more curled; hair spreads sparsely over junction of pubes
Stage IV	Hair resembles adult in type; distribution still considerably smaller than in adult. No spread to medial surface of thighs
Stage V	Adult in quantity and type with distribution of the horizontal pattern
Stage VI	Spread up linea alba: "male escutcheon"

Modified from Tanner JM: *Growth at adolescence,* ed 2, 1962, Blackwell Scientific Publications.

---

required for the prepubertal child unless there is vaginal bleeding, laceration requiring suturing, or strong suspicion of a foreign body. The child should be sedated if such examination is required.

Multiple studies have shown that a high percentage of children with documented sexual abuse have no physical findings.[3] For example, oral-genital contact and fondling do not cause physical trauma. The anus is made to allow large objects to easily pass with care and lubrication, so signs of abuse may not be evident. Physical findings are usually nonspecific and require a good history to determine significance. Legal and social systems are often unwilling to protect children unless evidence exists of physical trauma.

Anorectal examination is performed with the child in a lateral decubitus position. Observe for rugae symmetry of verge tissue. Gently separate the buttocks and inspect for tears, fissures, bruising, or abrasions and sphincter tone. Holding traction can prevent blood flow from the anus, resulting in venous pooling, which can be mistaken for bruising.

Explain actions with a soft, reassuring voice throughout the examination to keep children informed and to decrease anxiety. Remind children that they are in charge, so if anything hurts, the examiner will stop and together they will decide a different way to do things. When the examination is over, reassure them that their "bottom is okay," and then give them a chance to ask questions.

Table 49-3	HUFFMAN STAGES
STAGE	DESCRIPTION
Stage 1 (0 to 2 months)	Postneonatal regression—external genitalia is highly estrogenized due to mother's hormones; hymen pink, thick, and moist.
Stage 2 (2 months to 7 years)	Early childhood—little estrogen evident; hymen thin; wispy, lacelike vascular pattern; sticky and painful to touch.
Stage 3 (7 to 11 years)	Late childhood—estrogen increase begins; changes in hymen directly correlated to increase in estrogen; hymen begins to thicken and take on a scalloped edge.
Stage 4 (11 to 12 years)	Premenarche—rapid pubertal changes occurring; hymen thickens, is redundant, pinkish-white, and not as sensitive to touch; physiologic white discharge.

From Giardino AP et al: *A practical guide to the evaluation of sexual abuse in the prepubertal child,* Newberry Park, Calif, 1992, Sage.

Table 49-4	PREPARING THE CHILD FOR MEDICAL EXAMINATION
QUESTIONS/ CONCERNS	HELPFUL RESPONSES
Do you know why you're here today?	To make sure your body is okay. We are going to look in your eyes, ears, nose, throat, mouth, where you go tee-tee (private area), and your skin all over. (Justify why they must undress.)
What is that big machine?	That is called a colposcope or big flashlight. It helps us see little bitsy things. The camera lets us take pictures. Do you think you could take some pictures for us? (Let child use long shutter cord to take pictures.)
Explain culture collection	We all have germs on our hands. They are also all over your body. I'm going to use a "bug-collector" (Dacron swab) to see if we can catch some germs, and if we do, let's feed them this chocolate bug food (modified Thayer-Martin culture medium for *Neisseria gonorrhoeae*) and give them some orange bug drink (*Chlamydia* culture medium).

Specimen Collection

For prepubertal females, use saline-moistened Dacron swabs to obtain cultures from the vagina, pharynx, and rectum for *N. gonorrhoeae* and the endocervix and rectum for *Chlamydia trachomatis*. Obtain wet preparation, potassium oxide (KOH) slide, and Gram's stain for vaginal discharge and viral cultures if herpes is suspected. If there is a history

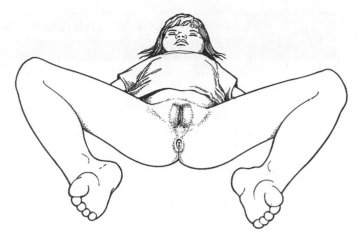

FIGURE 49-13 Frog-leg position for evaluation.

of penile-genital contact, obtain a serum pregnancy test. If the patient can tolerate a speculum, obtain a Pap smear.

In males culture the urethra, rectum, and pharynx for *N. gonorrhoeae,* and the rectum and urethra (if there is a discharge) for *C. trachomatis*. Obtain a Gram's stain of any discharge from male or female victims of acute assault or in which the perpetrator has a high risk for STDs. Obtain hepatitis B surface antigen, Venereal Disease Research Laboratory or rapid plasma reagin test (repeat in 12 weeks), and HIV antibody test (repeat in 6 months). See Table 49-7 for medical management of STDs.

Documentation

Child protection services rely heavily on the medical record; however, many child protective service workers admit they cannot read the writing, understand the terminology, or discern the significance of findings or lack of findings in these records. Health care providers have a responsibility to disseminate information in an understandable manner to law enforcement, child protective service workers, and the judicial system. Document findings accurately and precisely. Use quotation marks, draw pictures, and write clearly and legibly. Avoid statements such as "hymen intact" or "has not been sexually abused" because these statements are ambiguous, and children with normal examinations may have been sexually abused. Samples of documentation are provided in Figure 49-14. Opening paragraphs should describe the examination; the last paragraph provides significance of the examination. This format communicates findings and allows better understanding of the medical report and facilitates more informed decisions. Monteleone[10] classified sexual abuse physical findings into categories along with their significance (Table 49-5). No "gold standard" for true significance of physical findings exists; however, this classification has the approval of many experts in the field.

EMOTIONAL ABUSE

Emotional abuse encompasses psychologic, mental injury, or verbal abuse. This can be defined as acts or the lack of

Table 49-5	CLASSIFICATION OF SEXUAL ABUSE PHYSICAL FINDINGS
CATEGORY	**FINDINGS**
Category 1: Normal appearing examination Majority (60% or more) of abused children fall into this category	Mounds, clefts, bands, septal remnants, bumps, and mild urethral dilation
Category 2: Nonspecific findings of sexual abuse Often seen in children who have not been sexually abused	Condylomata (children younger than 2 years), hymenal thickening, erythema, increased vascularity, rounding of hymenal edges, labial adhesions, narrowing of hymen, enlargement of hymenal opening, increased pigmentation, venous pooling in anus
Category 3: Specific Suspicious/highly suspicious for sexual abuse	Hymenal/vaginal tears or scars, herpes type 2, *Chlamydia trachomatis* (outside the newborn period), reflex anal dilatation >2 cm with no stool in the vault, hymenal attenuation (narrowing <2 mm or flat), perianal skin tags outside the midline, PID
Category 4: Conclusive of sexual abuse For children younger than 12 years, as well as older children	*Neisseria gonorrhoeae* (nonneonatal), *Treponema pallidum* (syphilis—nonneonatal), sperm, pregnancy, HIV (nonneonatal and no history to explain occurrence), may be sexually active

Modified from Monteleone JA, Brouder AE: *Child maltreatment: a clinical guide and reference,* St. Louis, 1994, GW Medical Publishing.
PID, Pelvic inflammatory disease; *HIV,* human immunodeficiency virus.

Table 49-6	CONDITIONS MISTAKEN FOR SEXUAL ABUSE
FINDINGS	**POSSIBLE CAUSES**
GENITAL	
Accidental trauma	Straddle injury with labia majora/minora affected; hymen unaffected
Lichen sclerosis	Dermal condition, skin is atrophic and easily traumatized; hymen not affected
Urethral prolapse	Often associated with bleeding; seen in African-American females ages 4 to 8 years
Congenital malformations	Midline failure to fuse; along median raphe
Hemangioma	May bleed and be mistaken for trauma
ANUS	
Inflammatory bowel disease	Crohn's disease may be accompanied by fissures, fistulas, tags, or abscess; usually appears in older children and accompanied by fever, weight loss, and stooling problems
Hemorrhoids	Rare; question intraabdominal venous congestion
Anal abscess associated with neutropenia	Possible leukemia
Perianal streptococcal infection	Painful erythematous rash

Modified from Berkowitz CD: Child sexual abuse, *Pediatr Rev* 13(12):443, 1992.

acts that cause or could possibly cause serious cognitive, behavioral, emotional, or mental disorders. Caregivers that use extreme measures of discipline such as locking a child in a closet or less severe acts such as habitual belittling or scapegoating are sufficient to warrant child protection interven-tion. Emotional abuse is almost always found with every form of child maltreatment.[12] Verbal abuse is one of the most common forms of emotional abuse.[6]

OTHER ISSUES RELATED TO CHILD ABUSE AND NEGLECT

Multidisciplinary Teams and Sexual Assault Nurse Examiners

Child abuse and neglect issues are complex and require the expertise of many professionals. Many hospitals and communities have adopted a multidisciplinary approach, using a core team with a health care provider (physician or nurse practitioner), social worker, and team coordinator. A consulting team may include a child psychiatrist, developmental specialist, psychologist, public health coordinator, adult psychiatrist, and attorney. Professionals who can offer opinions on a case-by-case basis include family physicians, public health nurses, child protection workers, police officers, mental health therapists, guardians ad litem, foster parents, county attorneys, and teachers.

A cooperative approach has decreased the incidence of reabuse, serious injury, and child death and consistently ensured that hospitals fulfill the legal mandate to report suspected abuse. Consistent use of trained experts increases case findings and reporting within the community while focusing treatment on the entire family. A team approach also provides expert collection of forensic evidence and court testimony, ensures continuing education across disciplines, and decreases burnout for professionals in this field. An interdisciplinary approach appears to be extremely successful but does have drawbacks, such as high salaries and communication. Without effective communication among team members, there is a chance for conflict. However, strong di-

Table 49-7 INITIAL TREATMENT OF SEXUALLY TRANSMITTED DISEASES IN CHILDREN

STD	TREATMENT

Neisseria gonorrhoeae	Less than 45 kg
	    Ceftriaxone 25-50 mg/kg IV or IM (single dose)
	Greater than 45 kg
	    Cefixime 400 mg PO (single dose) *or*
	    Ceftriaxone 125 mg IM (single dose) *or*
	    Ciprofloxacin 500 mg PO (single dose) *or*
	    Ofloxacin 400 mg PO (single dose) *or*
	    Azithromycin 1 gm PO (single dose) *or*
	    Doxycycline 100 mg PO BID for 7 days

Chlamydia trachomatis	Less than 45 kg
	    Erythromycin 50 mg/kg/day divided into 4 equal doses daily for 10-24 days
	Greater than 45 kg but less than 8 years
	    Azithromycin 1 g orally (single dose)
	Greater than 8 years
	    Doxycycline 100 mg BID for 7 days *or*
	    Azithromycin 1 g orally (single dose)

Trichomonas	Prepubertal
	    Metronidazole 15 mg/kg/day with a maximum of 250 mg TID for 7 days
	Pubertal
	    Metronidazole 2 gm PO (single dose) *or*
	    Metronidazole 250 mg PO TID for 7 days

Bacterial vaginosis	Metronidazole 35-50 mg per kg of body weight in three divided doses daily.
Herpes genitalis	Acyclovir 400 mg PO TID for 7 to 10 days *or* Acyclovir 200 mg PO five times per day for 7 to 10 days *or* Famciclovir PO TID for 7 to 10 days *or* Valacyclovir 1 gm PO BID for 7 to 10 days
Chancroid (*Haemophilus ducreyi*)	Azithromycin 1 gm PO (single dose) *or* Ceftriaxone 250 mg IM (single dose) *or* Ciprofloxacin 500 mg PO BID for 3 days *or* Erythromicin base 500 mg PO QID for 7 days
Primary syphilis	Benzathine penicillin 50,000 units/kg IM up to adult dose of 2.4 million units in a single dose

Data from Centers for Disease Control and Prevention: 2002 Guidelines for treatment of sexually transmitted diseases, *MMWR* 51(RR-6):51, 2002.

rection and coordination can overcome these and other obstacles.

Sexual Assault Nurse Examiners

The Sexual Assault Nurse Examiner (SANE) program began in 1977 in Minneapolis and has now grown to more than 116 programs nationwide. The primary mission of a SANE program is to "meet the needs of the sexual assault victim by providing immediate, compassionate, culturally sensitive and comprehensive forensic evaluation and treatment by trained, professional nurse experts within the parameters of the individual's State Nurse Act, the SANE Standards of the International Association of Forensic Nurses, and the individual agency policies." The SANE is responsible for performing the entire sexual assault evidentiary examination. This includes the perineal exam, collection of forensic evidence, STD prevention, pregnancy risk evaluation and interception, crisis intervention and referrals for follow-up care.[14]

Testifying for Child Abuse and Neglect Cases

Health care providers are often the first professionals who become aware of child abuse; therefore, the quality of documentation is critical to future prosecutorial decisions. The medical record and the health care professional who examined the child will almost certainly be involved if the case goes to court. Consequently, effective communication skills are essential for charting, obtaining history, handling parents, and interacting with investigators and attorneys. Physician testimony is not considered hearsay, so doctors are allowed to testify as to what the child told them during a medical examination.

If you do receive a subpoena and have never testified, contact the attorney. Find out what is expected from your testimony and discuss what you can and cannot say. If you are called as a material witness, there is an expectation to "tell what you observed." An "expert" witness is required to prepare and support expert knowledge with current scientific

A

Clinic Note

NAME: Female Child   DOB: 00/00/00
MR#   000000   DOV: 00/00/00

This child was examined in the frog leg supine position. This is a Tanner stage 1 female with unestrogenized female genitalia. The labia majora and minora are well formed and without acute or chronic signs of trauma. The hymen has a crescentic orifice, with a thin velamentous border. The vestibular surface and posterior fourchette do not demonstrate any acute or chronic signs of injury. There is no abnormal degree of redness.

The external anal verge tissues have a symmetric rugal pattern, normal sphincter tone, normal response to traction, and no post-inflammatory pigment change.

IMPRESSION: Class 1 - Normal These are findings which have been noted in non-abused, prepubertal children. These physical findings do not preclude the possibility of sexual abuse.

_____   _____
Health Care Examiner   Date

_____   _____
Exam Assistant   Date

B

Clinic Note

NAME: Female Child   DOB: 00/00/00
MR#   000000   DOV: 00/00/00

This child was examined in the frog leg supine position. This is a Tanner stage 1-2 female with unestrogenized female genitalia. The labia majora and labia minora are well formed and without acute signs of trauma. Posterior labial adhesions are present. The hymen is poorly visualized due to the labial adhesions. The vestibular surface and posterior fourchette do not demonstrate any acute or chronic signs of injury. There is no abnormal degree of redness. We did not obtain cultures at this time.

IMPRESSION: Class 2 - Nonspecific Labial Adhesions - These findings are nonspecific and may be seen in both abused and non-abused children. We prescribed premarin cream and will re-examine this child in approximately one month.

_____   _____
Health Care Examiner   Date

_____   _____
Exam Assistant   Date

C

Clinic Note

NAME: Female Child   DOB: 00/00/00
MR#   000000   DOV: 00/00/00
         This child was examined in the frog leg supine position. This is a Tanner stage 1 female with unestrogenized female genitalia. The labia majora and minora are well formed and without acute or chronic signs of trauma. The hymen has a crescentic orifice, with a thin velamentous border. There are intravaginal ridges at 3, 4, and 6 o'clock. The area of hymen adjacent to the intravaginal ridge at 6 o'clock has a diameter which is less than 1 mm. This does not appear to be a deformation associated with the intravaginal ridge. The vestibular surface and posterior fourchette do not demonstrate any acute or chronic signs of injury. There is no abnormal degree of redness.
         The external anal verge tissues have a symmetric rugal pattern, normal sphincter tone, normal response to traction, and no post-inflammatory pigment change.

IMPRESSION: Class 3 - Specific for Sexual Abuse
There is a minimal amount of hymenal tissue adjacent to the intravaginal ridge at 6 o'clock. This is abnormal and suggestive of penetrating injury.

_____   _____
Health Care Examiner   Date

_____   _____
Exam Assistant   Date

D

Clinic Note

NAME: Female Child   DOB: 00/00/00
MR#   000000   DOV: 00/00/00
         This child was examined in the frog leg supine position. This is a Tanner stage 1 female with unestrogenized female genitalia. The labia majora and minora are well formed and without acute or chronic signs of trauma. The hymen has a crescentic orifice, with a thin velamentous border. There is a complete transection of the hymen at 5:30. This extends to the vaginal floor, and no hymenal tissue is present in this area. The vestibular surface and posterior fourchette do not demonstrate any acute or chronic signs of injury. There is no abnormal degree of redness. Microscopic exam of wet prep found

sperm to be present.

         The external anal verge tissues have a symmetric rugal pattern, normal sphincter tone, normal response to traction, and no post-inflammatory pigment change. A small fissure is present at 12 o'clock.

IMPRESSION: Class 4 - Conclusive of Sexual Abuse
These findings are diagnostic of blunt force penetrating trauma to the hymen. The most common cause of this type of blunt force penetrating trauma in pre-pubertal girls is sexual abuse. The small anal fissure is a nonspecific finding and may or may not be associated with sexual abuse.

_____   _____
Health Care Examiner   Date

_____   _____
Exam Assistant   Date

FIGURE 49-14   Documentation samples. **A,** Class 1—Normal. **B,** Class 2—Nonspecific. **C,** Class 3—Specific for sexual abuse. **D,** Class 4—Conclusive of sexual abuse.

literature. The National Center for Prosecution of Child Abuse provides a hotline for more information on how to focus the examination for children who have been sexually abused (contact number is 703-739-0321).

Child Death Review Teams

The past 10 years have seen an increased focus on child deaths resulting from abuse and neglect. The National Center on Child Abuse and Neglect found a 49% increase in reports of child death since 1985. In 1997 an estimated 1200 child fatalities from abuse were reported—more than 90% of these children were younger than 5 years and more than 40% were infants younger than 1 year. Children vulnerable to serious or fatal abuse are those least visible to the community, educational programs, and protective services.

Child death review teams grew from an effort to determine how and why children were dying. In 1983, a tiny infant was beaten and eventually starved to death. A Los Angeles deputy sheriff mapped more than 52 contacts with 10 agencies. Investigations of drug abuse, domestic violence, reports of suspicious injuries, and drunken brawls were conducted; however, no agency knew the other was involved, and no one saw a need to remove the infant. From that meeting, a small group of professionals began to meet, share records, and make team decisions. Teams stood together, faced judges returning children to abusive settings, and started asking questions about siblings. Michael Durfee, a child psychiatrist, pressed for child death review teams across the country. Because of Durfee's efforts, most states have designated teams to review child deaths.

The death of a child in an ED is usually unexpected and sudden. Health care providers need to be sensitive to the family's needs while trying to obtain a history and conduct an examination to determine cause of death. After the death has been called, provide the family an opportunity to view and hold the child. Every ED should have written policies and procedures accompanied by checklists (Box 49-5) that should be followed in the event of a child's death. The medical examiner and child's private caregiver should be notified of the death. Autopsies should be required on suspicious, obscure, or otherwise unexplained deaths.[2] Community resources should be offered for grief counseling. Hospital resources such as critical incident stress debriefings should be made available to all caregivers who have been emotionally stressed by a child's death.[1]

Prevention

Precursors to physical maltreatment include excessive parental physical discipline, failure to provide basic necessities such as food and a safe home, and unobtainable goals set by parents. Programs for prevention of child abuse and neglect typically focus on physical abuse, centering on the parent, parenting skills, and damaging practices. Pilot programs such as home visiting and increased public awareness have decreased physical abuse of children in some areas. Changing attitudes and modifying behaviors require 6 to 12 months. To successfully reduce physical abuse and neglect within diverse populations, preventive services should begin before or shortly after birth of the first child—through support of effective child-rearing skills. Prevention efforts should tie the child's developmental level to parent enhancement education. Parents must observe and be able to model desired parental behaviors. Child safety can depend on the parent's ability to take advantage of social programs and obtain assistance as needed. All prevention programs must recognize and accept cultural differences.

Current sexual abuse prevention focuses on the child.[12] The child is given the responsibility for saying "no." Classroom education teaches "good touches" and "bad touches" and who the child should tell if someone tries to hurt him or her. But what if the abuser is the child's mom or dad? Sexual abuse is convoluted; secrecy is a large component of manipulation. Effective prevention programs should stress community involvement, self-confidence, and the child's cognitive abilities.

SUMMARY

Child abuse and neglect are complex, life-threatening situations. Medical professionals who work with children must speak out for abused children. No one agency or discipline

can be solely responsible for protection of children. The community, law enforcement, child protection workers, mental health counselors, legislators, educators, health care providers, and the judicial system must work together to remove barriers to identification, treatment, and prevention of child abuse and neglect.

BOX 49-5 CHECKLIST FOR CHILD DEATH IN THE EMERGENCY DEPARTMENT

Obtain a complete history (medical, family, social)
Describe the circumstances of death (especially when SIDS is suspected):
  Position in which the child was put to sleep
  Type of bed and bedding
  Did child sleep alone or cosleep
  What and when was child last fed
  Position child found and by whom
  Clothing child was wearing
  Temperature of room
Core temperature upon arrival to ED
Perform a complete physical examination (head to toe including eyes, skin, and genitalia)
Photograph any bruises or wounds if present
Review prior medical records
Skeletal survey
Laboratories such as cultures, drug screen, and routine blood studies
Grief support for family and ED staff
Autopsy (documentation of circumstances and blood should accompany body to morgue)

SIDS, Sudden infant death syndrome; *ED,* emergency department.

References

1. American Academy of Pediatrics: Care of children in emergency department: guidelines for preparedness, *Pediatrics* 107(4):777, 2001.
2. American Academy of Pediatrics: Committees on Child Abuse and Neglect and Community Health Services: investigation and review of unexpected infant and child deaths, *Pediatrics* 99(104):1158, 1998.
3. American Academy of Pediatrics: Guidelines for the evaluation of sexual abuse in children, *Pediatrics* 103(1):186, 1999.
4. American Academy of Pediatrics: shaken baby syndrome: rotational cranial injuries (policy statement), *Pediatrics* 108(1):206, 2001.
5. Bonner BL, Crowe SM, Logue MD: Fatal child neglect. In Dubowitz H: *Neglected children: research, practice, and policy,* Thousand Oaks, Calif, 1999, Sage.
6. Emergency Nurses Association: *Emergency nursing core curriculum,* ed 5, Des Plaines, Ill, 2000, The Association.
7. Emergency Nurses Association: *Emergency nursing pediatric course provider manual,* ed 2, Des Plaines, Ill, 1998, The Association.
8. Giardino AP et al: *A practical guide to the evaluation of sexual abuse in the prepubertal child,* Newberry Park, Calif, 1992, Sage.

9. Herman-Giddens ME, Brown G, Verbiest S et al: *Underascertainment of child mortality in the United States,* JAMA 282(5):463, 1999.

10. Monteleone JA, Brodeur AE: *Child maltreatment: a clinical guide and reference,* St. Louis, 1994, GW Medical Publishing.

11. Peddle N, Wang C: *Current trends in child abuse prevention, reporting, and fatalities: the 1999 fifty state survey (2002),* National Center on Child Abuse Prevention Research. Retrieved February 21, 2002 from the World Wide Web: www.preventchildabuse.org.

12. Prevent Child Abuse America: *Total estimated cost of child abuse and neglect in the United States.* Retrieved February 21, 2002 from the World Wide Web: www.preventchildabuse.org.

13. U.S. Department of Health and Human Services, Office for Victims of Crime: *Sexual assault nurse examiner development and operation guide,* Washington DC, 2000 U.S. Government Printing Office.

14. U.S. Department of Health and Human Services: *Child maltreatment 1998: reports from the state to the national child abuse and neglect data system,* Washington DC, 2000 U.S. Government Printing Office.

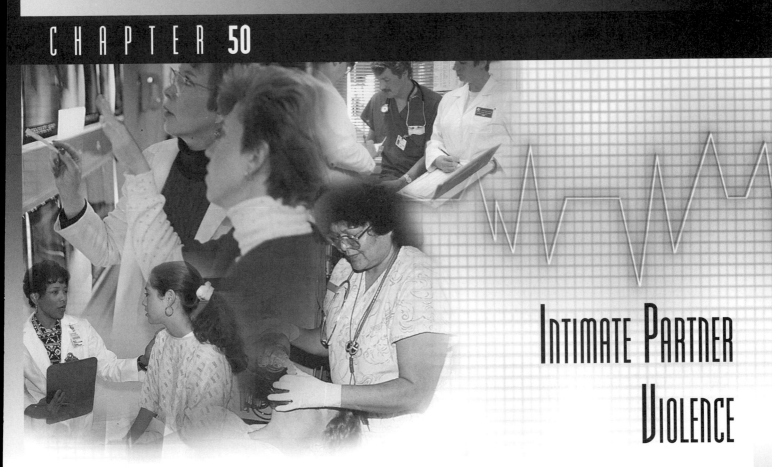

CHAPTER 50

INTIMATE PARTNER VIOLENCE

SUE MOORE

Intimate partner violence (IPV) is actual or threatened physical or sexual violence or psychologic or emotional abuse.[3,11] Other terms for IPV include domestic violence, spouse abuse, courtship violence, and wife beating. Legally, IPV includes various nonphysical actions in addition to actual physical violence. Most state laws define specific acts that constitute IPV (Box 50-1). Victims of partner abuse in heterosexual and homosexual relationships are most frequently female. The defining factors in these relationships are power and control. The perpetrator creates fear in the victim to exert control. This is most often a pattern in which a male is exerting power over a female. IPV is also reported in same-sex and transgender relationships. Women who live with chronic partner abuse live in chronic fear. The focus of this chapter is violence and psychologic or emotional abuse. Sexual assault is discussed in detail in Chapter 54, child abuse in Chapter 49, and elder abuse in Chapter 51.

HISTORY

The United States has a violent history. The pioneer fought for his family, protecting his wife and children. Until recently laws implied that a man owned his family. The wife and children were his possessions, and what he did with them was a private matter. He protected his family; therefore, the family should be grateful and subservient.

Our society has a high tolerance for violence. This is dramatically illustrated in a multitude of violent scenes on television and in the movies. Acceptance of certain forms of violent behavior is ingrained in the American value system.

Cultural beliefs that lead to partner abuse exist in the United States today. Many men and women believe a woman should be subservient to a man. They may believe the man suffers so much stress in his work life or from various personal events that he is justified in "taking it out" on his wife. Many people are unwilling to invade the privacy of the home, even though what occurs is against the law.

Only in the past few years has IPV become a societal issue. Sadly, many people still do not believe that it is a problem. A number of judges continue to sentence men to "a slap on the wrist" for beating their wives. Many people, men and women, blame the victim by believing she did something to warrant the abuse or by asking, "Well, why doesn't she just leave?"

PREVALENCE

Each year in the United States, approximately 1.5 million women and 834,700 men are physically assaulted or raped by an intimate partner.[46] Women between 16 and 24 years of age showed the highest per capita rate of IPV (19.4 per 1000 women).[2] An exact number of IPV incidents is difficult to obtain because many are never reported. IPV is one of the most underreported crimes in the United States. Approximately 2000 women die each year at the hands of men who say they love them. More women die from IPV than

Box 50-1 ACTS OF INTIMATE PARTNER VIOLENCE

Battery or actual physical violence
Assault or the threat of violence
Compelling the other person by force or threat of force to perform an act from which he or she has a right to refrain or to refrain from an act that he or she has a right to perform
Sexual assault
Knowing, purposeful, or reckless course of conduct to harass the other
Kidnapping
False imprisonment
Unlawful entry of the other's residence, or forcible entry against the other's will if there is a reasonable, foreseeable risk of harm to the other from the entry
Stalking

Box 50-2 REASONS WOMEN REMAIN IN AN ABUSIVE SITUATION

She has few if any friends. When a woman leaves, she leaves her house, neighbors, and frequently her friends because they are probably also his friends. If the abuser has behaved in a typical manner, he has narrowed her circle of friends to those he considers acceptable and who will not accept her if she leaves.
She fears loss of her children. If she has children, her husband, even though convicted of spouse abuse, can gain custody of the children. He is often the one with a job and house and is frequently very charming in court. If the woman leaves her children with the abuser, he may turn his anger toward them and she will not be there to protect them.
The victim's family may not support her decision. Because of religious beliefs, they may insist she stay and make the marriage work. More commonly, they do not want to be in a position where they have to support and protect her. Family members may simply not believe her.
She loves the abuser. Typically, after an explosive episode of abuse, the perpetrator is repentant and treats the victim very kindly. She finds herself forgiving him and believing him when he says it will not happen again.
The abuser becomes more violent if she threatens to leave or actually does so. Most murders related to domestic abuse happen after the partner has tried to leave the relationship. Some abusers do not become physically violent until the victim leaves; then he begins stalking her. As many as half of all batterers threaten to retaliate, and more than 30% inflict further assaults while they are under prosecution.

from automobile crashes, rapes, and muggings combined. Fifty-three percent of homicides in 1998 related to IPV were committed by spouses.[22] Most women are not killed by strangers. At every age in the life span, females are more likely to be sexually or physically assaulted by their father, brother, family member, neighbor, boyfriend, husband, partner, or ex-partner than by a stranger or anonymous assailant.

Prevalence of IPV in the lesbian, gay, bisexual, and transgender population has been reported as high as 40%.[2,21] A 1997 study by the National Coalition of Anti-Violence Programs documented 3327 cases with 52% reported by men and 48% by women.[21] The numbers represent a startling 41% increase from the previous year; however, most experts generally agree the actual incidence is probably higher. There is some suggestion that gay IPV may be greater than heterosexual IPV given the acceptance of male contact and the involvement of two males in the couple.[21]

Surveys of emergency patients present quite a range in the prevalence of IPV. Studies show that 19% to 54% of women and 8.5% to 28% of men who visit EDs have suffered some form of partner abuse in their lives. The number of female emergency patients currently in abusive relationships is 13% to 19%. Between 2% and 9% of women who come to the ED have complaints directly related to IPV.[3-7,9,11,17,18] Even with the small percentage of visits to the ED directly for injuries related to IPV, it is estimated that 458,096 ED visits for women and 65,253 ED visits for men are for injuries sustained during IPV.[26]

THE VICTIM

Predicting precisely who may be a victim of IPV is not possible. Any person can be in an abusive relationship. Several studies of ED patients have attempted to identify risk factors associated with IPV. It has been very difficult to do because victims of IPV come from all walks of life.

Many women do not experience physical violence in a relationship until they become pregnant. The unborn child

may be perceived as a threat to the abuser, as someone coming between the partners, someone who takes away the woman's attention. Many spontaneous abortions and preterm deliveries are related to physical abuse.

IPV victims tend to visit EDs more often than nonvictims do, most often for complaints not directly related to IPV. There is no predictable pattern to these complaints. The only difference in disorders between victims and nonvictims is that victims have significantly more psychiatric presentations and a greater incidence of attempted suicide and alcohol-related problems.[23] Women in violent relationships may come to the ED with complaints related to depression or gastrointestinal disorders. All "frequent flyer" patients (i.e., those patients who present to the ED repeatedly) should be viewed through a filter of IPV. They may be using the ED as an escape from the home or may unconsciously develop physical complaints as legitimate reasons for requesting help.

The question health care providers ask most frequently is, "Why does she stay?" The answer is that leaving can be the most dangerous thing to do. The most common reasons why a woman stays are described in Box 50-2. The victim lives every day with a degree of fear. After years of such conditions, self-esteem suffers, and the woman develops "learned helplessness." The woman may reach a point where saving herself or her children is no longer conceivable. Fortunately, most women do not get to that point; many do eventually leave.

Signs Indicating a Woman Is Ready to Leave

Women who fight back during the assault and those who develop a consistently uncaring attitude toward their partners are more likely to leave. As with quitting an addiction, the victim rehearses many times before she is successful. She may rehearse packing up and leaving while her spouse is at work, only to return and put everything away before he returns home. She may actually move out of the home several times, only to return when the abuser apologizes and begs her to return or threatens increased violence toward her or her children.

Not all victims are pleasant people who easily gain our feelings of pity. Many are substance abusers who can be hostile toward emergency staff and to their significant others. They may have come to the relationship with psychiatric disorders or substance abuse problems or they may develop them in the fearful environment. The bottom line, however, is that no one deserves to be hit. Every victim of IPV deserves information that can help her protect herself or himself.

THE BATTERER

The abuser creates a web of power and possessiveness. His or her response to challenge or disappointment is to blame someone else: if the abuser is driven to beat his or her partner, the partner made him do it through her thoughtlessness, infidelity, sloppiness, stupidity, or any other negative descriptor. If the batterer does enter therapy, he most likely will spend his first sessions explaining why his partner made him abuse her. In counseling it has been found that about 40% of batterers acknowledge their recent assaults and less than 20% admit to using severe tactics, even after they are convicted.

Counseling is not enormously effective. More than 25% of convicted batterers engage in physical violence within 1 or 2 years of counseling. Arrest does stop the violence, at least while the batterer is incarcerated. Some batterers say that arrest is what finally caught their attention.

The typical picture of an abuser is the man who will not allow his wife to answer any questions in the ED and will not allow her to be alone with the nurse. However, it is just as likely that the batterer will be very charming toward nursing staff and appear very compassionate toward his spouse, allowing her to interact normally. He may communicate his control to the spouse with very subtle gestures and expressions that only the victim, after years of living in fear, can perceive.

Alcohol and other drugs of abuse play a large role in IPV. In some cases, both partners may be substance abusers.[23] The strongest predictor for acute injury from IPV is a history of alcohol or other drug abuse by the abuser.[10,12,14,15] Alcohol eliminates inhibitions. A person inclined to violence finds it easier to commit aggressive acts while intoxicated. Methamphetamines and, to a lesser degree, cocaine, can alter thought processes and cause paranoia, which may be aimed at the partner. Despite this, mind-altering substances are not an excuse for violent behavior. Many people who use drugs do not beat their spouses. The tendency for violence must already exist.

Spouse abuse is not a disease or addiction. The batterer abuses because he thinks he has the right to do so and because he can get away with it. He must first see the need to change his behavior and then learn alternative ways to deal with frustration.

THE ROLE OF THE EMERGENCY NURSE

In 1992 the Massachusetts Medical Society developed the acronym RADAR, which identifies steps in screening and intervention for IPV. Box 50-3 describes the RADAR process.

Routine Screening

Privacy is essential for the patient interview. Questions should not be asked in a public place, such as a centrally located triage desk or waiting room. The patient should not be questioned in the presence of a possible abuser.

Routine screening is recommended by the Emergency Nurses Association and American College of Emergency Physicians. One study found that, before implementing routine screening, only 0.4% of emergency patients were identified as victims of IPV. After screening was implemented, 14.2% of patients were identified as victims. Only 1.3% of emergency patients questioned refused to answer.[19]

Many EDs have implemented routine screening. It has not always been easy. Even after staff education and implementation of protocols, compliance can be minimal.[1,16] The most effective way to increase compliance with routine screening protocols may be to change the structure of the ED record so that health care providers are reminded.[24,39]

A brief screening instrument asking three questions has been very effective in identifying victims of IPV. The questions are:
1. Have you been hit, kicked, punched, or otherwise hurt by someone within the past year? If so, by whom?
2. Do you feel safe in your current relationship?
3. Is there a partner from a previous relationship making you feel unsafe now?[8]

The first question is nearly as sensitive and specific as the combination of the three questions.[8] In the busy ED setting, the first question may be asked at triage. Positive answers can be investigated further after the patient is in the treatment area.

Ask Directly, Kindly, Nonjudgmentally

Only 25% of victims say they would divulge information regarding IPV without being asked directly.[13] Nurses must overcome their own feelings of discomfort and learn to ask every patient. At first nurses can feel very awkward, but as with any new skill, the more it is practiced the easier it becomes.

The emergency nurse may become suspicious because of physical and behavioral findings. These findings should be the basis for a more focused assessment. Suggested questions include, "I notice you have bruises on your face. Has someone hit you?" or "Your husband seems very anxious. Did he hurt you?" As with all patient communication, the emergency nurse should assess the patient's level of education, trust, sobriety, and anxiety and then plan the approach accordingly.

Many patients who do not volunteer information about abuse will deny it when asked. If the patient does deny it or becomes angry, the emergency nurse should let the patient know that the door is always open and that if the patient changes his or her mind he or she can always return to the ED for help.

Surveys of patients in violent relationships and those not in violent relationships show that most patients are grateful to health care providers who inquire about violence and abuse in relationships and do not consider this line of inquiry offensive or intrusive. Victims have been interviewed regarding their experiences in the ED. Half of the women interviewed reported negative experiences in the ED, such as feeling humiliated, being blamed for their abuse, having abuse minimized, and not being identified as victims of IPV. The ED should be a sanctuary, a safe place to go for help, where the victim can look forward to support, not humiliation. Many victims assume that health care personnel do not want to help them unless they are planning to leave their abusers. Their assumption is right. It is important to communicate that you understand how difficult it can be to leave and that there are resources available to her even if she stays in the relationship.

The emergency nurse must have a high index of suspicion and be alert for physical and behavioral clues. Many behavioral clues related to IPV are the same as those for child abuse. The patient may wait several hours or days before seeking help for her injuries. She may hope to avoid embarrassment or the need to lie about her injuries, or the perpetrator may prevent her from leaving home. The patient may have a history of several injuries, telling the nurse that she is clumsy or stupid and frequently falls or bumps into things. She may bypass closer EDs so personnel do not get suspicious of her frequent visits. The given mechanism of injury may not fit physical findings.

As with child abuse the victim may have bruises, fractures, and other injuries in various stages of healing. Most victims of IPV do not present for treatment of their injuries. The emergency nurse must be alert for injuries unrelated to the chief complaint. Box 50-4 describes injuries suggestive of IPV.

Document Your Findings

Documentation on the medical record can be very helpful to a victim when it can be used as evidence in court. The notes should be very specific. The clearer the information, the less likely the nurse will have to appear in court to explain them. Include photographs if possible—these are valuable evidence. Documentation should include items listed in Box 50-5. The nurse who practices in a state with mandatory reporting must report any documented suspicions. Documentation should note that the crime was reported to the appropriate law enforcement authority.

The nurse who practices in a state where there is no mandatory reporting of IPV is free to chart any suspicions. Documentation should include that the patient was asked if she wanted to report the crime and what the patient said in reply. Even if a patient denies physical abuse, the nurse should chart findings and the suspicion that the findings do not fit the history and may indicate battery. If the victim changes her mind later, a chart in evidence that says her injuries implied abuse will go a long way to help her case. The nurse should also document any referrals or resources given to the patient and the patient's reaction to the information.

Assess Safety

If a patient presents with a chief complaint of battery, the first pieces of information to obtain are the current location of the batterer, whether he has access to a weapon, and whether he is under the influence of drugs or alcohol. Ask if law enforcement personnel have been notified and if the abuser has been apprehended. If the abuser is not in custody,

---

Box 50-5   DOCUMENTATION

Quote the patient directly; use quotation marks.
Record the patient's description of the incident.
Ask the name of the abuser and document it.
Record injuries on a body map.
Relate injuries to the type of weapon used, if possible.

Box 50-6   ESSENTIAL ITEMS FOR RAPID ESCAPE

Identification papers, birth certificate, social security card, and income tax forms so he or she can apply for assistance
Extra set of car and house keys
Emergency money
List of emergency phone numbers
A few days' clothing
Clothing and supplies for each child
Essential medications for him or her and the children

Box 50-7   NATIONAL RESOURCES ON DOMESTIC VIOLENCE

National Toll-Free Hotlines: (800) 799-SAFE
National Resource Center on Domestic Violence:
  (800) 537-2238
Health Resource Center on Domestic Violence:
  (800) 313-1310
Centers for Disease Control and Prevention: (770) 488-5259
  http://www.cdc.gov/nccdphp/drh/wh_violence.htm

---

determine if he knew the patient was coming to the ED. It is important to maintain safety for the patient, nurse, and others in the ED. If it is possible that the perpetrator will follow the victim, notify security and move the patient to a safe place.

After treatment, if the patient decides to return home, the nurse can help her make an emergency action plan. Several local IPV programs have implemented a "911 phone" plan. The victim is provided with a donated cellular phone so she can call 911 if she is in immediate physical danger. Encourage her to pack a suitcase with essential items for rapid escape (Box 50-6). The suitcase should be kept at a neighbor's or relative's home.

Review Options and Provide Referrals

Provide the patient with information about IPV resources in the community. Local IPV support groups can provide a great deal of information for emergency nurses. If local groups are not available, national organizations (Box 50-7) can provide information regarding state and local resources, as well as posters and leaflets for the ED.

Most patients are aware that battering one's partner is against the law. They may not be aware that more subtle acts such as threats of bodily harm, false imprisonment, harassment, or forcing someone to perform acts against his or her will are also against the law. Frequently, discussion of these issues is the first step in providing the patient information on IPV.

The patient should be given a phone number he or she can call 24 hours a day to get help. The nurse may offer pamphlets or cards with phone numbers. Patients may refuse cards or phone numbers because it may not be safe to bring home material that deals with IPV. If the patient will not take any material, give the number of the ED or the name of a local IPV organization to him or her to look up in the phone book.

Reassure the patient that he or she is not to blame for the battering. Many patients assume they have done something to incite the beating and are sure they can prevent further beatings if they simply behave in the appropriate manner. This is absolutely untrue. The pattern of abuse will continue until an outside intervention stops it.

If the patient is receptive, discuss the effect partner abuse has on children. Many women may not be motivated to leave for themselves but may be willing to leave for the sake of their children. Much research has shown that violence travels in family lines. If children witness abuse or are victims of abuse, they are much more likely to become abusers.[10,20] If the abuser is not already hitting the children, chances are very good that he or she will soon do so.

The best place to display posters and provide pamphlets on IPV is in the treatment room or bathrooms. The waiting room is too public, and the victim may have to walk in front of several people, including the perpetrator, to get the information. Treatment rooms and bathrooms provide the patient a chance to read a pamphlet in private, even if she is not able to take it home.

After the patient decides to seek treatment for his or her injuries, the next decision is whether to report the crime. In a few states reporting is mandatory. Be sure you tell the patient that the crime will be reported. If the choice belongs to the patient, the emergency nurse can help the patient decide whether to report the crime by discussing the consequences if it is reported and if it is not.

Only occasionally does a patient immediately and permanently leave the batterer, though he or she may be promising to do so while in the ED. When intervening in IPV, the nurse must not use the "did she leave him" factor as a determinant of effectiveness. Most patients do not leave after the first few episodes. Years later, the patient may use the information the nurse provided. Survivors report that simple acknowledgment and a nonjudgmental attitude helped them enormously in the emergency setting.

If the patient has decided not to go home, the nurse should help him or her explore resources. Most shelters do not automatically accept all comers if they have safe alternatives. Does the patient have relatives or friends who will accept him or her? Does he or she have financial resources for traveling to friends or relatives out of town? Are there children still at home who must be protected?

The immediate plan usually involves protection for the patient and children. After the patient has formed a plan, he or she needs access to a phone to implement it. Long-term needs center around legal assistance, employment, and housing. The ED is not the best place to make plans for meeting these needs.

LEGAL ISSUES

Mandatory reporting laws specifically for IPV have been enacted in several states. There is a great deal of controversy associated with mandatory reporting. Many advocates for victims of IPV do not want mandatory reporting because they fear that it will deter visits to the ED for necessary medical care. The first question many victims of IPV ask is "Will you have to call the police?" At the least, victims want to avoid the shame. At the worst, victims are placed at risk for retribution. One study found that 39% of victims say they would not disclose IPV if they knew that ED personnel were required to report it.[13]

Supporters of mandatory reporting feel that IPV is a crime, as is child abuse, and that perpetrators should be dealt with as other violent criminals are. They feel mandatory reporting can relieve the victim from the onus of reporting. The victim has no choice; therefore, he or she cannot be blamed.

Many episodes of IPV are already reported, even in states with no mandatory reporting law. Unfortunately, these are usually the most serious episodes because all states require reporting any injuries secondary to firearms, knives, or other weapons and "grave injuries" incurred as a result of criminal acts.

In some states mandatory reporting laws have been in place for a few years, with mixed results. One study found that, despite these laws, the incidence of medical personnel reporting IPV to law enforcement did not increase.[26] Surveyed emergency and primary care physicians reported that they would not comply with the law if the patient objected to reporting.[24]

A controversial area of law surrounds the ED's responsibility to protect the patient. Should a victim, even at his or her request, be discharged home when emergency care providers know that IPV, in most cases, escalates and therefore the patient may be in serious danger? Unfortunately, there is no clear answer to this dilemma.

Patients in abusive situations who present with communicable diseases that must be reported to the health department may be put in danger when the health department contacts his or her partner. The patient should always be told when a reportable disease has been diagnosed, so he or she can take protective action, if necessary.

If they decide to leave the relationship, victims should obtain civil protective orders. Local IPV organizations are usually well informed regarding the process and can help the victim through these legal steps. Protection orders in themselves tend to be fairly useless because they are difficult to enforce and batterers routinely ignore them. Their most ef-

fective use is in court. If a victim can show his or her abuser violated a protective order, he or she has a better case.

SUMMARY

IPV is prevalent in today's society and is frequently seen in the ED. About 16% of all female patients seen in the ED are in abusive relationships. Emergency nurses have an obligation to provide these patients useful information should they decide to leave the relationship at that time or later. Most patients do not leave immediately. Patients are best served by acknowledging the problem and supporting their decisions in a nonjudgmental manner.

References

1. Allert CS, Chalkley C, Whitney JR et al: Domestic violence: efficacy of health care provider training in Utah, *Prehosp Disaster Med* 12(1):52, 1997.
2. Broaddust T, Merrill G: *Annual report on lesbian, gay, bisexual, transgender violence,* San Francisco, 1998, National Coalition of Anti-Violence Programs.
3. Centers for Disease Control and Prevention: *Intimate partner fact sheet* (2001), Atlanta, Ga, CDC. Retrieved September 25, 2001 from the World Wide Web: http://www.cdc.gov/ncipc/factsheets/ipvfacts.htm.
4. Dearwater SR, Coben JH, Campbel JC: Prevalence of intimate partner abuse in women treated at community hospital emergency departments, *JAMA* 280(5):433, 1998.
5. Dienemann J, Trautman D, Shahan J et al: Developing a domestic violence program in an inner-city academic health center emergency department: the first 3 years, *J Emerg Nurs* 25(2):110, 1999.
6. Ernst AA, Nick TG, Weiss SJ et al: Domestic violence in an inner-city ED, *Ann Emerg Med* 30(2):190, 1997.
7. Fanslow JL, Norton RN, Spinola CG: Indicators of assault-related injuries among women presenting to the emergency department, *Ann Emerg Med* 32(3 pt 1):341, 1998.
8. Feldhaus KM, Koziol-McLain J, Amsbury HL: *JAMA* 277(17):1400, 1997.
9. Geary FH, Wingate CB: Domestic violence and physical abuse of women: the Grady Memorial Hospital experience, *Amer J Obstet Gynecol* 181(1)S17, 1999.
10. Gondolf E: Characteristics of batterers in a multi-site evaluation of batterer intervention systems, *Minnesota Center Against Violence and Abuse electronic clearinghouse.* Retrieved January 21, 2001 from the World Wide Web: http://www.mincava.umn.edu/papers/gondolf/batchar.htm
11. Greenfeld L et al, editors: Violence by intimates: analysis of data on crimes by current or former spouses, boyfriends, and girlfriends, *Bureau of Justice Statistics Factbook,* NCJ-167237, Washington, DC, 1998, U.S. Department of Justice.
12. Grisso JA, Schwarz DF, Hirschinger N et al: Violent injuries among women in an urban area, *New Engl J Med* 341(25):1927, 1999.
13. Hayden SR, Barton ED, Hayden M: Domestic violence in the emergency department: how do women prefer to disclose and discuss the issues? *J Emerg Med* 15(4):447, 1997.
14. Kyriacou DN, Anglin D, Taliaferro E et al: *New Engl J Med* 341(25):1892, 1999.
15. Kyriacou DN, McCabe F, Anglin D et al: Emergency department-based study of risk factors for acute injury from

domestic violence against women, *Ann Emerg Med* 31(4): 502, 1998.

16. Larkins GL, Hyman KB, Mathias SR et al: Universal screening for intimate partner violence in the emergency department: importance of patient and provider factors, *Ann Emerg Med* 33(6):669, 1999.

17. McGrath ME, Hogan JW, Peipert JF: A prevalence survey of abuse and screening for abuse in urgent care patients, *Obstet Gynecol* 91(4):511, 1998.

18. Mechem CC, Shofer FS, Reinhard SS et al: History of domestic violence among male patients presenting to an urban emergency department, *Acad Emerg Med* 6(8):786, 1999.

19. Morrison LJ, Allan R, Grunfeld A: Improving the emergency department detection rate of domestic violence using direct questioning, *J Emerg Med* 19(2):117, 2000.

20. National Clearinghouse on Child Abuse and Neglect Information: *In harm's way: domestic violence and child maltreatment.* Retrieved January 21, 2001 from the World Wide Web: http://www.calib.com/nccanch/pubs/otherpubs/harmsway.htm.

21. Niolan R: *Domestic violence in gay and lesbian couples, gay and lesbian resources.* Retrieved February 23, 2002, from the World Wide Web: www.pschypage.com/learning/library/gay/gayvio.html.

22. Rennison CM, Welchan S: *Intimate partner violence,* Bureau of Justice Statistics, special report, Washington, DC, 2000, U.S. Department of Justice.

23. Roberts GL, Lawrence JM, O'Toole BI et al: Domestic violence in the emergency department: I. Two case-control studies of victims, *General Hosp Psychiatry* 19(1):5, 1997.

24. Rodriguez MA, McLoughlin E, Bauer HM et al: Mandatory reporting of intimate partner violence to police: views of physicians in California, *Amer J Public Health* 89(4):575, 1999.

25. Sachs CJ, Peek C, Baraff LJ: Failure of the mandatory domestic violence reporting law to increase medical facility referral to police, *Ann Emerg Med* 31(4):448, 1998.

26. Tjaden P, Thoennes N: *Extent, nature, and consequences of intimate partner violence: findings from the National Violence Against Women Survey,* Washington, DC, 2000, U.S. Department of Justice, Office of Justice Programs.

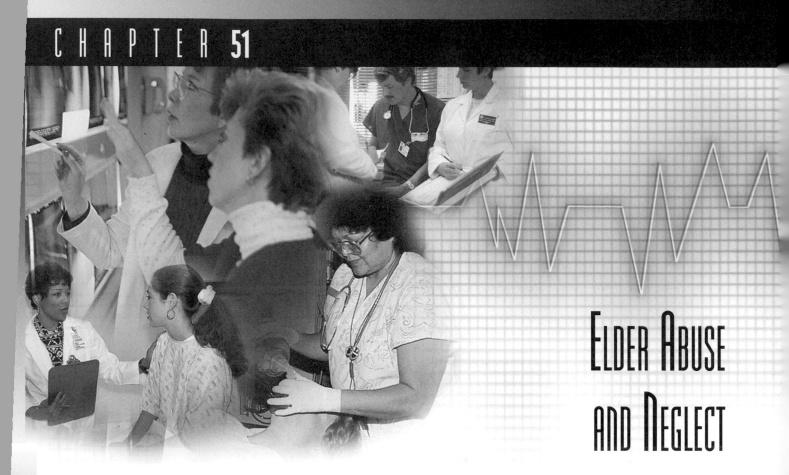

ELDER ABUSE AND NEGLECT

NANCY STEPHENS DONATELLI

Elder abuse and neglect take different forms; however, the common denominator is harm or threatened harm to the health or welfare of the elderly.[2] Abuse and neglect of the elderly have increased steadily as the number of older adults requiring care has increased. Caregivers for this group are sandwiched between careers, families, and changing health care insurance that does not provide custodial care. Abuse is found among all racial, ethnic, and socioeconomic backgrounds.[6]

The life span of the average American is increasing, whereas the U.S. birth rate has declined. More people require care, but fewer people are available to provide care. Consequently, elder abuse is expected to increase at an alarming rate.

Elder abuse and neglect have been defined by the American Medical Association as "actions or the omission of actions that result in harm or threatened harm to the health or welfare of the elderly." Seven primary categories of elder mistreatment—physical abuse, neglect, self-neglect, psychologic or emotional abuse, abandonment, violation of personal rights, and financial abuse—are described in Table 51-1.[3]

Obtaining a clear, accurate picture of demographics surrounding elder abuse is difficult. Significant shame and embarrassment are associated with this problem, so abused individuals may keep the problem within the family to decrease further embarrassment. Results of groundbreaking research were released in September 1998 in the National Elder Abuse Incidence Study. This study provides for the first time national incidence estimates of elder abuse. This landmark study conducted by the National Center on Elder Abuse at the American Public Human Services Association and the Maryland-based social science and survey research firm, Westat, contains the most up-to-date information on elder abuse, neglect, and self-neglect. In this study data were gathered through a nationally representative sample of 20 counties in 15 states. Sampling used two sources: (1) reports from local Adult Protective Service agencies and (2) reports from "sentinels," defined as "specially trained individuals in a variety of community agencies having frequent contact with older persons."[7] Study findings confirm commonly held theories that officially reported cases of abuse are only the "tip of a much larger iceberg."

The best national estimate is that a total of 551,011 elderly people, age 60 and over, experienced abuse, neglect or self-neglect in domestic settings in 1996. The study further concluded from these figures that almost four times as many elders could have been victims of abuse, neglect, or self-neglect, which was not reported.[7]

Our oldest elders (80 and older) are abused and neglected at 2 to 3 times their proportion of the elderly population.[7] It was predicted that by the year 2000 the fastest growing age-group would be those individuals age 95 and older.[5]

Making up about 58% of the total national elderly population in 1996, female elders were more likely to be victims of all categories of abuse, except abandonment. Elders unable to care for themselves were more likely to suffer abuse.

Table 51-1	PRIMARY CATEGORIES OF ELDER MISTREATMENT
CATEGORY	**DESCRIPTION**
Physical abuse	Pain, injury, or physical confinement; an act of violence that results in bodily harm or mental distress; includes sexual abuse
Neglect	Deliberate refusal to meet basic needs; withholding assistance vital to performance of activities of daily living or behavior that causes mental anguish
Self-Neglect	Behaviors of an elderly person that threaten his or her own health or safety. Victims are usually depressed, confused, or extremely frail. Excluded are situations in which a mentally competent older person makes a conscious and voluntary decision to engage in acts that threaten his or her health or safety[9]
Psychologic/Emotional abuse	Verbal aggression, intimidation, and humiliation; threats to deprive the elder of property or services, place in a nursing home, remove financial support; unreasonable demands; deliberately ignoring the person
Violation of personal rights	Deprivation of inalienable rights (i.e., personal liberty, personal property, free speech, privacy, voting)
Financial abuse	Unauthorized use of money or goods for personal gain; includes petty theft, material exploitation, or declaration of the elder as incompetent to confiscate property; failure to pay bills
Abandonment	Desertion of an elderly person by an individual who has physical custody or otherwise has assumed responsibility for providing care for an elder or by a person with physical custody of an elder[9]

In descending order of frequency, substantiated types of maltreatment were physical abuse, abandonment, emotional or psychologic abuse, financial or material abuse, and neglect.[7]

The perpetrator is a family member in almost 9 of 10 incidents of domestic elder abuse and neglect. Adult children are responsible for almost half of elder abuse and neglect. Spouses represented the second largest group of perpetrators. Overall men were perpetrators of abuse and neglect 52.2% of the time.[9] The age category with the most perpetrators was the 41 to 59 age-group. About three fourths of the domestic elder abuse perpetrators were white and less than one fifth were black.[9] Other minority groups accounted for only 2% of the total.[7]

An area of elder maltreatment that is quickly coming to the forefront is known as "gray murders." The expectancy that an elderly person will die is such a fact of life that details are often not questioned. Homicide related to elder abuse has long been overlooked. Since 1960 the rate of homicide in those 65 years of age or older has increased.[4] Box 51-1 describes risk factors associated with elder abuse.

ORIGIN OF THE PROBLEM

Four main theories may explain elder abuse: role theory, transgenerational theory, psychopathology theory, and stressed caregiver theory.

Role Theory

As the parent ages and becomes more childlike, the child must assume a parental role. The elder who once helped the child must now take orders from that child. The psychologic impact of this role reversal is significant for both generations. When role conflicts are present, the potential for abuse increases substantially.

Box 51-1	RISK FACTORS ASSOCIATED WITH ELDER ABUSE

Advanced age
Greater dependency on the caregiver increases risk for abuse
Alcohol or drug abuse in the elder or caregiver
Child abuse by the parent may lead to a role reversal where the child now abuses the parent
History of abuse is a great risk for future abuse in the same setting
Caregiver inexperience
Economic stress
Caregiver mental illness
Caregiver stress from effects of "the sandwich generation" (i.e., being squeezed between demands of dependent parents and dependent children)
Lack of support systems or practical help for the caregiver
Sudden, unwanted, or unexpected dependency of the elder on the caregiver
Cramped living conditions

Transgenerational Theory

The underlying philosophy of transgenerational theory is that violence is a learned behavior. If a child grows up in a family in which aggressive behavior is a part of life, the child exhibits similar behavior. If the parent abused the child, then the child as the caregiver abuses the parent in retribution.

Psychopathology Theory

Altered impulse control caused by psychologic problems such as mental illness or drug or alcohol dependence places the elder at greater risk for abuse. The typical abuser is a middle-age, white woman who lives with the victim, is an alcohol or drug addict, and has long-term financial problems and high stress levels. The abuser perceives the victim as the source of this stress.

Stressed Caregiver Theory

This is one area in which the nurse providing long-term care for the elderly can abuse the elderly as easily as the family caregiver. Caregivers under stress have limited amounts of internal resources. Stress associated with the health care environment and stress in the individual's personal and family life may lead the caregiver to express stress through mistreatment of the elderly. Women may also find themselves in the caretaker role for their spouse's parents.

SIGNS AND SYMPTOMS

The emergency nurse should always remember that despite rising concerns about elder abuse, there are no uniform comprehensive definitions of the term. Identification of elder abuse is easy only in cases where outright battering is visible.[1]

Elder abuse cannot be assessed quickly or easily from a cluster of signs and vague presenting symptoms. Keen awareness when performing the physical examination is essential to identify elder abuse.[1] Potential indicators of abuse are described in Box 51-2.

Each category of abuse or neglect is associated with distinct diagnostic and clinical findings (Table 51-2). Almost one half of the cases of substantiated abused and neglected elderly were individuals who were not physically able to care for themselves. Excluding abandonment, female elders were more likely to be victims of all other categories of abuse.[7] The elder person's history should be obtained from several sources whenever possible. Interactions between the caregiver and the elder should be carefully observed. The patient may be fearful or agitated in the presence of the caregiver or may appear passive and compliant. The caregiver may use harsh words and tone when speaking to the patient or say demeaning things to the elder. Assess the patient's mental status carefully.

When assessing the patient, observe carefully for signs of malnourishment. Note the presence of old and new bruises. Bruises on the upper aspects of both arms suggest the patient has been held tightly and shaken. Bruises on the trunk suggest beating with fists. Bruises on the wrists or ankles occur when the patient has been tied down. Cigarette burns on the skin may be present. Old, healed burns appear as skin discolorations. (Photographs of bruises, lacerations, and other injuries should be obtained to document type and extent of injuries.)

Alopecia secondary to repeated pulling and tugging of the person's hair is another significant finding.[8] Blows to the eyes can cause dislocation of the lens, subconjunctival hemorrhage, or retinal detachment. Whiplash injuries are seen after repeated, violent shaking. Consider the possibility of sexual abuse. Difficulty walking or sitting may be a subtle sign, whereas bruises or lacerations of the inner thighs or genitalia are more overt signs. Pain or itching in the genital area may indicate a sexually transmitted disease. Multiple decubiti without interventions suggest neglect. Be alert to the implication that "old people always get bed sores."

Box 51-2 CLUES TO ELDER ABUSE

Pattern of "health care shopping"
Series of missed appointments
Previous unexplained injuries
Presence of old and new bruises
Poor personal hygiene
Sexually transmitted diseases
Extreme mood changes
Depression
Fearfulness
Excessive concern with health care cost

Table 51-2 CLINICAL FINDINGS WITH ELDER ABUSE

TYPE OF ABUSE	CLINICAL FINDINGS
Physical	Bruises, welts, lacerations, fractures, burns, rope marks; medication overdose, inadequate medication; unexplained venereal disease or genital infection
Neglect	Dehydration, malnutrition, decubitus ulcers, poor personal hygiene, lack of compliance with medication regimens
Psychologic abuse	Berated verbally, harassed, intimidated, threatened punishment or deprivation; elder treated like an infant; isolated from family, friends, or activities
Psychologic neglect	Elder left alone for long periods; ignored or given the silent treatment; failure to provide companionship, changes in routine, news, or information
Financial or material abuse	Denial of a home for the elder; stolen money or possessions; coercion of the elder to sign contracts, assign durable power of attorney, purchase goods, or change the elder's will
	Lack of substantial care in the home despite adequate financial resources; patient confused about or unaware of financial situation or suddenly transfers assets to a family member

ASKING THE RIGHT QUESTIONS

When screening for elder abuse, the patient and suspected abuser should be interviewed separately. Begin with general questions about the patient's perception of safety in the home.

- Do you feel safe where you live?
- Do you need help taking care of yourself?
- Who prepares your meals?
- Who handles your checkbook?
- How many people are living in your home?

More specific questions about maltreatment might include the following:

- Do you have frequent disagreements with your caregiver?
- When you disagree, what happens?
- Are you ever physically hurt or confined to your room?
- Do you ever have to wait long periods for food or your medicine?
- Has anyone ever failed to answer your request for help?

When talking with the suspected abuser, empathy and an understanding approach go a long way in obtaining information about the patient's care environment. Try to identify specific issues that may present problems resulting from the patient's diagnosis. For example, close monitoring for skin breakdown in a patient with dementia and frequent episodes of incontinence is a challenge. In talking with this patient's caregiver you might say, "Caring for your father in this stage of his dementia must be a real challenge at times. Do you ever feel overwhelmed with the responsibility? How do you deal with it?" It is essential to avoid confrontation in this phase of the assessment.

INTERVENTION

Access is a major issue in assessment and intervention for alleged abuse or neglect of the elderly. The competent elder has the right to make his or her own personal care decisions. The elder may choose to stay in the abusive situation despite all efforts to effect a change. Victims of abuse often have both positive and negative feelings toward their abusers. Such ambivalence makes separation from the abuser difficult for the abuse victim.

The Older Americans Act of 1965 and its 1987 Amendment require each state to identify agencies involved in recognizing and treating abused, neglected, and exploited elders and to determine the need for appropriate services. Although all 50 states have adult protection legislation, mandatory reporting laws vary from state to state. Emergency nurses should be familiar with the reporting requirements for their specific state. The Older Americans Act Amendment of 2000 is the most recent reauthorization legislation. It provides for the first time critical and much-needed support for families caring for loved ones who are ill or disabled. This program includes respite care for family members struggling to care for older relatives at home and other needed services.

The primary goal of intervention is to protect the patient from immediate and future harm. A secondary—and equally important goal of intervention—is to break the cycle of mistreatment. The well-being of the abused individual must be considered concurrently with coping ability of the abuser.

Elder abuse is divided into two broad categories with regard to intervention in family-mediated abuse and neglect.[1] First are cases in which the elder has physical or mental impairment and is dependent on the family for daily care needs. The second group comprises individuals with minimal needs or care needs overshadowed by pathologic behavior of the caregiver. Potential intervention strategies include referrals to community agencies for continual monitoring of the situation, support services to decrease caregiver stress, close health care follow-up to prevent switching to another health care provider, reports to adult protective services with removal of the individual from a harmful environment, or use of 24-hour supervision through a home health agency.

Care needs of elders in the home increase over time; however, resources of the family in terms of psychosocial and financial reserves do not always increase at the same rate. Intervention requires a multidisciplinary team approach. Such a team is able to assess aspects of the situation such as physical injury, mental status, competency, financial irregularities, legality, treatment, assistance, protection, or prosecution. When there is a high degree of suspicion for elder abuse, consult social services or the responsible agency in your area. When appropriate, contact a home health agency to make an initial home assessment. In acute situations the elder may require shelter or protective care.

SUMMARY

The American population is living longer. As baby boomers enter their senior years, there are more and more seniors with increasing health problems who require assistance to perform simple activities of daily living. Caregivers are trapped between demands of a young family, career, and aging parents.

As children we are taught to honor our mothers and fathers and to respect and care for the elderly. The notion of frail elderly human beings facing a life of fear and pain caused by someone they love and trust is beyond our comprehension. Likewise, understanding the frustration, fear, and sadness of the person who has gone from being a child cared for and nurtured by a parent to being the adult caring for that parent as one would a small child is also difficult to accept. For health care professionals to successfully diagnose and treat elder abuse, a nonjudgmental, open, and caring attitude toward all those involved is essential.

References

1. All AC: A literature review: assessment and intervention in elder abuse, *J Gerontol Nurs,* 25, 1994.

2. Collins KA, Bennett AT, Hanzlick R. Elder abuse and neglect, *Arch Intern Med,* 2000, 160(11). Retrieved February 22, 2002 from the World Wide Web: http://archinte.gma-assn.org.

3. Elder Abuse Center: The basics: what is elder abuse? Retrieved February 22, 2002 from the World Wide Web: http://www.elderabusecenter.org.

4. Falzon AL et al: A 15 year retrospective review of homicide in the elderly, *J Forensic Sci* 43(2):371, 1998.

5. Hogstel MO et al: Elder abuse revisited, *J Gerontol Nurs* 25(7):10, 1999.

6. Jogerst GJ et al: Community characteristics associated with elder abuse, *J Amer Geriatr Soc* 48(5):513, 2000.

7. National Center on Elder Abuse at the American Public Health Services Association: National elder abuse incidence study, executive summary. (September 1998) Retrieved February 22, 2002 from the World Wide Web:http://www.aoa.gov/abusereport/default.htm.

8. National Institute of Justice (2000). Elder justice: medical forensic issues concerning abuse and neglect (draft and report). Retrieved February 22, 2002 from the World Wide Web: http://www.ojp.usdoj.gov.

9. U.S. Department of Justice: Elder abuse and neglect, statistical overview. Retrieved February 22, 2002 from the World Wide Web: http://www.djp.usdoj.gov.

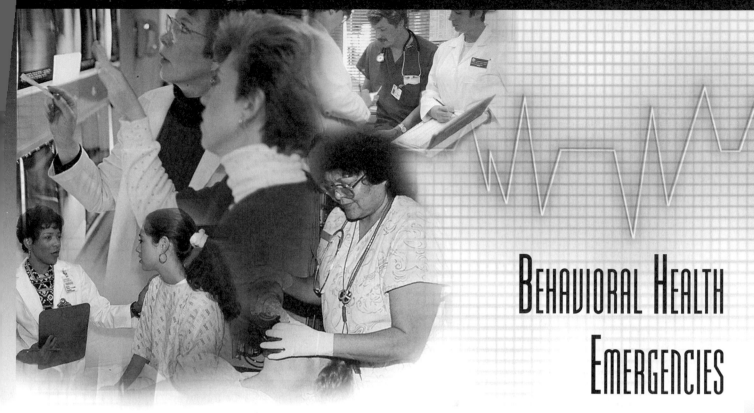

BEHAVIORAL HEALTH EMERGENCIES

STEVEN A. WEINMAN,
LORENE NEWBERRY

Psychosocial emergencies take many forms in the emergency department (ED). These patients may arrive in the ED with severe dysfunction of behavior, mood, thinking, or perception that represents a significant threat to life, daily living, or psychologic integrity. Severity is related to the patient's ability to function and adapt, but also depends on the person's support systems. Working with this type of patient requires patience, understanding, and flexibility. Comprehensive discussion of psychiatric emergencies is beyond the scope of this chapter. Therefore material presented herein focuses on those conditions seen more often in the ED—anxiety, panic disorder, depression, and schizophrenia. Anorexia nervosa and bulimia are also discussed.

ANXIETY

Anxiety is a complex feeling of apprehension, fear, and worry often accompanied by pulmonary, cardiac, and other physical sensations.[12] Types of anxiety disorders are listed in Box 52-1. Severe anxiety is seen in the ED most often as patients with panic attacks and panic disorders. Approximately 20% to 30% of individuals with panic disorders have persistent symptoms up to 10 years from the time of initial diagnosis and treatment. In some cultures panic attacks may involve fear of witchcraft or magic. Panic disorders have a bimodal distribution; one peak occurs in late adolescence, and a second, smaller peak occurs in the person's mid-30s. Phobic disorders, obsessive-compulsive disorders, and generalized anxiety disorder (GAD) tend to occur in late adolescence or the early 20s.[33] Panic disorder is discussed in greater detail later in this chapter.

A heightened physiologic response and elevated catecholamine levels play an important role in the normal physiologic response of the body to stress and anxiety. It has been hypothesized that disturbances in the cerebral cortex play a pathologic role in anxiety. The data specifically cite the limbic system (hypothalamus, septum, hippocampus, amygdala, cingulate), other neural bodies (thalamus, locus caeruleus, medial raphe nuclei, dental or interpositus nuclei of the cerebellum), and connections between these structures.[5]

Three neurotransmitters are associated with anxiety—norepinephrine, gamma-aminobutyric acid (GABA), and serotonin.[5] The efficacy of benzodiazepines in treating anxiety has implicated GABA in the pathophysiology of anxiety disorders. Drugs that affect norepinephrine such as tricyclic antidepressants and monoamine oxidase inhibitors are efficacious in treatment of several anxiety disorders. Data regarding serotonin are limited.

Assessment

Anxiety in its most severe form can be quite debilitating. The condition is categorized as mild, moderate, severe, or panic disorder. Organic illness, medications, drug abuse, and obvious psychotic causes of an anxious state must be ruled

---

Box 52-1 TYPES OF ANXIETY DISORDERS

Panic disorder with agoraphobia
Panic disorder without agoraphobia
General anxiety disorder
  Persistent fear, worry, or tension in the absence of panic attacks
  Disabling persistent worry out of proportion to impact of the feared event; typically revolves around routine life circumstances
  Occurs frequently with mood disorders such as major depression
  Tremulousness, shaking, insomnia, irritability, and restlessness noted
  Muscle tension, cold clammy hands, dry mouth, diaphoresis, nausea, diarrhea, urinary frequency
Obsessive-compulsive disorder
Phobic disorders
  Social phobia
  Specific phobia
  Agoraphobia without panic disorder
Posttraumatic stress disorder
Acute stress disorder
Anxiety disorder
  Related to general medical condition
Substance abuse anxiety disorder
Panic attacks
  Recurrent episodes of spontaneous, intense periods of anxiety
  Usually last less than 1 hour
  Often in significant distress

Box 52-2 DIFFERENTIAL DIAGNOSES IN ANXIETY DISORDERS

Alcohol and substance abuse
Angina
Congestive heart failure or pulmonary edema
Costochondritis
Depression or suicidal ideation
Hyperthyroidism, thyroid storm, Grave's disease
Hyperventilation syndrome
Hypoglycemia
Mitral valve prolapse
Myocardial infarction
Neoplasms (brain)
Neuropathies
Pneumonia
Pneumothorax
Pulmonary embolism
Schizophrenia
Tachydysrhythmias (sinus, atrial, junctional, and ventricular)
Toxicities (benzodiazepam, sympathomimetic, thyroid hormone)
Withdrawal syndromes

Evaluation of mental status can be especially helpful in distinguishing functional disorders from organic disorders. Assessment should include the following:

- Level of consciousness
- Affect
- Behavioral observation
- Speech pattern
- Level of attention
- Language comprehension
- Memory, calculation, and judgment

Anxiety states are associated with increased prevalence of other physical illnesses. Avoid falsely attributing somatic symptoms of anxiety to other medical conditions. Box 52-2 reviews potential differential diagnoses to be considered in patients with suspected anxiety disorders.

Laboratory tests to rule out physical illness include a complete blood count (CBC) with differential, serum chemistry profile, pregnancy test, and serum or urine screens for drugs. Specific serum endocrine panels are also available to diagnose illnesses such as hyperthyroidism. Cardiopulmonary disorders such as pneumonia, congestive heart failure, and pneumothorax can be ruled out through physical assessment and a chest x-ray. An electrocardiogram can identify tachydysrhythmias and myocardial infarction as the etiology of palpitations and other symptoms.

While remaining vigilant for life-threatening illness, emergency nurses should reassure patients suffering from anxiety. Place the patient in a calm, quiet room for formal evaluation. Rhythmic breathing, imagery techniques, and hypnotic suggestion have been used for patients with anxiety.

Treatment

Acute anxiety has been effectively treated with the passage of time, social support, and a short course of fast-acting

---

out and documented before treatment of anxiety. Patients require ED treatment for anxiety when they are in such an acutely anxious state that they pose a danger to themselves and others in the immediate vicinity. A thorough medical and psychiatric history is critical. Documentation should include any changes in behavior and somatic symptoms such as headaches, dizziness, disorientation, confusion, and syncope. Family and significant others are reliable sources of history for the patient with acute anxiety. Previous psychiatric illnesses and any current medical problems should be documented. Identify any agents that can cause anxiety (e.g., caffeine, nicotine, prescribed drugs, over-the-counter medications, illicit drugs, alcohol). Thorough physical assessment is required to identify potential life-threatening illnesses. The clinician should focus on signs and symptoms of anxiety; however, organic etiologies should be eliminated first. Diagnostic studies are used to rule out physical causes of anxiety such as metabolic disorders. Needle marks indicate illicit drug involvement, whereas hepatomegaly, ascites, and spider angioma suggest alcohol abuse.

A patient with a classic panic attack will experience at least four of the following symptoms—palpitations, diaphoresis, tremulousness, shortness of breath, chest pain, dizziness, nausea, abdominal discomfort, fear of injury or going crazy, derealization (perception of altered reality), and depersonalization (perception that one's body is surreal).

anxiolytics, preferably a benzodiazepine.[17] In chronic anxiety psychotherapy and anxiolytics are the recommended course. Chronic anxiety often requires a comprehensive approach using psychotherapy, counseling, and a wider spectrum of anxiolytics (e.g., benzodiazepines, buspirone, antidepressants). Short-acting benzodiazepines in parenteral form are most useful for acute treatment. Benzodiazepines should only be prescribed in motivated and cooperative individuals with reliable follow-up arrangements. Beta-blockers do not reduce intrinsic anxiety but may be beneficial in treatment of associated tachycardia. Buspirone may be initiated in the ED after consultation with a psychiatrist or the patient's primary care physician. Antidepressants have well-known pharmacologic profiles and could be useful in the patient with concomitant depression and anxiety. They have demonstrated benefit as adjunct agents in the treatment of GAD. Antidepressants have been relegated to long-term outpatient use for other chronic anxiety disorders.

Anxiety disorders are often chronic illnesses and require follow-up psychiatric intervention for successful treatment. Any patient with anxiety who presents with suicidal ideation, homicidal ideation, or acute psychosis require emergent psychiatric consultation.[23] Some studies report the failure rate for diagnosing anxiety disorders as high as 50%.[34] This can result in overutilization of health care resources and increased morbidity and mortality rates for anxiety disorders and comorbid medical conditions. Listening to the patient and allowing expression of concern makes the patient feel safe.

PANIC DISORDERS

Understanding panic disorder (PD) is important for emergency nurses because patients with PD frequently present to the ED with various somatic complaints. As many as 70% of PD patients are unrecognized, so very few are referred to mental health professionals for appropriate follow-up.[4] These patients have a fourfold higher risk of alcohol abuse and eighteenfold higher risk of suicide than the general population. Some studies do suggest panic disorder itself is not a risk factor for suicide in the absence of other risks such as affective disorders, substance abuse, eating disorders, and personality disorders. Serious medical problems—such as asthma—cardiac dysrhythmia, or metabolic disturbances—such as hypoglycemia, hypoxia, and thyroid storm—can mimic panic attack. After exclusion of somatic disease and other psychiatric disorders, confirmation of the diagnosis with a brief mental status screening examination and initiation of appropriate treatment and referral is time- and cost-effective in patients with high rates of medical resource utilization.

PD appears to be a genetically inherited neurochemical dysfunction that involves autonomic imbalance, increased adenosine receptor function, increased cortisol, diminished benzodiazepine receptor function and disturbances in serotonin, norepinephrine, GABA, dopamine, cholecystokinin,

---

Box 52-3 DIFFERENTIAL DIAGNOSES IN PANIC DISORDER

Angina and myocardial infarction (e.g., dyspnea, chest pain, palpitations, diaphoresis)
Cardiac dysrhythmia (e.g., palpitations, dyspnea, syncope)
Mitral valve prolapse
Pulmonary embolus (e.g., dyspnea, hyperpnea, chest pain)
Asthma (e.g., dyspnea, wheezing)
Hyperthyroidism (e.g., palpitations, diaphoresis, tachycardia, heat intolerance)
Hypoglycemia or hyperglycemia
Pheochromocytoma (e.g., headache, diaphoresis, hypertension)
Hypoparathyroidism (e.g., muscle cramps, paresthesias)
Transient ischemic attack
Seizure disorder
Drug toxicity (e.g., stimulants, hallucinogens)

---

and interleukin-1-beta. Some theorize that PD may represent a state of chronic hyperventilation and carbon dioxide (CO_2) receptor hypersensitivity.

Positron emission tomography (PET) scanning has demonstrated increased flow in the right parahippocampal region of panicky patients. Magnetic resonance imaging (MRI) has demonstrated smaller temporal lobe volume despite normal hippocampal volume in these patients. In experimental settings symptoms can be elicited in panic subjects by hyperventilation, inhalation of CO_2, caffeine consumption, or intravenous infusions of sodium lactate, cholecystokinin, isoproterenol, or flumazenil.

Other conditions found in the patient with PD include depression, obsessive-compulsive disorder, specific phobias, social phobia, agoraphobia (fear of being unsafe in public settings), irritable bowel syndrome, migraine, mitral valve prolapse, and alcohol and drug abuse. Lower oxygen consumption and exercise tolerance than the general population has been identified in patients with PD.

Symptoms of PD create a significant hindrance in lifestyle for many patients. Those with agoraphobia may be unable to travel alone, be in crowds, malls, or on public transportation. Unemployment, depression, substance abuse, and suicide are also common. Studies have found PD present in 30% of patients with chest pain and normal angiograms, 5% to 40% of asthmatics, 15% of headache patients, 20% of epilepsy patients, 8% to 15% of patients in alcohol treatment programs, and 10% of patients in primary care settings.[14]

Panic attacks may be triggered by injury, surgery, illness, interpersonal conflict, or personal loss. Use of stimulants such as caffeine, decongestants, cocaine, and sympathomimetics (e.g., amphetamine) can precipitate panic attacks in susceptible individuals.[14] Box 52-3 highlights differential diagnoses that should be ruled out in patients with suspected PD. Bouts of panic can also occur in certain settings, such as stores and public transportation, especially in patients with agoraphobia.

> **Box 52-4   SYSTEMIC MANIFESTATIONS OF PANIC DISORDER**
>
> Palpitations, trembling, shaking, sweating
> Shortness of breath or feeling of smothering or choking
> Chest pain or discomfort, nausea, or abdominal distress
> Dizzy, unsteady, lightheaded, or faint
> Derealization (feeling of unreality)
> Depersonalization (being detached from oneself)
> Fear of dying and of losing control or going crazy (some
>   authors describe a variant of panic disorder without fear)
> Paresthesias (numbness or tingling sensations)

Assessment

Patients in the throes of a panic attack complain of sudden onset of fear or discomfort, typically peaking in 10 minutes. Attacks are associated with a constellation of systemic symptoms (Box 52-4).

During an acute episode patients have the urge to flee or escape—they experience a strong sense of impending doom as though they are dying from a heart attack or suffocation. Other symptoms include headache, cold hands, diarrhea, insomnia, fatigue, intrusive thoughts, and ruminations. Patients with PD have recurring episodes of panic with fear of recurrent attacks causing significant behavioral changes (avoiding situations or locations) and worry about implications of the attack or its consequences (e.g., losing control, going crazy, dying). Attacks can lead to changes in personality traits, characterized by increasing passivity, dependence, or withdrawal.

Assessment should include precipitating events, suicidal ideation or plan, phobias, agoraphobia, obsessive-compulsive behavior, and involvement of alcohol, illicit drugs, and medications with stimulatory effects (e.g., caffeine). Determination of a family history of panic or other psychiatric illness is indicated.

Patients with PD may manifest any one of several physical symptoms. They appear anxious and may have cool, clammy skin. Heart rate and respiratory rate are usually elevated; however, blood pressure and temperature are usually normal. Hyperventilation may be difficult to detect by observing breathing because respiratory rate and tidal volume may appear normal.

Room air pulse oximetry values are normal to high-normal; however, arterial blood gas analysis is indicated to rule out the presence of acid-base abnormalities. Hypoxemia with hypocapnia or a widened A-a gradient should raise the possibility of pulmonary embolus in the patient who appears to be having a panic attack. Laboratory studies that may be helpful in excluding other medical disorders include serum electrolytes to exclude hypokalemia and acidosis; serum glucose to exclude hypoglycemia; cardiac markers in patients suspected of acute coronary syndromes; hemoglobin in patients with near-syncope; thyroid-stimulating hormone in patients suspected of hyperthyroidism; and urine toxicology screen for amphetamines, cocaine, and phencyclidine in patients suspected of intoxication.[29]

Chest x-rays are useful in excluding various causes of dyspnea. An electrocardiogram (ECG) should be inspected for signs of ventricular pre-excitation (short PR and delta wave) and long QT interval in patients with palpitations and for ischemia, infarction, or pericarditis patterns in patients with chest pain—conditions that share symptomatology with or may precipitate a panic attack.

Treatment

Patients presenting to the ED that appear anxious but also complain of chest pain, dyspnea, palpitations, or near-syncope should be treated as they clinically present. Place the patient on oxygen and monitor pulse oximetry, ECG, and frequent vital signs. PD patients require frequent reassurance and explanation; many may benefit from social service intervention after more serious organic causes of symptoms are ruled out. A major component of therapy involves education that the symptoms are neither from a serious medical condition nor from mental deficiency, but rather from a chemical imbalance in the fight-or-flight response.

The ED staff should listen, remain empathic, and be nonargumentative with these patients. Statements such as "It's nothing serious" and "It's related to stress" can be misinterpreted as implying lack of understanding and concern. Intravenous medication (e.g., Ativan, 0.5 mg intravenously [IV] every 20 minutes) may be necessary in PD patients who, as a result of subsequent poor impulse control, pose a risk to themselves or to those around them.[10] PD patients are best served by referral to a qualified mental health professional who can establish constructive rapport with the patient and follow his or her needs on a long-term basis before beginning anxiolytic medications.

Aside from IV medications required to treat acute anxiety states in the ED, the use of pharmacotherapy for panic disorder patients should, in most instances, be deferred to the psychiatrist following the patient long-term. Benzodiazepines are optimal for ED and outpatient abortive therapy because of their immediate antipanic effects.[35] Selective serotonin reuptake inhibitors (SSRIs) are becoming first-line preventive agents in PD, with tricyclic antidepressants (TCAs) and monoamine oxidase inhibitors (MAOIs) used in refractory cases. Coexisting disorders may influence medication choice (e.g., MAOIs, clonazepam, and SSRIs for social phobia; SSRIs or Anafranil for obsessive-compulsive disorder; TCAs for depression).[10] Beta-blockers, clonidine, and buspirone, although promising in theory, have had poor efficacy in PD.[36]

Institution of treatment for PD in the ED is appropriate in a very limited subset of PD patients. Those who are very motivated, cooperative, and possess an understanding of the psychologic nature of their disorder and whose symptoms are elicited as a response to temporary stress are good candidates. In such cases pharmacotherapy with an oral benzodiazepine for no longer than 1 week may be appropriate.

Inpatient treatment is necessary in patients with suicidal ideation and a suicide plan, serious alcohol or sedative withdrawal symptoms, or when potential medical disorders warrant admission (e.g., unstable angina, acute myocardial ischemia). Follow-up with a chemical dependence treatment specialist should be arranged when indicated. All discharged PD patients should be referred to a psychiatrist, psychologist, or other mental health professional.

DEPRESSION

Depression is a potentially life-threatening mood disorder that afflicts up to 10% of the population.[12,25] This holistic disorder affects the body, feelings, thoughts, and behaviors. Considerable pain and suffering significantly affect the individual's ability to function. It is important to note that depression also adversely affects significant others, sometimes destroying family relationships or work dynamics between the patient and others. The economic cost of depressive illness is estimated at $30 to $44 billion a year in the United States alone. The human cost cannot be overestimated. As many as two thirds of the people suffering from depression do not realize they have a treatable illness and therefore do not seek treatment. A real ignorance exists on the part of the public and many health care providers as to the legitimacy of this mental illness.

An estimated 5% to 20% of people will experience depression at some time in their life. Mortality of depression is measurable and is the direct result of suicide, the ninth leading cause of death in the United States.[1] Almost all those who kill themselves intentionally have a diagnosable mental disorder with or without substance abuse.[18] Ironically, substance abuse is often the result of attempted self-treatment for symptoms of depression. The majority of suicide attempts are expressions of extreme distress, not bids for attention.[2]

The etiology of depression is multifactorial but is thought to involve changes in receptor-neurotransmitter relationships in the limbic system of the brain. The condition may be due to biologic, physiologic, genetic, or psychosocial factors. Medications (prescription, over-the-counter, recreational, and herbals) should also be considered. Serotonin and norepinephrine are the primary neurotransmitters involved, although dopamine has also been related to depression. A family history of depression is common. Bipolar disorder has a prominent depressive phase but is a different clinical entity from depression.

Assessment

Depression is often difficult to diagnose because it can manifest in many different forms. Box 52-5 highlights the symptoms of depression. To establish the diagnosis of major depression, a patient must express at least one primary symptom and at least five secondary symptoms. Such disturbances must be present almost daily for at least 2 weeks; however, symptoms can last for months or years. The indi-

---

Box 52-5   **SYMPTOMS ASSOCIATED WITH DEPRESSION**

PRIMARY SYMPTOMS

Persistent sadness
Loss of pleasure in usual activities (anhedonia)

SECONDARY SYMPTOMS

Feel helpless, guilty, or worthless
Crying, hopeless, or persistently pessimistic
Fatigue or decreased energy
Loss of memory, concentration, or decision-making capability
Restless, irritable
Sleep disturbances
Change in appetite or weight
Physical symptoms that do not respond to treatment (especially pain and gastrointestinal complaints)
Thoughts of suicide, death, or suicide attempts
Poor self-image (e.g., self-reproach)

Box 52-6   **PSYCHOMOTOR SIGNS OF DEPRESSION**

Psychomotor retardation or agitation (e.g., slowed speech, sighs, long pauses)
Slowed body movements, even to the extent of motionlessness or catatonia
Pacing, wringing hands, and pulling on hair
Preoccupation
Lack of eye contact
Tearfulness
Self-deprecatory manner
Memory loss, poor concentration, and poor abstract reasoning

---

vidual may experience significant personality changes during this period, making it difficult for others to feel charitable toward the sufferer. Some symptoms are so disabling they interfere with the ability to function from day to day. In severe cases patients may be unable to eat or leave their beds. Box 52-6 highlights psychomotor symptoms of depression. Episodes may occur only once in a lifetime, may be recurrent, or chronic and longstanding. Occasionally symptoms are precipitated by life crises or other illnesses, whereas at other times depression can occur at random. Clinical depression often occurs concurrently with other medical illnesses and worsens the prognosis for these illnesses.

In addition to depression, alcohol and substance abuse, impulsiveness, and certain familial factors are highly associated with risk for suicide.[18] Familial factors include history of mental illness or substance abuse, suicide, family violence of any type, and separation or divorce. Other risk factors include prior suicide attempts, presence of a firearm in the home, incarceration, and exposure to suicidal behavior of family members, peers, celebrities, or even highly publicized fictional characters.

Box 52-7   DIFFERENTIAL DIAGNOSES IN DEPRESSION

Alcohol or substance abuse
Chronic fatigue syndrome
Electrolyte disturbances of sodium, magnesium, phosphorus
Hypothermia
Liver failure
Medication side effects
Medication abuse or overdose
Medication interactions (especially in the elderly)
Metabolic disorders of the parathyroid, pituitary, or thyroid
Myxedema coma
Renal failure (acute or chronic)
Vitamin deficiency
Withdrawal syndrome

Box 52-8   LABORATORY STUDIES IN PATIENTS WITH DEPRESSION

Complete blood count
Electrolytes, including calcium, phosphate, magnesium
Blood urea nitrogen and creatinine
Calcium
Serum toxicology screen
Thyroid function tests

The emergency nurses's responsibility when caring for a patient with depression is to maintain a high index of suspicion for the diagnosis, especially in populations at risk for suicide. Primary at-risk populations include young adults and the elderly; however, depression and suicide can occur in any age group, including children.[28] Depression should be suspected as an underlying factor in drug overdose (including alcohol), self-inflicted injury, or intentionally inflicted injury when the assailant is known to the victim. In any such patient, screening for diagnostic symptoms of major depression and suicide is essential.

When a patient has contemplated or attempted suicide, the patient should be carefully asessed to determine the presence of suicidal ideation and accessible means and plans.[15] Psychiatric evaluation should occur only after this screening evaluation is complete and all acute medical complications are addressed.

Treatment

Depression is a clinical diagnosis; however, symptoms associated with depression may be the result of medications, metabolic disorders, and other nutritional abnormalities. Assessment and treatment of the person with depression should rule out various treatment conditions. Box 52-7 lists differential diagnoses for the patient with depression. Laboratory tests are primarily used to rule out other diagnoses such as renal failure, hypoglycemia, and drug toxicity (Box 52-8). Additional diagnostic studies include computed tomography (CT), MRI, and electroencephalogram to rule out organic brain syndrome or other central nervous system (CNS) problems. Inpatient care is recommended when there is significant concern for the patient's safety.

SCHIZOPHRENIA

Insanity, psychosis, madness . . . regardless of how it is labeled, schizophrenia is a chronic psychotic disorder with onset typically in adolescence or young adulthood. Schizophrenia results in fluctuating, gradually deteriorating, or relatively stable disturbances in thinking, behavior, and perception. These disturbances include the presence of both positive and negative symptoms. Positive symptoms include delusions, hallucinations, and disorganized speech and behavior; negative symptoms include poverty of speech, flattened affect, and social withdrawal.

Current diagnostic requirements are met if the syndrome continues for at least 6 months with at least 1 month in which active symptoms are present and these symptoms result in significant impairment of occupational and social functioning. Other schizophrenia-related disorders have a milder, less global, or more transient course, but share strong familial association with schizophrenia.

The causes of schizophrenia are multifactorial and include genetically inherited brain abnormalities or embryonic developmental insult, perhaps in concert with psychosocial stressors. Hallucinogenic or sympathomimetic drug abuse is a frequent precipitating or contributing factor. Psychosocial stresses may interact with the etiology and expression of the disorder.

Schizophrenia is now conceptualized as a broad syndrome expressed by a heterogeneous group of brain disorders rather than as a single disease entity. In addition, schizophrenia is viewed as the most severe end of a spectrum of schizophrenia-related disorders. Although placed in the category of "functional" psychiatric disorders, schizophrenia is primarily associated with abnormalities of brain neurochemistry and neuroanatomy.

Schizophrenics occupy up to 25% of all hospital psychiatric beds at any given time.[25] The condition is devastating, with a profound effect on family and the patient's social and occupational life. Premature death may result from poor health maintenance, substance abuse, poverty, and homelessness. Onset of symptoms is insidious in about half of all patients. The prodromal phase can begin years before the full-blown syndrome. It is characterized by losses of previously achieved functioning in home, society, and occupation (e.g., poor school or work performance, deterioration of hygiene and appearance, decreasing emotional connections with others, behaviors considered odd for this individual).

Gradual onset predicts a more severe and chronic illness course, whereas abrupt onset of hallucinations and delusional, bizarre, or disorganized thinking in previously functioning patients can lead to better intermediate and long-term outcome. Such patients arrive in the ED in a psychotic crisis requiring acute management, often without having

---

Box 52-9 DIFFERENTIAL DIAGNOSES IN SCHIZOPHRENIA

Central nervous system infection
Delerium, dementia, and amnesia
Depression
Neuroleptic malignant syndrome
Panic disorder
Personality disorder
Poisonings or toxicity
Hallucinogenic mushrooms
Hallucinogens
Phencyclidine
Stimulants
Sympathomimetics

Box 52-10 COMMON BEHAVIORAL MANIFESTATIONS OF SCHIZOPHRENIA

Delusions: Bizarre or illogical false beliefs that often have a paranoid, grandiose, persecutory or religious flavor; or false interpretation of normal perceptions
Hallucinations: Typically auditory (visual or tactile strongly suggest organic etiology), often involving malevolent or taunting voices commenting on the patient's actions or character, often with sexual flavor; giving commands (command hallucinations); two or more voices discussing or arguing with each other; audible thoughts; thought withdrawal (feeling that thoughts are being removed from head); thought broadcasting or thought interference by outside agent
Disorganized speech: Tangential, incoherent, rambling; neologisms (new word creation); loosening of associations
Grossly disorganized or catatonic behavior

---

been previously diagnosed with a psychiatric illness. They present diagnostic dilemmas regarding organic versus psychiatric etiology and primary psychotic versus affective disorder that may be further complicated by the presence of alcohol or drug intoxication.

Because of the variability of symptom expression and diagnostic requirements of chronicity, the diagnosis of schizophrenia in the ED should be provisional at best. As a diagnosis-by-exclusion, schizophrenia must be distinguished from the numerous psychiatric and organic disorders that also lead to psychotic behaviors. Box 52-9 lists differential diagnoses for schizophrenia.

Assessment

The most common etiologies for severe mental status changes in the ED are organic, not psychiatric. They include medications, drug intoxication, drug withdrawal syndromes, and general medical illnesses causing delirium.[18] The presence of an affective disorder (e.g., major depression, bipolar disorder, schizoaffective disorder) must be excluded. Conditions that can be mistaken for schizophrenia have very different prognoses and therapies. In addition, an organic etiology (e.g., drug intoxication, medical illness) must be ruled out. Commonly, problems with antipsychotic medications are the chief complaint. Medical illness can cause or complicate a psychotic process. Obtain a complete medication history; many commonly prescribed medicines can cause psychotic reactions.

Psychiatric and organic illness can coexist and interact at the same time in the same patient. Acute psychiatric symptoms and difficulty obtaining a reliable history can mask serious organic illness. A brief medical clearance examination is limited in usefulness and is insufficient to rule out organic etiologies. History obtained in the ED may relate to a complication of treatment (medication side effects) or crisis arising from socioeconomic factors secondary to schizophrenia, such as poverty, homelessness, social isolation, and failure of support systems. Box 52-10 reviews common behavioral manifestations of schizophrenia.

Information should be elicited about the actual or potential likelihood for acts of violence. Acutely psychotic patients presenting to the ED place other patients and staff in danger. A paranoid schizophrenic, in response to delusions and command hallucinations, can be extremely dangerous and unpredictable. Identify threats made to others, expressions of suicidal intent, and possession of weapons at home or on the person.

The schizophrenic patient may be wildly agitated, combative, withdrawn, or severely catatonic. Conversely, they may appear rational, cooperative, and well controlled. Blunting of affect may be noted or the person may be subtly odd, unkempt, or grossly bizarre in manner, dress, or affect. Physical examination with attention to vital signs, pupillary findings, hydration status, and mental status should be performed. Diagnostic evaluation is required when organic etiology or drug intoxication may be related to mental status changes.

Pay particular attention to fever (tachycardia can be a sign of neuroleptic malignant syndrome), heat stroke (antipsychotics inhibit sweating), and other medical illness. Look for dystonia, akathesia, tremor, and muscle rigidity. Tardive dyskinesia is a common, often irreversible sequela of long-term (and sometimes brief) antipsychotic use. The condition is characterized by uncontrollable tongue thrusting, lip smacking, and facial grimacing. Mental status is usually normal with sensorium clear and the person oriented to person, place, and time. Assess attention, language, memory, constructions, and executive functions.

Treatment

There are no specific laboratory findings diagnostic of schizophrenia; however, some studies may be necessary to rule out organic causes for psychosis or to uncover complications of schizophrenia and its treatment. Blood levels of certain psychiatric drugs, specifically lithium and mood-stabilizing antiseizure medications, can confirm compliance or indicate toxicity. Serum alcohol and toxicology tests can be useful when substance abuse is suspected. A finger stick glucose test is a rapid, inexpensive method of ruling out a diabetic emergency masquerading as an exacerbation of a psychotic illness. Similarly, oxygen saturation can disclose hypoxia as a potential cause of behavioral or CNS disturbances. Electrolytes may reveal hyponatremia secondary to water intoxication (psychogenic polydipsia), which is common in undertreated or refractory schizophrenia.

A CT scan and MRI scan can disclose abnormalities of brain structure and function in the schizophrenic patient. Although they are of interest for research, such studies have very narrow clinical relevance.

Evolving from the efficacy of modern antipsychotic medications and the subsequent widespread budget cutting of psychiatric services over the past two decades, deinstitutionalization of the schizophrenic patient has had a major impact on emergency nursing. The schizophrenic patient is now a frequent visitor to the ED, with problems ranging from disease exacerbation, medication noncompliance, or side effects to medical and socioeconomic crises arising from substance abuse, poverty, homelessness and failed support systems.

Care for the schizophrenic patient in the ED may be limited to diagnosis and treatment of an urgent or nonurgent medical complaint. In some patients brief medical evaluation before psychiatric, crisis intervention, or social service consultation is adequate. For others, evaluation and treatment of a psychiatric drug adverse reaction is necessary. Physical and chemical restraint is indicated when the patient represents an immediate threat to self or others and alternatives have failed. Box 52-11 highlights current guidelines for use of restraint or seclusion in the ED. Figure 52-1 provides a sample restraint or seclusion flowsheet for use in the ED.

Crisis liaison teams, typically made up of clinical social workers, psychologists, or psychiatric nurses, are available in many EDs 24 hours a day through the hospital or local psychiatric agencies. Psychiatry consultation should be used as soon as organic processes are ruled out to correctly diagnose or safely treat a severely disturbed schizophrenic patient.

Antipsychotic medications (previously referred to as neuroleptics or major tranquilizers), have revolutionized the treatment of and prognosis for schizophrenia. These agents block dopamine receptors in the brain, whereas newer atypical agents also affect serotonin transmission. The newer agents (e.g., risperidone, clozapine, olanzapine, quetiapine) are less likely to produce dystonia and tardive dyskinesia and more likely to improve negative symptoms. However, with the possible exception of clozapine, they are no more effective than traditional agents (e.g., haloperidol, fluphenazine) in the treatment-resistant patient. Benzodiazepines also have a role in schizophrenia, especially for emergency care of the acutely psychotic patient. Anticholinergic medications are used to counteract dystonic and Parkinsonian side-effects (extra-pyramidal symptoms [EPS]) of antipsy-

Box 52-11 RESTRAINT OR SECLUSION GUIDELINES

Restraint or seclusion should be used only when other alternatives have been exhausted or when there is an immediate threat to life.

Reasons for restraint or seclusion should be documented, specifying immediate threat to life or failure of other methods.

Orders must be time-specific. "Restrain as needed" and "restrain for the duration of the visit" are not acceptable orders.

Continuous face-to-face observation is required for the first hour of restraint or seclusion. Remote observation by camera is not acceptable.

Safety and well-being must be assessed every 15 minutes after the first hour.

chotics, particularly higher potency agents which are less sedating but more likely to produce EPS.

Schizophrenia is a chronic and disabling illness. Fewer than 20% of patients recover fully from a single psychotic episode; a few have little or no recovery from the first episode and persist with chronic, pervasive psychotic illness. Approximately 60% will recover sufficiently to lead functional lives but only 50% of those will be employed. Approximately 30% remain severely and permanently handicapped with 10% being chronically hospitalized. Rapid and aggressive medication therapy of acute psychotic episodes is correlated with better overall prognosis.

ANOREXIA NERVOSA

Anorexia nervosa is an eating disorder characterized by severe weight loss to the point of significant physiologic consequences. Diagnostic criteria include the following:

- Intense fear of obesity despite slenderness
- Overwhelming body-image perception of being fat
- Weight loss of at least 25% from baseline or failure to gain weight appropriately (resulting in weight 25% less than would be expected from the patient's previous growth curve)
- Absence of other physical illnesses to explain weight loss or altered body-image perception
- At least 3 weeks of secondary amenorrhea or primary amenorrhea in a prepubescent adolescent[24]

Associated physical characteristics include excessive physical activity, denial of hunger in the face of starvation, academic success, asexual behavior, and history of extreme weight loss methods (e.g., diuretics, laxatives, amphetamines, emetics). Psychiatric characteristics include excessive dependency needs, developmental immaturity, behavior favoring isolation, obsessive-compulsive behavior, and constriction of affect. Patients with anorexia nervosa generally fall into two categories—those with extreme food restriction and those with food binge and purge behavior.

Anorexia nervosa is thought to result from psychologic, biologic, and societal stresses involving sexual development

WELLSTAR Health System

Emergency Services
Restraint/Seclusion Flowsheet

☐ Cobb   ☐ Kennestone
☐ Douglas ☐ Paulding

Patient Sticker

Reason for Restraint/Seclusion	Type Restraint	Seclusion	Patient/Belongings
☐ Self-Harm ☐ Harm to Others/Surroundings Other behavior(s):	☐ Soft ☐ Non-disposable ☐ 2pt ☐ 4pt ☐ Safety Vest	Room _____ ☐ Camera	Searched as appropriate ☐ Patient ☐ Belongings Items removed: _____

Less Restrictive Measures   ☐ Contraindicated – Immediate Restraint Required

☐ Utilized without success (Talking down, family at bedside, security in attendance)

Signature of RN Initiating Restraint or Seclusion: _____

Given to ☐ Family ☐ Security

PHYSICIAN RESTRAINT/SECLUSION ORDERS – NO PRN ORDERS ALLOWED.

☐ Restrain patient _____ hrs (<24).[1]   ☐ Restrain patient 24 hrs.[1]   ☐ Seclude adult _____ hrs (<4).[2]   ☐ Seclude adolescent (9-17) ___ hrs (<2).[2]
☐ Seclude child <9 for one hour only.[2]

Time _____   Date _____   MD Signature: _____

Time	Face to Face Observation may be done by an RN, LPN, NCA, HCW, or security personnel.	Comments	Initials
	Placed in Seclusion or Restraint – Continuous Face-to-Face Observation Begins		
	First Hour of Seclusion or Restraint finished – Continuous Face-to-Face Observation Ends		

Time	Seclusion, 4pt, Non-disposable[3] Safety, Visual Q 15 minutes	2 point restraints[3] Safety, Visual Q 30 minutes	Complete on Restraints and Seclusion[3]			Complete for Restrained Patients[3]			Comments	Initials
			LOC Q2hr	Fluids Q 2hr	Toilet Q 2hr	Circulation Q 2hr	ROM Q 2hrs	Release Q 2 hrs		

Restraints and/or Seclusion Discontinued

☐ Reassessed – patient continues to need restraint. (Reassess at least every 8 hours for restraints– more often if condition improves.)

☐ Reassessed – patient continues to need seclusion. (Reassess according to time limits for specified by order.)

☐ Documentation continued on next page.   ☐ Patient transferred. Documentation to continue on inpatient restraint flow sheet.

[1] Physician must assess patient for continued restraint at the end of the time frame identified in the original order.

[2] Physician must assess patient & write new seclusion orders – adults every 4 hrs, adolescents (9 – 17) every 2 hrs, children < 9 every hr.

[3] Behavior codes for above assessment are listed on back.

Initials	Signature/Title	Initials	Signature/Title	Initials	Signature/Title

ITEM #2096 WS00097   WHITE - Medical Record Copy   PINK - ER Charge Nurse Copy   (Rev. 11/00)

FIGURE 52-1   Sample restraint or seclusion flowsheet for use in the emergency department. (Courtesy Wellstar Emergency Services.)

at puberty. There is a high incidence of premorbid anxiety disorder in prepubescent patients who subsequently develop anorexia nervosa. The patient's altered body image results in a perception of fatness. Attempts to correct this flaw through food restriction or progressive purging lead to progressive starvation. Modern preoccupation with slenderness and beauty is believed to contribute greatly to the mindset of slenderness in girls and young women.

Anorexia malnutrition causes protein deficiency and disrupts multiple organ systems. Other nutritional deficiencies including hypoglycemia, severe loss of fat stores, and multiple vitamin deficiencies follow.

Cardiovascular effects of anorexia include atrial and ventricular tachydysrhythmias, bradycardia, orthostatic hypotension, and shock. Renal aberrations lead to decreased glomular filtration rate, elevated blood urea nitrogen, edema, metabolic acidosis, hypokalemia, and hypochloremic alkalosis resulting from vomiting. Gastrointestinal findings include constipation, delayed gastric emptying, gastric dilation and rupture, dental enamel erosion, esophagitis, and Mallory-Weiss tears. Bone marrow suppression leading to platelet, erythrocyte, and leukocyte abnormalities have been reported.

Anorexia nervosa occurs in approximately 1 of 100 adolescent females and is most frequently found in middle- and upper-class families. Recent studies suggest there is no increased incidence in anorexia nervosa over the last four decades. There does appear to be a familial component to the disease.

Suspect anorexia in patients presenting with extreme weight loss and history of food refusal, amenorrhea, dehydration in an otherwise healthy individual, flat affect, or near-catatonic behavior. Patients may be depressed, so the risk of suicide should be carefully assessed. Obtain a mental health history because there is a strong association with depression and substance abuse.

Box 52-12	**DIFFERENTIAL DIAGNOSES IN ANOREXIA NERVOSA**

Adrenal insufficiency or adrenal crisis
Alcohol and substance abuse
Ketoacidosis (alcoholic and diabetic)
Anemia
Anxiety
Bowel obstruction (large and small)
Conversion disorder
Chronic infection
Depression or suicidal ideation
Diabetes (type 1 and 2)
Gastroenteritis
Hyperthyroidism, thyroid storm, Grave's Disease
Inflammatory bowel disease
Malabsorption syndromes
Malignancy
Metabolic acidosis
Pediatrics, dehydration
Schizophrenia
Shock

Assessment

The most striking physical attribute in patients with moderate to severe anorexia is their cachectic appearance. Physical examination may reveal hypothermia, peripheral edema, and thinning hair.[16] Behaviorally, these patients have a flat affect and display psychomotor alterations. Physical and behavioral symptoms also occur in other conditions so it is important to rule out potentially treatable causes (Box 52-12).

A CBC may reveal normocytic, normochromic anemia resulting from bone marrow suppression from starvation. Serum chemisitries often indicate varying degrees of hypokalemia from laxative abuse. In addition, dehydration can cause significant electrolyte abnormalities including hyponatremia. Hypocalcemia from dietary deficiency of calcium or associated protein deficiency also occur. Beta-human chorionic gonadotropin can determine when pregnancy is the cause of vomiting and electrolyte abnormalities. Urinalysis is used to rule out urinary tract infections, dehydration, or renal acidosis. Positive fecal occult blood suggests esophagitis, gastritis, or repetitive colonic trauma from laxative abuse and a bleeding disorder or severe protein malnutrition. Serum erythrocyte sedimentation rate and thyroid function tests are unlikely to alter ED management but may be ordered to rule out inflammatory or endocrine pathologic processes.

An ECG should be obtained because anorexia can precipitate several heart rhythm disturbances. Recognized ECG changes include nonspecific ST and T wave abnormalities, atrial or ventricular tachydysrhythmias, idioventricular conduction delay, heart block, nodal rhythms, ventricular escape, premature ventricular contractions, and prolonged QTc interval. These abnormalities are attributable to starvation, ipecac toxicity, electrolyte, and neuroendocrine abnormalities.

Rib fractures from repetitive vomiting in the presence of hypocalcemia do occur, so a chest x-ray should be obtained. Cardiomegaly from ipecac toxicity or malnutrition has been noted in many patients. Electrolyte disturbances or malnutrition can lead to development of an ileus, so abdominal x-rays are often obtained.

Treatment

Care in the ED may include rehydration, correction of electrolyte abnormalities, and appropriate referral for continuing medical and psychiatric treatment.[31] Consultations with psychiatry and adolescent medicine specialists are recommended for inpatient care and to facilitate outpatient follow-up care.

No specific medications have been shown to alleviate the disordered body-image characteristic of anorexia. For nutritional therapy, forced feedings with total parenteral nutrition or tube feedings may be used to replace nutrients, stabilize nutrient deficiency syndromes, and alter mood when the patient becomes nutritionally replenished.

BULIMIA

Bulimia nervosa is an eating disorder characterized by eating binges followed by self-induced vomiting, laxative or diuretic abuse, prolonged fasting, or excessive exercise.[7] The patient with binge eating exhibits the following characteristics:

1. Eating, in a discrete period of time (e.g., within any 2-hour period), an amount of food that is definitely larger than most people would eat during a similar period of time under similar circumstances.
2. A perceived lack of control over eating during the episode (i.e., a feeling that one cannot stop eating or cannot control what or how much one is eating).

Some patients with anorexia nervosa also manifest bulimia; however, patients with bulimia have a normal weight or are overweight. Recurrent inappropriate compensatory behavior is used to prevent weight gain (e.g., self-induced vomiting; misuse of laxatives, diuretics, enemas, or other medication; fasting; excessive exercise). Binge eating and inappropriate compensatory behaviors occur at least twice a week for 3 months on average.[13] Self-evaluation is unduly influenced by body shape and weight.

Bulimia nervosa is categorized as purging type when the person regularly engages in self-induced vomiting or misuse of laxatives, diuretics, or enemas. If other inappropriate compensatory behaviors, such as fasting or excessive exercise, are used without self-induced vomiting or misuse of laxatives, diuretics, or enemas, the diagnosis is bulimia nervosa, nonpurging type. Individuals who binge eat without regular use of characteristic inappropriate compensatory behaviors of bulimia nervosa are included under the category of eating disorders not otherwise specified.

It has been reported that 5% to 35% of women ages 13 to 20 years have a history of bulimia. Other investigators have reported the prevalence of bulimia as 1.5% in young girls, whereas partial syndromes or mild variants of the disorder occur in 5% to 10% of young women.[9] Symptoms of bulimia, such as isolated episodes of binge eating and purging, have been reported in up to 40% of college women. Anorexia and bulimia nervosa may be increasing in incidence, although increased reporting of cases resulting from greater medical and public awareness of the disorders over the past two decades cannot be discounted.[20]

Bulimia nervosa is a chronic disorder with a waxing and waning course.[13] Mortality rates are not known. Comorbid conditions associated with bulimia nervosa include affective disorders, personality disorders, anxiety disorders, substance abuse, and adverse events related to aggression or poor impulse control.[27,33]

The vast majority (90% to 95%) of patients with bulimia nervosa are women. Eating disorders also occur frequently among men who participate in sports with a weight requirement (e.g., wrestling) or in whom low body fat is important (bodybuilders).[8] As in anorexia, a morbid fear of obesity is the overriding psychologic preoccupation in bulimia nervosa. Bulimia, however, is more frequent in people with a history of obesity. The common behavior of dieting may be related to the development of bulimia. Bulimia may occur after an episode of anorexia nervosa or substance abuse. Self-loathing and disgust with the body are even more severe in bulimia than in anorexia nervosa.

Binges may occur habitually or may be triggered sporadically by unpleasant feelings of anger, anxiety, or depression. Food deprivation (i.e., dieting) also plays a role in inducing bingeing. Guilt and dysphoria are common feelings after binges; however, some patients find these binges themselves soothing.

Binges are typically followed by efforts to prevent weight gain. Generally, patients attempt to prevent weight gain by self-induced vomiting; however, ingestion of ipecac syrup is occasionally used to prevent weight gain. Laxative or diuretic misuse is also common, although these substances almost exclusively produce fluid loss rather than calorie loss. Individuals may display extreme caloric restriction between episodes, exhibit wide fluctuations in weight, or become obese.

Although the act of self-induced vomiting may occur only occasionally and may be of little consequence, a chronic pattern may develop leading to poor overall health, decreased muscle strength, dental erosion, serious electrolyte abnormalities, cardiac arrhythmias, or death. Electrolyte abnormalities resulting from vomiting may be compounded by those from laxative-induced diarrhea or diuretic use. Chronic laxative (phenolphthalein) overdose has been reported. Menstrual irregularities may be caused by weight fluctuations, nutritional deficiency, or emotional stress.[24]

Deaths related to bulimia are believed to result from cardiac arrhythmias. Gastric or esophageal rupture, Mallory-Weiss tear, pneumomediastinum, and postbinge pancreatitis have resulted from gorging and vomiting, and may be life threatening.[21] Diet pills can cause hypertension and cerebral hemorrhage when taken in excess. Ipecac-related deaths have been reported, probably resulting from emetine cardiotoxicity in conjunction with electrolyte imbalances.[21]

Assessment

Common complaints include muscle weakness, cramps, dizziness, carpopedal spasm, hematemesis, abdominal pain, chest pain, heartburn, sore throat, or menstrual irregularity. Unrecognized bulimia nervosa has been associated with perioperative cardiac dysrhythmias.[32] Patients are characteristically young and female. Males with bulimia often have a history of participation in sports with weight requirements.[8] Patients may admit to use of diuretics for edema but often deny self-induced vomiting or laxative use. Caffeine, pseudoephedrine, phenylpropanolamine (now off the market), ginseng, thyroid replacement preparations, ma huang, and other "cleansing" or "dieters" herbs may be used in an attempt to increase metabolic rate and calorie loss. Many "natural" or herbal remedies thought to be completely safe actually contain substances that increase blood pressure or promote electrolyte imbalance.

Vital signs may be normal. Tachycardia and hypotension, when present, suggest volume depletion, whereas hypertension should raise the suspicion of stimulant use. Physical examination may reveal signs of dehydration and erosion of tooth enamel with or without frank caries. A callus resulting from repetitive contact with the upper teeth during self-induced vomiting may be found on the dorsal surface of the

Box 52-13 DIFFERENTIAL DIAGNOSES IN BULIMIA

Caustic infections
Esophageal perforation, rupture, or tear
Esophagitis
Gastroenteritis
Hyperemesis gravidarum
Mediastinitis
Munchausen syndrome

Box 52-14 POTENTIAL COMPLICATIONS OF BULIMIA

Electrolyte abnormalities resulting from vomiting but may be compounded by those from laxative-induced diarrhea or diuretic use
Chronic laxative abuse may lead to dependence and constipation; phenolphthalein poisoning resulting from laxative overdose has been reported
Menstrual irregularities resulting from weight fluctuations, nutritional deficiency, emotional stress, and possible loss of estrogen stores
Substance abuse
Complications of purging include gastric or esophageal rupture, Mallory-Weiss tear, pneumomediastinum, or postbinge pancreatitis
Central nervous system events include hypertension, cerebral hemorrhage, and death from diet pills
Ocular complications include subjunctival hemorrhage, detached retina, and retinal hemorrhage

index and long finger of the patient's dominant hand. Alopecia, hypertrichosis, and nail fragility are other common skin findings.[16]

Weight is frequently normal or above normal with the remainder of the physical examination usually normal. Specific complications, however, may be found on examination of the abdomen (e.g., epigastric tenderness, guaiac-positive stools), chest (e.g., Hamman crunch resulting from air in the mediastinal space from an esophageal tear), or extremities (e.g., edema). These symptoms can be found with other conditions, so care should be taken to rule these out. Box 52-13 lists the differential diagnoses for bulimia.

Research is ongoing regarding the potential role of other chemical mediators in the pathogenesis of eating disorders. Significantly higher rates of sexual assault and aggravated assault among women with bulimia nervosa support the hypothesis that victimization may contribute to development or maintenance of the disease.

Obtain electrolytes even in patients with normal weight. Hypokalemia, hypomagnesemia, and metabolic alkalosis secondary to compulsive vomiting are confirmatory for bulemia. Sodium and chloride levels may be decreased. In patients who abuse laxatives but are not vomiting, hypokalemia is associated with metabolic acidosis, whereas hypocalcemia is caused by loss of bicarbonate and calcium in diarrheal stool. Diuretic abuse can decrease serum sodium and potassium levels and increase uric acid and calcium levels.

Urinary findings vary with the degree of vomiting or laxative-induced diarrhea, diuretic use, and volume status. Findings also depend on whether the condition is acute or chronic. If abdominal pain is present, serum lipase and amylase measurements are used to screen for pancreatitis. Gastric rupture should be ruled out with an upright chest x-ray. Pneumomediastinum secondary to esophageal rupture may also be evident. If hematemesis or melena has been reported, placement of a nasogastric tube may be indicated. A pregnancy test should be obtained in all female patients of childbearing age.

Treatment

Emergency nurses should anticipate and be prepared to intervene for the complications of bulimia, including volume depletion, electrolyte abnormalities, esophagitis, Mallory-Weiss tear, esophageal or gastric rupture, pancreatitis,

arrhythmias, or adverse effects of medication (e.g., ipecac, appetite suppressants). Associated illnesses, including depression, anxiety disorders, and substance abuse, put patients at risk for other illness and injury. Directly question patients regarding suicidal ideation.

For patients unable to halt the dangerous sequence of dieting, bingeing, and purging, admission may be necessary to break the cycle. Psychiatric hospitalization may be necessary for patients with severe depression and suicidal ideation, weight loss greater than 30% over 3 months, failure to maintain outpatient weight contract, or family crisis. Medical admission is warranted for patients with significant metebolic disturbance or other physical complication of bingeing or purging, such as Mallory-Weiss tear, esophageal rupture, or pancreatitis.

Treatment usually combines individual psychotherapy with a cognitive-behavioral approach, group or family therapy, and pharmacotherapy.[19] The pharmacotherapy of bulimia nervosa is based on two models—seizure disorder and affective disorder. Medications include thiamin, multivitamins, and magnesium. Antidepressants have been reported to reduce binge eating, vomiting, and depression.[11] They may improve eating habits although their impact on body dissatisfaction remains unclear. There are a number of potential complications associated with bulimia (Box 52-14).

Patients should be educated about the risks of using diet pills, amphetamines, and energy pills and diet teas that claim to be natural. These often contain herbal forms of caffeine and ephedrine and have been associated with hypertension, cerebral vascular accident, and death. Phenylpropanalamine, the most common ingredient in both over-the-counter diet pills and decongestants, has been taken off the market because of the fear of severe hypertension leading to stroke and other serious pathology (especially in females).

Patients with serious eating disorders often mistrust health care professionals, whom they see as being interested only in refeeding them or making them lose their will so they become fat. Education about body weight regulation and the effects of starvation, vomiting, and laxatives on bodily functions may be helpful. Discussion of issues of self-esteem is important, especially how basing self-worth entirely on body size leads to forcing oneself to be something that is not natural.

MUNCHAUSEN SYNDROME

Patients with factitious illnesses cause unique difficulties for ED staff. Patients who present with overt demonstrable symptoms that prove factitious, such as with Munchausen syndrome, are particularly challenging and fascinating. Munchausen syndrome, is named for Baron von Munchausen (1720-1797), a wanderer widely known for his dramatic but untruthful stories.[3] The pathophysiology behind Munchausen remains unknown. Patients with this syndrome have associated personality disorders such as poor impulse control, self-destructive behavior, or borderline or passive-aggressive personality traits.

Classically, patients with Munchausen syndrome are male. There is a subset of women who reproduce a single set of symptoms instead of a constellation of different symptoms found in the average patient with Munchausen syndrome. The women in this subset exhibit less evidence of personality dysfunction than the average patient with Munchausen syndrome. They also have a strong tendency to form personal bonds with a single health care professional such as a physician or nurse practitioner. The classic patient with Munchausen syndrome almost always jumps from primary care provider to primary care provider and hospital to hospital.

The incidence of Munchausen syndrome peaks in young-to-middle age adults but has been reported in patients of all ages (i.e., childhood through old age). It is also important to note that pediatric Munchausen syndrome is not the same disease as Munchausen syndrome by proxy (Box 52-15).[25]

Patients arrive with dramatic presentations of apparently severe illnesses. Reported symptom patterns are often quite plausible, subjective, and parallel a textbook presentation. A history of extensive surgical and inpatient workups for a variety of diseases, workups that span multiple hospitals and cities, and notable vagueness or inconsistency in the details of the medical problems should raise a red flag of suspicion toward Munchhausen syndrome. Evidence of pathologic lying in areas other than presenting symptoms is also consistent with this illness.

The physical findings that patients with Munchausen syndrome display are inconclusive and typically subjective in nature. In an effort to obtain hospitalization and an invasive workup, patients with Munchausen syndrome have mimicked nearly every severe disease that generates physical findings and symptoms. Again the key emphasis is that symptoms are typically subjective and difficult to verify by physical assessment or diagnostics.[6]

In distinguishing Munchausen syndrome from other factitious illnesses, the lack of etiology of this syndrome is a

---

Box 52-15	MUNCHAUSEN SYNDROME BY PROXY (MSBP)

MSBP is a syndrome in which an adult simulates or creates symptoms in a child to receive an ill-defined secondary gain from the child's hospitalization. MSBP is child abuse and must be dealt with when it is suspected. The abuser is very attentive to the child's health care needs and appears very caring to those around him or her. The abuser is usually the primary caregiver. Because of the dangerous nature of the varied means used to create factitious symptoms, mortality rate is significant: estimates range from 5% to 50%.

---

key issue. Conversion and somatoform disorders are driven by a secondary gain. Treating the underlying stressor often can alleviate presenting symptoms. In contrast, a patient with Munchausen syndrome actively seeks hospitalization and invasive painful procedures simply to undergo them.

Depending on symptoms displayed, essentially any lab test used in the ED may be indicated in evaluation of patients with Munchausen syndrome. The same principle also applies to the use of imaging studies. If the purported condition is severe enough, or the technique used to mimic organic illness has produced sufficient pathology in and of itself, any or all of the procedures in the purview of the ED may become necessary for care of the patient.

Initial care and stabilization of patients with Munchausen syndrome is driven by presenting symptoms, coupled with any untoward side effects of the practices used by the patient to simulate or induce symptoms. If in doubt, consult the appropriate specialist for the purported illness, and seek admission to the hospital.

Drugs that may be proposed for a patient with Munchausen syndrome fall into two categories—drugs used to treat the presenting symptoms and antipsychotic medications to treat the underlying condition. The first category is necessarily vast because patients with Munchausen syndrome have portrayed nearly every disease known to medicine. To date, there is no evidence that antipsychotic drugs have had any effect on the course or prognosis of Munchausen syndrome.

If the diagnosis of Munchausen syndrome is quite clear, psychiatric consultation and referral should be offered to the patient even if admission for the patient's medical problems is declined. The patient nearly always declines such referrals, and such refusal should be documented in the patient's record. Very often the patient will leave against medical advice if they believe they have been discovered.

SUMMARY

Psychosocial conditions found in the ED are varied and challenging (Box 52-16). Regardless of presenting symptoms it is important for the emergency nurse to treat the patient with empathy and respect while protecting the patient and others from harm.

Box 52-16	**NURSING DIAGNOSES FOR PSYCHOSOCIAL EMERGENCIES**

Anxiety
Communication, Impaired verbal
Coping, Ineffective
Injury, Risk for
Thought processes, Disturbed
Violence, Risk for self-directed

References

1. Angst J, Angst F, Stassen HH: Suicide risk in patients with major depressive disorder, *J Clin Psychiatry* 60(suppl 2):57, 1999.
2. Apter A, Horesh N, Gothelf D: Relationship between self-disclosure and serious suicidal behavior, *Compr Psychiatry* 42(1):70, 2001.
3. Asher R: Munchausen's syndrome, *Lancet* 1:339, 1951.
4. Ballenger JC, Davidson JR, Lecrubier Y et al: Consensus statement on panic disorder from the International Consensus Group on Depression and Anxiety, *J Clin Psychiatry* 59(suppl 8):47, 1998.
5. Brawman-Mintzer O, Lydiard RB: Biological basis of generalized anxiety disorder, *J Clin Psychiatry* 58(suppl 3):16, 1997.
6. Bretz SW, Richards JR: Munchausen syndrome presenting acutely in the emergency department, *J Emerg Med* 18(4):417, 2000.
7. Brewerton TD, Dansky BS, Kilpatrick DG: Which comes first in the pathogenesis of bulimia nervosa: dieting or bingeing? *Int J Eat Disord* 28(3):259, 2000.
8. Carlat DJ, Camago CA, Herzog DB: Eating disorders in males: a report on 135 patients, *Am J Psychiatry* 154(8):1127, 1997.
9. Corcos M, Flament MF, Giraud MJ: Early psychopathological signs in bulimia nervosa: a retrospective comparison of the period of puberty in bulimic and control girls, *Eur Child Adolesc Psychiatry* 9(2):115, 2000.
10. den Boer JA: Pharmacotherapy of panic disorder: differential efficacy from a clinical viewpoint, *J Clin Psychiatry* 59(suppl 8):30, 1998.
11. El-Giamal N, de Zwaan M, Bailer U: Reboxetine in the treatment of bulimia nervosa: a report of seven cases, *Int Clin Psychopharmacol* 15(6):351, 2000.
12. eMedicine.com: *Emergency medicine* (2001). Mental health emergencies. Retrieved February 21, 2002 from the World Wide Web: http://www.emedicine.com.
13. Fairburn CG, Cooper Z, Doll HA: The natural course of bulimia nervosa and binge eating disorder in young women, *Arch Gen Psychiatry* 57(7):659, 2000.
14. Fleet RP, Marchand A, Dupuis G et al: Comparing emergency department and psychiatric setting patients with panic disorder, *Psychosomatics* 39(6):512, 1998.
15. Gliatto MF, Rai AK: Evaluation and treatment of patients with suicidal ideation, *Am Fam Physician* 59(6):1500, 1999.
16. Glorio R, Allevato M, DePablo A: Prevalence of cutaneous manifestations in 200 patients with eating disorders, *Int J Dermatol* 39(5):348, 2000.
17. Hales RE, Hilty DA, Wise MG: A treatment algorithm for the management of anxiety in primary care practice, *J Clin Psychiatry* 58(suppl 3):76, 1997.
18. Harwitz D, Ravizza L: Suicide and depression, *Emerg Med Clin North Am* 18(2):263, 2000.
19. Hay PJ, Bacaltchuk J: Psychotherapy for bulimia nervosa and binging (Cochrane Review), *Cochrane Database Syst Rev* 4:CD000562, 2000.
20. Hetherington MM: Eating disorders: diagnosis, etiology, and prevention, *Nutrition* 16(7-8):547, 2000.
21. Keel PK, Mitchell JE: Outcome in bulimia nervosa, *Am J Psychiatry* 154(3):313, 1997.
22. Kreipe RE, Birndorf SA: Eating disorders in adolescents and young adults, *Med Clin North Am* 84(4):1027, 2000.
23. Lagomasino I, Daly R, Stoudemire A: Medical assessment of patients presenting with psychiatric symptoms in the emergency setting, *Psychiatr Clin North Am* 22(4):819, 1999.
24. Morgan JF: Eating disorders and reproduction, *Aust NZ J Obstet Gynaecol* 39(2):167, 1999.
25. Polli GE, Engman-Lazear S: Mental health emergencies. In *Emergency nursing core curriculum*, ed 5, Philadelphia, 2000, WB Saunders.
26. Rickels K, Schweizer E: The clinical presentation of generalized anxiety in primary-care settings: practical concepts of classification and management, *J Clin Psychiatry* 58(suppl 11):4, 1997.
27. Ringskog S: Somatic complications in anorexia and bulimia nervosa, *Lakartidningen* 96(8):882, 1999.
28. Rives W: Emergency department assessment of suicidal patients, *Psychiatr Clin North Am* 22(4):779, 1999.
29. Roy-Byrne P, Stein M, Bystrisky A et al: Pharmacotherapy of panic disorder: proposed guidelines for the family physician, *J Am Board Fam Pract* 11(4):282, 1998.
30. Schatzberg AF: New indications for antidepressants, *J Clin Psychiatry* 61(suppl 11):9, 2000.
31. Schulze U, Neudorfl A, Krill A et al: Follow-up and treatment outcome of early anorexia nervosa, *Z Kinder Jugendpsychiatr Psychother* 25(1):5, 1997.
32. Suri R, Poist ES, Hager WD: Unrecognized bulimia nervosa: a potential cause of perioperative cardiac dysrhythmias, *Can J Anaesth* 46(11):1048, 1999.
33. von Ranson KM, Kaye WH, Weltzin TE: Obsessive-compulsive disorder symptoms before and after recovery from bulimia nervosa, *Am J Psychiatry* 156(11):1703, 1999.
34. Zajecka J: Importance of establishing the diagnosis of persistent anxiety, *J Clin Psychiatry* 58(suppl 3):9, 1997.
35. Zun LS: Panic disorder: diagnosis and treatment in emergency medicine, *Ann Emerg Med* 30(1):92, 1997.

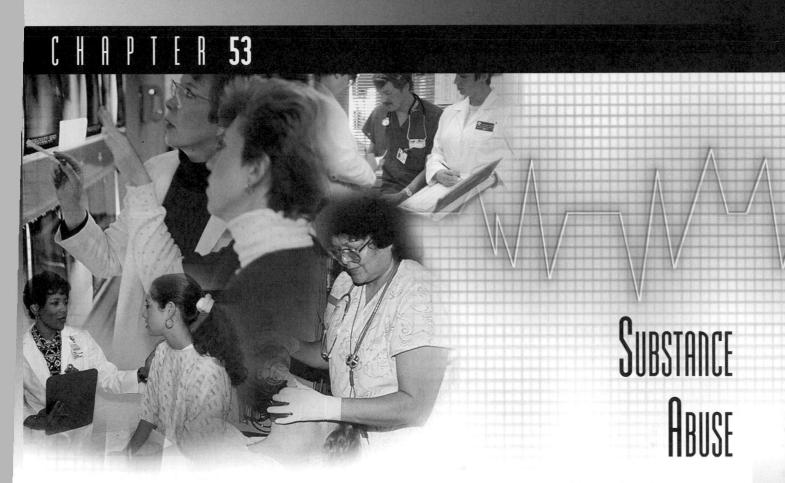

CHAPTER 53

SUBSTANCE ABUSE

DIANA M. LOMBARDO

Substance abuse has reached crisis proportions in the United States. And, regrettably, the problem will only get worse.[20] Drugs have invaded every social level and stratum of our society, including schools and the workplace. According to Drug Abuse Resistance Education, almost one in five workers uses dangerous drugs regularly on the job, including health care workers. Effects of drugs in the workplace center around three key areas: absenteeism, work habits, and interpersonal relations. Law enforcement authorities estimate that two thirds of all serious crimes can be linked to drug abuse. The National Institute on Drug Abuse estimates that 25% of the 4 million babies born annually in the United States are affected by drugs and alcohol. The National Association for Families and Addiction Research and Education estimates that 15% of all babies born in the United States in 1995 will test positive for illicit drugs. In the face of such overwhelming data, society, particularly health care providers, must learn the facts about drugs and substance abuse.

Substance abuse refers to the inappropriate use of prescription drugs or use of illicit substances. Regardless of legal status, substance abusers generally fall into five categories (Table 53-1). For the purposes of this chapter, specific information is presented on alcohol, cocaine, designer drugs, and heroin. The reader is encouraged to seek other sources for a more comprehensive discussion of prescription drug abuse.

ADDICTION

Researchers have discovered evidence that some alcoholics are genetically predisposed to alcoholism; however, scientists have not been able to determine if drug abusers have a genetic predisposition. Some drug abusers say they feel normal after substance abuse rather than euphoric. This may indicate that drug abuse has a biologic basis in certain individuals.

Drugs exert a powerful control on behavior because they act directly on the primitive brainstem and the limbic structure. If you do something pleasurable, the message received reinforces the behavior responsible for the pleasure. Understanding this process makes it easier to understand addiction.

Drug addiction is a biologically based disease that alters the pleasure center and other aspects of the brain via the neurotransmitter dopamine. Dopamine connects neurons through the dendrite synaptic junction to a receptor site. When a neurotransmitter couples with a receptor, as with a key fitting into a lock, the biochemical process in that neuron is activated. This process, called chemical neurotransmission, allows a receptor neuron to connect with other neurons. Heroin mimics the effects of this natural neurotransmitter (dopamine), whereas substances such as lysergic acid diethylamide (LSD) block receptors and prevent natural transmission. Cocaine interferes with the process of neurotransmission by preventing release of

Table 53-1	SUBSTANCES OF ABUSE
CATEGORY	**EXAMPLES OR STREET NAMES**
Cannabis	Marijuana, pot, grass
Stimulants	Crack, amphetamines, cocaine
Depressants	Sedatives, hypnotics, tranquilizers, alcohol
Narcotics	Morphine, heroin, meperidine, fentanyl
Hallucinogens	Psychedelic drugs, PCP, LSD

Box 53-1   FACTS ABOUT TOBACCO ABUSE

46.5 million American adults smoked in 1999.
25.7% of men and 21.5% of women smoked in 1999.
4.5 million adolescents between ages 12 and 17 smoke.
American Indians/Alaska natives have the highest prevalence of smoking—40.8% of the population.
Smoking prevalence is greatest in those living below the poverty line (33.1%).
More than 6000 persons less than 18 years of age try their first cigarette each day.
Adolescents who become daily smokers before age 18 increased 77% from 1988 to 1996.
9.2% of middle school students smoke.
2.7% of middle school students use smokeless tobacco.

dopamine. Phencyclidine (PCP) interferes with the way messages proceed from the surface receptors into the cell interior.

The biologic basis for addiction is the repeated process of altering chemical neurotransmission. Repeated use of these drugs can and will affect the brain on a permanent basis. Addiction begins when the pleasure circuit is repeatedly stimulated. The pleasure circuit is activated in a variety of ways, depending on the drug of choice. Heroin activates the opiate receptors, whereas cocaine allows dopamine to accumulate in the synapses, where it is released. Increasing amounts of dopamine at the synapses lead to euphoria.

SPECIFIC SUBSTANCES

Emergencies related to substance abuse may be acute or chronic. The patient may come to the emergency department (ED) in acute withdrawal, severe drug intoxication, or seeking help for addiction. This chapter focuses on addiction rather than acute drug intoxication. Refer to Chapter 43 for comprehensive discussion of drug overdose, intoxication, and other toxicologic emergencies.

Tobacco

Tobacco use includes cigarettes, pipes, cigars, and smokeless tobacco. Novel tobacco use includes the use of clove cigarettes. In addition to the previously mentioned substances of abuse, many individuals abuse tobacco, steroids, and some natural stimulants available in health food stores. It is beyond the scope of this text to describe all potential substances of abuse; however, the use of tobacco does warrant brief discussion.

Tobacco abuse is related to a multitude of health care problems, including cardiovascular disease, lung cancer, bronchitis, and many more. Box 53-1 highlights a few facts about this common addiction. Ironically, tobacco abuse is also common in the health care community. The emergency nurse should recognize the broad effects of tobacco abuse and provide pertinent education to the patient and family.

Cocaine

Approximately 1.5 million Americans 12 years of age and older were chronic cocaine users in 1997. Adults between ages 18 and 25 years had the highest rate of use.[19,21] Teens become addicted to cocaine in 15.5 months, whereas adults

take more than 4 years to develop a serious cocaine problem. Crack, the smokable form of cocaine, was introduced to the drug scene in 1986. Slightly more than 3% of eighth graders reported using crack at least once in their lifetime. The high is 10 times more powerful than that caused by snorting the drug. The associated rush or euphoria lasts only 5 to 10 minutes, which encourages more frequent use, so greater dependency develops. Many individuals addicted to cocaine say they continued to use in an attempt to experience the rush of their first time.

Cocaine can be snorted, smoked, or injected. Injecting cocaine and other drugs carries the added risk of contracting human immunodeficiency virus (HIV). Effects of cocaine on the cardiovascular system include chest pain, myocarditis, cardiomyopathy, endocarditis, ventricular arrhythmias, aortic dissection, hypertension, cerebrovascular accident, and myocardial infarction (MI). MI is the most commonly reported cardiovascular consequence of cocaine use. The first reported MI related to recreational or illegal drugs occurred in 1982. Other effects of cocaine are excitation, increased alertness, increased heart rate, increased blood pressure, loss of appetite, insomnia, dilated pupils, runny nose, and nasal congestion. In some situations cocaine can trigger paranoia. Cocaine is an extremely strong stimulant, which may lead to seizures, cardiac and respiratory arrest, and even stroke. Long-term use of cocaine causes mucous membranes of the nose to disintegrate. Heavy cocaine use can actually cause the nasal septum to collapse. Despite views to the contrary, cocaine does not improve performance. Use can lead to loss of concentration, irritability, loss of memory, loss of energy, anxiety, and a loss of interest in sex.

Cocaine is also an issue in pregnancy. Literature supports the fact that cocaine, as with other drugs, can increase the risk of prematurity, stillbirth, low birth weight, central nervous system damage, and uterine rupture. Concomitant use of alcohol increases these risks and contributes to long-term development problems. Table 53-2 summarizes effects of maternal cocaine use on mothers and fetuses or babies.

Table 53-2 EFFECTS OF MATERNAL COCAINE USE ON MOTHERS AND FETUSES OR BABIES

SYSTEM	EFFECTS ON MOTHER	EFFECTS ON FETUS OR BABY
Neurologic	Seizures Neural damage* Insomnia	Increased irritability Increased startle response Difficult to console Tremors Jittery
Ocular	Retinal crystals causing flashes of light called snow lights	Eye defects*
Respiratory	Shortness of breath Lung damage, if smoked Nasal membrane burns and lesions Respiratory paralysis in overdose	Increased respiratory rate Abnormal ventilatory patterns Increased risk for sudden infant death syndrome*
Cardiovascular	Acute hypertension Angina Arrhythmias Tachycardia Palpitations Cerebral artery injury or cerebrovascular accident Cardiac failure	Intrauterine growth retardation Tachycardia Cerebral artery injury/infarction* Acute hypertension*
Gastrointestinal	Sore throat Hoarseness Anorexia leading to weight loss and malnutrition	Diarrhea Poor tolerance for oral feeding Prune-belly syndrome*
Renal		Hydronephrosis*
Reproductive	Increased uterine contractility Abruptio placentae Spontaneous abortion Premature labor Stillbirth	Cryptorchidism*

*Suspected but not established.

It is not uncommon for a substance abuser to use more than one drug. This polysubstance abuse creates additional problems and often jeopardizes the health of the user. The most frequently used substance in association with cocaine or crack is alcohol; however, barbiturates, marijuana, and tranquilizers are often taken with or immediately after cocaine or crack. Combining cocaine or crack with heroin, called "speedballing," can be deadly. Reports from the National Institute on Drug Abuse indicate increasing use of cocaine or crack with a hallucinogenic drug such as PCP, a space ball. Another combination that is extremely deadly is freebasing, which is the process of converting street cocaine to pure form by removing some of the cutting agents. The result is a more powerful drug that reaches the brain in seconds. The high occurs rapidly, but the euphoria disappears quickly, so the user has a craving to freebase again and again.

Life-threatening emergencies related to cocaine include chest pain, MI, seizures, severe hypertension, and stroke. Management of these life-threatening emergencies is no different in the patient who uses cocaine than in other patients with these problems. Recognition of cocaine as a causative agent is not essential to manage these patients in the ED; however, long-term management must address the issue of substance abuse. Other cocaine-related problems include ag-

Table 53-3 DESIGNER DRUGS

CHEMICAL NAME	STREET NAME
Phencyclidine	Angel dust, dust, peace pill, Captain Crunch
Methamphetamine	Ice, meth, crank, speed, crystal
1-Methyl-4-phenyl-4-propionoxy-piperidine	MPPP
Methylenedioxy-amphetamine	Ecstasy, MDA, E, X, XTC, love, Adam
Lysergic acid diethylamide	LSD, acid, Mickey Mouse, paper acid, blotter acid
Mescaline	Peyote
Psilocybin	Magic mushrooms
Dimethyltryptamine	DMT

itation, paranoia, and epistaxis. There is an increased risk for injury to self and others with these patients. Decrease stimulation and monitor the patient carefully.

Designer Drugs

Designer drugs are synthetically produced from a mixture of substances. Examples include PCP, methamphetamine, LSD, mescaline, psilocybin, and many others. Table 53-3 lists some designer drugs and their most common street names. Crystallized methamphetamine has been tried by 1% to 3% of all high school students. Honolulu police estimate that methamphetamine may be involved in almost 70% of spousal abuse cases within their jurisdiction. More than 100 deaths on the West Coast have been linked to MPPP. One drop of MPPP is strong enough to kill 50 people. Dimethyltryptamine is a hallucinogen used to soak tobacco or marijuana.

Phencyclidine

PCP is a hallucinogen that alters reality, touch, hearing, smell, taste, and visual perceptions. These effects may lead to serious bodily injury to the user. Chronic and long-term use can cause permanent changes in cognitive ability, memory, and fine motor function. Pregnant women who use PCP often deliver babies with visual, auditory, and motor disturbances.

The patient under the influence of PCP may be extremely violent with an increased risk for harm to self and others. Decrease stimulation in these patients and monitor carefully for escalating violence.

Lysergic Acid Diethylamide

LSD, a hallucinogen developed in 1938, has recently become popular in the adolescent and young adult population.[22] It comes as a tablet or liquid (which is sold on squares of blotter paper). Effects are primarily sensory and emotional. Colors, sounds, and smells are greatly intensified. The user may hear or feel colors and all sounds. The effects can be erratic and combined with hallucinations that can be pleasurable or terrifying. Psychosis has been reported.

Heroin

Heroin treatment admissions increased by 200% or more in six U.S. states with an increase between 100% and 199% in 11 other states from 1993 to 1999.[20] Intravenous heroin use increases risk of HIV, hepatitis, skin abscesses, phlebitis, and bacterial endocarditis. Heroin may be intentionally used with cocaine to enhance the rush or high. The heroin dealer

may also cut the heroin with other substances such as strychnine, PCP, and others.

Heroin is an opiate that affects the pleasure center, causing physical dependence. Any attempt to stop using the drug causes severe, painful withdrawal symptoms including watery eyes, runny nose, yawning, loss of appetite, tremors, panic, chills, sweating, nausea, muscle cramps, and insomnia. Elevated blood pressure, pulse, respiratory rate, and temperature occur as withdrawal progresses. Heroin causes shallow breathing, pinpoint pupils, nausea, panic, insomnia, and a need for increasingly higher doses of the drug.

The heroin addict may present to the ED in acute withdrawal, after an overdose, or with problems related to intravenous drug injection. The patient in acute withdrawal is treated symptomatically with antianxiety agents, antihypertensive agents, and in some cases, administration of methadone. Acute heroin intoxication is treated with administration of naloxone, ventilatory support, and intravenous fluids when appropriate. Naloxone administration can precipitate severe withdrawal in some patients, so careful monitoring is essential.

RAVES

Raves are all-night dance parties attended by youths, sometimes in excess of 20,000 teenagers.[27] Rave parties are an international phenomena with loud techno music,[2] typically held in large abandoned or rented warehouses, and are advertised by word of mouth. Liberal use of drugs has caused concern and scrutiny of raves. Drugs that have gained much of the attention because of these raves include ecstasy (3,4-methylenedioxymethamphetamine), GHB (gamma-hydroxybutyrate), and ketamine (Table 53-4).[2,27]

The estimated age of rave attendees is between 15 and 25 years of age. Many ravers perceive rave events as safe havens for outcasts, nerds, and computer geeks.[27] Not all ravers use drugs, but many illicit drugs are available. Alcohol is absent because it is believed to incite aggression and violence.

The literature supports the fact that rave attendees have required clothing that includes baseball caps, T-shirts with logos, baggy pants, running shoes, knapsacks, barrettes, in-

Table 53-4	DRUGS ASSOCIATED WITH RAVE		
DRUG	STREET NAME	CLINICAL FEATURE	TOXICITIES
Ecstasy	E, X, XTC, love	Heightened perception and sensual awareness, mydriasis, sympathomimetic, bruxism, jaw tension, ataxia	Dysrhythmias, hyperthermia, rhabdomyolysis, DIC, hyponatremia, seizures, death
MDMA	Adan		
Ketamine	Kit-kat, special K, vitamin K	Nystagmus, increased tone, purposeful movements, amnesia, hallucinations, sympathomimetic	Loss of consciousnes, respiratory depression, catatonia, highly addictive
GHB	G, liquid grievous bodily harm, Georgia home boy	Agitation, nystagmus, ataxia, sedation, amnesia, hypotonia, vomiting, muscle spasm	Seizures, apnea, sudden reversible coma with abrupt awakening and violence, bradycardia

DIC, Disseminated intravascular coagulation.

fant toys, beads, plastic chains, and infant soothers.[27] According to the literature, this form of dressing for ravers states their lack of pretension and open acceptance of themselves and their community. Androgynous dress diminishes distinctions based on physical attractiveness and sexual orientation,[27] supporting ravers' need for acceptance.

Ecstasy

Ecstasy is a synthetic amphetamine derivative that was originally developed as an appetite suppressant in 1914.[2,27] Ecstasy is unique in that it produces stimulant and hallucinogenic effects[2,27] and is potentially life threatening. As with other street drugs, ecstasy is a combination of other illicit drugs with numerous recipes used to produce it. A new variation called herbal ecstasy is composed of ephedrine or pseudoephedrine and caffeine from the kola nut. Ecstasy comes as a tablet, powder, or capsule and in virtually any color. Imprints may or may not be present. The drug is primarily taken orally or snorted but can also be injected or taken rectally. There has been a 71% increase in ecstasy use in adolescents. The butterfly is the universal symbol for ecstasy and appears on drug paraphernalia used at raves. These include cigarettes and other products that do not actually contain ecstasy.

Ecstasy is one of several date rape drugs—drugs used to facilitate sexual assault. These drugs in combination with alcohol increase feelings of sexual disinhibition and arousal; this heightened sense of sexuality, coupled with short-term narrow cognitive focus, increases the likelihood that sexual assault will occur.[25] Patients crave touch and experience a heightened sensuality, giving rise to many of the names for ecstasy such as "love" and the "hug drug". Other effects include hyperthermia, hypertension, tachycardia, and ataxia.

Use of ecstasy in adolescents is an increasing concern; there has been a 71% increase in teen ecstasy use since 1999.[23] Increased use may be due to availability of the drug, as well as its intoxicating effects. All night raves are where many users are introduced to this drug. The drug is packaged as capsules or pills with a cost to the user of $7 to $30 per pill or capsule. Another factor that may contribute to increased use is duration of the effects. An ecstasy high can last up to 24 hours.

Gamma-Hydroxybutyrate

Gamma-hydroxybutyrate (GHB) is a putative neurotransmitter, structurally related to gamma-aminobutyric acid and glutamic acid, which has been the subject of investigation since 1960. More recently GHB has been introduced in clinical practice for management of alcoholism.[1] GHB is a naturally occurring metabolite that produces a biphasic dopamine response and triggers release of an opiate-like substance that mediates sleep cycles, temperature regulation, cerebral glucose metabolism and blood flow, memory and emotional control, and crosses the blood brain barrier.[1,2,3,27] There is no antidote for GHB overdose, and treatment is restricted to nonspecific supportive care to include ventilatory support and atropine for persistent bradycardia.[1,2,3,16]

Ketamine

Ketamine is rapid-acting dissociative anesthetic that provides hypnotic, analgesic, and amnesic effects with minimal respiratory depression. Onset of action when given as an intramuscular injection is 6 minutes. The person appears to be in a coma with the eyes open. The first priority in the management of adverse effects of ketamine ingestion is protecting the airway.

INHALANTS

Use of inhalants is more likely to occur in younger adolescents, with higher use for eighth graders. Inhalants are substances of first use for many with thousands available, including solvents, glues, paints, gasoline, and aerosols.[13,26] Inhalants are cheap, usually free if found at home, easily available, and readily used.[13] Huffing refers to direct inhalation or inhaling deeply from a chemical-soaked cloth within a paper bag.[13] Inhalants can have immediate and extremely deleterious consequences, including death. Short-term symptoms include palpitations, delirium, respiratory distress, dizziness, and headaches. Frostbite injury in the roof of the mouth has been noted with use of some substances. Prolonged use can lead to irreversible brain damage, muscle weakness, nosebleeds, sensory disturbances, arrhythmias, kidney and liver damage, cognitive problems, and violent behavior.[17] Boys and girls are at equal risk for use of inhalants.[13]

ALCOHOLISM

Between 13 and 16 million people require treatment for alcoholism or drugs in any given year, but only 3 million receive care.[10] Sixty percent of the American population has a drink at least once a month. There are 10.5 million alcoholics in America; 17.5 million others abuse alcohol. Accidents involving drunk drivers account for 45.1% of all traffic deaths. This translates to 1 death every 30 minutes or more than 100,000 deaths per year. Two of five Americans will be involved in an alcohol-related car accident in their lifetime. One to three babies out of every 1000 births are born with fetal alcohol syndrome.[14]

Alcoholism is one of the most serious public health problems in the United States today. Among the 18.3 million adult heavy drinkers, 12.1 million have one or more symptoms of alcoholism, an increase of 8.2% since 1980.

Comorbidity of substance abuse and mental illness exacerbates symptoms and often leads to treatment noncompliance, greater depression, and likelihood of suicide, incarceration, family friction, and higher services use and cost.[10]

Alcoholism is defined as a primary or chronic disease with genetic, psychosocial, and environmental factors influencing development and manifestation. The disease is often progressive and fatal and is characterized by impaired control over drinking, preoccupation with the drug alcohol despite adverse consequences, and distortions in thinking, most notably denial.[4,10,11]

Alcohol consumption affects all organs of the body but the most significant is the central nervous system.[13] Alcohol depresses inhibitory control mechanisms, leading to apparent stimulation, which has a major effect on neurotransmittors of the brain. Alcohol intake results in diminished judgment and impulsiveness that leads to risky and reckless behaviors. Excessive intake can lead to severe impairment, respiratory compromise, blackouts, unconsciousness, and death.

Every patient whom you suspect has been drinking or who responds positively to drinking alcohol when questioned should be screened by the CAGE test. The CAGE test is an easy and effective way to determine if someone has a drinking problem (Box 53-2). The test has a 70% sensitivity and a 90% specificity.

Effects of Ethanol on Body Systems

Cardiovascular

Alcohol initially depresses myocardial contractility and causes peripheral vasodilatation, resulting in a mild drop in blood pressure with a compensatory increase in heart rate and cardiac output.[4] Increase of three or more drinks a day results in hypertension and dysrhythmias. There is an association between cerebrovascular accidents and alcoholism, especially within 24 hours of heavy drinking.[3,4] Holiday heart syndrome refers to ventricular or atrial dysrhythmias that occur after an episode of binge drinking. Paroxysmal tachycardia is the most common.[4] Conversely, one to two drinks per day over long periods may decrease cardiovascular death by increasing high-density lipoproteins.[4]

Central Nervous System

After a few drinks, rapid eye movement sleep is affected, leading to a more rapid than normal alternation between sleep stages and deficiency in deep sleep. Peripheral neuropathy is noted in 5% to 15% of the cases as a result of thiamine deficiency.[3,4] Wernicke's and Korsakoff's syndromes are caused by thiamin deficiency. Korsakoff's syndrome presents with profound anterograde amnesia. Alcoholics can show severe cognitive problems and impairment in recent and remote memory for weeks to months.[4] Almost every psychiatric syndrome can be seen during heavy drinking or subsequent withdrawal.

Gastrointestinal System

Acute alcohol intake can result in inflammation of the esophagus and stomach. Esophagitis can cause epigastric distress and gastritis, the most frequent cause of gastrointestinal bleeding in heavy drinkers.[3,4] Violent vomiting can result in a Mallory-Weiss tear. Most gastrointestinal symptoms are reversible; however, two complications of chronic alcoholism, esophageal varices secondary to cirrhosis-

| Box 53-2 | **CAGE SCREENING** |

C: Have you ever felt the need to cut down on your drinking?
A: Have you ever felt annoyed by criticism of your drinking?
G: Have you ever felt guilty about your drinking?
E: Have you ever felt the need for an eye-opener in the morning?

induced portal hypertension and atrophy of gastric cells, may be irreversible.[4]

Alcoholics commonly develop acute or chronic pancreatitis. In the liver, alcohol is the preferred fuel. Glyconeogenesis is impaired and lactate production increases, and there is an increase in fat accumulation within liver cells resulting from decreased oxidation of fatty acids in the citric cycle.[4] With repeated exposure to alcohol, more severe changes in the liver function are likely to occur. Hepatitis and cirrhosis are due to repeated exposure to alcohol. Icterus, bruising, spider angiomata, and hepatomegaly are common findings in people that abuse alcohol.

Genitourinary System

Initially, modest intake of alcohol can increase sexual drive in men and simultaneously decrease erectile function. However, men with chronic alcoholism exhibit testicular atrophy that is irreversible, with concomitant loss of sperm cells.[4]

In women with chronic alcoholism, amenorrhea, decreased ovarian size, infertility, and spontaneous abortions have been reported.[4] Alcohol abuse during pregnancy is responsible for fetal alcohol syndrome.

Hematopoietic System

Anemia is a common finding in the person with severe alcoholism. Mild thrombocytopenia and an elevated MCV are also seen in alcoholics.[3,4] Alcohol affects platelets and their ability to clump or stick to each other. Consequently, these patients may bleed more easily and longer from even minor cuts.

Skin

Findings seen in people who abuse alcohol include distal extremity hair loss, facial telangiectases, rosacea, seborrheic dermatitis, skin atrophy, and superficial infections.

Other Effects of Ethanol

Chronic intake and abuse of alcohol cause various nutritional deficiencies, increased risk for fractures resulting from alterations in calcium metabolism, modest but reversible decrease in T4, and a marked decrease in T3.[4]

Alcohol and Aging.   Decreased lean body mass related to aging affects distribution of alcohol, therefore, the elderly have an increased peak alcohol concentration with any given dose of alcohol.[11,24] Drug absorption is affected by delayed gastric emptying and fluctuation in drug clearance, and drugs with narrow therapeutic indexes such as warfarin or anticonvulsants can have hazardous consequences.[11,24] Alco-

Box 53-3	SYMPTOMS OF ALCOHOL WITHDRAWAL

Restlessness, irritability, anxiety, agitation
Anorexia, nausea, vomiting
Tremor, elevated heart rate, increased blood pressure
Insomnia, intense dreaming, nightmares
Impaired concentration, memory, judgment
Increased sensitivity to sounds, alteration in tactile sensations
Delirium—disorientation to time, place, and situation
Hallucinations—auditory, visual, or tactile
Delusion—usually paranoid
Grand mal seizures
Elevated temperature

Data from The National Clearinghouse for Alcohol & Drug Information, 1997.

hol intake can affect adherence to treatment, and medication regimens may be entirely abandoned.

Alcohol Withdrawal. Individuals with severe alcoholism experience withdrawal when their serum ethanol drops below the patients normal level. Symptoms may be mild during the early hours of withdrawal and can progress to full-blown delirium tremems within days. Box 53-3 highlights symptoms of alcohol withdrawal. It is important to note that symptoms occur when there is a drop below the person's normal level, not necessarily when there is no alcohol in the person's system.

In younger alcoholics tremors usually begin 8 to 12 hours after the last drink and peak in 24 to 36 hours.[11,24] In older alcoholics it is not unusual to see the effects of withdrawal delayed, with symptoms starting several days after cessation. Confusion rather than tremor is often the predominant clinical sign. Hallucinations in the elderly are usually tactile; delirium tremens is a late manifestation of withdrawal that occurs 2 to 10 days after cessation of drinking.[11,24]

Acute treatment of alcohol withdrawal includes a safe environment and treatment of nutritional and electrolyte deficiencies. Benzodiazepines have proven effective and are the drugs of choice because of their rapid onset and their short- and long-term effects. Lorazepam is preferred for individuals with liver dysfunction because it does not depend on hepatic metabolism for clearance. The literature supports use of long-term benzodiazepines; however, there is controversy in use of short- and long-term benzodiazepines. Antipsychotic medications such as thioridazine or haloperidol[12] are sometimes used; however, they must be prescribed with care because they can lower the seizure threshold.[4]

NURSING CONSIDERATIONS

Emergency nurses should continue to educate themselves and others about the effects of substance abuse. Drug abuse knows no social boundaries; therefore, emergency nurses should be meticulous in assessment of patients seen in the ED. Obtain a detailed history and observe the patient for be-

haviors or physical symptoms that indicate drug use or abuse. Table 53-5 summarizes the effects of the most common illegal drugs. If you suspect the patient is abusing drugs, report your findings to the physician managing the patient's care so that appropriate testing or screening can be initiated. Ensure a safe environment for the patient, visitors, and personnel working in the ED.

The potential for violence increases in individuals under the influence of drugs. Increased injury severity and increased length of hospital stay occur in the presence of drug abuse. Patients often present for treatment of injuries associated with high-risk behavior such as assaults, penetrating trauma, blunt trauma, and sexually transmitted diseases rather than the drug abuse. Treat potentially life-threatening injuries and then evaluate the patient for drug-related problems. Patients with acute signs and symptoms of abuse need medical intervention for the effects of the drug taken. Consultation or referral to a drug treatment center is indicated for substance abuse treatment after the patient is medically cleared.

SUMMARY

Every day, ambulances and police cars race through neighborhoods because someone has been injured in a drug-related incident. Drugs in schools and the workplace will significantly affect the future of society. Violence and crime have increased tremendously in the past decade and continue to be a major health concern. The most powerful weapon in the war on drug abuse is knowledge. One of the major challenges for all health care providers will be incorporating rapidly developing scientific knowledge of substance abuse into practice and public policies, policies that will improve outcomes of substance abuse. These patients present a variety of psychologic, emotional, and physiologic changes. Box 53-4 provides a brief list of nursing diagnoses that apply to these patients.

Box 53-4	NURSING DIAGNOSES FOR SUBSTANCE ABUSE

Anxiety
Fear
Injury, Risk for
Poisoning, Risk for
Sensory perception, Disturbed

Table 53-5 **ILLEGAL DRUGS AND THEIR EFFECTS**[15]

DRUGS	STREET NAME	SIGNS OF USE	OVERDOSE	ROUTE TAKEN
Cocaine/Crack cocaine	Coke Crack Snow Dust Blow Girl Rock Freebase rocks	Excitation Increased alertness Increased heart rate Increased blood pressure Insomnia Runny nose Nasal congestion Dilated pupils	Agitation Increase in body temperature Hallucinations Seizures Possible death	Snorted Smoked (freebased) Injected
Amphetamines/ Methampheta-mines	Crank Ice Meth Speed Crystal Ecstasy	Excitation Increased alertness Increased heart rate Increased blood pressure Insomnia Runny nose Nasal congestion Dilated pupils	Agitation Increase in body temperature Hallucinations Seizures Possible death	Swallowed Snorted Smoked Injected
Heroin	Smack Stuff Horse Dope Boy	Excitation Drowsiness Respiratory depression Constricted pupils Nausea	Respiratory depression Seizures Coma Clammy skin Possible death	Injected Smoked Snorted
Phencyclidine	PCP Angel dust Hog Loveboat	Illusions and hallucinations Poor perception of time and distance	Psychosis Longer, more intense "trip" episodes "Awake" coma Bizarre behavior Violence Possible death	Oral Injected Snorted Smoked
Lysergic acid diethylamide	LSD Acid Mickey Mouse Paper acid Blotter acid Green/Red dragon	Illusions and hallucinations Poor perception of time and distance	Psychosis Longer, more intense "trip" episodes Violence Possible death	Oral
Marijuana	Weed Grass Pot THC Acapulco gold Joint Roach	Difficulty concentrating Euphoria Short-term memory loss Dilated pupils Loss of depth perception Disciplinary problems Increased appetite Disoriented	Fatigue Paranoia Possible psychosis	Oral Smoked

References

1. Addolorato G, Cibin M, Caputo F: γ-Hydroxybutric acid in the treatment of alcoholism: dosage factioning utility in nonresponder alcoholic patients, *Drug Alcohol Dependence* 7, 1998.

2. Adlaf EM, Smart RG: Party subculture or dens of doom? An epidemiological study of rave attendance and drug patterns among adolescent students, *J Psychoactive Drugs* 29(2):193, 1997.

3. Bailes B: What perioperative nurses need to know about substance abuse, *AORN J* 68(4):611, 1998.

4. Braunwald E, Hauser S, Fauci A et al: *Harrison's principles of internal medicine,* ed 15, New York, 2001, McGraw-Hill.

5. Centers for Disease Control and Prevention: Cigarette smoking among adults—United States, 1999, *MMWR Highlights* 50(40), 2001.

6. Centers for Disease Control and Prevention: *Health effects of smoking among young people.* Retrieved February 24, 2002 from the World Wide Web: www.cdc.gov/tobacco/research.

7. Centers for Disease Control and Prevention: Incidence of cigarette smoking among U.S. teens. Retrieved February 24, 2002 from the World Wide Web: www.cdc.gov/tobacco/research.

8. Centers for Disease Control and Prevention: Tobacco use among middle and high school students: national youth tobacco survey, *MMWR Highlights* 49(3), 2000.

9. Centers for Disease Control and Prevention: Trends in cigarette smoking among high school students—United States, 1991-1999, *MMWR Highlights* 49(3), 2000.

10. Department of Health and Human Services: *Changing the conversation: a national plan to improve substance abuse treatment,* Washington, DC, 2000, The Department.

11. Fingerhood M: Substance abuse in older people, *Geriatrics* 48(8):985, 2000.

12. Galloway GP, Frederick SL, Staggers FE Jr et al: Gammahydroxybutyrate: an emerging drug of abuse that causes physical dependence, *Addiction* 92(1):89, 1997.

13. Hogan MJ: Diagnosis and treatment of teen drug use, *Adolesc Med* 84(4):927, 2000.

14. National Clearinghouse for Alcohol and Drug Information: *Alcohol, tobacco, and other drugs and pregnancy and parenthood.* Retrieved February 24, 2002 from the World Wide Web: www.health.org.

15. National Clearinghouse for Alcohol and Drug Information: *Drugs of abuse.* Retrieved February 24, 2002 from the World Wide Web: www.health.org.

16. National Clearinghouse for Alcohol and Drug Information: *GHB.* Retrieved February 24, 2002 from the World Wide Web: www.health.org.

17. National Clearinghouse for Alcohol and Drug Information: *Inhalants.* Retrieved February 24, 2002 from the World Wide Web: www.health.org.

18. National Clearinghouse for Alcohol and Drug Information: *Ketamine: a fact sheet.* Retrieved February 24, 2002 from the World Wide Web: www.health.org.

19. National Clearinghouse for Alcohol and Drug Information: *The OASIS report: cocaine treatment admissions decrease: 1993-1999.* Retrieved February 24, 2002 from the World Wide Web: www.health.org.

20. National Clearinghouse for Alcohol and Drug Information: *The OASIS report: heroin treatment admissions increase: 1993-1999.* Retrieved February 24, 2002 from the World Wide Web: www.health.org.

21. National Institute on Drug Abuse, Research Report Series: *Cocaine abuse and addiction.* Retrieved February 24, 2002 from the World Wide Web: www.nida.gov/researchreports/cocaine.

22. National Institute on Drug Abuse, Research Report Series: *Hallucinogens and dissociative drugs.* Retrieved February 24, 2002 from the World Wide Web: www.nida.gov/researchreports/cocaine.

23. Partnership for a Drug-Free America: *The partnership attitude tracking study.* Retrieved February 24, 2002 from the World Wide Web: www.health.org.

24. Rigler SK: Alcoholism in the elderly, *Am Fam Physician* 61(6):1710, 2000.

25. Slaughter L: Involvement of drugs in sexual assault, *J Reprod Med* 45(5):425, 2000.

26. Tweed SH: Intervening in adolescent substance abuse, *Nurs Clin North Am* 33(1):29, 1998.

27. Weir E: Raves: a review of the culture, the drugs and the prevention of harm, *Can Med Assoc J* 162(13):1843, 2000.

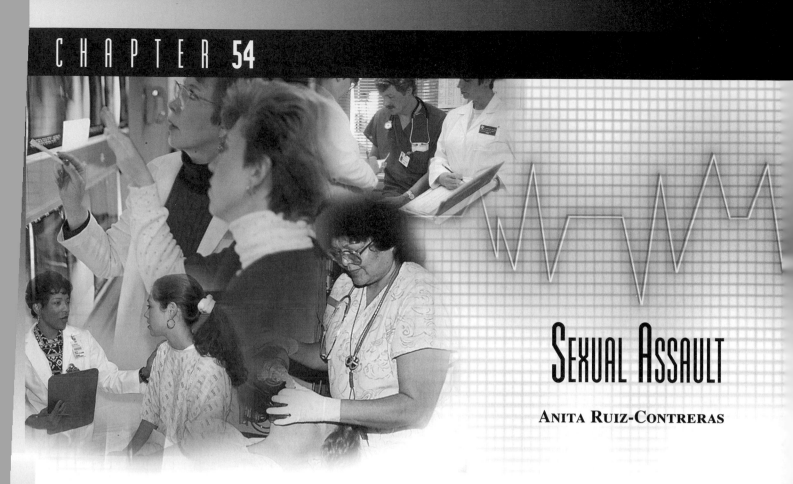

CHAPTER 54

SEXUAL ASSAULT

ANITA RUIZ-CONTRERAS

At some point, emergency care providers encounter patients who have been sexually assaulted. Each of us will care for a patient, know someone close to us, or experience the horror ourselves. Sexual assault is not defined by gender, social level, ethnic origin, religious affiliation, or culture lines.[9]

One of four women will be sexually assaulted in their lifetime.[5] The Uniform Crime Reports from the Federal Bureau of Investigation (FBI) do not maintain statistics on sexual assault of males, although the numbers of reported assaults on males are increasing.[7,8,16] A review of data for assaults from 1991 through 1996 found that approximately two thirds of assaults occurred between 6 PM and 6 AM, with over half of all assaults in the victim's home.[11] Thirty-four percent of victims during this period were under the age of 12 years.[11]

Sexual assault is one of the most feared and least understood crimes. Of all the choices made in our lives, the most intimate choices are sexual. In a sexual assault this choice is taken away. Sexual assault is not a crime of passion. In a classic study of more than 600 sex offenders, Amir[1] was one of the first to describe rape as a crime of power and control. Groth[12] interviewed more than 500 sexual "aggressors" and found power and anger described as motivating factors. Sex is used by the rapist as a tool to control and humiliate the victim. Sexual assault involves a wide range of behaviors with the common characteristic of unwanted sexual contact.[10] Both psychologic coercion and physical force are part of sexual assault.

SEXUAL ASSAULT PATIENTS ARE SURVIVORS

Survivor is a common term used for patients who have been sexually assaulted. The patient who has experienced sexual assault has lived through a life-threatening event. Use of the term victim denotes helplessness and hopelessness. The term survivor has more of a positive, empowering connotation. Use of "survivor" as an identifying term can be helpful when counseling patients. However, some professionals working in the area of sexual assault treatment do not use the term because it is felt that it may minimize or take away from the devastation of the actual event.

MYTHS AND MISCONCEPTIONS

Common myths such as "victims are women wearing suggestive clothing" or "a woman cannot be raped by an acquaintance" have long ago been dispelled. Regrettably, other myths remain prevalent. The media often portrays women as secretly wanting to be raped, which is the so-called "rape fantasy." When an individual fantasizes, he or she selects the players, the setting, and the sexual acts. In sexual assault all choice is taken away. This myth confuses sex and rape. Sex becomes the tool used by the rapist to degrade and humiliate the victim. Emergency nurses can use their knowledge regarding myths and misconceptions when counseling patients and families to dispel these beliefs and help begin the process of healing.

The patient may arrive with expectations about the hospital and the staff that are based on misconceptions. The patient, law enforcement officer, and emergency nurse may also have long-held beliefs based on misconception. It is important for health care professionals to examine their own attitudes regarding survivors of sexual assault.[10] Myths and misconceptions surrounding sexual assault harm the patient and hamper development of a trusting relationship with the emergency nurse.

RAPE TRAUMA SYNDROME

In a landmark study of 94 rape victims, Burgess and Holmstrom[4] first identified rape-trauma syndrome, a cluster of symptoms experienced by survivors of sexual assault. Symptoms include somatic, behavioral, and psychologic reactions. The framework of rape-trauma syndrome includes recognition of the long-term reorganization a survivor goes through when recovering from the assault. Reorganization may take weeks or even years. There is recognition of differences in lifestyle choices made by individuals, in which lifestyles are not judged but seen as normal for that person. Prostitutes who normally charge for sexual services can be raped. A wife, a husband, a boyfriend, or a girlfriend can be raped. Many people are raped by someone they know. In a 1999 study almost 7 of 10 sexual assault victims stated that the offender was an intimate, other relative, a friend, or an acquaintance.[3]

It is also important to remember that men can be victims of sexual assault. Male sexual assault may be one of the most underreported of all groups. Myths surrounding male sexual assault include beliefs that it only happens in prison or that homosexuality is a causative factor. Lipscomb et al,[9] in a study of 99 adult male victims of sexual assault, found no statistically significant difference between incarcerated and nonincarcerated victims. All people are potential victims regardless of sexual orientation. Men are raped for the same reason women are raped: power, control, and humiliation. The male survivor needs the same level of compassion and recognition as any other patient who has been sexually assaulted.

Rape-trauma syndrome is an approved nursing diagnosis and can be used to plan nursing care. The initial hospital experience can have a major affect on the acute phase of the sexual assault survivor's recovery. When interacting with the sexual assault victim, it is essential for the emergency nurse to develop a trusting relationship. As with any patient, a calm, confident approach facilitates this process. Listen to the patient and explain what will happen during the examination. Show concern for the patient's experience. Specific questions that require the patient to relive the assault are not needed. Determining the presence of physical trauma that requires immediate treatment is the initial priority. The extent of emotional injury cannot be estimated. Each person's response to a sexual assault is different. Individuals may laugh, cry, tell a joke, or become catatonic. Patients may blame themselves for fighting back or for not fighting back.

Inform the patients that their actions helped get them through the ordeal, regardless of what action was taken. Patients may believe they caused the rape by accepting the ride or opening the door. Remind these patients that they did not cause the assault. Patients need to hear that they have the right to decide what to do with their own bodies and that no one has the right to hurt them.

THE SEXUAL ASSAULT SURVIVOR IN THE EMERGENCY DEPARTMENT

Evaluation of the sexual assault survivor in the emergency department (ED) requires planning, development of specific policies and procedures, and staff education. The goal is to provide sensitive, individualized care for each person in a manner that ensures adherence to legal and regulatory requirements. Staff should be knowledgeable of state laws and regulations regarding sexual assault. A standard documentation form or protocol may be required by local or state policy. For example, the California State Medical Protocol for the Examination and Treatment of Sexual Assault Victims must be used by all California hospitals and health care practitioners who perform examinations on survivors of sexual assault.[5] If hospitals do not wish to comply, they must develop a referral protocol with a hospital that does comply. For each case, a standard documentation form is used with copies for law enforcement, the criminalistic laboratory, and the hospital. The protocol outlines the steps of examination including evidence collection, laboratory testing, medications, and follow-up care.

Sexual Assault Response Teams

For more than 20 years, specialized teams of nonphysician medical providers have been responsible for performing sexual assault medical and legal examinations.[2] The teams identified as sexual assault response teams (SART) or suspected abuse response teams consist of a nurse examiner, rape crisis advocate, and law enforcement personnel. Nurses with specialized training are identified as sexual assault/abuse nurse examiners (SANE). These individuals are usually on call and respond when a sexual assault victim arrives at an identified hospital. The SART programs train registered nurses to obtain patient histories, conduct evidentiary exams, provide sexually transmitted disease (STD) prophylaxis and pregnancy prevention, and ensure follow-up care. The proliferation of these programs across the United States is evidence of their effectiveness. SANE personnel become the medical and legal experts in the field of sexual assault. Offices of the district attorney in areas with established programs have found that SANE personnel are competent, well-informed courtroom witnesses.

Development of a specialized team is the ideal; however, hospitals without specialized programs can still treat sexual assault victims effectively. Individual hospitals can train all ED nurses or an identified number of nurses to care for sexual assault survivors during their work hours. Identified personnel may conduct the complete evidentiary examination independently or in conjunction with a physician. The nurse acts as a patient care coordinator, ensuring adherence to established procedures.

The Examination Begins

Sexual assault survivors should receive an emergent priority behind patients experiencing an acute life-threatening event. The patient should be immediately placed in a safe, secure room. A medical screening examination should be performed to rule out an emergency medical condition. A nurse should be instructed to remain with the patient throughout the ED visit to provide continuity and decrease repetition of data. The patient should be allowed a support person such as a family member, friend, or representative from a rape crisis center. Asking "Who can I call for you?" allows the patient to think of a name, whereas asking "Is there someone I can call for you?" is often followed by a "No" answer. Rape crisis advocates are an integral part of any sexual assault treatment program. If available, a rape crisis advocate should be available whenever the SART is called to the hospital.

Consent

By obtaining consent, the nurse begins to develop a therapeutic relationship with the patient. The examination of a sexual assault survivor has been called "another rape." The goal of the hospital or clinic experience is to cause as little additional stress as possible. All interactions should be handled with sensitivity and understanding. Every effort should be made to ensure that the patient has the opportunity to make informed choices about medical care. Patients must be informed if the hospital is required to notify law enforcement. The hospital may be required to report; however, the patient has the right to decide whether he or she wishes to speak with law enforcement. It has been found that women assaulted by a partner are significantly less likely to report sexual assault to police or seek medical care.[8] The *FBI Unified Crime Reports 2000* stress that the relationship of the patient and offender does not affect classification of the crime. Patients should be informed of the nurses' and the hospitals' reporting responsibility. The patient may wish to speak to an advocate before talking to hospital staff or the law enforcement officer. Law enforcement officers today are well prepared to deal sensitively with survivors of sexual assault. The nurse should ensure that the patient is well informed and understands the examination process. Consent should be obtained for medical treatment including evidentiary examination and photographs. The patient must understand that the evidence collected will be used for prosecution of the accused rapist if a report is made. Many patients are not ready to file a report with law enforcement, even with treatment in the ED. One study of 337 sexual assault victims found only 62% were certain they wanted to file such a report.[14]

Patient history
Time and date of assault
Surroundings
Body orifices penetrated
Use of any foreign objects
Other sexual acts
Injuries incurred during the assault
Activities after assault such as urination, showering, or douching
Recent gynecologic treatment or surgery
History of consensual intercourse within the last 72 hours

History

A standard form should be used to gather the patient's history. This history helps the nurse decide on the type of evidence collection required. Examinations performed within 72 hours of the assault are more likely to yield evidence of assault[8]; however, this time frame should not negate performing examinations on individuals assaulted beyond the 72-hour time frame. Evidence of sexual assault has been found after many days.[5] When questioning the patient, the patient does not need to describe the assault in specific minute-by-minute detail. Pertinent areas for questioning are summarized in Box 54-1. Questions should be asked in a manner understood by the patient. Translate medical terms into everyday language. History taking may be delayed when the patient's emotional response to questioning makes it impossible to ascertain the information. Documentation should be completed legibly and clearly. If this case is called to court, the nurse may be asked to discuss what was written in the record. The nurse must be able to understand what he or she wrote months or even years after it was written, so the nurse should be write it in such a manner that it can be explained to the jury.

Potential use of various date rape drugs (e.g., Rohypnol, GHB, ketamine) should be assessed while obtaining other historical data. This data helps the SANE or other examiner determine the need for drug screening. Assaults with these agents are referred to as drug-facilitated sexual assaults.

Physical Examination and Evidence Collection

Collection of various laboratory tests should be accomplished early to allow for pregnancy test results. A negative pregnancy test is needed to administer medication for prevention of pregnancy. The patient's clothing is collected and placed in paper rather than plastic bags for evaluation at the local crime laboratory. Use of plastic allows body fluids and other trace evidence to deteriorate more quickly. A head-to-toe physical assessment is completed to assess for all injuries. Documentation of any injuries should include color and size of injuries such as bruises, abrasions, lacerations or avulsions. Use of body figures on the documentation tool

Table 54-1 EVIDENTIARY REQUIREMENTS FOR SEXUAL ASSAULT

ITEM	DESCRIPTION
Clothing	Note condition of the clothing. Place each piece of clothing in a separate paper bag.
Fingernail scrapings	Collect when indicated. Hold each hand over a piece of paper. Using wooden sticks, scrape under each nail.
Skin	Scan body with Wood's lamp. Collect dried and moist secretions using cotton-tipped swabs. Collect a control swab from same area of the body.
Oral cavity	Collect if oral penetration occurred within the last 6 hours. Collect 2 swabs from oral cavity and 1 swab from area around the mouth.
Reference sample—oral	With clean forceps, place clean gauze or cotton pledget under the tongue.
External genitalia	Examine with Wood's lamp. Collect dried material and matted hair. Swab areas of fluorescence with a moistened cotton-tipped applicator.
Pubic hair	Local requirements may include samples of body and facial hair or head hair. Comb pubic hair and then place in evidence envelope. Cut up to 40 pubic hairs from different perineal areas per local guidelines.
Vagina	Collect 3 separate swabs/slides from the vaginal pool. Prepare 1 wet mount slide and 2 dry mount slides. Examine wet mount for motile or nonmotile sperm.
Penis	Collect dried secretions using 2 swabs. Collect 1 swab from the urethral meatus and 1 swab from the glans and shaft. Examine the penis and scrotum for injury.
Rectum	Collect dried secretions using 2 rectal swabs. Collect 2 separate swabs/slides. Do 2 dry mount swabs. Examine buttocks, perianal skin, and anal folds for injury. Anoscopic or proctoscopic examination may be indicated.
Other evidence such as foreign material or dried secretions	When dried secretions are collected using a moistened cotton-tipped swab, a control sample should be taken from the same area of the body

Modified from the Office of Criminal Justice Planning: *California state medical protocol for examination of sexual assault and child sexual abuse victims,* State of California, 1987.

can assist in recording this data. A Wood's lamp or other ultraviolet light is used to identify semen on the patient's skin. Semen appears as an orange or blue-green color on the skin. The fluorescent area should be swabbed with a moistened cotton-tipped applicator. A control swab should then be taken from area of the body adjacent to where the swab was taken. Caution should be taken when reporting Wood's lamp findings because other materials such as lint also fluoresce. Oral swabs are taken for evidence of semen and as a reference sample. Reference samples include saliva, blood, semen, pubic hair, and body hair. These reference samples are compared to specimens from potential suspects. Table 54-1 lists essential evidentiary requirements.

For the female patient, the pelvic examination begins with a gross visual examination. Photographs are then used to detect and document genital trauma.[6] Colposcopic photographs have become standard as part of the pelvic or genital evaluation. The colposcope provides binocular vision, magnifies the area by 5 to 30 times, and can take photographs.[10] Lenahan[6] found that the colposcope improved detection of genital trauma when compared with gross visualization alone. The external genitalia is examined for signs of injury or foreign materials. Documentation should indicate if the injury is apparent without use of the colposcope. Injuries should be described by size, appearance, and location.

Pubic hair is combed to look for foreign hairs. A representative number of the patient's pubic hairs are cut close to the skin for comparison. During the pelvic examination, swabs and slides are taken from the vaginal pool. Historically, baseline testing for chlamydia and gonorrhea has also

Table 54-2 LABORATORY TESTING FOR SEXUAL ASSAULT

AREA OF BODY PENETRATED	RECOMMENDED TESTS
Oral	Culture for gonorrhea; blood test for syphilis
Vaginal	Culture for gonorrhea, chlamydia; blood test for Hepatitis C and syphilis; pregnancy testing
Penile	Culture for gonorrhea, chlamydia; blood test for Hepatitis C and syphilis
Rectal	Culture for gonorrhea, chlamydia; blood test for Hepatitis C and syphilis

been performed. Recently, some established programs have stopped performing these tests because each patient is offered prophylactic antibiotic treatment.

Rectal examination includes colposcopy, swabs, slides, and baseline testing for STDs (as indicated by local policy). The perianal area should be cleansed after taking vaginal/penile specimens to avoid contamination from vaginal or perianal drainage.[8] Table 54-2 summarizes laboratory testing for sexual assault. All swabs and slides must be labeled to identify the patient and the source. After they are collected, swabs or slides should be placed in a drying box with cool airflow. Drying swabs and slides also prevents deterioration of evidence. Testing of swabs and slides is done by a criminalistic laboratory in the hope of linking evidence to potential suspects. Current methods of deoxyribonucleic acid

Table 54-3 MEDICATION PROPHYLAXIS IN SEXUAL ASSAULT		
POTENTIAL PROBLEM	**NO PENICILLIN ALLERGY**	**PENICILLIN ALLERGY**
Gonorrhea, chlamydia, syphilis* in nonpregnant patient	Cefixime 400 mg PO as stat dose, then doxycycline 100 mg PO BID for 7 days	Spectinomycin 2 gm IM, then doxycycline 100 mg PO BID for 7 days
Gonorrhea, chlamydia, syphilis* in pregnant patient	Cefixime 400 mg PO stat dose, then erythromycin 500 mg PO QID for 7 days	Spectinomycin 2 gm IM, then erythromycin 500 mg PO QID for 7 days
Pregnancy†	Ovral 2 tablets PO and 2 tablets in 12 hr	

From Sexual Assault Response Team: *Standardized procedure: medication administration, sexual assault victims,* San Jose, 1996, Santa Clara Valley Medical Center.
PO, By mouth; *BID,* twice daily; *QID,* four times a day.
*Efficacy against syphilis not proven.
†Give only after obtaining negative pregnancy test.

(DNA) typing allow detection of semen donor type beyond the 72-hour time frame. Detection has occurred as many as 5 to 6 days after a sexual assault. Special care must be taken by the nurse to prevent any contamination of evidence collected. All equipment that comes in contact with evidence must be clean. The nurse should limit handling of evidence and take care not to leave any of his or her own DNA on the evidence. This can be facilitated by using gloves and by not talking over the evidence.

Chain of Custody

To maintain validity of evidence collected, the nurse must be able to verify the whereabouts of all evidence. A chart can be used to indicate that evidence was taken from the patient by the nurse and then given to the law enforcement officer. All transfers of evidence must be logged to show that evidence was transferred from one person to another, with each transfer dated and timed. The best practice is to keep transfers of evidence to a minimum. If a drying box is used, it should have a lock that is closed and opened only by the nurse.

Postexamination

A shower and clean clothing should be available for the patient after the sexual assault examination. Ideally, the hospital maintains a closet with clean, new or used clothing. If desired by the patient, medication should be provided for prevention of pregnancy and STD (Table 54-3). Consent for pregnancy prevention should be obtained after a negative pregnancy test result and after the patient is informed of associated risks. A specific postcoital consent form should be used. Prophylaxis for HIV is not yet routine for all sexual assault victims; however, programs in California, New York, and Vancouver (B.C.) do offer the option to all patients.[16]

Follow-up Care

Patients should be rechecked in 10 days to 2 weeks. Referral to a gynecologist or nearby clinic is essential—cultures for chlamydia and gonorrhea can be obtained at this time. At the follow-up appointment, timelines for human immunodeficiency virus testing can be discussed. Many established specialized teams include follow-up care as part of their overall program.

LEGAL ASPECTS

When the case goes to court, the nurse may be called as a witness to describe what the nurse did and saw. In some situations the nurse may be qualified by the judge as an expert, which allows the nurse to give opinion and conclusions. Each encounter with a sexual assault patient has the potential for becoming a court case. In court the nurse is not there to represent one side or the other. The nurse may receive a subpoena from the district attorney's office or a defense attorney representing the accused. In preparation for court the nurse should review the patient's medical record. The nurse should also have a professional curriculum vitae that can be reviewed by both attorneys and should be prepared to describe his or her education, experience, and sexual assault training. The nurse may need to explain the SART process to the jury. Attire in the courtroom should be professional. In most cases the nurse will be excluded from the courtroom until he or she is called in for actual testimony. It is most important to answer questions in a calm, confident manner. Box 54-2 provides clues to answering questions while on the witness stand.

SUMMARY

In an expanded role, emergency nurses are uniquely suited to act as sexual assault nurse examiners or as coordinators of care for a sexual assault survivor. However, if this role is not identified in the nurse's institution or state, it is still vital that the emergency nurse be knowledgeable about local or state protocol. The emergency nurse should care for the patient in a supportive, nonthreatening, nonjudgmental manner. The ED visit can significantly affect the emotional recovery of the sexual assault survivor. Box 54-3 lists pertinent nursing diagnoses for these patients.

Box 54-2   TIPS FOR BEING A WITNESS

Listen to the complete question.
Respond to the question by facing the jury.
Tell the truth.
Remain calm.
Be objective.
Avoid becoming defensive or angry.
Be prepared to spell and define medical terms.
Ask for clarification of any questions you do not understand.
Answer only the question you are asked.
Ask the judge for permission to speak if you feel an explanation is needed.
Wait to answer until the judge has ruled on an objection.
Say "I don't know" confidently if you don't know.

Box 54-3   NURSING DIAGNOSES FOR SEXUAL ASSAULT

Anxiety
Fear
Pain
Powerlessness
Rape-trauma syndrome

References

1. Amir M: *Patterns of forcible rape,* Chicago, 1971, University of Chicago Press.
2. Antognoli-Toland P: Comprehensive program for examination of sexual assault victims by nurses: a hospital-based project in Texas, *J Emerg Nurs* 11(3):132, 1985.
3. Bureau of Justice Statistics: *Characteristic of crime, 2001,* U.S. Department of Justice. Retrieved February 22, 2002 from the World Wide Web http://www.ojp.usdoj.gov/bjs/cvict_c.htm.
4. Burgess AW, Holmstrom LL: Rape-trauma syndrome, *Am J Psychiatry* 131:981, 1974.
5. California Medical Training Center: *Training on the California medical protocol for the examination of sexual assault and child sexual abuse victims,* Sacramento, Calif, 2001, California Medical Training Center.
6. Ernoehazy W, Murphy-Lavoie H: Sexual assault, *emedicine* 3(1), 2002.
7. Federal Bureau of Investigation: *Uniform crime reports: Crime in the United States, 2000,* Washington, DC, 2000, U.S. Department of Justice.
8. Feldhaus KM: Lifetime sexual assault prevalence rates and reporting practices in an emergency department population, *Ann Emerg Med* 36(1):23, 2000.
9. Giardono AP: *Sexual assault: victimization across the life span,* Maryland Heights, Mo, 2002, GW Medical Publishing.
10. Girardin B et al: *Color atlas of sexual assault,* St. Louis, 1997, Mosby.
11. Greenfeld LA: *Sex offenses and offenders: an analysis of data on rape and sexual assault,* Washington, DC, 1997, Bureau of Justice Statistics.
12. Groth AN: *Men who rape: the psychology of the offender,* New York, 1979, Plenum Press.
13. Ledray LE: The clinical care and documentation for victims of drug-facilitated sexual assault, *JEN* 27(3):301, 2001.
14. Ledray LE: *Sexual assault nurse examiner (SANE): development and operation guide,* Washington, DC, 1999, Office for Victims of Crime, U.S. Department of Justice.
15. Moe I, Grau A: HIV prophylaxis within a treatment protocol for sexual assault victims: rationale for the decision, *JEN* 27(5):511, 2001.
16. Pinto N: Gender differences in rape reporting, *Sex Roles: A Research Journal,* 1999.

Index

Airway—cont'd
  management of
    in burn patient, 355
    in spinal trauma, 268-269
    in maxillofacial trauma assessment, 366-367
    obstruction of, by foreign body in pediatric patient, 726-727
    stabilization of
      in pediatric trauma patient, 383
      for transport, 100
    upper, obstruction of, in smoke inhalation, 57*f*, 355, 356*f*
AKA. *See* Alcoholic ketoacidosis (AKA)
Albuterol (Proventil, Ventolin)
  for asthma in pediatric patient, 728*t*
  for pulmonary conditions, 436*t*
Alcohol(s)
  toxicity from, 650-651
  trauma and, 215-216
  withdrawal of, medications for, 591*t*
Alcoholic ketoacidosis (AKA), 585, 587-588
Alcoholism, 793-795
Alkalosis
  causes of, 137*t*
  metabolic, characteristics of, 509*f*
  respiratory, characteristics of, 509*f*
Allen's test, 133-134, 135*f*
  procedure for, 134*b*
All-terrain vehicle collisions, mechanism of injury in, 226
Alteplase (Activase), in acute myocardial infarction management, 476*t*
Altitude
  changes in, effects on patient, 106*t*
  flow rates and, 112*t*
  partial pressure of ambient oxygen and, 105*t*
Ambulation, assisted, 346
Aminophylline
  for asthma in pediatric patient, 728*t*
  for pulmonary conditions, 437*t*
Amiodarone (Cordarone), in cardiopulmonary resuscitation, 459*t*
Amitriptyline (Elavil)
  cardiopulmonary arrest induced by, 455*t*
  in pain management, 167*t*
Amniotic fluid embolism, 716-717
Amphetamines, effects of, 796*t*
Amputations, traumatic, 322-323
Anaerobic bacterial pneumonias, causes, characteristics, clinical manifestations, and complications of, 433*t*
Analgesia, systemic, 164-165
Analgesics in pain management, 159-160, 163
Anaphylactic shock, 512-513
Anaphylaxis, in pediatric patient, 734-735
Anemia, 637-638
  dilutional, in pregnancy, 411
Anesthesia, for wound management, 148-149
Aneurysm(s), aortic, 502-503
  dissecting, chest pain in, characteristics of, 469*t*
  patient assessment in, 485-486
  patient management in, 503
Angina
  in acute coronary syndrome evaluation, 465-466
  differential diagnosis of, 467*t*
  Ludwig's, 682
Angiography, in renal trauma, 309
Angiomatosis, bacillary, AIDS and, 608*t*
Angioplasty, coronary, percutaneous transluminal, in acute myocardial infarction management, 474-475
Angular impact in motorcycle crash, 225
Animal bites, 146, 147
  rabies prophylaxis for, 153-155
Anion gap, 575
  calculation of, 577*b*

Anistreplase (Eminase), in acute myocardial infarction management, 476*t*
Ankle
  dislocation of, 341, 344*f*
  fractures of, 334, 335*f*
  veins of, 115, 117*f*
Anorexia nervosa, 782-784
Ant sting, 625*t*, 631
Anterior cord syndrome, 275
Anterior segment of eye, assessment of, 693
Anthrax, symptoms and care related to, 199*t*
Anthrax pneumonia, causes, characteristics, clinical manifestations, and complications of, 432*t*
Antiallergy medications, ocular, 697*t*
Antibacterials, ocular, 697*t*
Antibiotics, in pediatric trauma management, 392
Anticholinergics, for pulmonary conditions, 437*t*
Antidepressants, tricyclic
  cardiopulmonary arrest induced by, 455*t*
  toxicity from, 649-650
Antidiuretic hormone (ADH)
  in homeostatic autoregulation, 551-552
  inappropriate, syndrome of, 598-600
  in response to shock, 507
  in water balance regulation, 569
Antidotes, 645
Antiseptic solutions, 142*t*
Antivenin therapy for snakebite, 628
Antiviral agents, ocular, 697*t*
Anus, anatomy of, 539
Anxiety, 775-777
  assessment of, 775-776
  chest pain in, characteristics of, 470*t*
  differential diagnosis of, 776*b*
  treatment of, 776-777
  types of, 776*b*
Aorta
  anatomy and physiology of, 296
  aneurysm of (*See also* Aneurysm, aortic)
  dissecting, chest pain in, characteristics of, 469*t*
  rupture of, 291
  thoracic, 280
Apgar score, 713, 714*t*
Appalachians, cultural beliefs of, 24
Appendicitis, 540-541
  in pediatric patient, 738
Appendix, variable position of, 540*f*
Arabics, cultural beliefs of, 24
Arachnid bites, 629-630
ARDS. *See* Adult respiratory distress syndrome (ARDS)
Arm, upper
  fracture of, 328
  veins of, 115, 116*f*
Arrhythmia, sinus, 482
Arsenic poisoning, 653
Arterial blood gases (ABGs)
  analysis of, specimen collection for, 133-135
  results of, 136-137
  values for, 137*t*
Arteritis, temporal, 521
Artery(ies)
  blood specimen collection systems for, 133-135
  brachial, specimen collection from, 133, 134*f*
  coronary, in myocardial infarction, 466*t*
  femoral, specimen collection from, 133, 134*f*
  injuries to, 319-320, 321*t*
  radial, specimen collection from, 133-135
Arthropod bites and stings, 625-626*t*
Asbestosis, agents, description, and complications of, 427*t*
Asians, touch during physical examination and, 89*b*